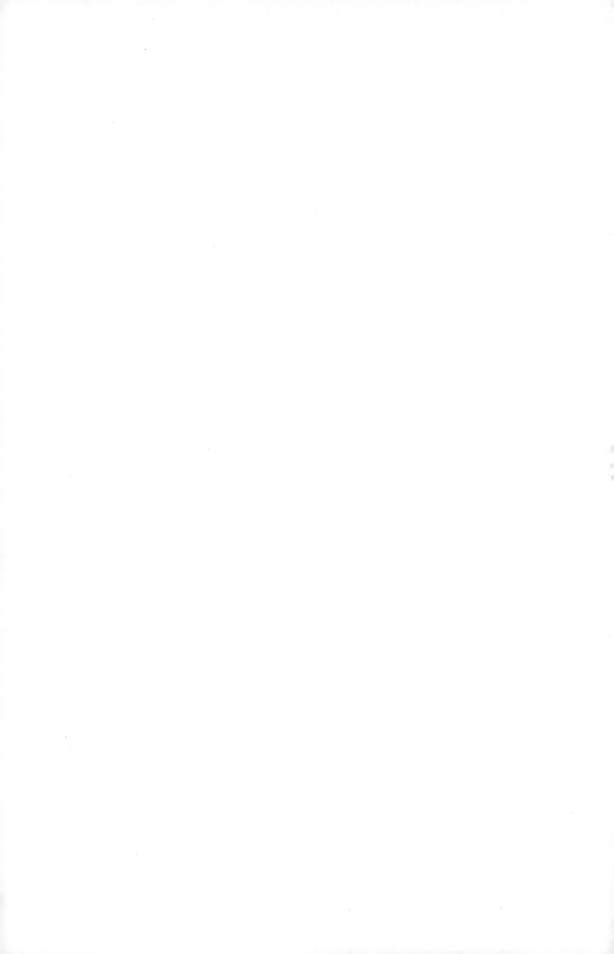

Principles
of
Neurotoxicology

NEUROLOGICAL DISEASE AND THERAPY

Series Editor

WILLIAM C. KOLLER

Department of Neurology
University of Kansas Medical Center
Kansas City, Kansas

Principles
of
Neurotoxicology

edited by
Louis W. Chang
University of Arkansas for Medical Sciences
Little Rock, Arkansas

Marcel Dekker, Inc.   **New York•Basel•Hong Kong**

Library of Congress Cataloging-in-Publication Data

Principles of neurotoxicology / edited by Louis W. Chang.
    p. cm. — (Neurological disease and therapy ; 26)
  Includes bibliographical references and index.
  ISBN 0-8247-8836-2 (alk. paper)
  1. Neurotoxicology. I. Chang, Louis W. II. Series: Neurological
disease and therapy ; v. 26.
  [DNLM: 1. Nervous System Diseases—chemically induced. 2. Toxins–
–adverse effects. 3. Central Nervous System—drug effects.
4. Peripheral Nervous System—drug effects. 5. Fetal Development–
–drug effects. 6. Behavior—drug effects. W1 NE33LD v.26 1994 /
WL 100 P95675 1994]
RC347.5.P75 1994
616.8'047—dc20
DNLM/DLC
for Library of Congress   94-7435
                                                  CIP

The publisher offers discounts on this book when ordered in bulk quantities. For more information, write to Special Sales/Professional Marketing at the address below.

This book is printed on acid-free paper.

Marcel Dekker, Inc.
270 Madison Avenue, New York, New York 10016

Current printing (last digit):
10 9 8 7 6 5 4 3 2 1

PRINTED IN THE UNITED STATES OF AMERICA

Series Introduction

Neurotoxicology has become of increasing importance to clinicians and basic scientists alike. Toxins tell us a great deal about neuronal mechanisms, in both health and disease—especially neurological disease, which can be caused by a variety of toxins.

This book is divided into five parts. Neurotoxicology of the central nervous system is discussed in four introductory chapters (Part I), neurotoxicology of the peripheral nervous system is discussed in six chapters addressing basic principles (Part II), and behavioral neurotoxicology is discussed in five chapters covering laboratory assessment and presenting a model in clinical diseases (Part III). Part IV is dedicated to biochemical and molecular neurotoxicology. A chapter on cell signaling shows that neural cell death is almost certainly related to neurotoxicity. The chapter on excitotoxicity will be of particular interest to neurologists. The discussion of oxidative stress and the role of ion channels in neurotoxicity introduces important mechanisms of potential cell death. The last section, Part V, is dedicated to developmental nerve toxicology. Its chapters deal with the basic principles of neurotoxicology and the role of toxins in developmental disorders.

Neurologists and cytologists in general will find the mechanisms of cell death of interest. *Principles of Neurotoxicology*, in keeping with this series in which basic science is blended with clinical knowledge, is an important book for all clinicians who take care of patients with neurological disease.

William C. Koller

Preface

Neurotoxicology may be considered as the science that deals with the adverse effects and mechanisms of chemicals and injurious agents on the nervous system. As a science, it can be viewed as the "offspring" of neuroscience and toxicology. Like its parents, neurotoxicology is multifaceted and multidisciplinary in nature, encompassing the many facets of neuroscience: neuroanatomy, neurophysiology, neurochemistry and biochemistry, neurocytology, neurobehavioral sciences, and neuropathology, as well as the interdisciplinary nature of toxicology: pharmacology, biochemistry/molecular biology, general toxicology, and cell biology and pathology.

Over one-third of the toxic chemicals surveyed by the U.S. Environmental Protection Agency are known to be neurotoxic, and the list is rapidly increasing with the implementation of more sensitive screening techniques. With the increased awareness of and attention to environmental, occupational, and mental health, the field of neurotoxicology has also grown rapidly. Indeed, neurotoxicology has matured independently from its parents, neuroscience and toxicology. With the increasing importance of this discipline, substantial publications, including several textbooks, were published in the past decade. Most of these textbooks were devoted to the toxic consequences of specific neurotoxicants with minimal emphasis on the fundamental principles and basic concepts on the "science" of Neurotoxicology. When I was asked to organize a "new" neurotoxicology book, it became apparent to me that it would be impossible to prepare a single volume that would provide the readers with a full-bodied presentation on the broad information in the field of neurotoxicology today.

The present volume, therefore, represents the first step in covering the fundamental principles and basic concepts in modern Neurotoxicology. It is divided into five sections, covering the five major areas in neurotoxicology: the central nervous system (CNS), the peripheral nervous system (PNS), behavioral neurotoxicology, biochemical/molecular neurotoxicology, and developmental neurotoxicology. An internationally recognized scientist in each of these specialized areas of neurotoxicology was invited to assist me in the planning and organization of these sections including selecting key topics to be covered and inviting chapter contributors for those topics. I am most fortunate that Drs. Mohamed B. Abou-Donia, Hugh A. Tilson, Stephen C. Bondy, and William Slikker, Jr., agreed to serve in this capacity and provided me with excellent advices and assistances.

The present volume focuses on the fundamental principles and concepts of neurotoxicology to give the reader a better understanding of the bases of toxic effects and mechanisms of neurotoxic events. Such neurotoxicological principles and concepts will be exemplified and illustrated with specific neurotoxicants. We believe that this volume will provide readers with a solid foundation of neurotoxicology as a whole. The "effects and mechanisms" of specific neurotoxicants and agents will be covered in greater detail in the next volume to follow.

The field of neurotoxicology will continue to surge into the future. This volume, together with those to follow, represents the combined efforts of the scientitists in neurotoxicology to carry this discipline forth into a new era. With the 21st century around the corner, we hope that these volumes will serve as the foundation and stepping-stone to new challenges. I extend my deepest thanks to all my distinguished colleagues who have put their faith and efforts into this ambitious project.

Louis W. Chang

Contents

Contributors

Mohamed B. Abou-Donia, Ph.D. Professor, Pharmacology and Neurobiology, and Deputy Director of the Toxicology Program, Department of Pharmacology, Duke University Medical Center, Durham, North Carolina

James David Adams, Jr., Ph.D. Associate Professor, Department of Molecular Pharmacology and Toxicology, University of Southern California School of Pharmacy, Los Angeles, California

Jane Adams, Ph.D. Assistant Professor, Department of Psychology, University of Massachusetts, Boston, Massachusetts

Judy L. Aschner, M.D. Assistant Professor, Department of Pediatrics, Albany Medical College, Albany, New York

Michael Aschner, Ph.D. Associate Professor, Department of Pharmacology and Toxicology, Albany Medical College, Albany, New York

William D. Atchison, Ph.D. Professor, Pharmacology and Toxicology, and Director, Neuroscience Program, Department of Pharmacology and Toxicology, Michigan State University, East Lansing, Michigan

Melvin L. Billingsley, Ph.D. Professor, Pharmacology, and Director, Macromolecular Core Lab, Department of Pharmacology, Pennsylvania State University College of Medicine, Hershey, Pennsylvania

Jacob J. Blum, Ph.D.   James B. Duke Professor of Physiology, Department of Cell Biology, Division of Physiology and Cellular Biophysics, Duke University Medical Center, Durham, North Carolina

Stephen C. Bondy, Ph.D.   Professor, Department of Community and Environmental Medicine, Irvine Occupational Health Center, University of California, Irvine, California

Thomas W. Bouldin, M.D.   Professor, Department of Pathology, University of North Carolina at Chapel Hill, Chapel Hill, North Carolina

Louis W. Chang, Ph.D.   Professor, Departments of Pathology, Pharmacology, and Toxicology, and Director of Experimental Pathology Program, University of Arkansas for Medical Sciences, Little Rock, Arkansas

Deborah A. Cory-Slechta, Ph.D.   Associate Professor, Department of Environmental Medicine, University of Rochester School of Medicine and Dentistry, Rochester, New York

Lucio G. Costa, Ph.D.   Professor and Director, Toxicology Program, Department of Environmental Health, University of Washington, Seattle, Washington

Stephen A. Daniel, Ph.D.   Associate Professor, Department of Psychology, Mercy College, Dobbs Ferry, New York

Hugh L. Evans, Ph.D.   Director, Laboratory of Neural Toxicology, Department of Environmental Medicine, New York University Medical Center, Tuxedo, New York

Jerry M. Farley, Ph.D.   Professor, Department of Pharmacology and Toxicology, University of Mississippi Medical Center, Jackson, Mississippi

Stephen C. Fowler, Ph.D.   Professor, Departments of Psychology and Pharmacology, University of Mississippi at Oxford, University, Mississippi

Jeffry F. Goodrum, Ph.D.   Research Scientist, Brain and Development Research Center and Department of Pathology, University of North Carolina at Chapel Hill, Chapel Hill, North Carolina

Ram P. Gupta, Ph.D.   Assistant Research Professor, Department of Pharmacology, Duke University Medical Center, Durham, North Carolina

Ing K. Ho, Ph.D.   Professor and Chairman, Department of Pharmacology and Toxicology, University of Mississippi Medical Center, Jackson, Mississippi

Jean M. Jacobs, Ph.D., FRCPath   Reader in Experimental Neuropathology, Department of Neuropathology, Institute of Neurology, London, England

Mary Jeanne Kallman, Ph.D.   Research Scientist, Toxicology Research Labs, Lilly Research Laboratories, A Division of Eli Lilly and Company, Greenfield, Indiana

Harold K. Kimelberg, Ph.D.   Research Professor, Division of Neurosurgery, and Professor, Pharmacology and Toxicology, Albany Medical College, Albany, New York

Lori K. Klaidman, B.A.   Research Laboratory Technician, Department of Molecular Pharmacology and Toxicology, University of Southern California School of Pharmacy, Los Angeles, California

Laura A. Lagunowich, Ph.D.   Scientist, Drug Safety Evaluations, Regeneron Pharmaceuticals, Inc., Tarrytown, New York

Ellen J. Lehning, Ph.D.   Research Associate, Department of Anesthesiology, State University of New York at Stony Brook, Stony Brook, New York

Pat Levitt, Ph.D.   Professor, Department of Neuroscience and Cell Biology, Robert Wood Johnson Medical School, University of Medicine and Dentistry of New Jersey, Piscataway, New Jersey

Richard M. LoPachin, Ph.D.   Associate Professor, Department of Anesthesiology, State University of New York at Stony Brook, Stony Brook, New York

Charles F. Mactutus, Ph.D.   Associate Professor, Division of Pharmacology and Experimental Therapeutics, College of Pharmacy; Tobacco and Health Research Institute; and Graduate Center for Toxicology, University of Kentucky, Lexington, Kentucky

Pierre Morell, Ph.D.   Professor, Biochemistry and Biophysics, Brain and Development Research Center, University of North Carolina at Chapel Hill, Chapel Hill, North Carolina

E. Hazel Murphy, Ph.D.   Professor, Department of Anatomy and Neurobiology, Medical College of Pennsylvania, Philadelphia, Pennsylvania

Toshio Narahashi, Ph.D.   John Evans Professor of Pharmacology and Alfred Newton Richards Professor of Pharmacology, Department of Pharmacology, Northwestern University Medical School, Chicago, Illinois

James P. O'Callaghan, Ph.D.   Senior Research Scientist and Senior Science Advisor, Neurotoxicology Division, U.S. Environmental Protection Agency, Research Triangle Park, North Carolina

John W. Olney, M.D.   Professor, Departments of Psychiatry and Pathology, Washington University School of Medicine, St. Louis, Missouri

Karen Opello, M.S.   Research Associate, Department of Psychology, Rutgers University, Piscataway, New Jersey

Merle G. Paule, Ph.D.   Head, Behavioral Toxicology Laboratory, Division of Neurotoxicology, National Center for Toxicological Research/FDA, Jefferson, Arkansas

Gordon T. Pryor, Ph.D.   Director, Neuroscience Department, SRI International, Menlo Park, California

Michael C. Reed, Ph.D.   Professor, Department of Mathematics, Duke University, Durham, North Carolina

Kenneth Reuhl, Ph.D.   Professor, Department of Pharmacology and Toxicology, College of Pharmacy, Rutgers University, Piscataway, New Jersey

William Slikker, Jr., Ph.D.   Director, Division of Neurotoxicology, National Center for Toxicological Research/FDA, Jefferson, Arkansas

John M. Spitsbergen, Ph.D.   Research Assistant, Department of Urology, University of Virginia College of Medicine, Charlottesville, Virginia

Hugh A. Tilson, Ph.D.   Director, Neurotoxicology Division, U.S. Environmental Protection Agency, Research Triangle Park, North Carolina

Charles V. Voorhees, Ph.D.   Professor, Department of Pediatrics and Environmental Health, University of Cincinnati, and Children's Hospital Research Foundation, Cincinnati, Ohio

Thomas J. Walsh, Ph.D.   Department of Psychology, Rutgers University, New Brunswick, New Jersey

Bernard Weiss, Ph.D.   Professor, Department of Environmental Medicine and Dentistry, University of Rochester School of Medicine and Dentistry, Rochester, New York

Foreword

It is difficult to define exactly what constitutes neurotoxicology, for ideas vary as to what it should comprehend. Perhaps a useful definition would be "the study of the adverse effects of chemical agents upon the structure or function of nervous tissue." For some this might seem too narrow a definition, for it excludes the use of cells of neural origin and might be considered also to exclude behavioral studies where true "damage" may be less in evidence. However, it is a good working definition as it recognizes, by implication, that the subject of neurotoxicology must be regarded as part of several disciplines. The subject has, indeed, been playing an unrecognized part in the scientific process within a number of biological disciplines for a long while. Thus, biochemists, such as Warburg and Peters, have for many decades used the effects of chemical agents in the test tube as well as in the whole animal in their studies of the complexities of tissue respiration. Physiologists have employed, with striking results, venoms and other biological products to analyze the details of the bioelectric phenomena that characterize the function of nerve fibers. Pharmacologists have, perhaps, long regarded toxicity as the nonbeneficial side of their subject, but none would ignore the further understanding these effects bring to pharmacological mechanisms. Of course, experimental neuropathologists rarely regard themselves as neurotoxicologists, but they have contributed greatly to our understanding of the cellular mechanisms of toxic damage to the nervous tissue. The nervous system of humans being so often inaccessible for study, the use of experimental animals has by necessity come to provide the models now extensively exploited to further our understanding of the mechanisms of neurological disease.

What this means, however, is the neurotoxicology as a newly emerging discipline is something more than the sum of all the components mentioned in the definition given earlier. It must, in fact, because of the complexity of nervous tissue, be a *multidisciplinary* study of the effects of neurotoxic chemicals. It is therefore essential that the physiologist engaged in neurotoxicology must become familiar with the biochemistry and pathology of the neurotoxic problem, and, at the same time, the biochemist and morphologist must do likewise. While scientists in different disciplines may not necessarily be steeped in the technology possessed by their colleagues, their experience and learning should be such that they can critically assess the conclusions of their colleagues without those feelings of insecurity that all too often overwhelm "trespassers" in another field of study. Neurotoxicology cuts across the artificial divisions and barriers that normally separate academic subjects. In neurotoxicology these barriers need to be broken down if proper judgment about mechanisms, chemical interactions, "risk factors," and other important practical aspects of the subject is to be justly exercised.

For these reasons, this volume that Professor Louis Chang is editing so masterfully, covering the entire field of neurotoxicology, is greatly welcomed. The subject has "come of age," and, as the number of sections in this volume testify, there is an explosion of knowledge in progress produced by a desire to understand how the environment, both natural and as altered by humans, might influence adversely the functions and structure of nervous tissue.

When I look at the list of subjects covered in this volume, it is pleasing to know that the subject of neurotoxicology has finally matured from being merely a part of the better known and longer established subject of toxicology. It has, in fact, become a subject in its own right, just as neuropathology has grown and become independent from general pathology. Indeed, in several enlightened academic institutions departments of neurotoxicology now exist. Just as with neuropathology, those working in neurotoxicology must possess not only the stuff of toxicology, but that of neurobiology and neuroscience as well. The special properties of the neuron and the glia, both cells with unique qualities, how they interact, and how they are organized to generate the prime functions of the brain are all features central to understanding the specific problems that may be posed by neurotoxic agents. The general toxicologist is often not aware just how different *toxicology* has become from *neurotoxicology,* and how much an understanding of the latter stems from knowledge of the special biology of neural tissue. Thus, the generalist would not be expected to be aware of the necessity and value of using immunocytochemical techniques now readily available and in constant use in neuropathological laboratories for cell identification and recognition of critical macromolecules. The traditional haematoxylin and eosin section can no longer stand on its own, but has come to be only the first of a number of probes designed to localize and define the nature of a lesion, including good perfusion-fixation and step-serial sectioning and a battery of immunocytochemical reactions. These are now mandatory before beginning any informed discussion of functional/structural correlations or forming hypotheses for further biochemical and functional studies.

The important development in neurotoxicology is perhaps in the area of mechanism of toxicity, for without an understanding of this, any advances in the other aspects must be largely empirical. Presently, we have reached a stage of understanding for many agents at which we can identify the tissue or cells most at risk, and we may have some understanding as to how the metabolic lesion brings this about, although more often than not, this is far from clear.

We are, however, on the threshold of a new and very exciting era of comprehension of metabolic processes that is already altering our attitude toward natural diseases, and this will be increasingly valuable to neurotoxic problems. Thus, the identification of gene mutations in certain hereditary diseases is leading us to the possibility of correcting these defects. Equally the absorption of a toxic chemical can lead to the specific impairment of protein functions—be they enzymes, receptors, or cytoskeletal structures within cells—

and how these cells will necessarily react by the induction or suppression of other functions. We see this sequence taking place in neurons when an axon is cut and the whole metabolic machinery of the cell within a few hours changes from that of its definitive adult state to one in which the need to regenerate new protoplasm is paramount. The capacity of cells-at-risk to react to the intoxicated state by the induction of compensatory metabolic processes could well determine whether they will survive. It should thus be possible to monitor changes in the protein products of immediate-early genes that initiate the sequence of changes within the cell. Early warning signs of this type would be of value for determining sensitivity of individual neuron types, probably at much lower exposure levels than are presently possible. By the same token, by in vitro hybridization and Northern blotting techniques it should be possible to determine changes in metabolic activity of critical components in affected metabolic pathways, thereby giving insight into the reasons for the selective vulnerability of one cell type or another. These are only two aspects of the new data gained by the techniques of molecular biology coming from the rapid advances in neurobiology. They will have significant and growing influence on the future of neurotoxicology and particularly on the assessment of risk, which is of such social and public importance.

We cannot ignore the pathological importance of locally released excitotoxic substances and the potential toxicity of locally uncontrolled release of free radicals or other substances in playing primary as well as secondary roles in the development of neurotoxic brain damage. Both classes of pathogenetic agents have become central not only to understanding how nervous tissue damage takes place in a wide variety of acute neurological conditions but also to a search for means of therapeutic intervention. The high oxygen and energy utilization of nervous tissue is a permanent threat to the integrity of its cellular components, and anything that interferes with the finely balanced built-in protective mechanisms endangers tissue survival. Already, the use of free radical scavengers and of excitotoxic antagonists and blocking agents is beginning to mitigate the effects of vascular insufficiency in various forms of stroke and reduce the size of the final lesion. As might perhaps be expected, many neurotoxic agents disturb this finely balanced metabolic protective system and will lead to local lesions where the oxygen tension and the energy utilization are greatest. Operating on this hypothesis, it has been possible to modulate the damage by reducing neuronal activity. There may be other ways of influencing both the localization and the severity of such neurotoxic damage. Certainly it should be possible to use free radical scavenging agents as positive therapeutic substances as well as agents to protect in suitable circumstances. Clearly prevention is better than cure, and the availability of a rational means to combat the toxicity is a desirable aim in neurotoxicology. May this remain uppermost in the minds of those engaged in this field of research.

It seems a long while from the time of Dr. Donald Hunter's pioneering clinical investigations into the causation of industrial diseases, but in the 1930s and 1940s serious industrial disease was rife and there was little understanding as to how it came about. Anyone who knew Dr. Hunter could not but be stimulated by his vigorous enthusiasm and his undying hope that the workplace should be made safe for the workers. He also taught that there was a need not only to prevent these disasters but also to understand how they came about. Now, 50 years later, it can be truly said that much has been achieved, but while the incidence of industrial illness has markedly declined because of more effective regulation of industries and a growing understanding as to how these illnesses occurred, there is still anxiety in many people's minds—not just about the health of factory workers, but also about the health of the general population being set at risk by constant exposure to atmospheric pollutants, processed food, chemically treated clothing, and similar hazards, some of which we may be quite unaware. The problem appears increasingly to be the slow absorption of chemicals that may conceivably have subtle, long-term effects on the nervous system. The suspicion is there, but the facts are lacking, and the problem is that we all too often have no satisfactory way of assessing where the truth lies. Only by the ever finer dissection of cellular and metabolic lesions, from the known to the unknown, and by more sophisticated probing into the health and function of tissues at risk can we arrive at a greater understanding. That is the ultimate way that neurotoxicology will have to go. It is a considerable challenge, but then the genius of mankind is the acceptance of such a challenge.

J. B. Cavanagh
Institute of Psychiatry
London, England

Part I
Neurotoxicology of the Central Nervous System
Introductory Overview

\Louis W. Chang

University of Arkansas for Medical Sciences
Little Rock, Arkansas

The central nervous system (CNS) is perhaps the most complex organ system. The nerve cells or groups of cells greatly vary in morphology, function, and characteristics from one region of the CNS to another. The complex interactions of these nerve cells (neurons) with one another, with their supporting cells or elements, and with their environments frequently puzzle and challenge biological scientists and medical practitioners. The probing of the "secrets" of the nervous system is now formally recognized as neuroscience, through which the structure, function, and chemical bases of the nervous system are explored via various approaches such as neuroanatomy, neurocytology, neurophysiology, neurobehavioral science, neurochemistry, neurobiochemistry, and molecular neurobiology.

Neurotoxicology may be simply defined as the scientific study of the adverse effects on the nervous system of chemicals or environmental agents. The principal objectives of neurotoxicology are therefore the study of the metabolism of neurotoxicants, the exploration and identification of their toxic effects, the characterization of lesion development, and the search for biochemical and molecular mechanistic bases of neurotoxicity. All these objectives are firmly based on clear understanding of the basic neuroscience of the "normal" nervous system. Thus, one may consider neurotoxicology as an independent science that branches from the trunk of toxicology and is deeply rooted in neuroscience. It is with this thought that the first chapter in this section is devoted to the basic principles and concepts of neuroscience, neurocytology, and neuropathology. Information in this chapter will serve as the stepping stone and first gateway for many students of neurotoxicology to the many chapters in this volume as well as to those volumes to follow.

The nervous system is well "protected" by a biological system from the general vascular circulation. In the CNS, this system is known as the blood-brain barrier (BBB), and in the peripheral nervous system it is referred to as the blood-nerve barrier (BNB). These systems are important in the regulation of nerve tissue metabolism in relationship to the circulatory blood supplies. Their normal structures and functions, as well as their dysfunction under the influences of certain chemicals, will be presented and discussed by Dr. Jean Jacobs. One of the unique functions and capabilities of the nervous system, particularly the CNS, is its capacity for cell-cell or cell–end organ communications. These communications are accomplished by signal transmission (via neurotransmitters) and signal reception (via neuroreceptors). These important principles and concepts will be presented and discussed by Professors Jerry M. Farley and I. K. Ho. The disturbance of these systems by chemicals will certainly precipitate dysfunction of the nervous system.

Neurocytoskeletal elements, including neurotubules and neurofilaments, are no longer viewed simply as organelles that provide "skeletal support" to the neurons and their processes. These elements are now found to be vital to the functions and survival of nerve cells. Many neurotoxic chemicals, such as heavy metals and organic solvents, are known to disrupt these elements, leading to various degenerative and functional changes in the nervous system. Consideration of these elements in relationship to neurotoxicity in the nervous system will be given by Professor M. B. Abou-Donia in Part II of this volume.

The most frequently misunderstood and neglected elements in the CNS are perhaps the glial cells. It used to be believed that the functions of the glial cells are "supportive": astrocytes for "connective" support and scar formation after injury (not unlike the fibroblasts in systemic connective tissue) and oligodendrocytes for myelination of axons in the CNS. While that notion concerning oligodendrocytes may still be by and large true, the functions of astrocytes are now much better defined and recognized. The role of astrocytes in neurometabolisn and repair as well as their relationships to neuronal damage during neurotoxic conditions will be discussed in a chapter by Dr. Michael Aschner and colleagues.

The focus of this volume is on basic principles and current concepts in neurotoxicology. Throughout this section and other sections in this volume, these principles and concepts are discussed in terms of neuroscience, neurobiology, neuropathology, and neurotoxicology. They are "illustrated" through selected neurotoxic conditions. Detailed consideration of toxic effects and the mechanisms of specific neurotoxicants or agents will be presented in the volume *Handbook of Neurotoxicology* to be published by Marcel Dekker, Inc.

1

Introduction to Basic Principles of Neurocytology and General Concepts on Neurotoxicopathology

Louis W. Chang
University of Arkansas for Medical Sciences
Little Rock, Arkansas

INTRODUCTION

The nervous system is perhaps the most complex biological system. It consists of interconnecting networks of heterogeneous cell groups. The variable activities and functions of the nerve cells respond to chemical challenges in an immensely diverse manner. Each component of the nerve cell may react differently to the same chemical. Likewise, chemicals, depending on their toxicological characteristics, may have selective action on a specific component of the neuron (e.g., axon or dendrite, neurofilaments or synaptic terminal).

Because of the complexity of the nervous system in morphological cytoarchitecture, metabolism, and function, a basic understanding of neuroscience should be considered a prerequisite for the study and understanding of neurotoxicology. This chapter serves to introduce the basic principles, concepts, and terminologies of neurocytology and neurotoxicopathology, on which much of the discussion of various aspects of neurotoxicology in the following chapters and sections in this volume will be based.

One of the unique characteristics of the nervous system is the capacity of nerve cells to communicate with each other and with other cells. In the 19th century, a controversy developed concerning how nerve cells interconnect and intercommunicate. The "reticular theory" suggested that there was a protoplasmic continuity between various nervous elements. A noted Spanish neuroanatomist, Santiago Ramón y Cajal (1852–1934), first proposed that nerve cells are contiguous but not continuous. In Cajal's "neuron theory," nerve cells were anatomical entities forming intercommunicating networks. After the birth of the neuron theory, modern techniques continued to verify that the central nervous system is composed of a variety of nerve cells and supporting glial elements. The nerve cells intercommunicate with each other via multiple processes and synaptic contacts. Detailed consideration of the basic structures and functions of the nerve cells and their supporting elements is available in standard neuroscience texts. Therefore, only the essence of these aspects will be included in this chapter.

Neurotoxicity may be simply defined as adverse effects on the structural, biochemical, and functional intergrity of the nervous system. While different neurotoxic agents may have different actions and effects on the nervous system, certain basic alterations of neurons are common and underlie many toxic injuries to nerve cells. These general aspects of neurotoxic alterations will also be presented in this chapter.

BASIC STRUCTURE AND FUNCTION OF NEURONS

Basic Morphology of Neurons

There is a wide range of sizes and shapes of neurons (Fig. 1). Despite their differences in morphological appearance, most, if not all, neurons share certain common structural features: prominent nuclei, neuronal processes (axons and dendrites), synapses, cytoskele-

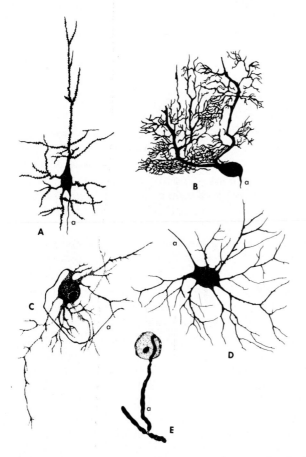

Figure 1 Variety of forms of neurons with tremendously diversified morphological appearances. (A) Pyramidal neuron (cerebral cortex). (B) Purkinje neuron (cerebellar cortex). (C) Sympathetic postganglionic neuron. (D) Motoneuron (spinal cord). (E) Sensory neuron (dorsal root ganglia). a = axon. (From Willis and Grossman, 1973.)

tal elements (neurotubules and neurofilaments), Nissl substance, and cytoplasmic organelles (Fig. 2).

Most neurons have a large nucleus (karyon) with a prominent nucleolus. The cytoplasmic area (perikaryon) is the metabolic site of the nerve cell. Many large neurons contain masses of chromophilic material called Nissl substance. This substance corresponds to areas of rough endoplasmic reticulum and clusters of polyribosomes seen on electron microscopy. This material is involved in protein synthesis in the nerve cells. The proteins produced (including enzymes and secretory materials) may be utilized by the neuron or be transported through the axonal process for secretion.

The perikaryon also contains the cytoplasmic skeletal systems: neurotubules and neurofilaments. The neurotubules, which have diameters of 200–400 Å, are known to be involved in axoplasmic flow and the transport of secretory products in the neuronal processes. The neurofilaments have a diameter of 80–100 Å. The precise function of these filaments in the nerve cells, aside from cytoskeletal support, is still not fully understood.

Most neurons are highly "polarized" in such a way that one pole receives information

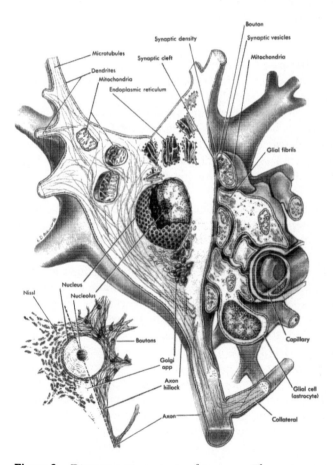

Figure 2 Diagrammatic anatomy of a neuron. The main neuronal organelles consist of large nuclei with prominent neucleoli, neurotubules, neurofilaments, rough endoplasmic reticulum, mitochondria, and Golgi apparatus. The neuronal surface may be in contact with synaptic terminals and enwrapped by astrocytic processes. (From Willis and Grossman, 1973.)

and the opposing pole transmits information to another nerve cell or to a receptor organ. The receptive pole is termed the dendritic pole and the transmitting pole is the axonal pole (portion) of the cell.

Axonal Portion of the Neuron

The major process of a neuron is the axon. An axon may give off branches near the cell body (axon collaterals) that end synaptically on nearby nerve cells. The main part of the axon may travel a long distance as fiber tract in the central nervous system or through a peripheral nerve to synapse with another neuron or on an effector cell. Golgi type I neurons are those with long axons and are the primary nerve cells of the neuronal pool. Golgi II neurons are usually smaller neurons with short axons. They are also known as internuncial neurons, with axons terminating on nearby neurons.

The axon has its origin at the axonal hillock of the nerve cell. The axonal hillock contains no organized Nissl bodies and only a few ribosomes. Bundles of neurotubules pass through the axonal hillock into the axon. The axon proper characteristically contains no ribosomes; furthermore, there are usually more neurofilaments than neurotubules in the axon. Some agranular (smooth) endoplasmic reticulum may be found in the axon. Not all axons are ensheathed by myelin, and not all myelinated axons have the same amount of myelin sheath.

Most of the protein needed by the axon to maintain its structural integrity and renew its synaptic transmitters is produced in the perikaryon of the neuron. The protein produced is transported down the axon from the neuronal body by axoplasmic flow. However, some protein may be polymerized in situ within the axon from small polypeptides and amino acids. Axoplasmic flow is now believed to be associated with the neurotubules in the axon. Although a majority of the axoplasmic flow is away from the neuronal body, evidence shows that reverse axoplasmic flow also exists. Two major components of axoplasmic flow have been identified: a slow flow that carries soluble proteins and a fast component that transports primarily amino acids and polypeptides.

Nerve impulses are produced by an electrochemical reaction within the nerve membrane. The propagation of the impulse along the axon is caused by a spread of ionic current that depolarizes neighboring areas of the membrane and so triggers the nerve impulse at each point along the membrane. The nerve impulse may also be considered as a sequence of alterations in membrane potential. This series of potential changes is called the action potential, which is produced by a sudden increase in membrane permeability to sodium ions followed by potassium ions.

The most characteristic part of the axon is the synaptic terminal or transmitting portion of the axon. At the fine structural level, the transmitting synaptic complex reveals three distinctive features. This triad consists of a presynaptic bulb with accumulation of synaptic vesicles, a specialization of membranes at the synaptic interface to form sticky attachment plaques, and increased electron-density accumulation under the postsynaptic membrane. The synapse represents the "communicating contact point" from the neuron. The major neurotransmitters include acetylcholine, norepinephrine, serotonin, γ-aminobutyric acid, glutamic acid, histamine, glycine, and substance P. Depending on the neurotransmitter, a neuron may be excitatory, inhibitory, or involved in various trophic actions.

Receptive (Dendritic) Portion of the Neuron

The receptive pole of the nerve cell is the geometrical dendritic zone of the neuron. Much of the difference in various types of neurons depends on the complexity and branching of the dendrites. Small neurons usually have a simple receptive zone. Large neurons, such as the cerebellar Purkinje cells, have an elaborate and branching dendritic formation. The receptive portion of a neuron is designed to respond to various bioelectrical or chemical stimuli and to integrate converging inputs from other neurons.

Dendrites may vary from none to many in a neuron. While they may have only a short extension from the neuronal cell body as compared with axons, dendrites may branch repetitively to form a characteristic arborization. This is best illustrated with the Purkinje cell of the cerebellum (Fig. 3).

The cytoplasm of dendrites may contain all the organelles found in the neuronal cytoplasm, including polyribosomes and rough endoplasmic reticulum. Characteristically, there are large numbers of neurotubules in dendrites.

Small protrusions, known as dendritic spines, are found on the branches of the dendritic processes. These spines serve as synaptic attachments. Thus they may be considered synaptic receptors of the nerve cells. However, the main dendritic surface as well as the neuronal body surface can also receive synaptic terminals without the spines.

In various toxic situations, such as mercury intoxication or alcoholism, there may be an atrophy or reduction of the dendritic spines, dendritic branches, and dendritic arborization (Fig. 4).

SUPPORTING CELLS IN THE NERVOUS SYSTEM

The major supporting cells in the central nervous system (CNS) include astrocytes, oligodendrocytes, and microglia. Collectively, they are known as the glial cells of the CNS

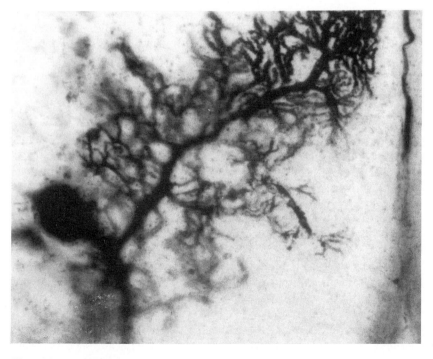

Figure 3 Cerebellar cortex, human, rapid Golgi stain. Note the elaborate dendritic arborization of a Purkinje cell (×400.)

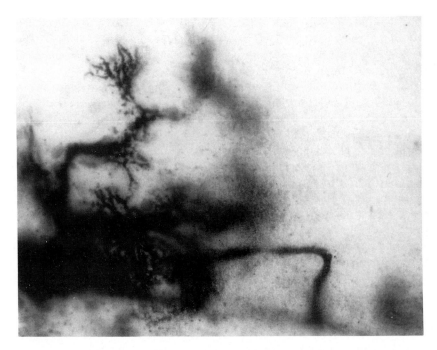

Figure 4   Cerebellar cortex, human, fetal Minamata disease (methylmercury poisoning), rapid Golgi stain. Extensive destruction of the dendritic branches of the Purkinje cell was noted. (×400.)

(Fig. 5). Ependymal cells, which are ciliated cuboidal epithelium lining the surfaces of the ventricular system of the brain and the central canal of the spinal cord, are also considered a supporting cell type of the CNS. The two main supporting cells of the peripheral nervous system are the satellite cells in the peripheral ganglia and the Schwann cells in the peripheral nerves.

Astrocytes

There are two types of astrocyte, protoplasmic and fibrous. It is generally believed that these are probably varieties of the same kind of cell. Protoplasmic astrocytes are more abundant in the white matter, while the fibrous astrocytes are more abundant in the gray matter. Morphologically, there are many processes extending from the astrocytes, giving them a star-like appearance (thus the term "astrocytes," star-like cells) (Fig. 6). The most characteristic feature of astrocytes is the abundance of glial filaments in the cytoplasm and processes of the cells.

Astrocytes, especially those in the gray matter, are found to interpose between the blood vessels and the nerve cells, with distended endings of processes encircling cerebral capillaries and with other processes covering the neuronal surface. The perivascular foot processes of astrocytes are a component of the blood-brain barrier, which selectively discriminates substances entering the CNS. Thus one may consider the blood-brain barrier and astrocytes the first gateway-control to the neurons. Many chemicals, such as certain heavy metals, are known to alter the astrocytes and the blood-brain barrier, leading to serious consequences in the nervous system (see Chapters 2 and 4 in this volume).

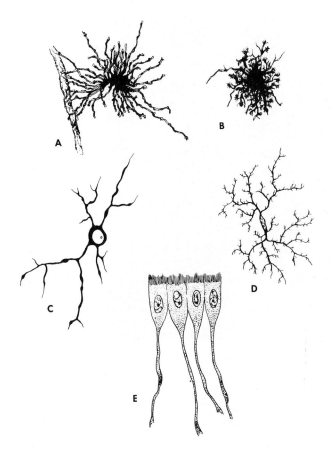

Figure 5 Different types of supporting neuroglial cells of the central nervous system. (A) Fibrous astrocyte. (B) Protoplasmic astrocyte. (C) Oligodendrocyte. (D) Microglia. (E) Ependymal cell. (From Willis and Grossman, 1973.)

The astrocytes are also important cell elements responding to damage to the CNS. These cells may proliferate, enlarge, and form glial scars. This repair process in the CNS is known as gliosis.

Oligodendrocytes

Oligodendrocytes are the glial cells responsible for the production of myelin sheaths around axons in the central nervous system. Some oligodendrocytes are situated adjacent to the neuronal cell bodies and are known as satellite or perineuronal cells. Unlike astrocytes, oligodendrocytes do not have abundant glial filaments but are rich in rough endoplasmic reticulum. Under the light microscope, oligodendrocytes appear to have smaller and denser nuclei than astrocytes. Each oligodendrocyte is known to have the ability to myelinate several axons or segments of an axon by multiple processes (Fig. 7).

Microglia

Microglia, unlike astrocytes and oligodendrocytes, which are ectodermally derived, arise from the mesoderm. They may be considered the macrophages of the CNS. Reacting to

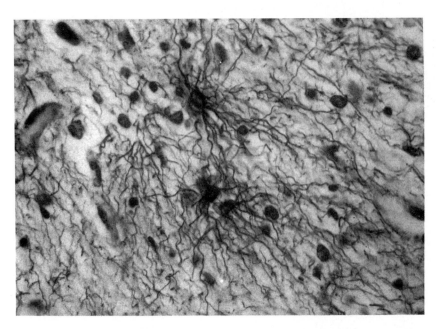

Figure 6   Cerebral cortex, human, Holzer stain. The astrocytes displayed many radiating processes, giving the cells a "star" appearance. (×400.)

CNS injuries, these cells proliferate, enlarge, and become phagocytic. Cellular debris may be found inside their enlarged cytoplasm. In this condition, they are referred to as glitter cells.

Schwann Cells and Myelin

Schwann cells are the cell type that is responsible for myelination of axons (nerve fibers) in the peripheral nervous system. With injury to the nerve fiber, Schwann cells may also display phagocytic activities (Chang and Hartmann, 1972a). Unlike oligodendrocytes, each Schwann cell can myelinate only a single internodal segment of one axon. Unmyelinated axons in the peripheral nervous system are usually also embedded in or surrounded by the cytoplasm of the Schwann cells.

The main function of the myelin sheath is to enhance the velocity of conduction of nerve impulses along the axon. Analyses by x-ray diffraction have revealed that the myelin sheath is composed of concentric layers of radially oriented lipid molecules sandwiched between tangentially oriented protein molecules. Electron microscopy has further demonstrated the structural conformation of the myelin membranes as a continuous spiral.

The myelin sheath, however, has two kinds of discontinuity: the nodes of Ranvier and the clefts of Schmidt-Lanterman. The nodes of Ranvier are junctional areas between two myelinating cells. There is a fairly free channel from the extracellular space to the nodal membrane. Ionic exchanges across the axonal membrane for nervous conduction are believed to take place at these nodes. The clefts of Schmidt-Landerman are formed by the intrusion of cytoplasm of the supporting cell between myelin lamellae. The cleft forms a

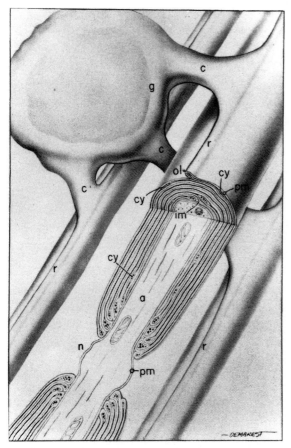

Figure 7   Diagrammatic representation of an oligodendrocyte (g) forming myelin sheaths (r) around several axons (a) by multiple processes (c). Also shown are node of Ranvier (n), axonal plasma membrane (pm), "trapped" glial cytoplasm (cy), inner mesaxon (im), and outer loop of glial plasma membrane (ol). (From Bodian, 1967.)

spiral channel connecting the cytoplasm external to the sheath with that internal to the sheath. It plays an important role in the transport of metabolites and nutrients through the myelin sheaths. The general structures of the node of Ranvier and cleft of Schmidt-Lanterman are diagramatically represented in Fig. 8.

When the cytoplasm of the myelinating cell totally encircles the axon, the opposing cytoplasmic membranes may fuse to form the mesaxon. The mesaxon elongates and continues to encircle the axon. The electron density of the apposing outer layer of the cell membrane is less than that of the apposing inner layer of the membrane. This results in an alteration of major dense lines and interperiod lines (Fig. 9). The electron-lucid zone between the dense lines represents the lipid component of the membranes.

Various toxic chemicals, such as acetyl ethyl tetramethyl tetralin (AETT), triethyltin (TET), and inorganic lead, are selective in inducing damage to the myelin sheaths. These phenomena will be discussed in Chapters 8 and 21.

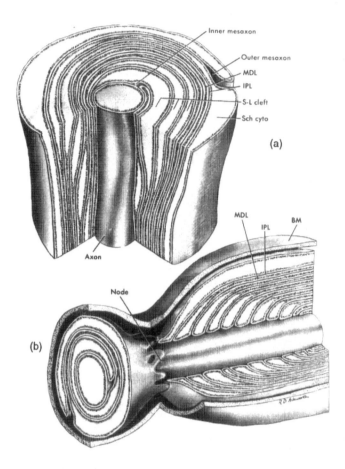

Figure 8 Diagrammatic representation of the (a) Schmidt-Lanterman cleft and (b) the node of Ranvier in the myelin sheath of a peripheral nerve. Shown are the Schmidt-Lanterman cleft (S-L cleft), Schwann cell cytoplasm (Sch cyto), major dense line (MDL), interperiod line (IPL), and basement membrane (BM). (From Willis and Grossman, 1973.)

GENERAL ASPECTS AND PATHOLOGICAL CLASSIFICATIONS OF NEUROTOXICITY

Neuropathology is one of the most important aspects of modern neurotoxicology. The two main objectives of neuropathology, morphologically speaking, are 1.) to identify the loci of the lesion produced (e.g., Ammon's horn of the hippocampus) and 2.) to define the cell types involved and the characteristics of the damage (e.g., cellular swelling and vacuolation or necrosis of the CA_3 pyramidal neurons of Ammon's horn). Thus neuropathology, when performed properly, helps to provide information on the form toxic lesions occurred and where, when, and sometimes even how they occur. This information may be used as an "indicator" or marker for the assessment of the neurotoxic agent in question or may be used to correlate with other data (e.g., neurophysiological, behavioral, and biochemical changes) for better understanding of the toxic actions and mechanisms of the chemicals involved.

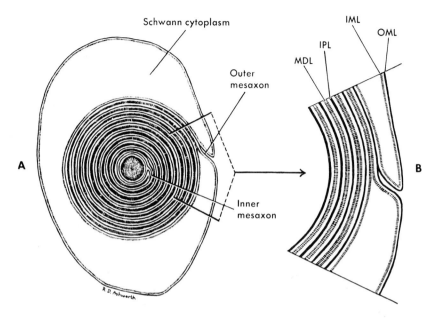

Figure 9   Structure of myelin sheath and formation of the major dense line and interperiod line. MDL = major dense line; IPL = interperiod line; IML = inner membrane lamella; OML = outer membrane lamella. (From Willis and Grossman, 1973.) The drawing in *B* is an enlargement of the portion of *A* indicated by the broken lines.

While the basic anatomy and function of neurons (nerve cell bodies and their processes) and the supporting cells are covered in the above section of this chapter, this section will be devoted to the most commonly seen histopathology in neurotoxic situations involving the neurons, their processes, and some of the supporting elements.

Toxic injuries of the nervous system may be classified in accordance with the components of involvement as nueronopathy, axonopathy, dendropathy, and myelinopathy. These toxic conditions will be discussed in detail in following chapters in this volume. Therefore, only the general concepts of these phenomena are presented in this chapter.

PATHOLOGY OF THE NEURON (NEURONOPATHY)

The basic functional unit of the nervous system is the neuron. As stated earlier, one group or type of neurons in one locus may be very different in size and morphology from those in other loci. The large neurons, such as those found in the hippocampal Ammon's horn, are pyramidal-shaped nerve cells with prominent nuclei and cytoplasmic Nissl substance. Small nerve cells, such as the granule cells in the fascia dentata of the hippocampus, are round, with small nuclei and minimal cytoplasm. Furthermore, different neuronal groups have different functions. Thus, one may expect different reactions and different degenerative changes to be induced in different groups of nerve cells by similar assaults. These changes may or may not be reversible. If the injury was too severe for recovery, eventual neuronal degeneration and neuronal death will occur. Pathological changes involving the neuronal body are termed neuronopathy.

The basic categories of neuronopathy may be outlined as follows.

Central Chromatolysis

Central chromatolysis is a neuronal reaction occurring primarily as a response to injury of the axon. Therefore, it is also referred to as "axonal reaction" (Fig. 10). This reaction is typically seen in large neurons with prominent Nissl substance, such as the anterior horn motoneuron or the large brain stem neurons. It takes place approximately 48 hours following injury and may reach its climax in about 2 to 3 weeks.

In this reaction, the neuronal cell body becomes slightly distended (rounded), with a dissolution of the Nissl substance in the cytoplasm. This disappearance of Nissl substance usually begins around the nucleus (and is thus called "central chromatolysis") (Fig. 11) and eventually involves the entire cell. The nucleus also moves away from the axonal hillock and acquires an eccentric position at the peripheral margin of the cell (Figs. 12 and 13). With electron microscopy, disintegration of the rough endoplasmic reticulum (Nissl substance) can be demonstrated (Fig. 14). If the cell manages to recover, the Nissl substance will gradually reaggregate, usually starting around the nucleus.

Examples of this type of neuronopathy are seen in the dorsal root ganglion neurons after methylmercury intoxication (Chang and Hartmann, 1972b; Chang, 1982), in the brain stem neurons of rats following alkyl lead poisoning (Walsh et al., 1986; Chang, 1987) and in the spinal ganglion neurons after podophyllotoxin poisoning (Chang et al., 1992).

Peripheral Chromatolysis

Peripheral chromatolysis represents a neuronal attempt to compensate for a noxious assault. Nerve cells with peripheral chromatolysis show a slight reduction in neuronal size and a

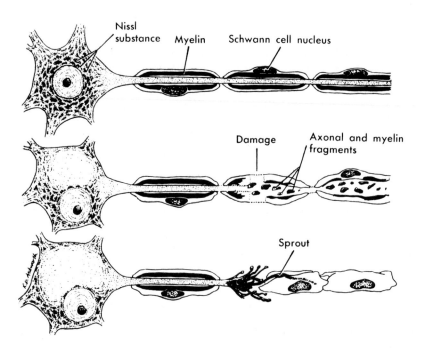

Figure 10 Axonal reaction. Axonal injuries induce a neuronal response (chromatolysis) and an axonal degeneration (Wallerian degeneration). If the neuron survives the injury, axonal spouting from the axonal end may occur in an attempt at axonal regeneration. (From Willis and Grossman, 1973.)

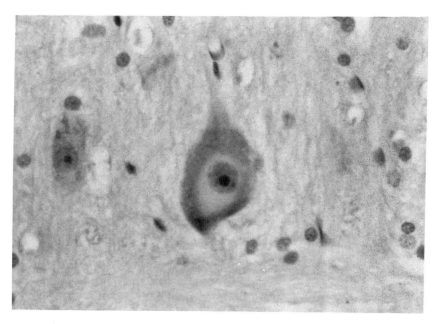

Figure 11 Brain stem, rat, trimethyllead intoxication, hematoxylin-eosin stain. Early chromatolysis (disappearance of Nissl substance) began around the nucleus of the neuron and is thus termed central chromatolysis. (×400.)

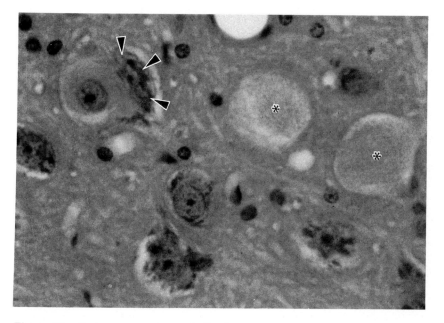

Figure 12 Brain stem, rat, trimethyllead intoxication, hematoxylin-eosin stain. Remnants of Nissl substance (arrowheads) were still observable at the periphery of a neuron undergoing chromatolysis. Two other neurons (asterisks) showed total disappearance of their Nissl substances. (×400.)

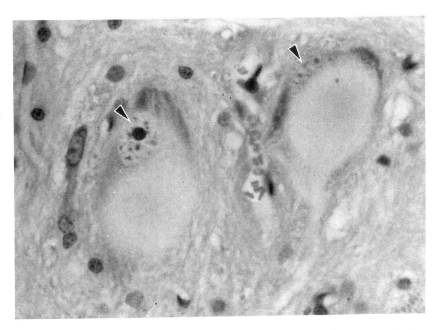

Figure 13 Brain stem, rat, trimethyllead intoxication, hematoxylin-eosin stain. Extensive chromatolytic neurons showing no stainable Nissl substance and eccentric nuclei (arrowheads). (×400.)

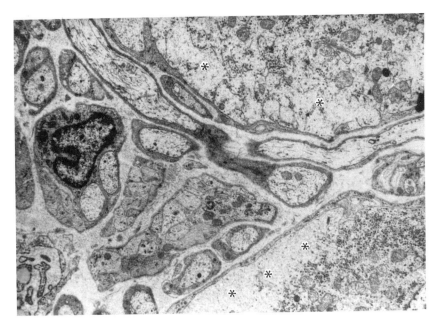

Figure 14 Dorsal root ganglion neuron, rat, methyl mercury poisoning. Disruption and disappearance of the rough endoplasmic reticulum (Nissl substance) (asterisks) in two neurons were demonstrated. (×6500.)

depletion of Nissl granules in the periphery zone of the cytoplasm. Heavy aggregation (hyperchromatic) of Nissl substance, however, can be observed around the nucleus, which remains in the center of the cell. A good example of this type of neuronal change can be observed in the anterior horn motoneurons in cases of progressive muscular atrophy or muscular degeneration.

Neuronal Atrophy and Degeneration

"Atrophy" denotes a reduction of cellular size. Simple atrophy of neurons is most commonly seen in a reduction of neuronal metabolism or function that may lead to eventual degeneration and death of the neuron. This phenomenon may be observed in certain vitamin deficiency states, chronic ischemia, chronic intoxication, or sytemic degeneration such as amyotrophic lateral sclerosis.

The nerve cell body often shrinks in size and becomes hyperchromatic or sclerotic without showing the reaction of chromatolysis (Fig. 15). Axonal or neuronal degeneration such as swelling or vacuolation may also be associated with this type of alteration. This kind of neuronal and axonal change is best exemplified in acute toxic peripheral neuropathy, such as acrylamide intoxication (Blakemore and Cavanagh, 1969; Prineas, 1969; Spencer and Schaumburg, 1976).

Injuries to some axons within the CNS may initially induce neuronal swelling and central chromatolysis of the nerve cells, but these alterations are later followed by eventual

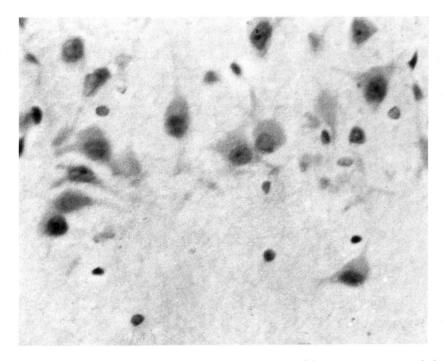

Figure 15 Hippocampal Ammon's horn, CA3, pyramidal neurons, rat, trimethyltin intoxication, hematoxylin-eosin stain. The nerve cells appeared to be hyperchromatic and reduced in size (atrophic). (×400.)

atrophy of the nerve cell bodies. This type of biphasic reaction is referred to as Gudden's atrophy. This phenomenon can be seen in the neurons of the inferior olives following axonal changes in the olivocerebellar tract.

Transsynaptic atrophy or degeneration may also occur in neurons following damage to the axons that make synaptic contact with them. An example of this phenomenon is atrophy or degenerative changes of the nerve cells in the external geniculate nuclei as a result of lesions in the optic nerve or optic tract. On the other hand, lesions may also be induced in neurons (e.g., Ammon's horn CA_3 neurons) as a result of transsynaptic hyperexcitation from presynaptic neurons (e.g., the granule cells of the fascia dentata). This toxic phenomenon can be seen in trimethyltin intoxication (Chang, 1986, 1990a,b). Similar neuronal damage may be produced by other neuroexcitotoxins under different conditions (Olney, 1980; also see Chapter 17).

Neuronal Swelling and Vacuolation

Cellular swelling is one of the most common and early changes of cellular injury. The neuron is not an exception. Neuronal swelling is the result of water accumulation in the cytoplasm of the nerve cell, yielding a distended and enlarged neuron. This condition is also known as edematous change and reflects a disturbance of the electrolyte balance system (mitochondrial function, ATP-system, Na^+-pump, plasma membrane integrity, etc.) of the nerve cell (Powell et al., 1980). Sodium ions and water flux into the cell, giving the cell a lucid and "watery" appearance. The nucleus, however, remains centrally located in most cases (Fig. 16).

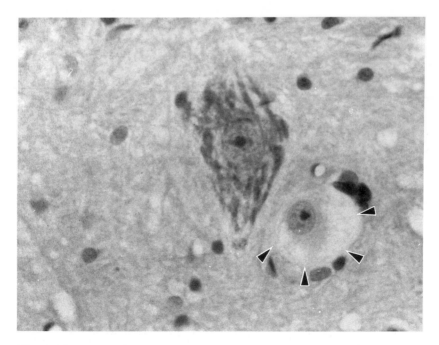

Figure 16 Anterior horn motoneuron, rat, trimethyllead poisoning, hematoxylin-eosin stain. An edematous neuron (arrowheads) acquired a lucid, watery appearance. A normal neuron with well-stained Nissl substance was also present. (×400.)

Routine paraffin sections (10 nm thick) with hematoxylin-eosin (H & E) staining may demonstrate floccular cytoplasm in the edematous neurons (Fig. 17). Thin plastic sections (1–2 nm), however, reveal a lacy cytoplasm with vacuoles within these nerve cells (Fig. 18). With the aid of electron microscopy, distended cisternae of the rough endoplasmic reticulum (RER) can be observed (Figs. 19 and 20). These distentions of the RER are believed to be a mechanism to isolate and to contain the increased water in the cytoplasm. Swelling of the mitochondria may also occur (Figs. 21 and 22). Continued enlargement and distention of the RER cisternae and swollen mictochondria will give rise to cytoplasmic vacuoles in the nerve cells observable by light microscopy. Extensive edematous changes of the nerve cells will eventually lead to hydropic or vacuolar degeneration of the cell. This type of neuronal change may be found in acute toxic situations such as those seen in the brain stem neurons or anterior horn cells of the spinal cord of mice under the toxic influence of trimethyltin (Chang et al., 1983, 1984).

Neurofibrillary Degeneration

Neurofibrillary degeneration is a special form of neuronal degeneration. A special histochemical technique (Bielschowsky method) reveals thickening and tortuosity of fibrils within the neuronal cytoplasm of the involved nerve cells. This type of degeneration is commonly seen in human patients with Alzheimer's disease, senile dementia, and Parkinsonism–dementia of Guam. Neurons in the frontal and temporal cortices as well as in the hippocampus are most frequently affected. This accumulation of neurofibrils in the nerve cells is referred to as neurofibrillary tangles in the neurons.

In neurotoxic situations, such as aluminum poisoning, similar, though not necessarily identical, fibrillary accumulation is induced in many neurons of the cerebral cortex and hippocampus (Fig. 23) (Klatzo et al., 1975; Wisniewski et al., 1977). Different alterations of

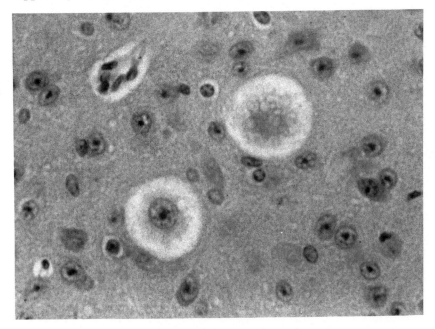

Figure 17 Brain stem, mouse, trimethyltin poisoning. Two edematous neurons appeared to be distended (rounded), with floccular cytoplasm. Note the centrally situated nucleus. (×400.)

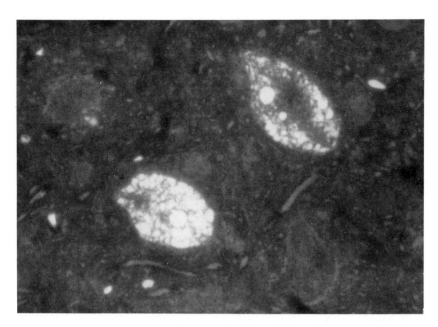

Figure 18 Spinal cord, mouse, trimethyltin poisoning, thin epoxy-embedded section stained with toluidine blue stain. Lacy cytoplasms with small vacuoles were revealed in the edematous neurons. (×400.)

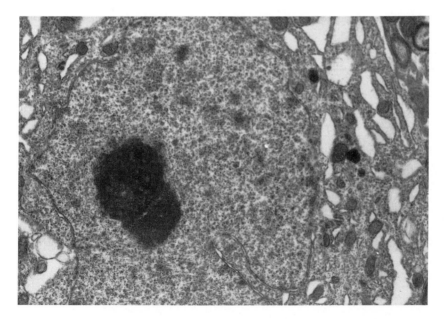

Figure 19 Brain stem neuron, mouse, trimethyltin intoxication. Distention of the rough endoplasmic reticulum and Golgi apparatus represented the early stage of edematous change in the neuron. (×4500.)

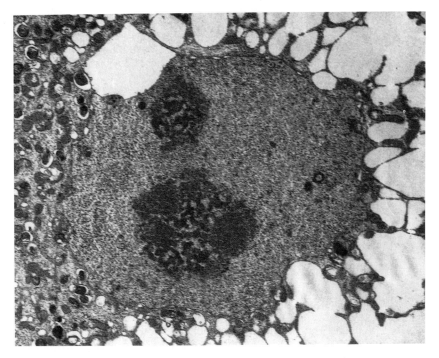

Figure 20 Brain stem neuron, mouse, trimethyltin intoxication. In severe edematous conditions, the neuronal membrane systems (endoplasmic reticulum and Golgi apparatus) were extensively distended by the intracellular fluid to give the cell a vacuolated honeycomb appearance. (×4500.)

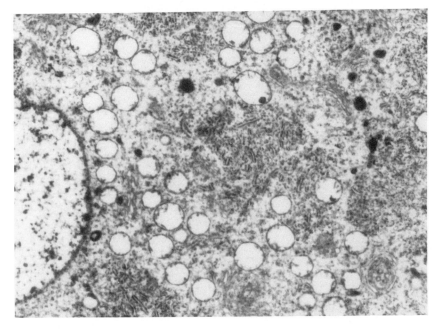

Figure 21 Spinal ganglion neuron, rat, Kepone intoxication. Multiple cytoplasmic vacuoles, measuring approximately 1 micron in diameter, were observed. (×3500.)

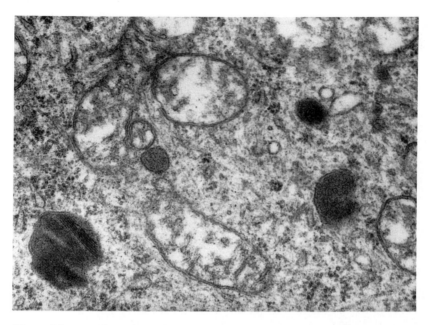

Figure 22 Spinal ganglion neuron, rat, Kepone intoxication. Close examination of the neuron, as illustrated in Fig. 21, revealed that these vacuolar structures were edematous (swollen and distended) mitochondria. Some mitochondria would rupture to form large cytoplasmic vacuoles. (×11,500.)

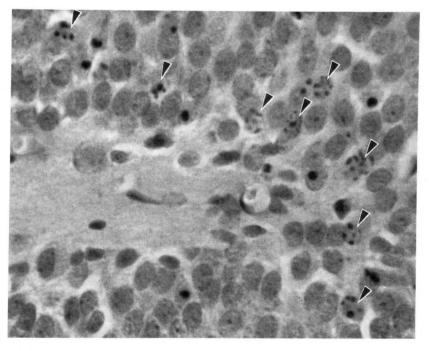

Figure 23 Hippocampus, rat, aluminum intoxication, Bielchowsky's stain. Heavy bundles of argentophilic filaments were found in the cytoplasm of a neuron (arrowheads). (×650.)

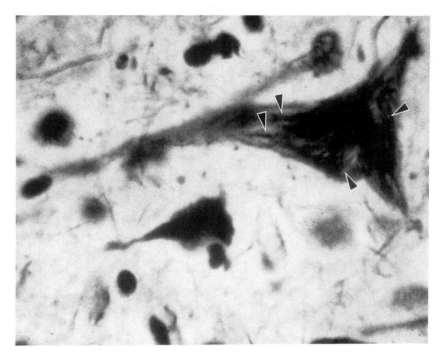

Figure 24 Fascia dentata, mouse, trimethyltin intoxication, hematoxylin-eosin stain. The pyknotic neurons (arrowheads) displayed highly condensed nuclei and eosinophilic cytoplasm. (×400.)

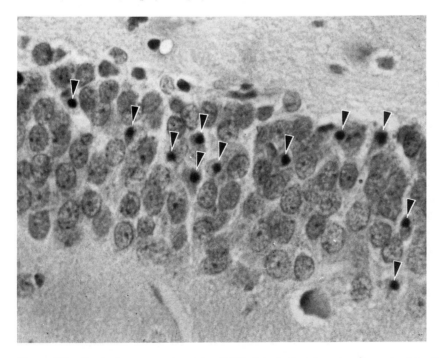

Figure 25 Fascia dentata, mouse, trimethyltin intoxication, hematoxylin-eosin stain. Neuronal necrosis in the form of pyknosis and karyorrhexis (arrowheads) was induced in the granule cell layer. (×400.)

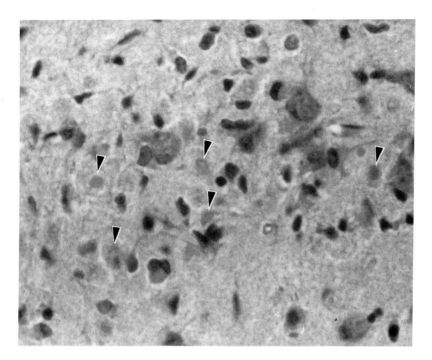

Figure 26   Pyriform cortex, rat, trimethyltin intoxication, hematoxylin-eosin stain. Neuronal necrosis with rapid lysis or fading of the nuclei (karyolysis) was observed (arrowheads). (×400.)

cytoskeletons (neurotubules and neurofilaments) also occur in other neurotoxic conditions such as those associated with organolead (Chang, 1987), β,β′-iminodipropionitrile (IDPN) (Chou and Hartmann, 1964, 1965), podophyllotoxin (Chang et al., 1992), and other neurotoxic compounds (Seppalainen and Halatia, 1980; Spencer et al., 1980b). Details of these phenomena will be discussed in other chapters in this volume and will not be elaborated here.

Neuronal Necrosis

Neuronal necrosis (neuronal death) can be recognized morphologically by nuclear changes in the nerve cell. Such change consists of condensation of the nuclear chromatin (pyknotic nucleus) with highly eosinophilic cytoplasm (Fig. 24). These cells are also referred to as pyknotic cells. Occasionally, fragmentation of the nuclei (karyorrhexis) (Fig. 25) or total dissolution and disappearance of the nuclei (karyolysis) may also occur. Because of a lack of nuclei in these cells, they are sometimes referred to as "ghost cells" (Fig. 26).

Pyknotic changes of neurons are most frequently seen in acute neuronal poisoning (e.g., fascia dentata neurons in trimethyltin intoxication) (Chang et al., 1982a,b) and in anoxia. It must be emphasized that there is a time lapse of 8 to 12 hours following cell death ("biological cell death") before such morphological change ("morphological cell death") can be detected by light microscopy.

PATHOLOGY OF NEURONAL PROCESSES

The neuronal processes, including the axon (myelinated or unmyelinated) and dendrites, are important functional structures of a nerve cell. Specific or selective damage to these structures by various toxicants or by disease states is frequent. Familiarity with these pathological changes is important to the understanding of the toxic action or disease involvement that induces such changes.

Wallerian Degeneration

Wallerian degeneration is secondary degeneration of the axon and its myelin sheath when they are disconnected from the nerve cell body or after the nerve cell body dies from direct injury (Fig. 10).

In this process, the axon becomes swollen, varicose, and irregularly shaped. The associated myelin sheath also breaks down, usually beginning at the nodes of Ranvier, and forms a series of ellipsoid structures enclosing fragments of the degenerating axon. Lipids derived from the breakdown of myelin will eventually be removed by macrophages.

Axonopathies

Pathological changes primarily involving axons, with or without associated myelin sheath changes, may be grouped together and referred to an axonopathies. According to the segment of the axon involved, axonopathy may be further classified as proximal and distal axonopathy (see Chapters 6 and 7).

Proximal Axonopathy

Proximal axonopathy involves selective degeneration of the proximal axon, which includes the axonal hillock, the initial segment, and the proximal portion of the axon (Griffin and Price, 1980; Asbury and Brown, 1980). The most important and characteristic change is the formation of giant axonal swellings with accumulation of neurofilaments. This type of degenerative change is typically seen in motor neuron diseases such as human amyotrophic lateral sclerosis (ALS) and hereditary canine spinal muscular atrophy (HCSMA). Giant axonal swellings are also observed in β,β'-iminodipropionitrile (IDPN) intoxication (Fig. 27) and in hexacarbon neuropathy (Fig. 28).

In IDPN intoxication, light-microscopic examination shows large, swollen structures. These structures are argentophilic and represent enlarged portions of the proximal axons that are filled with massive accumulations of neurofilaments (Chou and Hartmann, 1964, 1965). The accumulation of neurofilaments in the proximal axons is found to be associated with an impairment of the slow component of the axoplasmic transport system (Mendell and Sahenk, 1980).

Distal Axonopathy

Distal axonopathy is characterized by degenerative changes primarily involving the distal portion of the axon (Lowndes and Baker, 1980; Sabri and Spencer, 1980; Sumner, 1980). The neuronal cell body (perikaryon) is usually not involved and remains morphologically intact. If the involvement is confined to the CNS, this process is referred to as central-distal axonopathy (Fig. 29), as in certain malnutritional conditions (Albee et al., 1987; Mattsson et al., 1988) or in clioquinol poisoning (Schaumburg and Spencer, 1980). When both the central and peripheral nervous systems are involved (e.g., motor fibers of the sciatic nerve), the condition is referred to as central-peripheral or peripheral-distal axonopathy. These phenomena can be exemplified in carbon disulfide and acrylamide intoxications (Seppalainen and Halatia, 1980; Le Quesne, 1980). Although in most situations the neuronal perikaryon is not involved, in late stages of the intoxication, changes may

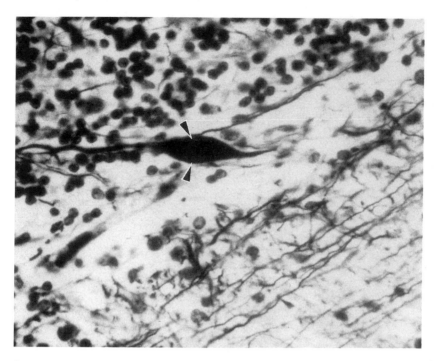

Figure 27   Cerebellum, rat, IDPN intoxication, Bielschowsky's stain. Axonal balloon (arrowheads) was observed. (×400.)

extend into the entire length of the axon and may even induce secondary changes in the perikaryon. This "retrograde" degenerative phenomenon is referred to as "dying-back axonal degeneration" (Prineas, 1969).

Although the precise pathogenetic mechanism for this type of degeneration is still unclear, it has been suggested that in distal axonopathies, the metabolism or mechanism required for maintenance of normal axonal integrity may be disrupted by toxic substances. Distal axonopathy displays characteristic internodal axonal swelling with massive accumulation of axonoplasmic elements, particularly neurofilaments, suggesting a disturbance in axonal metabolism and possibly also in the axoplasmic flow mechanism.

Details on various aspects of toxic axonopathy will be presented in Chapters 6 and 7 and will not be discussed further in this chapter.

Dendritic Changes (Dendropathy)

Although axonopathies are extensively studied by neurotoxicopathologists, toxic changes of the dendrites have received much less attention. This lack of investigation is most likely related to the fact that dendrites are not readily visible in routine histological preparations (H&E-stained paraffin sections). Elaborate and special techniques (e.g., rapid Golgi technique) are required for such investigation (Fig. 3).

Dendritic changes in Purkinje neurons, such as atrophy and reduction of organized secondary and tertiary branches of the dendritic aberration, have been observed in alcoholism, in lead intoxication (McConnell, 1983), and in chronic mercury poisoning

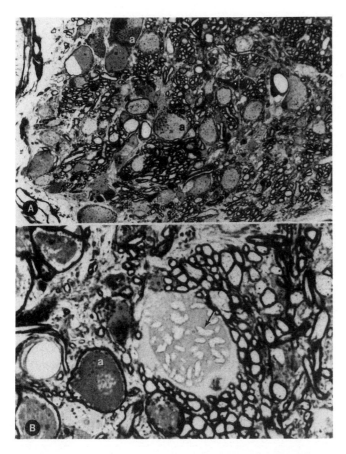

Figure 28 (A) Medulla oblongata, rat, hexacarbon intoxication, thin epoxy section with toluidine blue staining. Giant axonal swellings (a) were observed. (×220.) (B) Giant axonal swelling (→) observed in an aging rat. (×2000.) (From Spencer et al., 1980a.)

(Chang et al., 1977a,b; Chang, 1984; Chang and Annau, 1984) (Fig. 4). Dendrites in the developing brain are most vulnerable to such toxic influences.

MYELINOPATHY

"Myelinopathy" refers primarily to destruction of the myelin sheaths of the axons. Poor development or underdevelopment of the myelin sheaths as a result of exposure to toxic substances during critical developmental periods of the nervous system is termed dysmyelination. Myelin sheaths formed under these averse conditions may be thinner (hypomyelination) than those in normal animals, may have irregular internodal distances, and may show abnormalities or degenerative changes in the myelin sheaths and node of Ranvier (Fig. 30). This type of change can be exemplified in mice exposed to toxicants such as methylmercury (Chang et al., 1977a,b; Chang and Annau, 1984; Chang 1984) and triethyltin (Watanabe, 1977; Veronesi and Bondy, 1986) during early developmental stages of life.

Destruction of well-developed myelin is referred to as demyelination. This process may

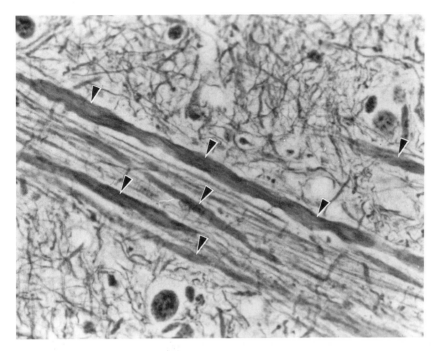

Figure 29 Brain stem, rat, protein-deficient diet. Axonal swellings (arrowheads) in the fiber tract were demonstrated. (×400.)

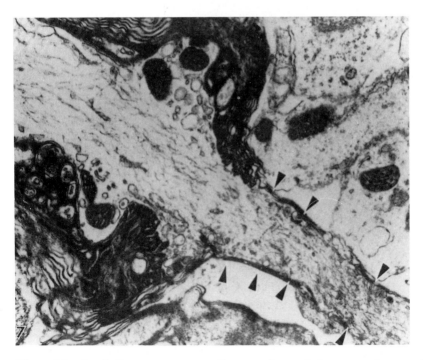

Figure 30 Cerebellum, mouse, prenatally exposed to methyl mercury, Segmental hypomyelination of the myelin sheath (arrowheads) with abnormal node of Ranvier in a nerve fiber was observed. (×25,000.)

involve the central axons, peripheral nerves, or both (Cammer, 1980; Rasminsky, 1980). Neurotoxic agents such as TET (Watanabe, 1980; Wenger et al., 1986; McMillan et al., 1986; Chang, 1990a), lead (Krigman et al., 1980), and AETT (Spencer et al., 1980a) will induce such patterns of change. Myelin bubbling, swelling, fragmentation, and breakdown are frequent changes in these conditions (Fig. 31). Myelin sheath destruction, frequently internodal or segmental as best exemplified in lead poisoning, occurs in peripheral nerves. In TET poisoning, swelling or edematous change of the central white matter (myelin sheath) without significant axonal involvement is observed (Figs. 32 and 33).

Myelinopathy should be distinguished from secondary myelin degeneration, as seen in Wallerian degeneration, which results from nerve cell or axonal damage. Mechanisms for the induction of myelin destruction are different for different toxic compounds. Removal of the myelin debris and lipid by-products by macrophages or Schwann cells and attempts at remyelination or repair (particularly in the peripheral nervous system) may be observed in late stages of the intoxication. For further discussions, please refer to Chapters 8 and 21.

CONCLUDING REMARKS

The nervous system is perhaps the most complex of all mammalian biological systems. The heterogeneity of the nerve cells, the varied components (axons, dendrites, synaptic

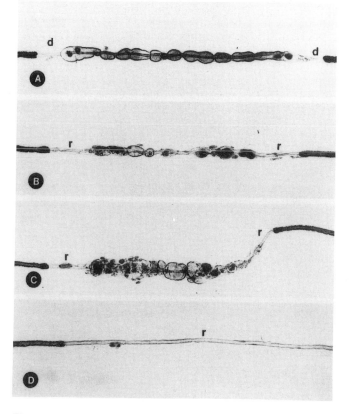

Figure 31 Tibial nerve, rat, acetyl ethyl tetramethyl tetralin poisoning, nerve fiber teasing technique. (A–C) Internodal bubbling of the myelin and paranodal demyelination. (D) Remyelination attempt. (d) area of demyelination; (r) area of remyelination. (From Spencer et al., 1980b.)

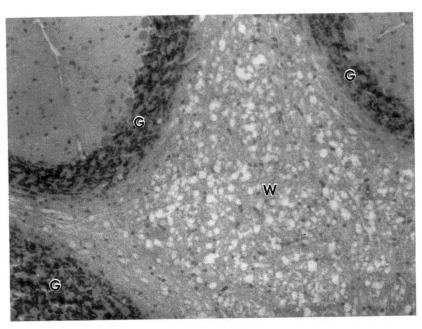

Figure 32 Cerebellum, rat, triethyltin intoxication, hematoxylin-eosin stain. Vacuolar, edematous change in the white matter (W) was observed. G = granule cell layer. (×250.)

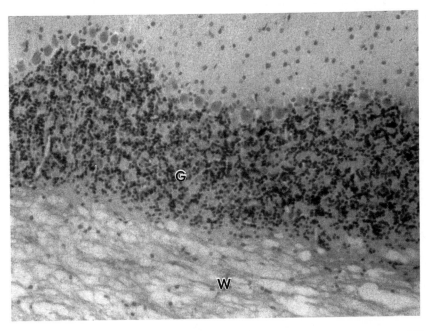

Figure 33 Cerebellum, rat, triethyltin intoxication, hematoxylin-eosin stain. Bubbling of the central myelin (white matter) (W) was the result of edematous condition of the myelin sheath. The axons were usually not affected. G = granule cell layer. (×400.)

terminals, etc.) of the nerve cells, the complexity of the neuronal interconnecting circuitry, and the cell-cell interaction between neurons as well as between nerve cells and their supporting neuroglia make the study of neurotoxicology a formidable task.

With the heavy emphasis on "molecular" aspects of biological research in recent years, there is a tendency toward excessive narrowness in the training of future scientists. It will be a grievous error for students of neurotoxicology not to have a firm and broad-based knowledge of basic neuroscience. It is far better to view the "toxic situation" of the nervous system from the standpoint of a neuroscientist than to try to study "isolated" biological phenomena of the nervous system, under toxic conditions, without basic and comprehensive concepts of the biology and function of the nervous system as a whole.

As pathology (study of abnormal biological condition) is based on basic biological sciences (anatomy, cell biology, biochemistry, physiology, and molecular biology), neurotoxicology (study of the responses of and consequences for the nervous system in toxic situations) should be based on basic neurosciences (neuroanatomy, neurocytology, neurochemistry, neurophysiology, neurobehavioral sciences, and neuromolecular biology) coupled with basic knowledge of the pharmacology/toxicology of the toxic compound involved.

We have seen in this chapter that each group of neurons may react or respond to the same chemical very differently. Furthermore, each component of the nerve cell (axon, dendrite, neuroskeletal elements, etc.) may also be selectively attacked by chemicals. This phenomenon of "selective vulnerability" of the nervous system to chemicals has perplexed neurotoxicologists and neuropathologists for centuries. Although some neurotoxic situations (e.g., methylmercury intoxication) follow the basic principle of "dose-effect" relationship, denoting a direct correlation betweeen tissue distribution of the toxic substance involved and the loci of lesion development ("direct neurotoxicity"), many other neurotoxic situations (e.g., trimethyltin or lead intoxication) present no apparent correlation or dose-effect relationship of these two factors ("indirect neurotoxicity"). These concepts of direct and indirect neurotoxicity, as presented by Chang (1992), are two major aspects of neurotoxicology. The biological and chemical bases for selective deposits of toxic substances on specific or preferential loci of the nervous system, as seen in direct neurotoxicity, and the mechanisms underlying various forms of indirect neurotoxicity certainly deserve further investigation. Other phenomena of neurotoxicity such as "secondary neurotoxicity" (toxicity to the nervous system as a secondary result of primary changes in other organs, e.g., chronic renal or hepatic failure) and "delayed neurotoxicity" (development of neurotoxicity after a long latency period from time of exposure) are also challenging concepts of neurotoxicology. These phenomena and concepts will be further discussed in other chapters in this volume or in other volumes to follow.

It is important to recognize and to distinguish the various varieties of neurotoxicological and neuropathological phenomena (neuronopathies, axonopathies, etc.) so that the basic neurological consequences and biomolecular mechanisms of these phenomena can be better understood and more appropriately explored. The interrelationships of these phenomena are complex and should also be addressed in future studies.

REFERENCES

Albee RR, Matsson JL, Yano BL, Chang LW (1987). Neurobehavioral effects of dietary restriction. Neurotoxicol Teratol 9:203–12.
Asbury AK, Brown MJ (1980). The evolution of structural changes in distal axonopathoies. In:

Spencer PS, Schaumburg HH, eds. Experimental and clinical neurotoxicology Baltimore: Williams & Wilkins, 179–92.

Blackemore WF, Cavanaugh JB (1969). Neuroaxonal dystrophy occurring in an experimental dying back process in the rat. Brain 92:789–806.

Bodian D (1967). Neurons, circuits, and neuroglia. In: Quarton GC, Melnechuk T, Schmitt FO, eds. The neurosciences. New York: Rockefeller University Press, 6–23.

Brady RO (1975). The nervous system: I. The basic neurosciences. New York: Raven Press.

Cammer W. (1980). Toxic demyelination: biochemical studies and hypothetical mechanisms. In: Spencer PS, Schaumburg HH, eds. Experimental and clinical neurotoxicology. Baltimore: Williams & Wilkins, 239–56.

Chang LW (1982). Pathogenetic mechanisms of the neurotoxicity of methyl mercury. In Prasad KN, Vernadakis A, eds. Mechanisms of neurotoxic substances. New York: Raven Press, 51–66.

Chang LW (1984). Developmental toxicology of methyl mercury. In Kacew S, Reasor MJ, eds. Toxicology and the newborn. Amsterdam: Elsevier, 175–97.

Chang LW (1986). Neuropathology of trimethyltin: a proposed pathogenetic mechanism. Fund Appl Toxicol 6:217–32.

Chang LW (1987). Neuropathological changes associated with accidental or experimental exposure to organometallic compounds: CNS effects. In: Tilson HA, Sparber SB, eds. Neurotoxicants and neurobiological function—effects of organoheavy metals. New York: John Wiley & Sons, 81–116.

Chang LW (1990a). The neurotoxicology and pathology of organomercury, organotin, and organolead. J Toxicol Sci (Japan) 15(suppl IV):125–51.

Chang LW (1990b). Neurotoxicity of trimethyltin of the hippocampus: a hyperexcitatory toxicity. Korean J Toxicol 6:191–204.

Chang LW (1992). The concept of direct and indirect neurotoxicity and the concept of toxic metal/essential element interactions as a common biomechanism underlying metal toxicity. In: Isaacson RL, Jensen KF, eds. The vulnerable brain and environmental risks, vol. 2, toxins in food. New York: Plenum Press, 61–82.

Chang LW, Annau Z (1984). Developmental neuropathology and behavioral teratology of methyl mercury. In: Yanai J, ed. Neurobehavioral teratology. Amsterdam: Elsevier, 405–32.

Chang LW, Hartmann HA (1972a). Ultrastructural studies of the nervous system after mercury intoxication. II. Pathological changes in the nerve fibers. Acta Neuropathol 20:316–34.

Chang LW, Hartmann HA (1972b). Ultrastructural studies of the nervous system after mercury intoxication. I. Pathological changes in the nerve cell bodies. Acta Neuropathol 20:122–38.

Chang LW, Ruehl KR, Spyker JM (1977a). Ultrastructural study of the long-term effects of methyl mercury on the nervous system after prenatal exposure. Environ Res 13:171–85.

Chang LW, Ruehl KR, Lee GW (1977b). Electron microscopic evidence of degenerative changes in the developing nervous system as a result of in utero exposure to methyl mercury. Environ Res 14:414–23.

Chang LW, Tiemeyer TM, Wenger GR, McMillan DE (1982a). Neuropathology of mouse hippocampus in acute trimethyltin intoxication. Neurobehav Toxicol Teratol 4:149–56.

Chang LW, Tiemeyer TM, Wenger GR, McMillan DE, Reuhl KR (1982b). Neuropathology of trimethyltin intoxication. I. Light miscroscopy study. Environ Res 29:435–44.

Chang LW, Tiemeyer TM, Wenger GR, McMillan DE (1983). Neuropathology or trimethyltin intoxication. III. Changes in the brainstem neurons. Environ Res 30:399–411.

Chang LW, Wenger GR, McMillan DE (1984). Neuropathology of trimethyltin intoxication. IV. Changes in the spinal cord. Environ Res 34:123–34.

Chang LW, Yang CM, Chen CF, Deng JF (1992). Experimental podophyllotoxin (Bajiaolan) poisoning: I. Effects on the nervous system. Biomed Environ Sci 5:283–92.

Chou SM, Hartmann HA (1964). Anxonal lesions and waltzing syndrome after IDPN administration in rats. Acta Neuropathol 3:428–37.

Chou SM, Hartmann HA (1965). Electron microscopy of focal neuroaxonal lesions produced by β-β-iminodipropionitrile (IDPN) in rats. Acta Neuropathol 4:500–11.

Griffin JW, Price DL (1980). Proximal axonopathies induced by toxic chemicals. In: Spencer PS, Schaumburg HH, eds. Experimental and clinical neurotoxicology. Baltimore: Williams & Wilkins, 161–89.

Hong JS, Obie J, Chang LW (1984). Alterations of pituitary adrenal functions after chlordecone administration in adult rats. Fed Proc 43:805.

Klatzo I, Wisniewski H, Streicher E (1975). Experimental production of neurofibrillary degeneration. I. Light microscopic observations. Neuropathol Exp Neurol 24:187–209.

Krigman MR, Bouldin TW, Muskak P (1980). Lead. In: Spencer PS, Schaumburg HH, eds. Experimental and clinical neurotoxicology. Baltimore: Williams & Wilkins, 490–507.

Le Quesne PM (1980). Acrylamide. In: Spencer PS, Schaumburg HH, eds. Experimental and clinical neurotoxicology. Baltimore: Williams & Wilkins, 309–25.

Lowndes HE, Baker T (1980). Toxic site of action in distal axonopathies. In: Spencer PS, Schaumburg HH, eds. Experimental and clinical neurotoxicology. Baltimore: Williams & Wilkins, 193–205.

Mattsson JL, Albee RR, Eisenbrandt DL, Chang LW (1988). Subchronic neurotoxicity in rats of the structural funigant, sulfuryl fluoride. Neurotoxicol Teratol 10:127–33.

McConnell P (1983). Neurotoxic effects of lead: In: Dreosti IE, Smith RM, eds. Neurobiology of the trace elements, vol. 2: neurotoxicology & pharmacology. Clifton, New Jersey: Humana Press, 141–66.

McMillan ED, Chang LW, Ideumdia SO, Wenger GR (1986). Effects of trimethyltin and triethyltin on lever pressing, water drinking and running in an activity wheel: associated neuropathology. Neurobehav Toxicol Teratol 8:499–507.

Mendell JR, Sahenk Z (1980). Interference of neuronal processing and axoplasmic transport by toxic chemicals. In: Spencer PS, Schaumburg HH, eds. Experimental and clinical neurotoxicology. Baltimore: Williams & Wilkins, 139–60.

Olney JW (1980). Excitotoxic mechanisms of neurotoxicity. In: Spencer PS, Schaumburg HH, eds. Experimental and clinical neurotoxicology. Baltimore: Williams & Wilkins, 239–56.

Powell HC, Myers RR, Lampert PW (1980). Edema in neurotoxic injury. In: Spencer PS, Schaumburg HH, eds. Experimental and clinical neurotoxicology. Baltimore: Williams & Wilkins, 118–38.

Prineas J (1969). The pathogenesis of dying-back polyneuropathies. II. An ultrastructural study of experimental acrylamide intoxication in the cat. J Neuropathol Exp Neurol 28:596–616.

Quarton GC, Melnechuk T, Schmitt FO (1967). The neurosciences. New York: Rockefeller University Press.

Rasminsky M (1980). Physiological consequences of demyelination. In: Spencer PS, Schaumburg HH, eds. Experimental and clinical neurotoxicology. Baltimore: Williams & Wilkins, pp. 257–71.

Sabri MI, Spencer PS (1980). Toxic distal axonopathy: biochemical studies and hypothetical mechanisms. In: Spencer PS, Schaumburg HH, eds. Experimental and clinical neurotoxicology. Baltimore: Williams & Wilkins, 206–19.

Schaumburg HH, Spencer PS (1980). Clioquinol. In: Spencer PS, Schaumburg HH, eds. Experimental and clinical neurotoxicology. Baltimore: Williams & Wilkins, 395–406.

Seppalainen AA, Halatia M (1980). Carbon disulfide. In: Spencer PS, Schaumburg HH, eds. Experimental and clinical neurotoxicology. Baltimore: Williams & Wilkins, 356–73.

Spencer PS, Bischoff MC, Schaumburg HH (1980a). Neuropathological methods for the detection of neurotoxic disease. In: Spencer PS, Schaumburg HH, eds. Experimental and clinical neurotoxicology. Baltimore: Williams & Wilkins, 743–57.

Spencer PS, Foster GV, Sterman AB, Horoupian D (1980b). Acetyl ethyl tetramethyl tetralin. In: Spencer PS, Schaumburg HH, eds. Experimental and clinical neurotoxicology. Baltimore: Williams & Wilkins, 296–308.

Spencer PS, Schaumburg HH (1976). Central and peripheral distal axonopathy—the pathology of dying-back polyneuropathies. In: Zimmerman HM, ed. Progress in neuropathology, vol. III. New York: Grune & Stratton, 253–62.

Sumner AJ (1980). Physiological consequences of distal axonopathy. In: Spencer PS, Schaumburg HH, eds. Experimental and clinical neurotoxicology. Baltimore: Williams & Wilkins, 220–4.

Veronesi B, Bondy S (1986). Triethyltin-induced neuronal damage in neonatally exposed rats. Neurotoxicology 7:69–75.

Walsh TJ, McLamb RL, Bondy SC, Tilson HA, Chang LW (1986). Triethyl and trimethyl lead: effects on behavior, central nervous system morphology and concentrations of lead in blood and brain of rat. Neurotoxicology 7:21–34.

Watanabe I (1977). Effect of triethyltin on the developing brain of the mouse. In: Roizin L, Shiraki H, Grecevic N, eds. Neurotoxicology, vol. 1. New York: Raven Press, 317–26.

Watanabe I (1980). Organotins (triethyltin). In: Spencer PS, Schaumburg HH, eds. Experimental and clinical neurotoxicology. Baltimore: Williams & Wilkins, 545–57.

Wenger GR, McMillan DE, Chang LW (1986). Effects of triethyltin on responding of mice under a multiple schedule of food presentation. Toxicol Appl Pharmacol 8:659–65.

Willis WD, Grossman RG (1973). Medical neurobiology. St. Louis: C.V. Mosby.

Wisniewski HM, Korthals TK, Kopeloff LM, Ferszt R, Chusid JC, Terry RD (1977). Neurotoxicity of aluminum. In: Roizin L, Shiraki H, Grecevic N, eds. Neurotoxicology, vol. 1 New York: Raven Press, 313–15.

2

Blood-Brain and Blood-Nerve Barriers and Their Relationships to Neurotoxicity

Jean M. Jacobs
Institute of Neurology
London, England

THE BLOOD-BRAIN BARRIER

Introduction

The blood-brain barrier (BBB) is now a major specialty in neuroscience. The study of the BBB involves a wide range of disciplines and includes among its most recent advances the isolation of the cDNA of γ-glutamyl transpeptidase (γ-GT), a marker of brain endothelial cells whose characteristics largely determine the barrier properties of brain capillaries. The physiological function of this enzyme is not known, but studies of its gene expression are in progress (Zinke et al., 1992).

My approach to the blood-brain and blood-nerve barriers in this chapter is mainly that of a morphologist, and the topics discussed are those thought to be most relevant to the field of neurotoxicological pathology.

The Blood-Brain Barrier Concept

History

In the course of studies using acidic vital stains in the search for chemotherapeutic agents, Ehrlich (1885) noticed that when dye was injected intravenously, the brain remained unstained, although other organs took up the dye. Goldmann (1909) confirmed these observations using trypan blue. He showed, in a second set of experiments (Goldmann, 1913), that administration of the dye directly into the cerebrospinal fluid (CSF) resulted in deep staining of brain tissues, rapidly causing neurological symptoms and death. This important observation was used to counter later suggestions that tracer dyes failed to enter the brain because there was no space to accommodate it. This idea was based on early electron-microscopic evidence of an apparent absence of extracellular space in brain tissue.

The term "blood-brain barrier" (*Bluthirnschranke*) was first introduced by Lewandowsky (1900), who had used intravenous Prussian blue dye and shown its exclusion from the brain. It is now known that the dyes used in these experiments are bound to proteins, so the barrier demonstrated was in fact to a dye-protein complex.

At the time of Goldmann's experiments, the barrier between blood and nervous tissue appeared to be absolute for these acidic dyes, except for the choroid plexuses, which were stained, and these for a time came to be viewed as providing the only vascular route into the brain.

A study of the movement between blood and CSF of substances other than dyes followed (Stern and Gautier, 1921), and led to the conclusion that passage of substances from blood to brain tissue took place with CSF as an intermediate step, so that CSF alone provided the nutrient pool for central nervous system tissue. It was then pointed out that nervous tissue is vascularized by a rich capillary bed that, according to this theory, would appear to have no function (Walter, 1929).

Since then, many studies have shown the selectivity of the barrier, underlining the inappropriateness of the term "barrier," which implies an absolute exclusion. As early as the 1920s, it was found that morphine could enter the brain, but not curare (Stern and Gautier, 1922). Studies using dyes appeared to show that their exclusion from the brain was based on ionic selectivity, basic dyes crossing the barrier but acidic dyes being excluded. However, there were some exceptions to this rule, and it was later found that lipid-solubility was also an important factor, with lipid soluble dyes such as neutral red, toluidine blue, and Nile blue all able to cross the BBB.

The environment of the brain is regulated by the BBB so that it can remain independent of fluctuations in concentrations of substances normally present in the blood. It is also largely protected from exogenous substances. Selectivity of the BBB to circulating substances depends not only on lipid-solubility, but also on mechanisms of trans–endothelial cell passage. Carrier-mediated transfer is the means of transport of many classes of compounds, and the carrier systems, like those in other membranes, are stereospecific, saturable, and competitively inhibited by structurally similar compounds. D-glucose, the main nutrient of the brain, acidic amino-acids such as L-glutamate, and basic amino acids such as L-arginine are some of the compounds for which BBB carrier systems have been demonstrated.

In addition to its function as a structural barrier, the BBB also acts as an enzymatic barrier. Many transmitters and peptides have different functions in the systemic circulation as compared with the brain. For example serotonin, dopamine, epinephrine, and norepinephrine act as transmitters in the brain, but they act as hormones in the periphery. It is important that monoamines in the blood be prevented from entering the brain, and this is achieved by the presence of degrading enzymes in brain endothelial cells, which restrict not only endogenous neuroactive substances such as monoamines, but also potentially neurotoxic exogenous compounds.

An exception is MPTP (1-methyl-4-phenyl-1,2,3,6-tetrahydropyridine), which in rats is oxidized by monoamine oxidase B (MOA-B) at the enzyme barrier, with the eventual formation of the neurotoxic metabolite MPP+ (1-methyl-4-phenylpyridinium) (Kalaria et al., 1987). MPTP is a highly potent and selective dopaminergic neurotoxin when administered systemically, particularly in humans and subhuman primates, but not in rats. However, MPP+ directly infused into rat substantia nigra is neurotoxic.

The neurotoxicity of MPTP was first identified in drug addicts intravenously injecting illicit drugs containing this meperidine analogue (Ballard et al., 1985). The neurological symptoms were similar to those of Parkinson's disease, and there was clinical improvement following levodopa therapy. MPTP is now widely used as a model of Parkinson's disease.

On investigating the mechanism of action of MPTP, an unexpected finding was that it acted as a substrate for MOA-B, the resulting MPP^+ being actively accumulated by dopaminergic neurons and leading to the degeneration of these cells (Jenner, 1989). In animals susceptible to MPTP neurotoxicity, MOA-B is present in glial cells, probably astrocytes. The resistance of rats to the neurotoxic effects of MPTP may be associated with a difference in the major site of MOA-B, which appears to be at the level of the blood-brain interface, in brain endothelial cells (Kalaria et al., 1987).

Methods of Examination of the Blood-Brain Barrier

With the development, over the last 25 years, of an array of methods for examining barrier characteristics and transport properties, our understanding of the BBB has increased enormously. Morphological methods, in addition to the use of circulating organic dyes, include the use of electron microscopy for the identification of barrier sites, usually in combination with tracers of varied molecular size and weight such as ferritin (400,000 Da, diameter $\geq$ 100Å), horseradish peroxidase (40,000 Da, 50–60 Å), and colloidal and ionic lanthanum (139 Da, 1.15 Å). Studies at the ultrastructural level have also been used in assessing the role (if any) of vesicular transport.

Methods for quantitative in vivo measurement of BBB permeability and transport in experimental animals are available; many are based on the principle of delivery of a substance into the circulation and measurement of the fraction "extracted" from the blood in a single pass through the brain, or direct measurement of the concentration of the substance in the brain. Methods for measurement of BBB permeability and transport in humans are being developed; these include positron emission tomography (PET) using radiolabeled tracers, and magnetic resonance imaging (MRI). A comprehensive description of these methods has been published by Smith (1992).

Morphology of the Blood-Brain Barrier

Brain capillaries, with the exception of those in some specialized parts of the brain, differ from capillaries in other tissues. Their endothelial cells are joined by belts of tight junctions (zonulae occludentes) that form a complete barrier between the cells. Endothelial cells in other tissues may also be joined by tight junctions, but these are in patches (maculae occludentes) that do not close the intercellular clefts completely. When studied in freeze-fracture preparations, tight junctions are recognized as collections of ridges on the protoplasmic (P) face with complementary grooves on the external (E) face. The number and depth of ridges is said to be directly related to the "tightness" of the junction (Claude and Goodenough, 1973).

Another characteristic feature of nervous system endothelial cells is the relative paucity of vesicles or endocytotic invaginations (Reese and Karnowsky, 1967; Brightman and Reese, 1969) compared with endothelial cells from other tissues (Fig. 1). Vesicles have been regarded as providing the equivalent of large pores for macromolecular transport by fusing transiently to form transcellular channels (Renkin, 1964). An ultrastructural study of the distribution of a tracer, ferritin, in pits on luminal and abluminal faces of endothelial cells suggests that this may indeed be the mechanism for progression of ferritin (and other macromolecules) across the cells (Clough and Michel, 1981). However, the role of vesicular transport across endothelial cells has been, and remains, a controversial topic. Unequivocal evidence of the existence of a continuous channel created by the coalescence of vesicles, with openings at both surfaces, has not been demonstrated. However, tubules apparently formed from the fusion of vesicles have been observed in thick sections by high-voltage

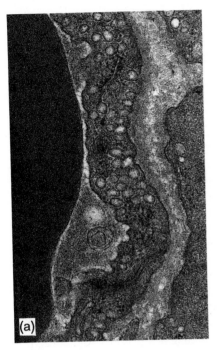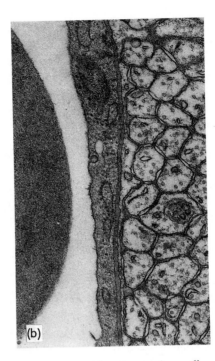

Figure 1   Electron micrographs of endothelial cells from (a) a rat muscle capillary showing large numbers of pinocytotic vesicles, and (b) rat cerebellum showing the paucity of pinocytotic vesicles. (×33,500.)

electron microscopy (Shivers and Harris, 1984). An alternative mechanism is that of a brief communication between a surface pit/vesicle and a second intracellular vesicle, allowing the transfer of a solute. After separation of the second vesicle, it hands on the solute to the next adjacent vesicle. As Brightman (1989) has pointed out, fixed tissue may not present a true representation of the living state. The process of fixation could be too slow to capture vesicles in the process of fusion and fission.

A basement membrane surrounds brain microvessels, separating the endothelial cells from the surrounding extracellular space. Basement membranes are composed of a complex including laminin, collagens, proteoglycans, and fibronectin. Although in the kidney the basement membrane is known to have a barrier function, preventing the passage of macromolecular plasma components such as albumin into the glomerular filtrate, it is not known whether it has a barrier function in the brain.

The Blood-Brain Barrier in the Immature Brain

The BBB is generally regarded as being less tight in the fetus and newborn. Evidence comes first from observations that certain circulating dyes stain the fetal brain but not the adult brain of a number of species (Stern and Peyrot, 1927). Second, the concentration of serum proteins is higher in the CSF of fetal than of adult brains (Cavanagh et al., 1983). Stewart and Hayakawa (1987) have suggested that in the developing brain, vascular proliferation is associated with leaky interendothelial junctions and therefore high nonspecific permeability. However, Saunders (1992) has recently reviewed the ontogenetic development of brain barrier mechanisms, and he points out that the barrier created by the tight junctions between cerebral endothelial cells develops at a very early stage of development. Naturally occurring proteins in plasma do not cross these immature vessels; the demonstration of "leakiness" of the barrier in experimental studies using dyes or horseradish peroxidase (HRP) is attributed to the use of excessive volumes or protein concentrations (see next section). Brain barrier mechanisms involving cerebral carriers or enzymes appear later in brain development.

Little seems to be known of the entry of drugs into the immature brain—a possible cause for concern in humans when they are used in the neonatal period (Saunders, 1992).

In a study of brain levels of paraquat, Corasaniti et al. (1991) found higher brain concentrations of this herbicide in very young (2-week-old) rats than in those 3 months of age.

Some of the amphiphilic drugs that induce lipidosis, such as triparanol, AY-9944, and perhexiline, are known to produce little change in the central nervous system (CNS) of adult animals. When administered during the first few weeks of life they cause lipidosis in many parts of the CNS (Drenckhahn and Lüllmann-Rauch, 1979).

Induction of the Blood-Brain Barrier

The topic of induction of the BBB has recently been reviewed by Abbott et al. (1992). The close association between astrocytes and brain capillaries led Davson and Oldendorf (1967) to suggest that astrocytes might be involved in induction of the barrier properties. A number of different experiments have now confirmed that this is the case. The earliest studies involved the grafting of brain tissue into nonbrain host tissues such as the iris. Vessels growing into the graft from the host tissues were found to have developed barrier properties. In the reverse experiment, nonbrain tissues grafted into the brain did not show barrier properties (Svengaard et al., 1975; Stewart and Wiley, 1981).

Tissue culture has been used to show that endothelial cells seeded onto a bed of astrocytes form long tubular strands resembling capillaries. When grown on plastic or thin collagen substrates, brain endothelial cells usually form a flat monolayer (Laterra et al., 1990; Minakawa et al., 1991; Laterra and Goldstein, 1991). Other coculture experiments showed that collagen-containing basement membrane was an important component in the induction process.

Studies on the development of the BBB show that in the mouse, early vascular invasion at E12–14 (when there are few perivascular glia) is by vessels which are permeable to HRP (Dermietzel and Krause, 1991). By E15, perivascular glia are more numerous and the vessels have become impermeable to HRP. At this time, the barrier-associated markers γ-GT and transferrin receptors appear in brain endothelium. Expression of the glucose transporter (GLUT-1) is another characteristic of brain capillaries as they develop tight junctions (Pardridge et al., 1990). Choroid plexus epithelium, which also has a barrier function, displays earlier expression of barrier markers than brain vessels (Dermietzel and Krause, 1991).

Blood-Ocular Barriers

The eye is part of the CNS, and barriers between this organ and its blood supplies have been reviewed and described by Kupersmith and Shakib (1989). The blood-aqueous barrier occurs at the blood vessels and the epithelium of the iris and ciliary body and regulates the exchange between blood and intraocular fluid. The more important blood-retinal barrier lies between retinal vessels and the retinal pigment epithelium, the site of the barrier being tight junctions between lateral surfaces of the pigment epithelial cells. The choroidal vessels are fenestrated and are even more permeable to albumin than kidney or muscle (Bill et al., 1980). In tracer studies, macromolecules such as trypan blue and HRP readily passed through these choroidal vessels but did not penetrate beyond the retinal pigment epithelium because of tight junctions between the epithelial cells (Shakib and Cunha-Vaz, 1966).

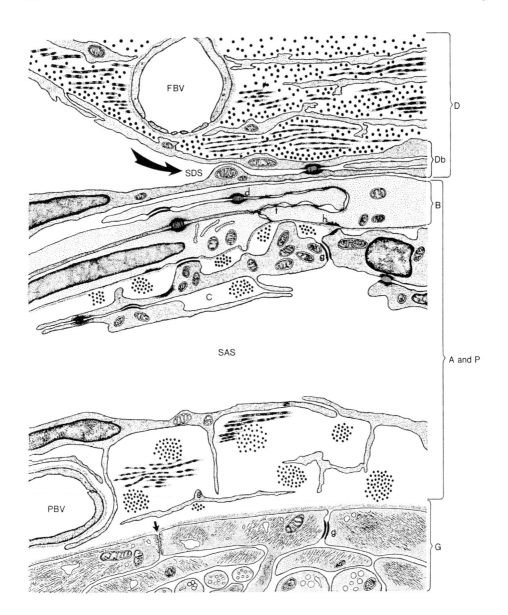

Figure 2   Diagram of the meninges and brain surface, based on examination of various mammals. Blood vessels in the dura (D) are fenestrated (FBV), while those in the subarachnoid space (SAS) are nonfenestrated (PBV). Processes of cells of the arachnoid barrier (B), lying superficial to the arachnoid and pia (A and P), are joined by tight junctions (t) creating a barrier between the two regions of differing vascular permeability. The cells of the astrocyte border junction (small arrow) forming the marginal glia (G) are joined by gap junctions (g). Dural border layer (Db) cells, separated by subdural space (SDS, large arrow), are joined by desmosomes (d). Hemidesmosomes (h) are present on the basement membrane-covered surface of the barrier layer cells. (From Nabeshima et al., 1975).

Meningeal Barrier

Early studies had shown that dyes used as vascular tracers, such as Evans blue–albumin, stained the dura covering the arachnoid membrane but did not penetrate into the CSF. The meninges consist of three membranes, the dura mater, the arachnoid, and the pia mater. Tracer studies with HRP, and ultrastructural studies including freeze-fracture techniques, have identified tight junctions between cells at the border of the arachnoid and the dura (Nabeshima et al., 1975). Blood vessels in the dura are sometimes fenestrated, but those in the subarachnoid space have tight junctions (Fig. 2).

BLOOD-NERVE BARRIER

Introduction

The blood-nerve barrier is formed by two components, the perineurium and the endoneurial blood vessels. Blood vessels in the epineurium are permeable; those in the endoneurium are impermeable. These two regions of differing vascular permeability are separated by another barrier created by the tight junctions that join lamellae of the perineurial sheath.

Permeability Studies

As in the brain, vascular permeability in peripheral nerves has been studied using many types of tracer. Early experiments made use of acid dyes that bind to albumin, such as Evans blue and trypan blue; these showed macroscopically that the dyes were generally excluded from brain and peripheral nerves, although dorsal root ganglia were stained blue. Microscopic examination of vascular permeability was studied by Olsson (1966, 1971) using albumin or gamma globulin labeled with fluorescent markers. More recent studies have made use of HRP and other tracers that can be visualized by light and electron microscopy. These studies have shown that epineurial blood vessels, like those in most other parts of the body, are permeable. Endoneurial vessels are relatively impermeable, although considerable variations have been reported in the degree of tracer leakage, due no doubt to the sensitivity of the methods used to identify the tracers. Species differences in endoneurial permeability have been described by Olsson (1967), with rabbit and guinea pig nerves showing more leakage than those of mice and rats. However, the amount of endoneurial capillary leakage is small compared, for example, with that of the epineurial vessels.

Ultrastructural studies of the permeability of peripheral nerves to HRP have shown that tight junctions between endoneurial endothelial cells block the passage of tracer from the blood, and tight junctions between perineurial cells prevent passage of HRP, which has leaked from the permeable epineurial blood vessels, into the endoneurium (Reese and Olsson, 1970) (Fig. 3).

Another approach to the study of the blood-nerve barrier has been the examination of constituents in the endoneurium. Poduslo et al. (1985) extracted endoneurial fluid from desheathed rat nerves and identified albumin as a major component of endoneurial fluid.

Van Lis and Jennekens (1977) used immunofluorescent techniques to show the presence and distribution of plasma proteins in human sural nerve biopsies from control and pathological nerves. Peroxidase-antiperoxidase (PAP) immunocytochemical methods were used by Leibert et al. (1985) to demonstrate the presence of proteins in the endoneurium of normal and pathological sural nerve biopsies. Mata et al. (1987) also

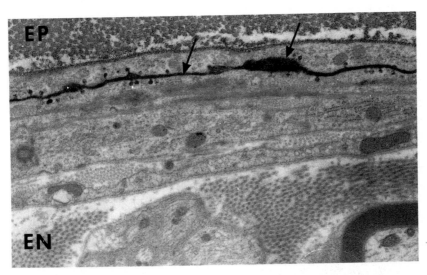

Figure 3   Electron micrograph of tibial nerve of a rat killed 5 minutes after intravenous injection of horseradish peroxidase (HRP). Tracer that has leaked from epineurial blood vessels is faintly present in the collagenous epineurial sheath (EP) and is more prominent in the space between outermost perineurial sheath cells (arrows) and in pinocytotic vesicles. No HRP is seen in the innermost layers of the perineurial sheath or in the endoneurium (EN). (×17,700.)

employed immunocytochemical methods in rat nerves to demonstrate serum albumin in the endoneurium. These findings all suggest that endoneurial vessels are normally permeable to plasma proteins, but to a variable degree. There is increased protein leakage in pathological conditions.

Morphology

The Perineurium

The perineurial sheath consists of layers of very attenuated perineurial cell processes, or lamellae, covered on both surfaces with a basement membrane, and separated by bundles of collagen. The number of lamellae varies according to the size of the fascicle, with as many as 15 layers around a large mammalian fascicle, diminishing to a single layer round the finest distal nerve branches. At unencapsulated nerve endings and at the neuromuscular junction, the perineurial sheath terminates with an open end.

Adjacent perineurial cells overlap or interdigitate, and are joined by tight junctions, which form the morphological basis of the perineurial barrier. Freeze-fracture studies of these tight junctions (Reale et al., 1975) reveal a series of ridges and complementary grooves on the fracture faces. The "tightness" of this type of junction appears to depend on the degree of complexity of the network of ridges and grooves.

A prominent feature of perineurial cells is the large number of pinocytotic vesicles that open onto external and internal surfaces; bundles of filaments within the cells may have a contractile function (Ross and Reith, 1969).

Early histochemical studies by Shanthaveerappa and Bourne (1962) showed that perineurial cells contain many phosphorylating enzymes and have a high level of adenosinetriphosphatase (ATPase) and creatine phosphate, providing evidence that the perineurium acts as a metabolically active diffusion barrier. The perineurial barrier is resistant to ischemia (Lundborg et al., 1973) and is unaffected by local administration of histamine, serotonin, and bradykinin (Söderfeldt et al., 1973); it is tight to tracers such as HRP, ferritin, and lanthanum salts applied to the external surface of nerves.

Perineurial permeability is incomplete in newborn rats and mice and is not fully developed until the end of the third postnatal week (Kristensson and Olsson, 1971).

The role of the blood-nerve barrier in regulating the microenvironment of the peripheral nerve has been reviewed by Rechthand and Rapoport (1987).

Endoneurial Blood Vessels

The endoneurial vasculature is composed largely of capillaries. Like capillaries in the brain, the endothelial cells of endoneurial capillaries are joined by tight junctions. There are no cells analogous to astrocytes in the peripheral nervous system, so the stimulus for induction of barrier properties in these capillaries is not known. Endoneurial capillaries differ from brain capillaries in the larger numbers of pinocytotic vesicles in the endothelial cells.

Blood-Muscle Spindle Barrier

The muscle spindle is surrounded by a capsule that is directly continuous with, and structurally similar to, the perineurium of the peripheral nerve. Muscle spindles of the anterior tibial nerve of mice were examined after intravenous injection of HRP (Dow et al., 1980). Although the capsule functions as a barrier to HRP, tracer was found in the polar regions of the spindle, probably as a result of spread through the open ends of the polar regions of the capsule. The equatorial region of the spindle remains free of tracer, because of both the barrier function of the capsule and an additional inner "capsule" consisting of fibroblast-like cells that take up HRP into their lysosomes.

REGIONS OF THE NERVOUS SYSTEM WITHOUT A BLOOD BARRIER

Morphology of Microvessels in Nonbarrier Regions

Microvessels in nonbarrier regions have been examined most thoroughly in the circumventricular organs and have been described by Gross (1992). Endothelial cells are joined by maculae occludentes, zones of tight junctions that only partially occlude the gap between adjacent cells, in contrast to the zonulae occludentes, or totally occluding tight junctions connecting brain endothelial cells. The nonbarrier endothelial cells contain large numbers of vesicles. Further differentiation of these endothelial cells occurs in the form of fenestrations—circular diaphragms, 5–6 nm thick and about 60 nm in diameter. Studies of the surface chemistry of fenestrations indicate that their luminal surfaces possess anionic sites. This suggests that the efflux of anionic plasma proteins would be limited or prevented, so that leakage across fenestrations is less than might be expected (Simionescu et al., 1981).

Circumventricular Organs

Circumventricular organs are illustrated in Fig. 4. They are regions containing cells that produce hormones or act as chemoreceptors or, in the case of the choroid plexus, produce CSF. Their capillaries allow the direct contact with plasma filtrates necessary for these functions. Most have unusually dense and permeable capillary networks.

The permeability of the vessels in these specialized regions of the brain has been studied quantitatively. Gross et al. (1986) found that the blood/tissue flux of a small amino

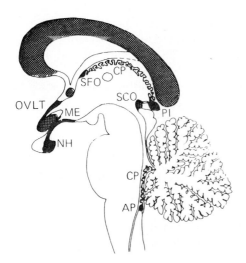

Figure 4 Diagram showing circumventricular organs (in solid black) projected on a median sagittal section of the human brain. AP = area postrema; ME = median eminence; NH = neurohypophysis; OVLT = organum vasculosum of the lamina terminalis; Pl = pineal body; SFO = subfornical organ; SCO = subcommisural organ; CP = choroid plexus. (From Weindl A.: Frontiers of neuroendocrinology. London: Oxford University Press, 1973.)

acid, α-aminoisobutyric acid, is 100–400 times faster across the fenestrated vessels of the subfornical organ than across barrier-type vessels in either gray or white matter.

In the regions of vascular permeability, the covering ependymal cells are joined by tight junctions to prevent leakage of plasma filtrates to the CSF (Reese and Brightman, 1968). In the choroid plexus, the choroidal epithelial cells are joined by tight junctions at their apical ends, creating a barrier between the choroidal stroma, with its fenestrated vessels, and the CSF (Fig. 5).

Optic Nerve

Small amounts of an intravenously administered tracer leak into the optic nerve because the barrier function of the optic nerve sheath is deficient at the lamina cribrosa (Olsson and Kristensson, 1973; Tso et al., 1975; Flage, 1977). Vessels in the connective tissues around the optic nerve are permeable, but the optic nerve sheath for the most part prevents diffusion of tracer into the nerve.

Olfactory Bulbs

Intravenous (and intranasal) HRP rapidly reaches the olfactory epithelium, passing through intercellular junctions to reach the olfactory bulbs of the CNS (Balin et al., 1986).

Brain Arterioles

Segments of some cerebral arterioles with an average diameter of 15 to 30 μm, situated mainly within sulci, and including both pial and parenchymal vessels, allow the passage of intravascular tracers such as HRP and ferritin (Westergaard and Brightman, 1973). The endothelial cells of all cerebral arterioles have many cytoplasmic vesicles and plasmalemmal pits, thus differing from the endothelial cells of typical brain capillaries. In the opinion of

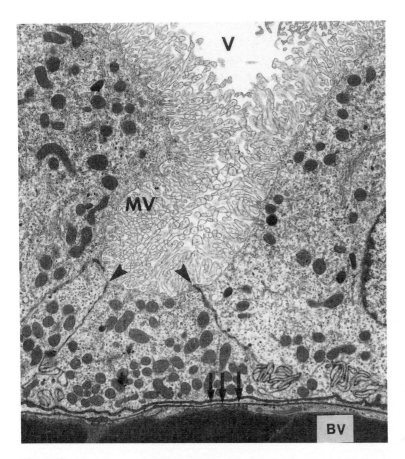

Figure 5 Electron micrograph of choroid plexus from a rat killed 5 minutes after intravenous injection of horseradish peroxidase (HRP). The blood vessel (BV) contains red cells and HRP that has passed through fenestrations (arrows), filling the stroma, occupying spaces between adjacent choroidal epithelial cells, and outlining the complex folding at the base of these cells. Tight junctions (arrowheads) at the apical poles of the cells prevent HRP from passing into the ventricle (V). MV = microvilli of choroidal epithelial cells. (×7,800.)

Westergaard and Brightman (1973), passage of protein across the "leaky" arterioles takes place by vesicular transport.

Dorsal Root and Autonomic Ganglia

Many early studies have shown gross staining of dorsal root ganglia following intravenous administration of Evans blue and trypan blue (e.g., Brightman et al., 1970), suggesting vascular leakage. Later studies using HRP showed the rapid appearance of intravenously injected tracer in dorsal root and autonomic ganglia (Olsson, 1971; Jacobs et al., 1976; Jacobs, 1977). Within 5 minutes of injection, HRP fills the gaps between satellite cells and ganglion cells; the adjacent ventral root contains no tracer (Fig. 6).

Leakage takes place through fenestrated blood vessels, which are found more frequently in autonomic (Fig. 7) than in dorsal root ganglia; HRP fills the space between

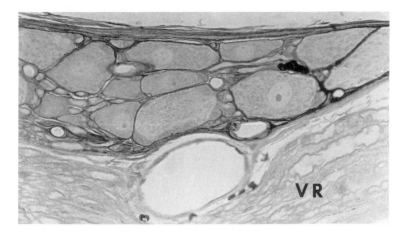

Figure 6   1-μm resin section through dorsal root ganglion and adjacent ventral root (VR) of a rat killed 5 minutes after intravenous injection of horseradish peroxidase. Tracer has filled the extracellular spaces between dorsal root ganglion cells but has been excluded from the ventral root. (×580.)

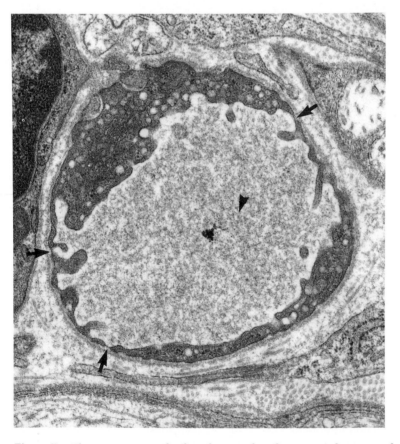

Figure 7   Electron micrograph of a celiac ganglion from a rat, showing endothelial cells of a small blood vessel, with several fenestrations (arrows). Numerous pinocytotic vesicles are seen in the endothelial cells. (×27,000.)

axons and satellite cell processes. A morphometric study has shown fenestrations in 12% of microvessel profiles in the superior cervical and 38% of those in the celiac mesenteric ganglia (Baker et al., 1989).

Myenteric Plexus

The myenteric plexuses are nerve networks lying between muscle layers of the gastrointestinal tract, extending from the smooth muscle part of the esophagus to the internal anal sphincter. Following intravenous injection into rats and guinea pigs, Jacobs (1977) found leakage of HRP between all elements forming the plexus—the nerve cells, the densely packed nerve cell processes, and glial cells. No blood vessels are to be found in the plexuses, and they are invested only by a basal lamina. Intravascular HRP rapidly leaks from permeable capillaries of the muscle layers in which the plexuses are embedded and readily permeates the nerve tissues.

The accessibility of the enteric plexus to circulating substances was demonstrated by the presence of silver (Rungby, 1986) and of amiodarone-induced inclusions (Costa-Jussà and Jacobs, 1985) within the nerve cells and processes of the plexus (see below). The presence of a blood–myenteric plexus barrier, similar to the blood-nerve and blood-brain barriers, has been described (Gershon and Bursztajn, 1978), although the findings in amiodarone and silver-localization studies (see below) do not support this.

Neuromuscular Junctions

At its terminal end, the axon of a motor nerve becomes closely apposed to the muscle cell surface, forming the neuromuscular junction. The nerve and muscle components are separated only by the basement membrane of the associated Schwann cell. Broadwell and Brightman (1976) have shown that circulating HRP, having readily leaked through permeable muscle capillaries, can enter the space between axon and muscle membranes, the basement membrane forming no barrier. Axon terminals at myoneural junctions pinocytose HRP, which is then transported retrogradely to the centrally located motor neuron cell bodies.

Figure 8 is taken from a study by Broadwell and Brightman (1976) and shows a dark field micrograph of a section at the level of the area postrema of a mouse after unilateral section of the hypoglossal nerve. The animal was killed 12 hours after intravenous injection of HRP. Peroxidase-labeled cell bodies in the hypoglossal nucleus are present on one side only, the unlabeled cells corresponding to the side of the ligated nerve. The area postrema, a region lying outside the blood-brain barrier, shows heavy labeling.

Retrograde transport along motor fibers from their endings in muscle to anterior horn cells has been suggested as a route for a number of toxic substances. One of the earliest examples of this mode of entry of a toxin into the nervous system is that of tetanus toxin (Price et al., 1975). Once within the anterior horn cells, the toxin has been demonstrated to pass transsynaptically to internuncial neurons (Dumas et al., 1979), where it blocks the release of inhibitory transmitters. This is likely to be the cause of the reflex spasms characteristic of this disease.

The experimental injection of diphtheria toxin into muscle and its retrograde transport to motor nerve cells has been used to study the mechanisms of cell damage to these cells (Sears et al., 1983). Similar types of study have been performed using the drug doxorubicin (see below) (Bigotte and Olsson, 1983). Silver may also enter motor neurons by this route (see below).

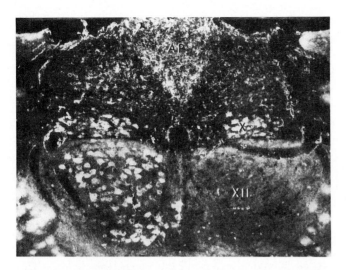

Figure 8 Dark field light micrograph of a section of medulla from a mouse with unilateral section of the hypoglossal nerve, killed 12 hours after intravenous injection of horseradish peroxidase (HRP). Tracer is present in the area postrema (AP) and labels cell bodies in the hypoglossal nuclei (XII) on the left side; there is no labeling of cells on the right side, since section and ligation of the associated nerve prevents the retrograde transport of HRP from leaked HRP at the neuromuscular endings. (×75.) (From Broadwell and Brightman, 1976.)

Studies in the etiology of motor neuron disease have investigated the possibility of the retrograde transport of a potentially toxic substance from the periphery, along motor nerves. Lead has long been a candidate for such a role, and many studies are reported on this important topic. In a review paper, Mitchell (1987) concludes that a syndrome closely resembling that of amyotrophic lateral sclerosis (ALS) may sometimes be seen in patients exposed to lead. However, there are many cases of ALS in which there has been no history of exposure to lead.

In order for retrograde transport to take place, substances require specific properties, in particular, an affinity for binding sites on the membrane of the nerve terminal. These will permit uptake into the nerve and subsequent transport within the axon (Stoeckel et al., 1977).

Broadwell and Brightman (1976) also describe uptake of HRP from sensory endings afferent to muscle spindles, shown by HRP labeling of cell bodies in the mesencephalic nucleus of nerve V. Although Dow et al. (1980) found the equatorial (sensory) region of the spindle to be protected from HRP leakage, it is possible that the high concentrations of HRP used in the studies by Broadwell and Brightman (1976) led to some intracapsular leakage into the sensory regions of the capsule.

MECHANISMS CAUSING INCREASED VASCULAR PERMEABILITY IN BRAIN AND NERVE

Breakdown of the Blood-Brain Barrier

Experimental manipulation of the BBB is a topic of increasing interest, but in general it lies outside the scope of this chapter and will therefore be mentioned only briefly.

Breakdown of the BBB can be induced experimentally, and methods to achieve reversible modification of the barrier have been investigated with the aim of enhancing delivery of therapeutic agents that would otherwise be prevented from reaching the brain. However, some antitumor drugs, such as cisplatin and doxorubicin, are associated with unacceptable neurotoxicity, precluding their use in methods that bypass the BBB.

The potential use of tumor-associated hybridoma-produced antibodies in the study and treatment of brain tumors has also been a stimulus for investigating methods of opening the BBB, since antibodies are normally excluded. This important topic has been reviewed by Neuwelt and Barnett (1989).

Methods that seem to be most successful in increasing brain vascular permeability are based on osmotic opening of the barrier and include the use of hyperosmolar solutions of the inert sugars mannitol and arabinose; bile salts at low concentrations seem to cause BBB opening in the rat without any apparent damage to cerebral endothelium. These and many other methods are discussed by Greig (1989), Neuwelt and Barnett (1989), and Greenwood (1992).

Increased Vascular Permeability Due to Peripheral Nerve Fiber Damage

Peripheral nerve fiber degeneration is associated with a breakdown of the blood-nerve barrier. Many experimental studies have shown that degeneration caused by nerve crush or transection is associated with an increase in vascular permeability, quite apart from the breakdown in the barrier at the lesion site. Olsson (1966) used serum albumin labeled with a fluorescent dye as a tracer, in rats, to show a wave of increased permeability throughout the nerve distal to the lesion. Mellick and Cavanagh (1968) showed that, in the chicken, the spread of leakage of radioiodinated albumin distal to a nerve lesion occurred at the same rate as regeneration of axons. Sparrow and Kiernan (1981) confirmed these findings in the rat sciatic nerve. They also showed that when nerve regeneration is prevented following nerve transection, breakdown of the blood-nerve barrier persists. Bouldin et al. (1991) studied permeability changes in several experimental models. In mice fed with tellurium, a demyelinating neuropathy was associated with vascular tracer leakage for a few weeks. Return of the barrier function probably corresponded to remyelination.

Alterations of vascular permeability in these experimental situations are due to changes in endoneurial endothelial cells rather than to the perineurial barrier functions. The basis of the increased endoneurial capillary permeability has been less thoroughly studied than the results of these changes. Using HRP, de la Motte and Allt (1976) studied capillaries in nerves with degenerating fibers after nerve transection and found evidence of increased vesicular transport across the endothelium, without opening of the tight junctions. Occasional fenestrated endoneurial capillaries have been described in neuropathies, but these probably are not an important factor in explaining increased permeability. Sparrow and Kiernan (1981) suggest that release of vasoactive substances by degenerating axons may cause increased vascular permeability, although the mechanism of "leakage" is not discussed.

In a study of the blood-nerve barrier in a mouse mutant (twitcher) that develops a demyelinating neuropathy (J. M. Jacobs, unpublished observations) it was noted that increased vascular permeability was associated with the beginning of myelin breakdown, the appearance of myelin debris, and the entry of macrophages into the nerve. The passage of macrophages between endothelial cells must, even if only transiently, break the barrier at these sites. Oaklander et al. (1987) found labeling of endoneurial endothelial cells with tritiated thymidine 1 day after nerve section. Proliferation of these cells may also be associated with a temporary breakdown of the barrier function.

These findings have some practical importance in relation to the potential exposure of peripheral nerve fibers to circulating toxic substances. Patients with a naturally occurring, or possibly subclinical, neuropathy may be more susceptible to drugs such as amiodarone (see below). Even the slow but inexorable aging process affecting nerve fibers, causing degeneration and demyelination (Jacobs and Love, 1985), may predispose the older patient to toxic neuropathies.

CENTRAL NERVOUS SYSTEM NEUROTOXICITY

Many neurotoxic substances are lipophilic and readily cross the blood-brain barrier; these include a number of organic metals such as tetraethyl- and tetramethyllead, triethyl- and trimethyltin, methylmercury, and organic arsenic. The neurotoxic effects are selective and are not obviously related to the blood-brain barrier. In the case of mercury it is known that mercury ions affect the transport of amino acids across the BBB, but is not clear how these metabolic effects are related to the selective pathology caused by this organic metal (see below).

Certain trace elements are essential for normal brain development (e.g., zinc), but little is known of the uptake mechanism involved (see Saunders, 1992). Iron is an essential metal that is transported by transferrin via receptors on the abluminal surface of cerebral endothelial cells. These trace metals have not been associated with neurotoxicity.

Aluminum, bismuth, manganese, and thallium are examples of metals associated with encephalopathy. Each causes a different pattern of damage that, again, is not related to the BBB.

A number of drugs and environmental neurotoxic substances are noted for their effects on the peripheral nervous system; except after gross exposure, their effect on the CNS, apart from regions without a BBB, is less obvious; these include acrylamide, organophosphorus compounds, colchicine, vincristine, and dapsone. Others are discussed in detail below. Exceptions include the drug amphotericin B, used in the treatment of fungal infections, and causing a diffuse cerebral leukoencephalopathy with relative preservation of axons. However, it has been suggested that prior total-body irradiation may have increased blood-brain barrier permeability to the drug; and uncontrolled infection of the nervous system may have also altered vascular permeability.

Methotrexate is a chemotherapeutic agent reported to cause widespread CNS demyelination after systemic injection; again, this is usually combined with cerebral irradiation. Intraventricular or intrathecal administration will bypass the BBB and may also cause leukoencephalopathy. Jacobs and Le Quesne (1992) give more details of these substances.

NEUROTOXIC SUBSTANCES WITH SELECTIVE EFFECTS ON REGIONS OF THE NERVOUS SYSTEM WITHOUT BLOOD BARRIERS

Cadmium

Cadmium is not reported to be neurotoxic to humans, although experimental studies show it to cause damage to the nervous system of rats, rabbits, guinea pigs, hamsters, and mice, in general only affecting regions without a blood barrier. In neonate rats, radiolabeled cadmium given intraperitoneally or intravenously was found autoradiographically in cerebral blood vessels and in the choroid plexus (Valois and Webster, 1987). In studies in adult rats, Arvidson (1986) found [109]Cd to accumulate only in regions of the CNS without BBBs, such as the choroid plexus, the pineal gland, and the hypophysis. These findings would suggest that although a functional blood-brain barrier has been demonstrated in immature brains (see above), the barrier is less "tight" to cadmium in immature than in adult animals. Interestingly, Arvidson (1986) also found uptake of [109]Cd into the olfactory bulbs, the iris, and the ciliary body and choroid of the eye, which suggests that these are all sites without a BBB. Workers exposed to cadmium in an industrial setting are reported to develop anosmia, and Arvidson has suggested that this may be related to its effects on the olfactory bulb.

In the peripheral nervous system, Arvidson and Tjalve (1986) found the highest concentrations of [109]Cd in the dorsal root and autonomic ganglia, known sites of vascular permeability.

Once cadmium has gained entry to either the central (Gabbiani et al., 1967a; Webster and Valois, 1981) or peripheral nervous system (Gabbiani et al., 1967b), its primary effect is on blood vessels, which show vacuolization and thinning of endothelial cells and widening of interendothelial gaps, leading to hemorrhagic lesions and secondary damage to neural elements. The cause of this selective effect is not known.

An unexplained finding is the apparent sparing of the celiac ganglion from vascular lesions although the superior cervical ganglia were affected (Arvidson, 1980). Conversely, there were vascular changes in the sciatic nerve of adult rats, a site with a blood nerve barrier.

Cisplatin

Cisplatin was introduced as a chemotherapeutic agent in 1972. Neurotoxicity is a major dose-limiting factor. Cisplatin may represent another example in which the selective toxicity to sensory ganglion cells (and possibly autonomic ganglion cells) is due to vascular permeability in these ganglia.

Clinically, the neuropathy is almost exclusively sensory. Many cases have been reported (e.g. Gastaut and Pellissier, 1985; Dewar et al., 1986; Amiel et al., 1987; Daugaard et al., 1987). In one case (Rosenfeld and Broder, 1984) autonomic symptoms were described and there was clinical evidence (Lhermitte's sign) suggesting dorsal column involvement in others (Dewar et al., 1986; Walther et al., 1987). Postmortem examination of one case confirmed degeneration of nerve fibers in posterior columns and loss of dorsal root ganglion cells (Amiel et al., 1987).

Gregg et al. (1992) measured platinum levels in neural tissues of 21 patients who had been treated with cisplatin; these were highest in dorsal root ganglia. Low levels of platinum were found in the spinal cord despite marked fiber degeneration in the posterior columns. Similar findings were described by Thompson et al. (1984) and suggest that selective neurotoxicity is a consequence of differential tissue distribution.

Experimental studies in rats (Clark et al., 1980) and ferrets (Montpetit et al., 1988a) have shown that cisplatin causes a sensory peripheral neuropathy. In the ferret experiment (Montpetit et al., 1988a) platinum concentrations were high in dorsal root ganglia, far lower in peripheral nerves, and lowest of all in the brain. In the rat CNS Clark et al. (1980) described axonal degeneration in the long tracts of the spinal cord and in the retrolaminar optic nerve. Axons are described as being focally enlarged with neurofilaments, which may suggest a direct effect on the axons rather than the sensory nerve cells (Clark et al., 1980). However, Tomiwa et al. (1986) and Cavaletti et al. (1982) described changes in the nuclei of rat dorsal root ganglion cells suggesting that these cells are the primary target of cisplatin.

Silver

Silver compounds are generally thought to be of low toxicity. Early studies on the distribution of exogenous silver in the CNS had indicated that it was selectively deposited in regions without a blood-brain barrier (Wislocki and Leduc, 1952) and in the basement membranes of cortical arterioles (Scott and Norman, 1980). The toxic effects of silver, in both humans and experimental animals exposed to the metal, have been mainly assessed in terms of the symptomatic reaction evoked. In humans, paralysis, convulsions, loss of coordination, and cerebellar ataxia have been reported, symptoms that suggest a more generalized effect than one related only to regions without a BBB.

Rungby and Danscher (1983a) exposed young adult rats to silver salts, either as a single intraperitoneal injection or in drinking water over several months. After absorption, silver is transported as a complex with plasma proteins, transferrin probably being a major vehicle (Matuk et al., 1981). Using methods for visualization of silver based on a photographic development technique, Rungby and Danscher (1983a) studied its localization in the CNS. The most intense silver staining occurred in regions without a BBB (area postrema, subfornical organ, pineal body, choroid plexus). Otherwise, heavy loading of silver was found in motor neurons in the brain stem and spinal cord. This was possibly due to uptake of silver, complexed with protein, from neuromuscular endings and its retrograde transport to the motor neurons, a process previously demonstrated to occur by Danscher (1982). Another site of silver accumulation was in neurons of the deep cerebellar nuclei and in the red nucleus. Only after extensive exposure was silver found, and then only in small amounts, in the cerebral cortex, hippocampus, and other regions of cerebral gray matter.

Exposure of pregnant rats to silver resulted in the deposition of silver in the choroid plexus and meninges of the offspring; the pattern of silver localization within the brain was similar to that found in silver-exposed adults rats (Rungby and Danscher, 1983b).

The distribution of silver deposition in the peripheral nervous system was studied following administration of silver salts to mice (Rungby, 1986). Silver was visualized by light microscopy in paraffin and resin sections (Danscher, 1981); its inherent electron density indicates its presence when examined by electron microscopy. Silver was found particularly in those parts of the peripheral nervous system without blood barriers, including dorsal root ganglia and the ganglion cells and glia of the myenteric plexus. There was much deposition of silver in satellite cells in the dorsal root ganglia. In peripheral nerves, silver was seen frequently in the epineurium and perineurium, mostly in association with basal laminae; it was relatively less common in the endoneurium, where it was seen in some Schwann cells. Intracellular silver was seen in structures identified as lysosomes.

Doxorubicin

Doxorubicin (Adriamycin) is an anthracycline compound used in antitumour therapy. It inhibits DNA-directed mRNA synthesis by intercalating between base pairs of nuclear DNA (Di Marco, 1975). In humans, a hydroxylated derivative of doxorubicin, called daunorubicin (rubidomycin) has been reported to cause degeneration of intracardiac neurons and dorsal root ganglion cells (Smith, 1969) but there are no reports of human neurotoxicity of doxorubicin.

Doxorubicin has been used in a number of experimental studies in rats and mice. The drug has a characteristic orange-red fluorescence when excited by ultraviolet light, and therefore the localization of the drug in cell nuclei can be studied by cytofluorescence microscopy. This has shown staining of all regions of the nervous system that lie outside a blood-brain (Bigotte et al., 1982a) or blood-nerve barrier (Bigotte et al., 1982b), which is maximal by 15 min following intravenous injection. The brain regions showing nuclear fluorescence are shown in Table 1. No drug-induced fluorescence was identified in brain parenchyma outside these regions.

The first pathological studies on doxorubicin (Cho, 1977) had shown neuronal degeneration in sensory ganglion cells, beginning with nuclear changes. Morphological changes were demonstrated in brain regions without a BBB, including the neurohypophysis, median eminence, and area postrema (Bigotte and Olsson, 1983). Neuronal degeneration was seen in the area postrema, and degenerate axon terminals were observed in the neurohypophysis and median eminence, with nuclear changes in glial cells.

If the BBB is opened by giving mannitol, intravenous doxorubicin causes cellular changes in the cerebral cortex, caudate nucleus, and putamen similar to those produced in dorsal root ganglion cells (Kondo et al., 1987).

Another method of circumventing the blood brain barrier is intramuscular injection, when there is degeneration of the associated motor neurons because of the retrograde axonal transport of doxorubicin (Bigotte and Olsson, 1982).

Amiodarone

Amiodarone, a diiodinated benzofuran derivative, is an amphiphilic drug used in the treatment of cardiac arrhythmias. In humans, peripheral neuropathy is an important side effect. Like other amphiphilic drugs, amiodarone induces the formation of cytoplasmic inclusions. In the case of amiodarone, this is due to inhibition of lysosomal phospholipases (Heath et al., 1985) leading to the accumulation of phospholipid-drug complexes within lysosomes. The lamellated or occasionally crystalline inclusions are useful markers for the presence of the drug.

Table 1 Distribution of Doxorubicin-Induced Nuclear Fluorescence at Various Intervals After Intravenous Injection into Mice

Central nervous system areas	Animal survival periods					
	15 sec	30 sec	1 min	15 min	1 h	24 h
Leptomeninges	−	−	−	−	−	−
Grey and white matter	−	−	−	−	−	−
Neurohypophysis	+++	+++	+++	+++	+++	−
Pineal gland	++	+++	+++	++	++	−
Subcommissural organ	−	−	−	−	−	−
Median eminence	+	++	+++	+++	++	+
Subfornical organ	+	++	+++	+++	++	−
Postremal area	+	++	+++	+++	+++	−
Choroid plexus	−	−	++	++	−	−
Optic nerve (lamina cribrosa)	−	−	++	++	−	−
Optic nerve sheath	+	++	+++	+++	−	−

− = no fluorescence; + = faint to easily visible fluorescence; ++ = intense fluorescence; +++ = very intense nuclear fluorescence.
Source: Bigotte et al., 1982a.

In humans, peripheral neuropathy has been reported in a number of papers (e.g., Kaeser et al., 1976; Pellissier et al., 1984; Jacobs and Costa-Jussà, 1985). The neuropathy is distal and symmetrical and may cause severe sensory and motor impairment. Because of the long elimination half-life of the drug, recovery is very slow following its discontinuation. Optic neuropathy has also been reported (Feiner et al., 1987; Nazarian and Jay, 1988).

The neuropathy is generally demyelinating in type, although in some cases there is severe loss of axons. In all cases the presence of drug-induced inclusions is reported, which are best identified by electron microscopy; they are visible by light microscopy in semithin resin sections but not in paraffin sections. High levels of iodine, a marker for the drug, have been found in nerve biopsies (Meier et al., 1979).

It is not clear why amiodarone should cause a neuropathy in humans. As described below, no neuropathy was induced in rats, because of the presence of a blood-nerve barrier. The blood-nerve barrier in humans may differ in its properties from that in the rat. Alternatively, other factors such as the presence of existing pathology in the nerve may alter the vascular permeability. Often, the patients who develop amiodarone-induced neuropathy are elderly, and there is evidence of nerve pathology with increasing age (Jacobs and Love, 1985).

In experimental studies on rats, amiodarone-induced inclusions were found only in parts of the nervous system without a blood-brain or blood-nerve barrier (Costa-Jussà and Jacobs, 1985). Regions studies included the area postrema, choroid plexus, sympathetic (Fig. 9) and dorsal root ganglia, and the myenteric plexus (Fig. 10). In ocular tissues there were large numbers of inclusions in the pigmented cells of the retina, and some axons in the prelaminar part of the optic nerve were distended with inclusions.

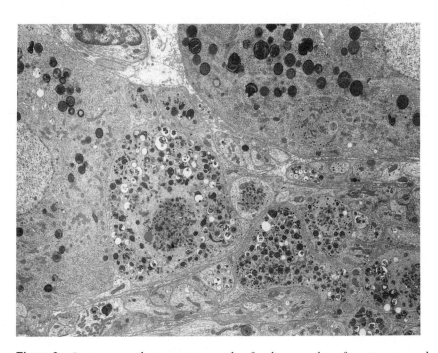

Figure 9 Low-power electron micrograph of celiac ganglion from a mouse dosed daily with amiodarone for 3 months. The nerve cell bodies contain many amiodarone-induced cytoplasmic inclusions, often with a lamellated appearance; several processes are filled with dense inclusions and appear to be degenerating. (×4200.)

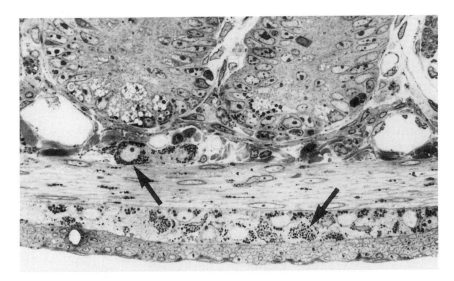

Figure 10 1-μm resin section of ileum from a rat dosed daily with amiodarone for 3 weeks. Neurons and processes with many dense, amiodarone-induced inclusions are seen in both myenteric and submucosal plexuses (arrows). Inclusions are also present in smooth muscle cells. (×600.)

No significant changes were seen in the peripheral nerves, because of the presence of a blood-nerve barrier, but when vascular permeability was increased by making a crush lesion, drug-induced inclusions were found in Schwann cells, endothelial cells, and macrophages. These inclusions soon disappeared, because the increased vascular permeability was only transient. There were some minor defects in myelination in the regenerated nerves.

In a recent experimental study, amiodarone was injected intraneurally into the rat tibial nerve, bypassing the blood-nerve barrier (Santoro et al., 1992). Effects were dose-related; high concentrations of the drug caused axonal degeneration and low concentrations produced a demyelinating lesion.

Other amphiphilic drugs are known to cause lipidosis in regions of the nervous system without a blood-brain barrier (Drenkhahn and Lüllmann-Rauch, 1979).

Pyridoxine

Pyridoxine is one of three interconvertible vitamers that form vitamin B_6. In its phosphorylated form, pyridoxine acts as a coenzyme in a large number of biological reactions. It is of particular importance in the brain, where it is involved as a coenzyme in the synthesis of neurotransmitters. Pyridoxine entry to the brain is carrier-mediated and is regulated so that it is difficult to increase amounts of pyridoxine in the brain (Spector, 1978a,b). Its entry into regions without a blood barrier, such as the dorsal root ganglia, appears to be uncontrolled, and in large doses it can produce a neurotoxic effect on these cells.

At the time of its introduction into clinical medicine, experimental studies had shown that large doses of pyridoxine administered to rats could cause degeneration in posterior columns because of effects on the sensory ganglion cells (Antopol and Tarlov, 1942). Later studies, mostly in dogs or rats, confirmed that large doses of pyridoxine caused a purely sensory neuropathy or neuronopathy (Krinke et al., 1980; Windebank et al., 1985; Montpetit et al., 1988b; Xu et al., 1989). Doses leading to degeneration of the ganglion cells will clearly cause degeneration of the associated axons. However, sublethal damage to the nerve cell bodies may result in a distal axonopathy affecting both central and peripheral axons.

Pyridoxine has been employed as a therapeutic agent in humans in a wide range of conditions, often involving the administration of large doses. Probably its most common use is in the premenstrual syndrome. Reports in the popular press and on television (in the United States) of the beneficial effects of vitamin megadoses has led to cases of self-medication, sometimes with large doses and for long periods.

The neurotoxic effects of pyridoxine in humans were first reported by Schaumburg et al. (1983), when long-term use of large doses was associated with development of a purely sensory neuropathy. Albin et al. (1987) described two cases of acute and severe sensory neuropathy following the use of very large doses of pyridoxine (one patient received 132 g over 3 days) as therapy for mushroom poisoning. Persistent and incapacitating sensory deficit was described in one of these patients after follow-up of several years (Albin and Albers, 1990). Further reports (Berger and Schaumburg, 1984; Parry and Bredesen, 1985) suggest that quite modest doses of pyridoxine may also be associated with neuropathy.

The specificity of neurotoxic effects of pyridoxine for dorsal root ganglion cells suggests that vascular permeability is a factor in determining this selectivity. Recent studies on pyridoxine neurotoxicity by Pires and Jacobs (unpublished) have shown that although there may be severe damage to dorsal root ganglion cells (Fig. 11), other regions without a blood barrier, such as the autonomic ganglia and the myenteric plexus of ganglion cells and processes, showed no significant change. In this instance, it may be that metabolic demands of the dorsal root ganglion cells, which support large volumes of axoplasm in both central and peripheral processes, may enhance the toxic effects of pyridoxine.

Methylmercury and Inorganic Mercury

Studies on a number of different species dosed with both methylmercury and inorganic mercury (see also next section) suggest a correlation between amounts of mercury present and lesions of dorsal root ganglion cells. Measurement of the amounts of ^{203}Hg in tissues of rats fed with isotopic methylmercury showed that dorsal root ganglia contained more ^{203}Hg than either cerebrum or cerebellum (Somjen et al., 1973). Similar findings were made after feeding with inorganic mercury. Morphological and biochemical studies confirm dorsal root ganglia as a site of selective damage (Chang and Hartmann, 1972a; Chang et al., 1972; Herman et al., 1973; Jacobs et al., 1975). Degenerative axonal changes have also been observed in autonomic ganglia and in the myenteric plexus of rats dosed with methylmercury (Jacobs, 1980); these regions also lie outside a blood barrier.

Glutamate

Glutamate is now recognized as the major excitatory neurotransmitter. It crosses the BBB by a carrier-mediated process and is present in the cytoplasm of most vertebrate neurons, both as an intermediate metabolic product and also in anionic form, contributing to the maintenance of the cellular environment. Glutamate in an extracellular situation is potentially neurotoxic, probably because of its prolonged depolarizing action at postsynaptic membranes, eventually leading to cellular edema and lysis. Any change involving glutamate

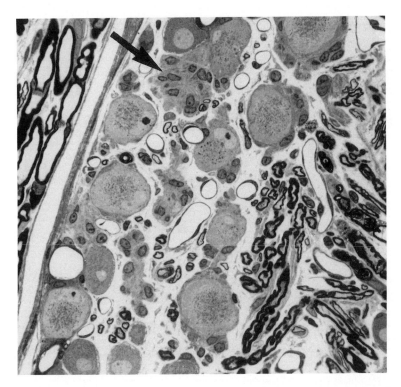

Figure 11   1-μm resin section of dorsal root ganglion from a rat dosed with pyridoxine. Many ganglion cells have eccentrically situated nuclei and contain collections of organelles. A group of satellite cells indicates the degeneration of a ganglion cell (arrow). Ventral root fibers to the left are normal. (×328.)

release from neurons, impairment of its uptake into neurons, or altered glutamate receptor function could lead to cell death as a result of excitotoxicity.

The neurotoxicity of systemically administered glutamate has long been recognized to be limited to regions lying outside the blood-brain barrier. Experimental studies have shown degenerative changes in neurons in circumventricular organs in several species including mice (Olney et al., 1977), primates (Olney and Rhee, 1978), and rats (Tóth et al., 1987). There is swelling of the neuronal cytoplasm and nuclear pyknosis (Fig. 12); swelling of dendritic processes is also a conspicuous feature. These changes are thought to be related to the excitotoxic action of glutamate. Transplacental neurotoxicity of glutamate was demonstrated by Tóth et al. (1987). When pregnant rats were given a single dose of glutamate during the last week of pregnancy, neuronal necrosis was seen in the area postrema of the adult rats and of 20- to 22-day embryos, although the fetal rats were far more sensitive to its effects. The BBB to glutamate in rats seems to be present by the last week of gestation.

The pathological changes invariably involve intracellular edema, the cells become shrunken, and the remains are rapidly phagocytosed by microglial cells.

The only evidence of glutamate neurotoxicity in humans is the "Chinese restaurant syndrome." Symptoms of facial and chest pain, burning sensations, and sometimes

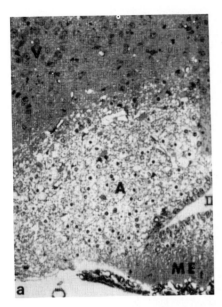 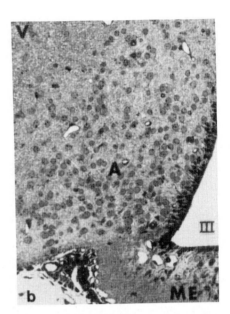

Figure 12 Sections through the hypothalamic region (arcuate nucleus [A] and median eminence [ME]), a site of vascular permeability, of (a) a 10-day-old mouse given a dose of monosodium glutamate 6 hours previously and (b) a control mouse of the same age. In (a) the neurons have greatly swollen cytoplasm and pyknotic nuclei. (×224.) (From Olney JW (1976) Brain damage and oral intake of certain amino acids. Adv Exp Med Biol 69:497–506.)

headache after eating Chinese food were found to be due to monosodium glutamate (MSG) added to the food as a flavor enhancer (Schaumburg et al., 1969).

Following recognition of the neurotoxicity of glutamate particularly to young experimental animals, the use of MSG in baby foods has been discontinued. The risks of adding MSG or glutamate (and aspartate) as protein hydrolysates to baby foods has been discussed by Olney (1980). Tóth et al. (1987) have drawn attention to the possibility of transplacental intoxication of human fetuses after consumption of glutamate-containing foods by the mother.

SUBSTANCES CAUSING GENERALIZED NEUROTOXICITY THROUGH DAMAGE TO BLOOD VESSELS OF THE NERVOUS SYSTEM

Inorganic Lead

Breakdown of the blood barrier occurs as a result of lead-induced damage to brain capillaries. This is probably the primary lesion in acute lead encephalopathy in humans, and it leads to brain swelling, which may be fatal. Capillaries may be dilated, narrowed, necrotic, or thrombosed, and endothelial cell swelling or "capillary activation" is described (Pentschew and Garro, 1966). The consequent extravasation of fluid disrupts the brain tissue, particularly the cerebellum, which develops a spongy appearance.

In experimental studies on the pathogenesis of lead encephalopathy in suckling rats, developing blood vessels were found to be the primary target, the cerebellum being more severely affected than other parts of the brain (Thomas et al., 1971; Press, 1977).

Hemorrhages and edema are seen in the cerebellum (Fig. 13). Studies using vascular tracers have shown increased permeability in lead-poisoned suckling rats (Pentschew and Garro, 1966; Press, 1985), but no permeability changes in adult rats or guinea pigs (Bouldin and Krigman, 1975).

The possible involvement of lead in the etiology of motor neuron disease, by its retrograde transport through motor nerves, is discussed above (see "Regions of the Nervous System Without a Blood Barrier; Neuromuscular Junctions").

Peripheral Neuropathy

In humans, exposure to inorganic lead, usually in an occupational setting, can cause a predominantly motor neuropathy. Although common in the 19th century, during the industrial revolution, lead neuropathy rarely occurs now.

Experimental studies of lead neuropathy have been made in the rat, with a view to discovering whether lead directly affects the blood-nerve barrier (Windebank et al., 1980).

Chronic feeding with lead carbonate causes segmental demyelination in peripheral nerves, and endoneurial edema is a feature of this neuropathy. Lead levels in peripheral nerves are significantly raised at an early stage of the neuropathy, before demyelination or endoneurial edema is evident (Windebank et al., 1980) and before changes in blood-nerve barrier function occur.

It appears that lead can pass through intact endoneurial blood vessels. Thus there is no evidence that lead neuropathy is related to direct toxic effects of lead on blood vessels, as is the case in lead encephalopathy.

Lefauconnier (1992) has reviewed transport of amino acids across the BBB and described methods of measurement. Modifications of amino acid transport have been sought in lead and mercury (see above) intoxication. In young rats given doses of lead lower than those required to produce encephalopathy, transport of alanine and phenylalanine was unchanged (Lefauconnier et al., 1980), but the permeability–surface area product

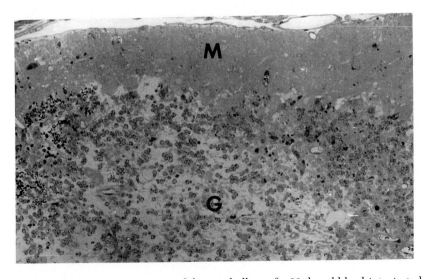

Figure 13 1-μm resin section of the cerebellum of a 26-day-old lead-intoxicated rat; diamino-ben-zidine staining shows the red cells as black structures. Hemorrhages are seen mainly in the granular layer (G), with a few extravasated cells in the molecular layer (M). Cells in the granular layer are separated by edema. (×125.)

for lysine and histidine was greater than that of controls in some regions of the cerebral hemisphere (Moorhouse et al., 1988). Lorenzo and Gewirtz (1977) found lower tryptophan extraction in 20- to 30-day-old rabbits.

Low levels of lead exposure in adult rats from birth did not affect tyrosine transport (Michaelson and Bradbury, 1982).

Methylmercury

Mercury is important as an environmental contaminant, and is most neurotoxic in its organic form. The short-chain alkyl compounds, particularly methylmercury, represent the greatest hazard. Methylmercury is highly lipid-soluble and is able to cross the BBB readily, causing irreversible damage (Chang and Hartmann, 1972b). The distribution of the CNS lesions is not related to blood vessel permeability. Chang (1980) has reviewed a number of studies identifying sites of localization of mercury in the CNS of experimental animals poisoned with methylmercury. Chang and Hartmann (1972c) together with more recent studies by Hargreaves et al. (1985), using a histochemical method involving silver precipitation (Danscher and Schroder, 1979), showed little evidence of correlation of the cellular affinity to mercury with the development of neuropathological changes.

In humans, intoxication with methylmercury is usually chronic, and CNS symptoms predominate. However, in a child accidentally given a large quantity of methylmercury, dorsal root ganglia were affected (T. Takeichi, 1976, unpublished observations).

Inorganic Mercury

Mercury vapor diffuses through the alveolar walls and peripheral capillaries, and a fraction crosses the BBB in an unoxidized form. Warfvinge et al. (1992) studied the localization of mercury in the brown Norwegian rat after exposure to mercury vapor, using a photoemulsion technique on formaldehyde-fixed paraffin sections (Suda et al., 1989). Mercury was distributed mainly in the neocortex, the basal nuclei, and cerebellar Purkinje cells, a pattern similar to that of inorganic mercury deposition following exposure to methylmercury (Möller-Madsen, 1990, 1991). This distribution is clearly not related to the BBB.

Mercury ions in high doses disturb transport of amino acids across the BBB (Hervonen and Steinwall, 1984). Inorganic mercury (mercuric chloride) at a concentration of 10^{-4} M almost completely inhibited the transport of cycloleucine and tryptophan (Pardridge, 1976). Marked inhibition of transport of alanine, phenylalanine, methyl-α-aminoisobutyric acid and glutamic acid was caused by 10^{-4} M mercuric chloride or methylmercury when tested on isolated microvessels (Tayarani et al., 1987). However, the mercurials also cause inhibition of ATPase activity, which would affect the sodium gradient at the abluminal surface, on which amino acid transport depends. Which of the two mechanisms, i.e. carrier transport or sodium gradient, is operative is uncertain. At lower doses, a sodium-independent system (the L-system, which is reactive with large neutral amino acids) allows mercury that is conjugated with L-cysteine to enter the brain (Aschner and Clarkson, 1988).

It is not clear how these metabolic changes might be related to the entry of mercury and to the pathological changes produced.

1,3-Dinitrobenzene

1,3-Dinitrobenzene causes symmetrical lesions in the rat brain stem (Philbert et al., 1987). Although glial cells were thought to be the primary target, it was noted that leakage of red cells into the Virchow-Robin spaces around arterioles was an early event in the pathogenesis of the lesion. A later study (Romero et al., 1991) showed that one of the first identifiable changes was an increase in blood flow, with the subsequent appearance of petechial hemorrhages, associated with microscopic evidence of arteriolar damage in regions known to become affected. At this time there were signs of early gliotoxicity.

While not immediately relevant to the BBB, 1,3-dinitrobenzene provides an example of neurotoxicity possibly related to its effects on the known presence of xanthine oxidase in the vascular bed of the brain, with "useless redox cycling" and the resulting free radical generation promoting damage to endothelial cells (Romero et al., 1991). It is suggested that the selectivity of the lesions may be due to local neuronal activity.

REFERENCES

Abbott NJ, Revest PA, Romero IA (1992). Astrocyte-endothelial interaction: physiology and pathology. Neuropathol Appl Neurobiol 18:424–33.

Albin RL, Albers JW, Greenberg HS, Townsend JB, Lynn RB, Burke JM, Alessi AG (1987). Acute sensory neuropathy-neuronopathy from pyridoxine overdose. Neurology 37:1729–32.

Albin RL, Albers JW (1990). Long-term follow-up of pyridoxine-induced acute sensory neuropathy-neuronopathy. Neurology 40:1319.

Amiel H, Gherardi R, Giroux C, Salama J, Bréau JL, Delaporte P (1987). Cisplatin neuropathy: seven observations one of which with post mortem study. Ann Med Interne 138:96–100.

Antopol W, Tarlov IM (1942). Experimental study of the effects produced by large doses of vitamin B6. J Neuropathol Exp Neurol 1:330–6.

Arvidson B (1980). Regional differences in severity of cadmium-induced lesions in the peripheral nervous system in mice. Acta Neuropathol 49:213–24.

Arvidson B (1986). Autoradiographic localization of cadmium in the rat brain. Neurotoxicology 7:89–96.

Arvidson B, Tjalve H (1986). Distribution of [109]cadmium in the nervous system of rats after intravenous injection. Acta Neuropathol 69:111–6.

Aschner M, Clarkson TW (1988). Uptake of methylmercury in the rat brain: effects of amino acids. Brain Res 462:31–9.

Baker DM, Santer RM, Blaggan AS (1989). Morphometric studies on the microvasculature of pre- and paravertebral sympathetic ganglia in the adult and aged rats by light and electron microscopy. J Neurocytol 18:647–60.

Balin BJ, Broadwell RD, Salcman M, El-Kalliny M (1986). Avenues for entry of peripherally administered protein to the central nervous system in mouse, rat, and squirrel monkey. J Comp Neurol 251:260–80.

Ballard PA, Tetrud JW, Langston JW (1985). Permanent human parkinsonism due to 1-methyl-4-phenyl-1,2,3,6-tetrahydropyridine (MPTP). Seven cases. Neurology 35:949–56.

Berger A, Schaumburg HH (1984). More on neuropathy from pyridoxine abuse. N Engl J Med 311:986–7.

Bigotte L, Arvidson B, Olsson Y (1982a). Cytofluorescence localization of adriamycin in the nervous system I. Distribution of the drug in the central nervous system of normal adult mice after intravenous injection. Acta Neuropathol 57:121–9.

Bigotte L, Arvidson B, Olsson Y (1982b). Cytofluorescence localization of adriamycin in the nervous system II. Distribution of the drug in the somatic and autonomic peripheral nervous systems of normal adult mice after intravenous injection. Acta Neuropathol 57:130–36.

Bigotte L, Olsson Y (1982). Retrograde transport of doxorubicin (adriamycin) in peripheral nerves of mice. Neurosci Lett 32:217–21.

Bigotte L, Olsson Y (1983). Cytotoxic effects of adriamycin on the hypoglossal neurons due to retrograde axonal transport of the drug. Acta Neuropathol 61:161–8.

Bill A, Tornquist P, Alm A (1980). Permeability of the intraocular blood vessels. Trans Ophthalmol Soc UK 100:332–6.

Bouldin TW, Krigman MR (1975). Acute lead encephalopathy in the guinea pig. Acta Neuropathol 33:185–90.

Bouldin TW, Earnhardt TS, Goines ND (1991). Restoration of blood-nerve barrier in neuropathy is associated with axonal regeneration and remyelination. J Neuropathol Exp Neurol 50:719–28.

Brightman MW (1989). The anatomic basis of the blood-brain barrier. Vol. 1 In: Neuwelt EA, ed. Implications of the blood-brain barrier and its manipulation. New York: Plenum, 53–83.

Brightman MW, Reese TS (1969). Junctions between intimately apposed cell membranes in the vertebrate brain. J Cell Biol 40:648–77.

Brightman M, Klatzo I, Olsson Y, Reese T (1970). The blood brain barrier to proteins under normal and pathological conditions. J Neurol Sci 10:215–39.

Broadwell RD, Brightman MW (1976). Entry of peroxidase into neurons of the central and peripheral nervous systems from extracerebral and cerebral blood. J Comp Neurol 166:257–78.

Cavaletti G, Tredeci G, Marmiroli P, Petruccioli MG, Barajon I, Fabbrica D (1992). Morphometric study of the sensory neuron and peripheral nerve changes induced by chronic cisplatin (DDP) administration in rats. Acta Neuropathol 84:364–71.

Cavanagh ME, Cornelis ME, Dziegielewska KM, Evans CAN, Lorscheider FL, Mollgard K, Reynolds ML, Saunders NR (1983). Comparison of proteins in CSF of lateral and IVth ventricles during early development of fetal sheep. Dev Brain Res 11:159–67.

Chang LW (1980). Mercury. In: Spencer PS, Schaumburg HH, eds. Experimental and clinical neurotoxicology. Baltimore: Williams & Wilkins, 508–26.

Chang LW, Hartmann HA (1972a). Ultrastructural studies of the nervous system after mercury intoxication. I. Pathological changes in the nerve cell bodies. Acta Neuropathol 20:122–38.

Chang LW, Hartmann HA (1972b). Blood-brain barrier dysfunction in experimental mercury intoxication. Acta Neuropathol 21:179–84.

Chang LW, Hartmann HA (1972c). Electron microscopic histochemical study on the localization and distribution of mercury in the nervous system after mercury intoxication. Exp Neurol 35:122–37.

Chang LW, Desnoyers PA, Hartmann HA (1972). Quantitative cytochemical studies of RNA in experimental mercury poisoning. I. Changes in RNA content. J Neuropathol Exp Neurol 32:489–501.

Cho ES (1977). Toxic effects of adriamycin on the ganglia of the peripheral nervous system—a neuropathological study. J Neuropathol Exp Neurol 36:907–15.

Clark AW, Parhad IM, Griffin JW, Price DL (1980). Neurotoxicity of cis-platinum: pathology of the central and peripheral nervous systems. Neurology 30:429.

Claude P, Goodenough DA (1973). Fracture faces of zonulae occludentes from "tight" and "leaky" epithelia. J Cell Biol 58:390–400.

Clough G, Michel CC (1981). The role of vesicles in the transport of ferritin through frog endothelium. J Physiol 315:127–42.

Corasaniti MT, Defilippo R, Rodino P, Nappi G, Nistico G (1991). Evidence that paraquat is able to cross the blood-brain barrier to a different extent in rats of various ages. Funct Neurol 6:385–89.

Costa-Jussà FR, Jacobs JM (1985). The pathology of amiodarone neurotoxicity. I Experimental studies with reference to changes in other tissues. Brain 108:735–52.

Danscher G (1981). Light and electron microscopic localization of silver in biological tissue. Histochemistry 71:177–86.

Danscher G (1982). Silver used as a marker of retrograde axonal transport. Neurosci Lett 10(suppl):5129.

Danscher G, Schroder HD (1979). Histochemical demonstration of mercury induced changes in rat neurons. Histochemistry 60:1–7.

Daugaard GK, Petrera J, Trojaborg W (1987). Electrophysiological study of the peripheral and central neurotoxic effects of cisplatin. Acta Neurol Scand 76:86–93.

Davson H, Oldendorf WH (1967). Transport in the central nervous system. Proc Roy Soc Med 60:326–8.

De la Motte DJ, Allt G (1976). Crush injury to peripheral nerve. An electron microscope study employing horseradish peroxidase. Acta Neuropathol 36:9–19.

Dermietzel R, Krause D (1991). Molecular anatomy of the blood-brain barrier as defined by immunocytochemistry. Int Rev Cytol 127:57–109.

Dewar J, Hunt H, Abernethy DA, Dady P, Haas LF (1986). Cisplatin neuropathy with Lhermitte's sign. J Neurol Neurosurg Psychiatry 49:96–9.

Di Marco A (1975). Adriamycin (NSC-123127): mode and mechanism of action. Cancer Chemother Rep 6:91–106.

Dow PR, Shinn SL, Ovalle WK (1980). Ultrastructural study of a blood–muscle spindle barrier after systemic administration of horseradish peroxidase. Am J Anat 157:375–88.

Drenckhahn D, Lüllman-Rauch R (1979). Drug-induced experimental lipidosis in the nervous system. Neuroscience 4:697–712.

Dumas M, Schwab ME, Baumann R, Thoenen H (1979). Retrograde transport of tetanus toxin through a chain of two neurons. Brain Res 165:354–7.

Ehrlich P (1885). Das Sauerstoff-Bedürfnis des Organismus. Berlin: Hirschwald.

Feiner LA, Younge BR, Kazmier FJ, Stricker BHC, Fraunfelder FT (1987). Optic neuropathy and amiodarone therapy. Mayo Clin Proc 62:702–17.

Flage T (1977). Permeability properties of the tissue in the optic nerve head of the rabbit and monkey: an ultrastructural study. Acta Ophthalmol 55:652–64.

Gabbiani G, Baic D, Deziel C (1967a). Toxicity of cadmium for the central nervous system. Exp Neurol 18:154–160.

Gabbiani G, Gregory A, Baic D (1967b). Cadmium-induced selective lesions of sensory ganglia. J Neuropathol Exp Neurol 26:498–506.

Gastaut JL, Pellissier JF (1985). Cisplatin-induced neuropathy. A clinical, neurophysiological and pathological study. Rev Neurol 141:614–26.

Gershon MD, Bursztajn S (1978). Properties of the enteric nervous system: limitation of access of intravascular macromolecules to the myenteric plexus and muscularis externa. J Comp Neurol 180:467–88.

Goldmann EE (1909). Die äussere und innere Sekretion des gesunden und gekranken Organismus im Licht der vitalen Färbung. Beitr Klin Chir 64:192–265.

Goldmann EE (1913). Vitalfärbung am Zentralnervensystem. Abh Preuss Akad Wiss Phys-Math 1:1–60.

Greenwood J (1992). Experimental manipulation of the blood-brain and blood-retinal barriers. In: Bradbury MWB, ed. Physiology and pharmacology of the blood-brain barrier. Heidelberg: Springer-Verlag, 459–486.

Gregg RW, Molepo JM, Montpetit VJA, Mikael NZ, Redmond D, Gadia M, Stewart DJ (1992). Cisplatin neurotoxicity: the relationship between dosage, time, and platinum concentration in neurologic tissues, and morphological evidence of toxicity. J Clin Oncol 10:795–803.

Greig NH (1989). Drug delivery to the brain by blood-brain barrier circumvention and drug modification. Vol I. In: Neuwelt EA, ed. Implications of the blood-brain barrier and its manipulation. New York: Plenum, 311–367.

Greig NH (1992). Drug entry into the brain. In: Bradbury MWB, ed. Physiology and pharmacology of the blood-brain barrier. Heidelberg: Springer-Verlag. 487–523.

Gross PM, Sposito NM, Pettersen SE, Fenstermacher JD (1986). Differences in function and structure of the capillary endothelium in grey matter, white matter and a circumventricular organ of the rat brain. Blood Vessels 23:261–70.

Gross PM (1992). Circumventricular organ capillaries. Prog Brain Res 91:219–34.

Hargreaves RJ, Foster JR, Pelling D, Moorhouse SR, Gangolli SD, Rowland IR (1985). Changes in the distribution of histochemically localized mercury in the CNS and in tissue levels of organic and inorganic mercury during the development of intoxication in methylmercury treated rats. Neuropathol Appl Neurobiol 11:383–401.

Heath MF, Costa-Jussà FR, Jacobs JM, Jacobson W (1985). The induction of pulmonary phospholipidosis and the inhibition of lysosomal phospholipases by amiodarone. Br J Exp Pathol 66:391–8.

Herman SP, Klein R, Talley FA, Krigman MR (1973). An ultrastructural study of methylmercury-induced sensory neuropathy in the rat. Lab Invest 28:104–18.

Hervonen H, Steinwall O (1984). Endothelial surface sulfhydryl-group in blood-brain barrier transport of nutrients. Acta Physiol Scand 121:343–51.

Jacobs JM, Macfarlane RM, Cavanagh JB (1976). Vascular leakage in the dorsal root ganglia of the rat studied with horseradish peroxidase. J Neurol Sci 29:95–107.

Jacobs JM (1977). Penetration of systemically injected horseradish peroxidase into ganglia and nerves of the autonomic nervous system. J Neurocytol 6:607–18.

Jacobs JM, Carmichael N, Cavanagh JB (1975). Ultrastructural changes in the dorsal root and trigeminal ganglia of rats poisoned with methyl mercury. Neuropathol Appl Neurobiol 1:1–19.

Jacobs JM (1980). Vascular permeability and neural injury. In: Spencer PS, Schaumburg, HH, eds. Experimental and clinical neurotoxicology. Baltimore: Williams & Wilkins, 102–17.

Jacobs JM, Costa-Jussà FR (1985). The pathology of amiodarone neurotoxicity. II. Peripheral neuropathy in man. Brain 108:753–69.

Jacobs JM, Love S (1985). Qualitative and quantitative morphology of human sural nerve at different ages. Brain 108:897–924.

Jacobs JM, Le Quesne PM (1992). Toxic disorders. In: Adams JH, Duchen LW, eds. Greenfield's neuropathology. 5th ed. London: Edward Arnold, 881–987.

Jenner P (1989). Clues to the mechanism underlying dopamine cell death in Parkinson's disease. J Neurol Neurosurg Psychiatry 52(suppl):22–8.

Kaeser HE, Ulrich J, Wuthrich R (1976). Amiodarone neuropathy. Praxis 65:1121–2.

Kalaria RN, Mitchell MJ, Harik SI (1987). Correlation of 1-methyl-4-1,2,3,6-tetrahydropyridine neurotoxicity with blood-brain monoamine oxidase activity. Proc Natl Acad Sci 84:3521–5.

Kondo A, Inoue T, Nagara H, Tateishi J, Fukui M (1987). Neurotoxicity of adriamycin passed through transiently disrupted blood-brain barrier by mannitol in the rat brain. Brain Res 177:347–60.

Krinke G, Schaumburg HH, Spencer PS, Surtees J, Thomann P, Hess, R (1980). Pyridoxine megavitaminosis produces degeneration of peripheral sensory neurons (sensory neuronopathy) in the dog. Neurotoxicology 2:13–24.

Kristensson K, Olsson Y (1971). The perineurium as a diffusion barrier to protein tracers. Differences between mature and immature animals. Acta Neuropathol 17:127–38.

Kupersmith MJ, Shakib M (1989). The blood-ocular barrier. In: Neuwelt EA, ed. Implications of the blood-brain barrier and its manipulation. Vol. 1. New York: Plenum Press, 369–390.

Laterra J, Guerin C, Goldstein GW (1990). Astrocytes induce neural microvascular endothelial cells to form capillary-like structures in vitro. J Cell Physiol 144:204–15.

Laterra J, Goldstein GW (1991). Astroglial-induced in vitro angiogenesis: requirements for RNA and protein synthesis. J Neurochem 57:1231–9.

Lefauconnier J.-M (1992). Transport of amino acids. In: Bradbury MWB, ed. Physiology and pharmacology of the blood-brain barrier. Heidelberg: Springer-Verlag, 117–150.

Lefauconnier JM, Lavielle E, Terrien N, Bernar DG, Fournier E (1980). Effect of various lead doses on some cerebral capillary functions in the suckling rat. Toxicol Appl Pharmacol 55:467–76.

Lewandowsky M (1900). Zur Lehre der Cerebrospinalflüssigkeit. Z Klin Med 40:480–94.

Liebert UG, Seitz RJ, Weber T, Wechsler W (1985). Immunocytochemical studies of serum proteins and immunoglobulins in human sural nerve biopsies. Acta Neuropathol 68:39–47.

Lorenzo AV, Gewirtz M (1977). Inhibition of [^{14}C]tryptophan transport into brain of lead exposed neonatal rabbits. Brain Res 132:386–92.

Lundborg C, Nordborg C, Rydevik B, Olsson Y (1973). The effect of ischemia on the permeability of the perineurium to protein tracers in rabbit tibial nerve. Acta Neurol Scand 49:287–94.

Mata M, Staple J, Fink DJ (1987). The distribution of serum albumin in rat peripheral nerve. J Neuropathol Exp Neurol 46:485–94.

Matuk Y, Ghosh K, McCulloch C (1981). Distribution of silver in eyes and plasma proteins of the albino rat. Can J Ophthalmol 16:145–50.

Meier C, Kauer B, Müller U, Ludin HP (1979). Neuromyopathy during chronic amiodarone treatment. J Neurol 220:231–9.

Mellick RS, Cavanagh JB (1968). Changes in blood vessel permeability during degeneration and regeneration in peripheral nerves. Brain 91:141–60.

Michaelson A, Bradbury M (1982). Effect of early inorganic lead exposure on rat blood-brain barrier permeability to tyrosine or choline. Biochem Pharmacol 31:1881–5.

Minakawa T, Bready J, Berliner J, Fisher M, Cancilla PA (1991). In vitro interaction of astrocytes and pericytes with capillary-like structures of brain microvessel endothelium. Lab Invest 65:32–40.

Mitchell JD (1987). Heavy metals and trace elements in amyotrophic lateral sclerosis. Neurol Clin 5:43–60.

Möller-Madsen B (1990). Localization of mercury in CNS of the rat. II. Intraperitoneal injection of methylmercuric chloride ($CH_3Hg\,Cl$) and mercuric chloride ($HgCl_2$). Toxicol Appl Pharmacol 103:303–23.

Möller-Madsen B (1991). Localization of mercury in CNS of the rat. III. Oral administration of methylmercuric chloride (CH^3HgCl). Fundam Appl Toxicol 16:172–87.

Montpetit VJA, Stewart D, Molepo JM, Mikhael N, Dancea S, Keaney MA (1988a). Cisplatinum neuropathy in ferrets: correlation of platinum concentration in neural tissues with sensory neuropathy. J Neuropathol Exp Neurol 47:312.

Montpetit VJA, Clapin DF, Tryphonas L, Dancea S (1988b). Alteration of neuronal cytoskeletal organisation in dorsal root ganglia associated with pyridoxine neurotoxicity. Acta Neuropathol 76:71–81.

Moorhouse SR, Carden S, Drewitt PN, Eley BP, Hargreaves RJ, Pelling D (1988). The effect of chronic low level lead exposure on blood-brain barrier function in the developing rat. Biochem Pharmacol 37:4539–47.

Nabeshima S, Reese TS, Landis DMD, Brightman MW (1975). Junctions in the meninges and marginal glia. J Comp Neurol 164:127–70.

Nazarian SM, Jay WM (1988). Bilateral optic neuropathy with amiodarone therapy. J Clin Neuro-Ophthalmol 8:25–8.

Neuwelt EA, Barnett PA (1989). Blood-brain disruption in the treatment of brain tumours: Animal studies. In: Neuwelt EA, ed. Implications of the blood-brain barrier and its manipulation. Vol. 2. New York: Plenum Press, 107–82.

Oaklander AL, Miller MS, Spencer PS (1987). Early changes in degenerating mouse sciatic nerves are associated with endothelial cells. Brain Res 419:39–45.

Ohara S, Ikuta F (1985). On the occurrence of the fenestrated vessels in Wallerian degeneration of the peripheral nerve. Acta Neuropathol 68:259–62.

Olney JW (1980). Excitotoxic mechanisms of neurotoxicity. In: Spencer PS, Schaumburg HH, eds. Experimental and clinical neurotoxicology. Baltimore: Williams & Wilkins, 272–94.

Olney JW, Rhee V (1978). Neurotoxic effects of glutamate on primate area postrema. (Abstract). J Neuropathol Exp Neurol 37:669.

Olney JW, Rhee V, Gubareff T (1977). Neurotoxic effects of glutamate on mouse area postrema. Brain Res 120:151–7.

Olsson Y (1966). Studies on vascular permeability in peripheral nerves I. Distribution of circulating fluorescent serum albumin in normal, crushed and sectioned rat sciatic nerve. Acta Neuropathol 7:1–15.

Olsson Y (1967). Phylogenetic variations in the vascular permeability of peripheral nerves to serum albumin. Acta Pathol Microbiol Scand 69:621–3.

Olsson Y (1971). Studies on vascular permeability in peripheral nerves. IV. Distribution of intravenously injected protein tracers in the peripheral nervous system of various species. Acta Neuropathol 17:114–26.

Olsson Y, Kristensson K (1973). Permeability of blood vessels and connective tissue sheaths in retina and optic nerve. Acta Neuropathol 26:147–56.

Pardridge WM (1976). Inorganic mercury: selective effects on blood-brain barrier transport systems. J Neurochem 27:333–5.

Pardridge WM, Boado RJ, Farrell CR (1990). Brain-type glucose transport (GLUT-1) is selectively localized to the blood-brain barrier. Studies with quantitative western blotting and in situ hybridization. J Biol Chem 265:18035–40.

Parry GJ, Bredesen DE (1985). Sensory neuropathy with low dose pyridoxine. Neurology 35: 1466–8.

Pellissier JF, Pouget J, Cros D, De Victor B, Serratrice G, Toga M (1984). Peripheral neuropathy induced by amiodarone chlorhydrate: a clinicopathological study. J Neurol Sci 63:251–66.

Pentschew A (1965). Morphology and morphogenesis of lead encephalopathy. Acta Neuropathol 5:133–60.

Pentschew A, Garro F (1966). Lead encephalo-myelopathy of the suckling rat and its implications on the porphyrinopathic nervous diseases. Acta Neuropathol 6:266–78.

Philbert MA, Nolan CC, Cremer JE, Tucker D, Brown AW (1987). 1,3-dinitrobenzene induced encephalopathy in rats. Neuropathol Appl Neurobiol 13:371–89.

Poduslo JF, Low PA, Nickander KK, Dyck PJ (1985). Mammalian endoneurial fluid; collection and protein analysis from normal and crushed nerves. Brain Res 332:91–102.

Press MF (1977). Lead encephalopathy in neonatal rats: morphological studies. J Neuropathol Exp Neurol 36:169–93.

Press MF (1985). Lead-induced permeability changes in immature vessels of the developing cerebellar microcirculation. Acta Neuropathol 67:86–95.

Price DL, Griffin J, Young A, Peck K, Stocks A (1975). Tetanus toxin: direct evidence for retrograde intraaxonal transport. Science 188:945–7.

Reale E, Luciano L, Spitznas M (1975). Freeze-fracture faces of the perineurial sheath of the rabbit sciatic nerve. J Neurocytol 4:261–70.

Rechthand E, Rapoport SI (1987). Regulation of the microenvironment of peripheral nerve: role of the blood-nerve barrier. Prog Neurobiol 28:303–43.

Reese TS, Brightman MW (1968). Similarity in structure and permeability to peroxidase of epithelia overlying fenestrated cerebral capillaries. (Abstract). Anat Rec 160:414.

Reese TS, Karnovsky MJ (1967). Fine structural localization of a blood-brain barrier to exogenous peroxidase. J Cell Biol 34:208–17.

Reese TS, Olsson Y (1970). The structural localization of a blood-nerve barrier in the mouse. (Abstract). J Neuropathol Exp Neurol 29:123.

Renkin EM (1964). Transport of large molecules across capillary walls. Physiologist 7:13–28.

Romero I, Brown AW, Cavanagh JB, Nolan CC, Ray DE, Seville MP (1991). Vascular factors in the neurotoxic damage caused by 1,3-dinitrobenzene in the rat. Neuropathol Appl Neurobiol 17:495–508.

Rosenfeld CS, Broder LE (1984). Cisplatin-induced neuropathy. Cancer Treatment Rep 68:659–60.

Ross MH, Reith EJ (1969). Evidence for contractile elements. Science 165:604–6.

Rungby J (1986). Exogenous silver in dorsal root ganglia, peripheral nerve, enteric ganglia and adrenal medulla. Acta Neuropathol 69:45–53.

Rungby J, Danscher G (1983a). Localization of exogenous silver in brain and spinal cord of silver exposed rats. Acta Neuropathol 60:92–8.

Rungby J, Danscher G (1983b). Neuronal accumulation of silver in brain of progeny from argyric rats. Acta Neuropathol 61:258–62.

Santoro L, Barbieri F, Nucciotti R, Battaglia F, Crispi F, Ragno M, Greco P, Caruso G (1992). Amiodarone-induced experimental acute neuropathy in rats. Muscle Nerve 15:788–95.

Saunders NR (1992). Ontogenetic development of brain barrier mechanisms. In: Bradbury MWB, ed. Physiology and pharmacology of the blood-brain barrier. Heidelberg: Springer-Verlag, 327–69.

Schaumburg HH, Byck R, Gerstl R, Mashman JH (1969). Monosodium L-glutamate: its pharmacology and role in the Chinese restaurant syndrome. Science 163:826–8.

Schaumburg H, Kaplan J, Windebank A, Vick N, Rasmis S, Pleasure D, Brown MJ (1983). Sensory neuropathy from pyridoxine abuse. A new megavitamin syndrome. N Engl J Med 309:445–8.

Scott T, Norman PM (1980). Silver deposition in arteriolar basal laminae in the cerebral cortex of argyric rats. Acta Neuropathol 52:243–6.

Sears TA, Pullen AP, Johnson IP (1984). Neuronopathy following retrograde axonal transport of diphtheria toxin. Proceedings of the international symposium on peripheral neuropathy, Nagoya, International Congress Series 662, Amsterdam, Excerpta Medica, 169–78.

Shakib M, Cunha-Vaz JG (1966). Studies on the permeability of the blood-retinal barrier. IV. Role of the junctional complexes of the retinal vessels on the permeability of the blood retinal barrier. Exp Eye Res 5:229–34.

Shanthaveerappa TR, Bourne GH (1962). The "perineurial epithelium," a metabolically active, continuous, protoplasmic cell barrier surrounding peripheral nerve fasciculi. J Anat 96:527–37.

Shivers RR, Harris RJ (1984). Opening of the blood-brain barrier in anolis carolinensis. A high voltage electron microscope study. Neuropathol Appl Neurobiol 10:343–56.

Simionescu N, Simionescu M, Palade GE (1981). Differentiated domains on the luminal surface of the capillary endothelium. I. Preferential distribution of anionic sites. J Cell Biol 90:605–13.

Smith B (1969). Damage to the intrinsic cardiac neurones by rubidomycin (daunorubicin). Br Heart J 31:607–9.

Smith QR (1992). Methods of study. In: Bradbury MWB, ed. Physiology and pharmacology of the blood-brain barrier. Heidelberg: Springer-Verlag, 23–52.

Söderfeldt B, Olsson Y, Kristensson K (1973). The perineurium as a diffusion barrier to protein tracers in human peripheral nerve. Acta Neuropathol 25:120–6.

Somjen CG, Herman SP, Klein RE, Brubaker PE, Briner WH, Goodrich JK, Krigman MR, Haseman JK (1973). The uptake of methyl mercury (Hg^{203}) in different tissues related to its neurotoxic effects. J Pharmacol Exp Ther 187:602–11.

Sparrow JR, Kiernan JA (1981). Endoneurial vascular permeability in degenerating and regenerating peripheral nerves. Acta Neuropathol 53:181–8.

Spector R (1978a). Vitamin B6 transport in the central nervous system. In vitro studies. J Neurochem 30:881–7.

Spector R (1978b). Vitamin B6 transport in the central nervous system. In vivo studies. J Neurochem 30:889–97.

Stern L, Gautier R (1921). Rapports entre le liquide céphalo-rachidien et la circulation sanguine. Arch Int Physiol 17:138–92.

Stern L, Gautier R (1922). Les rapports entre le liquide céphalo-rachidien et les éléments nerveux de l'axe cérébrospinal. Arch Int Physiol 17:391–448.

Stern L, Peyrot R (1927). Le fonctionnement de la barrière hematoencéphalique aux divers stades de développement chez les divers espèces animales. C R Soc Biol (Paris) 96:1124–6.

Stewart PA, Hayakawa EM (1987). Interendothelial junctional changes underly the developmental 'tightening' of the blood-brain barrier. Dev Brain Res 32:271–81.

Stewart PA, Wiley MJ (1981). Developing nervous system tissue induces formation of blood-brain barrier characteristics in invading endothelial cells: a study using quail-chick chimeras. Dev Biol 84:183–92.

Stoeckel K, Schwab M, Theonen H (1977). Role of gangliosides in the uptake and retrograde axonal transport of cholera and tetanus toxin as compared to nerve growth factor and wheat germ agglutinin. Brain Res 132:273–85.

Suda I, Eto K, Tokunaga H, Furusawa R, Suetomi K, Takahashi H (1989). Different histochemical findings in the brain produced by mercuric chloride and methyl mercury chloride in rats. Neurotoxicology 10:113–26.

list of small-molecular-weight neurotransmitters and the number of receptor subtypes they activate. The length of even this abbreviated listing demonstrates the difficulties inherent in determining the exact mechanism of action of a xenobiotic. More than 50 receptors have been demonstrated to exist. However, there are common features of synaptic transmission processes that permit generalization concerning the possible sites of action of xenobiotics.

GENERAL PHYSIOLOGY OF THE SYNAPSE

The synapse has both presynaptic and postsynaptic elements. The presynaptic neuron contains all the mechanisms necessary for the synthesis, storage, and release of neurotransmitter. The postsynaptic cell recognizes the neurotransmitter when it binds to the extracellular surface of a receptor protein. The binding energy of the neurotransmitter and receptor results in a conformational change of the receptor protein. The conformational change results in transmembrane signaling and the induction of intracellular responses. The nerve terminal for most smaller neurotransmitters contains the metabolic machinery for synthesis of the neurotransmitter. Once synthesized, the neurotransmitter is stored within the nerve terminal in concentrated form in small lipid vesicles. The lipid vesicles are recycled from the nerve terminal membrane after exocytosis has occurred. The vesicles may also be transported from the cell body prepackaged with neurotransmitter, as is the case for the larger peptides. The vesicles are specialized structures containing transport proteins that concentrate neurotransmitters and retain them within the vesicle. In order for neurotransmission to occur, the release of the contents of the vesicles into the synaptic cleft is necessary. For a more complete description of the processes to be discussed, books exist that cover these topics in detail (Cooper et al., 1991; Hille, 1992a; Howell et al., 1989; Kandel and Schwartz, 1983).

Each neurotransmitter has specific synthetic enzymes, although many structurally related transmitters have similar synthetic pathways (e.g., the catecholamines: dopamine, norepinephrine, and epinephrine). The synthesis of the neurotransmitter can be altered by xenobiotics. The filling or refilling of the vesicles is very important. Interference with the transport process into the vesicles can result in reduced neurotransmitter content of the nerve terminal, for example, as is the case for reserpine (Curzon, 1990). Storage of the neurotransmitter in vesicles protects the transmitter from destruction by cytosolic, mitochondrial, or other enzymes and maintains the transmitter in a concentrated, rapidly releasable form. In addition, the vesicle may contain other substances important for the uptake (adenosine triphosphate [ATP]) and storage (chromogranins, for instance, in the case of biogenic amines) of neurotransmitter, enzymes (e.g., dopamine-β-hydroxylase), and possibly another transmitter substance (e.g., enkephalins, vasoactive intestinal polypeptide). In particular, those neurotransmitters that can exist in an uncharged form, such as the biogenic amines, may "leak" from the nerve terminal through the neuronal membrane. This process is important in the action of some xenobiotics—for example, in amphetamine-induced displacement of norepinephrine.

The normal release of neurotransmitter results from the invasion of the nerve terminal by an action potential. The action potential in most nerves arises from sodium ion influx across the nerve membrane due to the opening of voltage-gated, sodium ion–selective channels in the axonal membrane. The sodium channels are both activated (gated open) by depolarization and closed by depolarization (inactivation). In addition, voltage-gated potassium channels open upon depolarization with a delay relative to the opening of the sodium channels. The opening of potassium channels causes repolarization of the membrane toward the Nernst

Table 1 Transmitters and Receptor Subtypes

Transmitter	Receptor types[a]	References
Acetylcholine	Muscarinic (5), nicotinic[b](>3)	Hulme, 1990; Schimerlik, 1989; Schimerlik, 1990; Lambert et al., 1992; Steinbach and Ifune, 1989
Epinephrine/norepineprhine	α_1 (3), α_2 (4), β_1, β_2, β_3	Lomasney et al., 1991; Strasser et al., 1992; O'Dowd et al., 1989; Roth et al., 1991
Dopamine	D_1, D_2	Cooper et al., 1991
γ-Aminobutyric acid	$GABA_A$, $GABA_B$	Cooper et al., 1991
Glutamate	Metabotropic (Quisqualate), ligand-gated[b] (NMDA, AMPA)[b]	Barnes and Henley, 1992
Histamine	H_1, H_2, H_3	Hill, 1990; Haaksma et al., 1990; Barnes, 1991
Serotonin	$5\text{-}HT_1$ (4), $5\ HT_{2-4}$	Sanders-Bush, 1990; Hoyer and Schoeffter, 1991; Schmidt and Peroutka, 1989
Adenosine, adenosine triphosphate	A_1, A_2, A, P P_2 (4)	Stone, 1991; O'Connor, 1992; Olah and Stiles, 1992; Burnstock, 1990

[a]The numbers in parenthesis give the number of subtypes within that group.
[b]These are multimeric proteins and can exist in many forms depending on the subunits.

equilibrium potential for potassium ions. As shown by Hodgkin and Huxley (Hodgkin and Huxley, 1952a, b, c), the activation of these channels results in a propagated depolarization, or action potential, down the axon. Inhibition of the action potential (as with tetrodotoxin) will result in decreases in neurotransmission, and prolongation of the action potential (for example, by 4-aminopyridine inhibition of potassium channels) results in an increase in release. The energy of the action potential is not sufficient to transfer information between cells that are separated by a cleft, such as those at most synapses. Therefore, in order to transfer this information, the action potential must be converted to another form, in this case the release of a chemical neurotransmitter.

The depolarization that represents the action potential causes the opening of voltage-gated calcium channels in the nerve terminal membrane. This opening permits the influx of calcium down its concentration gradient. This event leads to a series of biochemical reactions that induce or permit the close approach and fusion of the lipid vesicles with the interior of the plasma membrane. The vesicle then opens through the extracellular membrane surface, resulting in release of the contents of the vesicle into the synaptic cleft. This process is known as exocytosis.

The water-soluble contents of the vesicle are released during exocytosis. We will primarily discuss the effects of the classical neurotransmitters and the actions of xenobiotics on these processes. However, it should be remembered that the other substances released may be biologically active, particularly after the overexcitation that may occur during xenobiotic exposure. For example, one substance generally present in vesicles is ATP. It provides energy for the transport of transmitter into the vesicles. Adenosine triphosphate or its metabolites (e.g., adenosine diphosphate [ADP]) have been shown to interact with purinergic receptors (Burnstock, 1990; Cusack and Hourani, 1990; Stone, 1991). In addition, increasing evidence indicates that some nerves may co-store and, under some conditions, co-release more than one neurotransmitter (Klein and Thureson-Klein, 1990). For example, adrenergic nerves have two forms of vesicle, one electron-lucent and the other dense-cored. It has been suggested that these vesicles contain two different types of transmitter, norepinephrine and a peptide, enkephalin (Kong et al., 1990). Vasoactive intestinal polypeptide release has been closely linked to the release of acetylcholine from many cholinergic nerves (Barnes, 1988). The release of the contents of the vesicles may therefore activate multiple receptors and cellular pathways. Xenobiotics could alter these "secondary" processes to induce acute and, maybe more important, subacute effects only peripherally related to the primary neurotransmitter receptor interaction at the synapse.

After its release the neurotransmitter can 1.) diffuse away from the synapse and enter the circulation, 2.) be removed actively from the cleft, or 3.) interact with neurotransmitter receptors. The structure of synapses minimizes the diffusion of the transmitter from the cleft under normal conditions. This makes transmission more efficient by containing the transmitter within the limited area of the synaptic contact. The removal of the neurotransmitter must occur under normal conditions and does so by one of two general processes, the mechanism depending on the type of synapse involved. For cholinergic synapses, the enzyme AChE is synthesized within the effector cell and transported and tethered to the cell surface. It brings about the rapid hydrolysis of acetylcholine to inactive components, choline and acetate. The second general mechanism involves the active removal of the neurotransmitter by uptake processes located in both the presynaptic and the postsynaptic cell membranes. The biogenic amines and GABA are examples of neurotransmitters actively removed by uptake processes. Inhibition by xenobiotics of these processes leads to prolonged exposure of the postjunctional and prejunctional membrane to the actions of the neurotransmitter, resulting in overexcitation (or inhibition). Cocaine is a good example of a compound that inhibits the uptake of biogenic amines (Reith, 1988).

The third possible fate of the neurotransmitter is to bind to a neurotransmitter receptor imbedded within the postjunctional membrane of the effector cell. The receptor is a transmembrane protein that has on its extracellular surface a stereoselective binding site for the neurotransmitter. The binding energy of the neurotransmitter with the receptor is translated into a conformational change of the receptor. The conformational change brings about the transmembrane signaling of the information that was originally contained in the action potential of the presynaptic nerve.

Each neurotransmitter can activate one general class of receptor proteins. However, within that general class there will be subclassifications. For example, in most pharmacology texts adrenergic receptors have been subclassified into α and β receptors, and these subclasses have been further categorized as α_1, α_2, β_1, and β_2. It is now clear that even this subclassification is insufficient. As is shown in Table 1 there are at least three subtypes of α_1 receptors and four of α_2 receptors. In addition, many receptors are multimeric proteins consisting of multiple subunits. By "mixing and matching subunits," so to speak, the cell can produce numerous receptor subtypes. For example, the $GABA_A$ receptor consists of five subunit types, termed α, β, γ, δ, and ρ. It is known that there are at least 14 forms of the $GABA_A$ receptor subunits (Cutting et al. 1991; Levitan et al. 1988; Luddens et al. 1990; Malherbe et al. 1990; Pritchett et al. 1989; Shivers et al. 1989; Ymer et al. 1989a, 1989b). Thus by altering the subunit structure, it is theoretically possible for the cell to produce many forms of the $GABA_A$ receptor.

Receptors can be subdivided into two very general classifications: 1.) those that have an ion channel within the subunit structure of the receptor and 2.) those that mediate cellular events through the intracellular activation of second messenger production. The basic categories are shown schematically in Fig. 1a and b.

In Fig. 1a the schematic of a receptor-activated ion channel is shown. This type of receptor is best illustrated by the nicotinic acetylcholine receptor at the neuromuscular junction. This receptor consists of five subunits, α (2), β, γ, and δ (Steinbach and Ifune, 1989). The subunits are arranged in a circular barrel-stave configuration around a central pore (see Fig. 1a). The binding of acetylcholine to the α subunits brings about the opening of the ion channel. The channel is permeable to sodium, potassium, and calcium ions (Adams et al., 1980; Dwyer et al., 1980; Dwyer and Farley, 1984). Opening of the channel results in depolarization of the cell (the cell membrane potential becomes more positive) toward a reversal potential of about -10 to 0 mV. This potential is approached because the permeability of the channels to sodium and potassium is very similar and because the monovalent cation concentration is similar intracellularly and extracellulary. Once the depolarization reaches threshold for activation of voltage-gated sodium channels, an action potential occurs in the muscle cell.

Whether the activation of a receptor ion channel is excitatory or inhibitory depends on the ionic permeability of the channel. There are three possible consequences of activation of receptor ion channels on membrane potential; depolarization, hyperpolarization, or no change. Depolarization generally leads to an increased excitability of the postsynaptic cells; for example, the activation of nicotinic receptors at the neuromuscular junction. Depolarization may be caused by a net influx of cations into the cell, by a net efflux of chloride ions from the cell, or by a decrease in permeability of the cell to potassium ions. Hyperpolarization is caused by either a net influx of anions (chloride, as through $GABA_A$ channels) into the cell or a net efflux of cations from the cell (predominantly potassium). The changes in potential may enhance the excitability (depolarization) or inhibit

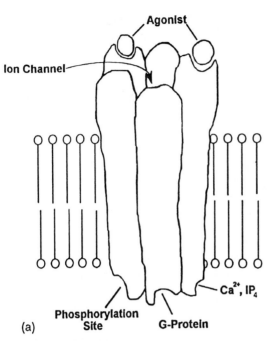

Figure 1 (a) A generalized ligand-gated ion channel type of receptor is illustrated. This type of transmembrane receptor protein is typically multimeric with a central pore. One or more stereoselective binding sites may exist for an agonist to bind with the receptor. The energy of binding causes a conformational change of the protein resulting in opening of the channel. The channel provides a site of interaction with xenobiotics. Although not shown, allosteric binding sites may also exist on the receptor. The intracellular face of the receptor may have one or more sites that can 1.) be phosphorylated, 2.) interact with a G protein subunit, or 3.) interact with a second messenger such as inositol tetrakisphosphate or Ca^{2+}. (b) A generalized schematic of a G protein–coupled receptor.

the activity (hyperpolarization) of the postsynaptic cell. However, it should be noted that increases in the permeability of the cell membrane reduce the input resistance of the postsynaptic cell, independently of the changes in potential, and thus the potential change caused by opening of other ion channels. For instance, if the reversal potential for an ion channel is equal to the resting membrane potential no change in potential will occur, but the conductance of the cell membrane will increase. This forms a low-resistance pathway for current flow through the cell membrane, resulting in smaller changes in membrane potential when other ion channels are active. This type of response can occur after activation of chloride-permeable channels, since chloride is distributed passively in most cells and thus is close to its electrochemical equilibrium potential at the resting potential of the cell.

The ion channel can also be viewed as a drug receptor. For example, ions do not just flow through the channel as through a pipe, but rather interact with the interior of the channel, binding to it, albeit with low affinity (Adams et al., 1981; Dwyer et al., 1980; Dwyer and Farley, 1984). The ion channel therefore provides another site of action of xenobiotics. A well-known example of interaction of a xenobiotic with a channel is the interaction of tetrodotoxin with the voltage-gated sodium channels in nerves. More information on the interaction of specific compounds with ion channels is available in several recent reviews (Narahashi, 1987, 1991, 1992; Wu and Narahashi, 1988).

Agonist

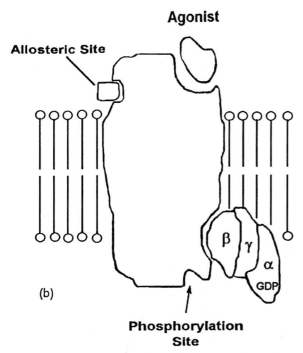

is illustrated. The receptor protein is often monomeric, with one or more binding sites for a neurotransmitter. There often exist allosteric sites on the protein with which xenobiotics can act. Neurotransmitter binding causes a transmembrane conformational change that induces the exchange of guanosine triphosphate for guanosine diphosphate on the α subunit of a G protein that is bound to the intracellular side of the receptor. Once the exchange has occurred the α subunit can dissociate and have effects. The βγ subunits may also activate cellular processes. The intracellular side of the receptor has phosphorylation sites. The phosphorylation sites are important in receptor regulation.

The second type of general receptor class illustrated in Fig. 1b typically does not form an ion channel through the membrane. The receptor is still activated by the binding of the neurotransmitter to the external binding site, but the conformational change induced causes the activation of a guanosine triphosphate (GTP)-binding protein at the interior surface of the cell membrane.

Several recent reviews discuss in detail the mechanism of the activation and possible sites of action of G proteins (Birnbaumer et al., 1990; Collins et al., 1992; Hille, 1992b; Kaziro et al., 1991; Milligan, 1992; Rodbell, 1992; Spiegel et al., 1992; Szabo and Otero, 1990). The receptor coupled G proteins represent a general class of proteins consisting of at least 3 or 4 families (G_s and G_i, for example). Each G protein consists of three subunits, α, β, and γ. The β and γ subunits are tightly coupled and do not dissociate; however, the α subunit and βγ subunit complex may dissociate on binding of the neurotransmitter to the receptor. Receptor activation initiates changes in the conformation of the G protein that cause the guanosine diphosphate (GDP) bound to the G protein complex to be exchanged with GTP. In the presence of magnesium, GTP can be hydrolyzed. After hydrolysis of the GTP, the α-GDP and βγ subunits reassociate. During the time that they are dissociated, the subunits interact with various cellular processes. Certain forms of the G proteins are also the site of action of xenobiotics that both activate (e.g., cholera toxin) and inhibit (e.g., pertussis toxin) the activity of the protein. Both cholera toxin and pertussis toxin ADP-ribosylate G proteins (Ui, 1984; West et al., 1985).

A large number of processes are activated or inhibited by the G proteins. For example, G protein G_p–mediated activation of phospholipase C brings about the production of inositol triphosphate (IP_3) and diacylglycerol (DAG) (Baron et al., 1989; Coburn and Baron, 1990; Majerus, 1992; Sterz et al., 1982). Inositol triphosphate has been shown to activate calcium channels in the endoplasmic reticulum that permit a rapid efflux of calcium from the endoplasmic reticulum into the cytosol (Ferris and Snyder, 1992). Increased intracellular calcium is linked to initiation of many events both at the surface membrane and throughout the cell. Inositol tetrakisphosphate (IP_4) has been proposed as activating ion channels in the cell membrane (Challiss et al., 1991; Downes and Macphee, 1990; Nahorski, 1990). Diacyglycerol, the other product, is known to activate protein kinase C, which can phosphorylate other proteins, bringing about their activation or inhibition (Downes and Macphee, 1990; Kirk, 1990; Nahorski, 1990).

G proteins (G_s and G_i) are also coupled with adenylate cyclase and guanylate cyclase, which convert ATP and GTP, respectively, to the cyclic monophosphates. The G_i family inhibits and the G_s family stimulates adenylate cyclase. The cyclic monophosphates are well known second messengers bringing about activation of numerous cellular events.

Some or all of these events may be altered by subacute exposure to xenobiotics. The subsequent sections will examine specific examples of how subacute exposure to a xenobiotic, an OP AChE inhibitor, could bring about alterations in the sensitivity to stimulation of two different systems: 1.) a simple system, muscarinic receptor activation of tracheal smooth muscle, and 2.) a complex system, the multiple interactive neural pathways in the CNS.

EXAMPLES OF SUBACUTE XENOBIOTIC ACTION: THE ORGANOPHOSPHATES

We will discuss the effects of subacute or chronic exposure to xenobiotics on synaptic function according to the following principle: *Subacute or chronic chemical insult to a neural element will result in changes in the neural element that will reduce the effects of the chemical insult*. A neural element may be a synapse or a neuronal circuit. The purpose of the following discussion is to examine more closely the specific changes that a subacute chemical insult may bring about in the normal responsiveness of a synapse. The difficulties inherent in a general discussion are 1.) that different xenobiotics at the same synapse could have the same overt action even though acting through different mechanisms, and may have different subacute actions; 2.) that at a single type of synapse, the response to subacute exposure will depend on the xenobiotic (e.g., subacutely, antagonists of muscarinic receptors can cause up-regulation of receptor number and agonists can cause down-regulation); 3.) that the physiology of the synapse is complex and there are numerous sites of action for compounds; and that 4.) a compound acting at a single site may have multiple effects on the function of the synapse that are only indirectly associated with the primary locus of action of the xenobiotic. These difficulties are mutliplied when alteration of the activity of one system affects the activity of other systems not directly acted on by the xenobiotic being studied. As an illustration, we will examine the subacute action of a xenobiotic (OP AChE inhibitors) on a relative simple system, tracheal smooth muscle muscarinic receptor–stimulated tension development.

ORGANOPHOSPHATE ACTIONS ON AIRWAY SMOOTH MUSCLE

When an animal is given an OP AChE inhibitor, cholinergic overstimulation results throughout the body. Airway constriction occurs, and when the airway smooth muscle's response to acetylcholine is examined in vitro, it is hypersensitive to acetylcholine when compared with control muscle (Mohan et al., 1988a, 1988b). However, after one and subsequent days of exposure of the animal to the OP AChE inhibitor, the sensitivity of the muscle in vitro to acetylcholine returns toward that of the control tissue. The return toward control sensitivity occurs despite the nearly complete absence of AChE activity in the muscle (Mohan et al., 1988a,b). What changes in the smooth muscle could have brought about the changes in sensitivity that must have occurred in the tissue to reduce the hyperresponsiveness to acetylcholine?

Figure 2 is a schematic of a synapse that shows some of the possible transduction processes initiated by receptor activation. By applying the principle stated earlier, we can predict that the sensitivity of the muscle in vitro to acetylcholine could be decreased in several ways. 1.) The number or subtypes of receptors available for activation by acteylcholine could be reduced or altered. 2.) The coupling of the receptor to the underlying intracellular events could be altered. 3.) The properties of the muscle may be changed so that the efficiency of receptor activation is altered.

Changes in Muscarinic Receptors

There are probably two types of muscarinic receptor in airway smooth muscle. The primary type appears to be an m_3 receptor (Yang et al., 1986, 1988) that is coupled through a G protein (G_p) to phospholipase C (Coburn and Baron, 1990). Activation of this receptor induces the formation of IP_3 and DAG. The rise in calcium initiated by IP_3 and the activation of protein kinase C by DAG bring about activation of cross-bridge cycling and

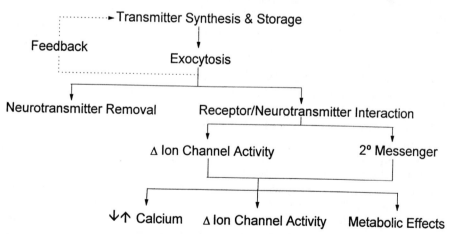

Figure 2 This diagram represents the basic processes that occur during chemical neurotransmission. When the action potential enters the nerve terminal and induces calcium influx the process of transmitter release is initiated. After release of the transmitter there are mechanisms for control of neurotransmitter release, removal of the neurotransmitter, and initiation of postsynaptic events through interaction of the neurotransmitter with receptor proteins in the effector cell. Each of the steps in the neurotransmitter pathway can be altered by xenobiotics after both acute and subacute exposure.

tension development (Forder et al., 1985; Hai and Murphy, 1989; Murphy, 1989; Park and Rasmussen, 1985; Rasmussen et al., 1990; Ratz and Murphy, 1987; Somlyo et al., 1990). The other muscarinic receptor subtype present appears to be the m_2 receptor, although this receptor has not been consistently observed (Barnes, 1990; Brichant et al., 1990; Haddad et al., 1991; Mak and Barnes, 1989; Roffel et al., 1988; Yang et al, 1991). The m_2 receptor acts through a G protein (G_i) to inhibit the formation of cyclic adenosine monophosphate (cAMP). Induction of tension is primarily dependent on activation of m_3 receptors (Brichant et al., 1990; Mak and Barnes, 1989). However, when muscarinic receptor number is determined using nonspecific ligands such as quinuclidynyl benzilate or atropine derivatives, all receptors will be measured without respect to subtype. If only one receptor subtype is altered by subacute treatment with OP AChE inhibitor, the changes in the receptor of interest may be either over- or underestimated if the proportion of the subtypes is not uniformly changed.

Decreased muscarinic receptor number occurs in swine airway smooth muscle after subacute treatment of the animal with diisopropylfluorophosphate (DFP) or another OP AChE inhibitor (Mohan et al., 1988b; Yang et al., 1988). Both surface and total (surface plus internalized) numbers are decreased after seven daily treatments with OP AChE inhibitors (Mohan et al., 1988b). Down-regulation of muscarinic receptors is a commonly observed phenomenon after subacute exposure to OP AChE inhibitors (Aas et al., 1987; Buckley and Heading, 1970; Cioffi and El-Fakahany, 1986a; Costa et al., 1981; Ehlert et al., 1980a,b; Emmelin, 1964; Foley and McPhillips, 1973; Gokhale et al., 1977; Levy, 1981; Lim et al., 1987; McPhillips, 1969; McPhillips and Dar, 1967; Olianas et al., 1984; Perrine and McPhillips, 1970; Sivam et al., 1983; Van Dongen and Wolthuis, 1989; Yamada et al., 1979; Yang et al., 1990). The receptors in airway smooth muscle appear to be primarily of the m_3 subtype, but others have shown that m_2 receptors are also present in other species (see above). The existence of a second subtype that does not appear to couple directly to tension development (m_2 receptors) may mask changes in receptor number of the subtype (m_3) that appears most important in tension development. As noted above, differential changes in receptor subtypes make correlation of changes in receptor density with end response difficult. Differential changes in the proportion of each muscarinic receptor subtype in the brain have been noted after treatment with atropine, a muscarinic antagonist (Wall et al., 1992). We have found that airway mucosa contains both m_1 and m_3 receptors and that the m_3 receptors are down-regulated to a greater extent than the m_1 receptors in this tissue (Farley and Dwyer, 1991). Therefore, care must be taken to determine the loss or increase in the particular subtype that is coupled with the end response being measured.

After seven daily treatments with DFP, muscarinic receptor number (total or cell surface) was reduced by 70–75%. The reduction in receptor number should result in decreased sensitivity to agonist. However, it has been found that at least 95% of the receptors in airway are spare receptors (Grandordy et al., 1986). Thus, even decreasing receptor number significantly might not greatly alter sensitivity of the tissue to acetycholine. However, without knowing whether the proportion of remaining m_2 and m_3 receptors changes during down-regulation, it is impossible to interpret these results further.

Changes in G Proteins

In addition, to the decrease in receptor number it was found that the binding properties of the muscarinic receptors had changed (Mohan et al., 1988a, 1988b). In control membrane homogenate preparations, the receptor existed in at least two forms with either a high or low affinity for carbachol (60% and 40%, respectively). The proportion of high- and low-affinity receptors was altered after seven daily DFP treatments of the animals to 25% and 75%, respectively. Assuming that the high-affinity form of the receptor is the active form, approximately 8% of the original number of receptors was in an active form after seven daily treatments. Thus the number of active receptors was reduced by more than 90%, a condition that would signify decrease sensitivity to acetylcholine. Addition of magnesium to the membrane homogenate from animals treated for 7 days completely restored the number of high- and low-affinity forms to the control levels (i.e., 60% and 40%). Magnesium alone had no effect on the proportion of high- and low-affinity receptors in control. This suggested that the changes in affinity might be related to changes in coupling of G proteins to the receptor or in the interaction of G proteins with magnesium, since magnesium is known to be important in G protein function. Changes in G proteins have been shown to occur with subacute treatment of animals with cocaine, opiates, and clonidine (Ammer et al., 1991; Attali and Vogel, 1989; Nestler et al., 1990). The changes may result from the expression of different forms of subunits within the G protein complex. Thus, the decreased number of receptors and altered coupling to G protein was consistent with decreased sensitivity to acetylcholine.

Other Changes in Muscle Function

Changes in muscarinic receptor binding were also accompanied by changes in muscle properties. It is known that in tracheal smooth muscle muscarinic receptor activation inhibits the activity of potassium channels (Kotlikoff, 1990; Saunders and Farley, 1992). It was observed that the membrane potential of muscles from animals treated for 7 days with OP AChE inhibitor was hyperpolarized by 5–7 mV from that of control muscle. The reason for the hyperpolarization is unknown, but may result from increased number or activity of the potassium channels in the muscle or from increased activity of an electrogenic ion pump. The inhibition of potassium channel activity will depolarize the cells and lead to calcium influx and muscle contraction. Thus OP AChE inhibitors would cause a sustained inhibition of potassium channels and depolarization of the tissue. Hyperpolarization of airway smooth muscle decreases the responsiveness to acetylcholine (Kume and Kotlikoff, 1991; Shieh et al., 1992). Presumably the decreased sensitivity to stimulation by acetylcholine and the subsequent inhibition of tension development is due to a decreased probability of opening of voltage-gated calcium channels. These are known to be present in airway smooth muscle and to participate in the transduction process for acetylcholine-induced tension by mediating increases in intracellular calcium (Kotlikoff, 1988; Worley and Kotlikoff, 1990).

Mechanisms Resulting in Decreased Sensitivity

How are these changes in the muscle brought about? In Fig. 3 proposed regulatory pathways are shown between 1.) receptor activation, 2.) metabolic processes that alter receptor function during the application of the agonist or other substance, and 3.) longer-term metabolic and genetic processes that alter receptor number or type, or alter the function of the tissue. Some of the terms used in the description of the changes involved in reduced receptor function or tissue response are desensitization, tachyphylaxis, sequestration (internalization), and down-regulation. The terms are not globally defined in the literature, and the specific meaning of each must be determined in the context of the paper

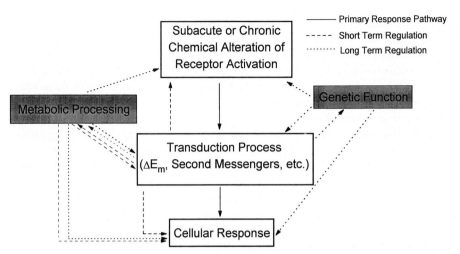

Figure 3   A diagram of possible mechanisms for the control of receptor function during subacute or chronic exposure to a xenobiotic. Both short-term and long-term homeostatic mechanisms are present for control of the receptor and transduction process. These changes return the sensitivity of the tissue toward that of control. Examples of short-term processes could be desensitization of the receptor and receptor internalization. Longer-term processes include up- or down-regulation of receptors that occurs through changes in metabolic and synthetic processes.

in which the term is used. Desensitization, for example, means one thing to a person writing about nicotinic receptor function (reversible shift of receptors to an agonist-insensitive pool) and something different to one writing about muscarinic receptor function (when the term is sometimes used to mean down-regulation, loss of receptors).

The mechanisms involved in the events described by these terms are separable. For example, Baumgold et al. (1989) demonstrated that sequestration and desensitization are not equivalent processes. Sequestration was shown to occur without desensitization (i.e., reduced cell response to stimulation in this case). We will use "desensitization" to refer to short-term reversible changes in receptor function. "Down-regulation" will refer to a loss of cell surface and total receptor number through increased metabolism of the receptors and/or decreased synthesis. Internalization is the removal of receptors from the cell surface by endocytosis of surface membrane. "Tachyphylaxis" is a general term describing a decreased response to continuous or repeated exposure to an agonist. No mechanism is implied in the use of this term.

When activated, the G protein/receptor complex dissociates, resulting in a decreased affinity of the receptor for agonist (Hulme, 1990; Lambert et al., 1992). In addition, the dissociation may uncover phosphorylation sites on the receptor, or the activated G protein may induce phosphorylation of the receptor. Phosphorylation of m_2 muscarinic receptors is known to occur and has been proposed to be important in desensitization and in down-regulation of the receptors (Collins et al., 1992). The enzymes that phosphorylate muscarinic receptors may be similar to the β-adrenergic receptor kinase (Collins et al., down-regulation of the receptors (Collins et al., 1992). The enzymes that phosphorylate muscarinic receptors may be similar to the β-adrenergic receptor kinase (Collins et al., 1992; Hulme, 1990), protein kinase A, or possibly protein kinase C (Collins et al., 1992). The continuous exposure of the receptor to agonist will increase the probability that the receptor can be phosphorylated and thus desensitized, internalized, or down-regulated. Similarly, the reduction of activity of the receptor by chronic inhibition would reduce the levels of the second messenger release within the cell that could lead to up-regulation of receptors. In this regard, Creazzo and Wrenn (1988) demonstrated that inhibition of protein kinase C resulted in an increase in muscarinic receptor (m_2) number in the heart. Under conditions where protein kinase C was active, m_2 receptor number decreased. Similarly, Liles et al. (1986) showed that activation of protein kinase C, either by muscarinic receptor activation or directly using a phorbol esther, led to rapid internalization of muscarinic receptors.

The second messengers that are released or produced intracellularly may also induce changes in the metabolism or expression of muscarinic receptors. The β-adrenoceptor has been studied best in this respect. It appears that cAMP can interact with the β-adrenoceptor and the genome through protein kinase A. The protein kinase phosphorylates the β-adrenoceptor, decreasing its activity, and also phosphorylates a protein that can stimulate transcription (cAMP response element binding protein [CREB]) at a region of DNA termed CRE (cAMP response element). A second area of DNA, the cAMP response element modulator (CREM), encodes for proteins similar in sequence to CREB that have a negative effect on transcription and thus could lead to down-regulation (Collins et al., 1992; Foulkes and Sassone-Corsi, 1992). The CRE may also be responsive to changes in calcium that occur after activation of receptors coupled to IP_3 formation (Collins et al., 1992; Sheng et al., 1990). Therefore, it is possible that the changes in receptor number observed in airway smooth muscle were brought about through similar mechanisms in which elevated second messenger levels caused changes in transcription resulting ultimately in reduction of receptor number.

It is also possible that other events further along in the transduction pathway, or one that is not necessarily associated with the end response being measured, are the driving forces behind the changes in tissue responsiveness. We will turn to developmental biology for an example of this. During the development of sympathetic neurons in culture, it is possible to switch them from adrenergic to cholinergic by altering their environment. Neurons that are chronically depolarized develop into adrenergic neurons, but if they are grown in medium that is conditioned by non-neuronal cells, they develop into cholinergic neurons (Grant and Landis, 1991). Adult tissue may not be as changeable as that of embryonic cells in culture, but the principle that long-term changes in cell function can be induced by changes in the environment is clearly true. For example, after subacute treatment of animals with OP AChE inhibitors, airway smooth muscle would be continuously depolarized. The depolarization could lead to changes in receptor and cellular function (Ferrante and Triggle, 1990).

Finally, channels, in a manner similar to receptors, are under feedback regulation to control their activity. In a recent review, Ferrante and Triggle (1990) discuss the regulation of voltage-dependent calcium channels after subacute administration of various chemicals in vivo and in vitro. These channels up- and down-regulate just like receptors. The channels down-regulate after chronic stimulation and up-regulate after chronic inhibition.

Therefore, even in the relatively simple system of airway smooth muscle, we conclude that subacute OP AChE inhibitor treatment causes 1.) decreased muscarinic receptor number, 2.) decreased or weakened coupling of the receptor to G proteins, and 3.) hyperpolarization of the muscle cells. The sum of these and most likely other events decreases the sensitivity of the muscle to stimulation by acetylcholine. However, this is only a superficial consideration of the effects of subacute OP AChE inhibitor exposure. There are many other possible changes that may occur in the tissue as well. For example, the muscle's sensitivity to increases in intracellular calcium and other second messengers may change, the mix of muscarinic receptor subtypes in the muscle may be altered, or the number of gap junctions may increase or decrease (Goto et al., 1978). We have focused on postsynaptic changes, but clearly presynaptic alterations in the neural control of airway smooth muscle activity also probably occur.

ORGANOPHOSPHATE ACTIONS ON NEURONAL PATHWAYS IN THE CENTRAL NERVOUS SYSTEM

The OP AChE inhibitors are classically viewed as operating through inhibition of AChE, with the subsequent accumulation of acetylcholine resulting in overstimulation of cholino-ceptors. This may be true after acute exposure to OP AChE inhibitors. However, after subacute exposure other neuronal systems are intimately involved in the adaptive changes in response to the chemical insult. In the following section we will examine the physiology of the GABA synapse and then discuss the actions of subacute OP AChE inhibitor treatment on the GABA neurons, followed by a more general discussion of the involvement of other pathways.

Overview of γ-Aminobutyric Acid Synapse

γ-Aminobutyric acid is one of the major inhibitory neurotransmitters found throughout the central nervous system (Cooper et al., 1991). It has been estimated that 25–50% of all synapses in the CNS use GABA as an inhibitory neurotransmitter (Young and Chu, 1990). γ-Aminobutyric acid is present in brain in concentrations of 1–10 mM. At the presynaptic site, GABA is formed by the decarboxylation of glutamic acid by the enzyme glutamic acid decarboxylase (GAD). Under physiological conditions, about 50% of the enzyme is active, with pyridoxal phosphate bound to the enzyme as cofactor. The synthesis of GABA is also regulated by product inhibition (Porter and Martin, 1984). The release of GABA from the presynaptic terminal upon nerve stimulation is calcium-dependent (Haycock et al., 1977). When GABA is released into the synaptic cleft, it can bind to pre- and post-synaptic receptors or be taken up by neuronal and glial cells. There are two types of GABA receptor: $GABA_A$ and $GABA_B$ (Bowery, 1989). Binding of GABA to $GABA_A$ receptors opens chloride channels and Cl^- ions pass through the membrane down their electrochemical gradient. The influx of chloride ions typically hyperpolarizes the membrane and also increases membrane conductance, both actions resulting in a decreased probability that the membrane will reach threshold for action potential initiation. Binding of GABA to $GABA_B$ receptor causes activation of a GTP-binding protein, which in turn initiates increased potassium channel conductance causing the neuron to hyperpolarize.

   The $GABA_A$ receptor is a membrane-spanning protein complex with a molecular weight of approximately 240,000 daltons (Mamalaki et al., 1989). The complex has binding sites for GABA, benzodiazepines, barbiturates, and channel-blocking convulsants, e.g., picrotoxin and t-butylbicyclophosphorothionate (TBPS). The $GABA_A$ receptors are heterooligomeric protein complexes that include multiple drug/agonist recognition sites (GABA, benzodiazepines, and barbiturates/convulsants) and a chloride ion channel (Vicini, 1991). The $GABA_A$ receptor complex consists of multiple subunits of different types (α, β, δ, γ, and ρ). Several isoforms of the subunits exist, and regionally the distribution of the isoforms is different. The functional significance of molecular heterogeneity is still unknown, but it is reasonable to believe that regional differences may result in pharmacologically diverse responses (Gallager and Tallman, 1990).

Recent cloning of cDNAs from several vertebrate species has demonstrated that functional $GABA_A$ receptor complexes can be formed from at least six different α subunits (Bateson et al., 1991; Olsen and Tobin, 1990; Schofield, 1989; Sequier et al., 1988), four β-subunits (Ymer et al., 1989b), two γ subunits (Prichett et al., 1989), a delta subunit (Shivers et al., 1989) and a ρ subunit (Cutting et al., 1991). The discovery of multiple forms of subunits suggests that pharmacological heterogeneity of the $GABA_A$ receptor may be due to the presence of different forms of the subunits in the receptor (Garrett et al., 1990). It has been shown that the distribution of mRNAs for the different types of subunits is uneven throughout the brain (Olsen and Tobin, 1990). For example, for the $GABA_A$ receptor, the α subunits in highest concentration in the cerebellum are α_1 and α_6. On the other hand, the cortex has a mixture of all of the different α subunits characterized to date with the exception of α_6. The cortex also possesses high levels of mRNA for both the γ_2 and the δ subunit. Additionally, phosphorylation of discrete sites on the receptor subunits by enzymes such as protein kinase A or protein kinase C (Browning et al., 1990) or tyrosine kinase (Pritchett et al., 1989) may be involved in regulation of the activity of the GABA-gated chloride channel (Chen et al., 1990). It is therefore likely that the types of subunits available to form the $GABA_A$ receptor complex and the phosphorylation of the subunits determine the properties of the receptor in a given area of the brain and its response to drug exposure. Conversely, exposure to a xenobiotic may lead to changes in the subunit composition of the receptor.

The inactivation of the chemical signal initiated by GABA occurs through uptake by a sodium-dependent transport system from the synaptic cleft into both neurons and glial cells. After the GABA is taken up into the cell, it is inactivated by the enzyme GABA:oxaloacetate aminotransferase (GABA-transaminase), which converts GABA to succinate semialdehyde. Succinate semialdehyde is rapidly converted to succinate by the enzyme succinate semialdehyde dehydrogenase, and returns to the Krebs cycle. The synthesis and degradation of GABA is usually referred to as the "GABA shunt." Xenobiotics may alter the activity of the GABA removal system.

Investigations of Multiple Systems Involved in the Action of Neurotoxic Chemicals

The complex interconnections of the nervous systems provide multiple systems that may be affected by neurotoxic chemicals. For instance, the toxicity of OP AChE inhibitors was found to be due to their irreversible inactivation of AChE, which produces long-lasting cholinergic overexcitation. Organophosphate acetylcholinesterase inhibitors elicit behavioral, neurological, and biochemical effects in both animals and humans. After long-term exposure, these compounds are known to induce changes in neuronal function. The neuronal changes result in development of tolerance to the behavioral effects of these agents. Evidence suggests that the tolerance may result from a subsensitivity that develops to acetylcholine. However, it is not well established that all of the toxic symptoms are due to alterations of cholinergic function. Other neurochemical changes may also be involved. Recent evidence has strongly implicated that noncholinergic systems, e.g., biogenic amines, glutamic acid, GABA, and cyclic nucleotides, play important roles in the initiation, continuation, and disappearance of OP AChE inhibitor–induced neurotoxicity. The study of DFP by Sivam et al. (1983) revealed that the numbers of both GABA and dopamine (DA) receptors were significantly increased after acute treatment, but that the increases were less prominent after chronic treatment. It has been reported that anticonvulsants, which are believed to act primarily via GABAergic mechanisms, block OP AChE inhibitor–induced convulsions (Lipp, 1973; Lundy and Magor, 1977; Rump et al., 1973). Lundy and Magor (1977) and Lundy et al. (1978) showed that small amounts of benzodiazepines, which are believed to act through enhancing GABAergic transmission (Olsen, 1981), totally abolished OP AChE inhibitor–induced convulsions, whereas the antimuscarinic agent atropine had no effect, even in high doses. These authors further showed that amino-oxyacetic acid (AOAA), which elevates GABA levels by inhibiting GABA-transaminase, also inhibited OP AChE inhibitor–induced convulsions. Kar and Martin (1972) suggested that paraoxon convulsions are related to GABA levels.in the CNS. Certain OP compounds cause convulsions and death but do not inhibit AChE (Bellet and Casida, 1976) and are believed to produce their effects by altering central GABA function (Bowery et al., 1976). Involvement of GABA in a variety of neuropsychiatric disorders including epilepsy and schizophrenia has been documented (Enna, 1981). The evidence, therefore, seems to indicate that GABA receptor activation may play a part in the acute effects of OP compounds.

The study by Sivam et al. (1983) also demonstrated that not only GABA$_A$ receptor density but also DA receptor density was increased after a single injection of DFP. Others have observed that DA levels are increased after acute DFP treatment (Glisson et al., 1974). On the other hand, mipafox was found to decrease DA levels after chronic administration (Freed et al., 1976). The increased motor activity of parkinsonism is known to be due to an imbalance of cholinergic and dopaminergic activity in the basal ganglia, i.e., increased cholinergic activity owing to DA deficiency (Heilbronn and Bartfai, 1978; Weiss et al., 1976). Striatal DA has an inhibitory effect on striatal neurons (Krnjevic and Phillis, 1963) and also reduces the spontaneous and cholinergic neuronal firing in the striatum (McGeer et al., 1975). It has been suggested that a delicate balance of dopaminergic (inhibitory) and cholinergic (excitatory) mechanisms maintains the normal function of striatum (Anden et al., 1966). The increases in striatal GABA and DA receptor densities observed after acute treatments with DFP gradually returned to control levels after cessation of treatment. Thus, the neurochemical imbalance produced as a result of acute inhibition of AChE may be partially counteracted by an acute increase in dopaminergic activity supported by an increase in GABAergic activity.

The results of these studies indicate an involvement of acetylcholine, DA, and GABA receptors in the effects of OP AChE inhibitors. It is suggested that the GABA and DA systems, singularly or in combination, counteract the enhanced cholinergic activity induced by OP compounds. Thus the primary site of action of a xenobiotic may bring about alterations in other systems with which that site is connected.

Alteration in Drug Susceptibility After Repeated Exposure to Neurotoxic Chemicals

It is well established that the nervous system changes its sensitivity to certain neurotoxic chemicals after exposure to a xenobiotic. For example, paraoxon and DFP are extremely potent inhibitors of AChE with rapid enzyme-aging action (Coult et al., 1966; Holmstedt, 1959). They cause CNS cholinergic overstimulation, including tremors, convulsions, chewing movements, and hind-limb abduction (Fernando et al., 1984, 1985a). These effects usually disappear within a few hours after a single dose of these agents, whereas the AChE activity gradually recovers over days (Fernando et al., 1985a). Muscarinic receptor antagonists such as atropine, effectively block the cholinergic neurotoxicity produced by anticholinesterase agents, DFP being a common example (Fernando et al., 1985b). On the other hand, if an antimuscarinic agent is given several hours after the administration of DFP, a characteristic form of hyperactivity results (Fernando et al., 1985b). It appears that after repeated exposure to neurotoxic chemicals, the vulnerability of a subject to drug exposure could be significantly modified.

Alteration in Synaptic Sensitivity

Modifications of the synaptic response to neurotransmitter is dependent on the nature of the agent and the conditions of exposure. The receptors for a particular neurotransmitter may be up-regulated (supersensitivity), or down-regulated (subsensitivity) or desensitized, by constant exposure to an antagonist or agonist for this neurotransmitter receptor, respectively. Subchronic or chronic administration of antagonists that block the action of neurotransmitters such as dopamine, norepinephrine, or acetylcholine produced an increase in the number of postsynaptic sites for the neurotransmitters (Ben-Barak and Dudai, 1980; Burt et al., 1977; Wolfe et al., 1978). For a complex receptor such as the $GABA_A$ receptor, alteration of one of the multiple binding sites may or may not change the nature of other binding sites. For example, subacute administration of bicuculline (an antagonist for the GABA-binding site of the $GABA_A$ receptor) significantly increases [^{3}H]muscimol binding in rat substantia nigra (Ito et al., 1988). In contrast, the antagonist binding of [^{3}H]SR 95531 was significantly decreased after subacute administration of bicuculline (Ito et al., 1992). However, subacute administration of bicuculline affected neither the K_d nor the B_{max} of [^{3}H]flunitrazepam and [^{35}S]TBPS bindings of the brain. These results suggest that GABA-binding sites of the $GABA_A$ receptors are up-regulated after subacute administration of bicuculline, with no change in benzodiazepine- and picrotoxin-binding sites. On the other hand, subacute administration of pentobarbital (which increases the probability of opening of the chloride ion channel of the $GABA_A$ receptor) significantly increased the convulsant binding of [^{35}S]TBPS. This suggests that after subacute exposure to xenobiotics, not only are the number of receptors regulated, but also the subunit structure may be modified or metabolic alteration of receptors may occur.

CONCLUSIONS

Subacute exposure to xenobiotics brings about numerous changes in complex neuronal systems such as the CNS or in relatively simple synaptic systems such as tracheal smooth muscle. The changes brought about by subacute exposure to xenobiotics go far beyond up- or down-regulation of neurotransmitter receptors, but also include changes in the subunit structure of proteins (e.g., receptors); G protein function; tissue function (e.g., change in ion channel density or properties); neuronal pathways secondarily affected by the primary action of the xenobiotic (e.g., GABA or DA neuronal function); and presynaptic proceesses (e.g., synthesis, uptake, and release of neurotransmitter). Although the possible number of changes that occur and may be studied are extensive, they all appear to be homeostatic, an attempt by the system to restore normal activity in the face of continuous insult. A study of the adaptive changes that result after subacute exposure to a xenobiotic can provide us with significant insight into the normal mechanisms operative in the system and the importance of each element of the system, in addition to an understanding of the long-term action of xenobiotics.

REFERENCES

Aas P, Veiteberg TA, Fonnum F (1987). Acute and sub-acute inhalation of an organophosphate induce alteration of cholinergic muscarinic receptors. Biochem Pharmacol 36:1261–6.

Adams DJ, Dwyer TM, Hille B (1980). The permeability of endplate channels to monovalent and divalent metal cations. J Gen Physiol 75:493–510.

Adams DJ, Nonner W, Dwyer TM, Hille B (1981). Block of endplate channels by permeant cations in frog skeletal muscle. J Gen Physiol 78:593–615.

Ammer H, Nice L, Lang J, Schulz R (1991). Regulation of G protein by chronic opiate and clonidine treatment in the guinea pig myenteric plexus. J Pharmacol Exp Ther 258:790–6.

Anden NE, Dahlstrom AL, Fuxe K, Larsson K (1966). Functional role of the nigro-neostriatal dopamine neurons. Acta Pharmacol 24:263–6.

Attali B, Vogel Z (1989). Long-term opiate exposure leads to reduction of the alpha$_{i-1}$ subunit of GTP-binding proteins. J Neurochem 53:1636–9.

Barnes JM, Henley JM (1992). Molecular characteristics of excitatory amino acid receptors. Prog Neurobiol 39:113–33.

Barnes PJ (1988). Airway neuropeptides. In: Barnes PJ, Rodger IW, Thomson NC, eds. Asthma: basic mechanisms and clinical management. London: Academic Press, 395–409.

Barnes PJ (1990). Muscarinic receptors in airways: recent developments. J Appl Physiol 68:1777–85.

Barnes PJ (1991). Histamine receptors in the lung. Agents Actions (suppl 33):103–22.

Baron CB, Pring M, Coburn RF (1989). Inositol lipid turnover and compartmentation in canine trachealis smooth muscle. Am J Physiol 256:C375–83.

Bateson AN, Harvey RJ, Wisden W, Glencorse TA, Hicks AA, Hunt SP, Barnard EA, Darlison MG (1991). The chicken GABA$_A$ receptor α_1 subunit: cDNA sequence and localization of the corresponding mRNA. Mol Brain Res 9:333–9.

Baumgold J, Cooperman BB, White TM (1989). Relationship between desensitization and seque-stration of muscarinic cholinergic receptors in two neuronal cell lines. Neuropharmacology 28:1253–61.

Bellet EM, Casida JE (1976). Bicyclic phosphorus esters: high toxicity without cholinesterase inhibition. Science 182:1135–6.

Ben-Barak J, Dudai Y (1980). Scopolamine induces an increase in muscarinic receptor level in rat hippocampus. Brain Res 193:309–13.

Birnbaumer L, Abramowitz J, Brown AM (1990). Receptor-effector coupling by G-proteins. Biochim Biophys Acta 1031:163–224.

Bowery NG (1989). GABA$_B$ receptors and their significance in mammalian pharmacology. Trends Pharmacol Sci 10:401–7.

Bowery NG, Collins JF, Hill RG, Pearson S (1976). GABA antagonism as a possible basis for the convulsant action of a series of bicyclic phosphorus esters. Proc Br Pharmacol Soc 4:435–536.

Brichant J-F, Warner DO, Gunst SJ, Rehder K (1990). Muscarinic receptor subtypes in canine trachea. Am J Physiol Lung Cell Mol Physiol 258:L349–54.

Browning MM, Bureau M, Dudek EM, Olsen RW (1990). Protein kinase C and cAMP-dependent protein kinase phosphorylate the beta subunit of the purified gamma-aminobutyric acid A receptor. Proc Natl Acad Sci USA 87:1315–8.

Buckley GA, Heading CE (1970). Tolerance to neostigmine. Br J Pharmacol 40:590P–1P.

Burnstock G (1990). Overview. Purinergic mechanisms. Ann NY Acad Sci 603:1–17.

Burt DR, Creese I, Snyder SH (1977). Antischizophrenic drugs: chronic treatment elevates dopamine receptor binding in brain. Science 196:326–8.

Challiss RA, Safrany ST, Potter BV, Nahorski SR (1991). Intracellular recognition sites for inositol 12,4,5-triphosphate and inositol 1,3,4,5-tetrakisphosphate. Biochem Soc Trans 19:888–93.

Chen QX, Stelzeter A, Kay AR (1990). GABA$_A$ receptor function is regulated by phosphorylation in acutely dissociated guinea-pig hippocampal neurons. J Physiol 420:207–21.

Cioffi CL, El-Fakahany EE (1986). Decreased binding of the muscarinic antagonist [^{3}H]N-methylscopolamine in mouse brain following acute treatment with an organophosphate. Eur J Pharmacol 132:147–54.

Coburn RF, Baron CB (1990). Coupling mechanisms in airway smooth muscle. Am J Physiol Lung Cell Mol Physiol 258:L119–33.

Collins S, Caron MG, Lefkowitz RJ (1992). From ligand binding to gene expression: new insights into the regulation of G-protein–coupled receptors. Trends Biochem Sci 17:37–9.

Cooper JR, Bloom FE, Roth RH (1991). The biochemical basis of neuropharmacology. New York: Oxford University Press.

Costa LG, Schwab BW, Hand H, Murphy SD (1981). Reduced [^{3}H]quinuclidinyl benzilate binding to muscarinic receptors in disulfoton-tolerant mice. Toxicol Appl Pharmacol 60:441–50.

Coult DB, Marsh BJ, Read G (1966). Dealkylation studies on inhibition of (AChE). Biochem J 98:869–73.

Creazzo TL, Wrenn RW (1988). Increased muscarinic receptor binding in heart membranes by an inhibitor of protein kinase C. FEBS Lett 242:175–7.

Curzon G (1990). How reserpine and chlorpromazine act: the impact of key discoveries on the history of psychopharmacology. Trends Pharamcol Sci 11:61–3.

Cusack NJ, Hourani SM (1990). Subtypes of P2-purinoceptors. Studies using analogues of ATP. Ann NY Acad Sci 603:172–81.

Cutting GR, Lu L, O'Hara BF, Kasch LM, Montrose-Rafizadeh C, Donovan DM, Shimada S, Antonarakis SE, Guggino WB, UhL GR, Kazazian HH Jr (1991). Cloning of the γ-aminobutyric acid (GABA) p1 cDNA: a GABA receptor subunit highly expressed in the retina. Proc Natl Acad Sci USA 88:2673–7.

Downes CP, Macphee CH (1990). Myo-inositol metabolites as cellular signals. Eur J Biochem 192:1–18.

Dwyer TM, Adams DJ, Hille B (1980). The permeability of the endplate channel to organic cations in frog muscle. J Gen Physiol 75:469–92.

Dwyer TM, Farley JM (1984). Permeability properties of chick myotube acetylcholine-activated channels. Biophys J 45:529–39.

Ehlert FJ, Kokka N, Fairhurst AS (1980a). Altered [^{3}H]quinuclidinyl benzylate binding in the striatum of rats following chronic cholinesterase inhibition with diispropylfluorophosphate. Mol Pharmacol 17:24–30.

Ehlert FJ, Kokka N, Fairhurst AS (1980b). Muscarinic receptor subsensitivity in the longitudinal muscle of the rat following chronic anticholinesterase treatment with diisopropylfluorophosphate. Biochem Pharmacol 29:1391–7.

Emmelin N (1964). Action of acetylcholine on the responsiveness of effector cells. Experientia 20:275.

Enna SJ (1981). GABA receptor pharmacology. Functional considerations. Biochem Pharmacol 30:907–13.

Farley JM, Dwyer TM (1991). Pirenzepine block of ACh-induced mucus secretion in tracheal submucosal gland cells. Life Sci 48:59–67.

Fernando JCR, Hoskins B, Ho IK (1984). Effect on striatal dopamine metabolism and differential motor behavioral tolerance following chronic cholinesterase inhibition with diisopropylfluorophosphate. Pharmacol Biochem Behav 20:951–7.

Fernando JCR, Hoskins B, Ho IK (1985a). Rapid induction of supersensitivity to muscarinic antagonist–induced motor excitation by continuous stimulation of cholinergic receptors. Life Sc 37:883–92.

Fernando JCR, Hoskins B, Ho IK (1985b). Variability of neurotoxicity of and lack of tolerance to the anticholinesterases Soman and Sarin. Res Commun Pharmacol Chem Pathol 48:415– 30.

Ferrante J, Triggle DJ (1990). Homologous and heterologous regulation of voltage-dependent calcium channels. Biochem Pharmacol 39:1267–70.

Ferris CD, Snyder SH (1992). Inositol 1,4,5-triphosphate–activated calcium channels. Ann Rev Physiol 54:469–88.

Foley DJ, McPhillips JJ (1973). Response of the rat ileum, uterus and vas deferens to carbachol and acetylcholine following repeated daily administration of a cholinesterase inhibitor. Br J Pharmacol 48:418–25.

Forder J, Scriabine A, Rasmussen H (1985). Plasma membrane calcium flux, protein kinase C activation and smooth muscle contraction. J Pharmacol Exp Ther 235:267–73.

Foulkes NS, Sassone-Corsi P (1992). More is better: activators and repressors from the same gene. Cell 68:411–14.

Freed VH, Martin MA, Fang SC, Kar PP (1976). Role of striatal dopamine in delayed neurotoxic effects of organophosphorous compounds. Eur J Pharmacol 35:229–32.

Gallager DW, Tallman JF (1990). Relationship of $GABA_A$ receptor heterogeneity to regional differences in drug responses. Neurochem Res 15:113–18.

Garrett KE, Saito N, Dumar RS, Abel MS, Ashton RA, Fujimori S, Beer B, Tallman JF, Vitek MP, Blume AJ (1990). Differential expression of γ-aminobutyric acid$_A$ receptor subunits. Mol Pharmacol 37:652–7.

Glisson SN, Karczmar AG, Barnes L (1974). Effects of diisopropylphosphorofluoridate on acetylcholine, cholinesterase, and catecholamines of several parts of rabbit brain. Neuropharmacology 13:623–31.

Gokhale VS, Bapat VM, Kanitkar SV, Kulkarni SD (1977). Altered sensitivity to acetylcholine during chronic administration of organophosphorus anticholinesterase (fenthion) in albino mice. Arch Int Pharmacodyn Ther 226:331–8.

Goto K, Westfall DP, Fleming WW (1978). Denervation-induced changes in electrophysiologic parameters of the smooth muscle of the guinea-pig and rat vas deferens. J Pharmacol Exp Ther 204:325–33.

Grandordy BM, Cuss FM, Sampson AS, Palmer JB, Barnes PJ (1986). Phosphatidylinositol response to cholinergic agonists in airway smooth muscle: relationship to contraction and muscarinic receptor occupancy. J Pharamcol Exp Ther 238:273–9.

Grant MP, Landis SC (1991). Unexpected plasticity at autonomic junctions. Environmental regulation of neurotransmitter phenotype and receptor expression. Biochem Pharmacol 41:323–31.

Haaksma EE, Leurs R, Timmerman H (1990). Histamine receptors: subclasses and specific subclasses. Pharmacol Ther 47:73–104.

Haddad E-B, Landry Y, Gies J-P (1991). Muscarinic receptor subtypes in guinea pig airways. Am J Physiol Lung Cell Mol Physiol 261:L327–33.

Hai C-M, Murphy RA (1989). Ca^{2+}, crossbridge phosphorylation, and contraction. Annu Rev Physiol 51:285–98.

Haycock JW, Levy WB, Cotman CW (1977). Pentobarbital depression of stimulus-secretion coupling in brain-selective inhibition of depolarization-induced calcium-dependent release. Biochem Pharmacol 26:159–61.

Heilbronn E, Bartfai T (1978). Muscarinic acetylcholine receptor. Prog Neurobiol 11:171–88.

Hill SJ (1990). Distribution, properties, and functional characteristics of three classes of histamine receptor. Pharamcol Rev 42:45–83.

Hille B (1992a). Ionic channels of excitable membranes. 2nd ed. Sunderland, Massachusetts: Sinauer Associates.

Hille B (1992b). G protein–coupled mechanisms and nervous signaling. Neuron 9:187–95.

Hodgkin AL, Huxley AF (1952a). Currents carried by sodium and potassium ions through the membrane of the giant axon of *Loligo*. J Physiol (Lond) 116:449–72.

Hodgkin AL, Huxley AF (1952b). The components of membrane conductance in the giant axon of *Loligo*. J Physiol (Lond) 116:473–96.

Hodgkin AL, Huxley AF (1952c). The dual effect of membrane potential on sodium conductance in the giant axon of *Loligo*. J Physiol (Lond) 116:497–506.

Hodgkin AL, Huxley AF, Katz B (1952). Measurement of current-voltage relations in the membrane of the giant squid *Loligo*. J Physiol (Lond) 116:424–48.

Holmstedt B (1959). Pharmacology of organophosphorus compounds. Pharamcol Rev 11:567–620.

Howell WH, Fulton, Ruch, Patton HD (1989). Textbook of Physiology excitable cells and neurophysiology. 21st ed., Philadelphia: W. B. Saunders.

Hoyer D, Schoeffter P (1991). 5-HT receptors: subtypes and second messengers. J Recept Res 11:197–214.

Hulme EC (1990). Muscarinic acetylcholine receptors: typical G-coupled receptors. Symp Soc Exp Biol 44:39–54.

Ito Y, Lim DK, Hayase Y, Murokoshi Y, Ho IK (1992). Effects of bicuculline on [^{3}H]SR 95531 binding in discrete regions of rat brains. Neurol Res 17:307–13.

Ito Y, Lim DK, Hoskins B, Ho IK (1988). Bicuculline up-regulation of GABA$_A$ receptors in rat brain. J Neurochem 51:145–52.

Kandel ER, Schwartz JH (1983). Principles of neural science. London: Elsevier/North Holland.

Kar PO, Martin MAJ (1972). Possible role of γ-aminobutyric acid in paraoxon induced convulsions. J Pharm Pharmacol 24:996–7.

Kaziro Y, Itoh H, Kozasa T, Nakafuku M, Satoh T (1991). Structure and function of signal-transducing GTP-binding proteins. Annu Rev Biochem 60:349–400.

Kirk CJ (1990). Recent developments in our understanding of the inositol lipid signalling system. Symp Soc Exp Biol 44:173–80.

Klein RL, Thureson-Klein AK (1990). Nueropeptide co-storage and exocytosis by neuronal large dense-cored vesicles: how good is the evidence? In: Osborne NN, ed. Current aspects of the neurosciences. New York: Macmillan, 220–52.

Kong JY, Thureson-Klein AK, Klein RL (1990). Are NPY and enkephalins costored in the same noradrenergic neurons and vesicles? Peptide 11:565–76.

Kotlikoff MI (1988). Calcium currents in isolated canine airway smooth muscle cells. Am J Physiol C793–801.

Kotlikoff MI (1990). Potassium currents in canine airway smooth muscle cells. Am J Physiol Lung Cell Mol Physiol 259:L384–95.

Krnjevic K, Phillis JW (1963). Iontophoretic studies of neurons in the mammalian cerebral cortex. J Physiol 165:274–304.

Kume H, Kotlikoff MI (1991). Muscarinic inhibition of single K$_{Ca}$ channels in smooth muscle cells by a pertussis-sensitive G protein. Am J Physiol Cell Physiol 261:C1204–9.

Lambert DG, Buford NT, Nahorski SR (1992). Muscarinic receptor subtypes: inositol phosphates and intracellular calcium. Biochem Soc Trans 20:130–5.

Levitan ES, Schofield PR, Burt DR, Rhee LM, Wisden W, Kohler M, Fujita N, Rodriguez HF, Stephenson A, Darlison MG, Barnard EA, Seeburg PH (1988). Structural and functional basis for GABA$_A$ receptor heterogeneity. Nature 335:76–9.

Liles WC, Hunter DD, Meier KE, Nathanson NM (1986). Activation of protein kinase C induces rapid internalization and subsequent degradation of muscarinic acetylcholine receptors in neuroblastoma cells. J Biol Chem 261:5307–13.

Lim DK, Fernando JCR, Hoskins B, Ho IK (1987). Quantitative assessment of tolerance development to diisopropylfluorophosphate. Pharmacol Biochem Behav 26:281–6.

Lipp JA (1973). Effect of benzodiazepine derivatives on Soman-induced seizure activity and convulsions in the monkey. Arch Int Pharmacodyn Ther 234:64–73.

Lomasney JW, Cotecchia S, Lefkowitz RJ, Caron MG (1991). Molecular biology of α-adrenergic receptors: implications for receptor classification and for structure-function relationships. Biochim Biophys Acta Mol Cell Res 1095:127–39.

Luddens H, Pritchett DB, Kohler M, Killisch I, Keinanen K, Monyer H, Sprengel R, Seeburg PH (1990). Cerebellar GABA$_A$ receptor selective for a behavioral alcohol antagonist. Nature 346:648–51.

Lundy PM, Magor GF (1977). Cyclic GMP concentrations in cerebellum following organophosphate administration. J Pharm Pharmacol 30:251–2.

Lundy PM, Magor GF, Shaw RK (1978). Gamma-aminobutyric acid metabolism in different areas of rat brain at the onset of Soman induced convulsions. Arch Int Pharmacodyn Ther 234:64–73.

Majerus PW (1992). Inositol phosphate biochemistry. Ann Rev Biochem 61:225–50.

Mak JCW, Barnes PJ (1989). Muscarinic receptor subtypes in human and guinea pig lung. Eur J Pharmacol 164:223–30.

Malherbe P, Sigel E, Baur R, Persohn E, Richards JG, Mohler H (1990). Functional expression and sites of gene transcription of a novel α subunit of the $GABA_A$, receptor in the rat brain. FEBS Lett 260:261–5.

Mamalaki C, Barnard EA, Stephenson FA (1989). Molecular size of gamma-aminobutyric acid receptor purified from mammalian cerebral cortex. *J Neurochem* 52:124–34.

McGeer EG, McGeer PL, Grewaal DS, Singh VK (1975). Striatal cholinergic interneurons and their relation to dopaminergic nerve endings. J Pharmacol 6:143–52.

McPhillips JJ (1969). Subsensitivity of the rat ileum to cholinergic drugs. J Pharmacol Exp Ther 166:249–54.

McPhillips JJ, Dar Mohammed S (1967). Resistance to the effect of carbachol on the cardiovascular system and on the isolated ileum of rats after subacute administration of an organophosphorus cholinesterase inhibitor. J Pharmacol Exp Ther 156:507–13.

Milligan G (1992). Multiple heterotrimeric guanine nucleotide binding proteins: roles in the determination of cellular signalling specificity. Biochem Soc Trans 20:135–40.

Mohan PM, Yang CM, Dwyer TM, Farley JM (1988a). Contractile responses of tracheal smooth muscle in organophosphate-treated swine: II. Effects of antagonists. J Auton Pharmacol 8:107–17.

Mohan PM, Yang CM, Saunders HM, Dwyer TM, Farley JM (1988b). Contractile responses of the tracheal smooth muscle in organophosphate treated swine: I. Agonist changes. J Auton Pharmacol 8:93–106.

Murphy RA (1989). Special topic: contraction in smooth muscle cells. Introduction. Annu Rev Physiol 51:275–83.

Nahorski SR (1990). Receptors, inositol polyphosphates and intracellular Ca^{2+}. Br J Clin Pharmacol 30(suppl 1):23S–26S.

Narahashi T (1987). Nerve membrane ion channels as the target site of environmental toxicants. Env Health Pers 71:25–9.

Narahashi T (1991). Transmitter-activated ion channels as the target of chemical agents. Adv Exp Med Biol 287:61–73.

Narahashi T (1992). Nerve membrane Na^+ channels as targets of insecticides. Trends Pharmacol Sci 13:236–41.

Nestler EJ, Terwilliger RZ, Walker JR, Sevarino KA, Duman RS (1990). Chronic cocaine treatment decreases levels of the G protein subunits G_{ialpha} and G_{oalpha} in discrete regions of rat brain. J Neurochem 55:1079–82.

O'Connor SE (1992). Recent developments in the classification and functional significance of receptors for ATP and UTP, evidence for nucleotide receptors. Life Sci 50:1657–64.

O'Dowd BF, Lefkowitz RJ, Caron MG (1989). Structure of the adrenergic and related receptors. Annu Rev Neurosci 12:67–83.

Olah ME, Stiles GL (1992). Adenosine receptors. Annu Rev Physiol 54:211–25.

Olianas MC, Onali P, Schwartz JP, Neff NF, Costa E (1984). The muscarinic receptor adenylate cyclase complex of rat stratium: desensitization following chronic inhibition of acetylcholinesterase activity. J Neurochem 42:1439–43.

Olsen RW (1981). GABA-benzodiazepine-barbiturate receptor interactions. J Neurochem 37:1–13.

Olsen RW, Tobin AJ (1990). Molecular biology of $GABA_A$ receptors. FASEB J 4:1469–80.

Park S, Rasmussen H (1985). Activation of tracheal smooth muscle contraction: syngergism between Ca^{2+} and activators of protein kinase C. Proc Natl Acad Sci USA 82:8835–9.

Perrine SE, McPhillips JJ (1970). Specific subsensitivity of the rat atrium to cholinergic drugs. J Pharmacol Exp Ther 175:496–502.

Porter TG, Martin DL (1984). Evidence for feedback regulation of glutamate decarboxylase by gamma-aminobutyric acid. J Neurochem 43:1464–7.

Pritchett DB, Sontheimer H, Shivers BF, Ymer S, Kettenmann H, Schofield PR, Seeburg PH (1989). Importance of a novel $GABA_A$ receptor subunit for benzodiazepine pharmacology. Nature 338:582–5.

Rasmussen H, Haller H, Takuwa Y, Kelley G, Park S (1990). Messenger Ca^{2+}, protein kinase C, and smooth muscle contraction. Prog Clin Biol Res 327:89–106.

Ratz PH, Murphy RA (1987). Contributions of intracellular and extracellular Ca^{++} pools to activation of myosin phosphorylation and stress in swine carotid media. Circ Res 60:410–21.

Reith MEA (1988). Cocaine receptors on monoamine transporters and sodium channels. In: Clouet D, Asghar K, Brown R, eds. Mechanisms of cocaine abuse and toxicity, NIDA research monograph 88 Washington, DC: U.S. Government Printing Office.

Rodbell M (1992). The role of GTP-binding proteins in signal transduction: from the sublimely simple to the conceptually complex. Curr Top Cell Reg 32:1–47.

Roffel AF, Elzinga CRS, Van Amsterdam RGM, De Zeeuw RA, Zaagsma J (1988). Muscarinic M_2 receptors in bovine tracheal smooth muscle: discrepancies between binding and function. Eur J Pharmacol 153:73–82.

Roth NS, Lefkowitz RJ, Caron MG (1991). Structure and function of the adrenergic receptor family. Adv Exp Med Biol 308:223–38.

Rump S, Grudzinska E, Edelwejn Z (1973). Effects of diazepam on epileptic-form patterns of bioelectrical activity of the rabbit's brain induced by fluorstigmine. Neuropharmacol 12:813–17.

Sanders-Bush E (1990). Adaptive regulation of central serotonin receptors linked to phosphoinositide hydrolysis. Neuropsychopharmacology 3:411–6.

Saunders H-MH, Farley JM (1992). Pharmacological properties of potassium currents in swine tracheal smooth muscle. J Pharmacol Exp Ther 260:1038–44.

Schimerlik MI (1989). Structure and regulation of muscarinic receptors. Annu Rev Physiol 51:217–27.

Schimerlik MI (1990). Structure and function of muscarinic receptors. Prog Brain Res 84:11–19.

Schmidt AW, Peroutka SJ (1989). 5-Hydroxytryptamine receptor "families." FASEB J 3:2242–9.

Schofield PR (1989). The GABA receptor: molecular biology reveals a complex picture. Trends Pharamcol Sci 10:476–8.

Sequier JM, Richards JG, Malherbe P, Price GW, Mathews GW, Mohler H (1988). Mapping of brain areas containing RNA homologous to cDNAs encoding the alpha and beta subunits of the rat $GABA_A$ gamma-aminobutyrate receptor. Proc Natl Acad Sci USA 85:7815–9.

Sheng M, McFadden G, Greenberg ME (1990). Membrane depolarization and calcium induce c-fos transcription via phosphorylation of transcription factor CREB. Neuron 4:571–82.

Shieh C-C, Petrini MF, Dwyer TM, Farley JM (1992). Cromakalim effects on acetylcholine-induced changes in cytosolic calcium and tension in swine trachealis. J Pharmacol Exp Ther 260:261–8.

Shivers BD, Killisch I, Sprengel R, Sontheimer H, Kohler M, Schofield PR, Seeburg PH (1989). Two novel $GABA_A$ receptor subunits exist in distinct neuronal populations. Neuron 3:327–37.

Sivam SP, Norris JC, Lim DK, Hoskins V, Ho IK (1983). Effect of acute and chronic cholinesterase inhibition with DFP on muscarinic, dopamine, and GABA receptors of the rat striatum. J Neurochem 40:1414–21.

Somlyo AV, Kitazawa T, Horiuti K, Kobayashi S, Trentham D, Somlyo AP (1990). Heparin-sensitive inositol trisphosphate signaling and the role of G-proteins in Ca^{2+}-release and contractile regulation in smooth muscle. Prog Clin Biolog Res 327:167–82.

Spiegel AM, Shenker A, Weinstein LS (1992). Receptor-effector coupling by G proteins: implications for normal and abnormal signal transduction. Endocr Rev 13:536–65.

Steinbach JH, Ifune C (1989). How many kinds of nicotinic acetylcholine receptors are there? Trends Neurosci 12:3–6.

Sterz R, Hermes M, Peper K, Bradley RJ (1982). Effects of ethidium bromide on the nicotinic acetylcholine receptor. Eur J Pharmacol 80:393–9.

Stone TW (1991). Receptors for adenosine and adenine nucleotides. Gen Pharmacol 22:25–31.

Strasser RH, Ihl-Vahl R, Marquetant R (1992). Molecular biology of adrenergic receptors. J Hypertension 10:510–16.

Szabo G, Otero AS (1990). G protein mediated regulation of K^+ channels in heart. Annu Rev Physiol 52:293–305.

Ui M (1984). Islet activating protein, pertussis toxin: a probe for functions of the inhibitory nucleotide regulatory component of adenylate cyclase. Trends Pharamcol Sci 5:277–9.

Van Dongen CJ, Wolthuis OL (1989). On the development of behavioral tolerance to organophosphates. I: Behavioral and biochemical aspects. Pharamcol Biochem Behav 34:473–81.

Vicini S (1991). Pharmacologic significance of the structural heterogeneity of the $GABA_A$ receptor–chloride ion channel complex. Neuropsychopharmacology 4:9–15.

Wall SJ, Yasuda RP, Li M, Ciesla W, Wolfe BB (1992). Differential regulation of subtypes m1–m5 of muscarinic receptors in forebrain by chronic atropine administration. J Pharmacol Exp Ther 262:584–88.

Weiss BL, Forster G, Kupfer DJ (1976). Cholinergic involvement in neuropsychiatric syndromes. In: Goldberg AM, Hanin I, eds. Biology of cholinergic function. New York: Raven Press, 603–17.

West RE Jr, Moss J, Vaughn M, Lui T, Lui T-Y (1985). Pertussis toxin–catalyzed ADP-ribosylation of transducin. J Biol Chem 260:14428–30.

Wolfe BB, Harden K, Sporn JR, Molinoff PB (1978). Presynaptic modulation of beta adrenergic receptors in rat cerebral cortex after treatment with antidepressants. J Pharmacol Exp Ther 207:446–57.

Worley JF III, Kotlikoff MI (1990). Dihydropyridine-sensitive single calcium channels in airway smooth muscle cells. Am J Physiol Lung Cell Mol Physiol 259:L468–80.

Wu CH, Narahashi T (1988). Mechanism of action of novel marine neurotoxins on ion channels. Annu Rev Pharmacol Toxicol 28:141–61.

Yamada S, Okudaira H, Hayashi E (1979). An alteration in sensitivity to cholinergic agents on guinea-pig ilea and atria after repeated administration of an organophosphate and an antagonism by a carbamate. Arch Int Pharmacodyn Ther 241:32–44.

Yang CM, Chou S-P, Sung TC, Chien H-J (1991). Regulation of functional muscarinic receptor expression in tracheal smooth muscle cells. Am J Physiol Cell Physiol 261:C1123–9.

Yang CM, Dwyer TM, Mohan PM, Ho IK, Farley JM (1990). Down regulation of muscarinic receptors in the striatum of organophosphate treated swine. Toxicol Appl Pharmacol 104:375–85.

Yang CM, Farley JM, Dwyer JM (1986). Biochemical characteristics of muscarinic cholinoreceptors in swine tracheal smooth muscle. J Auton Pharmacol 6:15–24.

Yang CM, Mohan PM, Dwyer TM, Farley JM (1988). Changes in affinity states during down regulation of muscarinic receptors in tracheal smooth muscle of organophosphate-treated swine. J Auton Pharmacol 8:79–91.

Ymer S, Draguhn A, Kohler M, Schofield PR, Seeburg PH (1989a). Sequence and expression of novel $GABA_A$ receptor a subunit. FEBS Lett 258:119–22.

Ymer S, Schofield PR, Draguhn A, Werner P, Kohler M, Seeburg PH (1989b). $GABA_A$ receptor beta subunit heterogeneity, functional expression of cloned cDNAs. EMBO J 8:1655–70.

Young AB, Chu D (1990). Distribution of $GABA_A$ and $GABA_B$ receptors in mammalian brain: potential targets for drug development. Drug Dev Res 21:161–7.

4

The Role of Glia in Central Nervous System Induced Injuries

Michael Aschner, Judy L. Aschner, and Harold K. Kimelberg
Albany Medical College
Albany, New York

INTRODUCTION

The working brain evokes images of the excitable neurons that endow the central nervous system (CNS) with the capacity to convey and process information. It may, therefore, come as a surprise that approximately 50% of the brain volume consists of nonexcitable cells. The largest class of these is the neuroglia, and among the most significant of the neuroglial cells are the astrocytes and oligodendrocytes.

Over the past 15 years, the functions of astrocytes and oligodendrocytes have begun to be delineated (for reviews see Aldridge 1958, 1977, 1978; Althans and Seifert, 1987; Kimelberg and Norenberg, 1989; Aschner et al., 1990; Aschner et al., 1991; Auer, 1991, Murphy, 1993). The prevailing view that astrocytes function predominantly as passive physical support for neurons is rapidly fading. Oligodendrocytes, which until recently were known only as the brain myelinating cells, are currently credited with additional functions such as the maintenance of K^+ levels within the white matter of the CNS (Barres et al., 1988). It is now clear that to understand the normal and abnormal brain we must also understand the roles assumed by astrocytes and oligodendrocytes, for they function prominently not only in normal brain physiology and development, but also in the pathology of the nervous system.

The neuronal-glial functional partnership proposed by Hydèn (1961) has now been accepted, and evidence for the specific events in neuron-glia interactions can be found in several recent reviews, a testimony to the growing interest in these cells and their roles in the CNS. Aspects of the relationships between oligodendrocytes, myelin sheaths, and axons, as well as the role of astrocytes in scar formation, have been elegantly described by several authors (Althaus and Seifert, 1987; Fedoroff, 1986a,b,c; Hatten and Mason, 1986; Vernadakis, 1988) and will not be reviewed here; nor will the morphological expressions of intoxicants on oligodendrocytes and astrocytes be described. Rather, we intend to develop the concept of active participation of neuroglia, particularly the astrocytes, in both facilitatory and protective roles in CNS induced injuries. By careful examination of neuroglial cultures much has been learned not only about their normal functioning, but also about their role in neurotoxin-induced injuries. In this chapter we will discuss some of these roles and provide examples of studies that can be carried out using these cultures.

PROTECTIVE ROLES OF ASTROCYTES IN NEUROTOXIC INJURIES

Astrocytes are now implicated in both a defensive and a facilitatory role for many neurotoxic injuries. An example of the former is revealed by studies on glutamate homeostasis in the CNS. Astrocytes are known to occupy a critical position in the metabolism of glutamate, an important excitatory neurotransmitter (Martinez-Hernandez et al., 1977; Schousboe, 1981; Ramaharobandro et al., 1982). Brain damage during ischemia and other pathological states is thought to be partly due to the inappropriate release of this amino acid, which, through activation of excitatory amino acid receptors (Fig. 1), causes death of certain neurons (Olney, 1979; Simon et al., 1984; Faden et al., 1989). For some time, the origin of glutamate was assumed to be solely through release or failure of reuptake of the presynaptic nerve ending. However, since the late 1970s (Hertz, 1979) it has become apparent that astrocytes function prominently in glutamate metabolism, possessing a high-affinity uptake system for this neurotransmitter. Astrocyte uptake and metabolism of glutamate to glutamine by the enzyme glutamine synthetase (Norenberg, 1979; Schousboe, 1981) in the presence of ammonia functions critically in the control of extracellular glutamate levels (Fig. 1).

The symbiotic relationship between neurons and astrocytes in relation to glutamate was elegantly probed by Rosenberg and Aizenman (1989). Cortical cultures were compared for their sensitivity to glutamate toxicity. Exposure to glutamate at selected concentrations for 18–24 hours resulted in extensive and concentration-dependent neuronal death in astrocyte-poor cultures. The glutamate EC_{50} for killing of neurons in astrocyte-poor cultures was $1.9 \pm 0.6\ \mu M$ compared with $194 \pm 43\ \mu M$ in astrocyte-rich cultures. Thus, a 100-fold difference in susceptibility to glutamate toxicity distinguished neurons maintained in astrocyte-poor versus astrocyte-rich environments. Glutamate toxicity appeared to be mediated predominantly by N-methyl-D-aspartate (NMDA) receptors, since it was blocked by 2-amino-phosphonovaleric acid (APV), an NMDA antagonist (Fig. 1).

The difference in vulnerability to glutamate toxicity observed in conditions of poor and high enrichment of astrocytes is not the result of a difference in the magnitude of membrane currents induced by NMDA-receptor activation (Rosenberg and Aizenman, 1989), suggesting that it is due to the amount of glutamate that reacts with neuronal receptors. One explanation for the protective effect afforded by astrocytes could be a physical shielding by the latter of dendritic-membrane NMDA receptors, which may be more sensitive to the toxicity of glutamate, since dendrites appear to have a specific mechanism for large and persistent NMDA receptor–stimulated calcium influx (Connors et al., 1988). Perhaps a more likely explanation is the existence in astrocytes of a powerful astrocytic uptake system for glutamate that reduces the extracellular concentration of this amino acid (Schousboe, 1981). The lack of specific blockers for this uptake vs. release (Kimelberg et al., 1989) makes resolution of this question difficult. Whatever the mechanism, the experiments with astrocyte-poor and astrocyte-enriched cultures show that these cells can attenuate glutamate neurotoxicity, at least in culture. Circumstances that alter astrocyte function, such as hypoxia, hypoglycemia, hepatic encephalopathy, and

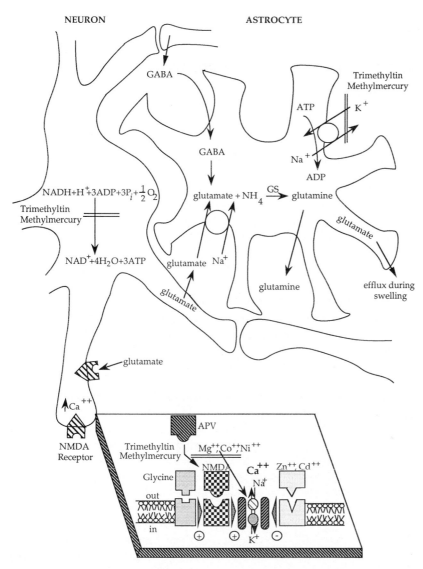

Figure 1 Schematic representation of excitotoxic-induced central nervous system injury. The astrocytic modulation of neurotoxicity depicted in the larger figure is described in the text. Inset: Diagrammatic representation of the NMDA receptor–ion channel complex. The NMDA agonist recognition site binds to glutamate, opening an ion channel that is permeable to Ca^{2+}, as well as Na^+ and K^+. The divalent cations magnesium, cobalt, and nickel block the ion channel at different sites in its interior. Heavy metals such as methylmercury and trimethyltin may lower the neuronal resting membrane potential to a point where the voltage-dependent Mg^{2+} blockade of the NMDA receptor is released, increasing calcium permeability through the ion channel complex. Positive allosteric regulation of the ion channel itself occurs via a glycine receptor, and negative allosteric regulation of the ion channel itself occurs via a binding site for zinc and cadmium. NMDA antagonists such as aminophosphonovalerate (APV), which is a polar, dipositive, mono-amino compound, bind to the NMDA receptor. GS = glutamine synthetase. (Partially adapted from Reynolds and Miller, Mol Pharmacol 1988; 33:581–4.).

metabolic poisoning, might therefore be expected to manifest themselves in increased glutamate-mediated neuronal injury and death.

FACILITATORY ROLE OF ASTROCYTES IN NEUROTOXIC INJURIES

The protection by astrocytes from glutamate-induced neural damage is but one example of how astrocytes fulfill a regulatory role aimed at maintaining a proper milieu for neuronal functions. However, it is now apparent that astrocytes may also be directly responsible for CNS damage.

The glutamate-glutamine pathway in astrocytes (Fig. 1) constitutes the site of a small glutamate pool in the brain that was originally described by Berl et al. (1961). The role of this pool in the etiology of brain injury has been the focus of numerous investigations. Release from this pool could occur as a result of swelling of astrocytes (Kimelberg et al., 1990). Swelling of isolated cells is known to lead to the release of glutamate (Fig. 1), aspartate, taurine, and several other amino acids as part of the regulatory process by which swollen cells regain their normal volume (Gilles et al., 1987).

The pathological conditions in which astroglial swelling is observed include traumatic CNS edema (Gerschenfeld et al., 1959), prolonged hypoxia (Yu et al., 1972), acute hypoxia with hypercapnia (Bakay and Lee, 1968), experimental (Barron et al., 1988) and human (Bullock et al., 1991) closed head injury, ischemia (Garcia et al., 1977; Jenkins et al., 1984), hypoglycemia and status epilepticus (Siesjo, 1981), and hepatic encephalopathy (Norenberg, 1981; Kimelberg et al., 1990). Cultured primary astrocytes have been shown to exhibit regulatory volume decrease after swelling in hypotonic media (Kimelberg and Frangakis, 1985), which is associated with reversible membrane depolarization (Kimelberg and O'Connor, 1988) and release of glutamate, aspartate, and taurine (Pasantes-Morales and Schousboe, 1988; Kimelberg et al., 1990). Aschner et al. (1990) observed swelling-induced efflux of amino acids (glutamate and aspartate) in primary astrocyte cultures treated with methylmercuric chloride (10^{-5} M). This efflux could be reversed by several anion transport blockers, such as 4-acetamido-4'-isothiocyanatostilbene-2,2'-disulfonic acid (SITS) and furosemide (Aschner et al., unpublished results). Increased release of glutamate and aspartate from preloaded astrocytes was also induced by 10^{-5} M trimethyltin (Aschner et al., 1991).

There is compelling evidence that astrocytes are involved in the etiology of heavy metal neurotoxicity. As early as 1966, Oyake et al. (1966) suggested that, in humans, methylmercury preferentially accumulates within astrocytes; this was further confirmed by Garman et al. (1975). Similarly, lead has been reported to concentrate in astrocytes (Holtzman et al. 1984; Tiffany-Castiglioni et al., 1989). Accordingly, the lead "sink hypothesis" was advanced, postulating that the resistance of the mature CNS to the development of lead encephalopathy is dependent on the capacity of astroglia to take up and sequester lead in nontoxic sites.

The clues linking astrocytes to methylmercury and trimethyltin neurotoxicity are numerous. Several studies allude to the sensitivity of Na^+-K^+-ATPase activity and ion permeability in astrocytes to both methylmercury and trimethylin (Aschner et al., 1990; Aschner et al., 1991). Both K^+ influx and efflux (as measured by $^{86}Rb^+$) are altered by exposure to methylmercury and trimethyltin concentrations as low as 10^{-5} M. The inhibition of K^+ influx appears to be due to inhibition of the ouabain-sensitive adenosine triphosphatase activated by Na^+ and K^+ (Na^+-K^+-ATPase), which drives the cation transport pump.

A generalized increased permeability to cations would be expected to depolarize the membrane potential and dissipate transmembraneous ion gradients, resulting in the inhibition of secondary active transport processes that are dependent on such gradients (Fig. 1). It is generally accepted that sodium gradients, dependent on the activity of Na^+-K^+-ATPase, provide the driving force for the transport of amino acids across cell membranes. A carrier with both sodium and substrate sites is required. Thus, one would predict that methylmercury and trimethyltin may effect a wide range of membrane transport systems secondary to sodium-pump inhibition and a subsequent rise in intracellular sodium (Fig. 1). This prediction is supported by observations of the inhibitory effect of both of these organometals on the Na^+-dependent L-glutamate and D-aspartate uptake in astrocytes (Aschner et al., 1990; Aschner et al., 1991). The transport of L-glutamate in astrocytes has been shown to diminish when the cells are depolarized (Kimelberg et al., 1989) and when the Na^+ electrochemical gradient is reduced. The mechanisms associated with the inhibitory effect of the organometals may be related to a direct inhibition of coupled transport secondary to a reduction of active sodium efflux or to an increase in passive sodium permeability, or both.

Both methylmercury and trimethyltin potently depress mitochondrial respiration (Aldridge, 1958, 1977, 1978; Webb, 1966). This, in turn, may lower the resting membrane potential of neurons to a point where the voltage-dependent Mg^{2+} blockade of the NMDA receptor is released (Fig. 1), enabling glutamate, aspartate, and perhaps other excitatory amino acids to act persistently on neurons, opening their ion channels and triggering a degenerative cascade (Nolan and Brown, 1989; Novelli et al., 1988). Since the NMDA receptor ion channel is permeable to calcium, deleterious calcium-triggered intracellular processes may ensue, initiated by excitatory activity at NMDA receptors (Auer, 1991; Benveniste and Diemer, 1988; Dux et al., 1987; Simon et al., 1984).

Astrocytes may be an additional source for the release of the excitatory amino acids glutamate, aspartate, and taurine, and perhaps other neurotoxins, such as quinolinic acid (Whetsell et al., 1988), which could contribute to excitotoxin-induced injuries within the CNS. In pathological states, release of excitatory amino acids may be massive and general, and indeed the failure of volume regulation, as indicated by the persistence of astrocytic swelling under these conditions in situ (Kimelberg and Ransom, 1986), may be accounted for by the release of these volume-regulatory substances from intracellular compartments. Abnormally high levels of stimulation of excitatory amino acid receptors on the surface of adjacent neurons can trigger a destructive cascade of events that can kill neurons en masse (Olney, 1979; Simon et al., 1984; Faden et al., 1989).

It is now also established that 1-methyl-4-phenyl-1,2,3,6-tetrahydropyridine (MPTP) selectively destroys the nigrostriatal dopaminergic neurons in humans, subhuman primates, and lower animals (Burns et al., 1983; Heikkila et al., 1984; Langston et al., 1984). The molecular mechanism of MPTP toxicity is only partially understood. Conversion of MPTP to 1-methyl-4-phenylpyridinium ion (MPP^+) is required for toxicity (Yang et al., 1988). 1-Methyl-4-phenyl-1,2,3,6-tetrahydropyridine is not neurotoxic when its conversion to MPP^+ is blocked by monoamine oxidase type B (MAO-B) inhibition (Chiba et al., 1984; Heikkila et al., 1984; Langston et al., 1984). Astrocytes in situ are MAO-B–positive by immunocytochemistry (Levitt et al., 1982). Their importance in the conversion of MPTP to MPP^+ has been shown in vitro (Marini et al., 1989; Ransom et al., 1987). Indeed, astrocytic cultures display a time-dependent production of MPP^+ when exposed to the parent compound MPTP. The current understanding of MPTP-induced neurotoxicity involves diffusion of nonoxidized MPTP into the brain, where it is metabolized by the

MAO-B isoenzyme to MPP^+, which presumably occurs in astrocytes and MAO-B–containing neurons. In turn, MPP^+ released from astrocytes and neurons by an as yet unknown route is concentrated in nigrostriatal neurons by uptake on the dopamine transporter. The mechanisms of its toxicity may involve free radical formation (Shina et al., 1986) or inhibition of mitochondrial respiration supported by NADH-linked substrates (Nicklas et al., 1985; Vyas et al., 1986; Poirier and Barbeau, 1985).

Since the phenotypic expression of MPTP-induced neurotoxicity involves, at least in part, astrocytic metabolism, one can test the dependence of MPTP-induced nigrostriatal neuronal death on astrocytes in situ. One such approach employs the astrocyte-selective toxicity of α-aminoadipic acid (α-AAD), a 6-carbon chemical analogue of glutamate. This toxin displays no degenerative effects on other cell types, including neurons, oligodendroglia, microglia, and endothelial cells, but specifically destroys astrocytes cocultured with neurons, as well as astrocytes in situ. Recently, Takada et al. (1990) demonstrated that co-injections of MPTP and α-AAD into the intra–substantia nigra pars compacta protected neurons from the toxicity that results from MPTP administration alone. Neurotoxicity of MPTP may also depend on more than intra-astrocytic oxidation of the parent compound to MPP^+; in vivo, the injury may be potentiated by astrocytic damage (non-α-AAD damage) and the subsequent release of excitatory amino acids.

Astrocytes have also been implicated in a variety of degenerative neurological disorders. Huntington's disease, for example, has been associated with elevated CNS levels of quinolinic acid (Schwarcz et al., 1983; Schwarcz et al., 1984; Schwarcz et al., 1988b; Beal et al., 1990), a normal by-product of the metabolism of the amino acid tryptophan. Quinolinic acid excites neurons by specifically interacting with the NMDA receptor (Young et al., 1988). At high doses, particularly after intrahippocampal injections, quinolinic acid causes convulsions and neurodegenerative changes that are remarkably similar to those observed in human temporal lobe epilepsy (Dam, 1980; Schwarcz et al., 1984). The enzyme that synthesizes quinolinic acid, 3-hydroxyanthranilate oxygenase (3-HAO), is present predominantly, or perhaps even exclusively, in astrocytes (Schwarcz et al., 1988a). Astrocytes are also implicated in the enzymatic degradation of quinolinic acid, carried out by quinolinic acid phosphoribosyltransferase (QPRT) (Du et al., 1990). Any abnormality in either of these enzymes, or increased release or decreased uptake of these substances, could produce a surplus of the toxic quinolinic acid in the extracellular fluid, leading to the death of specific neurons. An overabundance of quinolinic acid could act at a presynaptic receptor to induce the release of a neurotransmitter that binds to a postsynaptic NMDA receptor, or quinolinic acid could itself bind to NMDA receptors on target neurons, causing neuronal degeneration. It has been established that quinolinic acid can bind and stimulate certain excitatory amino acid receptors and reproduce some of the effects of Huntington's disease in monkey brains, killing and sparing neurons in the same pattern as seen in affected human brains. This raises the possibility that the genetic flaw in Huntington's disease is expressed as an alteration in homeostatic mechanisms that modulate quinolinic acid synthesis and degradation in astrocytes.

Astrocytes also play a fundamental part in the pathophysiology of several CNS diseases that arise from primary disorders lying completely outside the CNS. This is exemplified in patients with severe cirrhosis or with Reye's syndrome who develop hepatic encephalopathy. The precise mechanisms by which liver disease adversely affects the CNS are not well understood. There is some indication that the inability of the liver to detoxify toxins leads to high plasma levels of ammonia, mercaptans, and short-chain fatty acids. In many patients who succumb to hepatic encephalopathy, the only observable brain pathology is the appearance of aberrant astrocytes with large nuclei and few fibers. These altered cells are known as Alzheimer's type II astrocytes (Norenberg, 1981). These changes can be mimicked in astrocytic tissue cultures (Gregorios et al., 1985a,b), where cytoplasmic granularity and vacuolization are proportional to the concentration and duration of ammonia treatment. Other studies by Olson et al. (1989) have demonstrated an inhibition of astrocytic volume regulation in hypo-osmotic medium by the fatty acid octanoate. The volume decrease is correlated with a decrease in basal and ouabain-sensitive oxygen consumption, an uncoupling of mitochondrial electron transport, and a decrease in the content of astrocytic ATP. Thus, it would appear that agents implicated in the etiology of brain edema in Reye's syndrome may alter the energy metabolic state and the cell volume regulatory function of astrocytes. Whether altered brain ion and water homeostasis is associated with the concomitant release of excitotoxins from swollen astrocytes treated with ammonia or fatty acids awaits further studies.

Ammonia-induced astrocyte toxicity can further aggravate neurotoxicity by impeding the detoxification of glutamate through inhibition of its conversion to glutamine (Fig. 1). The conversion of glutamate to glutamine by astrocytes is thought to be the brain's primary means of protection against the accumulation of high ammonia concentrations in the extracellular fluid (Norenberg, 1981). Astrocytic injury by high ammonia levels may result in the inability of astrocytes to concentrate and convert glutamate to glutamine, which would further contribute to both ammonia and glutamate accumulation in the extracellular fluid. The result could be a synergistic destruction of the CNS, first by high ammonia levels, followed by excitotoxic damage from high extracellular glutamate levels.

ASTROCYTES: A LINK BETWEEN THE CENTRAL NERVOUS SYSTEM AND THE IMMUNE SYSTEM

The long-standing view that the brain is insulated from the effects of the immune system is now being challenged as a result of the elegant in vitro work of Adriano Fontana and his colleagues (Fierz et al., 1985; Fontana and Fierz, 1985; Fontana et al., 1986; Schnyder et al., 1986; Malipiero et al., 1990) showing that astrocytes have the capability to participate in immune responses of the CNS. Astrocytes have also been implicated in the etiology of autoimmune disorders such as multiple sclerosis (Massa et al., 1987; Massa, 1989).

Invasion of tissues with activated T lymphocytes constitutes an essential element of the local inflammatory response of the CNS to viral diseases (Hasek et al., 1977). Upon treatment of primary astrocyte cultures derived from newborn mice with lipopolysaccharide (LPS, *E. coli*), astrocytes are found to secrete interleukin-1 (IL-1) (Fontana et al., 1982). Intracerebral synthesis of IL-1 has been implicated as a prerequisite to intracerebral T cell activation, primarily because IL-1 enhances the production of IL-2 and expression of IL-2 receptors on T cells (Fontana et al., 1987). Astrocytes may therefore assume an important role in immune-mediated processes within the CNS (Fig. 2).

Astrocytes have also been considered as antigen-presenting cells (APCs), i.e., cells with the ability to present antigens to lymphocytes, on the basis of studies with primary astrocyte cultures (Erb et al., 1986; Fontana et al., 1987; Frei et al., 1987; Frei et al., 1988). The study of the capacity of astrocytes to function as APCs has been facilitated by the development of myelin basic protein (MBP)-specific T lymphocyte lines from mice or rats immunized with MBP in complete Freund's adjuvant. Astrocytes from Lewis rats cocultured with a syngenic, MBP-specific, Ia-restricted T cell line of Lewis rat origin stimulate T cell proliferation, the process being antigen-specific and restricted to the major

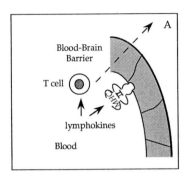

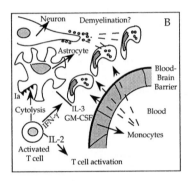

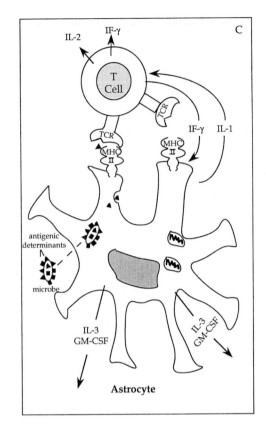

Figure 2   Schematic of potential roles of astrocytes in immune-mediated responses. Note that astrocytes (B and C) express class II major histocompatibility complex gene products and can present antigens to T cells. Activated T cells, in turn, produce a number of lymphokines that have diverse effects on systemic monocytes. For further details refer to the text. GM-CSF = granulocyte-macrophage colony stimulating factor; IL-1 = interleukin 1; IL-2 = interleukin 2; IFN-γ = interferon-γ; TCR = T cell receptors.

histocompatibility complex (MHC) (Fontana et al., 1984). During such cocultivation of T cells and astrocytes, the latter are induced by the preactivated T cells to express MHC type II molecules (also termed Ia antigens) (Fontana et al., 1984; Fierz et al., 1985). Furthermore, interferon-γ (IFN-γ)-containing supernatants of lectin-stimulated spleen cells can induce murine astrocytes in culture to express Ia antigens (Hirsch et al., 1983), underscoring the dependence of astrocytes as APCs on the presence of Ia-inducing signals, such as IFN-γ. Induction of Ia expression on astrocytes is sensitive to stimulators of protein kinase C (PKC), since phorbol myristate acetate (PMA) (Nishizuka, 1984) is capable of strongly inducing Ia expression (Massa and ter Meulen, 1987). The Ca^{2+} ionophore A23187, at the minimal dose required for Ca^{2+} influx in other cell systems (Zawalich et al., 1983; Nishizuka, 1984) has the same effect on Ia induction as LPS and PMA, suggesting that Ca^{2+} mobilization may play a role in astrocytic Ia induction, possibly through indirect stimulation of PKC (Massa and ter Meulen, 1987).

   A prominent feature of inflammatory and degenerative diseases of the CNS is the accumulation of macrophages, recruited from circulating blood monocytes and from CNS macrophages (Fig. 2B). Although the signals leading to this accumulation are poorly understood, it is now believed that astrocytes function prominently in such processes. Astrocytes have been recently shown to secret an IL-3-like factor (Fig. 2C) that induces growth of cultured mouse peritoneal exudate cells (PECs) and brain tissue macrophages (Frei et al., 1985; Frei et al., 1986). Astrocytes also secrete granulocyte-macrophage colony-stimulating factor (GM-CSF) (Fig. 2C), as evidenced by induction of colony formation in bone marrow cells and growth of FDC-P1 cells (Malipiero et al., 1990). These effects can be neutralized with antibodies to GM-CSF, but not to anti-IL-3. Granulocytes-macrophage colony-stimulating factor is a cytokine necessary for growth and differentiation of macrophages and has been found to lead to an accumulation of macrophages at the site of inflammatory lesions. Granulocyte-macrophage colony-stimulating factor enhances a number of functional activities of mature macrophages, such as their phagocytic, cytotoxic, and microbicidal activities. Granulocyte-macrophage colony-stimulating factor produced locally by astrocytes may therefore provide an essential element for recruitment and activation of macrophages. Using Northern blots, Malipiero and colleagues (1990) have also demonstrated the presence of the mRNA for GM-CSF in cultured astrocytes. It would therefore appear that after the initial penetration of T cells into the CNS, astrocytes could further support the intracerebral T cell activation process.

A well-reproduced laboratory model for the CNS autoimmune disease multiple sclerosis is experimental allergic encephalomyelitis (EAE). As early as 1933, Rivers et al. (1933) noted that monkeys that were injected with a rabbit brain extract developed encephalitis characterized by destruction of the white matter. Aided by development of MBP-specific T lymphocyte lines, EAE can be reproducibly induced by injecting homogenized brain tissue of MBP from one animal into another (Ben-Nun et al., 1981; Zamvil et al., 1985). Experimental allergic encephalomyelitis represents an Ia-restricted delayed-type hypersensitivity (DTH) reaction, in which the injection of MBP triggers an immune response, leading to the destruction of healthy CNS tissue. In search of a phenotypic marker determining genetically controlled susceptibility to DTH reactions in the brain, the EAE model was used to compare the IFN-γ induction of Ia molecules on astrocytes and macrophages cultured from rat and mouse strains that are susceptible and resistant to this disease (Massa et al., 1987). Focusing on Ia expression, because DTH reactions to self or foreign antigens are largely mediated by lymphocytes restricted to class II (Ia) antigens of the MHC, it was revealed that Lewis rats (fully susceptible to injection of foreign MBP) and brown Norway rats (fully resistant to injected MBP) are very different in their response. Astrocytes cultured from Lewis rats express much higher levels of constituitive Ia than astrocytes cultured from brown Norway rats. Hyperinduction of Ia by the susceptible Lewis rats was also shown to be astrocyte-specific, since peritoneal macrophages of susceptible and resistant strains showed the same Ia induction profile. In addition, the structural damage caused by EAE was greatly lessened by antibodies to the class II molecules. In view of these findings it was postulated that pathological DTH reactions may represent a two-step phenomenon. The first step involves the ability of strain-specific Ia molecules to associate physically with the DTH-eliciting antigens, and the second step involves the strain-specific ability to express abnormally high levels of Ia molecules on tissue-specific cells (Massa et al., 1987).

The blood-brain barrier plays a major role in separating the brain from the blood, thus lowering the chances of mutual communication and restricting the intracerebral invasion of cellular elements of the immune system. There is no doubt, however, that in the course of some forms of encephalitis, such as multiple sclerosis, tissue damage is due to an immune-mediated response; the damage may represent a T cell–mediated cellular immune reaction initiated by activated T helper cells (Fontana et al., 1987). Endothelial cells may play a critical role in the initiation of immune responses within the CNS in the course of a systemic antiviral immune response. They may take up antigens transported from the brain parenchyma to the luminal surface of endothelial cells. These antigens may be identified by lymphocytes passing through the brain vasculature (Fig. 2A). Interaction between lymphocytes and endothelial cells may culminate in the disruption of endothelial tight junctions. Once antigen-specific T cells adhere to brain capillaries and are able to invade the brain parenchyma, astrocytes could further support intracerebral T cell activation (Fig. 2C) by the elaboration of IL-1 (McCarron et al., 1985). Having arrived in the brain parenchyma, the future of the intruding T cells may depend on 1). the presence of the antigen toward the T cells that have been sensitized, 2.) the capacity of the T cells to release IFN-γ, and 3.) the amount of Ia being induced by IFN-γ on antigen-presenting cells within the tissue (Fontana et al., 1987).

Although controversy still exists about which cells are the "real" APCs in the CNS, recent data from rats (Vaas and Lassmann, 1990) and humans (Lampson and Hickey, 1986) suggest that astrocytes can indeed express MHC type II antigens in vivo. While such expression is also common to microglia, several lines of evidence favor the view that astrocytes are more significant than microglia in this regard. First, astrocytes in the adult CNS far outnumber the microglia and are therefore more immediately accessible for antigen-presenting functions. Second, in vitro studies demonstrate that the amount of Ia expressed on IFN-γ–treated astrocytes correlates with the in vivo susceptibility of the CNS to immune-mediated encephalitis.

As schematically shown in Fig. 2B, once activated, the T helper cells may cause disruption of homeostatic functions provided by neuroglia, including known metabolic cooperation between the astrocytes, oligodendrocytes, and neurons (Sun and Wekerle, 1986). Release of IL-2 from astrocytes (Fig. 2B) may lead to further intracerebral T cell activation and the secretion of factors such as IFN-γ, the latter enhancing the phagocytic activity of macrophages involved in tissue injury (Fig. 2B). T cell products such as IL-2 may even contribute to the development of astrocytic scarring and remyelination, since IL-2 receptors have been identified on oligodendrocytes (Merrill et al., 1984; Saneto et al., 1986), and T cell products as well as IL-1 have been found to stimulate astrocytic growth in culture (Fontana et al., 1981; Giulian and Lachman, 1985). Recruitment and expansion of cells of the macrophage lineage may be achieved by chemotactic factors for monocytes released in the tissue and by T cell–derived macrophage colony stimulating factors such as GM-CSF and IL-3, or by an IL-3-like factor produced by activated astrocytes (Fig. 2B and C). Increased oxidation potential, phagocytic capacity, and secretion of proteolytic enzymes may initiate a cascade of events resulting in tissue damage, accompanied, for example, by active demyelination (Fig. 2B). Therefore, one can envision multiple sclerosis, as well as other autoimmune diseases, as an overexpression of MHC class II genes by brain cells, in particular astrocytes, triggering a genetic susceptibility to these diseases by the enhancement of CNS immunogenicity in response to immune-triggering stimuli.

The literature is now replete with accounts of factors that exert inhibition on Ia expression in cultured astrocytes. It is known that astrocytes synthesize and release an α/β-type interferon (Tedeschi et al., 1986). This finding is important because IFN-β can significantly inhibit IFN-γ–induced Ia expression on human macrophages (Ling et al., 1985). Kishikawa et al. (unpublished results) have recently demonstrated that 48-hour pretreatment of neonatal rat primary astrocytes in culture with lead acetate can significantly inhibit the ability of concanavalin A to induce astrocytic Ia expression. The behavioral effects of lead in rodents (Golter and Michaelson, 1975) have led neurochemists to study the effects of lead exposure on catecholamine release (review by Silbergeld, 1982). Changes in catecholaminergic neurotransmission associated with lead exposure have been reported with increased turnover of norepinephrine (Golter and Michaelson, 1975), decreased levels of dopamine and norepinephrine (Satija et al., 1978; Silbergeld and Goldberg, 1975), and increased activity of tyrosine hydroxylase (Wince and Azzaro, 1978). It is tempting to speculate on these findings in the context of lead toxicity. It is now well established that astrocytes in culture express β-adrenergic receptors (Kimelberg, 1988). These appear to be mainly β_1 but may include β_2 receptor subtypes as well. Their activation results in large increases in the cellular cAMP content. The role of β-adrenergic receptors in mammalian astrocytes is of interest in relation to the expression of MHC class II antigens. Norepinephrine is known to inhibit IFN-γ–induced Ia antigen expression on cultured astrocytes via a β_2-adrenergic signal transduction pathway (Frohman et al, 1988). It is, therefore, feasible that initiation of intracerebrally mediated immune responses may be directly thwarted by the effect of lead on inhibitory modulators, such as norepinephrine, which can down-regulate MHC antigen expression (Frohman et al., 1988). Frohman et al. have elegantly demonstrated that when increasing concentrations of IFN-γ are added to astrocytes in culture, the ability of norepinephrine to block Ia expression in astrocytes is diminished. These in vitro results suggest that the brain also contains inhibitory norepinephrine mediators that play a pivotal role in the regulation of intracerebral immune responses by modulating the expression of MHC antigens on astrocytes, and that this can be by IFN-γ. These recent findings linking neurotoxins to CNS immune disorders make this an exciting area for further investigation.

CONCLUSIONS AND FUTURE DIRECTIONS

Evaluation of chemically-induced cytotoxicity, particularly in an heterogeneous system such as the brain, is often difficult to study in the intact animal because numerous factors (neural, hormonal, and hemodynamic) are not under experimental control. Clearly, a simplified model, such as tissue culture, is indispensable as an initial approach to understanding basic physiology and pathology. We owe much of the existing body of literature on the role of astrocytes in the neurotoxic effects of glutamate, methylmercury, trimethyltin, MPTP, ammonia, and inorganic lead to the availability of primary astrocyte cultures, and progress using cocultures with neurons in vivo is likely to continue. Astrocytes may provide an important link in the new focus of research on the interaction between the CNS and the immune system. Astrocytes appear to be capable of being sites where the future of potentially encephalitogenic T cells invading the brain parenchyma is decided. Thus, by using astrocyte cultures and extending experiments to astrocytic-neuronal cocultures and in vivo, we can now begin to experimentally affirm or deny which of their many proposed roles are likely to contribute to the etiology of CNS diseases. It will be some time, however, before we will know how "guilty" the astrocytes are in the etiology of neurodegenerative disorders.

ACKNOWLEDGEMENT

Preparation of this manuscript and the authors' work described therein were supported in part by NIEHS grant 05223 and USEPA 819210, awarded to MA, NINDS grants 19492 and 23750, awarded to HKK.

REFERENCES

Aldridge WN (1958). The biochemistry of organotin compounds, trialkyltins and oxidative phosphorylation. Biochem J 69:367–76.

Aldridge WN (1977). Oxidative phosphorylation. Halide-dependent and halide-independent effects of triorganotin and triorganolead compounds on mitochondrial functions. Biochem J 168:353–64.

Aldridge WN (1978). In: Gielen M, Harrison PG, eds. The organometallic and coordination chemistry of germanium, tin, and lead. Vol. 9 Tel Aviv: Freundt, 9–30.

Althaus HH, Seifert W, eds (1987). Glial-neuronal communication in development and regeneration. Berlin: Springer-Verlag.

Aschner M, Eberle NB, Miller K, Kimelberg HK (1990). Interactions of methylmercury with rat primary astrocyte cultures: inhibition of rubidium and glutamate uptake and induction of swelling. Brain Res 530:245–50.

Aschner M, Gannon M, Kimelberg HK (in press). Interactions of trimethyl tin (TMT) with rat primary astrocyte cultures: altered uptake and efflux of rubidium, L-glutamate and D-aspartate. Brain Res.

Auer RN (1991). Excitotoxic mechanisms, and age-related susceptibility to brain damage in ischemia, hypoglycemia and toxic mussel poisoning. Neurotoxicology 12:541–6.

Bakay L, Lee JC (1968). The effect of acute hypoxia and hypercapnia on the ultrastructure of the central nervous system. Brain 91:697–706.

Barres BA, Chun LLY, Corey DP (1988). Ion channel expression by white matter glia: I. Type 2 astrocytes and oligodendrocytes. Glia 1:10–30.

Barres BA, Chun LLY, Corey DP (1990). Ion channels in vertebrate glia. Annu Rev Neurosci 13:441–74.

Barron KD, Dentinger MP, Kimelberg HK, Nelson LR, Bourke RS, Keegan S, Mankes RF, Cragoe EJ, Jr (1988). Ulstrastructural features of brain injury model in cat. I. Vascular and neurological changes and the prevention of astroglial swelling by a fluorenyl(aryloxy) alkanoic acid derivative. Acta Neuropathol 75:295–307.

Beal MF, Matson WR, Swartz KJ, Gamache PH, Bird ED (1990). Kynurenine pathway measurements in Huntington's disease striatum: evidence for reduced formation of kynurenic acid. J Neurochem 55:1327–39.

Ben-Nun A, Wekerle H, Cohen IR (1981). The rapid isolation of clonable antigen-specific T lymphocyte line capable of mediating autoimmune encephalomyelitis. Eur J Immunol 11:195–9.

Benveniste H, Diemer NH (1988). Early postischemic ^{45}Ca accumulation in rat dentate hilus. J Cereb Blood Flow Metabol 8:713–9.

Berl S, Lajtha A, Waelsch H (1961). Amino acid and protein metabolism. J Neurochem 8:186–97.

Bullock R, Maxwell WL, Graham DI, Teasdale GM, Adams JH (1991). Glial swelling following human cerebral contusion: an ultrastructural study. J Neurol Neurosurg Psychiatry 54:427–34.

Burns RS, Chiueh CC, Markey SP, Ebert HM, Jacobowitz DM, Kopin IJ (1983). A primate model of parkinsonism: selective destruction of dopaminergic neurons in the pars compacta of the substantia nigra by 1-methyl-4-phenyl-1,2,3,6-tetrahydropyridine. Proc Natl Acad Sci USA 80:4546–50.

Chiba K, Trevor AJ, Castagnoli N (1984). Metabolism of the neurotoxic tertiary amine MPTP by brain monoamine oxidase. Biochem Biophys Res Commun 120:574–8.

Connors JA, Wadman WJ, Hockberger PE, Wong RKS (1988). Sustained dendritic gradients of Ca^{2+} induced by excitatory amino acids in CA1 hippocampal neurons. Science 240:649–53.

Dam AM (1980). Epilepsy and neuron loss in the hippocampus. Epilepsia 21:617–29.

Du F, Okuno E, Whetsell WO Jr, Köhler C, Schwarcz R (1990). Distribution of quinolinic acid phosphoribosyltransferase in the human hippocampal formation and parahippocampal gyrus. J Comp Neurol 295:71–82.

Dux E, Mies G, Hossmann K-A, Siklós L (1957). Calcium in mitochondria following brief ischemia of gerbil brain. Neurosci Lett 78:295–300.

Erb P, Kennedy M, Hagmann, I, Wassmer P, Huegli G, Fierz W, Fontana A (1986). Accessory cells and the activation and expression of different T cell functions. In: Feldmann M, McMichael A, eds. Regulation of immune gene expression. Clifton, New Jersey: Humana Press, 187.

Faden AI, Demediuk P, Panter SS, Vink R (1989). The role of excitatory amino acids and NMDA receptors in traumatic brain injury. Science 244:798–800.

Fedoroff S (1986a). In: Fedoroff S, Vernadakis A, eds. Astrocytes: development, morphology, and regional specialization. Vol. 1. Orlando, Florida: Academic Press.

Fedoroff S (1986b). In: Fedoroff S, Vernadakis A, eds. Astrocytes: biochemistry, physiology and pharmacology of astrocytes. Vol. 2. Orlando, Florida. Academic Press.

Fedoroff S (1986c). In: Fedoroff S, Vernadakis A, eds. Astrocytes: cell biology and pathology of astrocytes. Vol. 3. Orlando, Florida: Academic Press.

Fierz W, Endler B, Reske K, Wekerle H, Fontana A (1985). Astrocytes as antigen presenting cells: I. Induction of Ia antigen expression on astrocytes by T cells via immune interferon and its effect on antigen presentation. J Immunol 134:3785–93.

Fontana A, Fierz W (1985). The endothelium-astrocyte immune control system of the brain. Springer Sem Immunopathol 8:57–70.

Fontana A, Erb P, Pircher H, Zinkernagel R, Weber E, Fierz W (1986). Astrocytes as antigen-presenting cells. Part II: Unlike H-2K-dependent cytotoxic cells H2Ia-restricted T cells are only stimulated in the presence of interferon-gamma. J Neuroimmunol 12:15–28.

Fontana A, Fierz W, Wekerle H (1984). Astrocytes present myelin basic protein to encephalitogenic T-cell lines. Nature 307:273–6.

Fontana A, Kristensen F, Dubs R, Gemsa D, Weber E (1982). Production of prostaglandin E and interleukin 1–like factors by cultured astrocytes and C-6 glioma cells. J Immunol 129:2413–9.

Fontana A, Frei K, Bodmer S, Hofer E (1987). Immune-mediated encephalitis: on the role of antigen presenting cells in brain tissue. Immunol Rev 100:185–201.

Fontana A, Otz U, De Weck AL, Grob PJ (1981). Glial cell stimulating factor (GSF): a new lymphokine. Part 2. Cellular sources and partial purification of human GSF. J Neuroimmunol 2:73–81.

Frei K, Siepl C, Groscurth P, Bodmer S, Schwerdel C, Fontana A (1987). Antigen presentation and tumor cytotoxicity by interferon-γ treated microglial cells. Eur J Immunol 17:1271–8.

Frei K, Siepl C, Groscurth P, Bodmer S, Fontana A. (1988). Immunobiology of microglial cells. Ann NY Acad Sci 540:218–27.

Frei K, Bodmer S, Schwerdel C, Fontana A (1985). Astrocytes of the brain synthesize interleukin 3–like factors. J Immunol 135:4044–7.

Frei K, Bodmer S, Schwerdel C, Fontana A (1986). Astrocyte-derived interleukin 3 as a growth factor for microglia cells and peritoneal macrophages. J Immunol 137:3521–7.

Frohman EM, Vayuvegula B, Gupta S, van den Noort S (1988). Norepinephrine inhibits γ interferon–induced major histocompatibility class II (Ia) antigen expression on cultured astrocytes via β2-adrenergic signal transduction mechanisms. Proc Natl Acad Sci USA 85:1292–6.

Garcia JH, Kalimo H, Kamijyo Y, Trump BF (1977). Cellular events during partial cerebral ischemia. 1. Electron microscopy of feline cerebral cortex after middle-cerebral-artery occlusion. Virchows Arch B Cell Pathol 25:191–206.

Garman RH, Weiss B, Evans HL (1975). Alkylmercurial encephalopathy in the monkey; a histopathologic and autoradiographic study. Acta Nuropathol 32:61–74.

Gerschenfeld HM, Wald F, Zadunaisky A, DeRobertis EDP (1959). Function of astroglia in water-ion metabolism of the central nervous system. Neurology 9:412–25.

Gilles R (1987). Volume regulation in cells of euryhaline invertebrates. In: Gilles R, Bolis L, Kleinzeller A, eds. Current topics in membranes and transport. Vol. 30. New York: Academic Press, 205–47.

Giulian D, Lachman LB (1985). Interleukin-1 stimulation of astroglial proliferation after brain injury. Science 228:497–9.

Golter M, Michaelson IA (1975). Growth, behavior and brain catecholamines in lead-exposed neonatal rats: a reappraisal. Science 187:359–61.

Gregorios JB, Mozes LW, Norenberg L-OB, Norenberg MD (1985). Morphologic effects of ammonia on primary astrocyte cultures. I. Light microscopic studies. J Neuropathol Exp Neurol 44:397–403.

Gregorios JB, Mozes LW, Norenberg MD (1985). Morphologic effects of ammonia on primary astrocyte cultures. II. Electron microscopic studies. J Neuropathol Exp Neurol 44:404–14.

Hasek M, Chutna J, Sládecek M (1977). Immunological tolerance and tumor allografts in the brain. Nature 268:68–9.

Hatten ME, Mason CA (1986). Neuron-astroglia interactions in vitro and in vivo. Trends Neurosci 9:168–74.

Heikkila RE, Hess A, Duvoisin RC (1984). Dopaminergic neurotoxicity of 1-methyl-4-phenyl-1,2,3,6-tetrahydropyridine in mice. Science 244:1451–3.

Hertz L (1979). Functional interactions between neurons and astrocytes. I. Turnover and metabolism of putative amino acid neurotransmitters. Prog Neurobiol 13:277–323.

Hirsch M-R, Wietzerbin J, Pierres M, Goridis C (1983). Expression of Ia antigens by cultured astrocytes treated with gamma-interferon. Neurosci Lett 41:199–204.

Holtzman D, DeVries C, Nguyen H, Olson J, Bensch K (1984). Maturation of resistance to lead encephalopathy: cellular and subcellular mechanisms. Neurotoxicology 5:97–124.

Hydèn H (1961). Satellite cells in the nervous system. Sci Am 205:62–70.

Jenkins LW, Becker DP, Coburn TH (1984). A quantitative analysis of glial swelling and ischemic neuronal injury following complete cerebral ischemia. In: Go KG, Baethmann A, eds. Recent progress in the study and therapy of brain edema. New York: Plenum Press, 523–37.

Kimelberg HK, ed. (1988). Glia cell receptors. New York: Raven Press.

Kimelberg HK, Pang S, Treble DH (1989). Excitatory amino acid–stimulated uptake of ^{22}Na$^+$ in parimary astrocyte cultures. J Neurosci 9:1141–9.

Kimelberg HK, Ransom BR (1986). Physiological and pathological aspects of astrocytic swelling. In: Fedoroff S, Vernadakis A, eds. Astrocytes: cell biology and pathology of astrocytes. Vol. 3. Orlando, Florida: Academic Press, 129–66.

Kimelberg HK, Frangakis MV (1985). Furosemide- and bumetanide-sensitive ion transport and volume control in primary astrocyte cultures from rat brain. Brain Res 361:125–34.

Kimelberg HK, O'Connor ER (1988). Swelling-induced depolarization of astrocyte membrane potentials. Glia 1:219–24.

Kimelberg HK, Goderie SK, Higman S, Pang S, Waniewski RA (1990). Swelling-induced release of glutamate, aspartate, and taurine from astrocyte cultures, J Neurosci 10:1583–91.

Kimelberg HK, Norenberg MD (1989). Astrocytes. Sci Am 260:66–76.

Kishikawa H, Lawrence D, Aschner M. Unpublished results.

Lampson LA, Hickey WF (1986). Monoclonal antibody analysis of MHC expression in human brain biopsies: tissue ranging from "histologically normal" to that showing different levels of glial tumor involvement. J Immunol 136:4054–62.

Langston JW, Forno LS, Rebert CS, Irwin I (1984). Selective nigral toxicity after systemic administration of 1-methyl-4-phenyl-1,2,3,6-tetrahydropyridine (MPTP) in the squirrel monkey. Brain Res 292:390–4.

Levitt P, Pintar JE, Breakfield XO (1982). Immunocytochemical demonstration of monoamine oxidase B in brain astrocytes and serotonergic neurons. Proc Natl Acad Sci USA 79:6385–9.

Ling PD, Warren MK, Vogel SN (1985). Antagonistic effect of interferon-β–induced expression of Ia antigen in murine macrophages. J Immunol 135:1857–63.

Malipiero UV, Frei K, Fontana A (1990). Production of hemopoietic colony-stimulating factors by astrocytes. J Immunol 144:3816–21.

Marini AM, Schwartz JP, Kopin IJ (1989). The neurotoxicity of 1-methyl-4-phenylpyridinium in cultured cerebellar granule cells. J Neurosci 9:3665–72.

Martinez-Hernandez A, Bell KP, Norenberg MD (1977). Glutamine synthetase: glial localization in brain. Science 195:1356–8.

Massa PT, ter Meulen V, Fontana A (1987). Hyperinducibility of Ia antigen on astrocytes correlates with strain-specific susceptibility to experimental autoimmune encephalopathy. Proc Natl Acad Sci USA 84:4219–23.

Massa PT (1989). Sites of antigen presentation in T cell mediated demyelinating diseases. Res Immunol 140:196–201.

Massa PT, ter Meulen V (1987). Analysis of Ia induction on Lewis rat astrocytes in vitro by virus particles and bacterial adjuvants. J Neuroimmunol 13:259–71.

McCarron RM, Kempski O, Spatz M, McFarlin DE (1985). Presentation of myelin basic protein by murine cerebral vascular endothelial cells. J Immunol 134:3100–3.

Merrill JE, Kutsunai S, Mohlstrom C, Hofman F, Groopman J, Golde DW (1984). Proliferation of astroglia and oligodendroglia in response to human T cell–derived factors. Science 224:1428–30.

Nicklas WJ, Vyas I, Heikkila RE (1985). Inhibition of NADH-linked oxidation in brain mitochondria by 1-methyl-4-phenylpyridine, a metabolite of the neurotoxin, 1-methyl-4-phenyl-1,2,3,6-tetrahydropyridine. Life Sci 36:2503–8.

Nishizuka Y (1984). The role of protein kinase C in cell surface signal transduction and tumor promotion. Nature 308:693–8.

Nolan CC, Brown AW (1989). Reversible neuronal damage in hippocampal pyramidal cells with triethyllead: the role of astrocytes. Neuropathol Appl Neurobiol 15:441–57.

Norenberg MD (1979). The distribution of glutamine synthetase in the central nervous system. J Histochem Cytochem 27:469–75.

Norenberg MD (1981). The astrocyte in liver disease. In: Fedoroff S, Hertz L, eds. Advances in cellular neurology. Vol. 2. New York: Academic Press, 304–38.

Novelli A, Reilly JA, Lysko PG, Henneberry RC (1988). Glutamate becomes neurotoxic via the N-methyl-D-aspartate receptor when intracellular energy levels are reduced. Brain Res 45:205–12.

Olney JW (1979). Excitotoxic amino acids and Huntington's disease. In: Chase TN, Wexler NS, Barbeau A, eds. Advances in neurology. Vol. 23. New York: Raven Press, 609–24.

Olson JE, Holtzman D, Sankar R, Lawson C, Rosenberg R (1989). Octanoic acid inhibits astrocyte volume control: implications for cerebral edema in Reye's syndrome. J Neurochem 52:1197–1202.

Oyake Y, Tanaka M, Kubo H, Cichibu H (1966). Neuropathological studies on organic mercury poisoning with special reference to the staining and distribution of mercury granules. Adv Neurol Sci 10:744–50.

Pasantes-Morales H, Schousboe A (1988). Volume regulation in astrocytes: a role for taurine as an osmoeffector. J Neurosci Res 20:505–9.

Poirier J, Barbeau A (1985). 1-methyl-4-phenylpyridinium–induced inhibition of nicotinamide adenosine dinucleotide cytochrome C reductase. Neurosci Lett 62:7–11.

Ramaharobandro N, Borg J, Mandel P, Mark J (1982). Glutamine and glutamate transport in cultured neuronal and glial cells. Brain Res 244:113–21.

Ransom BR, Kunis DM, Irwin I, Langston JW (1987). Astrocytes convert the parkinsonism inducing neurotoxin, MPTP, to its active metabolite, MPP$^+$. Neurosci Lett 75:323–8.

Rivers TM, Sprunt DH, Berry GP (1933). Observations on attempts to produce acute disseminated encephalomyelitis in monkeys. J Exp Med 58:39–53.

Rosenberg PA, Aizenman E (1989). Hundred-fold increase in neuronal vulnerability to glutamate toxicity in astrocyte-poor cultures of rat cerebral cortex. Neurosci Lett 103:162–8.

Saneto RP, Altman A, Knobler RL, Johnson HM, de Vellis J (1986). Interleukin 2 mediates the inhibition of oligodendrocyte progenitor cell proliferation in vitro. Proc Natl Acad Sci USA 83:9221–5.

Satija MK, Seth TD, Tandon DS (1978). Dopamine and noradrenaline levels in the brains of lead and zinc poisoned rats. Toxicology 10:13–16.

Schnyder B, Weber E, Fierz W, Fontana A (1986). On the role of astrocytes in polyclonal T cell activation. J Neuroimmunol 10:209–18.

Schousboe A (1981). Transport and metabolism of glutamate and GABA in neurons and glial cells. Int Rev Neurobiol 22:1–45.

Schwarcz R, Whetsell WO, Mangano RM (1983). Quinolinic acid: an endogenous metabolite that produces axon-sparing lesions in rat brain. Science 219:316–8.

Schwarcz R, Foster AC, French ED, Whetsell WO Jr, Köhler C (1984). Current topics II. Excitotoxic models for neurodegenerative disorders. Life Sci 35:19–32.

Schwarcz R, Tamminga CA, Kurlan R, Shoulson I (1988a). Cerebrospinal fluid levels of quinolinic acid in Huntington's disease and schizophrenia. Ann Neurol 24:580–2.

Schwarcz R, Okuno E, White RJ, Bird ED, Whetsell WO (1988b). 3-Hydroxyanthranilate oxygenase activity is increased in the brains of Huntington's disease victims. Proc Natl Acad Sci USA 85:4079–81.

Shina BK, Singh Y, Krishna G (1986). Formation of superoxide and hydroxyl radicals from 1-methyl-4-phenylpyridinium ion (MPP$^+$): reductive activation by NADPH cytochrome P-450 reductase. Biochem Biophys Res Commun 135:583–8.

Siesjo BK (1981). Cell damage in the brain: a speculative synthesis. I Cereb Blood Flow Metab 1:155–85.

Silbergeld EK (1982). Neurochemical and ionic mechanisms of lead neurotoxicity. In: Prasad KN, Vernadakis A, eds. Mechanisms of action of neurotoxic substances. New York: Raven Press, 1–23.

Silbergeld EK, Goldberg AM (1975). Pharmacological and neurochemical investigations of lead-induced hyperactivity. Neuropharmacology 14:31–44.

Simon RP, Swan JH, Griffiths T, Meldrum BS (1984). Blockade of N-methyl-D-aspartate receptors may protect against ischemic damage in the brain. Science 226:850–2.

Sun D, Wekerle H (1986). Ia-restricted encephalitogenic T lymphocytes mediating EAE lyse autoantigen-presenting astrocytes. Nature 320:70–2.

Takada M, Li ZK, Hattori T (1990). Astroglial ablation prevents MPTP-induced nigrostriatal neuronal death. Brain Res 509:55–61.

Tedeschi B, Barrett JN, Keane RW (1986). Astrocytes produce interferon that enhances the expression of H-2 antigens on a subpopulation of brain cells. J Cell Biol 102:2244–53.

Tiffany-Castiglioni E, Sierra EM, Wu J-N, Rowles TK (1989). Lead toxicity in neuroglia. Neurotoxicology 10:417–44.

Vass K, Lassmann H (1990). Intrathecal application of interferon gamma. Progressive appearance of MHC antigens within the rat nervous system. Am J Pathol 137:789–800.

Vernadakis A (1988). Neuron-glia interrelations. Int Rev Neurobiol 30:149–225.

Vyas I, Heikkila RE, Nicklas WJ (1986). Studies on the neurotoxicity of 1-methyl-4-phenyl-1,2,3,6-tetrahydropyridine: inhibition of NAD-linked substrate oxidation by its metabolite, 1-methyl-4-phenylpyridinium. J Neurochem 46:1501–7.

Webb JL (1966). Mercurials. In: Webb JL, ed. Enzyme and metabolic inhibitors. Vol. 2. New York: Academic Press, 729–1070.

Whetsell WO Jr, Kohler C, Schwarcz R (1988). Quinolinic acid: a glia-derived excitotoxin in the mammalian central nervous system. In: Norenberg MD, Hertz L, Schousboe A, eds. The biochemical pathology of astrocytes. New York: Alan R. Liss, 191–202.

Wince, L, Azzaro AJ (1978). Neurochemical changes of the central dopamine synapse following chronic lead exposure. Neurology 4:382.

Yang S-C, Johannessen JN, Markey SP (1988). Metabolism of [^{14}C]MPTP in mouse and monkey implicates MPP$^+$, and not bound metabolites, as the operative neurotoxin. Chem Res Toxicol 1:228–33.

Young AB, Greenamyre JT, Hollingsworth Z, Albin R, D'Amato C, Shoulson I, Penney JB (1988). NMDA receptor losses in putamen from patients with Huntington's disease. Science 241: 981–3.

Yu MC, Bakay L, Lee JC (1972). Ultrastructure of the central nervous system after prolonged hypoxia. II. Neuroglia and blood vessels. Acta Neuropathol 22:235–44.

Zamvil S, Nelson P, Trotter J, Mitchell D, Knobler R, Fritz R, Steinman L (1985). T-cell clones specific for myelin basic protein induce chronic relapsing paralysis and demyelination. Nature 317:355–8.
Zawalich W, Brown C, Rasmussen H (1983). Insulin secretion: combined effects of phorbol ester and A23187. Biochem Biophys Res Commun 117:448–55.

Part II
Neurotoxicology of the Peripheral Nervous System
Introductory Overview

Louis W. Chang
University of Arkansas for Medical Sciences
Little Rock, Arkansas

Mohamed B. Abou-Donia
Duke University Medical Center
Durham, North Carolina

One of the unique features of the neuron is the existence of the axon, through which nerve impulses and signal conductance can be propagated and transmitted. Certain neurotoxicants are known to injure the axons. In such conditions, the term "axonopathy" is frequently used. In this section, three chapters are devoted to chemically induced injuries to the nerve fibers (neuropathies and axonopathies). In Chapter 5, "Models of Axonal Transport," by Blum and Reed, these authors discuss the importance of axonal transport (axoplasmic flows) in the maintenance of the axon and the neuron and instances in which neuropathies might arise from derangement of the axonal transport systems. Mathematical models are presented for these transport systems. Applications of these models for the understanding of certain neuropathies are also discussed. In Chapter 6, "Axonopathy," Drs. Gupta and Abou-Donia discuss the phenomena of and current concepts concerning proximal and distal axonopathies. The toxic chemicals inducing these neuropathological conditions are reviewed and discussed. In the following chapter, "Involvement of Cytoskeletal Proteins in Chemically Induced Neuropathies," the same authors explore and discuss in greater detail the biomolecular mechanisms involved in the induction of neurocytoskeletal protein alterations by various chemicals, in both the nerve cell bodies and the axons.

Many axons are myelinated. In the peripheral nervous system, myelination is accomplished by the Schwann cells. Demyelination syndromes occur as a result of direct injuries to the myelin sheaths or to the Schwann cells. In Chapter 8, "Toxicant-Induced Demyelinating Neuropathy," Bouldin and Goodrum present and discuss the various forms of demyelinating neuropathy, and the pathology and toxicology related to these neurotoxic conditions. In the following chapter, "Schwann Cell-Axon Interactions," by LoPachin and Lehning, further consideration is given to the close interrelationship between the Schwann cells and the axons. The relevance of interruption of such relationships to neuropathy is also discussed.

One of the most important portions of the peripheral nervous system is the neuromuscular junction. At this synaptic junction, neural communication with the end-organ (muscle) takes place. Yet this important site has frequently been ignored in neurotoxicology texts. In the final chapter of this section, "The Neuromuscular Junction as a Target for Neurotoxicity," Drs. Atchison and Spitsbergen present a detailed discussion of the basic principles and toxic consequences of the neuromuscular junctions. The morphological, physiological, and biochemical bases of these synaptic junctions are presented. The various toxic chemicals and toxic consequences related to neuromuscular toxicity are also discussed.

This section presents a general conception and basic principles of peripheral neurotoxicity and neuropathy, covering the axons, axonal transports, axonal components (microtubules and microfilaments), the myelin sheaths, the Schwann cells, and the end-synaptic junctions.

5

Models of Axonal Transport: Application to Understanding Certain Neuropathies

Jacob J. Blum and Michael C. Reed
Duke University
Durham, North Carolina

INTRODUCTION

Although protein synthesis in neurons occurs in dendrites (for references, see Sheetz and Martenson, 1991) as well as in the soma, it is generally agreed that all the proteins and lipids found in the nerve axon are synthesized in the soma. Thus, both during growth and after the axon has reached its final length, all components of the axon must be transported from the soma, in some cases for distances of 1 m or more. Membrane-bound organelles such as secretory vesicles, mitochondria, and multivesicular bodies are transported along microtubules (Allen et al., 1985) at speeds ranging from about 200–400 μm/min for vesicles to 50 μm/min for mitochondria (Brady and Lasek, 1982). Transport in the anterograde direction, i.e., from the soma toward the distal end of the axon, is powered by an adenosine, triphosphate (ATP)-driven motor termed kinesin; transport in the retrograde direction is powered by a cytoplasmic dynein (see, e.g., Schroer and Sheetz, 1990). All other material,[a] i.e., the filamentous components of the axoplasm and associated proteins, move in the anterograde direction at speeds about two orders of magnitude slower than the fast transport system (Brady and Lasek, 1982).

The slow transport system appears to comprise two major components: SCa, the slower component, contains the neurofilament triplet, and several other proteins such as tubulin, neurofilament-associated protein, fodrin, and the tau protein. SCb, the faster-moving component, contains "soluble" proteins such as glycolytic enzymes, calmodulin, and actin- and myosin-like enzymes (Baitinger and Willard, 1987, and references therein).

---

[a] There are two reports that a slow retrograde transport sytem may be present in axons. Fink and Gainer (1980) and Cena et al. (1984) observed slow retrograde transport of proteins that may be albumin and calmodulin, respectively.

Presumably it is the interaction between myosin and the actin microfilaments that power the slow transport system, but other possibilities have been envisaged (Sheetz and Martenson, 1991).

There is now considerable evidence that a number of neuropathies arise from derangements of the fast and slow axonal transport systems (see, e.g., Schlaepfer, 1987; Griffin and Watson, 1988). Mathematical models for these systems are useful for several reasons. The development of a model requires a careful formulation of the underlying hypotheses about mechanism. The model, once formulated, can be used to test the relationships between the elements of these complex systems. Successful fits to extant data with such models permit estimates of the ranges of some important biological parameters of the system, while unsuccessful fits force a reevaluation of the hypotheses about the underlying mechanisms.

In Sections 2 and 3 of this review, we briefly present the essential elements of our models for fast and slow axonal transport, respectively. The application of these models to understanding certain neuropathies is presented in Section 4.

A MODEL FOR FAST TRANSPORT

Let $P(x,t)$ be the concentration of free organelles of a specific type at position x along the axon at time t; $E(x,t)$ the concentration of free kinesin (or, for retrograde transport, of free cytoplasmic dynein); and $T(x,t)$ the concentration of free binding sites along the microtubules. An organelle may interact with n kinesins to form an organelle-kinesin complex.

$$P + nE \rightleftharpoons P \cdot nE \tag{1}$$

This complex may then interact with n free binding sites on a microtubule to form the complex $Q = P \cdot nE \cdot nT$.

$$P \cdot nE + nT \rightleftharpoons P \cdot nE \cdot nT \tag{2}$$

Thus the organelles have three states: free; bound to kinesins; and bound via their kinesins to a microtubule. In this third state it is assumed that the organelle is translocated at constant velocity, V_0, along the microtubule. We note that organelles bound to microtubules are sometimes stationary, presumably because the kinesin is not activated. In the present treatment we ignore this state; when information on the regulation of kinesin activity becomes available, the model can be extended to include this state.

It is useful to consider a typical experiment in which a radioactive substance is injected into the soma. The substance is used in the synthesis of a particular class of compounds such as proteins or lipids, and the labeled organelles subsequently enter the axon on the transport mechanism. For purposes of our discussion here we assume that the axon is locally at equilibrium, i.e., that the total amount of each of the constituents remains constant in time at each space point, x, along the axon. In order to solve the partial differential equations that correspond to the propagation of radioactivity down the axon, one must also specify the amount of radioactivity entering the axon per unit time. Further details and the partial differential equations are discussed in detail in Blum and Reed (1985). Computer simulations of the equations show a great variety of shapes of radioactive profiles, depending on the rate constants, the local concentrations of organelles and kinesins, and other parameters of the system. In general, the radioactivity propagates as a wave with a slowly spreading wave front, consistent with many experiments in the literature. The factors that determine the shape and sharpness of the propagating wave have been analyzed by Blum and Reed (1988) and Reed et al. (1990).

The model as formulated thus far ignores deposition, sequestration, and leakage of the transported material, but these processes can easily be added (Reed and Blum, 1986). For example, the vesicles (or material such as lipids or proteins within the vesicles) may become immobilized by insertion into or attachment onto the inner surface of the plasma membrane. Let M(x,t) denote the concentration of immobilized material. Then

$$P(x,t) \overset{k_m}{\to} M(x,t) \tag{3}$$

describes the insertion process, assuming that it is a first order process with rate constant k_m. The insertion of channel proteins into axonal membranes, either uniformly along the length as might occur in unmyelinated axons or primarily at the nodes of Ranvier in myelinated axons, is an example of such a process (Ritchie and Rogart, 1977; Wood et al., 1977; Armstrong et al., 1987).

Proteins or lipids that have been inserted into a membrane may undergo further processing. The material may be partially degraded in organelles moving in either direction (Snyder, 1989). We again assume that this occurs according to a first-order process and that the degraded material, whose concentration is denoted by D(x,t), may then enter the retrograde transport system and be transported at a constant velocity back toward the soma.

$$M(x,t) \overset{k_d}{\to} D(x,t) \tag{4}$$

Proteins or lipids may also leave the neuron. This can occur either by leakage from organelles and diffusion out of the neuron (rate constant k_{l1}) or by leakage of membrane-bound material (rate constant k_{l2}), according to suitable rate equations.

This model accounts qualitatively for the general shapes of a variety of experimentally derived curves of radioactivity versus distance as a function of time after injection of a radioactive precursor, including experiments with ligation and cold blocks. It has also been used to obtain quantitative information for the specific case of lipid transport and the effects of acrylamide on the deposition of glycoproteins (see below). Toews et al. (1983, 1988) examined the kinetics of transport of phosphatidylcholine (PC), phosphatidylethanolamine (PE), cholesterol, and diphosphatidylglycerol (DPG) along rat sciatic nerve. It was possible to obtain theoretical profiles that closely matched the experimental profiles for each of the four lipid classes examined (Blum et al., 1992). Many parameters were the same in all four cases; the parameters that were different provided useful information on differences in deposition, leakage, etc. for the four lipid classes in sciatic nerve axons. For example, Fig. 1A and B shows the experimental and theoretical profiles obtained for DPG. The values of k_1, k_2, k_3, and k_4 are large enough to ensure rapid equilibration of the binding and desorption reactions relative to the speed of translocation of the organelles along the microtubules, and thus the wave fronts are sharp (Blum and Reed, 1988). The value of V_0 = 0.6 cm/hr is approximately half the value for PE and PC (see Blum et al., 1992), consistent with a slower rate of translocation for mitochondria as compared with smaller vesicles (Brady and Lasek, 1982). The values of kl_{l1} and k_{l2} are both zero, indicating that there is no significant leakage of DPG from the mitochondria. The rate constant, kl_m, for deposition of DPG is larger than that for PC. In lobster axons it has been observed that mitochondria localized close to the plasma membrane are often stationary (Forman et al., 1987). This is

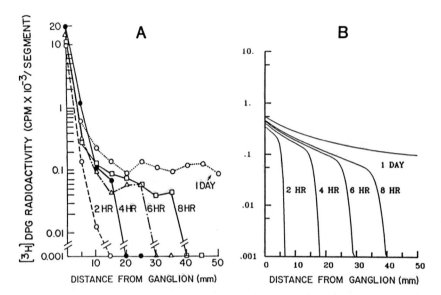

Figure 1 Experimental and theoretical curves for labeled DPG. (A) The distribution of labeled diphosphatidylglycerol (DPG) in the dorsal root ganglion and sciatic nerve of the rat at various times after the injection of [2-^{3}H]glycerol into the L-5 ganglion. (From Fig. 3 of Toews et al., 1983.) (B) The theoretical curves derived from the model using the following parameter values: $k_1 = k_3 = 20$; $k_2 = k_4 = 10$; $k_m = 13$; $k_d = 10$; $m_0 = 0.3$; $V_0 = 0.6$ cm/hr. For further discussion, definition of other units, etc., see Blum et al., 1992.

equivalent to deposition, since the DPG in such mitochondria has been effectively removed from the fast transport system. Thus the model suggests that a similar situation may occur in rat sciatic nerve. The value of $k_d = 10$ hr^{-1}, the first-order rate constant for removal of DPG via the fast retrograde system, is very much larger than k_d for PC, PE, or cholesterol (each < 0.1 hr^{-1}), consistent with observations that mitochondria move in both the fast retrograde and the fast anterograde systems (Forman, et al., 1987; Takenaka et al., 1990).

It has been suggested that the mitochondrial membrane contains multiple sites capable of interacting with the force-generating motors (Martz et al., 1984). For the simulations shown in Fig. 1, the value of n was 2. A comparably good fit to the data was obtained with n = 3 and n = 4 (unpublished data). There are, however, noticeable differences in the precise shape of the curves, so that if more extensive data were available, an estimate of the effective in situ value of n might be obtained.

The experimental profiles for PE are very different from those for DPG; at each time at which the nerve was examined the profile of PE decays exponentially along the axon. The PC profiles are intermediate between those of DPG and PE. Toews et al. (1983) suggested that the difference was due to a much larger rate of deposition of PE, and, to a lesser extent, of PC, compared with that of DPG. This was confirmed, and quantitative estimates of the parameter values were obtained by using the model (Blum et al., 1992). We note also that the model calculations suggest that both PE and PC (but not cholesterol or DPG) are transported at two fast anterograde rates (about 0.6 to 1.0 cm/hr and also at a slower rate of 0.2 cm/hr), consistent with observations that different classes of synaptic vesicles and other membrane-bounded organelles travel at disparate speeds in this range (see, e.g., Morin et al., 1991).

A MODEL FOR SLOW TRANSPORT

Whereas kinesin and cytosolic dynein are the engines for fast anterograde and fast retrograde transport, respectively, the engine(s) for slow transport is unknown. Indeed, it is not known whether SCa and SCb, whose composition varies between different axons even in the same species (Oblinger et al., 1987), are powered by the same or different mechanochemical enzymes. Although considerable evidence supports the view that the entire axonal cytoskeleton moves as a unit (Lasek, 1986), this view has been challenged (Lewis and Nixon, 1988) and reaffirmed (Lasek, Paggi, and Katz, submitted for publication; personal communication). Given these uncertainties, which we shall deal with in more detail below, it might appear that developing a kinetic model would be premature. One of the advantages of such an approach, however, is that it may allow a very diffuse body of information, such as that on various neuropathies, to be organized in a coherent fashion. Furthermore, one can investigate the underlying mechanisms by generating hypotheses and testing predictions (both by experiment and by machine computation). Before describing our model for slow transport we briefly review the properties of the major structural components of the system, microtubules (MTs) neurofilaments (NFs), and microfilaments (MFs). For a more extensive discussion of the cytoskeletal elements see Burgoyne (1991).

Microtubules

Miller et al. (1987) observed two populations of MTs in lobster axons, one type acting as architectural elements, the other acting as the preferred type for vesicle transport by the fast transport system. Tashiro et al. (1984) also described two types of MT in the sensory fibers of rat sciatic nerve, one type migrating with NFs in SCa, the other type migrating more rapidly. Indeed, Denoulet et al. (1989) have shown that several isoforms of tubulin are present in rat sciatic nerve motor axons, and that these are distributed differently between the cytoskeletal MTs and the soluble tubulin fractions. The relative amount of certain isotubulins is greater in SCb than in SCa. In human nerves, organelles have a unique speed/position pattern on any given MT, and this pattern is not necessarily related to the pattern on adjacent (< 0.5 μm separation) MTs (Lynn et al., 1986). In addition to variation between adjacent microtubules, there is considerable evidence that individual microtubules are not uniform along their length. Sahenk and Brady (1987) provide evidence that axonal MTs consist of a cold-stable inner segment with cold-labile regions at each end. Baas and Black (1990), using nocodazole sensitivity as a criterion, estimate that at least 40% of the MTs in an axon are composite, with a stable detyrosinated domain directly continuous with a labile tyrosinated domain. In the model to be described below, these and other complexities, such as possible post-transitional modifications that may occur as the microtubules move along the axon (Brown et al., 1982) or the presence of membrane-specific isoforms (Hargreaves and Avila, 1985) are ignored, and only two types of tubulin, designated as TA and TB, are included.

Neurofilaments

In mammalian neurons, neurofilaments are comprised three subunits with SDS-PAGE–apparent molecular weights of 210, 170, and 68 kD (NF-H, NF-M, and NF-L, respectively) in ratios that vary somewhat depending on species (Scott et al., 1985). NF-L appears to form the core of each filament. NF-M and NF-H are not present at all stages of neuron development, and probably mediate interactions with other NFs and with MTs. The heavy component, NF-H, is a major component of the cross-bridges between NFs in axons. NF-H, NF-M, and NF-L are phosphorylated in vivo. Phosphorylation of the head region favors diassembly, while phosphorylation of the tail region may regulate filament interactions (Black and Lee, 1988; Shaw, 1991). During early postnatal development NF-H is not present. When it appears, it is incorporated rapidly into the neurofilaments. Both before and after the appearance of NF-H, there is a proximo-distal gradient of NF content along the axon, the highest concentrations being closest to the soma (Schlaepfer and Bruce, 1990). Although the ratio of NF-H:NF-M:NF-L remains essentially constant along the length of the axon, there is ample evidence that the phosphorylation state of each component changes with distance from the soma (e.g., Lewis and Nixon, 1988; Toyoshima et al., 1988). Indeed, in mouse optic axons there are four NF-H variants differing only in the degree of phosphorylation. These variants are distributed differently along the length of these axons (Lewis and Nixon, 1988; see also Sihag and Nixon, 1990). Lewis and Nixon (1988) suggest that changes in the phosphorylation state may be one factor in determining the rate of incorporation of the moving neurofilaments into a stationary portion of the cytoskeleton, evidence for which is summarized by Nixon (1987). The model for slow transport shown in Fig. 2 does not include the deposition of NF into a stationary phase, but this could be done straightforwardly as in the model for fast transport. The scheme is also oversimplified in that it accounts only for the formation of NF dimers, whereas, in fact, the NF filaments may interact with one another to form an interconnected network.

Microfilaments

Actin is generally transported at least as fast as any other component of SCb. It comprises about 6% of the total protein in axoplasm extruded from the squid giant axon, and about 60% of this actin appears to be polymerized in MF (Morris and Lasek, 1984), most of which are less than 1 μm in length (Fath and Lasek, 1988). Microfilaments of the inner axonal cytoskeleton are organized in longitudinally arranged columns, and tend to cluster near MTs (Fath and Lasek, 1988). In the model described below, the underlying motive force is provided by an "engine", E, for example, an actin filament that is driven by myosin. A mechanochemical enzyme termed dynamin has been reported to mediate sliding between

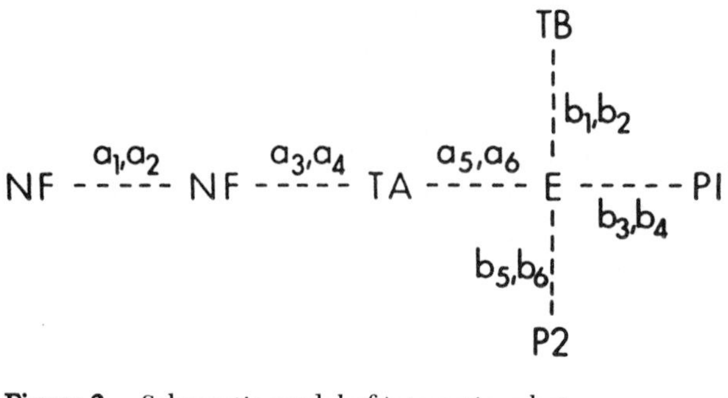

Figure 2   Schematic model of interactions between components of SCa and SCb. The pairs of rate constants shown are the forward and reverse constants for each interaction. The dashed lines indicate the reversible bonds that may form between these elements. a_1, a_3, a_5, b_1, b_3, b_5 are association rate constants. a_2, a_4, a_6, b_2, b_4, b_6 are the corresponding rate constants for dissociation. TA and TB are two types of microtubules. (From Blum and Reed, 1989).

microtubules isolated from calf brain (Shpetner and Vallee, 1989), and it is also possible that this enzyme acts as the engine or that more than one engine is involved in moving different subportions of the cytoskeletal network. Indeed, two populations of actin microfilaments are present in the giant axons of squid (Fath and Lasek, 1988). In the model of fast transport described in Section 1, MFs play no role, since at present the nature of their influence on the fast transport system is unknown.

A Model for Slow Transport

We have developed a simple prototypical model that incorporates the major structural components described above in order to investigate whether reversible binding and translocation mechanisms (such as those used for fast transport) can account for the essential features of SCa and SCb. The model also includes the "soluble" cytoplasmic proteins such as fodrin, calmodulin, glycolytic enzymes, butylcholinesterase, heat shock proteins, and others that are transported in a coherent fashion in SCb (Garner and Lasek, 1982; Cancalon, 1979; Baitinger et al., 1983; Couraud et al., 1982; Tytell and Barbe, 1987; Baitinger and Willard, 1987; Petrucci et al, 1991). We assume that the slow transport system is driven by an "engine", E, for example, an actin microfilament–myosin complex. The other components of the slow transport system are assumed to form reversible bonds either with E or with each other as shown in Fig. 2. Each component is stationary unless attached to E (either directly or indirectly), in which case it moves at a constant velocity, V_0. In the model, the two types of microtubule bind directly to E, but neurofilaments bind only via TA. Neurofilament-neurofilament interaction is also allowed but only to the extent of the formation of dimers. The numerous cytoplasmic proteins are represented by P_1 and P_2, which bind directly to the engine, E. It is known that various glycolytic enzymes and other cytoplasmic proteins bind to actin in a relatively nonspecific way (see, e.g., Walsh and Knull, 1988; Roberts and Somero, 1989, and references therein). The partial differential equations whose simulations describe the shape and speed of the concentration profiles to be expected from both continuous labeling and pulse labeling experiments are presented in detail in Blum and Reed (1989). Figure 3 shows the results of a simulation at 40 and 100 days after a pulse labeling of the proteins in the soma. Each labeled protein moves as a slowly spreading constant velocity pulse. It is noteworthy that although we have assumed a single motile element, the profiles have separated into two groups corresponding to SCa and SCb. This arises because of the relatively weak binding of TA to E compared to the stronger binding of P_1 and P_2 to E. Neurofilaments are transported more slowly than TA, consistent with experimental data, because they interact with E only through TA. It is also noteworthy that the cytoplasmic proteins and TB form a coherent group in SCb. This remains true whether they all bind directly to E (as shown in Figure 3) or indirectly, e.g. P_1 binds to P_2, which binds to E. The speeds of the SCa and SCb pulses depend on the rate constants and on the concentrations of TA, TB, E, and NF. As discussed in Blum aznd Reed (1989), this can account for the differences in speeds and relative composition of SCa and SCb observed in different axons.

Recent evidence shows that in sciatic nerves of 4-week old rats, the two forms of tubulin are transported as a single wave with a speed of about 2 mm/day. By 7 weeks, however, most of the insoluble form of tubulin is associated with neurofilaments, and these proceed at a rate of about 1.5 mm/day, typical of SCa. The remaining tubulin, largely the soluble form, moves at 3 mm/day, typical of SCb (Tashiro and Kamiya, 1991). As we have mentioned above, the speed of the wave in the model depends on the association and dissociation rate constants of the various components. Thus one can see how these changes in transport rates could occur if the rate constants for interaction between NF and TA, TA and E, and TB and E change in suitable directions during maturation. We shall see below that this model can also be used to gain insight into some of the changes in slow transport that occur in certain neuropathies.

NEUROPATHIES CAUSED BY PHARMACOLOGICALLY ACTIVE CHEMICALS

In the models for fast and slow transport developed above, the rates of transport and deposition, shapes of profiles, etc., depend only on the concentrations of the various components and the rate constants governing their interactions. A neurotoxicant can affect these interactions by simply altering one or more of the rate constants. A neurotoxicant can also affect concentrations by altering rates of synthesis in the soma, or by altering interactions that in turn change the effective local concentrations. In both models we explicitly assumed that when a component is attached to the motile element it moves at a constant velocity, thus ignoring the fact that mechanical impediments may play a significant role. For example, an organelle moving along a microtubule may be blocked by a cross-link between two elements of the slow transport system. The number of such cross-links will depend on the local rate constants and concentrations of the cytoskeletal elements involved, which may be appreciably altered by present or prior exposure to neurotoxicants. The resulting increases in concentrations can in turn further affect the mechanical properties of the system. Eventually, this may lead to large-scale morphological changes such as those seen in various peripheral neuropathies. In the following, we use our models of fast and slow transport as guides to understanding the chemical effects of neurotoxicants and the likely mechanical consequences. Expansion of the model to include mechanical interactions will require much more knowledge of the local organization of the cytoskeletal system (e.g. the distribution of cross-links, interaction of the cytoskeleton with the axolemma, etc.).

2,5-Hexanedione

2,5-Hexanedione (2,5-HD) produces distal (dying-back) axonopathy after single or repeated application to exposed rat sciatic nerves (Politis et al., 1980). The morphological sequence of events is similar to that observed after exposure to acrylamide, carbon disulfide, and 3,4-dimethyl-2,5-hexanedione (DMHD) (Graham et al., 1982; Anthony et al, 1983, and references therein). In some nerves, neurofilamentous masses pass along the axons to their terminals, whence they subsequently disappear, presumably because of proteolysis (Paggi and Lasek, 1984; Zalewska et al., 1986; Nixon et al., 1986). In other tracts, especially in the longer peripheral nerves, the filamentous masses accumulate, generally at constrictions at nodes of Ranvier (Cavanagh, 1982). These masses contain numerous high-molecular-weight polypeptides that are immunoreactive to antibodies against NF-H, NF-M, and NF-L (Lapadula et al., 1986; Karlsson et al., 1991). Neurons treated with DMHD develop neurofilamentous masses more proximaly than 2,5-HD-treated neurons, presumably because of the greater rate and extent of cross-link formation, both in vitro and in vivo, by DMHD (Anthony et al., 1983; Graham et al., 1984; DeCaprio and O'Neill, 1985). Depending on the dose, the schedule of drug administration, and the kinds of nerves examined, both acceleration *and* deceleration of slow axonal transport have been observed. Thus Griffin et al. (1984) observed that a 5-day pretreatment of young rats with DMHD reduced the rate of transport of NF proteins in SCa by as much as 90%, whereas tubulin and other components of SCb were only modestly retarded. In rats treated with 2,5-HD, which is less effective in forming pyrrole-mediated cross-links than DMHD, the transport rates of NF and of two other polypeptides in SCa in optic axons were increased, again with little change in the rate of transport of SCb components (Monaco et al., 1985). Similar results were obtained in motor and sensory axons in rat sciatic nerve, and it was also shown that fast anterograde transport was not altered (Braendegaard and Sidenius, 1986a). After sufficiently long exposure to 2,5-HD there was, however, a significant reduction in the rate of fast retrograde transport that did not appear to be due to any delay in "turnaround" at the nerve terminals (Braendegaard and Sidenius, 1986b). Studies with 3-acetyl-2,5-hexanedione, which forms protein-bound pyrroles but does not lead to cross-link formation, show that it does not cause an acceleration of SCa transport rate or any accumulation of NF-filled axonal swellings (St. Clair et al., 1988; Pyle et al., 1992). Thus cross-linking of neurofilaments appears to be an essential component of at least some of the neurotoxic effects of the γ-diketones and, perhaps, of several other neurotoxicants, as will be described below.

In Fig. 3 we have seen that pulse labeling of the soma can lead to the formation of separate SCa and SCb waves that propagate along the axon. Suppose an axon was exposed to a neurotoxicant such as 2,5-HD (or DMHD) that markedly increased NF-NF interactions. The dotted line in Fig. 4 shows that this would cause an increase in the speed of NF transport in SCa, as observed. This comes about because as the number of NF-NF aggregates increases, a larger number of NF molecules will be transported even though the number of NF-TA bonds may remain the same. Of course, in the simple model shown in Fig. 2, only dimer formation is depicted. A more realistic model would include the formation of NF-NF aggregates of various sizes and their mechanical properties. As the degree of cross-linking (covalent or noncovalent) increases and the NF aggregates become larger and larger, they would tend to interfere with one another and a slowing of transport would occur. Furthermore, large-diameter axons tend to have deeply constricted nodes of Ranvier (Cavanagh, 1982), where, since the neurofilamentous aggregates would come into close proximity with one another, one would expect increased interaction because of the local increase in NF concentration, and, therefore, increased blockage of fast axonal transport and the initiation of the dying-back process. Since axonal diameter is correlated with NF content (Lasek et al., 1983b; Hoffman et al., 1985; Parhad et al, 1987a), this would be especially noticeable in large-diameter axons. Thus the model can account for both the acceleration of NF transport at short times and low doses of 2,5-HD and the deceleration at long times and high doses.

With compounds such as DMHD, which is much more reactive than 2,5-HD, such "logjams" would occur in the proximal regions of the axon. Unless experiments were performed with low doses of DMHD on relatively long axons, one might observe only the decrease in NF transport rate resulting from blockage. It would be interesting to ascertain whether at low-dose DMHD regimens, an increase in the NF transport rate at short times would occur. A comparable experiment has been performed, using 3-methyl-2,5-hexanedione (MHD), a diketone that is a structural "average" between 2,5-HD and DMHD. When rats were treated with MHD, the NF accumulations occurred sufficiently far from the axon hillock to allow NF transport to be measured (Monaco et al., 1990). The finding that the rate of NF transport was accelerated led Monaco et al. to suggest that pyrrolation of crucial lysine residues of NF proteins would disrupt interactions with the MT network, thereby allowing NF to move more rapidly. However, the predictions of the model show that an increase in NF-NF interactions would also lead to an acceleration of NF transport, and in view of the capacity of the neurotoxic diketones to form cross-links (covalent or

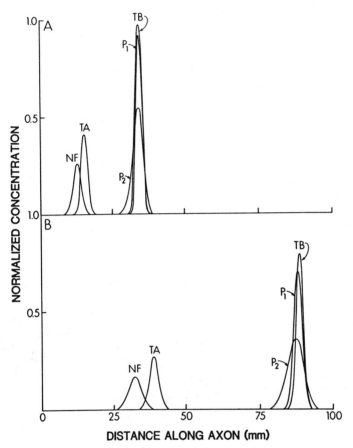

Figure 3   Coherent transport of proteins in SCa and SCb. In each of these simulations the axonal length was 100 mm, pulse labeling at the soma was of 3 days duration, and the speed V_0 of the actin microfilaments was 1 mm/day (not shown). Panels A and B show the results obtained at 40 and 100 days respectively. The total local concentrations (labeled plus unlabeled) were $E = 1.0$, TA = 0.2, NF = 0.2, TB = 0.03, $P_1 = 0.1$, $P_2 = 0.2$. The rate constants for SCa were $a_1 = 10$, $a_2 = 2$, $a_3 = 10$, $a_4 = 0.1$, $a_5 = a_6 = 30$. Those for SCb were $b_1 = 30$, $b_2 = 3$, $b_3 = 15$, $b_4 = 1.5$, $b_5 = 3$, $b_6 = 0.3$. Radiolabeled concentrations shown on the ordinate were normalized by dividing each by the (constant) total local concentration of that species. (From Blum and Reed, 1989.)

noncovalent), it is possible that this is the cause of the observed acceleration of NF transport in the region of the axon before the formation of neurofilamentous masses.

Recently, experiments were performed in which rats were pretreated with 2,5-HD and then ^{35}S-methionine was injected into the eye and the rate of transport of NF in the optic nerve was measured (Pyle et al., 1992). The finding that NF transport was faster in axons from the pretreated rats than in axons from untreated rats and about as fast as in optic axons in rats treated with 2,5-HD starting at the time of injection of ^{35}S-methionine suggests that the acceleration of NF transport is a secondary response of the axon to the initial 2,5-HD injury rather than a consequence of the ongoing presence of 2,5-HD. Although an increase in SCa transport rate could occur if the neuronal response to 2,5-HD was to synthesize more NF per unit time (see Fig. 3 of

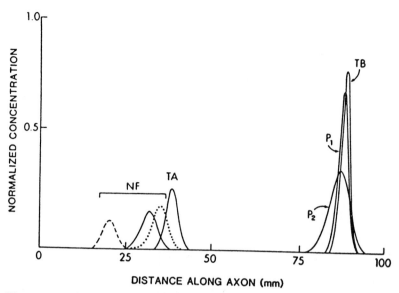

Figure 4 The effect of neurotoxicants that alter NF-NF or NF-TA interactions on the speed of neurofilament transport. The solid line shows the same simulation as in Figure 3B. The dotted line shows the speedup of the NF pulse caused by a neurotoxicant that increases NF-NF binding 1000-fold ($a_1 = 50$, $a_2 = 0.01$), with all other rate constants and concentrations the same as in Fig. 3. The dashed line shows the slow-down of the NF pulse caused by a neurotoxicant that increases the dissociation rate constant of NF-TA by a factor of ten; $a_4 = 1$, and all other parameters as in Fig. 3. The pulses of TA, TB, P_1, and P_2 were not appreciably affected by these neurotoxicants, so the corresponding dashed and dotted lines coincide with the solid lines.

Blum and Reed, 1989), this is not likely to be the underlying mechanism, since there was a significant *decrease* in the amount of labeled NF-H in the 2,5-HD treated groups (Pyle et al., 1992). There are two fundamentally different ways in which a long-lasting effect of pretreatment with 2,5-HD could be explained within the framework of the present model. One hypothesis might be that 2,5-HD pretreatment causes long-lasting changes in the synthesis or post-translational modification of NF isozymes such that their interaction with TA after they enter the axon is increased. An alternative hypothesis is that cross-linking during the pretreatment with 2,5-HD alters some axonal proteins so that they become effectively stationary and that these stationary complexes enhance the NF-NF or NF-TA interactions.

As mentioned above, 2,5-HD had little effect on the rate of fast anterograde transport. Single injections of 2,5-HD do, however, reduce the quantity of fast-transported protein by about 42–51% without significantly inhibiting the rate of protein synthesis (Sickles, 1989b). This suggests interference with the loading of vesicles onto the fast transport system in the region of the axon hillock, i.e., an effect outside the scope of the present model. Although 2,5-HD had little effect on fast anterograde transport, it did cause a slowing of fast retrograde transport. One possible mechanism for this inhibition might be formation by 2,5-HD of cross-links within the dynein motor, reducing V_1 and/or reducing the rate constants for the interaction between the dynein and the binding sites on the lamellar and multivesicular bodies that are transported in the fast retrograde system.

Acrylamide

Since acrylamide interacts with sulfhydryl, amino, and hydroxyl groups, almost any protein component of the slow and fast transport systems could be involved in the development of the distal axonopathy that results from exposure to this neurotoxicant. Although no obvious changes in MT, NF, or smooth endoplasmic reticulum were observed in earlier studies (Miller and Spencer, 1985; Spencer et al., 1985), radiolabeled NF-H and NF-M (and several other as yet unidentified proteins) are observed after injection of very low doses (200 µg/kg) of ^{14}C-acrylamide into mice (Carrington et al., 1990). Following a single high dose of acrylamide, there is a slight decrease in the rate of slow transport, and NFs begin accumulating in the proximal region of the axon, with the formation of local swellings (Gold, 1987). Whether this results from the formation of NF-NF cross-links remains to be determined. After repeated doses of acrylamide, when distal degeneration has begun, the proportion of NF in SCa is markedly reduced, and there is a decrease in diameter of the proximal axon (Gold, 1987). This reduction in caliber presumably reflects a secondary response of the soma, e.g., a decrease in synthesis and/or delivery of NF components to the axon (Lasek et al, 1983b; Parhad et al., 1987b).

In addition to the effect of acrylamide on slow transport, it is clear that it also inhibits fast retrograde transport, and, to a much lesser extent if at all, fast anterograde transport (Jakobsen et al., 1983; Miller and Spencer, 1985; Spencer et al., 1985; Moretto and Sabri, 1988; Sickles, 1989a). Since fast retrograde transport is inhibited before evident neuropathies appear, it is not apparent whether the same defect that leads to a decrease in the rate of slow transport is responsible for the inhibition of the fast retrograde system. Given that NF forms cross-links with MT (Tashiro et al., 1984), it is possible that abnormalities in this interaction could interfere with fast transport, although there is at present no reason to suppose that such a defect would selectively interfere with the retrograde as opposed to the anterograde system. If this were the mechanism, the model for fast transport (Section I) would have to be modified to include equations for the interactions of MT with NF. A more likely explanation for the inhibition of the fast retrograde system is that acrylamide preferentially reacts with cytosolic dynein as compared with kinesin. If this were shown to be the case, such information could easily be incorporated into the model. It has recently been shown that exposure of chick dorsal root ganglion explants to acrylamide reduced the frequency and mean velocity of both retrogradely and anterogradely transported vesicles, but not the maximum observed velocity (C. H. Martenson et al., personal communication). This suggests that acrylamide affects the rate constants for the interaction of dynein and kinesin with the vesicles rather than V_0, but sheds no light on why the retrograde system is affected much more than the anterograde system.

In addition to the effects just described, it has been suggested that acrylamide treatment also causes an increase in the deposition of axonally transported glycoproteins (but not of proteins in general) in rat sciatic nerve (Harry et al., 1989). To ascertain whether this interpretation was sufficient to explain the differences between the profiles obtained from control and acrylamide-treated rats, we used the fast transport model discussed above. Figure 5A shows the experimental profiles and Fig. 5B shows the best-fit theoretical profiles from the model. The parameters used to obtain the fit (see the figure legend) are identical in the control and acrylamide-treated cases except for a four-fold increase K_m, the rate constant for deposition of glycoproteins into stationary structures. This supports the interpretation of Harry et al. (1989) and strongly suggests

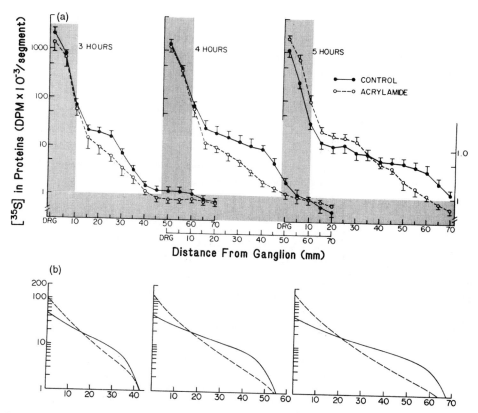

Figure 5 Experimental and theoretical profiles for glycoprotein transport in rat sciatic nerve. (a) The experimental profiles show the distribution of labeled glycoproteins in the dorsal root ganglion and sciatic nerve of control and acrylamide-treated rats at 3, 4, and 5 hours after injection of [³H]glucosamine. (From Fig. 3 of Harry et al., 1989; stippling added by us.) (b) The theoretical profiles were obtained using the fast transport equations described in the text. Units on the abscissa and the ordinate are the same as for the experimental curves. Typical experimental profiles increase markedly as one approaches the soma because of the large pool of injected radioactivity there. Since the model deals only with the material after it has entered the axon proper, no attempt was made to fit the first 10 mm of the experimental profiles. Thus, the simulation profiles for distances between 0 and 10 mm from the ganglion show what would be measured in the absence of the soma pool. We have also ignored the small values (below 10^3 DPM/segment) at the leading edge of each experimental curve, since these may arise from non-specific leakage. For ease of comparison with the theoretical curves, we have stippled these regions on the experimental profiles.

In the simulation, the following parameter values were used for both control and acrylamide-treated rats: $k_1 = k_3 = 2.5$; $k_2 = k_4 = 1.0$; $n = 2$; $k_d = 0.0$; $V_0 = 1.9$. The values of k_m were 0.2 and 0.8 for the control and the acrylamide-treated rats, respectively. Units are the same as in Fig. 1.

that the primary effect of acylamide on fast anterograde transport is an increase in the deposition of glycoproteins carried by organelles in the fast transport system. If comparable data existed for proteins carried by the slow transport system, further insights into the effects of acrylamide might be obtained. In particular, one might be able to investigate the interplay between the slow and fast transport systems in the presence of acrylamide.

β,β′-Iminodipropionitrile

β,β′-Iminodipropionitrile (IDPN), whether injected intraperitoneally or directly into a nerve bundle, slows the transport of NF all along the axon without interfering with either fast anterograde or fast retrograde transport (Griffin et al., 1978). Within a few days after the injection of IDPN, proximal swellings occur and progressively enlarge, as occurs after 2,5-HD or DMHD treatment (Griffin et al., 1984; Sayre, et al., 1985). Of particular interest is the observation that after IDPN treatment the microtubules, smooth endoplasmic reticulum, and actin microfilaments tend to associate in the center of the axon, whereas the NFs localize primarily in the periphery (Papasozomenos et al., 1982; Griffin et al., 1983a,b; Papasozomenos and Payne, 1986). This segregation of NFs in the periphery is not unique to IDPN treatment; it has also been observed to occur shortly after 2,5-HD treatment (Griffin et al., 1983a; Griffin and Watson, 1988) and after DMHD treatment (Genter et al., 1987). In so far as IDPN interferes with the NF-TA interaction and also increases NF-NF interactions (Fig. 2), a reduction in the rate of transport of NF and the subsequent formation of proximal swellings is expected in the model. The relocation of the NFs to the periphery, however, is not within the scope of the present model. It should be pointed out that even in normal axons, the NFs are not distributed at random throughout a given cross-section of the axon. Ordered lattice-like regions are present and there is a distinct helical organization (Lasek et al., 1983a). The distribution of interneurofilament distances is roughly Gaussian and decreases only slightly (from 44.1 to 39.3 nm) in IDPN-treated axons (Parhad et al, 1987a). Thus the primary effect of IDPN may be on NF-TA interactions, rather than on NF-NF interactions. Clearly, much more work on the precise nature of the interaction of IDPN with NF will be required before an understanding of the reasons for their movement to the periphery are understood. Although Griffin et al. (1978) did not observe any slowing of either the fast anterograde or the retrograde transport systems, Sickles (1989b) reported a slight decrease in the rate of fast anterograde transport after a single injection of IDPN, and Fink et al. (1986) reported a marked inhibition of fast retrograde transport in rat sciatic nerve. As pointed out by Fink et al. (1986), Griffin et al. (1978) measured retrograde transport from the nerve terminal, whereas Fink et al. measured it from the midregion of the axon to the cell body. If transport from the terminal was not affected but transport from the axon through the proximal NF swellings was inhibited, this would explain the different observations. Thus, a primary role for IDPN as an inhibitor of slow transport is well established, but it is not clear whether the inhibition of fast retrograde transport is a primary or secondary effect. Treatment with IDPN and increasing age are similar in that in both cases the rate of transport of NF in SCa decreases and the degree of phosphorylation of NF increases (Watson et al., 1989). Several protein kinases appear to be involved in the phosphorylation of NF-M (Sihag and Nixon, 1990; Floyd et al., 1991), but the consequences of phosphorylation on the interactions of NF with themselves or with other proteins are as yet unknown. Further studies will be required to ascertain the causal interrelations between the IDPN-induced slowing of NF transport and the increased degree of NF phosphorylation. Since there is a diminishing proximo-distal gradient of NF along axons (Schlaepfer and Bruce, 1990) as well as a progressive change in their state of phosphorylation (Nixon and Lewis, 1986), it is clear that the assumption of a homogeneous axon in the model shown in Fig. 3 is an oversimplification. When the kinases, phosphatases, and proteases that are involved have been further characterized in a single nerve so that their activities as a function of location along the axon are better understood, it will be desirable to include such nonlinearities in the model.

NEUROPATHIES CAUSED BY GENETIC OR UNKNOWN FACTORS

Diabetic Neuropathy

About 25% of diabetics develop symptoms of peripheral neuropathy (Medori et al., 1985, and references therein). Two models have been widely used to study various aspects of diabetic neuropathy. Injection of streptozotocin (STZ) into mice or rats destroys the pancreatic islets within a day, so that the exact time of onset of diabetes is known. Use of animals with recessive mutations (e.g., db/db mice or BB rats) that lead to the spontaneous formation of diabetes yield similar results (Medori et al., 1985, 1988). Nonenzymatic glycosylation of peripheral nerve proteins (Vlassara et al., 1981) may affect interactions between proteins and hence affect the rate of transport. Vitadello et al. (1983) examined the rates of transport of four isozymes of acetylcholinesterase. Two of the isozymes (G4 and A12), which travel in the fast anterograde system, were not affected in db/db mice, but isozymes G1 and G2, which travel in the slow system, were reduced in the late phase of neuropathy, at which time axonal dwindling (i.e., decreasing diameter with increasing distance from the soma) was evident. This is consistent with (but not proof of) a decreased rate of slow transport, as is the finding of a reduced rate of transport of three glycolytic enzymes (Medori et al., 1988). Although fast anterograde transport is not affected by diabetes, the fast retrograde transport of glycoproteins and of ^{125}I-labeled nerve growth factor (NGF) is inhibited (Jakobsen et al. 1981). This defect in retrograde transport of NGF was already evident 3 days after STZ treatment, i.e., before the development of structural lesions, and did not worsen at later times when axonopathy was present (Schmidt et al., 1985). There was no evidence for retardation of NGF at the sites of the lesions, a finding consistent with the view that extensive cross-linking does not occur. The inhibition of the fast retrograde but not fast anterograde system suggests a diabetes-induced alteration in cytosolic dynein and/or in the surface of the retrogradely transported vesicles, but this remains to be investigated. Both Jakobsen et al. (1983) and Schmidt et al. (1985) observed an inhibition of proteins transported in SCa and SCb, though the primary effect of the diabetes appears to be on SCa, particularly NF (see also Macioce et al., 1989). Larsen and Sidenius (1989) showed that the amount of NF-H (but not of NF-M or NF-L) in the axon is decreased after STZ treatment, presumably because of a decreased rate of synthesis. They suggested that the decreased synthesis of NF-H leads to the observed slowing of the rate of transport of NF-M and NF-L, but this appears to conflict with evidence that developing axons with no NF-H have the highest rates of NF transport. Clearly much more detailed studies of the transport rates (as opposed to amount of synthesis) of individual proteins in SCa and SCb, coupled with analysis of the degree of glycosylation of those proteins, will be required before further understanding of the mechanism responsible for the slowing of SCa and/or SCb can be achieved.

Amyotrophic Lateral Sclerosis

In control nerves from patients with no known neuropathy, the mean translocation speed of organelles moving in the anterograde direction is about 1.5 μm/sec, and the distribution is approximately symmetrical about the mean (Breuer et al., 1987). In nerves from patients with severe wasting and weakness of hand muscle function due to amyotrophic lateral sclerosis (ALS), the distribution of anterograde speeds is bimodal, with a majority of the organelles moving at about 1.5–2.0 μm/sec, and a sizable minority moving at about 3.5 μm/sec. The percentage of small round organelles was considerably larger in nerves from

ALS patients than in those from controls. If small organelles move faster in both the control and ALS nerves, this alone could explain the bimodal distribution in ALS patients. Such an explanation raises the question why the smaller organelles move faster. One possibility would be that they bind kinesin more tightly than larger organelles and hence have a higher probability of interacting with sites on the microtubules. In addition, the smaller may encounter fewer barriers. Studies of kinesin-binding to isolated vesicles of this size class from control and ALS nerves could, in principle, test this possibility. The cause of the proximal NF swellings in ALS is at present unknown, though several possibilities have been suggested (Gold, 1987).

Other Neuropathies

There are, of course, a number of other neuropathies caused by toxicological agents or by disease that appear to involve one or more of the axonal transport systems. For example, both acute and chronic exposure to ethanol causes a decrease in axonal transport (McLane, 1987). An increase in the degree of phosphorylation of NF-H accompanied by a decrease in NF-associated protein phosphatase activity occurs in NF obtained from the spinal cord of rats after chronic ethanol ingestion (Guru et al., 1991). SCa is slower in hypothyroid rats than in euthyroid controls, while hyperthyroidism may cause an increased rate of clearance (e.g., loss of protein via deposition or leakage or degradation) in the proximal axon (Sidenius et al., 1987). A single dose of di-n-butyl-dichlorovinyl-phosphate slows the rate of retrograde transport in nerves of hens before the development of clinical neuropathy (Moretto et al., 1987). When more detailed data become available on these neuropathies, it should be possible to use the models presented above to obtain insight into the underlying processes.

   A characteristic feature of giant axonal neuropathy in humans is the occurrence of focal axonal enlargements due to the accumulation of NF. In this disease, the minimum separation between NF ranges from 12 to 30 nm instead of 20 to 60 nm as in controls. Some axons were devoid of NF, and contained an increased density of MT, which, however, did not run longitudinally (Donaghy et al., 1988). These authors raise the possibility that a post-translational modification of NF-H could explain its failure to protrude normally as the side arm of neurofilaments.

   Although transport studies in goldfish optic nerves (Alpert et al., 1980) and garfish olfactory nerves (Cancalon, 1982) support the view (Lasek, 1986) that the cytoskeleton is transported as a unit after nerve transection, this may not be the case for mammalian nerves. When sciatic nerves of a strain of mice that undergo slow Wallerian degeneration following transection were examined, a gradual redistribution of cytoskeletal elements occurred, and NF accumulated at both the proximally and distally severed ends of an axonal segment (Glass and Griffin, 1991). Furthermore, as observed in both 2,5-HD-, DMHD-, and IDPN-treated axons and in giant axonal neuropathy, NFs and MTs tend to form separate domains. Glass and Griffin (1991) point out that since this pattern of MT and NF segregation, with the formation of NF aggregates, occurs in the axotomized nerve in the absence of any neurotoxic agent, the reorganization of the cytoskeletal elements may not require cross-linking. It is worth emphasizing that in the present model for slow transport (Fig. 2), all the interactions occur via reversible binding, and our use of the term cross-linking does not necessarily refer to the formation of covalent links; the effects of neurotoxic agents, axotomy, or disease-induced axonopathy may be interpreted within the framework of the present model whether or not covalent cross-links are formed. When more information becomes available on the factors that control NF-NF interactions, it should be possible to modify the model shown in Fig. 2 to include a much more realistic representation of the NF interactions with one another (and with MTs), and thus further improve the usefulness of the model as a guide to interpreting the differences between various neuropathies.

ACKNOWLEDGMENTS

We are grateful to Dr. D. D. Carr for modeling the effect of acrylamide on glycoprotein deposition and to Drs. D. C. Anthony and C. H. Martenson for a number of useful criticisms of the manuscript. This work was supported by NIH grant R01 NS25191 and NSF grant DMS8822449.

REFERENCES

Allen RD, Weiss DG, Hayden JH, Brown DT, Fujiwake H, Simpson M (1985). Gliding movement of and bidirectional transport along single native microtubules from squid axoplasm: evidence for an active role of microtubules in cytoplasmic transport. J Cell Biol 100:1736–52.

Alpert RM, Grafstein B, Edwards DL (1980). Slow axonal transport in goldfish optic axons. Soc Neurosci Abs 6:83.

Anthony DC, Boekelheide K, Anderson CW, Graham DG (1983). The effect of 3,4-dimethyl substitution on the neurotoxicity of 2,5-hexanedione. Toxicol Appl Pharmacol 71:372–82.

Armstrong R, Toews AD, Morrel P (1987). Axonal transport through nodes of Ranvier. Brain Res 412:196–9.

Baas PW, Black MM (1990). Individual microtubules in the axon consist of domains that differ in both composition and stability. J Cell Biol 111:495–509.

Baitinger C, Cheney R, Clements D, Glicksman M, Hirokawa N, Levine J, Meiri K, Simon C, Skene P, Willard M (1983). Axonally transported proteins in axon development, maintenance, and regeneration. Cold Spring Harbor Symp Quant Biol 48:791–802.

Baitinger C, Willard M (1987). Axonal transport of synapsin I like proteins in rabbit retinal ganglion cells. J Neurosci 7:3723–35.

Black MM, Lee VMY (1988). Phosphorylation of neurofilament proteins in intact neurons: demonstration of phosphorylation in cell bodies and axons. J Neurosci 8:2296–3305.

Blum JJ, Carr DD, Reed MC (1992). Theoretical analysis of lipid transport in sciatic nerve. Biochim Biophys Acta 1125:313–320.

Blum JJ, Reed MC (1985). A model for fast axonal transport. Cell Motility 5:507–27.

Blum JJ, Reed MC (1988). The transport of organelles in axons. Math Biosci 90:233–45.

Blum JJ, Reed MC (1989). A model for slow axonal transport and its application to neurofilamentous neuropathies. Cell Motility Cytoskel 12:53–65.

Brady ST, Lasek RJ (1982). Axonal transport: a cell biological method for studying proteins that associate with the cytoskeleton. Meth Cell Biol 25:365–98.

Brady ST, Lasek RJ, Allen RD, Yin HL, Stossel TP (1984). Gelsolin inhibition of fast axonal transport indicates a requirement for actin microfilaments. Nature 310:56–8.

Braendegaard H, Sidenius P (1986a). Anterograde components of axonal transport in motor and sensory nerves in experimental 2,5-hexanedione neuropathy. J Neurochem 47:31–7.

Braendegaard H, Sidenius R (1986b). The retrograde fast component of axonal transport in motor and sensory nerves of the rat during administration of 2,5-hexanedione. Brain Res 378:1–7.

Breuer AC, Lynn MP, Atkinson MB, Chou SM, Wilbourn AJ, Marks KE, Culver JE, Fleegler EJ (1987). Fast axonal transport in amyotrophic lateral sclerosis: an intra axonal organelle traffic analysis. Neurology 37:738–48.

Brown BA, Nixon RA, Marotta CA (1982). Posttranslational processing of tubulin during axoplasmic transport in CNS axons. J Cell Biol 94:159–64.

Burgoyne RD, ed. (1991). The neuronal cytoskeleton. New York: Wiley-Liss.

Cancalon P (1979). Subcellular and polypeptide distributions of slowly transported proteins in the garfish olfactory nerve. Brain Res 161:115–30.

Cancalon P (1982). Slow flow in axons detached from their pericaria. J Cell Biol 95:989–92.

Carrington CD, Lapadula DM, Dulak L, Friedman M, Abou Donia MB (1990). In vivo binding of ^{14}C-acrylamide to proteins in the mouse nervous system. Neurochem Int 18:191–7.

Cavanagh JB (1982). The pattern of recovery of axons in the nervous system of rats following 2,5-hexanediol intoxication: a question of rheology? Neuropathol Appl Neurobiol 8:19–34.

Cena V, Garcia AG, Gonzalez-Garcia C, Kirpekar SM (1984). Orthograde and retrograde axonal transport of calmodulin in a cat noradrenergic neurone. Br J Pharmacol 82:143–9.

Couraud JY, Di Giamberardino L, Hassig R (1982). Slow axonal transport of the molecular forms of butyrylcholinesterase in a peripheral nerve. Neuroscience 7:1015–21.

De Caprio AP, O'Neill EA (1985). Alterations in rat axonal cytoskeletal proteins induced by in vitro and in vivo 2,5-hexanedione exposure. Toxicol Appl Pharmaol 78:235–47.

Denoulet P, Filliatreau G, de Nichaud B, Gros F, Di Giamberardino L (1989). Differential axonal transport of isotubulins in the motor axons of the rat sciatic nerve. J Cell Biol 108:965–71.

Donaghy M, King RHM, Thomas PK, Workman JM (1988). Abnormalities of the axonal cytoskeleton in giant axonal neuropathy. J Neurocytol 17:197–208.

Fath KR, Lasek RJ (1988). Two classes of actin microfilaments are associated with the inner cytoskeleton of axons. J Cell Biol 107:613–21.

Fink DJ, Gainer H (1980). Retrograde axonal transport of endogenous proteins in sciatic nerve demonstrated by covalent labelling in vivo. Science 208:303–5.

Fink DJ, Purkiss D, Mata M (1986). β,β′-iminodinitropropionitrile impairs retrograde axonal transport. J Neurochem 47:1032–8.

Floyd CA, Grant P, Gallant PE, Pant HC (1991). Principal neurofilament associated protein kinase in squid axoplasm is related to casein kinase I. J Biol Chem 266:4987–94.

Forman DS, Lynch KJ, Smith AS (1987). Organelle dynamics in lobster axons: anterograde, retrograde, and stationary mitochondria. Brain Res 412:96–106.

Garner JA, Lasek RJ (1982). Cohesive axonal transport of the slow component complex of polypeptides. J Neurosci 2:1824–35.

Genter MB, Szakal-Quin G, Anderson GW, Anthony DC, Graham DG (1987). Evidence that pyrrole formation is a pathogenic step in γ-diketone neuropathy. Toxicol Appl Pharmacol 87:351–62.

Glass JD, Griffin JW (1991). Neurofilament redistribution in transected nerves: evidence for bidirectional transport of neurofilaments. J Neurosci 11:3146–54.

Gold BG (1987). The pathophysiology of proximal neurofilamentous giant axonal swellings: implications for the pathogenesis of amyotrophic lateral sclerosis. Toxicology 46:125–39.

Graham DG, Anthony DC, Bockelheide K (1982). In vitro and in vivo studies of the molecular pathogenesis of n-hexane neuropathy. Neurobehav Toxicol Teratol 4:629–34.

Graham DG, Szakal Quin G, Priest JW, Anthony DC (1984). In vitro evidence that covalent cross-linking of neurofilaments occurs in diketone neuropathy. Proc Natl Acad Sci USA 81:4979–82.

Griffin JW, Anthony DC, Fahnestock KE, Hoffman PN, Graham DG (1984). 3,4-Dimethyl 2,5-hexanedione impairs the axonal transport of neurofilament proteins. J Neurosci 4:1516–26.

Griffin JW, Fahnestock KE, Price DL, Cork LC (1983a). Cytoskeletal disorganization induced by local application of β,β′-iminodinitropropionitrile and 2,5-hexanedione. Ann Neurol 14:55–61.

Griffin JW, Fahnestock KE, Price DL, Hoffman PN (1983b). Microtubule-neurofilament segregation produced by β,β′-iminodipropionitrile: evidence for the association of fast axonal transport with microtubules. J Neurosci 3:557–66.

Griffin JW, Hoffman PN, Clark AW, Carroll PT, Price DL (1978). Slow axonal transport of neurofilament proteins: impairment by β,β'-iminodipropionitrile administration. Science 202:633–5.

Griffin JW, Watson DF (1988). Axonal transport in neurological disease. Ann Neurol 23:3–13.

Guru GC, Shetty KT, Shankar SK (1991). Effect of chronic ethanol ingestion on phosphate content of neurofilament proteins and neurofilament-associated protein phosphatase in rat spinal cord. Neurochem Res 16:1193–7.

Hargreaves AJ, Avila J (1985). Localization and characterization of tubulin-like proteins associated with brain mitochondria: the presence of a membrane specific isoform. J Neurochem 45:490–6.

Harry GJ, Goodrum JF, Bouldein TW, Toews AD, Morrell P (1989). Acrylamide-induced increases in deposition of axonally transported glycoproteins in rat sciatic nerve. J Neurochem 52:1240–7.

Hoffman PN, Griffin JW, Gold BG, Price DL (1985). Slowing of neurofilament transport and the radial growth of developing nerve fibers. J Neurosci 5:2920–9.

Jakobsen J, Brimijoin S, Sidenius P (1983). Axonal transport in neuropathy. Muscle Nerve 6:164–6.

Jakobsen J, Brimijoin S, Skau K, Sidenius P, Wells D (1981). Retrograde axonal transport of transmitter enzymes, fucose labelled protein, and nerve growth factor in streptozotocin diabetic rats. Diabetes 30:797–803.

Karlsson JE, Rosengren LE, Haglid KG (1991). Quantitative and qualitative alterations of neuronal and glial intermediate filaments in rat nervous system after exposure to 2,5-hexanedione. J Neurochem 57:1437–44.

Lapadula DM, Irwin RD, Suwita E, Abou Donia MB (1986). Cross linking of neurofilament proteins of rat spinal cord in vivo after administration of 2,5-hexanedione. J Neurochem 46:1843–50.

Larsen JR, Sidenius P (1989). Slow axonal transport of structural polypeptides in rat, early changes in streptozotocin diabetes, and effect of insulin treatment. J Neurochem 52:390–401.

Lasek RJ (1986). Polymer sliding in axons. J Cell Sci 5(suppl):161–79.

Lasek RJ, Metuzals J, Kaiserman Abramof IR (1983a). Cytoskeletons reconstituted in vitro indicate that neurofilaments contribute to the helical structure of axons in developing and regenerating nervous systems. New York: Alan R. Liss. pp. 1–18.

Lasek RJ, Oblinger MM, Drake PF (1983b). Molecular biology of neuronal geometry: expression of neurofilament genes influences axonal diameter. Cold Spring Harbor Symp Quant Biol 68:731–44.

Lewis SE, Nixon RA (1988). Multiple phosphorylated variants of the high molecular mass subunit of neurofilaments in axons of retinal cell neurons: characterization and evidence for their differential association with stationary and moving neurofilaments. J Cell Biol 107:2689–2701.

Lynn MP, Atkinson MB, Breuer AC (1986). Influence of translocation track on the motion of intra-axonally transported organelles in human nerve. Cell Motility Cytoskel 6:339–46.

Macioce P, Filliatreau G, Figliomeni B, Hassig R, Thiery J, Di Giamberardino L (1989). Slow axonal transport impairment of cytoskeletal proteins in streptozotocin-induced diabetic neuropathy. J Neurochem 53:1261–7.

Martz D, Lasek RJ, Brady ST, Allen RD (1984). Mitochondrial motility in axons: membranous organelles may interact with the force generating system through multiple surface binding sites. Cell Motility 4:89–101.

McLane JA (1987). Decreased axonal transport in rat nerve following acute and chronic ethanol exposure. Alcohol 4:385–9.

Medori R, Autilio-Gambetti L, Monaco S, Gambetti P (1985). Experimental diabetic neuropathy: impairment of slow transport with changes in axonal cross sectional area. Proc Natl Acad Sci USA 82:7716–20.

Medori R, Jenich H, Autilio-Gambetti L, Gambetti P (1988). Experimental diabetic neuropathy: similar changes of slow axonal transport and axonal size in different animal models. J Neurosci 8:1814–21.

Miller MS, Spencer PS (1985). The mechanisms of acrylamide axonopathy. Annu Rev Pharmacol Toxicol 25:643–66.

Miller RH, Lasek RJ, Katz MJ (1987). Preferred microtubules for vesicle transport in lobster axons. Science 235:220–2.

Monaco S, Autilio-Gambetti L, Zabel D, Gambetti P (1985). Giant axonal neuropathy: acceleration of neurofilament transport in optic axons. Proc Natl Acad Sci USA 82:920–4.

Monaco S, Wongmongkolrit T, Shearson CM, Patton A, Schaetzle B, Autilio-Gambetti L, Gambetti P, Sayre LM (1990). Giant axonopathy characterized by intermediate location of axonal enlargements and acceleration of neurofilament transport. Brain Res 519:73–81.

Moretto A, Lotti M, Sabri MI, Spencer PS (1987). Progressive deficit of retrograde axonal transport is associated with pathogenesis of di n-butyl dichlorvos axonopathy. J Neurochem 49:1515–22.

Moretto A, Sabri MI (1988). Progressive deficits in retrograde axon transport precedes degeneration of motor axons in acrylamide neuropathy. Brain Res 440:18–24.

Morin PJ, Liu N, Johnson RJ, Leeman SE, Fine RE (1991). Isolation and characterization of rapid transport vesicle subtypes from rabbit optic nerve. J Neurochem 56:415–27.

Morris J, Lasek RJ (1984). Monomer polymer equilibria in the axon: direct measurement of tubulin and actin as polymer monomer in axoplasm. Cell Biol 98:2064–76.

Nixon RA (1987). The axonal transport of cytoskeletal proteins: a reappraisal. In: Smith RS, Bisby MA, eds. Axonal transport. New York: Alan R. Liss, 175–200.

Nixon RA, Lewis SE (1986). Differential turnover of phosphate groups on neurofilament subunits in mammalian neuron in vivo. J Biol Chem 261:16298–301.

Nixon RA, Quackenbush R, Vitto A (1986). Multiple calcium activated neutral proteinases (CANP) in mouse retinal ganglion cell neurons: specificities for endogenous neuronal substrates and comparison to purified CANP. J Neurosci 6:1252–63.

Oblinger MM, Brady ST, McQuarrie IG, Lasek RJ (1987). Cytotypic differences in the protein composition of the axonally transported cytoskeleton in mammalian neurons. J Neurosci 7:453–62.

Paggi P, Lasek RJ (1984). Degradation of purified neurofilament subunits by calcium-activated neutral protease: characterization of the cleavage products. Neurochem Int 6:589–97.

Papasozomenos SC, Payne MR (1986). Actin immunoreactivity localizes with segregated microtubules and membranous organelles and in the subaxolemmal region in the β,β′-iminodipropionitrile axon. J Neurosci 6:3483–91.

Papasozomenos SC, Yoon M, Crane R, Autilio-Gambetti L, Gambetti P (1982). Redistribution of proteins of fast axonal transport following administration of β,β′-iminodipropionitrile: a quantitative autoradiographic study. J Cell Biol 95:672–5.

Parhad IM, Clark AW, Griffin JW (1987a). Effect of changes in neurofilament content on caliber of small axons: the iminodipropionitrile model. J Neurosci 7:2256–63.

Parhad IM, Clark AW, Griffin JW (1987b). The effect of impairment of slow transport on axonal caliber. In: Smith RS, Bisby MA, eds. Axonal transport. New York: Alan R. Liss, 263–77.

Petrucci TC, Macioce P, Paggi P (1991). Axonal transport kinetics and post-translational modification of synapsin I in mouse retinal ganglion cells. J Neurosci 11:2938–46.

Politis MJ, Pellegrino RG, Spencer PS (1980). Ultrastructural studies of the dying back process, V. Axonal neurofilaments accumulate at sites of 2,5-hexanedione application: evidence for nerve fiber dysfunction in experimental hexacarbon neuropathy. J Neurocytol 9:505–16.

Pyle SJ, Amarnath V, Graham DG, Anthony DC (1992). The role of pyrrole formation in the alteration of neurofilament transport induced during exposure to 2,5-hexanedione. J Neuropathol Exp Neurol 51:451–58.

Reed MC, Blum JJ (1986). Theoretical analysis of radioactivity profiles during fast axonal transport: effects of deposition and turnover. Cell Motility Cytoskel 6:620–7.

Reed MC, Venakides S, Blum JJ (1990). Approximate travelling waves in linear reaction-hyperbolic equations. SIAM J Appl Math 50:167–80.

Ritchie JM, Rogart RB (1977). The density of sodium channels in mammalian myelinated nerve fibers and the nature of the axonal membrane under the myelin sheath. Proc Natl Acad Sci USA 74:211–5.

Roberts SJ, Somero GN (1989). Properties of the interaction between phosphofructokinase and actin. Arch Biochem Biophys 269:284–94.

Sahenk Z, Brady ST (1987). Axonal tubulin and microtubules: morphologic evidence for stable regions on axonal microtubules. Cell Motility Cytoskel 8:155–64.

Sayre LM, Autilio-Gambetti L, Gambetti P (1985). Pathogenesis of experimental giant neurofilament-ous axonopathies: a unified hypothesis based on chemical modification of neurofilaments. Brain Res Rev 10:69–83.

Schlaepfer WW (1987). Neurofilaments: structure, metabolism and implications in disease. J Neuropathol Exp Neurol 46:117–29.

Schlaepfer WW, Bruce J (1990). Neurofilament proteins are distributed in a diminishing proximo-distal gradient along rat sciatic nerve. J Neurochem 55:453–60.

Schmidt RE, Plurad SB, Saffitz JE, Grabau GG, Yip HK (1985). Retrograde axonal transport of ^{125}I-nerve growth factor in rat ileal mesenteric nerves: effect of streptozotocin diabetes. Diabetes 34:1230–40.

Schroer T, Sheetz M (1990). Functions of microtubule based motors. Annu Rev Physiol 53:629–52.

Scott D, Smith KE, O'Brien BJ, Angelides KJ (1985). Characterization of mammalian neurofilament triplet proteins. J Biol Chem 260:10736–47.

Shaw G (1991). Neurofilament Proteins. In: Burgoyne RD, ed. The neuronal cytoskeleton. New York: Wiley-Liss, 185–214.

Sheetz MP, Martenson CN (1991). Axonal transport: beyond kinesin and cytoplasmic dynein. Curr Opin Neurobiol 1:393–8.

Shpetner HS, Vallee RB (1989). Identification of dynamin, a novel mechanochemical enzyme that mediates interactions between microtubules. Cell 59:421–32.

Sickles DW (1989a). Toxic neurofilamentous axonopathies and fast anterograde axonal transport. I. The effects of single doses of acrylamide on the rate and capacity of transport. Neurotoxicology 10:91–102.

Sickles DW (1989b). Toxic neurofilamentous axonopathies and fast axonal transport. II. The affects of single doses of neurotoxic and non-neurotoxic diketones and iminodiproprionitrile (IDPN) on the rate and capacity of transport. Neurotoxicology 10:103–12.

Sidenius P, Nagel P, Larsen JR, Boye N, Laurberg P (1987). Axonal transport of slow component a in sciatic nerves of hypo- and hyperthyroid rats. J Neurochem 49:1790–5.

Sihag RK, Nixon RA (1990). Phosphorylation of the amino terminal head domain of the middle molecular mass 145 kDa subunit of neurofilaments. J Biol Chem 265:4166–71.

Snyder RE (1989). Loss of material from the retrograde axonal transport system in frog sciatic nerve. J Neurobiol 20:81–94.

Spencer PS, Miller MS, Ross SM, Schwab BW, Sabri MI (1985). Biochemical mechanisms underlying primary degeneration of axons. In: Lajtha A, ed. Handbook of neurochemistry. Vol. 9. New York: Plenum Press, 31–66.

St. Clair MBG, Amarnath V, Moody MA, Anthony DC, Anderson CW, Graham DG (1988). Pyrrole oxidation and protein cross linking as necessary steps in the development of diketone neuropathy. Chem Res Toxicol 1:179–85.

Takenaka T, Kawakami T, Hikawa N, Gotoh H (1990). Axoplasmic transport of mitochondria in cultured dorsal root ganglion cells. Brain Res 528:285–90.

Tashiro T, Komiya Y (1987). Organization of cytoskeletal proteins transported in the axon. In: Smith RS, Bisby MA, eds. Axonal transport. New York: Alan R. Liss, 201–21.

Tashiro T, Komiya Y (1991). Maturation and aging of the axonal cytoskeleton: biochemical analysis of transported tubulin. J Neurosci Res 30:192–200.

Tashiro T, Kurokawa M, Komiya Y (1984). Two populations of axonally transported tubulin differentiated by their interactions with neurofilaments. J Neurochem 43:1220–5.

Toews AD, Armstrong R, Roy R, Gould RM, Morell P (1988). Deposition and transfer of axonally transported phospholipids in rat sciatic nerve. J Neurosci 8:593–601.

Toews AD, Saunders BF, Blaker WD, Morell P (1983). Differences in the kinetics of axonal transport for individual lipid classes in rat sciatic nerve. J Neurochem 40:555–62.

Toyoshima I, Yamamoto A, Satake M (1988). Processing of neurofilament proteins from perikaryal to axonal type. Neurochem Res 13:621–4.

Tytell M, Barbe MF (1987). Synthesis and axonal transport of heat shock proteins. In: Smith RS, Bisby MA, eds. Axonal transport. New York: Alan R. Liss, 473–92.

Vitadello M, Filliatreau G, Dupont JL, Hassig R, Gorio A, Di Giamberardino L (1983). Altered axonal transport of cytoskeletal proteins in the mutant diabetic mouse. J Neurochem 45:860–8.

Vlassara H, Brownlee M, Cerami A (1981). Nonenzymatic glycosylation of peripheral nerve protein in diabetes mellitus. Proc Natl Acad Sci USA 70:5190–2.

Walsh JL, Knull HR (1988). Heteronomous interactions among glycolytic enzymes and of glycolytic enzymes with actin: effects of poly (ethylene glycol). Biochem Biophys Acta 952:83–91.

Watson DF, Griffin JW, Fittro KP, Hoffmann PN (1989). Phosphorylation-dependent immunoreactivity of neurofilaments increases during axonal maturation and iminodipropionitrile intoxication. J Neurochem 53:1818–29.

Wood JG, Jean DH, Whitaker JM, McLaughlin BJ, Albers RW (1977). Immunocytochemical localization of the sodium potassium activated ATPase in knifefish brain. J Neurocytol 6:571–81.

Zalewska T, Kanje M, Edstrom A (1986). A calcium activated neutral protease in the frog nervous system which degrades rapidly transported axonal proteins. Brain Res 381:58–62.

6
Axonopathy

Ram P. Gupta and Mohamed B. Abou-Donia
Duke University Medical Center
Durham, North Carolina

AXONOPATHY

The fundamental unit of the nervous system is the nerve cell, or neuron. While neurons have many of the same structural features and cellular organelles found in other cells of the body, they are unique in that they also have axons and dendrites. Neurotransmitters, after synthesis in the neuronal perikaryon, travel through the axon and are secreted at the synapses. These specialized chemical messengers interact with other neurons through the dendrites and participate in communication processes. Axons and dendrites transport in both directions cytoskeletal proteins (e.g., neurofilaments, tubulin, microtubule associated proteins (MAPs)), enzymes, and many other proteins that are essential for the maintenance of the axon and the cell body. Unlike dendrites, the axon of the cell is a single fiber and carries impulses to other parts of the nervous system, muscle fibers, or secretory cells.

Although all cells of the body can be adversely affected by toxic substances, the nervous system is particularly vulnerable because of its special functions and its low turnover (very limited capacity to regenerate). Many industrial chemicals, pesticides, foods, food additives, therapeutic drugs, and metals have been found to be neurotoxic and to result in axonopathy. Toxic substances can alter both the structure and the function of the cells. Structural changes include damage to the cell body or subcellular organelles within it (neuropathy), damage to the axons (axonopathy), or damage to the myelin sheaths (myelinopathy). However, neuropathy is also used as a general term denoting functional disturbances or pathological changes in the peripheral nervous system. Besides neurotoxic agents, certain drugs, diseases, malnutrition, and genetic defects also produce axonopathy in experimental animal and human subjects.

PROXIMAL AXONOPATHY

Proximal axonopathy is characterized by accumulation of neurofilaments close to the cell body and results in axonal swellings in the first proximal internodes of large sensory and motor axons. This is produced by certain heritable factors (Asbury, 1979) or chronic exposure to neurotoxic chemicals (Griffin et al., 1983). β,β'-Iminodipropionitrile (IDPN) induces accumulation of neurofilaments in the proximal part and depletion in the distal parts of axons (Griffin et al., 1983). However, there is no degeneration of neurons in IDPN-treated rats. Aluminum salts and 3,4-dimethyl-2,5-hexanedione also produce accumulation in proximal axons, but differ from IDPN in that they also cause degeneration of nerve cells (Banks and Kastin, 1989, Sayre et al., 1985). It was originally believed that proximal axonopathy and distal axonopathy were manifestations of two mutually exclusive pathogenetic mechanisms. Distal axonopathy comprises accumulation of neurofilaments in the distal parts of axons. Later studies, however, showed that substitution of methyl groups in 2,5-hexanedione, forming 3-methyl-2,5-hexanedione and 3,4-dimethyl-2,5-hexanedione, resulted in accumulation of neurofilaments closer to the cell body. Thus 3,4-dimethyl-2,5-hexanedione treatment had an effect similar to that of treatment with IDPN (Sayre et al., 1985).

β,β'-Iminodipropionitrile

Injection of IDPN (Fig. 1) into a variety of animal species produces a characteristic syndrome consisting of hyperactivity, lateral and vertical head and neck movements, random circling, increased locomotor activity, and increased startle response. This syndrome has been designated ECC syndrome (excitation, circling, and choreiform head and neck movements) (Selye, 1957). Rats administered 0.05% IDPN in drinking water for 2 months exhibit the intoxication symptoms described above. Histochemical studies using monoclonal antibodies show enhanced immunostaining of enlarged axons, large spheroids in the spinal cord, and dorsal root ganglia of intoxicated animals. Similarly, immunoblotting analysis reveals enrichment of the three neurofilament proteins NF-H, NF-M, and NF-L in the homogenates of dorsal root ganglia and of proximal motor and dorsal nerve roots, and depletion of all three NFs in distal nerve roots and in sciatic nerves (Carden et al., 1987). Immunoblots show uniform increase in three neurofilament proteins in the aggregates without change in their ratio or state of phosphorylation, suggesting that alteration in the phosphorylation state of neurofilaments is not required for their accumulation in proximal axons (Carden et al., 1987).

Gold and Austin (1991) studied the effect of a single injection of IDPN (2 g/kg) followed by 0.1% IDPN in drinking water or by tap water alone. The number of dorsal root ganglion (DRG) cells immunostained with monoclonal antibodies against phosphorylated NFs (anti-pNF) increased in 1–5 days, and the increase was maintained in animals given continuous IDPN treatment but was followed by a significant decrease in 3–5 weeks in the group given a single injection of IDPN (Gold and Austin, 1991). Neuropathological lesions include axonal swelling of unmyelinated axons with little change occurring in the perikaryon in the brain stem. Axonal swelling is also observed in the proximal axons of the cervical and lumbar spinal cord, accompanied by occasional axonal degeneration in high-dose males (Schulze and Boysen, 1991). Quick-freeze, deep-etch electron microscopy

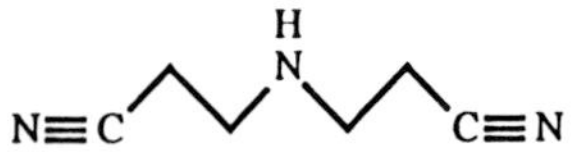

Figure 1   Structure of β,β'-iminodipropinoitrile (IDPN).

shows that microtubles form bundles in the central region of axons, that neurofilaments are segregated to the periphery, and that most membrane-bound organelles are associated with microtubules and not with neurofilaments (Hirokawa et al., 1985).

Some of the metabolites of IDPN have also been studied for their neurotoxicity. The metabolite dehydro-IDPN (Fig. 2) produces only occasional temporary hind limb paralysis in rats, with no symptoms of permanent effect at a dose 50% higher than standard. However, the metabolite hydroxy-IDPN (HOIDPN) (Fig. 2) consistently produces behavioral and neuropathological effects at 250 mg/kg (one-eighth of the standard IDPN dose) (Jacobson et al., 1987; Morandi et al., 1987). However, the increase in the neurotoxicity of IDPN in carbon tetrachloride–treated rats (Llorens and Crofton, 1991) and the direct interaction of IDPN with neurofilaments (Eyer et al., 1989) also suggest that IDPN per se is neurotoxic.

Axonopathy induced by IDPN is associated with defective slow axonal transport. In sciatic nerves, which are rich in neurofilaments, neurofilament transport is reduced by 75–90% and tubulin and actin transport by 25–50% (Parhad et al., 1986). IDPN also retards the rate of fast anterograde axonal transport, but only at a higher dose of the chemical, 4 g/kg i.p. (Sickles, 1989a). Retrograde transport is more sensitive to IDPN intoxication, since an acute reduction in this transport is obserbed at a dose of IDPN of 2 g/kg i.p. (Fink et al., 1986).

Amyotrophiic Lateral Sclerosis

Amyotrophic lateral sclerosis (ALS) is a progressive disease of unknown etiology ultimately characterized by neuronal loss and axonal degeneration in motoneurons and consequent paralysis (Parhad et al., 1992). The major neuropathological feature of ALS is the presence of large neurofilamentous swellings in the proximal axons (Sasaki et al., 1989, 1990). Proximal axonal swellings morphologically identical to those observed in ALS are found in IDPN-treated animals. Although there is no loss of neurons or axons in these animals, the IDPN model provides an opportunity to examine the influence of provimal axonal swellings on various features of ALS, e.g., electrophysiological functions and axonal transport of cytoskeletal proteins.

DISTAL AXONOPATHY

Distal axonopathy (central-peripheral distal axonopathy, dying-back neuropathy) is the most common form of axonopathy in the central and peripheral nervous system and is ascribed to exogenous toxins (many drugs, industrial and environmental chemicals), metabolic disorders (uremia, diabetes, porphyria, endocrine disorders), deficiency of vitamins (thiamine, pyridoxine), and genetic defects. It is marked by accumulation of mainly neurofilaments (neurofilamentous axonopathy) or vesicular material and irregular microtu-

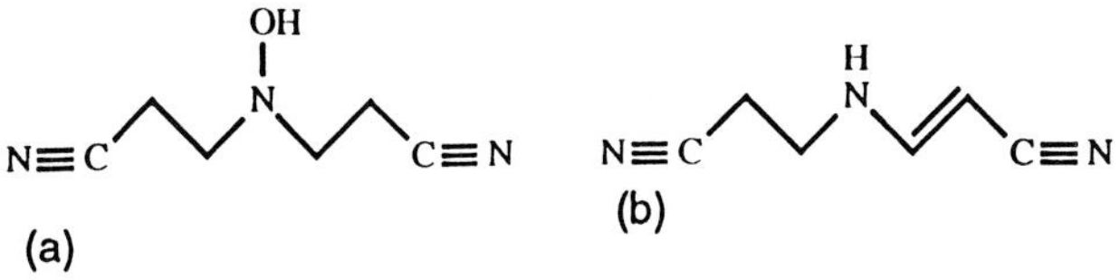

Figure 2   Structures of (a) hydroxy-IDPN (HOIDPN) and (b) dehydro-IDPN.

bules (tubulovesicular axonopathy) in the initial stages and wallerian-like degeneration after some weeks in the distal parts of axons. Wallerian degeneration consists of total degeneration of axon and myelin distal to the injury.

Neurofilamentous Axonopathy

Acrylamide

Acrylamide (Fig. 3) is an industrial chemical to which humans are exposed in grouting operations, in preparation of acrylamide gels in laboratories, and through leakage of monomers from polyacrylamide used in the purification of drinking water. The exposed workers develop numbness, limb pain, peeling of skin, and sweating of hands (Bachmann et al., 1992). Adult rats injected with acrylamide monomer (50 mg/kg, i.p.) develop hind-limb paresis, and distal motor nerve conduction velocity is decreased (Brismar et al., 1987). Similarly, rats treated with acrylamide (30 mg/kg, i.p.) for 3 weeks become unusually nervous and hyperactive toward the end of the second week (10–11 days). Their hind limbs begin to splay widely by the 10th day, and this splaying is obvious in all the animals by the 14th day of treatment. The animals progressively lose control of their hind limbs during the third and fourth weeks, and their forelimbs become ataxic. Some improvement in the movement of hind limbs is observed by the end of the fifth week, 2 weeks after the termination of treatment (Cavanagh, 1982).

Repeated exposure to acrylamide produces central-peripheral distal axonopathy in experimental animals. Widespread swelling occurs almost simultaneously in motor and sensory nerve endings in the peripheral nervous system after about 7 days of treatment with acrylamide as described above. The motor terminals become club-shaped, and sensory endings are grossly thickened (Cavanagh, 1982). Microscopic changes in acrylamide-treated animals (10 or 30 mg/kg/day orally for 5 weeks) are typical of wallerian-like degeneration and characterized by increased/decreased diameter of axons; increased variation in argyrophilia of axons; disruption, fragmentation, and distortion of axons; and dilation and fragmentation of myelin sheaths. Some sections show an increased number of macrophages. The lesions are observed in the white matter of the cervical and lumbar spinal cord; the gasserian and dorsal root ganglia; and the sciatic, tibial, and sural nerves. The most severe changes are found in the large fibers of the tibial and sural nerves of animals given high doses. Brain regions are not markedly affected (Schulze and Boysen, 1991).

Chronic administration of acrylamide produces proximal atrophy in virtually all sensory fibers of lumbar dorsal root ganglia despite the presence of some intact distal axons. Proximal atrophy of axons without degeneration of distal parts becomes more evident when animals are given a single higher dose of acrylamide (75 mg/kg, i.p.) followed by lower doses (30 mg/kg, i.p.) for 4 days. At day 5, sensory fibers in L5 dorsal root ganglia are significantly smaller in caliber and less circular up to 2 mm from the DRG, while degeneration is not present in the distal portions of either centrally (dorsal root) or

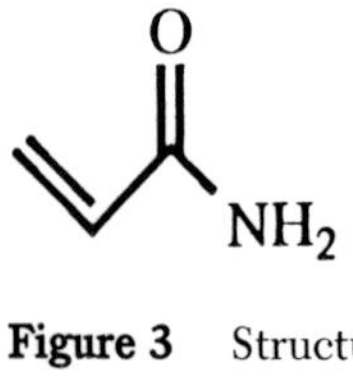

Figure 3   Structure of acrylamide.

peripherally (sciatic nerve) projecting sensory fibers (Gold et al., 1992). Electron micros-copy shows that reduction in caliber is due to decreased neurofilament content. On the other hand, primary afferent terminals in muscles of the hind feet are packed with neurofilaments. It is suggested that proximal atrophy of axons is not initiated by degeneration of distal axons, but by the inhibition of retrogradely transported target-de-rived "trophic" signal to the neuronal perikaryon (Gold et al., 1992). Acrylamide neuro-toxicity also produces changes in DRG cell bodies, and some of these alterations take place before swellings and degenerations are visible in the axons (Jones and Cavanagh, 1986).

Immunohistochemical study shows marked accumulation of 68-kDa NF in the distal part of the basket cell axons connected to the Purkinje cells. Some of the parallel fibers are also stained by anti–68-kDa NF in the molecular layer of cerebellum of acrylamide-treated rats. No difference is observed in the perikarya of nerve cells in the cerebrum of control and treated animals. Many axons are swollen and strongly immunostained for 68-kDa NF in the lumbar region of the spinal cord. The motoneurons in the spinal cord do not show any alteration in immunoreactivity to anti-NF on acrylamide treatment. The axons in the tibial nerve are also swollen segmentally and strongly stained with all three anti-NFs, particularly anti–68-kDa NF (Hashimoto et al., 1988).

Acrylamide is readily absorbed from the gastrointestinal tract on oral administration and is distributed uniformly in the body, and renal and hepatic elimination is completed in about 24 hr (Dearfield et al., 1988). Acrylamide undergoes mixed-function oxidation to form an epoxide, glycidamide (Fig. 4). Both acrylamide and glycidamide are further metabolized through conjugation with glutathione (Sumner et al., 1992). Pretreatment of rats with phenobarbital, *trans*-stilbene oxide, or dichlorodiphenyltrichloroethane (DDT) results in earlier onset of toxicity signs and subsequent development of acrylamide-induced hind-limb paralysis (Srivastava et al., 1985). The results suggest that some metabolite of acrylamide, probably glycidamide, is more neurotoxic than the parent chemical acrylamide. Recent studies have demonstrated that glycidamide produces neurotoxicity similar to that of acrylamide (Abou-Donia et al., 1993). The delaying effect of cobalt chloride pretreatment on acrylamide neurotoxicity is consistent with the above hypothesis. The direct comparison of acrylamide and glycidamide, however, shows acrylamide to be more neurotoxic than glycidamide (Costa et al., 1992), and another metabolite of acrylamide, 2-hydroxyethyl acrylate (HEA) (Fig. 4), affects weight and some behavioral measures but does not produce distal axonopathy similar to that produced by acrylamide.

An acute dose of acrylamide (75 mg/kg, i.p.) decreases neurofilament transport and subchronic treatment (30 mg/kg, i.p.) with acrylamide produces an overall increase in neurofilament transport (Gold et al., 1985). A single dose of acrylamide inhibits fast anterograde transport by 9.3–20.8%, but a greater inhibitory effect is seen in the quantity of the transported proteins (Sickles, 1989b). Retrograde transport of proteins is even more sensitive to a single dose of acrylamide (Miller and Spencer, 1984).

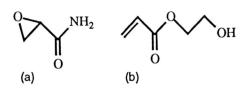

(a)   (b)

Figure 4 Structures of (a) glycidamide and (b) 2-hydroxyethyl acrylate.

Hexacarbons (n-Hexane, Methyl n-Butyl Ketone)

n-Hexane, methyl *n*-butyl ketone, 2,5-hexanedione (Fig. 5) are considered together, since the first two solvents are metabolized to 2,5-hexanedione, which is responsible for most of the neurotoxic effects of the parent chemicals. *n*-Hexane is widely used as a solvent in lacquers and glues, and as a glue thinner. The most common complaint in less severe cases is numbness of the toes and fingers, and the more severe cases involve weight loss, weakness, anorexia, abdominal pain, and cramp in the lower extremities. The patients also have difficulty in pinching, grasping objects, and stepping over curbs. Rats treated with 1% 2,5-hexanedione show signs of weakness in the hind limbs in 2 weeks and are almost paralyzed in 6 weeks (Backstrom and Collins, 1987).

Electron-microscopic examination of nerves from mild cases may not reveal any difference from control animals, but nerve samples from moderate or severe cases show paranodal giant axonal swellings accompanied by myelin retraction. These swellings consist of 10-nm-diameter neurofilaments and are identical to the abnormalities observed in experimental animals (Spencer et al., 1980). Giant axonal swellings in rats consists of 10-nm neurofilaments and, sometimes, clustered neurotubules, mitochondria, and smooth endoplasmic reticulum (Spencer and Schaumberg, 1977). Rats treated with *n*-hexane or methyl *n*-butyl ketone show swellings in the distal part of the axons on the proximal side of the nodes of Ranvier. The large myelinated fibers in tibial nerve branches exhibit multifocal giant axonal degeneration before similar changes appear in much longer plantar nerve fibers (Spencer and Schaumburg, 1976). This pattern is different from that observed with acrylamide, in which both type of fiber are equally vulnerable. The degeneration in *n*-hexane–, methyl *n*-butyl ketone–, or 2,5-hexanedione–treated rats does not begin at the distal end and proceed toward the cell perikaryon, as the term "dying back" would apply. On the contrary, degeneration is initiated by paranodal giant axonal swellings that begin in a multifocal pattern on the proximal side of multiple nodes of Ranvier (Spencer and Schaumburg, 1976).

Immunohistological studies show axonal swellings in many regions of the central, peripheral, and sympathetic nervous system, and the axonal swellings contain larger amounts of neurofilaments and lesser amounts of tubulin in comparison with control animals (Backstrom and Collins, 1987).

Hexacarbons such as *n*-hexane and methyl *n*-butyl ketone are metabolized to the neurotoxic chemical 2,5-hexanedione through intermediates such as 2-hexanol, 2,5-hexanediol, and 5-hydroxy-2-hexanone. 2,5-Hexanedione then reacts with the primary amino group of lysine in proteins and forms pyrrole (Fig. 6). The latter undergoes autooxidation and cross-links cytoskeletal proteins (Krasavage et al., 1980; Lapadula et al., 1986: DeCaprio and Fowke, 1992).

The location of accumulation of neurofilaments depends on the nature of the chemical.

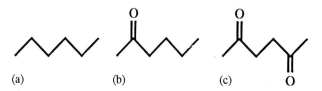

(a)   (b)   (c)

Figure 5   Structures of (a) *n*-hexane, (b) methyl *n*-butyl kenone, and (c) 2,5-hexanedione.

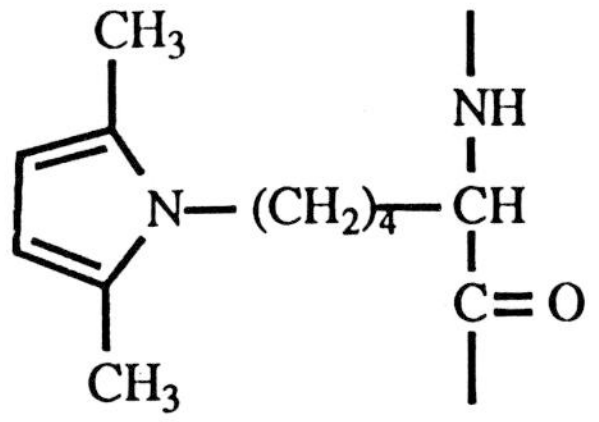

Figure 6 Structure of pyrrole adduct with protein (substituted pyrrole adduct with lysine ε-amino group of protein).

Treatment with 2,5-hexanedione or 3-methyl-2,5-hexanedione results in accummulation of neurofilaments in the distal part or midpart of the axon, respectively. There is an increase in the rate of neurofilament transport, in both cases, in the proximal region of swelling. The transport of tubulin is not altered in 2,5-hexanedione–treated rats (Monaco et al., 1989). It is suggested that an increase in the rate of neurofilament transport in the proximal axon and a progressive decline toward the distal end, with accumulation of neurofilaments in the distal part of the axon, may be responsible for atrophy of the proximal axon and axonal swelling (Monaco et al., 1989). Hexacarbon axonopathy suggests that cross-linking of neurofilaments is essential for the alteration of neurofilament transport and development of neurotoxicity, since 3-acetyl-2,5-hexanedione (AcHD), which forms pyrrole adducts more readily than 2,5-hexanedione but is unable to cross-link neurofilaments, is not able to change the rate of neurofilament transport or produce neurotoxicity (Pyle et al., 1992). It is suggested that fast anterograde and retrograde transport of proteins is associated with axonal degeneration, since IDPN, which does not change fast axonal transport, results in the accumulation of neurofilaments in the axon but not in its degeneration. 2,5-hexanedione intoxication, which is associated with the degeneration of distal axons, results in the reduction of fast anterograde axonal transport (18–25%) and, to an even greater degree, of retrograde transport (50–63%) (Sickles, 1989a). Sickles (1992) studied the roles of the neuronal perikaryon and axon in the reduction of fast axonal transport by exposing both regions of the dorsal root ganglion separately to a 2,5-hexanedione solution. The results show that exposure of the axon, not of the cell body, is required to reduce fast axonal transport.

Carbon Disulfide

Carbon disulfide is used in the production of viscose rayon fibers and cellophane films. It is also used in agriculture, as it is a major component of fumigant mixtures. Chronic exposure to low carbon disulfide levels (10–40 ppm) results in prolonged motor nerve conduction in the lower limbs, and exposure to higher levels (170 ppm) for 4–6 months produces numbness and weakness in the distal part of the lower extremities accompanied by diminished sensitivity to pin prick, touch, and vibration. Upper limbs are also involved on continued exposure (Vigliani, 1954; Vasilescu, 1972). A similar distal neuropathy is produced in experimental animals by an inhalation procedure. This is characterized by hind-limb weakness and decreased nerve conduction velocity (Knobloch et al., 1979).

Rats exposed to 800 ppm carbon disulfide (6 h/day, 5 days/week) for 90 days develop neurofilamentous axonal swellings in the distal parts of long fiber tracts of the spinal cord. There are numerous prominent swellings in the dorsal ascending sensory fibers of the cervical spinal cord. In contrast, rare swellings are seen in the dorsal corticospinal fibers in the cervical spinal cord and dorsal sensory fibers in the lumbar spinal cord. In the peripheral nervous system, the majority of changes are seen in the posterior tibial nerve. The sciatic nerve does not show axonal loss, and axonal swelling is seen only occasionally. Cross-sections of the muscular branches of the tibial nerve exhibit abundant large axonal swellings, axonal loss, and wallerian-like degeneration (Gottfried et al., 1985). The reduction in peripheral nerve conduction velocity is observed long before the appearance of histological lesions and is, therefore, a more sensitive indicator of neurotoxicity (Colombi et al., 1981). The axonal enlargements in the optic tracts of carbon disulfide–treated rats are filled with disorganized filaments with occasional mitochondria and cisterns of smooth endoplasmic reticulum (Pappolla et al., 1987). Axonal swellings in the optic tracts of carbon disulfide–treated rats have been studied by immunostaining with anti-NFs (Pappolla et al., 1987). Immunostaining shows the presence of all three NFs in axonal swellings, and NF-H is phosphorylated.

Carbon disulfide produces axonopathy similar to that produced by hexacarbons (e.g., *n*-hexane, methyl *n*-butyl ketone, and 2,5-hexanedione), but cross-linking of proteins by carbon disulfide is still debatable. DeCaprio et al. (1992) demonstrated binding of carbon disulfide to the lysine-containing dipeptide and bovine serum albumin, but no evidence was available for the intermolecular cross-linking of protein by carbon disulfide. In contrast, Valentine et al. (1992) suggested a mechanism for the cross-linking of proteins by carbon disulfide and showed cross-linking of β-lactoglobulin after incubation for 24 h or more with carbon disulfide. Thus, cross-linking of proteins may also play a role in carbon disulfide–induced axonopathy. Carbon disulfide undergoes both nonenzymatic and enzymatic transformations. Oxidation by the mixed-function oxidase system and enzymatic desulfurization of carbon disulfide yields carbonyl sulfide (COS), CO_2, and electrophilic sulfur metabolites. These metabolites probably are responsible for the hepatotoxicity of carbon disulfide. The neurotoxic effect of carbon disulfide probably also involves the direct interaction of carbon disulfide with protein molecules (DeCaprio et al., 1992). Recent studies have shown that carbon disulfide inhalation results in neurotoxicity accompanied by Ca^{2+}/calmodulin-dependent kinase–mediated phosphorylation of neurofilaments and microtubule associated proteins-2 (Wilmarth et al., 1993).

Pappolla et al. (1987) carried out morphometric and axonal transport studies in the primary visual axons of carbon disulfide–treated rats. Axonal enlargements are absent in the optic nerve. The neurofilament content of the optic tract increases in a proximodistal direction, and the cross-sectional area of the axon proximal to the enlargement is decreased. However, no detectable degeneration is visible in the optic tract. Neurofilament transport (NF-M, NF-L) is markedly accelerated as in the case of 2,5-hexanedione–induced axonopathy, while there in no significant change in the transport of tubulin. The transport of actin also shows a moderate increase. Thus carbon disulfide and 2,5-hexanedione, which have different chemical properties, produce almost identical changes in slow transport and alter axonal cytoskeleton in a similar way.

Tubulovesicular Axonopathy

Dithiocarbamates

Dithiocarbamates and thiuram compounds (Oskarsson, 1987) (Table 1) (Fig. 7) are extensively distributed in the environment. They are used in agriculture as pesticides and fungicidas, as accelerators in the rubber industry, and as bacteriostatic and disinfectant agents (Howell and Edington, 1968; Oskarsson, 1987). Chickens treated with sodium

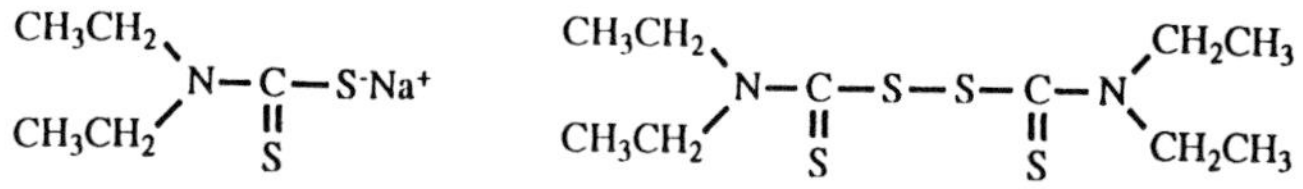

Figure 7 Structures of (a) sodium diethyldithiocarbamate and (b) tetraethylthiuram disulfide.

diethyldithiocarbamate (NaDDC) (Fig. 7) show marked degeneration of nerve fibers in the cerebellum, medulla, and spinal cord. Morphological changes are observed in the nerve fibers of ventral and lateral columns at different locations in the spinal cord. In contrast, the dorsal columns of the spinal cord are rarely affected. A well-defined tract of degenerated nerve fibers is found at the periphery of the medulla of all chickens. The damaged areas consist of ballooned myelin sheaths and eosinophilic swollen axons. Some swollen axons and fragmenting myelin sheaths are also seen in sections from the median, radial, and sciatic nerves of NaDDC-treated chickens (Howell and Edington, 1968). There is extensive damage to nerve fibers in the central nervous system, associated with wallerian-like degeneration rather than primary demyelination. The distrubition of lesions is similar to that observed in tri-*o*-cresyl phosphate (TOCP)-treated chickens and in chronic thiamine deficiency in pigeons.

Rasul and Howell (1973) studied the neurotoxic effects of NaDDC on 1-week-old and adult chickens. Chicks show lesions in the spinal cord after 18 weeks and ataxia after 25 weeks of treatment. Adult chickens, on the other hand, show lesions in 4 weeks and ataxia in 5 weeks. The nature of the lesions is, however, the same in both groups and consists of degeneration of long tracts of the spinal cord. The degenerated nerve fibers are visible in the adult cocks killed even 3 weeks after the termination of treatment, suggesting that irreversible metabolic disturbances are initiated in some neurons during the period of NaDDC treatment. However, the number of degenerated fibers decreases when the birds are allowed to survive for some time after 8 weeks of treatment (Rasul and Howell, 1974).

Organophosphorus Compounds

Organophosphorus compounds are widely used in agriculture and industry. Most of them have anticholinesterase activity, and those having a neurotoxic effect also inhibit neuropathy target enzyme (NTE). Neurotoxic organophosphorus compounds such as tri-*o*-cresyl phosphate (TOCP) (Fig. 8) are capable of producing neuropathy in humans (Smith et al., 1930; Abou-Donia et al., 1986) and in sensitive animals, and the signs of

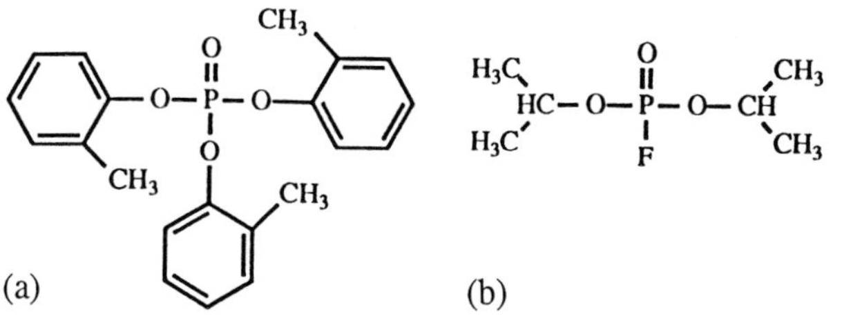

Figure 8 Structures of (a) tri-*o*-cresyl phosphate and (b) diisopropyl phosphorofluoridate.

neuropathy (e.g., ataxia, paralysis) appear in humans after several weeks of exposure. This has been designated organophosphorus compound–induced delayed neurotoxicity (OPIDN) and can be produced in 6–14 days after a single dose of the neurotoxic organophosphorus compounds TOCP (Patton et al., 1986) and diisopropyl phosphorofluoridate (DFP) (Fig. 8) (Carrington and Abou-Donia, 1988; Carrington et al., 1988). The disease is characterized by ataxia and paralysis, and neuropathologic lesions are seen as wallerian-type degeneration in the distal parts of large-diameter and long central and peripheral nerves (Cavanagh, 1964a,b; Abou-Donia et al., 1983, 1986b). Histopathological studies in cats show degeneration in the ascending tracts of the upper cervical levels and descending tracts of the lumbosacral spinal cord. The extent of damage depends on the dose of chemical and sensitivity of the animal species.

Electron microscopy reveals abnormal membranes arranged as vesicles, irregular tubules, and flattened cisterns in the mildly affected fibers (Prineas, 1969). The plasma membranes of the axons appears less clearly defined and somewhat irregular in the treated animals. In the severely affected animals, the axoplasm is generally rarefied and contains a few normal or abnormal constituents and finely granular material. Sometimes, severely degenerated fibers show compact masses of degenerated mitochondria, membranes, dense bodies, fine granular material, and aggregates of electron-dense particles. Myelin degeneration is seen only in severely affected axons (Prineas, 1969).

Saligenin cyclic-o-tolyl phosphate (Fig. 9) is the active metabolite of TOCP that is suggested as being responsible for the neurotoxic effects of TOCP. Saligenin cyclic-o-tolyl phosphate concentration is relatively low in tissue, probably because of its instability and high activity (Nomeir and Abou-Donia, 1984). TOCP is absorbed faster in rats than in chickens, a species sensitive to OPIDN. The peak level of ^{14}C from labeled TOCP is reached in most tissues in 12 h in rats and in 24 h in chickens. At this time (24 h), chicken brain, spinal cord, and sciatic nerve have 1.95-, 1.05-, and 1.22-fold ^{14}C radioactivity, respectively, as compared with rat tissues (Abou-Donia et al., 1986a). The rate of disappearance of TOCP is also slower in the chicken than in the rat, and that may contribute to the sensitivity of chickens to delayed neurotoxicity.

Organophosphorus compound–induced delayed neuropathy has been classified as type I and type II, depending on the characteristics of the neuropathy produced in the treated animals. For example, triphenyl phosphite (TPP) treatment produces axonal damage in the lateral columns of the spinal cord and peripheral nerves similar to that produced by TOCP or DFP (type I compounds). However TPP (type II) treatment also causes damage to axons in the brain and the gray matter of the spinal cord that is not observed in type II delayed neuropathy induced by TOCP and DFP (Carrington and Abou-Donia, 1988; Abou-Donia and Lapadula, 1990). Furthermore, type II OPIDN seems to have a shorter latent period than type I.

Fast and slow axonal transport has been studied in different species treated with organophosphorus compounds. Diisopropyl phosphorofluoridate and TOCP do not alter

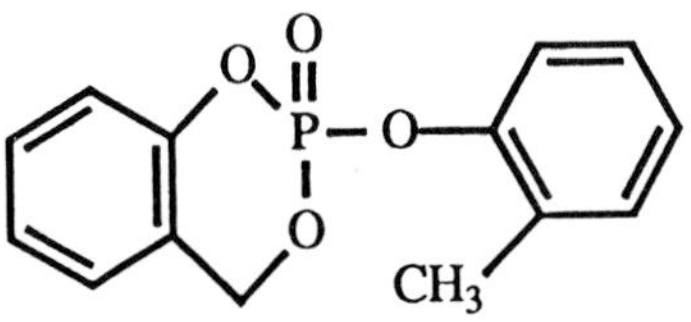

Figure 9   Structure of saligenin cyclic-o-tolyl phosphate.

slow axonal transport in chickens and cats, respectively (James and Austin, 1970; Pleasure et al. 1969). The effect on fast axonal transport is controversial, however, and increase, decrease, and no effect on fast transport have been reported by different investigators (Carrington et al., 1989; Bradley and Williams, 1973; James and Austin, 1970).

Diabetes and Hypoglycemia

Neuropathy contributes to increased morbidity and mortality in diabetic patients. It involves peripheral sensory and motor nerves, autonomic nerves, and often cranial nerves. Studies of streptozocin-induced diabetes show reduction in myelinated fiber size at both proximal and distal levels of peripheral nerves. The axonal atrophy seems to be more severe in the distal portions. The axonal atrophy is ascribed to the loss of neurofilaments in the axon. It is not clear whether the decrease in neurofilament is due to decrease in synthesis or supply of neurofilaments (Yagihashi et al., 1990). Britland and Sharma (1990) studied the development of proximal and distal nerves of control and streptozocin-diabetic rats. Experimental diabetes impairs the maturation of the sural nerve, and the effect is more severe in the proximal than in the distal part. The findings do not support the previous suggestions that experimental diabetes is mainly a dying-back axonopathy. Besides diabetes, hypoglycemia is also known to cause degeneration of axonal nerve fibers. However, hypoglycemia should be severe (< 1.5 mmol/L) and of long duration (≥ 12 hr) to induce axonopathy in animals (Yasaki and Dyck, 1991). Furthermore, peripheral nerves are more vulnerable to prolonged severe hypoglycemia in younger rats than in older rats (Yasaki and Dyck, 1990), since axonal degeneration is not inducible in older rats under the conditions described above. Axonal degeneration in hypoglycemic animals is not typical of distal polyneuropathy but of a focal or multifocal nature.

Acquired Immunodeficiency Syndrome

A variety of central and peripheral nervous system disorders have been reported in adults and children with the acquired immunodeficiency syndrome (AIDS). Axonal degeneration in the sural nerve and reduced conduction velocity in both motor and sensory nerves are observed even in patient with AIDS without symptoms or signs of peripheral neuropathy (Fuller et al., 1991). There is reduction in the density of myelinated fibers principally affecting the larger fibers. Patients with AIDS or AIDS-related complex show 1.) distal, predominantly sensory, peripheral neuropathy, 2.) chronic inflammatory demyelinating polyneuropathy, or 3.) acute inflammatory demyelinating polyneuropathy when examined by electrophysiological methods or nerve biopsy (Leger et al., 1989). Axonal degeneration and decrease in axonal population has been documented in the majority of patients with AIDS (Tenhula et al., 1992). Infants and children with AIDS show pathological changes predominantly in the corticospinal tract. There is a decrease in the number of axons, and axons are poorly myelinated. The deep cerebral white matter is attenuated, and in some cases there is marked infiltration of inflammatory and multinucleated giant cells (Dickson et al., 1989).

Hereditary Disorders

Several genetic disorders are known to be responsible for various forms of neuropathy, such as familial amyloid polyneuropathy, hereditary spastic paraparesis, hereditary distal spinal muscular atrophy, and X-linked dominant hereditary neuropathy. Familial amyloid polyneuropathy is classified into at least seven subtypes, and type I is the most common (Sobue et al., 1990). Distally accentuated axonal loss and marked axonal sprouting is the most prominent feature. The myelinated fiber population is severely diminished in the spinal nerves, and myelinated fibers are almost completely absent in the sciatic and tibial nerves. In hereditary spastic paraparesis, degeneration of the corticospinal tract decreases from the lower lumbar to cervical spinal cord, and degeneration of the posterior columns decreases from the upper cervical to lumbar spinal cord. There is also about 50% degeneration of spinocerebellar tracts in this disease (Bruyn, 1992). Patients with hereditary distal spinal muscular atrophy complain of pain in the upper legs, and a progressive motor weakness of the lower legs and feet is found in these patients (Frequin et al., 1991). Motor and sensory nerve conduction velocity and electromyography of the examined nerves are normal in this disease, and teased-fibers analysis also does not show any abnormality. However, axonal atrophy is indicated by too much thickness of some myelin sheaths in comparison with the axon diameter. An accumulation of mitochondrial, vesicular, and lamellar structure is also seen at the nodes of Ranvier and other areas. Axonal degeneration or demyelination is, however, not detectable in hereditary distal spinal muscular atrophy. X-linked dominant hereditary motor and sensory neuropathy is another form of hereditary neuropathy (Hahn et al., 1990). Males are more severely affected in this disease than females. Electrophysiological studies show substantial loss of distal motor and sensory nerves, and nerve biopsies demonstrate loss of myelinated and unmyelinated fibers, regenerating fibers, and secondary demyelination.

Drugs

A large number of drugs have been implicated in peripheral neuropathy. Neuropathy is the dose-limiting factor in the treatment with some drugs, such as vinca alkaloids (Olesen and Jensen, 1991). However, neuropathy is a rare complication of drug therapy. Drug-induced neuropathy is almost always dose-dependent, and the use of such drugs is restricted in patients with a risk of developing neuropathy. Thus, taxol produced predominantly sensory axonopathy in 16 of 60 patients in one study (Lipton et al., 1989). However, neuropathy is produced only at doses above 200 mg/m^2. The electrophysiological data suggested taxol-induced axonal degeneration and demyelination in these patients. Some other drugs that produce axonopathy are cyclosporine (Stanley and Pender, 1991), cisplatin (Cavaletti et al., 1992), methotrexate (Shibutani et al., 1989; Shibutani and Okeda, 1989), and D-amphetamine (Ryan et al., 1990; Molliver et al. 1990). Each of these drugs, however, produces neuropathy with characteristic symptoms because of their distinct modes of interaction with the central and peripheral nervous system. Some drugs produce axonopathy mainly by axonal demyelination rather than degeneration (e.g., cyclosporine).

Vitamin Deficiency and Protein-Calorie Undernutrition

Although thiamine (vitamin B$_1$) deficiency is generally associated with alcoholism, a thiamine-poor diet alone can also cause damage to the nervous system. Degeneration of long and large myelinated nerve fibers is consistenly observed in thiamine-deficient pigeons (Swank, 1940; Prineas, 1970). Disorders of peripheral nerves are also produced by deficiency of riboflavin (vitamin B$_2$), niacin (nicotinic acid, vitamin B$_3$), pyridoxine (vitamin B$_6$) and vitamin E (derivatives of tocol and tocotrienol). Vitamin deficiencies may occur as a result of some diseases, malabsorption, reaction with certain drugs, or destruction of vitamins during processing of food (Victor, 1975; Pallis and Lewis, 1974; Southam et al., 1991). The predominant morphological change in vitamine E–deficient rats is axonal dystrophy and degeneration in the rostral parts of the dorsal columns. Dystrophic changes consist of focal axonal swellings containing tubulovesicular structures. The latter are probably derived from smooth endoplasmic reticulum, mitochondria, dense lamellar bodies, neurofilaments, multifascicular bodies, and lysosomes (Southam et al., 1991).

Malnutrition is worldwide problem, and protein or protein-calorie undernutrition retards the growth of the central nervous system in the early part of life. Histological studies have shown reduced diameter of myelinated nerve fibers, retardation of myelination, segmental demyelination and remyelination, axonal degeneration, and shortened longitudinal growth of internodes. Motor and sensory nerve conduction are significantly impaired in children with protein-calorie undernutrition as well as in animals subjected to protein or protein-calorie deficiency (Chopra, 1991).

REFERENCES

Abou-Donia MB, Ibrahim SM, Corcoran JJ, Lack L, Friedman M, Lapadula DM (1993). Neurotoxicity of glycidamide, an acrylamide metabolite, following intraperitoneal injections in rats. J Toxicol Environ Health 39:101–18.

Abou-Donia MB, Jensen DN, Lapadula DM (1983). Neurologic manifestations of tri-*o*-cresyl phosphate delayed neurotoxicity in cats. Neurobehav Toxicol Teratol 5:431–42.

Abou-Donia MB, Lapadula DM (1990). Mechanisms of organophosphorus ester–induced delayed neurotoxicoty: type I and type II. Annu Rev Toxicol 30:405–40.

Abou-Donia MB, Suwita E, Nomeir AA (1986a). Absorption, distribution, and elimination of a single oral dose of [^{14}C]tri-*o*-cresyl phosphate in hens. Toxicology 61:13–25.

Abou-Donia MB, Trofatter LP, Graham DG, Lapadula DM (1986). Electromyographic, neuropathologic, and functional correlates in the cat as the result of tri-*o*-cresyl phosphate delayed neurotoxicity. Toxicol Appl Pharmacol 83:126–41.

Bachmann M, Myers JE, Bezuidenhout BN (1992). Acrylamide monomer and peripheral neuropathy in chemical workers. Am J Indus Med 21:217–22.

Backstrom B, Collins VP (1987). Cytoskeletal changes in axons of rats exposed to 2,5-hexanediol, demonstrated using monoclonal antibodies. Neurotoxicology 8:85–96.

Banks WA, Kastin AJ (1989). Aluminum-induced neurotoxicity: alterations in membrane function at the blood-brain barrier. Neurosci Behav Rev 13:47–53.

Bradley WG, Williams MH (1973). Axoplasmic flow in axonal neuropathies. I. Axoplasmic flow in cats with toxic neuropathies. Brain 96:235–46.

Brismar T, Hildebrand C, Tegner R (1987). Nodes of Ranvier in acrylamide neuropathy: voltage and electron microscopic analysis of rat sciatic nerve fibers at proximal levels. Brain Res 423:135–43.

Britland S, Sharma A (1990). A new perspective on myelinated nerve fiber pathology in experimental diabetes. Diabetes Res 5:69–75.

Bruyn RPM (1992). The neuropathology of hereditary spastic paraparesis. Clin Neurol Neurosurg 94(suppl):S16–18.

Carden MJ, Goldstein ME, Bruce J, Cooper HS, Schlaepfer WW (1987). Studies of neurofilaments that accumulate in proximal axons of rats intoxicated with β,β′-iminodipropionitrile (IDPN). Neurochem Pathol 7:189–205.

Carpenter, S (1968). Proximal axonal enlargement in motor neuron Disease. Neurology 18:841–51.

Carrington CD, Abou-Donia MB (1988). Triphenyl phosphite neurotoxicity in the hen: inhibition of neurotoxic esterase and of prophylaxis by phenylmenthylsulfonyl fluoride. Arch Toxicol 62:375–80.

Carrington CD, Brown HR, Abou-Donia MB (1988). Histopathological assessment of triphenyl phosphite neurotoxicity in the hen. Neurotoxicology 9:223–34.

Carrington CD, Lapadula DM, Abou-Donia MB (1989). Acceleration of anterograde axonal transport in cat sciatic nerve by diisopropyl phosphorofluoridate. Brain Res 476:179–82.

Cavaletti G, Tredici G, Marmiroli P, Petruccioli MG, Barajon I, Fabbrica D (1992). Morphometric study of the sensory neuron and peripheral nerve changes induced by chronic cisplatin (DDP) administration in rats. Acta Neuropathol 84:364–71.

Cavanagh JB (1964a). The significance of the "dying back" process in experimental animals and human neurological disease. Int Rev Exp Pathol 3:219–67.

Cavanagh JB (1964b). Peripheral nerve changes in ortho-cresyl phosphate poisoning in the cat. J Pathol Bacteriol 87:365–83

Cavanagh JB (1982). The pathokinetics of acrylamide intoxication: a reassessment of the problem. Neuropathol Appl Neurobiol 8:315–36.

Chopra JS (1991). Neurological consequences of protein and protein-calorie undernutrition. Crit Rev Neurobiol 6:99–117.

Colombi A, Maroni M, Picchi O, Rota E, Castano P, Foa V (1981). Carbon disulfide neuropathy in rats. A morphological and ultrastructural study of degeneration and regeneration. Clin Toxicol 18:1463–74.

Costa LG, Deng H, Gregotti C, Manzo L, Faustman EM, Bergmark E, Calleman CJ (1992). Comparative studies on the neuro- and reproductive toxicity of acrylamide and its epoxide metabolite glycidamide in the rat. Neurotoxicology 13:219–24.

Dearfield KL, Abernathy CO, Ottley MS, Brantner JH, Hayes PF (1988). Acrylamide: its metabolism, developmental and reproductive effects, genotoxicity, and carcinogenicity. Mut Res 195:45–77.

DeCaprio AP, Spink DC, Chen X, Fowke JH, Zhu M, Bank S (1992). Characterization of isothiocyanates, thioureas, and other lysine adduction products in carbon disulfide–treated peptides and protein. Chem Res Toxicol 5:496–504.

DeCaprio AP, Fowke JH (1992). Limited and selective adduction of carboxyl-terminal lysines in the high molecular weight neurofilament proteins by 2,5-hexanedione in vitro. Brain Res 586:219–28.

Delio DA, Fiori MG, Sharer LR, Lowndes HE (1985). Evolution of axonal swellings in cats intoxicated with β,β'-iminodipropionitrile (IDPN). Exp Neurol 87:235–48.

Dickson DW, Belman AL, Kim TS, Horoupian DS, Rubinstein A (1989). Spinal cord pathology in pediatric acquired immunodeficiency syndrome. Neurology 39:227–35.

Eyer J, Mclean WG, Leterrier J-F (1989). Effect of a single dose of β,β'-iminodipropionitrile in vivo on the properties of neurofilaments in vitro: comparison with the effect of iminodipropionitrile added directly to neurofilaments in vitro. J Neurochem 52:1759–65.

Fink DJ, Purkiss D, Mata M (1986). β,β'-Iminodipropionitrile impairs retrograde axonal transport. J Neurochem 47:1032–8.

Frequin STFM, Gabreels FJM, Gabreels-festen AAWM, Joosten EMG (1991). Sensory axonopathy in hereditary distal spinal muscular atrophy. Clin Neurol Neurosurg 93:323–6.

Fuller GN, Jacobs JM, Guiloff RJ (1991). Subclinical peripheral nerve involvement in AIDS: an electrophysiological and pathological study. J Neurol Neurosurg Psychiatry 54:318–24.

Gold BG, Austin DR (1991). Regulation of aberrant neurofilament phosphorylation in neuronal perikarya. III. Alterations following single and continuous β,β'-iminodipropionitrile administrations. Brain Res 563:151–62.

Gold BG, Griffin JW, Price DL (1985). Slow axonal transport in acrylamide neuropathy: different abnormalities produced by single-dose and continuous administration. J Neurosci 5:1755–68.

Gold BG, Griffin JW, Price DL (1992). Somatofugal axonal atrophy precedes development of axonal degeneration in acrylamide neuropathy. Arch Toxicol 66:57–66.

Gottfried MR, Graham DG, Morgan M, Casey HW, Bus JS (1985). The morphology of carbon disulfide neurotoxicity. Neurotoxicology 6(4):89–96.

Griffin JW, Fahnestock KE, Price DL, Cork LC (1983). Cytoskeletal disorganization induced by local application of β,β'-iminodipropionitrile and 2,5-hexanedione. Ann Neurol 14:55–61.

Hahn AF, Brown WF, Koopman WJ, Feasby TE (1990). X-linked dominant hereditary motor and sensory neuropathy. Brain 113:1511–25.

Hashimoto K, Kurosaka Y, Tanii H, Hayashi M (1988). Immunochemical studies of acrylamide-associated neuropathology. Toxicology 49:65–9.

Hirokawa N, Bloom GS, Vallee RB (1985). Cytoskeletal architecture and immunocytochemical localization of microtubule-associated proteins in regions of axons associated with rapid axonal transport: the β,β′-iminodipropionitrile-intoxicated axons as a model system. J Cell Biol 101:227–39.

Howell JM, Edington N (1968). The neurotoxicity of sodium diethyldithiocarbamate in the hen. J Neuropathol Exp Neurol 27:464–72.

Jacobson AR, Coffin SH, Shearson CM, Sayre LM (1987). β,β′-Iminodipropionitrile (IDPN) neurotoxicity: a mechanistic hypothesis for toxic activation. Mol Toxicol 1:17–34.

James KA, Austin L (1970). The effect of DFP on axonal transport of protein in chicken sciatic nerve. Brain Res 18:192–4.

Jones HB, Cavanagh JB (1986). The axon reaction in spinal ganglion neurons of acrylamide-treated rats. Acta Neuropathol (Berlin) 71:55–63.

Knobloch K, Stetkiewicz J, Wronska-Nofer T (1979). Conduction velocity in the peripheral nerves of rats with chronic carbon disulfide neuropathy. Br J Ind Med 36:148–52.

Krasavage WJ, O'Donoghue JL, DiVincenzo GD, Terhaar CJ (1980). The relative neurotoxicity of methyl n-butyl ketone, n-hexane and their metabolites. Toxicol Appl Pharmacol 52:433–41.

Lapadula DM, Irwin RD, Suwita E, Abou-Donia MB (1986). Cross-linking of neurofilament proteins of rat spinal cord in vivo after administration of 2,5-hexanedione. J Neurochem 46:1843–50.

Leger JM, Bouche P, Bolgert F, Chaunu MP, Rosenheim M, Cathala HP, Gentilini M, Hauw JJ, Brunet P (1989). The spectrum of polyneuropathies in patients infected with HIV. J Neurol Neurosurg Psychiatry 52:1369–74.

Lipton RB, Apfel SC, Dutcher JP, Rosenberg R, Kaplan J, Berger, A, Einzig AI, Wiernik P, Schaumberg HH (1989). Taxol produces a predominantly sensory neuropathy. Neurology 39:368–73.

Llorens J, Crofton KM (1991). Enhanced neurotoxicity of 3,3′-iminodipropionitrile following carbon tetrachloride pretreatment in the rat. Neurotoxicity 12:583–94.

Miller MS, Spencer PS (1984). Single doses of acrylamide reduce retrograde transport velocity. J Neurochem 43:1401–8.

Molliver ME, Berger UV, Mamounas LA, Molliver DC, O'Hearn E, Wilson MA (1990). Neurotoxicity of MDMA and related compounds: anatomic studies. Ann NY Acad Sci 600:649–61.

Monaco S, Autilio-Gambetti L, Lasek RJ, Katz MJ, Gambetti P (1989). Experimental increase of neurofilament transport rate: decrease in neurofilament number and in axon diameter. J Neuropathol Exp Neurol 48:23–32.

Morandi A, Gambetti P, Arora PK, Sayre LM (1987). Mechanism of neurotoxic action of β,β′-iminodipropionitrile (IDPN): N-hydroxylation enhances neurotoxic potency. Brain Res 437:69–76.

Nomeir AA, Abou-Donia MB (1984). Disposition of [^{14}C]tri-o-cresyl phosphate and its metabolites in various tissues of the male cat following a single dermal application. Drug Metab Dispos 12:705–11.

Olesen LL, Jensen TS (1991). Prevention and management of drug-induced peripheral neuropathy. Drug Safety 6:302–14.

Oskarsson A (1987). Comparative effects of ten dithiocarbamate and thiuram compounds on tissue distribution and excretion of lead in rats. Environ Res 44:82–93.

Pallis CA, Lewis PD (1974). The neurology of gastrointestinal disease. Philadelphia: W.B. Saunders.

Pappolla M, Penton R, Weiss HS, Miller CH Jr, Sahenk Z, Autilio-Gambetti L, Gambetti P (1987). Carbon disulfide axonopathy: another experimental model characterized by acceleration of neurofilament transport and distinct changes of axonal size. Brain Res 424:272–80.

Parhad IM, Griffin JW, Hoffman PN, Koves JF (1986). Selective interruption of axonal transport of neurofilament proteins in the visual system by β,β′-iminodipropionitrile (IDPN) intoxication. Brain Res 363:315–24.

Parhad IM, Oishi R, Clark AW (1992). GAP-43 gene expression is increased in anterior horn cells of amyotrophic lateral sclerosis. Ann Neurol 31:593–7.

Patton SE, Lapadula DM, Abou-Donia MB (1986). Relationship of tri-o-cresyl phosphate–induced delayed neurotoxicity to enhancement of in vitro phosphorylation of hen brain and spinal cord proteins. J Pharmacol Exp Ther 239:597–605.

Pleasure DE, Michler KC, Engel WK (1969). Axonal transport of proteins in experimental neuropathies. Science 166:524–5.

Prineas, J (1969). The pathogenesis of dying-back polyneuropathies. Part I. An ultrastructural study of experimental tri-ortho-cresyl phosphate intoxication in the cat. J. Neuropathol. Expt. Neurol. 28:571–97.

Prineas J (1970). Peripheral nerve changes in thiamine-deficient rats. An electron microscopic study. Arch Neurol 23:541–8.

Pyle SJ, Amarnath V, Graham DG, Anthony DC (1992). The role of pyrrole formation in the alteration of neurofilament transport induced during exposure to 2,5-hexanedione. J Neuropathol Exp Neurol 51:451–8.

Rasul AR, Howell JM (1973). A comparison of the effect of sodium diethyldithiocarbamate on the central nervous system of young and adult domestic fowl. Acta Neuropathol (Berlin) 24:68–75.

Rasul AR, Howell JM (1974). The effect of varying periods of administration and the cessation of administration of sodium diethyldithiocarbamate upon the central nervous system of domestic fowl. Acta Neuropathol (Berlin) 28:243–51.

Ryan LJ, Linder JC, Martone ME, Groves PM (1990). Histological and ultrastructural evidence that D-amphetamine causes degeneration in neostriatum and frontal cortex of rats. Brain Res 518:67–77.

Sasaki S, Maruyama S, Yamane K, Sakuma H, Takeishi M (1989). Swelling of the proximal axons in a case of motor neuron disease. Ann Neurol 25:520–2.

Sasaki S, Maruyama S, Yamane K, Sakuma H, Takeishi M (1990). Ultrastructure of swollen proximal axons of anterior neurons in motor neuron disease. J Neurol Sci 97:233–40.

Sayre LM, Autilio-Gambetti L, Gambetti P (1985). Pathogenesis of experimental giant neurofilamentous axonopathies: a united hypothesis based on chemical modification of neurofilaments. Brain Res Rev 10:69–83.

Schulze GE, Boysen BG (1991). A neurotoxicity screening for use in safety evaluation: effects of acrylamide and β,β'-iminodipropionitrile. Fund Appl Toxicol 16:602–15.

Selye H (1957). Lathyrism. Rev Can Biol 16:1–73.

Shibutani M, Okeda R (1989). Experimental study on subacute neurotoxicity of methotrexate in cats. Acta Neuropathol 78:291–300.

Shibutani M, Okeda R, Hori A, Schipper H (1989). Methotrexate-related multifocal axonopathy. Report of an autopsy case. Acta Neuropathol 79:333–5.

Sickles DW (1989a). Toxic neurofilamentous axonopathies and fast anterograde axonal transport: II. The effects of single doses of neurotoxic and non-neurotoxic diketones and β,β'-iminodipropionitrile (IDPN) on the rate and capacity of transport. Neurotoxicology 10:103–12.

Sickles DW (1989b). Toxic neurofilamentous axonopathies and fast anterograde axonal transport. I. The effects of single doses of acrylamide on the rate and capacity of transport. Neurotoxicology 10:91–102.

Sickles DW (1992). Toxic neurofilamentous axonopathies and fast anterograde axonal transport: IV. In vitro analysis of transport following acrylamide and 2,5-hexamedione. Toxicol Lett 61:199–204.

Smith MI, Elvove E, Frazier WH (1930). The pharmacological action of certain phenol esters, with special reference to the etiology of so called ginger paralysis. Pub Health Rep 45:2509–607.

Sobue G, Nakao N, Murakami K, Yasuda T, Sahashi K, Mitsuma T, Sasaki H, Sakaki Y, Takahashi A (1990). Type I familial amyloid polyneuropathy. A pathological study of the peripheral nervous system. Brain 113:903–19.

Southam E, Thomas PK, King RHM, Goss-Sampson MA, Muller DPR (1991). Experimental vitamin E deficiency in rats. Brain 114:915–36.

Spencer PS, Schaumburg HH (1976). Central-peripheral distal axonopathy–the pathology of dying-back polyneuropathies. In: Zimmerman H, ed. Progress in neuropathology. Vol. 3. New York: Grune and Stratton, 253–95.

Spencer PS, Schaumburg HH (1977). Ultrastructural studies of the dying-back process. III. The evolution of experimental peripheral giant axonal degeneration. J Neuropathol Exp Neurol 36:276–99.

Spencer PS, Schaumburg HH, Sabri MI, Veronesi B (1980). The enlarging view of hexacarbon neurotoxicity. CRC Crit Rev Toxicol 7:279–356.

Srivastava SP, Seth PK, Das M, Mukhtar H (1985). Effects of mixed-function oxidase modifiers on neurotoxicity of acrylamide in rats. Biochem Pharmacol 34:1099–102.

Stanley GP, Pender MP (1991). The pathophysiology of chronic relapsing experimental allergic encephalomyelitis in the Lewis rat. Brain 114:1827–1953.

Sumner SCJ, MacNeela JP, Fennell TR (1992). Characterization and quantitation of urinary metabolites of [1,2,3-^{13}C]acrylamide in rats and mice using ^{13}C nuclear magnetic resonance spectroscopy. Chem Res Toxicol 5:81–9.

Swank RL (1940). Avian thiamine deficiency. A correlation of the pathology and clinical behaviour. J Exp Med 71:683–702.

Tenhula WN, Xu S, Madigan MC, Heller K, Freeman WR, Sadun AA (1992). Morphometric comparison of optic nerve loss in acquired immunodeficiency syndrome. Am J Ophthalmol 113:14–20.

Valentine WM, Amarnath V, Graham DG, Anthony DC (1992). Covalent cross-linking of proteins by carbon disulfide. Chem Res Toxicol 5:254–62.

Vasilescu C (1972). Motor nerve conduction velocity and electromyogram in carbon disulfide poisoning. Revue Roumaine de Neurologie et de Psychiatrie 9:63–71.

Victor M (1975). Polyneuropathy due to nutritional deficiency and alcoholism. In: Dyck PJ, Thomas PK, Lambert EH, eds. Peripheral neuropathies. Vol. 2. Philadelphia: W.B. Saunders, 1030–66.

Vigliani EB (1954). Carbon disulfide poisoning in viscose rayon factories. Br Med J 11:235–44.

Wilmarth KR, Viana ME, Abou-Donia MB (1993). Carbon disulfide inhalation increases Ca^{2+}/calmodulin-dependent kinase phosphorylation of cytoskeletal proteins in the rat central nervous system. Brain Res (in press).

Yagihashi S, Kamijo M, Watanabe K (1990). Reduced myelinated fiber size correlates with loss of axonal neurofilaments in peripheral nerve of chronically streptozotocin diabetic rats. Am J Pathol 136:1365–73.

Yasaki S, Dyck PJ (1990). Duration and severity of hypoglycemia needed to induce neuropathy. Brain Res 531:8–15.

Yasaki S, Dyck PJ (1991). Spatial distribution of fiber degeneration in acute hypoglycemic neuropathy in rat. J Neuropathol Exp Neurol 50:681–92.

7

Involvement of Cytoskeletal Proteins in Chemically Induced Neuropathies

Mohamed B. Abou-Donia and Ram P. Gupta
Duke University Medical Center
Durham, North Carolina

INTRODUCTION

The function of the nervous system is to sense information from different parts of the body and from the outside world, and then to interpret and process this information and direct actions of different organs of the body. This is accomplished by storage of information as well as its transfer from one cell to another. Dendrites of the neuron receive stimuli from other cells and conduct impulses generated by the stimuli to the cell body (perikaryon). The axon of the cell is a single fiber that carries impulses to another part of the nervous system, a muscle fiber, or a secretory cell. Communications between neurons occur at the synapses, which are called electrical and chemical synapses. The human central nervous system (CNS) contains mainly chemical synapses. The chemical synaptic transmission is mediated through a number of distinct steps. These steps of transmission include transmitter synthesis and storage and transmitter release from the presynaptic terminal into the cleft between the neurons. The secreted transmitter binds to the receptors on the receiving cell, activates the receptor-associated channels, and is subsequently degraded and inactivated. The neurotransmitter is released when an action potential moves down an axon, enters the presynaptic terminal, and results in its depolarization. This depolarization causes opening of the voltage-dependent Ca^{2+} channels and movement of calcium into the terminal. The elevation of the free cytoplasmic calcium in the axon terminal leads to the discharge of neurotransmitter into the synaptic cleft. Neurotoxic chemicals interfere in signal transduction between the cells by modifying any of the processes mentioned above at the presynaptic terminal or postsynaptic membranes. Some neurotoxic chemicals alter the cytoskeletal proteins in the neuronal perikaryon or axon that are required for the anterograde and retrograde transport of essential proteins in the axon.

CELL BODY

Mercury

Mercury compounds are potent neurotoxic substances and have caused human poisoning worldwide. Methylmercury (MeHg) is highly neurotoxic and caused human poisoning in Japan in the 1950s and in 1964, and in Iraq in 1971. Intoxication with mercury sometimes occurs from that spread on the carpet, and the neurotoxicity due to dental amalgam, although controversial, is of great concern. Neurotoxicity due to amalgam is not limited to vapor inhalation and is suspected to result from the release of mercury from the amalgam and its distribution in the body, including the fetus of a pregnant woman (Verity, 1992). Methylmercury accumulates in freshwater fish and therefore constitutes an important source of exposure for humans. Recent studies suggest that MeHg can be demethylated in the brain to inorganic mercury. This could lead to the accumulation of inorganic mercury in the central nervous system (CNS) after long-term exposure to MeHg (Rossi et al., 1991).

Pathology of Intoxication

Neuropathological studies showed that there was dose-dependent degeneration of cortical and cerebellar neurons on prenatal exposure to MeHg (Annau and Cuomo, 1988). Even a single dose of 4 mg/kg administered on the fourth day of gestation to the mother had effect on 10–15% of the neurons. The developmental neurotoxic effects of MeHg in humans include reduced brain size, altered cytoarchitecture of the brain (presumably due to disruptions in neuronal migration), and a cerebral palsy–like syndrome in severe cases (Sager and Matheson, 1988). Lehotsky et al. (1988) examined the behavioral effect of prenatal methoxyethylmercury chloride (MEMC) exposure on rat pups. Rat dams were treated with different doses of MEMC (2.0, 0.62, 0.02 mg/kg daily) on days 7–15 of gestation. Treatment with MEMC did not cause any mortality of dams even at the highest dose given, 2.0 mg/kg. There was a high mortality rate (18%) of the offspring at this dose, even though some other characteristics were normal after birth. Ambulation increased significantly in 90-day-old pups. The so-called no-effect level was 0.02 mg/kg daily. Another study, by Lindstrom et al. (1991), in which rats were exposed to MeHg (3.9 mg/kg diet) during gestation as well as after birth up to 50 days postpartum, showed no general toxic effects or alterations in brain morphology as evaluated by cresyl violet histology. There was a slight increase in brain weight. However, there was a 117% increase in norepinephrine in cerebellum without any change in other brain regions. Thus long-term exposure may affect some specific transmitter-identified systems in the brain in the absence of any apparent neurotoxic effects.

Disruption of Microtubules and Intermediate Filaments

In vitro studies have shown that MeHg interacts with microtubules and causes their depolymerization (Abe et al., 1975). Incubation of MeHg with PtK_2 kidney epithelial cells also resulted in disruption of cytoplasmic microtubules and subsequent redistribution of vimentin filaments (Sager and Matheson, 1988). The effect was concentration-dependent, and microtubules appeared similar to "cold-stable" microtubules observed after exposure to low temperatures. The redistribution of vimentin was ascribed to the loss of microtubules, as has been shown for nocodazole and colcemid treatment. The MeHg treatment also affected the mitosis of cells. There was an increase in mitotic index at the lowest concentration tested and a decrease at higher MeHg concentrations. The number of multinucleated cells and cells containing fragmented nuclei also increased with MeHg treatment. The antimitotic effect of MeHg appeared to be due solely to the disruption of microtubules, since similar effects were observed on treatment with other antimicrotubule drugs.

Depolarization and Intracellular Calcium Concentration

A demonstrated effect of both MeHg and mercury has been the vulnerability of the functions of the presynaptic terminals. They increase the spontaneous release of neurotransmitter (Juang, 1976; Atchison and Narahashi, 1982; Minnema et al., 1989; Komulainen and Bondy, 1987) but block their evoked release from the terminals (Manalis and Cooper, 1975; Juang, 1976; Atchison and Narahashi, 1982; Traxinger and Atchison, 1987). This led to the determination of the effects of these neurotoxic chemicals on the depolarization of plasma and mitochondrial membranes of synaptosomes and on intracellular calcium concentration. Both mercurials (1–20 μM) produce a concentration-dependent increase in carbocyanine dye fluorescence after 5 min of exposure of the synaptosomes (Hare and Atchison, 1992), and this is independent of the calcium concentration of the medium. An increase in membrane-associated dye (3,3'-diethylthiadicarbocyanine iodide) fluorescence is an indicator of depolarization of membrane. Depolarization of synaptosomes induced by MeHg and Hg^{2+} is not affected by either lowering the Na^+ concentration of the medium or adding the Na^+ and Ca^{2+} channel blockers tetrodotoxin (TTX) and Co^{2+}, respectively, to the medium. Both mercurials depolarize synaptosomal plasma membrane at a concentration that has no effect on mitochondrial membrane potential, and Hg^{2+} at equimolar concentration shows more pronounced mitochondrial membrane depolarization than MeHg. The depolarization of membranes, however, does not involve movement of ions through voltage-dependent channels, since depolarization is not inhibited by the channel blockers TTX and Co^{2+} or in the absence of Ca^{2+} in the medium. It is suggested that depolarization of membrane potential by mercurials may be due to an increased nonselective cation conductance (Hare and Atchison, 1992; Arakawa et al., 1991). The mechanism of depolarization by mercurials may differ in other organs and species. For example, a combination of Co^{2+} and TTX, but neither agent alone, is able to block the depolarization of frog skeletal muscle (Miyamoto, 1983). The greater sensitivity of synaptosomal membrane to Hg^{2+} is probably due to less efficient penetration of Hg^{2+} than of MeHg through the plasma membrane, leading to its higher concentration at the surface (Nakada and Imura, 1982). In addition, Hg^{2+} has a higher affinity for thiol groups than MeHg (Carty and Malone, 1979). On the other hand, the greater neurotoxicity of MeHg is likely to be due to its lipophilic nature and greater ability to cross the blood-brain barrier as compared with Hg^{2+}.

Synaptosomal Plasma Membrane Potential

Kauppinen et al. (1989) determined the plasma membrane potential of synaptosomes from cerebral cortices of guinea pigs by ^{86}Rb diffusion and the mitochondrial membrane potential by the safranine method. In addition, the cytosolic free calcium concentration, $(Ca^{2+})_c$, was measured to assess the effect of depolarization. Methylmercury increases $(Ca^{2+})_c$ by 127 nM at a 30-μM concentration without significantly altering the resting plasma membrane potential of –67 mV. There is a significant increase in $(Ca^{2+})_c$ in the absence of calcium in the medium, although it is much lower than in the presence of 1 mM Ca^{2+}. Methylmercury at a 30-μM concentration inhibits mitochondrial respiration completely, but anaerobic glycolysis is increased three-fold. On the other hand, MeHg at a 100-μM concentration, which also inhibits glycolysis by 90%, increases $(Ca^{2+})_c$ by 882 nM, and plasma membrane is also depolarized to 36 mV. It is suggested that the increase in $(Ca^{2+})_c$ at 30 μM MeHg is at least partly due to the release of Ca^{2+} from the mitochondria. However, the increase in $(Ca^{2+})_c$ at 100 μM MeHg is due to the release of calcium from intracellular sources as well as its leakage through nonspecific ion channels, since increase in $(Ca^{2+})_c$ is insensitive to the voltage-dependent Ca^{2+} channel blocker verapamil (Komulainen and Bondy, 1987). Bondy and McKee (1991) measured the transmembrane potential of both rat brain (excluding cerebellum and pons-medulla) synaptosomes and mitchondria within the synaptosomes. There was dose-dependent diminution of transmembrane potential of both plasma membrane and mitochondria, but mitochondria showed greater sensitivity to the toxicant. It was suggested that the special vulnerability of mitochondrial membrane potential was due to disruption of oxidative phosphorylation as a result of the increase of intrasynaptosomal free Ca^{2+} concentration by the chemicals.

Block of Ca^{2+} Uptake by Synaptosomes

Although mercurials depolarize plasma and mitochondrial membranes of synaptosomes and also alter membrane potential, depending on the concentration of mercurials, they have been shown to inhibit the uptake of $^{45}Ca^{2+}$ by synaptosomes at rest and during depolarization (Hewett and Atchison, 1992; Shafer and Atchison, 1989). There is concentration-dependent inhibition of basal influx of $^{45}Ca^{2+}$. Basal influx was measured with 5 mM KCl in the medium, at which concentration there was no depolarization. On the other hand, influx of $^{45}Ca^{2+}$ during depolarization was measured under two conditions. The fast phase of influx was measured at 1 of K^+-induced depolarization, and the slow phase of influx was measured during the last 10 s of a 20-s period of depolarization. Both fast and slow influx of calcium is inhibited in a concentration-dependent manner, but there is a difference in the characteristics of inhibition depending on the nature of the mercurials (ethylmercury, MeHg, Hg^{2+}). The following conclusions were drawn from this study: 1.) The block of calcium uptake at resting potential is probably due to the specific block of calcium channels. 2.) High concentrations of mercurials, except dimethylmercury and *p*-chloromercuriphenylsulfonate, inhibited calcium influx at resting potential. 3.) A positive charge on the mercurials is essential to inhibit the influx of calcium. 4.) Organic mercurials (e.g., ethylmercury, MeHg) block influx of calcium in a noncompetitive and voltage-dependent manner. 5.) Divalent mercury, i.e., Hg^{2+}, blocks influx of calcium in a competitive and voltage-independent manner. 6.) The consequences of exposure to different mercurials depend not only on the quantity but also on their chemical structure, i.e., lipophilicity and charge.

Effect on Cell Signaling

Several studies show that mercury can interfere with growth stimulation and various components of signaling systems. Mercury bichloride ($HgCl_2$) can block specific binding to high-affinity receptor sites in the rat brain. Muscarinic and α-adrenergic receptors appear to be particularly sensitive to this toxicant. The stimulation of these receptors is coupled to phosphatidyl inositol breakdown, and $HgCl_2$ interferes with the phosphatidyl inositol/protein kinase C pathway: $HgCl_2$ inhibits protein kinase C at relatively low concentrations. It is suggested that this arrests the growth, division, and migration of neurons by altering the inositol phosphate signaling system. The effect of $HgCl_2$ on signal transduction has been studied in the neuroadrenergic cell line PC12. Mercury bichloride up to 0.5 μM did not affect the cytosolic Ca^{2+} levels in the unstimulated cells, but the cytosolic Ca^{2+} concentration increased with higher Hg^{2+} concentrations and was maximal at 2 μM Hg^{2+}.

This was due to enhanced Ca^{2+} entry through the voltage-operated channels, as increase in Ca^{2+} concentration could be prevented by pretreatment of PC12 cells with Ca^{2+} blockers. Most of the mercury was found to be associated with the membrane proteins when $^{203}HgCl_2$ was used at concentrations between 0.5 and 2 μM. The study suggested that the verapamil-sensitive Ca^{2+} channel was opened as a result of Hg^{2+} binding to the membrane site (Rossi et al., 1991).

The effect of $HgCl_2$ on the response of PC12 cells to hormone stimulation was also examined. Pretreatment of PC12 cells with 0.1–0.5 μM Hg^{2+} did not affect the intracellular Ca^{2+} signal produced by bradykinin but significantly increased the Ca^{2+} signal produced by the P_2-purinergic receptor agonist adenosine triphosphate (ATP). The induction of the Ca^{2+} signal was ascribed to the modification of voltage-operated Ca^{2+} channels at low Hg^{2+} concentration, <0.5 μM. The ATP-stimulated Ca^{2+} signal was ascribed to the modification of voltage-dependent Ca^{2+} channels at low Hg^{2+} concentration. In contrast to ATP, brady-kinin seems to increase cytosolic Ca^{2+} concentration through release from intracellular sources. Pretreatment of PC12 cells with higher Hg^{2+} concentrations (0.5–2 μM) decreased CA^{2+} signal induction by either hormone. This inhibition of hormone-induced Ca^{2+} signal was attributed to elevation of cytosolic Ca^{2+} concentration due to enhanced Ca^{2+} influx through voltage-dependent channels and inhibition of inositol phosphate production caused by interference with some proteins in the signal transduction pathway. The latter was supported by the finding that Hg^{2+} at higher concentrations caused a partial inhibition of agonist-stimulated inositol phosphate generation (Rossi et al., 1991). Preliminary studies indicated that a marked inhibition of cell growth occurred when cells were exposed to 1–2 μM Hg^{2+} for 10 min.

Inhibition of Glutamate Transport in Astrocyte Cells

Inhibition of glutamate transport is a potential indirect cause of excitotoxic damage by glutamate to the central nervous system. Acute exposure to 0.5 μM Hg^{2+} inhibited 50% of initial glutamate transport. Inhibition by Hg^{2+} was specific in that other divalent metals such as Al^{3+}, Pb^{2+}, Co^{2+}, Sr^{2+}, Cd^{2+}, and Zn^{2+} did not show inhibition up to a 10-μM concentration. The inhibition was reversible at a low Hg^{2+} concentration (0.5 μM) but progressively changed to slowly reversible when the concentration of Hg^{2+} (1–2 μM) and the period of treatment (1–3 hr) were increased. Hg^{2+} had no effect on 2-deoxyglucose at concentrations up to 1 μM. Uptake of 2-deoxyglucose uptake is an index of glucose utilization and reflects Na^+,K^+-ATPase activity, hexokinase activity, and membrane integrity. The results suggested that Hg^{2+} could impair glial glutamate transport at low concentrations that had no effect on some other vital cell functions (Brookes, 1988) and thereby produce an excitotoxic insult to neurons.

Aluminum

Aluminum Neurotoxicity

Aluminum is ubiquitous in the earth's crust. Its widespread occurrence makes it virtually impossible to avoid exposure to this metal ion. Aluminum is used in package materials and utensils. It is used in the aviation and automobile industries. Aluminum compounds, especially aluminum sulfate, are used in water purification in some countries. A number of aluminum compounds are used as drugs: aluminum hydroxide is administered as an antacid to treat stomach ulcers and as a phosphate binder to regulate phosphate levels in cases of renal deficiency (van der Voet et al., 1991). Aluminum is known to be neurotoxic to the CNS. Its role in the development of dialysis dementia is well established. This disease occurs in patients who are unable to eliminate aluminum because of renal dysfunction and is characterized by speech difficulties, electroencephalographic (EEG) changes, convulsions, dementia, myoclonus, and seizures (Banks and Kastin, 1989; Murray et al., 1991). However, high concentrations of aluminum have also been observed in elderly people with impaired coordination and memory in the absence of renal failure. Aluminum has also been associated with other neurological disorders, e.g., Alzheimer's disease, endemic amyotrophic lateral sclerosis, and parkinsoniam dementia of Guam. The relation between aluminum and Alzheimer's disease is based on the finding that elevated levels of aluminum are present in neurofibrillary tangles and senile plaques in comparison with similar regions of brains of aged-matched persons without Alzheimer's disease. Further support was obtained from animal experiments in which intraneuronal accumulation of dense bundles of filaments was observed on intracranial administration of soluble aluminum salts. The bundles of accumulated filaments were similar but not identical to the paired helical filaments found in Alzheimer's disease. Furthermore, oral administration of aluminum did not induce the neuropathological findings observed on parenteral adminis- tration, even though equivalent brain aluminum concentrations were achieved. Therefore, a correlation between aluminum exposure and development of Alzheimer's disease is still not conclusively established. However, it is possible that aluminum binds to the fibrillary tangles and accelerates the degeneration of neurons. Accumulation of aluminum has also been demonstrated in neurofibrillary tangles in parkinsoniam dementia of Guam. This disorder is characterized by brain atrophy and neurofibrillary degeneration, but without senile plaques (Murray et al., 1991). Administration of aluminum to laboratory animals induces encephalomyelopathy with degeneration of cerebral nerve cells, brain stem demyelination, and development of plaques and tangles.

Cation Metabolism Dysfunction by Aluminum Substitution

Alkaline earth cations such as calcium and magnesium are involved as labile complexes at various cellular levels. Aluminum, which forms more stable complexes with amino acids such as glutamic acid and aspartic acid, is able to replace calcium from the glutamate complex and cross the blood-brain barrier (BBB) (Deloncle and Guillard, 1990). However, another pathway has also been proposed for the entry of aluminum into the CNS. Aluminum binds to transferrin and enters tissues by a receptor-mediated endocytosis of the complex. Binding sites for transferrin have been found on brain endothelial cells and brain tissue (Banks and Kastin, 1989; Verity, 1992). It has been suggested that the replacement of calcium and magnesium by aluminum is involved in various disturbances in the brain and other organs. The replacement of calcium by aluminum in the bone mineral component generates weakness in bone structure, which has been shown to occur in patients with Alzheimer's disease and dialysis dementia. In acute aluminum intoxication, high levels of aluminum have been reported in bones and high levels of calcium in blood. Similarly, replacement of calcium in muscles affects the electrical conduction of myocardiac fibers, and cardiomyopathies have indeed been described in some hemodialyzed patients.

The most serious troubles might occur in neurons, in which both calcium and magnesium are involved in various functions. If aluminum crosses the BBB as glutamate complex, it will bind to the neurons rich in glutamate receptors in the hippocampus and amygdala. These regions are rich in glutamatergic neurons. Later, aluminum present in the neuron cytoplasm can replace calcium and magnesium and interfere with synaptic transmission, where calcium is involved in neurotransmitter release. Similarly, aluminum can also replace magnesium and disturb the transport of chemical species, which is linked to the magnesium-dependent polymerization/depolymerization of neurotubules. Aluminum can also link to neurofilament proteins through glutamic and aspartic amino acids and may be responsible for the three-dimensional structure observed in amyloid protein and neurofibrillary tangles. The presence of a protease-resistant core in paired helical filaments may also be the result of aluminum bound to amino acid carboxyl groups, since proteases are not able to disrupt these complexes. In addition, L-glutamic acid in the form of aluminum complex is not able to detoxify ammonia from neurons by producing L-glutamin, and accumulation of ammonia may cause the death of neurons and disrupt all related neuronal functions. This is consistent with the accumulation of ammonia and progressive loss of neurons in Alzheimer's disease (Deloncle and Guillard, 1990).

Inhibition of Calcium Influx

Besides displacing Ca^{2+} from receptors, especially glutamate receptors, aluminum has also been shown to inhibit the fast phase of Ca^{2+} influx in brain synaptosomes (Koenig and Jope, 1987). An inhibitory effect on voltage-dependent fast transport of Ca^{2+} was observed even at a 50-μM aluminum concentration in a depolarizing medium (50 mM K^+) and at a concentration above 500 μM in a low-K^+ medium. The inhibition of Ca^{2+} influx at high aluminum concentrations under nondepolarizing conditions is probably due to perturbations of the calcium channel or of the phospholipid domain near the channels. The inhibitory effect of aluminum on fast Ca^{2+} transport may be partly responsible for the neurotoxic effect of aluminum, since these channels are involved in the evoked release of neurotransmitters (Drapeau and Blaustein, 1983). There was no effect of aluminum on the depolarization-dependent slow phase of Ca^{2+} influx, since calcium influx decreased with increasing aluminum concentration under both depolarizing and nondepolarizing conditions. Thus there is no evidence to suggest that aluminum has any effect on the voltage-dependent slow phase of Ca^{2+} influx.

Accumulation of Neurofilaments

An encephalopathy may be induced in a rabbit experimental model by injection of aluminum salts into the cerebrospinal fluid. This is accompanied by formation of neuro-fibrillary tangles (NFTs) as a result of the accumulation of neurofilaments in the perikaryon, axons, and dendrites of large neurons. These include cells of the anterior horn of the spinal cord, pyramidal cells of the cortex, cells of the hippocampus, and cerebellar Purkinje cells. Ultrastructurally, these tangles contain straight 10-nm neurofilaments and are different in appearance from the paired helical neurofilaments (PHFs) of Alzheimer's disease. Biochemically, NFTs contain normal neurofilament triplet proteins of molecular weight 200, 160, and 68 kDa (van der Voet et al., 1991; Smitt and de Jong, 1989) that are, unlike PHFs, soluble in standard protein solvents. There is swelling in proximal axons and wallerian-type degeneration further down in the axon. Accumulation of neurofilaments was associated with reduction in the expression of mRNAs for 68-kDa neurofilament protein (NF-L) and tubulin, but the level of mRNA for actin was not altered. There was no reduction in mRNAs for NF-L and tubulin in dorsal root ganglia, which remained unaffected by aluminum administration (Muma et al., 1988). These experiments were carried out 7–14 days following intoxication, when accumulations of neurofilaments were prominent in the motor neurons. The mechanism of the reduction of NF genes is not known. The reduction of NF gene expression could be due to the direct interaction of aluminum with the genome or to accumulation of neurofilaments in the neuron. The accumulated neurofilament contained increased concentrations of normal neurofilament protein as well as abnormally phosohorylated neurofilament protein (Bizzi and Gambetti, 1986; Troncoso et al., 1986). Al- though the molecular mechanism of aluminum-induced neurofilament accumulation is not known, in vitro addition of aluminum and other multivalent cations can cause aggregation of purified NFs (Diaz-Nido and Avila, 1990; Troncoso et al., 1990). The tangles were nonreactive for microtubule associated proteins-2, tau, or different β-tubulin isotypes (Verity, 1992).

Depletion of Some Cytoskeletal Proteins

The concentration of cytoskeletal proteins has been assessed by immunoblotting as well as immunohistochemical methods in aluminum-treated rats (Johnson et al., 1992). The rats were given 0.3% aluminum in drinking water for 2–3 months, and this elevated the serum aluminum concentration eightfold. Oral aluminum intoxication decreased MAP-2 concentration in the hippocampus and brain stem in adult rats and in the cortex and brain stem in developing rats. Aluminum also decreased the concentration of spectrin, but only in the hippocampus. There was no effect on other cytoskeletal proteins, e.g., tubulin, tau, and neurofilament triplet. The reduction of MAP-2 was apparently not due to its increased proteolysis by calpain or cathepsin D, since in vitro addition of aluminum chloride had no effect on the proteolysis of MAP-2. This was in contrast to the observation that aluminum chloride inhibits Ca^{2+}-dependent and -independent degradation of mouse CNS neurofilament proteins (Shea et al., 1992). It is not yet known (1) whether aluminum directly reacts with the genome and interferes with the expression of mRNA, (2) whether increase in the concentration of cAMP and hence increased phosphorylation of some protein modifies MAP-2 mRNA transcription or translation, or (3) whether increased phosphorylation of endogenous MAP-2 occurring in response to aluminum exerts an inhibitory effect on the transcription or translation of MAP-2. However, decrease in the concentration of MAP-2 may alter the interactions of neuronal cytoskeletal proteins resulting in neuronal dysfunction and memory impairment.

Alteration in Cyclic Adenosine Monophosphate and Cyclic Guanosine Monophosphate Levels

Oral administration of aluminum (0.3% in drinking water) significantly elevated cyclic adenosine monophosphate (cAMP) levels in different brain rat brain regions. The effect on cyclic guanosine monophosphate (cGMP) was less widespread and depended greatly on the aluminum salt (citrate or sulfate) administered (Johnson and Jope, 1987). The increase in the concentrations of cAMP and cGMP is consistent with the increased phosphorylation of proteins, e.g., neurofilaments, in aluminum-treated animals (Bizzi and Gambetti, 1986; Johnson and Jope, 1988), since these second messengers act primarily by activating protein kinases. The mechanism of these increases is not known. Aluminum has been shown in vitro to interact with both stimulatory and inhibitory G proteins. Johnson (1988) examined the effect of a cholinergic agonist (pilocarpine), a dopaminergic agonist (apomorphine), and an adrenergic agonist (isoproterenol) on aluminum-treated rats. Pilocarpine-induced increases in cAMP and cGMP were significantly attenuated in aluminum-treated rats, whereas apomorphine-induced increase in cGMP was potentiated. Apomorphine had no effect on cAMP levels in tested brain regions. Isoproterenol treatment did not show any effect on cAMP concentration in brain regions, but the concentration of cAMP was significantly reduced in the cerebral cortex of aluminum-treated animals (Johnson, 1988). In contrast, in vitro treatment with isoproterenol enhanced cAMP levels in cerebral cortical slices, and this was potentiated by preincubation with aluminum chloride (Johnson et al., 1989). Incubation of cortical slices with aluminum chloride alone had no effect on cAMP concentration. Similar in vitro results were obtained on 2-chloroadenosine treatment. Both isoproterenol and 2-chloroadenosine activate stimulatory receptors coupled to adenylate cyclase in rat brain slices. It is suggested that aluminum may promote hormone receptor–stimulatory G-protein coupling, resulting in potentiation of agonist-induced increase in cAMP. This is consistent with the observation that aluminum showed potentiation effect at high concentrations of 2-chloroadenosine. Alternatively, aluminum may inhibit agonist-dependent guanosinetriphosphatase (GTPase) activity and thus increase the lifetime of the active GTP–α subunit complex. The potentiation of cAMP by aluminum in vitro may account for the increase in cAMP in aluminum-treated rats (Johnson and Jope, 1987), but it is not in conformity with the results obtained on isoproterenol treatment of aluminum-pretreated rats (Johnson, 1988).

Effects on Cholinergic Receptors

Reduced levels of choline acetyltransferase (ChAT) activity have been found in postmortem brains from patients with dialysis encephalopathy or Alzheimer's disease (Johnson and Jope, 1987). Therefore, it is important to examine the effects of aluminum administration on the activities of ChAT and related enzymes to reveal any relation between aluminum accumulation and decrease in ChAT in those diseases. Aluminum administration by intraperitoneal, intracisternal, or intracerebroventricular (i.c.v.) injections results in reduction of ChAT activity in different brain regions (Gulya et al., 1990; Yates et al., 1980; Simpson et al., 1985). Johnson and Jope (1987), however, did not find any effect on ChAT of i.c.v. injection of aluminum ions, and decrease in ChAT activity was not observed on aluminum sulfate administration in drinking water for 30 days (Connor et al., 1988). Intraperitoneal administration of aluminum caused reduction in nicotinic and muscarinic receptors in all the tested brain regions, whereas administration in drinking water showed increase in hippocampal but not in cortical muscarinic receptors. Thus, alterations in cholinergic receptors and enzymes seem to depend on the route of administration, duration of treatment, and rise in aluminum concentration in brain regions. The alterations observed in cholinergic receptor numbers or enzyme activities are probably not due to their direct interaction with aluminum ions, since 1.) no change was found in ChAT activity and receptor binding on in vitro treatment, as compared with their decrease on in vivo treatment, and 2.) there was alteration in acetylcholinesterase activity on in vitro treatment and not on in vivo treatment (Gulya et al., 1990). In contrast to brain tissue, cerebral microvessels consisting primarily of capillary segments showed enhanced binding of [^{3}H]quinuclidinayl benzilate on in vitro treatment with aluminum chloride (Grammas and Caspers, 1991). The decrease in ChAT activity and in nicotinic and muscarinic receptors on intraperitoneal injection of aluminum ions is consistent with similar findings in Alzheimer's disease. It is suggested that the decrease in cholinergic parameters in aluminum-treated animals and in Alzheimer's disease is the result of aluminum accumulation followed by neuronal degeneration.

Effect on Phosphoinositide Metabolism

Cholinergic muscarinic receptors activate phosphoinositide-specific phospholipase C (PLC), which hydrolyzes phosphoinositides into two second messengers, inositol trisphosphate (IP3) and diacylglycerol (DAG). Inositol trisphosphate stimulates calcium release from intracellular sources, and DAG activates protein kinase C. The rise in intracellular calcium concentration and activation of protein kinase C result in the phosphorylation of specific proteins and thereby control various cell functions including release of neurotransmitters, e.g., acetylcholine (Berridge and Irvine, 1989; Rana and Hokin, 1990; Candural et al., 1991). Any alteration in the concentration of muscarinic receptors by aluminum intoxication as noted above can disturb phosphoinositide metabolism and affect neuronal functions controlled by intracellular calcium and protein kinase C. The CNS muscarinic receptor activation is coupled to phosphoinositide hydrolysis via G proteins (guanine nucleotide–binding proteins). Aluminum in the form of fluoroaluminate (AlF_4^-) has been demonstrated to enhance phosphoinositide metabolism by activating specific G proteins (Candural et al., 1991). Aluminum-activated phosphoinositide metabolism differs from the muscarinic receptor–stimulated pathway in that the former is 1.) not potentiated by carbachol (a muscarinic agonist) or GTP(S), 2.) not inhibited by the GTP-binding antagonist GDP(S), and 3.) not inhibited by phorbol 12-myristate 13-acetate (PMA). On the other hand, AlF_4^--dependent stimulation of phosphoinositide metabolism in hepatocyte membranes is inhibited by GDP(S). It is suggested that AlF_4^- interacts with G protein at a site different from the GTP-binding site or may stimulate PLC directly (Candural et al., 1991). Inhibition of AlF_4^--stimulated activity in hepatocytes seems to lend support to the hypothesis that AlF_4^- interacts with G protein at a site different from the GTP(S)-binding site. Aluminum chloride also stimulated phosphoinositide metabolism of cerebral cortical membranes, but this was unexpectedly stimulated by the inhibitors GDP(S) and PMA, and the mechanism is not yet known. Thus aluminum seems to interact with phosphoinositide metabolism directly through specific G proteins and can modulate various neuronal functions.

CENTRAL AND PERIPHERAL AXONOPATHY

Proximal

β,β′-Iminodipropionitrile

β,β′-Iminodipropionitrile (IDPN) is a synthetic compound known to induce massive focal accumulation of neurofilaments almost exclusively in the proximal segments of motor and sensory axons. Although IDPN is not a chemical that is present in the environment and likely to produce polyneuropathy in humans, it provides a model to study the role of swelling formation in some diseases such as amyothophic lateral sclerosis (ALS), dyskinetic disorders, and other motor disorders. However, it is not a model for ALS, since IDPN treatment does not lead to degeneration of axons or neuronal cells or to several other symptoms observed in ALS patients (Smitt and de Jong, 1989).

Neurotoxicity. Repeated oral administration of IDPN produces neuropathological and behavioral changes in rats. Neuropathological lesions include axonal swelling (ballooning) of unmyelinated axons with little change in perikaryons in the brain stem and the cervical and lumbar spinal cord of rats (Schulze and Boysen, 1991). Little change is found in the tibial and sural nerves, and some axonal degeneration is noted in the proximal sciatic nerve of high-dose animals. The changes are most prominent in males and most severe in the lumbar spinal cord of treated animals. These proximal axonal swellings due to massive accumulation of neurofilaments are followed by depletion of neurofilaments in distal axons (axonal atrophy), but there is not wallerian-type degeneration. Quick-freeze, deep-etch electron microscopy has shown that microtubules form bundles in the central region of axons, that neurofilaments are segregated to the periphery, and that most membrane-bound organelles are associated with the microtubules and not neurofilaments (Hirokawa et al. 1985). Immunostaining shows that actin is codistributed with segregated microtubules in the central region and is also present in the subaxolemmal region (Papasozomenos and Payne, 1986). Significant alterations in behavioral performance are polyuria, postural changes, bizarre behavior, circling, and impaired aerial righting. The "waltzing syndrome," characterized by lateral head movements and circling, is now termed ECC syndrome (excitation, circling, and choreiform head and neck movements). The time course for developing behavioral deficits shows a dose-response relationship, with high-dose animals developing behavioral deficits before low-dose animals. There is also a sex difference, male rats being more severely affected. IDPN produces learning and memory deficits as shown by neurobehavioral tests such as repeated-trials active avoidance (AA) and passive avoidance (PA) conditioning. Rats treated with IDPN required more conditioning trials to become capable of the required performance (Peele et al., 1990).

Metabolism of IDPN. To understand the mechanism of IDPN neurotoxic action, it is necessary to know whether IDPN or its metabolite is responsible for IDPN neurotoxicity. The proposed metabolism of IDPN is shown in Fig. 1. The major metabolite of IDPN is cyanoacetic acid, and minor metabolites are β-aminopropionitrile (BAPN) and β-alanine (Morandi et al., 1987; Jacobson et al., 1987). Further attention has focused on the metabolites hydroxy-IDPN (HOIDPN) and dehydro-IDPN, and their neurotoxocity has been tested. Administration of dehydro-IDPN at 3 g/kg (50% higher than the standard dose used in studies) produced only occasional temporary hind limb paralysis in rats, with no symptoms of permanent neurotoxic effects, whereas HOIDPN at 250mg/kg (one-eighth

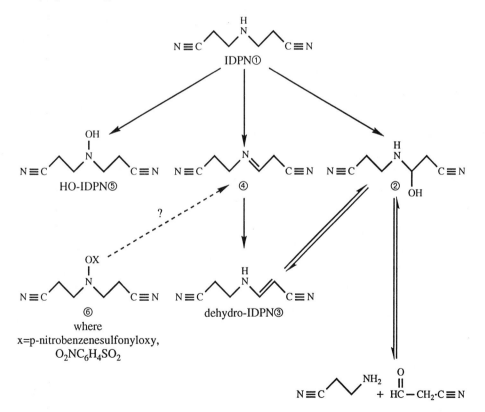

Figure 1 Proposed pathway for β,β′-iminodipropionitrile (IDPN) metabolism (adapted from Morandi et al., 1987).

of the standard IDPN dose) consistently produced the behavioral and neuropathologic effects found on IDPN intoxication. The results apparently indicate that HOIDPN may be the active metabolite of IDPN. The production of both morphological and behavioral aberrations by HOIDPN intoxication also support the hypothesis that this metabolite of IDPN may be responsible for both clinical and morphological symptoms. The chemical mechanism of HOIDPN is not clear. It is suggested that HOIDPN may undergo autoxidation to form a nitrone (Fig. 2), followed by other reactions.

A direct covalent modification of neurofilaments by IDPN or its metabolite is supported by the observation that both systemic administration of IDPN and its application directly to the neural tissue result in rapid dissociation of neurofilaments from microtubules. The segregated neurofilaments accumulate in the perimeter, and microtubules accumulate in the central axon. Llorens and Crofton (1991) studied the neurotoxicity of IDPN in carbon tetrachloride–pretreated rats. The administration of carbon tetrachloride was sufficient to impair IDPN biotransformation, and the effect was confirmed by pentobarbital sleeping

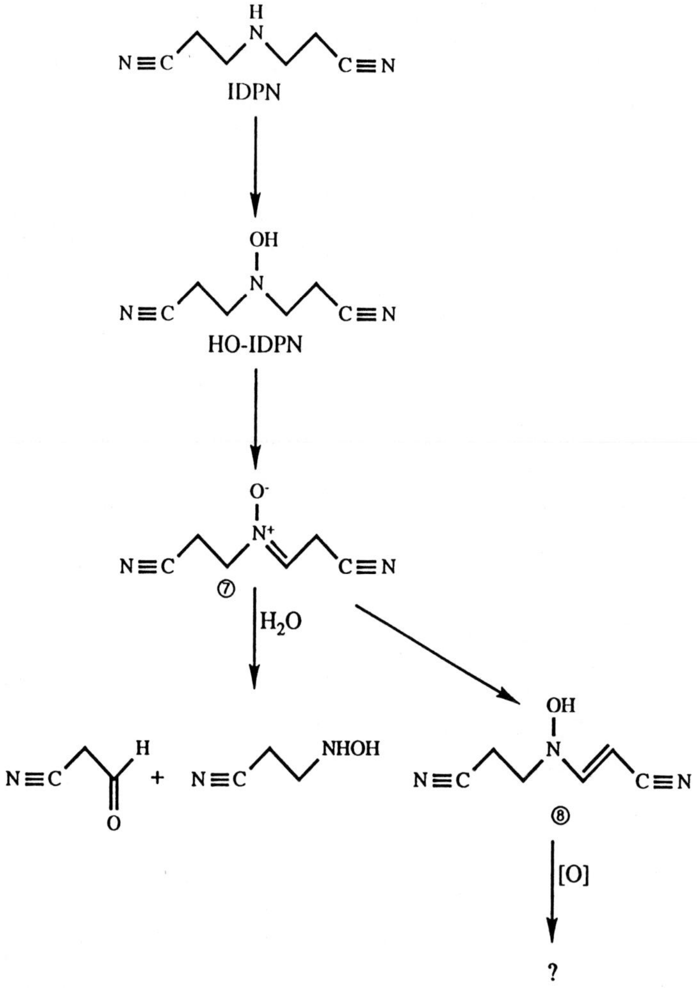

Figure 2 Proposed mechanism for the formation of nitrone (adapted from Morandi et al., 1987).

time. The results showed that the neurotoxicity produced by 100 mg/kg IDPN for 3 days in carbon tetrachloride–pretreated rats was equivalent to that produced by 200 mg/kg IDPN for 3 days without pretreatment. Furthermore, in vitro incubation of IDPN with bovine neurofilament preparation increases the preparation's viscosity at 1 and 2.5 mM and inhibits the reaction at higher concentrations, suggesting that IDPN per se may interact with neurofilaments and change their properties (Eyer et al., 1989).

Phosphorylation of Neurofilaments. The status of phosphorylation of neurofilaments has been studied in proximal axonal swellings and distal atrophic axons to reveal the mechanism of neurofilament accumulation in IDPN-treated animals and a number of human disorders (Carden et al., 1987; Gold and Austin, 1991). Accumulation of neurofilaments by a variety of neurotoxic chemicals suggests that covalent modification of neurofilaments may be the initial cause of their bundling in axons. Neurofilaments are extensively phosphorylated in axons and poorly phosphorylated in the normal neuronal perikarya. A single dose of IDPN (2 mg/kg) increased phosphorylated neurofilaments in L_4 and L_5 dorsal root ganglia but not in the anterior horn of the lumbar spinal cord (Gold and Austin, 1991). These proximal axonal swellings become smaller and slowly move down the axon with time after a single injection of IDPN. In contrast, the proximal axonal swellings persist close to the cell body if the rats are continuously treated with IDPN in their drinking water after the initial IDPN injection. The axons of both the anterior horn and dorsal root ganglia are strongly immunostained for phosphorylated neurofilaments in IDPN-treated animals as compared with untreated rats. The same pattern of immunostaining of neuronal perikarya and axons is observed after axotomy. These findings suggest that IDPN neuropathy produces an axotomy-like response in the neuronal cell body and axons without apparent degeneration. Although a direct effect of IDPN cannot be ruled out, it is suggested that phosphorylation of neurofilaments in the neuron arises from an impairment of retrograde transport through the promixal axonal swellings of a target-derived "trophic" signal. On the other hand, an increase in the concentration of phosphorylated neurofilaments and a decrease in the number of neurofilaments (axonal atrophy) in distal axons are ascribed to the reduced delivery of newly synthesized, poorly phosphorylated neurofilaments through proximal swellings. However, the accumulation of neurofilaments in proximal axons of the anterior horn without increase in phosphorylation is not clear. In contrast to axonopathy that is associated with decrease in neurofilament synthesis, IDPN treatment does not affect the expression of neurofilament mRNA in the spinal cord either qualitatively or quantitatively (Parhad et al., 1988).

Eyer et al. (1989) carried out in vitro phosphorylation of neurofilaments purified from control and IDPN-treated rats. There was no difference in the polypeptide composition of neurofilaments on SDS-polyacrylamide electrophoresis, and no covalent cross-linking of neurofilaments from control and treated rats was observed. Conversely, autophosphorylation of neurofilaments on in vitro incubation was higher in neurofilaments from IDPN-treated rats than in those from controls. In addition, neurofilaments from IDPN-treated rats showed a lower critical concentration and a greater rate of gelation on incubation at room temperature. In vitro incubation of IDPN with bovine neurofilaments also resulted in the increased phosphorylation of neurofilaments, suggesting the direct influence of IDPN on protein kinase activity. The results support the hypothesis that IDPN may interfere with assembly of neurofilaments and change their lateral interactions through their phosphorylation by neurofilament-associated protein kinases.

Fast and Slow Axonal Transport. Neurofilamentous axonal swelling observed in human motor neuron diseases or chemical-induced neuropathies is always associated with a defect in axonal transport of neurofilaments. The susceptibility of neurons to IDPN neurotoxicity depends on their neurofilament content. In sciatic nerves, which are rich in neuro-filaments, neurofilament transport velocity is reduced by 75–90% and tubulin and actin transport is retarded by 25–50%. In contrast, in the dorsal motor nucleus of the vagus nerve, which is devoid of neurofilaments, tubulin and actin transport is not affected. In the visual system, which has an intermediate amount of neurofilaments, there is 50% inhibition of neurofilament transport and no effect is observed on tubulin and tau transport (Parhad et al., 1986). Neurofilament transport in the sciatic nerve is inhibited even after a single injection of IDPN, but the inhibition is about 50%, with a possible halt of neurofilament transport for a short time after IDPN injection. The dose-response data indicate that the threshold lies between 0.5 and 1.0 mg/kg. An increase in IDPN dose to 1.5 mg/kg does not cause further retardation of neurofilament transport (Komiya et al., 1986). Treatment with IDPN also retards fast axonal transport, but only at higher concentrations, 2 and 4 mg/kg. There is no effect on fast transport at a dose of 1 mg/kg (Sickles, 1989a). The lack of effect on fast anterograde transport is supported by lack of consistent effect on tubulin transport by IDPN intoxication, since fast axonal transport is probably associated with the microtubule domain in the axon. Quick-freeze, deep-etch electron microscopy also shows segregation of microtubules from neurofilaments and the association of vesicles with the microtubules and not with neurofilaments (Hirokawa et al., 1985). However, there is inhibition of retrograde transport of cytoskeletal proteins on IDPN intoxication. This defect is observed in dorsal root ganglia as well as in motor neurons, although a significant difference is not found at early intervals in motor neurons (Fink et al., 1986). It is feasible that the defect in retrograde transport may contribute to the similarity of axonopathy produced by IDPN intoxication and by axotomy.

Role of Serotonin System. Chronic administration of IDPN produces the abnormalities termed ECC syndrome in rats and mice. Similar symptoms can be produced by a number of drugs including serotonin (5-HT) receptor agonists, dopamine (DA) agonists, opiate peptides, thyrotropin-releasing hormone or its analogues, and enkephalins (Cadet et al., 1988). In addition, 5-HT–induced dyskinesis as well as some aspects of the IDPN-induced syndrome can be inhibited by dopamine, serotonin, and α_1-noradrenergic receptor antagonists. Thus administration of ketanserin, a 5-HT_2 receptor antagonist, blocks the persistent lateral head shakes, vertical neck dyskinesias, and random circling induced by IDPN (Cadet et al., 1988). Dyskinesia induced by IDPN in rats resembles the idiopathic dyskinesia seen in humans. Both dopaminergic and serotonergic mechanisms have been suggested for this disease. There is a significant increase in 5-HT and 5-hydroxyindolacetic acid (5-HIAA) in the caudate nucleus and putamen and in the nucleus accumbens during IDPN treatment. The increase in 5-HT is supported by a decrease in 5-HT_2 receptors (Cadet et al., 1988) in the same organs. On the other hand, there is an increase in 5-HT_2 receptors in the frontal cortex, cingulate cortex, and claustrum in IDPN-treated animals (Cadet et al., 1987). Autoradiographic methods using $5\text{-}[^3\text{H}]\text{HT}$ binding showed and increase in 5-HT_1 receptors in the Ca3 field of the hippocampus and a decrease in other brain regions including the caudate nucleus and putamen and nucleus accumbens. These experiments support the involvement of 5-HT in the development of the IDPN-induced dyskinetic syndrome (Przedborski et al., 1990).

Role of Neurotensin and Opiate Receptors. The tridecapeptide neurotensin (NT) is widely distributed in the CNS and probably acts as a neurotransmitter. It interacts with the DA system in the CNS. Chronic treatment with IDPN decreases [^{3}H]NT binding in different brain regions such as layers I and III of the frontal and cingulate cerabral cortex, the rhinal sulcus, and the ventral tegmental area (Przedborski et al., 1989). It is suggested that decreased binding of [^{3}H]HT is attributable to down-regulation of NT receptors as a result of increased concentration of NT in these brain regions. Treatment with IDPN has been shown to affect sigma opiate receptors in the corpus striatum of rats. D-Ala-D-Leu-enkephalin ([^{3}H]DADLE) binding has revealed a 26% decrease in sigma opiate receptors in the striatum of IDPN-treated rats (Cadet and Rothman, 1986). Opiate receptors can modulate behaviors elicited by DA agonists and antagonists, are localized in regions of the brain such as the corpus striatum and globus pallidus, and participate in the control of normal movements. Naltrexone, an opiate-receptor antagonist, significantly reduces the hyperactivity and completely inhibits the dyskinetic neck movements of IDPN-treated mice (Cadet and Braun, 1986). The site of action of naltrexone is not known, since opiates can interact with both the DA and the norepinephrine (NE) systems. However, it is also possible that opiate receptors present in the brain are directly involved in eliciting hyperactivity.

Role of the Dopamine System. It has been suggested that the DA system is involved in dyskinesia, since administration of D-amphetamine, a DA agonist, causes an increase in the rate of circling and dyskinetic movements of IDPN-treated rats and these excerbations are antagonized by DA antagonists such as chlorpromazine, haloperidol, and pimozide (Ogawa et al., 1991; Cadet, 1989). Recent studies have shown marked alterations in dopamine and acetylcholine (ACh) levels in neurons. The concentration of DA is decreased in the frontal cortex, hippocampus, corpus striatum, hypothalamus, and hindbrain. In contrast, the concentration of DA metabolites is increased in the nucleus accumbens and the thalamus and midbrain, suggesting enhanced activity of the DA system in these brain regions. In other areas of the brain, both DA and its metabolites are decreased. There is no change in the density of D_2 receptors in the corpus striatum in IDPN-treated rats, but D_1 receptors are decreased in the corpus striatum, nucleus accumbens, and substantia nigra of IDPN-treated rats. Dyskinesia induced by IDPN is enhanced by the administration of L-dopa, which increases DA concentration, and inhibited by ceruletide, which inhibits DA release. However, dyskinesia is not aggravated by the DA agonists apomorphine and bromocriptine, but is transiently improved. Ogawa et al. (1991) studied the inhibition of IDPN-induced dyskinesia by ceruletide along with measurement of monoaminergic neurotransmitters and their metabolites such as 3,4-dihydroxyphenylacetic acid (DOPAC), homovanillic acid (HVA), and 5-hydroxyindoleacetic acid (5-HIAA). The abnormal ratio of (DOPAC + HVA)/5-HIAA, which is greater in the corpus striatum and smaller in the hippocampus of rats with IDPN-induced dyskinesia, returns to normal values after ceruletide treatment. It is suggested that an imbalance of two neuronal systems (dopaminergic, serotonergic) may play a major in the pathogenesis of dyskinesia (Ogawa et al., 1991). Acetylcholine (ACh) is decreased in the frontal cortex, hippocampus, nucleus accumbens, corpus striatum, thalamus and midbrain, and hypothalamus, and muscarinic ACh receptors (MCRs) are increased in striatum. The increase in MCRs in the corpus striatum is attributed to up-regulation resulting from the decrease in ACh in the corpus striatum.

Role of the Norepinephrine System. There is some evidence for the involvement of NE in IDPN-induced dyskinesia. Abnormalities induced by IDPN are antagonized by α_1-adrenoceptor antagonist, prazosin, and by the α_2 agonist clonidine in mice (Cadet, 1989).

Norepinephrine is markedly increased in the medulla, midbrain, and corpus striatum on day 7 of IDPN treatment but decreases to normal values on day 14. Similarly, increased binding of [³H]prazosin is found in the frontal cortex, cingulate cortex, and lateral geniculate nuclei in rats 2 weeks after the development of the IDPN syndrome. The increase in α_1-adrenoceptors may be related to the increased startle response seen in IDPN-treated animals, since blocking of these receptors with prazosin can decrease the startle response in rats. Cadet and Karoum (1988) also found transient changes in the metabolism of NE in the hypothalamus of IDPN-treated rats. There is a transient increase in NE metabolism on day 3 of treatment that reverts back to normal after some time. However, the ratio of NE/total DA is reversed in IDPN-induced dyskinesia, suggesting that alteration in this ratio may be related to the development of this disease.

Role of Calcium Channels. Chronic treatment with IDPN induces a complex motor syndrome associated with hyperactivity, increased startle response, lateral and vertical spasmodic head dyskinesias, and random circling. Administration of the dihydropyridine (DHP) calcium channel antagonist nifedipine has been shown to correct some of the abnormalities produced by IDPN. The most complete effect of drug is on circling, which is almost completely inhibited at higher doses of nifedipine (Cadet et al., 1988). Nifedipine is also able to inhibit phencyclidine (PCP)- and amphetamine-induced hyperactivity in mice. Later, Bangalore et al. (1991) found a significant inhibitory effect of other calcium channel antagonists such as verapamil and diltiazem on some symptoms of IDPN-induced dyskinesia. This suggests the involvement of the DHP-sensitive L class of voltage-gated calcium channels in IDPN-induced dyskinesia. There is no effect of IDPN treatment on the affinity (K_d) or density (Bmax) of [3H]PN 200-110 binding sites in the whole brain of mice, but a significant increase in Bmax in the corpus striatum and a decrease in K_d in the cortex is found in the binding sites for PN 200-110. In contrast, binding parameters of 1251-w-conotoxin are not changed in these brain regions in IDPN-treated mice. These results suggest that L-type rather than N-type channels are involved in this syndrome (Shafer and Atchison, 1991; Bangalore et al., 1991). However, a role of T and P calcium channels cannot be ruled out in the absence of availability of specific ligands for these channels. Since the calcium channel antagonists do not reduce IDPN-induced symptoms to the baseline level, it is certainly possible that other neurochemical factors are also involved in the development of this disorder.

Electrophysiological Abnormalities. The swellings due to accumulation of neurofilaments in proximal axons and atrophy of aions beyond swellings may be expected to influence electrophysiological characteristics of motor and sensory neurons. Studies have been performed in cats that were administered IDPN (50 mg/kg, i.p.) once a week for up to 35 weeks. The conduction velocities are significantly decreased in IDPN-treated cats in all motor unit types. However, the decrease in conduction velocity is greater in fast fatigable (FF) and fast with intermediate fatigability (FI) than in fatigue-resistant fast (FR) and slow (S) motor units (Delio et al., 1992). Delio and Lowndes (1989) studied the changes in excitability and frequency-current relationship on day 35 of IDPN-treatment in cats. The lumbar motoneurons (MNs) have increased thresholds for sustained discharge, tend to achieve higher discharge frequencies, and adapt less readily to continuous current. Seventy-five percent of normal MNs exhibit both primary and secondary firing ranges, whereas only 39% of MNs do so in IDPN-treated cats. In treated cats, MNs that exhibit both primary and secondary firing ranges require larger current strengths than normal cells. Repetitive firing on single stimulation is usually observed in treated cats. Repetitive firing occurs most prominently in fast MNs early in the neuropathy (Delio et al., 1989). At higher currents, MNs discharge doublet potentials interspersed with singlet responses. The second potential of the doublet responses is derived from the large delayed depolarization in treated animals. Similarly, most of the parameters of afterhyperpolarization (AHP) are significantly altered in affected MNs, such as reduction of peak amplitude, duration, and conductance. Duration of AHP is decreased as early as 7 days in all MNs, especially in type FF, FR, and S motoneurons. The incidence of electrical cross-talk between MNs has been measured at different intervals in IDPN-treated cats. An increase in the incidence of cross-talk is observed as early as 7 days of treatment, and the incidence increases with the duration of treatment (Delio et al., 1987). The frequency of recording also increases because of an increase in the number of affected neurons with increasing duration of treatment, but there is no increase in the incidence of cross-talk per recording. Many of the changes in electrophysiological parameters are the result of axonal swellings, which represent discontinuity in axonal diameter. For example, swellings act as a current sink, and, therefore, greater current strength is required to maintain the frequency-current relationship and for some other functions. The mechanism of cross-talk between motoneurons is not clear. It is suggested that there is an increase in extracellular K^+ concentration due to paranodal demyelination and abundance of voltage-sensitive K^+ channels, and that this increase in K^+ concentration is responsible for cross-talk between MNs (Delio et al., 1987).

Distal (Dying-Back)

Neurofilamentous Neuropathies

Acrylamide. Acrylamide is a neurotoxic industrial chemical. Its production has doubled in the past decade in United States and reached 140 million pounds in 1985 (Official Report, 1987, 1988). Humans are exposed to this chemical in industrial processes, in grouting operations, during preparation of acrylamide gels, and by leakage of monomers from polyacrylamide used in the purification of drinking water. The number of laboratory workers exposed to acrylamide in the preparation of polyacrylamide gels is estimated to be about 100,000 to 200,000 (Official Report, 1988). Acrylamide is also used as a soil stabilizer for the construction of dams, in foundations, in tunnels, in roadways, in the maintenance of tunnels and sewage-carrying pipes, and in the textile industry (Dearfield et al., 1988).

Neurotoxicity. Longer-term exposure to acrylamide causes various neurological symptoms such as numbness and tingling of fingers, tremors, and weakness and unsteadiness of legs in humans (Suzuki and Pfaff, 1973). Similar symptoms have been reported in experimental animals exposed to acrylamide. Rats treated with acrylamide 30 mg/kg, i.p., for 3 weeks become unusually nervous and hyperactive on inspection toward the end of the second week (10–11 days). Their hind limbs begin to splay more widely by the 10th day, and this is obvious in all animals by the 14th day of treatment. Also, when the animals are suspended by the tail, the hind legs do not outstretch, but move around till they clasp each other. There is no muscular weakness by this time, and the splay reflex, elicited by rapidly lowering the animal, is normal. The animals progressively lose control of their hind limbs during the third and fourth weeks, and their forelimbs become ataxic. Some improvement in the movement of the hind limbs is observed by the end of the fifth week, 2 weeks after the termination of treatment (Cavanagh, 1982).

Potentiation of neurotoxicity. Pretreatment of rats with phenobarbital, *trans*-stilbene oxide, or dichlorodiphenyltrichloroethane (DDT) results in earlier onset of toxicity signs and subsequent development of acrylamide-induced hind-limb paralysis. In contrast, cobalt chloride pretreatment delays the onset of development of hind-limb paralysis (Srivastava et al., 1985). The results suggest that acrylamide is metabolized to a more neurotoxic intermediate by the same cytochrome P-450 isozyme induced by these chemicals. That cytochrome P-450 and not P-448 is involved in the formation of a neurotoxic metabolite of acrylamide is supported by the fact that β-naphthoflavone pretreatment, which induces P-448, has no effect on acrylamide-induced neuropathy. The delaying effect of pretreatment with cobalt chloride (a depletor of cytochrome P-450) on acrylamide neurotoxicity is consistent with the involvement of mixed-function oxidase enzymes in acrylamide metabolism. Similarly, IDPN pretreatment has been shown to increase the susceptibility of rats to acrylamide toxicity, and pretreatment of rats with acrylamide for 4 weeks masks the development of proximal neurofilamentous swelling on IDPN treatment (Gold and Halleck, 1989).

Neurobehavioral effects. Various neurobehavioral tests have been used for assessing acrylamide-induced changes in neuronal functions. Miller et al. (1984) conducted the following tests after treating rats with 50 mg/kg, i.p., for 10 consecutive days: 1.) the presence of a withdrawal reflex in response to pricking the skin of the hind paw; 2.) the response to nociceptive heat by determining the latency to withdrawal of the tail from a 55°C water bath; 3.) the response to pressure by the use of von Frey's anesthesimeter; 4.) the duration of response when 50 μl of a 1% solution of Zingerone solution was placed in the eye of each animal (normal rats respond by intensely wiping the treated eye for approximately 10 sec); 5.) forepaw grip strength; and 6.) dropping foot-splay test. They also compared the ocular Zingerone test with the dropping foot-splay test at different cumulative doses of acrylamide. At a cumulative dose of 500 mg/kg, sensitivity to pressure by von Frey's anesthesimeter is increased by 40%, duration of response to Zingerone solution is increased by 260%, foot splay is increased by 46%, and forelimb grip strength is decreased by 64%. A significant difference in the sensitivity to Zingerone solution is detected at a cumulative dose of 150 mg/kg, whereas alterations in foot splay are not apparent until a cumulative dose of 225 mg/kg. Therefore, the ocular Zingerone test is suggested as a sensitive and simple technique for assessing the degree of intoxication by acrylamide (Miller et al., 1984).

Histopathology and electron microscopy. Repeated exposure to acrylamide produces central-peripheral distal axonopathy in experimental animals. Widespread swelling occurs almost simultaneously in motor and sensory nerve endings in the peripheral nervous system after about 7 days of treatment with acrylamide 30 mg/kg, i.p., for 3 weeks (Cavanagh, 1982). The motor terminals become club-shaped, and sensory endings are grossly thickened. These alterations slowly spread toward the proximal end in the subsequent weeks. Degeneration initially occurs in large sensory fibers but is abundant in sensory fibers in the limbs by 21 days of treatment. Motor nerve degeneration is comparatively minimal but can be seen in distal ends. Swelling and argyrophilia (silver staining with high affinity for neurofilaments) of terminals also occurs in the CNS, but it is initially seen in the gracile and cuneate nuclei. Later changes take place in the gray matter of the lumbar and cervical spinal cord and in mossy fibers of the cerebellum. In the last phase, all regions of the cerebellum are affected (Cavanagh, 1982). During the early phase of treatment, there is no wallerian degeneration of peripheral axons, but loss of Purkinje cells is evident from the cell counts and increasing number of necrotic cells (Cavanagh and Nolan, 1982). Glycidamide (2,3-epoxy-1-propanamide), an acrylamide metabolite, produced neurotoxicity and neuropathologic lesions similar to that of acrylamide following intraperitoneal injections in rats (Abou-Donia et al., 1993a).

Immunohistochemical methods have also been used to study the neuropathology of the CNS and peripheral nervous system (PNS) of acrylamide-treated rats (50 mg/kg, i.p., 8 days). There is no significant difference in the immunoreactivity of neurofilament protein (NF) in the cerebrum of control and treated rats. Similarly, no difference is observed in Purkinje cells in the cerebellum, but a marked neurofilament accumulation is seen in the distal part of basket cell fibers connected to the Purkinje cells. The cerebellar nucleus also show some cells and fibers with positive immunoreactivity for 68-kDa NF. In the lumbar region of the spinal cord, many axons are found swollen that are strongly stained for 68-kDa NF. Motoneurons do not show any difference in immunostaining. In the tibial nerve, many swollen axons showing strong immunoreactivity for all the three NFs, especially 68 kDa-NF, are evident along the entire length of axons in treated animals (Hashimoto et al., 1988). Thus, immunohistochemical methods using monoclonal anti-NF antibodies are useful in screening neurofilamentous changes in the CNS and PNS of intoxicated animals.

Degenerating terminal branches are evident in the soleus muscle neuromuscular junctions (NMJs) after only three doses of acrylamide (35 mg/kg) (DeGrandchamp and Lowndes, 1990), and there is proliferation of terminal sprouts after 3–5 doses of acrylamide. However, further treatment inhibits this proliferation, and it is less evident after 10 doses. The results suggest that pathological changes in terminal branches commence early and at very low doses of acrylamide, and that acrylamide does not prevent the initiation of regeneration, but causes degeneration of the maturing sprouts.

Swelling and degeneration of distal axons is also accompanied by axonal atrophy in the proximal region of dorsal root ganglia (Gold et al., 1992). Sensory fibers in the L4 and L5 dorsal root ganglia appear smaller in caliber and less circular in shape in comparison with age-matched control animals. Electron microscopy shows that there is also decreased neurofilament content in this part of the axon. It is suggested that this proximal atrophy is due to inhibition of the retrograde transport of some "trophic" signal to the perikaryon. Acrylamide treatment also affects the neuronal perikaryon in addition to promimal and distal axons.

Acrylamide neurotoxicity also produces changes in sensory and motor cell bodies, and some of these alterations take place before swellings and degenerations are visible in the axons. The changes in dorsal root ganglia include loss of Nissl substance from the central and peripheral perikaryon, nuclear eccentricity, nucleolemmal crenation, and enlarged and bizarre forms of mitochondria, with increased number of matrix granules consisting of calcium phosphate, depletion of neurofilaments, and cell shrinkage (Jones and Cavanagh, 1986). In contrast, the activity of the satellite cells is enhanced, suggesting their increased metabolic interaction with the neurons. Light microscopy reveals few changes in motoneuron perikarya on acrylamide intoxication. However, ultrastructural microscopy shows some cytological reorganization. A prominent feature is reduction in the size of Nissl bodies, and few Nissl bodies are seen more than 10 μm in length. Granular endoplasmic reticulum exists in small aggregates, and free ribosomes seem to be increased. There is also some decrease in Golgi complex and mitochondria in acrylamide-treated animals (Sterman and Sposito, 1985). The volume of the neocortex is significantly decreased, but the density of neurons is increased and the mean volume is decreased, resulting in an unchanged total number of neurons (Tandrup and Braendgaard, 1992). These results show that acrylamide also affects the perikarya of motoneurons and sensory neurons in addition to its toxic effects on the axons.

Acrylamide metabolism and interaction with proteins. Acrylamide is readily absorbed from the gastrointestinal tract on oral administration and is distributed uniformly in the body, without specific localization in any tissue. Absorption from the stomach is virtually complete by 3 h, and renal and hepatic elimination is complete in nearly 24 h. Acrylamide persists for a longer time in red blood cells, presumably by reacting with the sulfhydryl groups in the hemoglobin (Dearfield et al., 1989). The distribution appears to be similar in male mice and pregnant female mice. Acrylamide undergoes mixed-function oxidation to form the epoxide glycidamide, by the oxidation of the olefinic bond. The

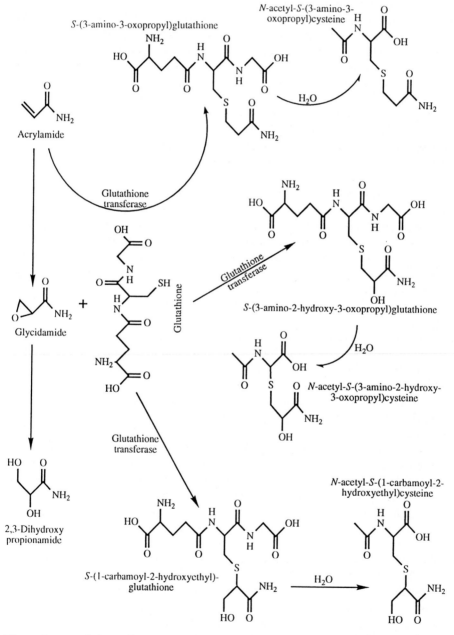

Figure 3   Metabolic pathways of acrylamide.

metabolites identified in rat and mouse urine are *N*-acetyl-*S*-(3-amino-3-oxopropyl)cysteine (I), *N*-acetyl-*S*-(3-amino-2-hydroxy-3-oxopropyl) cysteine (II), *N*-acetyl-*S*-(1-carbamoyl-2-hydroxy- ethyl)cysteine (III), glycidamide (IV), and 2,3-dihydroxypropionamide (V) (Sumner et al., 1992). These metabolites arise from direct conjugation of acrylamide with glutathione or from glycidamide (Fig. 3). The major metabolite is I, which is the result of direct reaction between acrylamide and glutathione. It accounts for 67% and 41% of total metabolite in rat and mouse urine, respectively. The epoxide glycidamide accounts for 6% and 17% of total metabolites in rat and mouse urine, respectively.

The rate of formation of glycidamide from acrylamide depends on the dose administered and is higher at low doses of acrylamide (Costa et al., 1992). The modulation of acrylamide neurotoxicity by inducers and inhibitors of cytochrome P-450 has produced varying results (Dearfield et al., 1988; Srivastave et al., 1985). The direct comparison of acrylamide and glycidamide, however, showed acrylamide to be more neurotoxic than glycidamide (Costa et al., 1992). Similarly, comparison of the neurotoxicity of acrylamide and of 2-hydroxyethyl acrylate (HEA) (Fig. 4) shows that HEA affects weight and some behavioral measures but does not produce distal axonopathy and neurobehavioral signs similar to those associated with acrylamide. The non-neurotoxicity of propionamide and absence of neuropathological changes induced by HEA reflects the importance of both the vinyl and amide groups of acrylamide for neurotoxicity.

Acrylamide and its metabolite glycidamide also react with the cysteine residue of proteins, e.g., hemoglobin, in addition to the main reaction with glutathione. The reaction between the cysteine amino acid of hemoglobin and acrylamide or glycidamide is shown by the identification of *S*-(2-carboxyethyl)cysteine or *S*-(2-carboxy-2-hydroxyethyl)cyteine residues upon acid hydrolysis of hemoglobin from acrylamide-treated animals (Calleman et al., 1990). Other studies have shown the reaction of acrylamide with cytoskeletal proteins also (Carrington et al., 1991; Lapadula et al., 1989).

Axonal transport. The molecular and cellular mechanisms of axonopathy are not clear, but it is suggested that atrophy, swelling, and/or degeneration of the axon is related to alteration of axonal transport resulting in the redistribution of cytoskeletal proteins. An acute dose of acrylamide (75 mg/kg) causes a mild increase in axonal diameter in the proximal portion of large myelinated fibers and a decrease (25%) in transport of NF (145 kDa), tubulin, and other slow-moving proteins. Despite the decrease in the transport of tubulin, there is no increase in the concentration of tubulin in the proximal axons. Subchronic treatment with acrylamide (30 mg/kg), on the other hand, results in different rates of transport for NF, tubulin, and actin (Gold et al., 1985). Tubulin and actin run at a faster rate in comparison with age-matched controls. The spectrum of velocities (front, peak, tail) of NF (145 kDa) is not altered, but there is an overall increase in the transport of NF because of a change in the formation of the peak. There is a marked decrease in the amount of NF in the axon. It is suggested that inhibition of slow transport on a single dose of acrylamide is due to the direct toxic effect of acrylamide on axonal transport,

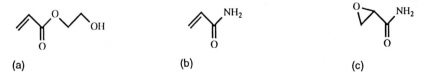

(a)   (b)   (c)

Figure 4 Chemical structures of (a) 2-;hydroxyethyl acrylate, (b) acrylamide, and (c) glycidamide.

whereas acceleration of axonal slow transport on subchronic exposure to acrylamide is the result of neuronal response to axonal injury. Axonal transport has also been studied in the rat optic system, where, in contrast with peripheral nerves, axons remain relatively intact even in advanced stages of acrylamide neuropathy. In this case, slow transport is reduced from 1.3 mm to 1 mm per day (Sabri and Spencer, 1990).

A single intraperitoneal injection of acrylamide inhibits fast anterograde transport by 9.3–20.8% in the sciatic nerve. However, a greater effect, 42.4–51.3%, is seen on the quantity of the transported protein. The decrease in transport is not due to inhibition of protein synthesis in intoxicated animals as determined by the incorporation of ^{3}H-leucine into total proteins (Sickles, 1989b). Both single and repeated administration of acrylamide also inhibits fast anterograde transport in the rat optic system (Sabri and Spencer, 1990). There is also a decrease (48%) in the quantity of transported protein. The inhibition of transport is, however, transient after a single injection of acrylamide. It remains depressed for 16 h and then recovers to normal levels in 24 h. Repeated injections of acrylamide followed by measurement of transport inhibition immediately after the injections show continuous compromise of fast transport (Sickles, 1991). Acrylamide (50 mg/kg, i.p.) treatment for 10 days produces change in the pattern of labeled proteins in both sensory and motor axons. The change in protein pattern, although less pronounced, is qualitatively similar to those in regenerating nerve cells after axotomy. Two-dimensional electrophoresis shows increased labeling of growth-associated protein 43 in acrylamide-treated rats. The change in protein pattern is seen after 10 days of treatment and not after 4 to 6 days, suggesting that the change in protein pattern may be due to an attempt by the nervous system to compensate for the injuries caused by acrylamide (Bisby and Redshaw, 1987). Recent studies show that acrylamide treatment has a greater effect on [^{3}H]glucosamine-labeled than on [^{3}H]methionine-labeled proteins. Control and acrylamide-treated rats show no difference in the distribution of [^{3}H]methionine-labeled proteins along the sciatic nerve 6 hr after labeling. In contrast, there is a marked paucity of [^{3}H]glucosamine-labeled proteins in the myelinated axons. It is suggested that this paucity of glycoprotein is due to either inhibition of glycosylation of proteins or the inhibition of transport of glycoproteins in the treated animals (Harry et al., 1992).

Acrylamide treatment (150 mg/kg or 300 mg/kg cumulative dose) decreases the retrograde transport of some proteins in the rat sciatic nerve (Logan and McLean, 1988). Two-dimensional electrophoresis of proteins accumulated in 18 hr in the sciatic nerve, immediately distal to the ligature, shows 14 proteins that are present in higher concentrations as compared with the contralateral control nerve (without a pair of ligatures) in normal animals. These are considered to be the proteins retrogradely transported in normal animals and accumulated distal to the ligature placed in the sciatic nerve. Four of these proteins fail to appear in animals treated with a cumulative dose of 150 mg/kg and eight in those treated with 300 mg/kg acrylamide. The deficit in retrograde transport is not due to reduced protein synthesis in the perikaryon of treated animals, since electrophoresis of proteins accumulated proximal to the ligature does not show any difference in protein pattern. This study shows that there is inhibition of transport of some proteins only and not of all the proteins that are retrogradely transported (Logan and McLean, 1988). Retrograde transport of proteins has also been studied in hens after single as well as repeated injections of acrylamide. A single injection of acrylamide (1.3 mmol/kg, i.p.) inhibits retrograde transport of ^{125}I-labeled tetanus toxin in both motor and sensory axons. The inhibitory effect is, however, transient and is not detectable after 35 h of dosing. Multiple doses of acrylamide increase the inhibitory effect on retrograde transport to the ventral spinal cord, which correlates with the progressive clinical signs of neuropathy. The accumulation of ^{125}I label in sensory neurons, however, is not statistically decreased (Moretto and Sabri, 1988). Thus acrylamide treatment exhibits an inhibitory effect on fast anterograde as well as retrograde transport, although its effect on slow axonal transport is not conclusive. Fast axonal transport may play an important role in axonal degeneration in acrylamide neuropathy.

Phosphorylation of cytoskeletal proteins. Studies have been performed on the phosphorylation status of cytoskeletal proteins, since aberrant phosphorylation can alter the interaction between cytoskeletal proteins and affect axonal transport in acrylamide-treated animals. Rats treated with acrylamide (50 mg/kg/day, i.p.) for 5 or 10 days show increased (20–40%) in vitro phosphorylation of NF-H (200 kDa) and NF-M (155 kDa) in the spinal cord (Howland and Alli, 1986). The phosphorylation of 70-kDa NF is decreased after treatment for 10 days, and no change is observed after 5 days of treatment. Increase in NF-H and NF-M phosphorylation is observed when rats exhibit marked splaying of hind limbs, and not after 5 days, when they show only mild splaying of hind limbs. Berti-Mattera et al. (1990) studied phosphorylation of sciatic nerve from acrylamide- and N,N'-methylenebisacrylamide (MBA)-treated rats by two methods: incorporation of $^{32}P_i$ by in vitro incubation of proximal and distal segments of sciatic nerve with $^{32}P_i$ and phosphorylation of homogenates of sciatic nerve with ^{32}P-ATP. Both treatments increased phosphorylation of some proteins of myelin origin and tubulin in proximal or distal segments of sciatic nerve on incubation with $^{32}P_i$. Phosphorylation of homogenates of sciatic nerve from acrylamide- and MBA-treated animals by ^{32}P-ATP also increased the phosphorylation of some proteins. However, increased phosphorylation of NF proteins was not observed in this study. In contrast, Reagan et al. (1993) have reported increased phosphorylation of all three NFs isolated from brains and spinal cords of acrylamide- and glycidamide-treated (0.7 mmol/kg, i.p.) rats. Animals treated with non-neurotoxic propionamide show no effect on phosphorylation of these proteins. The discrepancy in results may be due to the composition of the reaction mixture, since Reagan et al. (1993) performed phosphorylation of NFs in the presence of calcium and calmodulin. However, it is necessary to study the in vivo phosphorylation status of NFs in intoxicated animals, since results obtained from in vitro phosphorylation of NFs may not reflect the phosphorylation status of NFs in vivo. Dorsal root ganglia of the fifth lumbar level, L5, have been examined for phosphorylated and nonphosphorylated NFs using specific monoclonal antibodies. However, the monoclonal antibodies used were not able to distinguish unambiguously between phosphorylated NF-H and NF-M. Chronic treatment with acrylamide enhances the immunoreactivity of all three phosphorylated NFs in 20–30% of neuronal cell bodies and the glomerular regions of their axons. In contrast, a single high dose of acrylamide has no effect on the staining of phosphorylated NFs, even though it is capable of impairing slow axonal transport (Gold et al., 1988). It is suggested that increased immunoreactivity of phosphorylated NFs in chronically intoxicated animals may be not the result of direct action of acrylamide, but a secondary response to axotomy-like axonal injury or impairment of axonal transport, such as retrograde transport. An increase in phosphorylated NFs and MAP-2 has also been reported in the central and peripheral nervous system of acrylamide- and glycidamide-treated rats (Ibrahim and Abou-Donia, 1993).

Effect on energy metabolism and enzymes. A normal energy supply is essential for proper function of the brain and fast axonal transport. Therefore, it is important to study the production of energy and related enzymes in the central and peripheral nervous system. Acrylamide treatment, however, does not alter the concentration of phosphocreatine, ATP, ADP, AMP, glucose, and lactate in the whole brain, indicating no deficiency of high-energy phosphate compounds in the brain (Matsuoka and Igisu, 1992). Extension of these studies included determination of the respiration rate of brain mitochondria from acrylamide-treated animals. The major part of the ATP used in brain, 80%, is obtained by mitochondrial oxidative phosphorylation. Chronic treatment with acrylamide has not effect on the respiration of mitochondria isolated from the cortex, brain stem, and whole brain (Medrano and LoPachin, 1989; Sickles et al., 1990). However, both state 3 and state 4 of mitochondrial respiration supported by pyruvate/oxaloacetic acid are decreased in the cerebellum of acrylamide-treated animals, resulting in reduced ADP/O ration in this brain region (Medrano and LoPachin, 1989). Single as well as repeated injections of acrylamide also decrease the activity of the enzyme responsible for oxidation of NADH, NADH-tetrazolium reductase (NADH-TR), in rat soleus muscle motoneurons (Sickles and Goldstein, 1986). The latter have high NADH-TR activity. The NADH-TR activity of motoneurons with low oxidative metabolism is not affected. These results provide evidence in support of the role of energy metabolism in acrylamide-induced neuropathy.

Inhibition of glycolytic enzymes such as glyceraldehyde-3-phosphate dehydrogenase (GADPH), neuron-specific enolase (NSE), and phosphofructokinase, and of creatine kinase (CK), has been suspected to contribute to acrylamide-induced degeneration of axons. However, in vitro as well as in vivo studies using various non-neurotoxic and neurotoxic analogues of acrylamide have not produced conclusive results (Vyas et al., 1985; Sakamoto and Hashimoto, 1985). In vitro incubation of brain slices with acrylamide, acetamide (a non-neurotoxicant), and methylenebisacrylamide (a weak neurotoxicant) show selective inhibition of GADPH, NSE, and *N*-acetylglucosaminidase at low concentration of acrylamide. Similar doses of acetamide and methylenebisacrylamide do not have the same effects on the activity of these enzymes. Incubation of acrylamide with brain slices depletes glutathione, and addition of glutathione is capable of preventing acrylamide-induced inhibition of GADPH and lysosomal enzymes (Ravindranath and Pai, 1991). However, this model of brain slices requires testing of more non-neurotoxic and neurotoxic analogues of acrylamide.

Ornithine decarboxylase (ODC) activity in dorsal root ganglia is increased after axonal injury such as nerve crush. This enzyme converts ornithine into putrescine, which accepts the c_3 fragment from S-adenosylmethionine and forms polyamines. Polyamines are involved in protein elongation, RNA and DNA synthesis, and gene expression. The increase in ODC activity is ascribed to the arrival of a signaling molecule, nerve growth factor, that is transported from the site of injury to the cell body. The rise in activity of ODC is decreased in streptozocin-induced diabetes, which is associated with inhibition of retrograde axonal transport. Acrylamide treatment of rats with a cumulative dose of 150 or 300 mg/kg also decreases the ODC activity evoked by sciatic nerve crush, suggesting that acrylamide-induced axonopathy is associated with reduction of retrograde transport (Myall et al., 1990b).

Endogenous substances such as proteins, nucleic acids, oligosaccharides, lipids, and foreign compounds are hydrolyzed by lysosomal enzymes, and proteins are also digested by proteinases, especially in the axon terminals. Accumulation of neurofilaments occurs in terminals if proteinases are inhibited by inhibitors such as leupeptin. Subchronic treatment with acrylamide increases the activity of β-glucuronidase and cathepsin D in the brain, spinal cord, and sciatic nerve. The increase in activity is more marked in the sciatic nerve than in the brain or spinal cord (Srivastava et al., 1984). A single injection of acrylamide (50 mg/kg, i.p.) has no effect on these lysosomal enzymes. In contrast, an acute dose of acrylamide (150 mg/kg, i.p.) decreases the activity of β-glucuronidase in the brain and sciatic nerve (Ravindranath and Pai, 1991). The discrepancy in results may be due to difference in dosage or in time of killing of the animal after the acute dose of acrylamide. The results obtained in the latter study are, however, consistent with the in vitro inhibition of this enzyme by acrylamide in brain slices. Acrylamide treatment also reduces the activity of proteinases in the tibial nerve and spinal cord. The degradation of NF-L (68 kDa) on in vitro incubation at 37°C is inhibited in the tibial nerve and that of all three NFs in the spinal cord (Tanii et al., 1988). Analysis of NF-H and NF-M could not be carried out in the tibial nerve because of the paucity of these NFs in this tissue. The alteration in the activity of lysosomal enzymes in acrylamide-treated animals may be related to neuropathy in these animals.

Electrophysiological abnormalities. Intoxication with acrylamide also produces changes in various electrophysiological characteristics, along with morphological alterations. Brismar et al. (1987) treated rats three times a week with acrylamide (50 mg/kg). The animals were given a total of three or 10 injections and were used for the measurement of motor nerve conduction velocity (MNCV) in the sciatic nerve. Some fibers were also examined by the potential clamp technique. This technique shows specific changes in nodal function. There is a decrease in MNCV measured in vivo, but not in MNCV measured in vitro on the excised nerve. There is marked rise in K permeability that correlates with the increase in capacitance, and an increased leak conductance in some isolated myelinated sciatic fibers. The increase in capacitance may be related to deficiency in the insulation of the axon provided by myelin, and the increase in K permeability may be due to exposure of hidden K-channels on intoxication (Brismar et al., 1987).

Monosynaptic reflex (MSR), dorsal root reflex (DRR), and dorsal root potential (DRP) have been measured in cats after acute and chronic administration of acrylamide. Chronic administration of acrylamide depresses MSR and DRP and alters DRR, while acute administration increases MSR and DRR (Goldstein and Fincher, 1986). This increase is observed even at low doses of acrylamide, 5 mg/kg. The decrease in MSR on chronic treatment is attributed to an alteration in primary afferent terminal (PAT) function, although the exact nature of the dysfunction is not clear. It may be due to a decrease in the number of PATs because of degeneration or because of a change in storage or utilization of calcium. Changes in storage and utilization may also explain increases in MSR and DRR following acute acrylamide intoxication. It is suggested that depolarization of neuronal membranes, which can be expected before cell injury or death, may also contribute to increase of spinal reflexes after acute administration of acrylamide (Goldstein and Fincher, 1986). Further extension of this study included determination of DRP and DRR in cats treated with acrylamide (30 mg/kg/day) for 5 and 10 days. The cats were sacrificed after the last injection, and DRP and DRR were studied in spinal cord isolated in situ. There was no change in DRP evoked in cats treated for 5 days and control cats (De Rojas and Goldstein, 1987). However, DRR evoked from the sural nerve was not seen in the 10-day group and in only 20% of the 5-day group. Dorsal root reflex evoked from the medial gastrocnemius nerve was, however, much less sensitive in differentiating between control and treated groups.

Electroneuromyographic changes have been examined in a group of 71 workers occupationally exposed to acrylamide (Fengsheng et al., 1989). Electroneuromyographic tests included measurement of maximal MNCV of median, ulnar, and peroneal nerves, sensory nerve conduction velocity of the median, ulnar, and sural nerves, H-reflex from the soleus muscle, and ankle tendon reflex from the medial head of the gastrocnemius muscle. The latency of detectable ankle reflex was significantly prolonged in 48 acrylamide-exposed workers, including 25 workers with no clinical neurological findings. The latency of the ankle tendon reflex seems to be a more sensitive test for the early detection of acrylamide neurotoxicity in humans.

   Effect on receptors.   Some studies have been performed on the effects of acrylamide treatment on various receptors. Receptors on the cell plasma membrane or terminals control various functions of the cell and secretion of neurotransmitters. Single (100 mg/kg) and repeated (50 mg/kg, 10 days) exposure to acrylamide results in a significant increase in [^{3}H]spiroperidol binding to corpus striatum membranes, suggesting an increase in the affinity or number of DA receptors. Scatchard analysis shows an increase in the affinity of binding (K_d) and not in the number of binding sites (Bmax). The specificity of binding is shown by the fact that methylene bisacrylamide (a non-neurotoxic analogue of acrylamide) has no effect on [^{3}H]spiroperidolbinding (Srivastava et al., 1986). Khanna et al. (1992) studied the effect of acrylamide exposure on pregnant and nonpregnant rats with a low-protein diet. The rats were administered a low dose of acrylamide (2 mg/kg/day) orally from gestation day 6 to 17 and then sacrificed to study DA, muscarinic, and benzodiazepine receptor binding in different brain regions. The low-protein diet had no effect on the binding properties of these receptors in nonpregnant rats with or without exposure to acrylamide. A low dose of acrylamide was used in this study, since a large number of pregnant rats died at a dose of 3–10 mg/kg/day. The lack of effect of acrylamide treatment on [^{3}H]spiperone binding in nonpregnant rats is in contrast to the above results, where an increase in [^{3}H]spiroperidol binding was observed on giving a high dose of acrylamide. On the other hand, pregnant rats showed a decrease in [^{3}H]spiperone binding even without acrylamide treatment on a low-protein diet, and acrylamide treatment resulted in significant inhibition of all the studied receptors in pregnant rats on a low-protein diet. However, receptor bindings in pregnant rats with a normal protein diet are not altered by acrylamide treatment. The decrease in DA receptors in the corpus striatum may be attributed to a decrease in monoamine oxidase activity observed in these animals, which may lead to higher levels of DA in cells. Similarly, a decrease in muscarinic receptors in the cerebellum is probably due to decreased activity of acetylcholinesterase. The results show that acrylamide neurotoxicity may be considerably modified under different conditions such as pregnancy and malnutrition.

γ-Diketones. Aliphatic hexacarbon solvents, e.g., *n*-hexane, methyl *n*-butyl ketone, and methyl isobutyl ketone have been extensively used in industry. Chronic exposure to these solvents produces central-peripheral polyneuropathy in humans and experimental animals (Spencer et al., 1980). Major clinical outbreaks of peripheral neuropathy have occurred among "glue sniffers" (Spencer et al., 1980; Korokobin et al., 1975) and among industrial workers exposed to *n*-hexane and methyl *n*-butyl ketone (Ishii et al., 1972; Allen, 1980).

   Neurotoxicity.   The most common complaint in the least severe cases among industrial workers and glue sniffers is the onset of numbness of the toes and fingers, and the more severe cases involve weight loss, weakness, anorexia, abdominal pain, and cramps in the lower extremities. The patient also has difficulty in pinching, grasping objects, and steeping over curbs. Cases of pure motor neuropathy are unusual in industrial cases. Glue sniffers display a subacute, distal-to-proximal progression of weakness in the early course of disease and may rarely suffer from phrenic nerve paralysis. Neurotoxicity seems to be increased when other solvents are present along with *n*-hexane, since some mixtures containing a much lower concentration of *n*-hexane have produced neurotoxicity in abusers (Spencer et al., 1980).

   In experimental hexacarbon neuropathy, *n*-hexane, methyl *n*-butyl ketone, 2,5-

hexanediol, or 2,5-hexanedione (2,5-HD) per se is used to induce neuropathy in experimental animals, since 2,5-HD is the active metabolite responsible for the induction of this disease. In one study, rats treated with 1% 2,5-hexanediol showed the first sign of weakness after 2 weeks in the hind limbs, and the weakness progressed with time. Some rats were almost completely paralyzed in 6 weeks, but the forelimbs never became paralyzed, although they became weaker. All of the rats had clumsy gait and were unstable when nudged. The fur was discolored and mellowed (Backstrom and Collins, 1987). The neurotoxicity of *n*-hexane is increased when animals are treated with both *n*-hexane and the solvent methyl isobutyl ketone. This synergistic effect is ascribed to the induction of cytochrome P-450 by methyl isobutyl ketone, which enhances the metabolism of *n*-hexane to 2,5-HD (Abou-Donia et al., 1985b). Methyl isobutyl ketone produces only transient weakness in the legs, but it potentiates the neurotoxicity of other toxic chemicals (Abou-Donia et al., 1985a; Abou-Donia et al., 1991).

Neurobehavioral effects. Some neurobehavioral studies have been performed to evaluate the neurotoxic effect of 2,5-HD treatment. Ladefoged et al. (1989) monitored behavioral effects with the rotarod test, in which the rod was driven at a speed of 9 r.p.m. and the balance time was measured in 30-sec intervals. The balance time is significantly reduced in the third and fourth week of 2,5-HD treatment and is reduced from second week with exposure to 2,5-hexanedione plus acetone. The onset of behavioral deficiency during 2,5-HD treatment appears at about the same time as the first recorded reduction in peripheral motor nerve conduction velocity. Performance in the radial eight-arm maze was measured in control, 2,5-HD–treated, and acetone-treated rats during 6 and 7 weeks of exposure (Lam et al., 1991). The choice of a correct arm in this test involves higher CNS processes and is independent of PNS alterations. Acquisition but not performance of spatial learning was inhibited to a minor degree by 2,5-HD alone and significantly by combined treatment with 2,5-HD and acetone. This study shows that acetone potentiates 2,5-HD–induced neurotoxic effects in the CNS, but the underlying mechanisms and the site of action are not clear.

Histopathology and electron microscopy. Nerve biopsy samples from mild case are usually normal even when examined by electron microscopy. Samples from severe cases show paranodal giant axonal swellings accompanied by myelin retraction, and the swellings consist of neurofilaments of 10-nm diameter. These pathological features are identical to those observed in experimental animal models (Spencer et al., 1980).

The animals used to study central-peripheral neuropathy are treated with *n*-hexane, methyl *n*-butyl ketone, 2,5-hexanediol, or 2,5-HD for some time to induce polyneuropathy. The degeneration begins distally and with time spreads proximally in the CNS as well as the PNS, and this has led to the designation "dying-back polyneuropathy." There are also swellings in the distal part of axons on the proximal side of nodes of Ranvier. The large myelinated fibers situated in tibial nerve branches exhibit multifocal giant axonal degeneration before similar changes appear in the much longer plantar nerve fibers (Spencer and Schaumburg, 1976). This is in contrast to the situation in acrylamide-treated rats, in which these two fibers are equally vulnerable. Similarly, longer nerves seem to be more vulnerable than shorter nerves: the hind limb, containing longer nerves, is affected before and more severely than the forelimb, which has much shorter nerves. Furthermore, in hexacarbon-treated animals, degeneration does not start from the nerve terminal, but begins in a multifocal pattern on the proximal side of nodes of Ranvier in the distal part of axon, and that leads to terminal degeneration. The interface between the preserved proximal porter of the fiber and the distal degenerating part of the axon is frequently marked by a swollen axon. In the CNS, distal regions of long spinal nerve tracts undergo dying-back degeneration before shorter nerve tracts. The giant axonal swellings are observed in dorsal spinocerebellar tracts, ventrolateral tracts, pyramidal tracts, and the gracile nuclei before clinical manifestation of hexacarbon neuropathy (Spencer and Schaumburg, 1976, 1977). Electron microscopy revealed 10-nm neurofilaments and, sometimes, clustered microtubules, mitochondria, and smooth endoplasmic reticulum in the axonal swellings (Spencer and Schaumburg, 1977). Microtubules and mitochondria are also seen along the perimeter of swollen axons. Backstrom and Collins (1987) studied axonal changes in 2,5-hexanediol–treated rats using immunohistochemical methods and monoclonal antibodies. The axonal swelling in the CNS as well as the PNS contain large amounts of NFs. The swellings contain tubulin but to a lesser extent than the normal axon, suggesting partial removal of tubulin from these areas.

   Metabolism and cross-linking.   *n*-Hexane and methyl *n*-butyl ketone exert a neurotoxic effect through their metabolism to the γ-diketone 2,5-HD. *n*-Hexane and methyl *n*-butyl ketone undergo omega-1 oxidation by hepatic mixed-function oxidases to form the toxic metabolite 2,5-HD (Fig. 5) (Krasavage et al., 1980). The latter reacts with the primary amino group of lysine residues in proteins, e.g., NFs, and forms pyrroles. Pyrrole derivatives of proteins undergo autoxidation and yield pyrrole-pyrrole intramolecular or intermolecular cross-linked neurofilaments (Lapadula et al., 1986; DeCaprio and Fowke, 1992). Pyrrole-adduct is probably formed through intermediate imine and enamine,

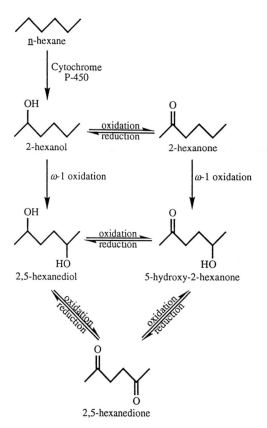

Figure 5   Metabolic pathways of *n*-hexane.

although the latter has not yet been detected (Fig. 6) (DeCaprio et al., 1987). Dicarbonyl spacing between ketone groups is important for neurotoxicity, since 2,6-heptanedione does not produce clinically detectable neuropathy, although it shows systemic toxicity and generalized wasting in treated animals. This also indicates the importance of cross-linking of neurofilaments for development of neuropathy. 2,6-Heptanedione rapidly reacts with ovalbumin but does not form cross-links between amino groups. The essential role of pyrrole in hexacarbon neuropathy is supported by increased neurotoxicity of 1.) dl-3,4-dimethyl-2,5-hexanedione (dl-DMHD) as compared with 2,5-HD and meso-3,4-dimethyl-2,5-hexanedione (meso-DMHD), and 2.) of 2,5-HD as compared with perdeuterio-2,5-HD ($[D^{10}]$-2,5-HD) (Boekelheide et al., 1988; DeCaprio et al., 1988). dl-DMHD forms pyrrole adduct at a greater rate than 2,5-HD and meso-DMHD, and 2,5-HD at a greater rate than $[D^{10}]$-2,5-HD. Similarly, 3,3-dimethyl-2,5-hexanedione, which is incapable of pyrrole

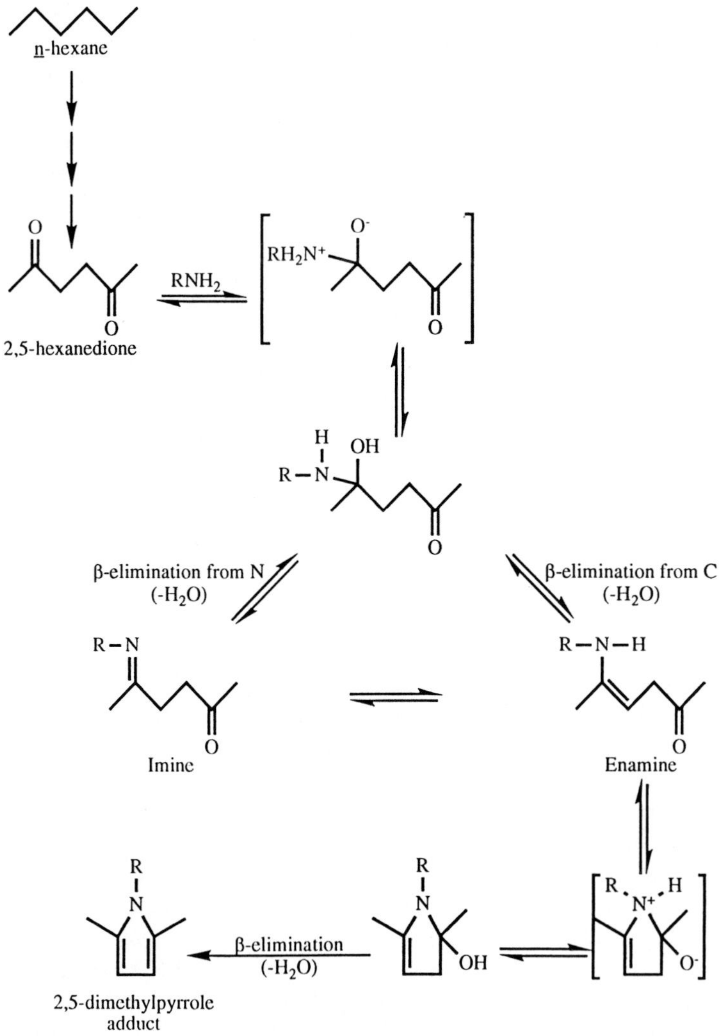

Figure 6 Proposed mechanism for the formation of dialkylpyrroles through intermediates imine and enamine.

formation, and some other γ-diketones (e.g., 3,4-diethyl-2,5-hexanedione, 3,4-isopropyl-2,5-hexanedione) that are slow in forming pyrrole adducts are nonneurotoxic (Boekelheide et al., 1988). That the pyrrole adducts undergo autoxidation before cross-linking the protein amino groups is supported by 1.) enhanced neurotoxicity of 2,5-HD with exposure to hyperbaric oxygen, which facilitiates autoxidation, and 2.) non-neurotoxicity of 3-acetyl-2,5-HD (AcHD), which results in massive formation of pyrrole derivatives but undergoes autoxidation with difficulty because of its high oxidation potential (Graham et al., 1991). Recent studies show that NF-H and NF-M have four to six times more binding sites for 2,5-HD than does NF-L, and 70–80% of binding sites are located in the tail region of NF-H and NF-M. The specific activities are 6.9, 4.7 and 1.3 mol/mol for NF-H, NF-M and NF-L, respectively (DeCaprio and Fowke, 1992). Therefore, pyrrole adduct is formed with only a small subset of lysine residues in the tail domain. The amino terminal binds with only 1 mol of 2,5-HD/mol of protein. The location of pyrrole adducts in the carboxyl-terminal region of heavy NFs is likely to alter interaction between NFs and other cytoskeletal proteins and to affect the anterograde transport of NFs in the axons.

Axonal transport. It is suggested that axonal swellings containing accumulated neurofilaments and wallerian-type degeneration of axons are linked to the alteration in axonal transport. The location of accumulation depends on the nature of chemical. For example, 2,5-HD treatment results in neurofilament accumulation in the distal parts of the axon, DMHD treatment in accumulation in the proximal part, and 3-methyl-2,5-HD treatment in accumulation in the midway axonal position (Monaco et al., 1990). Both 2,5-HD and 3-methyl-2,5-HD have been shown to accelerate neurofilament transport in the sections of axons proximal to the enlargement, and it is difficult to determine transport in the case of DMHD, since the accumulation of neurofilaments occurs very close to the cell body. Acceleration of neurofilament transport has been found in both the central (optic nerve) and the peripheral (sciatic nerve) nervous system. The transport of tubulin is not affected on 2,5-HD treatment (Monaco et al., 1989). However, there is a progressive decline in the velocity of neurofilament transport with increasing distance along the axons, resulting in decrease in the number and diameter of neurofilaments in the proximal axon and increase in both number and diameter of neurofilaments in the distal axons (Monaco et al., 1989). Axonal transport studies using 2,5-HD and AcHD suggest that cross-linking of neurofilaments is essential for alteration in axonal transport and neurotoxicity of the chemical. 3-Acety-2,5-HD forms pyrrole adducts more readily than 2,5-HD but is incapable of cross-linking the proteins. Treatment with AcHD neither alters neurofilament transport nor induces neurotoxicity (Pyle et al., 1992). Measurement of axonal transport after intrathecal injection of 2,5-HD shows a decrease in the velocity of neurofilaments in the sensory axons (Hammond-Tooke, 1992). In this case, axonal swellings were produced proximally in the spinal nerve roots of rats, and transport was measured in the axon down the swellings. Thus it appears that the axonal transport of neurofilaments is increased proximal to the swellings and decreased beyond it in γ-diketone–induced axonopathy.

It has been suggested that fast anterograde and retrograde transport are associated with axonal degeneration, since IDPN, which does not affect fast axonal transport, causes only accumulation of neurofilaments in proximal axons without degeneration. Treatment with 2,5-HD results in reduction of fast axonal transport by 18–25%, but the greater effect of treatment is observed in the quantity of protein transport, which is reduced by 50–63% (Sickles, 1989). A similar effect is observed with DMHD treatment. This decrease in transport is not due to decrease in synthesis of protein, since there is no decrease in leucine uptake or synthesis of protein during the period of experiment. The transport remains depressed for 16 h and then recovers to a normal level by 24 h. Repeated administration of 2,5-HD does not enhance reduction in the quantity of transported proteins, suggesting that 2,5-HD produces a transient and repeated compromise of fast axonal transport during treatment (Sickles, 1991). Sickles (1992) studied the role of the neuronal perikaryon and axon in the reduction of fast axonal transport capacity by exposing both regions of dorsal root ganglia separately to 2,5-HD. Exposure of the nerve fiber to 2,5-HD solution decreases the capacity for fast axonal transport, whereas exposure of the cell body to 2,5-HD has no effect on fast axonal transport, suggesting that neurotoxicants directly penetrate the nerve fiber and alter axonal transport.

Treatment with 2,5-HD and DMHD also affects retrograde fast axonal transport. A single injection of 2,5-HD produces a time-dependent decrease in retrograde transport in the mouse sciatic nerve (Sabri, 1992). The inhibition is maximal at 2–2.5 hr after toxin administration, and then retrograde transport returns to normal velocity. Similarly, subchronic treatment of rats with DMHD results in the inhibition of retrograde transport. Mice are refractory to even higher doses of DMHD. Treatment with 2,5-HD also decreases retrograde transport in rats. In this study, anterograde and retrograde build-up was determined in both motor and sensory nerves for short and long periods (6 and 14 hr) in 2,5-HD–treated rats. The rats were treated for 2–8 weeks. Motor nerves showed decrease in retrograde transport during both short and long accumulation intervals (Braendgaard and Sidenius, 1986). Sensory nerves, however, showed less severe damage in retrograde axonal transport during short (6-h) than during long (14-h) accumulation intervals. After the treatment was stopped, there was complete recovery of retrograde transport build-up for short accumulation times and an improvement, but not complete recovery, for long accumulation times. Furthermore, abnormalities in retrograde transport appeared in motor nerves after an accumulated dose of 4 g/kg, whereas sensory nerves showed a decrease after 6 g/kg.

Phosphorylation of proteins. Studies on the determination of phosphorylated neurofilaments along the dorsal and ventral roots show that the concentration of phosphorylated neurofilaments increases with increasing distance from the perikaryon, and this is also accompanied by a decrease in the rate of neurofilament transport down the axon. The concentration of phosphorylated neurofilaments also increases with maturity in normal animals (Watson et al., 1989). Treatment with 2,5-HD (0.5%) decreases the ratio of phosphorylated/nonphosphorylated neurofilaments in ventral roots, dorsal roots, and peripheral sensory nerves (Watson et al., 1991). This is consistent with the increase in neurofilament transport observed in the same nerves. Similarly, Lapadula et al. (1988) found decreased phosphorylation of neurofilaments in the spinal cords of 2,5-HD–treated animals on in vitro phosphorylation in the presence of trifluoperizine, and this decreased phosphorylation of neurofilaments is compatible with the results of Watson et al. (1991). However, some recent findings show increased concentrations of phosphorylated neurofilaments in the brain, spinal cord, and peripheral nerves on immunohistochemical analysis in 2,5-HD–treated animals (Huges et al., 1993). Similarly, there is increased in vitro incorporation of ^{32}P in 55-kDa and 180-kDa proteins in the proximal sciatic nerve of 2,5-HD–treated animals, and in 55-kDa, 180-kDa, and myelin proteins (P_o, P_1, P_r) of DMHD-treated animals (Horan et al., 1989). The increased phosphorylation of these proteins with 2,5-HD treatment is not consistent with the decreased concentration of phosphorylated neurofilaments in the dorsal and ventral roots observed by other investigators (Watson et al., 1991). However, it is feasible that conditions for in vitro ^{32}P incorporation may not be applicable to in vivo phosphorylation of proteins in the spinal cord.

Effect on energy metabolism and other enzymes. Axonal transport, especially fast axonal transport, is an energy-dependent process, and inhibition of enzymes that are related to energy production can interfere with axonal transport. 2,5-Hexanedione has been shown to inhibit state 3 respiration of brain mitochondria directly at 1-mM concentrations. Furthermore, all brain regions of 2,5-HD–treated rats show reduced pyruvate/oxaloacetate-supported state 3 respiration, and the brain stem also shows glutamate/malate-supported respiration in the isolated mitochondria (Medrano and LoPachin, 1989). It has been suggested that inhibition is specific, since the non-neurotoxic analogue 1,6-hexanediol has no inhibitory effect on mitochondrial respiration. Inhibition of pyruvate/oxaloacetate-supported and not glutamate/malate-supported respiration in some brain regions suggests pyruvate dehydrogenase as the possible site of 2,5-HD action, and inhibition of glutamate/malate-supported respiration in the brain stem indicates another site of action in the TCA cycle or electron transport chain.

2,5-Hexanedione is also capable of inhibiting GAPDH, an enzyme of the glycolytic pathway. It inhibits 25% and 55% of GAPDH activity at 1 and 5 mM concentrations, respectively, on in vitro incubation for 2 hr, and millimolar concentrations of 2,5-HD have been shown to be present in the blood of 2,5-HD–treated animals (Sabri, 1984). 2,4-Hexanedione, a non-neurotoxic analogue of 2,5-HD, has no inhibitory effect on this enzyme. Inhibition of GADPH is also seen in the sciatic nerve, but not in brain homogenates of 2,5-HD–treated animals. Inhibition of GADPH activity may assist in the inhibition of energy-dependent fast axonal transport, and the reduction of the rate and capacity of fast axonal transport has been implicated in axonal degeneration. The inhibitory effect may be more critical in the paranodal region, since the nodal region of a nerve fiber is a high energy–requiring site that is involved in the maintenance of transmembrane potential as well as axonal transport.

Activity of the enzyme ODC is increased after axotomy or other nerve injury. This enzyme catalyzes the conversion of ornithine to putrescine, which is converted into polyamines that are responsible for protein elongation and RNA and DNA synthesis and are probably related to changes in genetic expression. Dorsal root ganglia were used as a model for study and were removed from control or 2,5-HD–treated rats 24 hr after crush of the sciatic nerve (Myall et al., 1990a). Treatment with 2,5-HD reduced the increase in ODC activity in dorsal root ganglia observed after sciatic nerve crush of control rats. Similar results are obtained in other conditions (e.g., diabetes, vinca alkaloid treatment) where retrograde axonal transport is reduced. The effect is observed only in treated animals, and 2,5-HD has no direct effect on the activity of ODC. Inhibition of activity suggests that retrograde transport is impaired in hexacarbon-induced neuropathy.

Treatment with 2,5-HD also reduces the degradation of neurofilament protein by Ca^{2+}-activated proteinase (Tanii et al., 1988). This enzyme has been shown to be involved in the turnover of NF and in wallerian degeneration in peripheral nerves. Degradation of neurofilament proteins was measured by in vitro incubation of tibial nerves from control and treated rats in a medium containing Ca^{2+} ions. The degradation of 68-kDa NF is depressed not only in 2,5-HD–treated animals, but also on treatment with other neurotoxic chemicals such as acrylamide, N-hydroxymethylacrylamide, N-isopropylacrylamide, and methacrylamide, but not on treatment with the non-neurotoxic chemical diacetone acrylamide.

Electrophysiological abnormalities. Electrophysiological studies have been performed in the central as well as the peripheral nervous system to reveal more sensitive parameters for the early detection of chemical-induced neuropathies. Nachtman and Couri

(1984) determined MNCVs in the hind limbs of 2,5-HD–treated rats. There is no significant difference in distal MNCV (MNCV between popliteal space and plantaris tendon) and proximal MNCV (MNCV between sciatic notch and popliteal space) of control and 2,5-HD–treated rats, but there is a significant increase in distal latency in treated rats. The increase in distal latency is observed at a dose of 40 mM 2,5-HD in drinking water and not at a 20-mM concentration, suggesting a threshold level of the neurotoxic agent. The results also showed that neurotoxic effects are first observed in the distal axons. Similarly, decrease in MNCV is also observed when measured in the tails of 2,5-HD–treated rats (Ladefoged and Simonsen, 1989). The decrease in MNCV and neurobehavioral deficiency on rotarod performance appeared at the same time (3 weeks) in the latter study. Thomas et al. (1984) measured motor and sensory nerve conduction velocity in tibial, sural, and median nerves and somatosensory evoked potentials in lower and upper limbs of 2,5-HD-treated baboons. Treatment with 2,5-HD resulted in a marked decrease in motor and sensory nerve conduction velocity of baboons also.

Although decrease in nerve conduction velocity has been reported in many studies, the detection of nerve injury can be made at a much lower levels of 2,5-HD treatment by measuring certain other parameters in place of nerve conduction velocity. For example, there is significant reduction in peak conduction velocity and increase in action potential duration at relatively much lower concentrations of 2,5-HD in drinking water, when there is no change in the onset conduction velocity (Anderson and Dunham, 1984). The latter is the most commonly used method for measuring coduction velocity in peripheral nerves. Similarly, there is a shift in the neuroexcitability of the sciatic nerve as measured by the relative refractory period. This is indicative of both slower conduction and slower repolarization of the nerve membrane following excitation. There is also enhanced K^+-induced depolarization of the sciatic nerves of 2,5-HD–treated rats. This may be due to some disruptive effect of hexacarbon treatment on membrane Na^+,K^+-ATPase activity, since acute administration of ouabain also results in enhanced K^+-induced depolarization of the sciatic nerve. Thus, these sensitive electrophysiological methods are able to indicate axonal injury when there is no overt effect of neurotoxicity except decrease in the weight gain of treated animals (Anderson and Dunham, 1984). Neurotoxic effects of 2,5-HD treatment on the CNS have been studied by measuring auditory brain stem response (ABR) and somatosensory-evoked potentials (SEPs) in control and treated rats (Hirata, 1990). Delays in some components of ABR and SEPs reflect the neurotoxic effects of 2,5-HD on the auditory ascending tract in the brain stem and the ascending somatosensory pathway in the cortex of the CNS, respectively.

Carbon Disulfide

Carbon disulfide (CS_2) is an industrial solvent used in rayon production and as an organic synthetic precursor. It is also used in agriculture, as it forms a major component of fumigant mixtures. Occupational exposure to CS_2 is associated with several adverse effects such as neurotoxicity, atherosclerosis, cardiovascular disease, liver injury, and endocrine disturbances, but we will focus below only on the neurotoxic effects of this industrial solvent.

Neurotoxic Effects of Carbon Disulfide. Chronic CS_2 exposure produces a decrease in the conduction velocity of sensory fibers of the peroneal, median, and ulnar nerves (particularly in the digital segments) of workers, although conduction velocity in the motor fibers was still within normal limits (Vasilescu, 1976). The abnormalities could be revealed by neurological and neuropsychological examination, as well as by cerebral computed tomography. The latter showed cerebral atrophy in 13 of 16 exposed persons (Aaserud et al., 1988). Rayon factory workers exposed to high CS_2 concentrations showed clinical and electromyographic evidence of neuropathy even 10 years after exposure. Ten of 20 subjects showed decrease in motor conduction velocity of the slow fibers in peripheral nerves (Corsi et al., 1983).

Chronic CS_2 exposure of rats induced neurofilamentous axonal swellings in the distal parts of long fibers, including dorsal ascending sensory fibers and dorsal corticospinal fibers of the spinal cord (Gottfried et al., 1985). In the peripheral nerves, the predominent effect was found in the posterior tibial nerve and was marked by numerous paranodal and internodal swellings and ongoing wallerian degeneration. Ultrastructurally, axonal swellings in the peripheral nerves consisted of whorls of tightly packed neurofilaments and a decreased number of microtubules and were followed by degeneration. The myelin sheath at the swellings was either thin or contained large intramyelinic vacuoles indicative of more dramatic demyelination. At the neuromuscular junction, filamentous swellings of nerve terminals were followed by their degeneration, i.e., disappearance of preterminal axoplasmic microtubules, partial disappearance of synaptic vesicles, and even total disappearance of terminal axons, while the postsynaptic part of the neuromuscular junctions remained unimpaired (Jirmanova and Lukas, 1984; Gottfried et al., 1985; Juntunen et al., 1977). There was also segregation of axoplasmic organelles and cytoskeletal components, intrusion of Schwann cell processes into the axoplasm, increase in the cytoplasmic content of Schwann cells, and Schwann cell proliferation around swollen and demyelinated axons. However, the degeneration of nerves was also accompanied by some regeneration. The reduction in peripheral nerve conduction velocity was observed much before the appearance of histological lesions (Colombi et al., 1981).

Axonal Transport. Several neurotoxic chemicals such as 2,5-HD, CS_2, IDPN, and acrylamide alter axonal transport of cytoskeletal proteins, although the role of axonal transport in the pathogenesis of axonopathy is still not clear. Axonal transport of cytoskeletal proteins has been studied in visual axons of CS_2-treated rats (Pappolla et al., 1987). Transport of neurofilaments was signficantly accelerated in optic axons, and the cross-sectional area of the axon proximal to the swelling was reduced. All these findings are similar to those observed in 2,5-HD–treated rats. Neurofilaments increase in number in a proximodistal direction, and it is suggested that this is responsible for their accumulation in distal axons. Immunocytochemical staining showed that all three NFs were present in the enlargements. Transport of tubulin was not significantly affected, and that of actin showed a moderate increase in rate. The mechanism of alteration of neurofilament transport is not clear, although CS_2 has been shown to bind protein amino and sulfhydryl groups (DeCaprio et al., 1992; Valentine et al., 1992). Carbon disulfide may directly bind to cytoskeletal elements and alter their interactions by phosphorylation of the cytoskeletal proteins. Recently, CS_2 treatment has been shown to increase the phosphorylation of cytoskeletal proteins in rats (Wilmarth et al., 1993).

Carbon Disulfide Metabolism and Cross-Linking of Proteins. Carbon disulfide, like 2,5-HD, acrylamide, and IDPN, produces central-peripheral neuropathy marked by axonal accumulation of neurofilaments. 2,5-Hexanedione treatment induces intermolecular cross-linking of proteins including neurofilaments by forming pyrrole adducts of protein followed by autoxidation and coupling with other protein nucleophiles (DeCaprio and Fowke, 1992; Sayre et al., 1985). By contrast, cross-linking of proteins by acrylamide and IDPN has not been demonstrated, and that by CS_2 is still debatable. DeCaprio et al. (1992) found intramolecular but not intermolecular cross-linking of bovine serum albumin, whereas

Valentine et al. (1992) were able to find both types of cross-linking in bovine serum albumin. The reasons for this discrepancy are not clear. The reactions were, however, carried out at neutral pH with slightly different conditions. Intramolecular cross-linking decreases the mobility of protein under denaturing conditions (SDS (sodium dodecyl sulfate-polyacrylamide) and β-mercaptoethanol), while intermolecular cross-linking decreases mobility by producing proteins of high molecular weight.

Carbon disulfide undergoes both nonenzymatic and enzymatic transformations. Oxidation by the mixed-function oxidase system and desulfurization yields carbonyl sulfide (COS), CO_2, and atomic sulfur (DeCaprio et al., 1992; Bus, 1985). It is suggested that the last mediates hepatic toxicity. In contrast, the neurotoxic effects of CS_2 are probably the result of direct interaction of CS_2 with protein molecules by nonenzymatic reactions. Carbon disulfide reacts with protein amino and thiol nucleophiles and forms dithiocarbamates and trithiocarbamates. The other protein nucleophiles such as hydroxyls and imidazole nitrogen are relatively unreactive. It has been suggested that the known chelating property of dithiocarbamates inhibits various metalloenzymes in the CNS and disturbs energy metabolism. Trithiocarbamate is convertible into dithiocarbamates by reacting with a protein amino group. Dithiocarbamates are unstable at low pH (acid-labile) and release free CS_2. Dithiocarbamate is converted into the secondary products isothiocyanate and thiuram disulfide. The latter is not stable and undergoes oxidation to form isothiocyanate. Protein lysine ε-amino group reacts with isothiocyanate and forms N,N'-disubstituted thiourea, which is probably the final stable adduction product of CS_2 with protein. Dithiocarbamate esters that may form by the reaction of free thiols with isothiocyanates were not detectable in the reaction products (DeCaprio et al., 1992). This may be due to relatively low concentrations of thiol groups in comparison with protein amino groups. N,N'-Disubstituted ureas were also found in the reaction products with bovine serum albumin and may have formed through the intermediates monothiocarbamate and isocyanate. Thus, intermolecular and intramolecular cross-linked protein could be formed by this proposed mechanism, although evidence for the formation of intermolecular cross-linked protein is still inconclusive.

Carbon Disulfide Binding to Cytoskeletal Proteins. Carbon disulfide distribution and its binding with cytoskeletal protein can be studied by using either ^{35}S- or ^{14}C-labeled CS_2. Administration of labeled CS_2 per se shows that the very little CS_2 is taken up by the brain, and its observed distribution is very different when ^{35}S- or ^{14}C-labeled CS_2 is used for inhalation (Bergmann et al., 1984). Sulfur 35–labeled metabolites were initially concentrated in the liver and kidneys but were rapidly eliminated from the body. In contrast, ^{14}C-labeled metabolites were found in several organs including the liver and kidneys, and marked retention of nonextractable ^{14}C-labeled metabolites was seen in the liver and thyroid gland. High concentrations of labeled CS_2 were seen in body fat but not in brain lipids, suggesting that CS_2 neurotoxicity may not be related to the high affinity of CS_2 for lipids. In vivo studies showed greater incorporation of CS_2 sulphur than CS_2 carbon in spinal cord axons, and the axons had more labeling than spinal cord homogenate (Savolainen and Vainio, 1976). Similarly, isolation of neurofilaments from the spinal cord homogenate showed 2–3 times more labeling of the neurofilament proteins than the homogenate. Again, more CS_2 sulphur was detected in the neurofilaments than CS_2 carbon (Savolainen et al., 1977). High binding of CS_2 to neurofilament proteins may be related to alteration in neurofilament transport and neurofilament accumulation in axons.

Histochemical Studies on Enzymes. Histochemical assays in rat brain after chronic exposure to CS_2 revealed reduction in the activities of succinic dehydrogenase, acetylcholinesterase, arylsulfatases, and glutamic dehydrogenase, and not of monoamine oxidase, ATPase, and glucose 6-phosphatase (Dietzmann and Laass, 1977). Myoneural junctions of tibialis anterior muscles, however, did not show any change in acetylcholinesterase activity (Juntunen et al., 1977).

Synergistic Effect of Alcohol Administration. Combined treatment with CS_2 and alcohol did not induce a significant increase in ultrastructural changes in the hippocampus and cerebral cortex but caused more disturbance in myelin of the peripheral nerves. Ethanol further elevated the increase in β-glucuronidase activity observed in the hippocampus and cerebral cortex of CS_2-treated rats. It seems that increase in β-glucuronidase activity is a very early sign of disturbance in the CNS, as it appeared before any detectable histopathological alterations. β-Glucuronidase activity is a marker for glial cell injury. Ethanol administration did not affect the high-affinity synaptosomal uptake of L-glutamate and γ-aminobutyric acid, which are important neurotransmitters of the hippocampus and cerebral cortex. In the peripheral nerves, ethanol did not affect β-glucuronidase activity and cholesterol ester content (Opacka et al., 1986). There was, however, an increase in cholesterol ester and ester/free cholesterol ratio in the peripheral nerves when the rats were exposed to CS_2 for 12–15 months (Opacka et al., 1985) instead of 8 months (Opacka et al., 1986). Studies on behavioral alterations showed that alcohol did not change exploratory motor activity, behavior in the open field, and passive avoidance performance but affected the performance of CS_2-treated rats in avoidance acquisition tests. Thus ethanol seems to have adverse effect on the memory and learning ability of CS_2-exposed rats (Opacka et al., 1984).

Energy Metabolism in the Brain. Chronic exposure to CS_2 results in the inhibition of respiration and cytochrome oxidase activity in the rat brain. Tarkowski and Sobczak (1971) studied the effect of acute and long-term exposure to CS_2 on oxidation and phosphorylation processes in rat brain mitochondria. Acute exposure and long-term exposure showed similar effects on the studied mitochondrial functions, although the results were more significant when the rats were exposed to a single higher dose for 18 hr than with exposure to a lower dose for 5 hr daily for 10 months. Acute exposure showed partial uncoupling of oxidative phosphorylation, decreased P:O ratio, a lower ATP-P_i exchange, and a lower respiratory control index. The respiratory control index is the ratio of respiratory rate in state 3 to the rate in state 4. There was also a decrease in the ATPase activity of brain mitochondria. The comparison of results from acute and chronic CS_2 exposure showed that the observed disorders were not cumulative in nature and that a longer break in CS_2 exposure reduced its toxic effects. Thus CS_2 exposure interfered with the energy metabolism of brain mitochondria.

Synthesis of Amino Acids. Carbon disulfide exposure also affects the synthesis of amino acids from 2-^{14}C-glucose and 1-^{14}C-butyrate. Glutamate and γ-aminobutyrate concentrations were lower and glutamin concentration was higher in CS_2-treated rat brains (Tarkowski and Cremer, 1972). The decrease in glutamate was smaller and did not compensate for the increase in glutamine. Incorporation studies using labeled glucose did not indicate any impairment of glucose utilization based on label incorporation in glutamate and aspartate. The total incorporation of ^{14}C from ^{14}C-glucose into glutamate was the same in control and CS_2-treated rat brains, but specific activity was lower in the treated animals. By contrast, 1-^{14}C-butyrate incorporation showed higher specific activity of glutamine in the treated animals. Similarly, the specific activity of glutamine was less than that of glutamate on labeled glucose incorporation and higher than that of glutamate on labeled butyrate incorporation. This variation in the incorporation of glutamine from labeled glucose and butyrate is ascribed to the compartmentation of glutamine, whereby it is readily labeled from ^{14}C-butyrate and not from ^{14}C-glucose. There was a decrease in the incorporation of ^{14}C into γ-aminobutyrate from both labeled glucose and butyrate in CS$_2$-treated animals. It is suggested that this decrease is due to inhibition of glutamic acid decarboxylase by CS$_2$. The latter is known to inhibit pyridoxal phosphate–dependent enxymes. Glutamic acid decarboxylase activity was found to be slightly but significantly lower in the treated animals. Similarly, the increase in glutamine synthesis is ascribed to the higher production of ammonia in CS$_2$-treated rats. This is supported by the fact that infusion of cats with ammonia increased incorporation of ^{14}C from labeled bicarbonate into glutamine by at least 50%. Thus CS$_2$ exposure may alter the synthesis of specific amino acids and thereby brain amino acid composition.

Dithiocarbamates

Neurotoxicity. Dithiocarbamates are the half amides of dithiocarbamic acid and are widely used in agriculture as pesticides and fungicides. The widely used dithiocarbamates are sodium diethyldithiocarbamate (nabam), zinc diethyldithiocarbamate (zineb), manganese diethyldithiocarbamate (maneb), sodium dimethyldithiocarbamate, ferric dimethyl-dithiocabamate (ferbam), zinc dimethyldithiocarbamate (ziram), and tetramethylthiuram disulfide (thiram). They have also been used in inorganic analysis, as vulcanization accelerators, antioxidants, and enzyme inhibitors, and in the treatment of chronic alcoholism (Thorn and Ludwig, 1962). These compounds or their metabolites produce numerous disorders in the body, but we will consider only the neurotoxic effects in the central and peripheral nervous system. Oral administration of nabam to adult chickens produced fiber degeneration in the cerebellum, medulla, spinal cord, and peripheral nerves (Howell and Edington, 1968; Rasul and Howell, 1974). The birds suffered from ataxia after the appearance of fiber degeneration. Sodium dimethyldithiocarbamate produced similar lesions in cocks. Wallerian-like degeneration of axons was a prominent feature, rather than demyelination. The distribution of lesions in hens was similar to that produced by tri-*o*-cresyl phosphate (TOCP) in the same species. There were, however, some minor differences between TOCP- and nabam-induced neurotoxicity: nabam produced neurotox-icity only after repeated administration, and lesions were never seen in the dorsal columns of nabam-treated hens, which is not the case with TOCP (Rasul and Howell, 1973a). The nature of the lesions produced by nabam was similar in both 1-week-old chicks and adult chickens, but the latter were more susceptible to nabam (Rasul and Howell, 1973a). Treatment with ziram, ferbam, or thiram did not produce lesions in the CNS (Rasul and Howell, 1974). Similarly, S-2,3,3-trichloroallyl diisopropylthiocarbamate (triallate) treat-ment of hens did not result in histopathological lesions, although the birds became moribund after 30 days (Lapadula et al., 1990).

The neurotoxicity of dithiocarbamates has also been examined in the rat, mouse, and rabbit. Neurotoxicity occurred only in female rats fed a diet containing high levels of thiram and ferbam (Lee and Peters, 1976). The neurotoxic effects were characterized by ataxia and paralysis of the hind legs accompanied by demyelination, degeneration, and the presence of macrophages in the nerve bundles of the sciatic nerve. The PNS was the primary site of lesions and neurotoxic effect on rats was not deemed to be sex-dependent. Thiram was more neurotoxic than ferbam. The increased neurotoxicity in female rats was ascribed to higher intake of dithiocarbamates because of difference in body weight and feed consumption (Lee and Peters, 1976). However, no lesions were found in the brains of ferbam-fed or thiram-fed rats (Lee et al., 1978). Rasul and Howell (1973b) studied the subchronic effect of nabam on rabbits and found nerve fiber degeneration in the long spinal tracts, including the spinocerebellar and corticospinal tracts. Nabam-produced lesions were similar to those produced by organophosphorus compounds.

Effect on Metabolism. The mechanism of nabam-induced neurotoxicity is not known, but dithiocarbamates or their metabolites have been shown to inhibit a number of enzymes in the brain and other organs: succinic dehydrogenase (Keilin and Hartree, 1940; Reddy et al., 1990), monoamine oxidase (Yamada and Yasunobu, 1962), Na^+,K^+-ATPase (Srinivas et al., 1989), Mg^{2+}-ATPase (Babu et al., 1989), aldehyde dehydrogenase (Johansson et al., 1989), and dopamine-β-hydroxylase (Thuranszky et al., 1982). The inhibition of the last enzyme probably resulted in the increase of concentration of DA and decrease in NE in nabam- and thiram-treated rat brains. Na^+,K^+-ATPase, inhibited by dithiocarbamate (benthicarb), is reactivated by NE, and this shows that NE has a protective effect on this enzyme. Na^+,K^+-ATPase is involved in Na^+,K^+ transport across the membrane, and alteration in its activity leads to neuronal dysfunction. The deficiency in NE in intoxicated animals as noted above is likely to destabilize the enzyme. It has been suggested that the inhibition of rat brain superoxide dismutase by nabam reduces the time to the onset of grand mal seizures (ts) at high oxygen pressures (Puglia and Loeb, 1984). The CNS is the major target of oxygen toxicity when the inspired partial pressure exceeds 2.8 ATA (atmosphere absolute). This toxicity is manifested in experimental animal species as generalized motor seizures. It is suggested that inhibition of superoxide dismutase by nabam reduces the antioxidant defense mechanism and is partly responsible for reducing ts (Puglia and Loeb, 1984). Different results have, however, been obtained by other investigators. Faimen et al. (1971) reported protection against central nervous system toxicity in disulfiram-treated mouse. Disulfiram is reduced to nabam immediately after absorption. Since nabam is itself a sulfhydryl compound, it is possible that it entered the brain and was available as a sulfhydryl free radical scavanger. It seems that the potentiation or protection of CNS toxicity at high oxygen pressure by pretreatment with nabam depends on the time of pretreatment and the dose of dithiocarbamate.

Modulation of Neurotoxicity of Other Metals. Dithiocarbamates are potent chelators of polyvalent metals and, therefore, form complexes with metals and alter their distribution in the body. Dithiocarbamates or thiuram compounds have been shown to increase brain levels of thallium, copper, zinc, mercury, nickel, and cadmium (Oskarsson, 1987). It is suggested that the lipophilic nature of the complexes facilitates the transport of metals across the blood-brain barrier and cell membranes. The neurotoxicity and excretion of the metal in the presence of dithiocarbamates, however, depend on the complexed metal: 1.) Thiram was the most effective in enhancing lead accumulation in brain. It decreased the fecal and urinary excretion of lead and potentiated the neurotoxicity of lead (Oskarsson, 1987). 2.) Nabam increased the accumulation of copper in the brain but also increased its excretion. Nabam has been proposed as an effective treatment for Wilson's disease (Aaseth et al., 1979). There is, however, a possibility of enhanced neurotoxicity by accumulated copper in the brain. 3.) Nabam increased the accumulation of cadmium in the brain and decreased its excretion, but accumulation of cadmium complex did not enhance the neurotoxicity of cadmium. This was probably due to the stability of the cadmium complex with diethyldithiocarbamate.

Tubulovesicular

Organophosphorus Compounds

Many organophosphorus compounds are manufactured, and such compounds are widely used in agriculture and industry (Davis and Richardson, 1980; Murphy, 1986). More than 50,000 organophosphorus compounds have been synthesized and uses as plasticizers, insecticides, acaricides, fungicides, cotton defoliants, and "nerve gases" in warfare (Matsumura, 1976). In 1981 more than 396.5 million pounds of phosphorus-containing compounds were produced in the United States (Chemical Economics Handbook, 1983). Organophosphorus compounds have anticholinesterase activity, are capable of phosphorylating proteins by reacting with serine and threonine hydroxyl groups, and may interfere in the phosphorylation of protein kinases and other proteins by competing with ATP as the phosphoryl group donor.

Neurotoxicity. Although the immediate action of organophosphorus esters is the inhibition of acetylcholinesterase activity, some of these compounds also produce a neurodegenerative disorder known as organophosphorus ester–induced delayed neurotoxicity (OPIDN). Tri-*o*-cresyl phosphate was the first organophosphorus compound shown to produce neurotoxicity in humans, in 1899, and its effect on other sensitive species was subsequently demonstrated (Smith et al., 1930; Abou-Donia, 1986). As many as 20,000 people were paralyzed in the late 1920s during Prohibition in the United States after drinking "Ginger Jake," a tonic that had become contaminated with 2% TOCP. Since then other organophosphorus compounds have been implicated as OPIDN agents in humans (Abou-Donia and Lapadula, 1990) including mipafox (*N,N'*-diisopropyl phosphofluoramidate) (Bidstrup et al., 1953), leptophos (*O*-methyl *O*-4-bromo-3,5-dichlorophenyl phenylphosphonothioate) (Xintaras et al., 1978), EPN (*O*-ethyl *O*-4-nitrophenyl phenylphosphonothioate, Xintaras and Burg, 1980), and chlorpyrifos (*O,O*-diethyl *O*-(3,5,6-trichloro-2-pyridinyl) phosphorothioate) (Lotti et al., 1986). The skin is the most important port of entry into the body for organophosphorus compounds, since these chemicals are rapidly absorbed through the intact skin because of their high lipid solubility (Abou-Donia, 1979; 1983). Organophosphorus ester–induced delayed neurotoxicity is characterized by a 6- to 14-day delay before onset of ataxia and paralysis. Neuropathological lesions are seen as wallerian-type degeneration of the axon and myelin in the distal parts of the longest tracts in both the central and peripheral nervous systems (Cavanagh, 1964). An important feature of this neurodegenerative disorder is species susceptibility. Some sensitive species include humans, cows, chickens, cats, dogs, and water buffalo (Abou-Donia, 1981). By contrast, rats, mice, and rabbits show resistance to delayed neurotoxicity. In addition to species sensitivity, OPIDN is age-dependent, and chicks are not susceptible. The resistance of chicks is, however, not absolute. Ataxia can be produced in 40-day-old chicks by di-*n*-butyl-2,2-dichlorovinyl phosphate (DBDCVP, 5.0 or 10.0 mg/kg, s.c.) and DFP (2.0 mg/kg, s.c.), and neuropathic organophosphates inhibit neuropathy target esterase (NTE) in chicks in a manner similar to that seen in adult chickens (Peraica et al., 1993). The clinical picture in chicks is different from that of adult hens, and the former completely recover from ataxia. The adult chicken has been the animal model of choice for studying OPIDN.

Neuropathological Changes. Although all organophosphorus compounds with delayed neurotoxicity produce histopathological alterations in both the central and peripheral nervous system, each class of chemicals induces is own characteristic topography of damage.

The nature and extent of lesions also depend on the animal species and the duration of exposure.

Tri-*o*-cresyl phosphate produces histopathological lesions in the spinal cord and peripheral nerves of cats in a dose-dependent manner (Abou-Donia et al., 1986). When a single dose of TOCP (250 mg/kg) is applied to the unprotected shaved skin, there is no abnormality in the dorsal root ganglia and anterior horn cells. However, degeneration of axons and myelin in the cervical spinal cord is evident in the ascending tract, i.e., the spinocerebellar and posterior columns, and especially in the gracile tracts (Abou-Donia et al., 1983a, 1986). In the spinal cord, below the cervical levels, degeneration is present in the lateral columns, especially the descending tracts, i.e., the corticospinal tracts, in areas most distal from the cell bodies. In the lumbar region, lesions are seen in the ventral columns, i.e., the corticospinal tracts. Prineas (1969) studied the histopathological lesions in cell bodies and their processes in cats after single and multiple subcutaneous doses of TOCP. The mildly affected fibers contain abnormal membranes arranged as vesicles, irregular microtubules, and flattened cisterns. The plasma membrane of the axon appears less clearly defined and somewhat more irregular than usual. In severely affected fibers, the axoplasm is seen as rarefied, the normal constituents are absent or decreased in number, and the axoplasm contains zones of finely granular material and a few abnormal membranous materials. Sometimes, severely degenerated fibers contain compact masses of degenerate mitochondria, membranes, dense bodies, and aggregates of electron-dense particles. Myelin destruction is visible in axons only after 26 or more days of TOCP administration. Anterior horn cells show an increase in the amount of smooth endoplasmic reticulum in the peripheral cytoplasm, some loss of the normal arrangement of rough endoplasmic reticulum, and loosening of polyribosomes and individual ribosomes in the cytoplasm. In cats treated with TOCP for 7 or more days increasing amounts of neurofilaments and microtubules are found throughout the cytoplasm of both large and small neurons.

In TOCP-treated chickens, the higher brain and the gray matter of the spinal cord are spared, as seen by the light microscopy. In the CNS, axonal and terminal degeneration seems to be confined to the spinal cord, medulla, and cerebellum (Abou-Donia and Lapadula, 1990; Tanaka and Bursian, 1989). Axon degeneration is noted in the fasciculus gracilis at cervical levels of the spinal cord 2 weeks after exposure. The degeneration extends to the cervical part of the dorsal spinocerebellar tract, to the lumbar part of the medial pontine-spinal tract, and to lamina VII in the lumbar ventral horn in the third week after intoxication. In the medulla, moderate amounts of degeneration appear in the lateral vestibular, gracile, and external cuneate and lateral cervical nuclei at two weeks after TOCP treatment. In the cerebellum, moderate amounts of degeneration are visible in the deep cerebellar nuclei after 1 week and moderate mossy fiber degeneration is seen in the granular layers of cerebellar folia I–V after 3 weeks. Electron microscopy shows anomalous structural features in the white matter of the spinal cord as early as the first day of appearance of the clinical symptoms (Bischoff, 1970). In the initial stages, there appears a vacuolic dilatation and channel-like elongation of the normal vesicular elements of the smooth endoplasmic reticulum in the axoplasma. This is accompanied by the proliferation of vesicular structures, which ultimately form an almost condensed mass. Simultaneously, there occurs a diminution of the normal filamentous axonic organelles, which in part are matted or disintegrated into granular clusters. The myelin sheath disintegrates to whorls and ovoids only in the final stages of degeneration. The axoplasmic changes are more numerous at the presynaptic endings in the gray substance than in the white matter of the spinal cord. The severed nerve endings are markedly enlarged, and the most frequent structural abnormality is the accumulation and agglutination of proliferated vesicular elements. The tangled filamentous structures are also seen in presynaptic terminals, rich in condensed organelles, in some preparation from chickens with paresis (partial paralysis).

Distribution and Metabolism of Organophosphorus Compounds. The distribution and metabolism of organophosphorus compounds, e.g., TOCP and EPN (*O*-ethyl *O*-4-nitro-phenylphenylphosphonothioate), has been studied in various species (Nomeir and Abou-Donia, 1984; Abou-Donia et al., 1983b). Appreciable concentrations of saligenin cyclic-*o*-tolyl phosphate, which is the active metabolite of TOCP, are present in the plasma at all time points (0.5–10 days) in cats. Tri-*o*-cresyl phosphate is the major compound in the brain, spinal cord, and sciatic nerve, while the liver, kidneys, and lungs contain mostly the metabolites. Saligenin cyclic-*o*-tolyl phosphate concentration is relatively low in all the tissues, probably because of its instability and high reactivity (Nomeir and Abou-Donia, 1984). Radioactivity of [^{14}C]tri-*o*-cresyl phosphate applied on the back of the animal's neck disappears biexponentially from the dosing site, and 70% of the dose disappears in the first 12 hr (Nomeir and Abou-Donia, 1986). Similar studies were carried out in chickens and rats after an oral dose of [^{14}C]tri-*o*-cresyl phosphate (Abou-Donia et al., 1990a,b). Radioactive material is absorbed faster in the rat than in the hen, as indicated by the reaching of peak level of ^{14}C in 12 hr in the rat versus 24 hr in the hen. In addition, TOCP-derived radioactivity in the brain, spinal cord, and sciatic nerve is higher in the hen than in the rat (1.95-, 1.05-, and 1.22-fold, respectively). The disappearance of radioactive material from most tissues is also slower in the hen, suggesting that slower absorption and metabolism of TOCP in the hen may contribute to the sensitivity of this species to TOCP intoxication.

Esterases as Targets for Organophosphorus Ester–Induced Delayed Neurotoxicity. The immediate action of organophosphorus esters is the inhibition of esterases (Abou-Donia, 1981). Some of these compounds, e.g., insecticides and nerve gases, are potent inhibitors of acetylcholinesterase (AChE), an enzyme essential to the life of animals. Other organophosphorus compounds, e.g., the cotton defoliants DEF (*S,S,S*-tri-*n*-butyl phosphorothithioate) and the industrial chemicals, e.g., TOCP, are weak inhibitors of AChE but are strong inhibitors of pseudocholinesterase (butyrylcholinesterase, BUChE) (Abou-Donia et al., 1979; Abou-Donia, 1985a). However, subsequent studies revealed that some organophosphorus compounds inhibited these enzymes but were not neuropathic, while others induced delayed neurotoxicity in animals but did not have any inhibitory effect on these esterases. For instance, tetraethyl pyrophosphate (TEPP) and paraoxon are potent inhibitors of most esterases but are not neuropathic (Carrington, 1989), and mipafox is neuropathic at doses that have little effect on cholinesterase activity. In addition, the activity of these esterases returns to control values before the appearance of the clinical signs of neuropathy.

Studies of binding between hen brain and ^{32}P-DFP, however, finally revealed an esterase whose inhibition of activity does correlate with the development of delayed neurotoxicity. This enzyme, previously called neurotoxic esterase, has been redesignated neuropathy target esterase (NTE). All neuropathic organophosphorus esters have been shown to inhibit NTE irreversibly, and others organophosphorus esters that inhibit this enzyme reversibly do not produce delayed neurotoxicity (Carrington, 1989; Abou-Donia, 1981; Johnson, 1990). Irreversibility of inhibition of NTE activity is related to subsequent aging of NTE, which consists of transfer of a part of a molecule of bound organophosphate to some other place in the same molecule. Organophosphates that are able to inhibit NTE but cannot undergo aging are not able to produce delayed neurotoxicity in exposed animals. Such compounds are reversible inhibitors of NTE. Despite many correlations found in ex vivo assay of NTE in the tissue of exposed animals, a few anomalies have appeared in making this enzyme as the marker for polyneuropathy. For example, organophosphates inhibit NTE activity in chicks but are not able to produce delayed neurotoxicity in these animals, and NTE activity in hen brain returns to normal before any visual polyneuropathy occurs. However, recent studies are able to show that ataxia can be produced in chicks by some organophosphates and by post-treatment with phenylmethylsulfonyl fluoride (PMSF) (Peraica et al., 1993). Similarly, although NTE activity returns to normal in exposed hen brains, it persists for a very long time in the distal parts of sciatic nerves that undergo degeneration (Carrington and Abou-Donia, 1984; Carrington, 1989). It is suggested that the resistance of chicks to OPIDN is due to the faster recovery of their nervous system. Neuropathy target esterase 1.) represents approximately 6% of phenyl acetate hydrolyzing activity in hen brains, 2.) is a membrane-bound enzyme, 3.) has a molecular weight of 160 kDa, 4.) has a target size, as determined by irradiation inactivation, of a 105-kDa protein, and 5.) is transported at a fast axonal transport rate of about 100 mm/day in the sciatic nerve (Carrington, 1989).

     An important drawback for this enzyme is that a physiological role has not been assigned to its activity and that nothing is known of how the binding of organophosphate to this enzyme leads to OPIDN in sensitive species. Neuropathy target enzyme has now been purified, and it may be feasible in future to elucidate its amino acid sequence and distribution and function in the nervous system (Ruffer-Turner et al., 1992). It is hypothesized that the transfer of an alkyl or aryl group to a second site during the aging process or the negative charge left on the oxygen atom that is dealkylated may be responsible for the initiation of polyneuropathy (Carrington, 1989).

Protein Kinases as Targets for Organophosphorus Ester–Induced Delayed Neurotoxicity.
     Since organophosphorus compounds are effective phosphorylating agents, it is reasonable to assume that the initial event in the mechanisms of OPIDN is the phosphorylation of a serine or threonine group at the target site of the protein. Phosphorylation studies are prompted by two observations: 1.) the earliest ultrastructural changes in OPIDN are the aggregation and accumulations of the cytoskeletal neurofilaments, microtubules, and other structures (Prineas, 1969), and 2.) the structural state of cytoskeletal proteins is significantly affected by protein kinase–mediated phosphorylation (Saitoh et al., 1991). Protein phosphorylation is a post-translational modification of proteins that is involved in the expression of specific functions of various proteins, integration of extracellular signals, and maintainance of cellular homeostasis, functions, and survival.

     The post-translation modification of cytoskeletal proteins may occur through direct phosphorylation by organophosphates or by the modification of various protein kinases that are involved in the phosphorylation of cellular proteins. Exposure of hens to organophosphorus compounds such as TOCP and DFP has been shown to increase in vitro phosphorylation of proteins by Ca^{2+}/calmodulin-dependent protein kinase II (CaM kinase II) (Abou-Donia and Lapadula, 1989, 1990). Early studies were carried out on synaptosomal (P_2) membranes and synaptosomal cytosolic proteins from hen brains and spinal cords (Patton et al., 1983a,b, 1986; Abou-Donia et al., 1984). In some experiments, purified and enriched protein fractions containing α- and β-tubulins, MAP-2, neurofilament triplet proteins (NFs), or CaM kinase II were used to study alteration in phosphorylation in organophosphorus compound–treated animals (Suwita et al., 1986a,b; Lapadula et al., 1991, 1992). Recent studies also showed increased phosphorylation of exogenous protein substrates, e.g., MAP-2, α- and β-tubulin, NFs, and myelin basic protein (Abou-Donia et al., 1993b). Aberant phosphorylated neurofilament aggregations have been demonstrated in central and peripheral axons of hens treated with tri-*ortho*-cresyl phosphate (Jensen et al., 1992, Fig. 7).

TOCP-increased protein phosphorylation correlates with the criteria for OPIDN:

1. Clinical condition. Increased protein phosphorylation correlates with the onset and progress of clinical signs of OPIDN.
2. Test chemical. Only organophosphorus compounds capable of producing OPIDN, e.g., TOCP, DFP, and mipafox, increase protein phosphorylation, while the nondelayed neurotoxicants, parathion or tri-*p*-cresyl phosphate, do not.
3. Species sensitivity. Increased protein phosphorylation is observed in chickens and cats, but not in rats.
4. Sex. Both male and female chickens are sensitive to OPIDN and exhibit increased protein phosphorylation.
5. Age sensitivity. Chicks neither develop OPIDN nor show increased protein phosphorylation.
6. Protection by PMSF. Treatment with PMSF protects hens against OPIDN and does not affect phosphorylation.

Further studies on the mechanism of increased phosphorylation by the organophosphorus compound DFP show that increased phosphorylation by brain supernatant is not due to increased amount of the CaM kinase II. It appears that there is some modification or change in the comformation of CaM kinase II that is reflected by increased binding of ^{125}I-calmodulin to the enzyme (Abou-Donia et al., 1993). Increased phosphorylation of various cytoskeletal proteins in animals with OPIDN suggests that alteration in the phosphorylation state of cytoskeletal proteins resulting in change in conformation, interaction, stability, or transport may be involved in the production of delayed polyneuropathy by organophosphates.

Protection against Organophosphorus Ester–Induced Delayed Neurotoxicity. Neuropathy target esterase is considered to be the initial molecular target for OPIDN. Organophosphorus compounds that produce delayed neurotoxicity mostly inhibit 70–80% of this activity, and in some cases much more inhibition of the enzyme is required. Furthermore, inhibition of NTE is followed by an aging process that results in the further modification of the inhibited enzyme and makes its inhibition irreversible. The potency of a given NTE inhibitor to cause OPIDN depends on the chemistry of the residue left attached to NTE and its affinity for the enzyme. Organophosphorus and other compounds such as carbamates (e.g., phenyl N-benzyl-N-methyl carbamate), sulfonyl fluorides (e.g., phenylmethylsulfonyl fluoride), phosphinates (e.g., 4-nitrophenyl di-*n*-butylphosphinate), and organophosphorus esters (e.g., one of the isomers of soman) that strongly inhibit NTE activity, but with which the inhibited enzyme is not capable of undergoing the aging process, are not able to produce delayed neurotoxicity. In addition, prior treatment with these compounds results in inhibition of NTE activity and prevents NTE from reacting with the organophosphorus compounds that would produce delayed neurotoxocity. These compounds have been shown to completely or partially protect the animal from OPIDN (Carrington, 1989; Carrington and Abou-Donia, 1988; Johnson et al., 1988; Lotti, 1991). The efficacy of protection is related to the time between administration of the prophylactic agent and of the neurotoxicant, and their dosage and chemical structure (Galli and Mazri, 1988).

Administration of acetyl- or butylcholinesterases has also been used to provide protection from or delay the onset of delayed neurotoxicity induced by organophosphorus compounds (Doctor et al., 1991). In addition, endogenous carboxylesterase is also known to be capable of scavenging organophosphates (OPs). Experiments have been performed using three animal species and three different OPs. The results demonstrate 1.) that a linear correlation exists between blood levels of esterases and the protection afforded against neurotoxicants, 2.) that approximately 1 mol of enzyme is required to neutralize 1 mol of OP, and 3.) that such a procedure is sufficient to protect the animal against OPIDN without any supportive drugs. Thus the dose of OP, blood-level of esterase, ratio of circulating enzyme to OP challenge, and rate of reaction between them determine the efficacy of the enzyme as a pretreatment drug.

Pretreatment with the cytochrome P-450 inducers 3-methylcholanthrene (3-MC) and β-naphoflavone (β-NF) has also been shown to protect hens against delayed neurotoxicity produced by intravenous administration of TOCP (Konno et al., 1988). Pretreatment with phenobarbital has no effect on OPIDN, although all three P-450 inducers depress substantially the concentration of unaltered TOCP in the brain and plasma in 1 h after dosing. However, only β-NF pretreatment decreases TOCP concentration in the spinal cord, and none of the inducers affects the TOCP level in the sciatic nerve and adipose tissue. It seems that some of the cytochrome P-450s induced by 3-MC and β-NF are capable of converting TOCP into its active metabolite, saligenin cyclic-*o*-tolyl phosphate [2-(*o*-cresyl)-4H-1,3,2-benzodioxaphosphorane-2-one].

Potentiation of Organophosphorus Ester–Induced Delayed Neurotoxicity. Phenylmethylsulfonyl fluoride, which protects experimental animals from OPIDN when administered before neurotoxicant OPs, exacerbates the neurotoxic effect of the latter if given after the intoxication of the animal (Pope and Padilla, 1990). The potentiation effect of PMSF, administered 4 h after intoxication, has been observed on mipafox- and DFP-induced delayed neurotoxicity. Phenylmethylsulfonyl fluoride also elevates the neurotoxic effect of OPs in chicks (Peraica et al., 1993) and developing chickens (35, 49, and 70 days of age) (Pope et al., 1992) on post-treatment. Chickens treated with DFP alone show a marked age-related increase in OPIDN, but those given post-treatment with PMSF show more extensive clinical deficits. Post-treatment with PMSF has no potentiating effect if PMSF has also been administered before OP exposure. Since DFP treatment alone causes 90% or more of NTE inhibition, the potentiation effect of PMSF is probably not ascribable to further inhibition of NTE. It is suggested that PMSF, a serine proteinase inhibitor, may interfere with regenerating/repairing process for OPIDN that has been initiated by the OPs. Studies have indicated that serine proteinases are involved in the outgrowth of neurites associated with development and regeneration. Although DFP is also a serine proteinase inhibitor, DFP and PMSF are known to have differences in their specificities toward some proteins (Pope et al., 1992).

Pretreatment (7–15 days, 300 mg/kg/day) or chronic treatment (200 mg/kg/day) with *n*-hexane shows rapid development of ataxia after a single oral dose of TOCP (Pellin et al., 1987, 1988). The animals treated with only TOCP show slow and slight ataxia development, and those treated with *n*-hexane alone show reversible weakness and sedative effects. The time course of development of ataxia is similar to that of OPIDN, and histopathological lesions are similar to those observed in hexacarbon neuropathy (Pellin et al., 1987). *n*-Hexane pretreatment has no effect on NTE inhibition produced by a dose of 200 mg/kg/day of TOCP, although it does increase NTE inhibition from 40–50% to 60–70% with a lower dose of TOCP, 20 mg/kg/day (Pellin et al., 1988).

The neurotoxic effect of TOCP is also increased by pretreatment with the mixed-function oxidase inhibitor piperonyl butoxide (Veronesi, 1984). Similarly, treatment with cycloheximide, a protein synthesis inhibitor, increases the toxicity as well as the neurotoxicity of TOCP, depending on its time of administration (Gupta and Dettbarn, 1987). Rats treated with DFP (0.5 mg/kg/day, s.c.) exhibit signs of cholinergic toxicity in 3–5 days and then develop tolerance on further treatment of 6–14 days, as is evident from the disappearance of the described toxicity signs. Pretreatment with the nontoxic dose of cycloheximide (0.5 mg/kg/day, s.c.) from the beginning results in the death of rats after the fifth injection of TOCP. On the other hand, if cycloheximide is given to rats that have developed tolerance to TOCP, it results in the development of toxicity signs. Cycloheximide treatment also increases the inhibition of NTE in DFP-treated animals. The results obtained from the inhibition of [^{14}C]valine incorporation into the free amino acid pool and proteins suggest that cycloheximide potentiates DFP toxicity by inhibition of synthesis of proteins such as acetylcholinesterases, butyrylcholinesterases, and carboxylesterases.

Type I and II Organophosphorus Ester–Induced Delayed Neuropathy. Organophosphorus ester–induced delayed neuropathy has been classified as type I and type II (Abou-Donia and Lapadula, 1990), which are characterized by the following differences: 1.) Type I compounds (e.g., TOCP, DFP) have a pentavalent phosphorus atom, whereas type II compounds (e.g., triphenyl phosphite) have a trivalent phosphorus atom. 2.) Sensitivity of species is different for the two types of compound. Young chicks are not sensitive to a single dose of TOCP, although repeated doses of TOCP are able to induce type II OPIDN. On the other hand, 1-week-old chicks develop type II OPIDN on one or two subcutaneous injections of triphenyl phosphite (TPPi) (1000 mg/kg). 3.) Although in both type I and type II OPIDN neurological deficits are evident after the lapse of some time after intoxication, type II seems to have a shorter latent interval than type I. 4.) Although clinical signs of type I and type II OPIDN are indistinguishable quantitatively in the adult chicken, other species, e.g., cats, exhibit distinct signs characteristic of each syndrome. 5.) The morphology and distribution of neuropathologic lesions is different in the two types of OPIDN in species such as cats and monkeys. 6.) Prior treatment with PMSF completely or partially protects the animals from type I and type II OPIDN, depending on the subsequent dose of organophosphorus compound. However, in the case of type II OPIDN, prior treatment with PMSF enhances the neurotoxic effect of TPPi at a high dose of 1000 mg/kg, which does not happen with the larger doses of TOCP. 7.) Inhibition of NTE activity by TPPi (1000 mg/kg, s.c.) in the hen brain returned to 50% of control values after 14 days, whereas a dose of 1184 mg/kg of TOCP produced complete inhibition of brain NTE activity that persisted for 21 days. Similarly, maximum inhibition of NTE activity in the rat brain by TPPi is 39%, in comparison with 69% inhibition by TOCP in the rat brain (Abou-Donia and Lapadula, 1990). 8.) Triphenyl phosphite inhibits nicotine- and high potassium–induced catecholamine secretion by primary cultures of bovine adrenomedullary chromaffin cells in a time- and dose-dependent manner. In contrast, DFP and the nondelayed-type neurotoxic organophosphorus compound O,O-diethyl-O-4-nitrophenyl phosphate (paraoxon) have no effect on secretion in the presence of nicotine and significantly stimulate secretion of catecholamine in the presence of high potassium concentrations (Knoth-Anderson and Abou-Donia, 1993).

Axonal Transport. Polyneuropathy produced by neurotoxic agents such as acrylamide, carbon disulfide, *n*-hexane, and organophosphorus compounds is associated with wallerian-type degeneration in the distal parts of axons and axonal swelling due to accumulation of 10-nm neurofilaments or other cytoskeletal elements in the axoplasm. These pathological conditions have been attributed to disruption of the movement of cytoskeletal proteins in the axon. Normal transport is essential to maintain axonal diameter and integrity. The transport of proteins in different directions has been studied: 1.) fast and slow transport from motor neurons in the spinal cord to the sciatic nerve (Pleasure et al., 1969; James and Austin, 1970), 2.) fast and slow transport from dorsal root ganglia to the spinal cord (Pleasure et al., 1969), 3.) fast and slow transport from dorsal root ganglia to the peripheral branches of the sensory nerves (Bradley and Williams, 1973; Carrington et al., 1989), 4.) fast transport from the gastrocnemius muscle to dorsal root ganglia and the spinal cord (Moretto et al., 1987), and 5.) fast transport in the optic nerve (Reichert and Abou-Donia, 1980) James and Austin (1970) did not find any effect on fast or slow transport in DFP-treated chicken, and Pleasure et al. (1969) did not observe any effect on slow transport in TOCP-treated cats. Carrington et al. (1989) observed an increase in fast transport in DFP-treated cats, whereas Bradley and Williams (1973) observed an inhibition of fast transport in TOCP-treated cats. The reason for the discrepancy in their results is not clear, although there are some differences in the experimental protocols and the organophosphorus compounds used in the studies. Moretto et al. (1987) and Reichert and Abou-Donia (1980) found an inhibition of anterograde and retrograde fast transport in DBDCVP-treated hens and TOCP-treated rats, respectively. The results seems to show no effect on anterograde transport and an inhibition of retrograde transport in OPIDN. It is suggested that reduction in retrograde transport reduces the level of perikaryal anabolic activity and export of materials required for axon maintainance (Miller and Spencer, 1985). The latter could contribute to the degeneration of the distal part of the axon.

ACKNOWLEDGMENTS

Supported in part by National Institute of Environmental Health Science grants No. ESO 5071 and ESO 5154 National Institute for Occupational Safety and Health grant No. OHO 0823.

REFERENCES

Aaserud O, Gjerstad L, Nakstad P, Nyberg-Hansen R, Hommeren OJ, Tvedt B, Russell D, Rootwelt K (1988). Neurological examination, computerized tomography, cerebral blood flow and neuropsychological examination in workers with long-term exposure to carbon disulfide. Toxicology 49:277–82.

Aaseth J, Soli NE, Forre O (1979). Increased brain uptake of copper and zinc in mice caused by diethyldithiocarbamate. Acta Pharmacol Toxicol 45:41–4.

Abe T, Haga T, Kurokawa M (1975). Blockage of axoplasmic transport and depolymerization of assembled microtubules by methylmercury. Brain Res 86:504–8.

Abou-Donia MB (1985a). Biochemical toxicology of organophosphorus compounds. In: Blum K, Manzo L, eds. Neurotoxicology. New York: Marcel Dekker, 423–43.

Abou-Donia MB (1979). Pharmacokinetics and metabolism of a topically applied dose of O-4-bromo-2,5-dichlorophenyl O-methyl phenylphosphonothioate in hens. Toxicol Appl Pharmacol 51: 311–28.

Abou-Donia MB (1981). Organophosphorus ester–induced delayed neurotoxicity. Annu Rev Pharmacol Toxicol 21:511–48.

Abou-Donia MB (1983). Toxicokinetics and metabolism of delayed neurotoxic organophosphorus esters. Neurotoxicology 4:113–29.

Abou-Donia MB, Graham DG, Timmons PR, Reichert BL (1979). Delayed neurotoxic and late acute effects of S,S,S-tributyl phosphorotrithioate on the hen: effect of route of administration. Neurotoxicology 2:425–48.

Abou-Donia MB, Ibrahim SM, Corcoran JJ, Lack L, Friedman MA, Lapadula DM (1993a). Neurotoxicity of glycidamide, an acrylamide metabolite, following intraperitoneal injections in rats. J. Toxicol. Environ. Health 39:447–64.

Abou-Donia MB, Jensen DN, Lapadula DM (1983a). Neurologic manifestations of tri-o-cresyl phosphate delayed neurotoxicity in cats. Neurobehav Toxicol Teratol 5:431–42.

Abou-Donia MB, Lapadula DM (1989). Studies on the molecular pathogenesis of organophosphorus compound–induced delayed neurotoxicity (OPIDN). In: Narahashi T, Chambers JE, eds. Insecticide action. New York: Plenum Press, 205–18.

Abou-Donia MB, Lapadula DM (1990). Mechanisms of organophosphorus ester–induced delayed neurotoxicity. Type I and Type II. Annu Rev Pharmacol Toxicol 30:405–40.

Abou-Donia MB, Lapadula DM, Campbell G, Abdo KM (1985b). The joint neurotoxic action of inhaled methyl butyl ketone vapor and dermally applied o-ethyl o-4-nitrophenyl phenylphosphonothioate in hens: potentiating effect. Toxicol Appl Pharmacol 79:69–82.

Abou-Donia MB, Lapadula DM, Campbell G, Timmons PR (1985b). The synergism of n-hexane-induced neurotoxicity by methyl isobutyl ketone following subchronic (90 days) inhalation in hens: induction of hepatic microsomal cytochrome P-450. Toxicol Appl Pharmacol 81:1–16.

Abou-Donia MB, Nomeir AA, Bower JH, Makkawy HA (1990b). Absorption, distribution, excretion, and metabolism of a single oral dose of [^{14}C]tri-o-cresyl phosphate (TOCP) in the male rat. Toxicology 65:61–74.

Abou-Donia MB, Patton SE, Lapadula DM (1984). Possible role of endogenous protein phosphorylation in organophosphorus compound–induced delayed neurotoxicity. In Narahashi T, ed. Cellular and molecular neurotoxicology. New York: Raven Press, 265–83.

Abou-Donia MB, Reichert BL, Ashry MA (1983b). The absorption, distribution, excretion, and metabolism of a single oral dose of O-ethyl O-4-nitrophenyl phenylphosphonothioate in hens. Toxicol Appl Pharmacol 70:18–28.

Abou-Donia MB, Suwita E, Nomeir AA (1990a). Absorption, distribution, and elimination of a single dose of [^{14}C]tri-o-cresyl phosphate in hens. Toxicology 13:13–25.

Abou-Donia MB, Trofatter LP, Graham DG, Lapadula DM (1986). Electromyographic, neuropathologic, and functional correlates in the cat as the result of tri-o-cresyl phosphate delayed neurotoxicity. Toxicol Appl Pharmacol 83:126–41.

Abou-Donia MB, Viana ME, Gupta RP, Anderson JK (1993b). Enhanced calmodulin binding concurrent with increased kinase-dependent phosphorylation of cytoskeletal proteins following a single subcutaneous injection of diisopropyl phosphorofluoridate in hens. Neurochem Int 22:165–73.

Abou-Donia MB, Zhuohan HU, Lapadula DM, Gupta RP (1991). Mechanisms of joint neurotoxicity of n-hexane, methyl isobutyl ketone and o-ethyl o-4-nitrophenyl phenylphosphonothioate in hens. J Pharmacol Exp Ther 257:282–9.

Allen N (1980). Identification of methyl n-butyl ketone as the causative agent. In: Spencer PS, Schaumburg HH, eds. Experimental and Clinical Neurotoxicology. Baltimore: Williams and Wilkins, 834–45.

Anderson RJ, Dunham CB (1984). Electrophysiologic deficits in peripheral nerve as a discriminator of early hexacarbon neurotoxicity. J Toxicol Environ Health 13:835–43.

Annau Z, Cuomo V (1988). Mechanisms of neurotoxicity and their relationship to behavioral changes. Toxicology 49:219–25.

Arakawa O, Nakahiro M, Narahashi T (1991). Mercury modulation of GABA-activated chloride channels and non-specific channels in rat dorsal root ganglion neurons. Brain Res 551:58–63.

Atchison WD, Narahashi T (1982). Methylmercury-induced depression of neuromuscular transmission in the rat. Neurotoxicology 3:37–50.

Babu GRV, Reddy GR, Chetty CS (1989). Kinetics of Mg^{2+}-ATPase inhibition of benthiocarb and its recovery by oximes and L-cysteine in brain of albino rat (Wistar strain). Arch Int Physiol Biochim 97:205–9.

Backstrom B, Collins VP (1987). Cytoskeletal changes in axons of rats exposed to 2,5-hexanediol, demonstrated using monoclonal antibodies. Neuro toxicology 8:85–96.

Bangalore R, Hawthorn M, Triggle DJ (1991). Iminodipropionitrile-induced dyskinesia in mice: striatal calcium channel changes and sensitivity to calcium channel antagonists. J Neurochem 57:550–5.

Banks WA, Kastin AJ (1989). Aluminum-induced neurotoxicity: alterations in membrane function at the blood-brain barrier. Neurosci Behav Rev 13:47–53.

Bergman K, Danielsson BRG, d'Argy R (1984). Tissue disposition of carbon disulfide: I. Whole-body autoradiography of ^{35}S- and ^{14}C-labelled carbon disulfide in adult male mice. Acta Pharmacol Toxicol 54:141–50.

Berridge MJ, Irvin RF (1989). Inositol phosphate and cell signalling. Nature 341:197–205.

Berti-Mattera LN, Eichberg J, Schrama L, LoPachin RM (1990). Acrylamide administration alters protein phosphorylation and phospholipid metabolism in rat sciatic nerve. Toxicol Appl Pharmacol 103:502–11.

Bidstrup PL, Bonnell JA, Beckett AG (1953). Paralysis following poisoning by a new organic phosphorus insecticide (mipafox). Br Med J 1:1068–72.

Bisby MA, Redshaw JD (1987). Acrylamide neuropathy: changes in the composition of proteins of fast axonal transport resemble those observed in regenerating axons. J Neurochem 48:924–8.

Bischoff A (1970). Ultrastructure of tri-o-cresyl phosphate poisoning in the chicken. II. Studies on the spinal cord. Acta Neuropathol (Berlin) 15:142–55.

Bizzi A, Gambetti P (1986). Phosphorylation of neurofilaments is altered by aluminum intoxication. Acta Neuropathol (Berlin) 71:154–8.

Boekelheide K, Anthony DC, Giangaspero F, Gottfried MR, Graham DG (1988). Aliphatic diketones: influence of dicarbonyl spacing on amine reactivity and toxicity. Chem Res Toxicol 1:200–3.

Bondy SC, McKee M (1991). Disruption of the potential across the synaptosomal plasma membrane and mitochondria by neurotoxic agents. Toxicol Lett 58:13–21.

Bradley WG, Williams MH (1973). Axoplasmic flow in axonal neuropathies. I. Axoplasmic flow in cats with toxic neuropathies. Brain 96:235–46.

Braendgaard H, Sidenius P (1986). The retrograde fast component of axonal transport in motor and sensory nerves of the rat during administration of 2,5-hexanedione. Brain Res 378:1–7.

Brismar T, Hildebrand C, Tegner R (1987). Nodes of Ranvier in acrylamide neuropathy: voltage clamp and electron microscopic analysis of rat sciatic nerve fivers at proximal levels. Brain Res 423:135–43.

Brookes N (1988). Specificity and reversibility of the inhibition by HgCl$_2$ of glutamate transport in astrocyte cultures. J Neurochem 50:1117–22.

Bus JS (1985). The relationship of carbon disulfide metabolism to development of toxicity. Neuro toxicology 6:73–80.

Cadet JL (1989). The iminodipropionitrile (IDPN)-induced dyskinetic syndrome: behavioral and biochemical pharmacology. Neurosci Biobehav Rev 13:39–45.

Cadet JL, Braun TL (1986). Naltrexone inhibits the persistent spasmodic dyskinesia induced by chronic intraperitoneal administration of iminodipropionitrile (IDPN). Neuropeptides 8:87–91.

Cadet JL, Jackson-Lewis V, Fahn S (1988). The iminodipropionitrile (IDPN) model of persistent spasmodic dyskinesias: regional serotonin metabolism in rat brain. Brain Res 456:371–4.

Cadet JL, Karoum F (1988). Central and peripheral effects of iminodipropionitrile on catecholamine metabolism in rats. Synapse 2:23–7.

Cadet JL, Kuyatt B, Fahn S, De Souza EB (1987). Differential changes in ^{125}I-LSD-labeled 5-HT-2 serotonin receptors in discrete regions of brain in the rat model of persistent dyskinesias induced by iminodipropionitrile (IDPN): evidence from autoradiographic studies. Brain Res 437:383–6.

Cadet JL, Rothman RB (1986). Decreased striatal opiate sigma-receptors in the rat model of persistent dyskinesia induced by iminodipropionitrile. Neurosci Lett 72:84–6.

Cadet JL, Taylor E, Freed WJ (1988). The iminodipropionitrile (IDPN)-induced dyskinetic syndrome in mice: antagonism by the calcium channel antagonist nifedipine. Pharmacol Biochem Behav 29:381–5.

Calleman CJ, Bergmark E, Costa LG (1990). Acrylamide is metabolized to glycidamide in the rat: evidence from hemoglobin adduct formation. Chem Res Toxicol 3:406–12.

Candural SM, Castoldi AF, Manzo L, Costal LG (1991). Interaction of aluminum ions with phosphoinositide metabolism in rat cerebral cortical membranes. Life Sci 49:1245–52.

Carden MJ, Goldstein ME, Bruce J, Cooper HS, Schlaepfer WW (1987). Studies of neurofilaments that accumulate in proximal axons of rats intoxicated with , '-iminodipropionitrile (IDPN). Neurochem Path 7:189–205.

Carrington CD (1989). Prophylaxis and the mechanism for the initiation of organophosphorus compound–induced delayed neurotoxicity. Toxicology 63:165–72.

Carrington CD, Abou-Donia MB (1984). The correlation between the recovery rate of neurotoxic esterase activity and sensitivity to organophosphorus-induced delayed neurotoxicity. Toxicol Appl. Pharmacol 75:350–7.

Carrington CD, Abou-Donia MB (1988). Triphenyl phosphite neurotoxicity in the hen: inhibition of neurotoxic esterase and of prophylaxis by phenylmethylsulfonyl fluoride. Arch Toxicol 62:375–80.

Carrington CD, Lapadula DM, Abou-Donia MB (1989). Acceleration of anterograde axonal transport in cat sciatic nerve by diisopropyl phosphorofluoridate. Brain Res 476:179–82.

Carrington CD, Lapadula DM, Dulak L, Friedman M, Abou-Donia MB (1991). In vivo binding of [14C]acrylamide to proteins in the mouse nervous system. Neurochem Int 18:191–7.

Carty AJ, Malone SF (1979). The chemistry of mercury in biological systems. In: Nriagu JO, ed. Topics in environmental health, vol. 3. The biogeochemistry of mercury in the environment. New York: Elsevier/North Holland, 433–79.

Cavanagh JB (1964). The significance of the "dying back" process in experimental animals and human neurological disease. Int Rev Exp Pathol 3:219–67.

Cavanagh JB (1982). The pathokinetics of acrylamide intoxication: a reassessment of the problem. Neuropathol Appl Neurobiol 8:315–36.

Cavanagh JB, Nolan CC (1982). Selective loss of Purkinje cells from the rat cerebellum caused by acrylamide and the responses of β-glucuronidase and β-galactosidase. Acta Neuropathol (Berlin) 58:210–4.

Chemical Economics Handbook (1983). Lubricating oil additives. Menlo Park, California: SRI International.

Colombi A, Maroni M, Picchi O, Rota E, Castano P, Foa V (1981). Carbon disulfide neuropathy in rats. A morphological and ultrastructural study of degeneration and regeneration. Clin Toxicol 18:1463–74.

Connor DJ, Jope RS, Harrell LE (1988). Chronic, oral aluminum administration to rats: cognition and cholinergic parameters. Pharmacol Biochem Behav 31:467–74.

Corsi G, Maestrelli P, Picotti G, Manzoni S, Negrin P (1983). Chronic peripheral neuropathy in workers with previous exposure to carbon disulfide. Br J Indust Med 40:209–11.

Costa LG, Deng H, Gregotti C, Manzo L, Faustman EM, Bergmark E, Calleman CJ (1992). Comparative studies on the neuro- and reproductive toxicity of acrylamide and its epoxide metabolite glycidamide in the rat. Neurotoxicology 13:219–24.

Davis CS, Richardson RJ (1980). Organophosphorus compounds. In Spencer PS, Schaumburg HH, eds. Experimental and Clinical Neurotoxicity. Baltimore: Williams and Wilkins, 527–44.

Dearfield KL, Abernathy CO, Ottley MS, Brantner JH, Hayes PF (1988). Acrylamide: its metabolism, developmental and reproductive effects, genotoxicity, and carcinogenicity. Mut Res 195:45–77.

DeCaprio AP, Briggs RG, Jackowski SJ, Kim JC (1988). Comparative neurotoxicity and pyrrole-forming potential of 2,5-hexanedione and perdeuterio-2,5-hexanedione in the rat. Toxicol Appl Pharmacol 92:75–85.

DeCaprio AP, Fowke JH (1992). Limited and selective adduction of carboxyl-terminal lysines in the high molecular weight neurofilament proteins by 2,5-hexanedione in vitro. Brain Res 586:219–28.

DeCaprio AP, Jackowski SJ, Regan KA (1987). Mechanism of formation and quantitation of imines, pyrroles, and stable nonpyrrole adducts in 2,5-hexanedione-treated proteins. Mol Pharmacol 32:542–8.

DeCaprio AP, Spink DC, Chen X, Fowke JH, Zhu M, Bank S (1992). Characterization of isothiocyanates, thioureas, and other lysine adduction products in carbon disulfide–treated peptides and protein. Chem Res Toxicol 5:496–504.

DeGrandchamp RL, Lowndes HE (1990). Early degeneration and sprouting at the rat neuromuscular junction following acrylamide administration. Neuropathol Appl Neurobiol 16:239–54.

Delio DA, Fiori MG, Lowndes HE (1992). Motor unit function during evolution of proximal axonal swellings. J Neurol Sci 109:30–40.

Delio DA, Gold BG, Lowndes HE (1987). Cross talk between intraspinal elements during progression of IDPN neuropathy. Toxicol Appl Pharmacol 90:253–60.

Delio DA, Gold BG, Lowndes HE (1989). Axotomy-like electrophysiological alterations in spinal motoneurons in β,β′-iminodipropionitrile neuropathy. Toxicol Appl Pharmacol 99:207–15.

Delio DA, Lowndes HE (1989). Influence of proximal axonal swellings on rhythmic motoneuron firing. Toxicol Appl Pharmacol 101:27–35.

Deloncle R, Guillard O (1990). Mechanism of Alzheimer's disease: arguments for a neurotransmitter-aluminum complex implication. Neurochem Res 15:1239–45.

De Rojas TC, Goldstein BD (1987). Primary afferent terminal function following acrylamide: alterations in the dorsal root potential and reflex. Toxicol Appl Pharmacol 88:175–82.

Diaz-Nido J, Avila J (1990). Aluminum induces the in vitro aggregation of bovine cytoskeletal proteins. Neurosci Lett 110:221–6.

Dietzmann K, Laass W (1977). Histological and histochemical studies on the rat brain under conditions of carbon disulfide intoxication. Exp Path Bd 13, S. 320–327.

Doctor BP, Raveh L, Wolfe AD, Maxwell DM, Ashani Y (1991). Enzymes as pretreatment drugs for organophosphate toxicity. Neurosci Biobehav Rev 15:123–8.

Drapeau P, Blaustein MP (1983). Initial release of [^{3}H]dopamine from rat striatal synaptosomes: correlation with calcium entry. J Neurosci 3:703–13.

Eyer J, Mclean WG, Leterrier J.-F (1989). Effect of a single dose of β,β′-iminodipropionitrile in vivo on the properties of neurofilaments in vitro: comparison with the effect of iminodipropionitrile added directly to neurofilaments in vitro. J Neurochem 52:1759–65.

Faiman MD, Mehl RG, Oehme FW (1971). Protection with disulfiram from central and pulmonary oxygen toxicity. Biochem Pharmacol 20:3059–67.

Fink DJ, Purkiss D, Mata M (1986). β,β′-Iminodipropionitrile impairs retrograde axonal transport. J Neurochem 47:1032–8.

Galli A, Mazri A (1988). Protection against diisopropylfluorophosphate intoxication by meptazinol. Toxicol Appl Pharmacol 95:388–96.

Gold BG, Austin DR (1991). Regulation of aberrant neurofilament phosphorylation in neuronal perikarya: III. Alterations following single and continuous β,β′-iminodipropionitrile administration. Brain Res 563:151–62.

Gold BG, Griffin JW, Price DL (1985). Slow axonal transport in acrylamide neuropathy: different abnormalities produced by single-dose and continuous administration. J Neurosci 5:1755–68.

Gold BG, Griffin JW, Price DL (1992). Somatofugal axonal atrophy precedes development of axonal degeneration in acrylamide neuropathy. Arch Toxicol 66:57–66.

Gold BG, Halleck M (1989). Axonal degeneration and axonal caliber alterations following combined β,β′-iminodipropionitrile (IDPN) and acrylamide administration. J Neuropathol Exp Neurol 48:653–68.

Gold BG, Price DL, Griffin JW, Rosenfeld J, Hoffman PN, Sternberger NH, Sternberger LA (1988). Neurofilament antigens in acrylamide neuropathy. J Neuropathol Exp Neurol 47:145–57.

Goldstein BD, Fincher DR (1986). Paradoxical changes in spinal cord reflexes following the acute administration of acrylamide. Toxicol Lett 31:93–9.

Gottfried MR, Graham DG, Morgan M, Casey HW, Bus JS (1985). The morphology of carbon disulfide neurotoxicity. Neurotoxicology 6:89–96.

Graham DG, St. Clair MBG, Amarnath V, Anthony DC (1991). Molecular mechanisms of gamma-diketone neuropathy. Adv Exp Med Biol 283:427–31.

Grammas P, Caspers ML (1991). The effect of aluminum on muscarinic receptors in isolated cerebral microvessels. Res Commun Chem Pathol Pharmacol 72:69–79.

Gulya K, Rakonczay Z, Kasa P (1990). Cholinotoxic effects of aluminum in rat brain. J Neurochem 54:1020–6.

Gupta RC, Dettbarn WD (1987). Interaction of cycloheximide and diisopropylphosphorofluoridate (DFP) during subchronic administration in rat. Toxicol Appl Pharmacol 90:52–9.

Hammond-Tooke GD (1992). Slow axonal transport is impaired by intrathecal 2,5-hexanedione. Exp Neurol 116:210–7.

Hare MF, Atchison WD (1992). Comparative action of methylmercury and divalent inorganic mercury on nerve terminal and intraterminal mitochondrial membrane potentials. J Pharmacol Exp Ther 261:166–72.

Harry GJ, Morell P, Bouldin TW (1992). Acrylamide exposure preferentially impairs axonal transport of glycoproteins in myelinated axons. J Neurosci Res 31:554–60.

Hashimoto K, Kurosaka Y, Tanii H, Hayashi M (1988). Immunochemical studies of acrylamide-associated neuropathology. Toxicology 49:65–69.

He F, Zhang S, Wang H, Li G, Zhang Z, Li F, Dong X, Hu F (1989). Neurological and electroneuromyographic assessment of the adverse effects of acrylamide on occupationally exposed workers. Scand J Work Environ Health 15:125–9.

Hewett SJ, Atchison WD (1992). Effects of charge and lipophilicity on mercurial-induced reduction of $^{45}Ca^{2+}$ uptake in isolated nerve terminals of the rat. Toxicol Appl Pharmacol 113:267–73.

Hirata M (1990). Reduced conduction function in central nervous system by 2,5-hexanedione. Neurotoxicol Teratol 12:623–26.

Hirokawa N, Bloom GS, Vallee RB (1985). Cytoskeletal architecture and immunocytochemical localization of microtubule-associated proteins in regions of axons associated with rapid axonal transport: the β,β′-iminodipropionitrile-intoxicated axon as a model system. J Cell Biol 101:227–39.

Horan KL, Eichberg J, Berti-Mattera LN, LoPachin RM (1989). Hexanedione effects on protein phosphorylation in rat peripheral nerve. Brain Res 491:366–70.

Howell JM, Edington N (1968). The neurotoxicity of sodium diethyldithiocarbamate in the hen. J Neuropathol Exp Neurol 27:464–72.

Howland RD, Alli P (1986). Altered phosphorylation of rat neuronal cytoskeletal proteins in acrylamide induced neuropathy. Brain Res 363:333–9.

Huges CL, Wilmarth KR, Ibrahim S, Abou-Donia MB (1993). [^{14}C]2,5-hexanedione (2,5-HD) binds in vitro to rat brain and spinal cord cytoskeletal proteins and alters in vivo phosphorylation (abstr). Toxicologist 13:127.

Ibrahim S, Abou-Donia MB (1993). Increased immunoreactivity of MAP-2 and phosphorylated neurofilaments in central and peripheral nervous systems of rats treated with acrylamide and glycidamide (abstr). Toxicologist 13:128.

Ishii N, Herskowitz A, Schaumburg HH (1972). *n*-Hexane polyneuropathy: a clinical and experimental study. J Neuropathol Exp Neurol 31:198–210.

Jacobson AR, Coffin SH, Shearson CM, Sayre LM (1987). β,β′-Iminodipropionitrile (IDPN) neurotoxicity: a mechanistic hypothesis for toxic activation. Mol Toxicol 1:17–34.

James KAC, Austin L. (1970). The effect of DFP on axonal transport of protein in chicken sciatic nerve. Brain Res 18:192–94.

Jensen KF, Lapadula DM, Anderson JK, Haykal-Coates N, Abou-Donia MB (1992). Anomalous phosphorylated neurofilament aggregations in central and peripheral axons of hens treated with tri-*ortho*-cresyl phosphate (TOCP). J Neurosc Res 33:455–60.

Jirmanova I, Lukas E (1984). Ultrastructure of carbon disulfide neuropathy. Acta Neuropathol (Berlin) 63:255–63.

Johansson B, Petersen EN, Arnold E (1989). Diethylthiocarbamic acid methyl ester. A potent inhibitor of aldehyde dehydrogenase found in rats treated with disulfiram or diethyldithiocarbamic acid methyl ester. Biochem Pharmacol 38:1053–9.

Johnson GWV (1988). The effects of aluminum on agonist-induced alterations in cyclic AMP and cyclic GMP concentrations in rat brain regions in vivo. Toxicology 51:299–308.

Johnson GW, Jope RS (1987). Aluminum alters cyclic AMP and cyclic GMP levels but not presynaptic cholinergic markers in rat brain in vivo. Brain Res 403:1–6.

Johnson GV, Jope RS (1988). Phosphorylation of rat brain cytoskeletal proteins is increased after orally administered aluminum. Brain Res 456:95–103.

Johnson GV, Li X, Jope RS (1989). Aluminum increases agonist-stimulated cyclic AMP production in rat cerebral cortical slices. J Neurochem 53:258–63.

Johnson GVW, Watson AL Jr, Lartius R, Uemura E, Jope RS (1992). Dietary aluminum selectively decreases MAP-2 in brains of developing and adult rats. Neurotoxicology 13:463–74.

Johnson MK (1990). Contemporary issues in toxicology. Organophosphates and delayed neuropathy—is NTE alive and well? Toxicol Appl Pharmacol 102:385–99.

Johnson MK, Willems JL, De Bisschop HC, Read DJ, Benschop HP (1988). High doses of soman protect against organophosphorus-induced delayed polyneuropathy but tabun does not. Toxicol Appl Pharmacol 92:34–41.

Jones HB, Cavanagh JB (1986). The axon reaction in spinal ganglion neurons of acrylamide-treated rats. Acta Neuropathol (Berlin) 71:55–63.

Juang MS (1976). An electrophysiological study of the action of methylmercuric chloride and mercuric chloride on the sciatic nerve–sartorius muscle preparation of the frog. Toxicol Appl Pharmacol 37:339–48.

Juntunen J, Linnoila I, Haltia M (1977). Histochemical and electron microscopic observations on the myoneural junctions of rats with carbon disulfide induced polyneuropathy. Scand J Work Environ Health 3:36–42.

Kauppinen RA, Komulainen H, Taipale H (1989). Cellular mechanisms underlying the increase in cytosolic free calcium concentration induced by methylmercury in cerebrocortical synaptosomes from guinea pig. J Pharmacol Exp Ther 248:1248–54.

Keilin D, Hartree EF (1940). Succinic dehydrogenase–cytochrome system of cells. Intracellular respiratory system catalyzing aerobic oxidation of succinic acid. Proc R Soc B 129:277–306.

Khanna VK, Husain R, Seth PK (1992). Protein malnourishment: a predisposing factor in acrylamide toxicity in pregnant rats. J Toxicol Environ Health 36:293–305.

Knoth-Anderson J, Abou-Donia MB (1993). Differential effects of triphenylphosphite and diisopropyl phosphorofluoridate on catecholamine secretion from bovine adrenomedullary chromaffin cells. J Toxicol Environ Health 38:103–114.

Koenig ML, Jope RS (1987). Aluminum inhibits the fast phase of voltage-dependent calcium influx into synaptosomes. J Neurochem 49:316–20.

Komiya Y, Cooper NA, Kidman AD (1986). The long-term effects of a single injection of β,β′-iminodipropionitrile on slow axonal transport in the rat. J Biochem 100:1241–6.

Komulainen H, Bondy SC (1987). Increased free intrasynaptosomal Ca^{2+} by neurotoxic organometals: distinctive mechanisms. Toxicol Appl Pharmacol 88:77–86.

Konno N, Katoh K, Yamauchi T, Fukushima M (1988). The effects of drug metabolism inducers on the delayed neurotoxicity and disposition of tri-o-cresyl phosphate in hens following a single intravenous administration. J Toxicol Sci 13:17–30.

Korokobin R, Asbury AK, Sumner AJ, Neilsen SL (1975). Glue-sniffing neuropathy. Arch Neurol 32:158–62.

Krasavage WJ, O'Donoghue JL, DiVincenzo GD, Terhaar CJ (1980). The relative neurotoxicity of methyl n-butyl ketone, n-hexane and their metabolites. Toxicol Appl Pharmacol 52:433–41.

Ladefoged O, Haas U, Simonsen L (1989). Neurophysiological and behavioural effects of combined exposure to 2,5-hexanedione and acetone or ethanol in rats. Pharmacol Toxicol 65:372–5.

Lam HR, Larsen J-J, Ladefoged O, Moller A, Strange P, Arlien-soborg P. (1991). Effects of 2,5-hexanedione alone and in combination with acetone on radial arm maze behavior, the "brain-swelling" reaction and synaptosomal functions. Neurotoxicol Teratol 13:407–12.

Lapadula DM, Bowe M, Carrington CD, Dulak L, Friedman M, Abou-Donia MB (1989). In vitro binding of [^{14}C]acrylamide to neurofilament and microtubule proteins of rats. Brain Res 481:157–61.

Lapadula DM, Irwin RD, Suwita E, Abou-Donia MB (1986). Cross-linking of neurofilament proteins of rat spinal cord in vivo after administration of 2,5-hexanedione. J Neurochem 46:1843–50.

Lapadula DM, Johannsen F, Abou-Donia MB (1990). Absence of delayed neurotoxicity and increased plasma butrylcholinesterase activity in triallate-treated hens. Fundament Appl Toxicol 14:191–8.

Lapadula ES, Lapadula DM, Abou-Donia MB (1991). Persistent alterations of calmodulin kinase II activity in chickens after an oral dose of tri-*o*-cresyl phosphate. Biochem Pharmacol 42:171–80.

Lapadula ES, Lapadula DM, Abou-Donia MB (1992). Biochemical changes in sciatic nerve of hens treated with tri-*o*-cresyl phosphate: increased phosphorylation of cytoskeletal proteins. Neurochem Int 20:247–55.

Lapadula DM, Suwita E, Abou-Donia, MB (1988). Evidence for multiple mechanisms responsible for 2,5-hexanedione-induced neuropathy. Brain Res 458:123–31.

Lee C-C, Peters PJ (1976). Neurotoxicity and behavioral effects of thiram in rats. Environ Health Perspect 17:35–43.

Lee C-C, Russell JQ, Minor JL (1978). Oral toxicity of ferric dimethyldithiocarbamate (ferbam) and tetramethylthiuram disulfide (thiram) in rodents. J Toxicol Environ Health 4:93–106.

Lehotzky K, Szeberenyi JM, Ungvary G, Kiss A (1988). Behavioral effects of prenatal methoxyethyl-mercury chloride exposure in rat pups. Neurotoxicol Teratol 10:471–4.

Lindstrom H, Luthman J, Oskarsson A, Sundberg J, Olson L (1991). Effects of long-term treatment with methyl mercury on the developing rat brain. Environ Res 56:158–69.

Llorens J, Crofton KM (1991). Enhanced neurotoxicity of 3,3'-iminodipropionitrile following carbon tetrachloride pretreatment in the rat. Neurotoxicology 12:583–94.

Logan MJ, McLean WG (1988). A comparison of the effects of acrylamide and experimental diabetes on the retrograde axonal transport of proteins in the rat sciatic nerve: analysis by two-dimensional polyacrylamide gel electrophoresis. J Neurochem 50:183–9.

Lotti M (1991). The pathogenesis of organophosphate polyneuropathy. Crit Rev Toxicol 21:465–87.

Lotti M, Moretto A, Zoppellari R, Dainese R, Rizzuto N, Barusco G (1986). Inhibition of lymphocyte neuropathy target esterase predicts the development of organophosphate-induced delayed polyneuropathy. Arch Toxicol 59:176–9.

Manalis RS, Cooper GP (1975). Evoked transmitter release increased by inorganic mercury at the frog neuromuscular junction. Nature 257:690–1.

Matsumura F (1976). Toxicology of pesticides. New York: Plenum Press.

Matsuoka M, Igisu H (1992). Brain energy metabolites in mice intoxicated with acrylamide: effects of ischemia. Toxicol Lett 62:39–43.

Medrano CJ, LoPachin RM (1989). Effects of acrylamide and 2,5-hexanedione on brain mitochondrial respiration. Neurotoxicology 10:249–56.

Miller MJ, Miller MS, Burks TF, Sipes IG (1984). A simple sensitive method for detecting early peripheral nerve dysfunction in rat following acrylamide treatment. Neurotoxicology 5(2):15–24.

Miller MS, Spencer PS (1985). The mechanisms of acrylamide axonopathy. Annu Rev Pharmacol Toxicol 25:643–66.

Minnema DJ, Cooper GP, Greenland RD (1989). Effects of methylmercury on neurotransmitter release from rat brain synaptosomes. Toxicol Appl Pharmacol 99:510–21.

Miyamoto MD (1983). Hg^{2+} causes neurotoxicity at an intracellular site following entry through Na and Ca channels. Brain Res 267:375–9.

Monaco S, Autilio-Gambetti L, Lasek RJ, Katz MJ, Gambetti P (1989). Experimental increase of neurofilament transport rate: decrease in neurofilament number and in axon diameter. J Neuropathol Exp Neurol 48:23–32.

Monaco S, Wongmongkolrit T, Shearson CM, Patton A, Schaetzle B, Autilio-Gambetti L, Gambetti P, Sayre LM (1990). Giant axonopathy characterized by intermediate location of axonal enlargement and acceleration of neurofilament transport. Brain Res 519:73–81.

Morandi A, Gambetti P, Arora PK, Sayre LM (1987). Mechanism of neurotoxic action of β,β'-im-inodipropionitrile (IDPN): N-hydroxylation enhances neurotoxic potency. Brain Res 437:69–76.

Moretto A, Lotti M, Sabri MI, Spencer PS (1987). Progressive deficit of retrograde axonal transport is associated with the pathogenesis of di-n-butyl dichlorvos axonopathy. J Neurochem 49:1515–22.

Moretto A, Sabri MI (1988). Progressive deficits in retrograde axon transport precede degeneration of motor axons in acrylamide neuropathy. Brain Res 440:18–24.

Moser VC, Anthony DC, Sette WF, MacPhail RC (1992). Comparison of subchronic neurotoxicity of 2-hydroxyethyl acrylate and acrylamide in rats. Fund Appl Toxicol 18:343–52.

Muma NA, Troncoso JC, Hoffman PN, Koo EH, Price DL (1988). Aluminum neurotoxicity: altered expression of cytoskeletal genes. Mol Br Res 3:115–22.

Murphy SD (1986). Pesticides. In: Klaasen CD, Amdur MO, Doull J, eds. Casarett and Doull's toxicology, the basic science of poisons. 3rd ed. New York: Macmillan, 519–81.

Murray JC, Tanner CM, Sprague SM (1991). Aluminum neurotoxicity: A reevaluation. Clin Neuropharmacol 14:179–85.

Myall OT, Allen SL, McLean WG (1990a). The effect of 2,5-hexanedione on the induction of ornithine decarboxylase in the dorsal root ganglion of the rat. Neurosci Lett 114:305–8.

Myall OT, Allen SL, McLean WG (1990b). The effect of acrylamide on the reduction of ornithine decarboxylase in the dorsal root ganglion of the rat. Brain Res 523:295–7.

Nachtman JP, Couri D (1984). An electrophysiological study of 2-hexanone and 2,5-hexanedione neurotoxicity in rats. Toxicol Lett 23:141–5.

Nakada S, Imura N (1982). Uptake of methylmercury and inorganic mercury by mouse glioma and mouse neuroblastoma cells. Neurotoxicology 3:249–58.

Nomeir AA, Abou-Donia MB (1984). Disposition of [^{14}C]tri-o-cresyl phosphate and its metabolites in various tissues of the male cat following a single dermal application. Drug Metab Dispos 12:705–11.

Nomeir AA, Abou-Donia MB (1986). Studies on the metabolism of the neurotoxic tri-o-cresyl phosphate. Distribution, excretion, and metabolism in male cats after a single dermal application. Toxicology 38:15–33.

Official Report, Office of Drinking Water, U.S. Environmental Protection Agency, Washington, DC (July 1987) TR-832-104A. Final draft for the drinking water criteria document on acrylamide.

Official Report, Office of Toxic Substances, U.S. Environmental Protection Agency, Washington, DC (March 1988). Preliminary assessment of health risks from exposure to acrylamide.

Ogawa N, Haba K, Asanuma M, Mori A (1991). Long-lasting effect of ceruletide on dyskinesia and monoaminergic neuronal pathways in rats treated with iminodipropionitrile. Brain Res 556:271–9.

Ogawa N, Mizukawa K, Haba K, Sato H (1990). Neurotransmitter and receptor alterations in the rat persistent dyskinesia model induced by iminodipropionitrile. Eur Neurol 30(suppl 1):31–140.

Opacka J, Baranski B, Wronska-Nofer T (1984). Effect of alcohol intake on some disturbances induced by chronic exposure to carbon disulfide in rats. I. Behavioural alterations. Toxicol Lett 23:91–7.

Opacka J, Opalska B, Kolakowski J, Wronska-Nofer T (1986). Neurotoxic effects of the combined exposure to carbon disulfide and ethanol in rats. Toxicol Lett 32:9–18.

Opacka J, Wronska-Nofer T, Kolakowski J, Opalska B (1985). Effects of alcohol intake on some distrubances induced by chronic exposure to carbon disulfide in rats. II. Biochemical and ultrastructural alterations in the peripheral nerves. Toxicol Lett 24:171–7.

Oskarsson A (1987). Comparative effects of ten dithiocarbamate and thiuram compounds on tissue distribution and excretion of lead in rats. Environ Res 44:82–93.

Papasozomenos SC, Payne MR (1986). Actin immunoreactivity localizes with segregated microtubules and membranous organelles and in the subaxolemmal region in the β,β'-iminodipropionitrile axon. J Neurosci 6:3483–91.

Pappolla M, Penton R, Weiss HS, Miller CH Jr., Sahenk Z, Autilio-Gambetti L, Gambetti P (1987). Carbon disulfide axonopathy. Another experimental model characterized by acceleration of neurofilament transport and distinct changes of axonal size. Brain Res 424:272–80.

Parhad IM, Griffin JW, Hoffman PN, Koves JF (1986). Selective interruption of axonal transport of neurofilament proteins in the visual system by β,β′-iminodipropionitrile (IDPN) intoxication. Brain Res 363:315–24.

Parhad IM, Swedberg EA, Hoar DI, Krekoski CA, Clark AW (1988). Neurofilament gene expression following β,β′-iminodipropionitrile (IDPN) intoxication. Mol Brain Res 4:293–301.

Patton SE, O'Callaghan JP, Miller DB, Abou-Donia MB (1983a). The effect of oral administration of tri-o-cresyl phosphate on in vitro phosphorylation of membrane and cytosolic proteins from chicken brain. J Neurochem 41:897–901.

Patton SE, O'Callaghan JP, Miller DB, Abou-Donia MB (1983b). Changes in *in vitro* brain and spinal cord protein phosphorylation after a single oral administration of tri-o-cresyl phosphate to hens. J Neurochem 45:1567–77.

Patton SE, Lapadula DM, Abou-Donia MB (1986). The relationship of tri-o-cresyl phosphate–induced delayed neurotoxicity to enhancement of in vitro phosphorylation of hen brain and spinal cord proteins. J Pharmacol Exp Ther 239:597–605.

Peele DB, Allison SD, Crofton KM (1990). Learning and memory deficits in rats following exposure to 3.3′-iminodipropionitrile. Toxicol Appl Pharmacol 105:321–32.

Pellin MC, Vicedo JL, Vilanova E (1987). Sensitivity to tri-o-cresyl phosphate neurotoxicity of n-hexane exposed hens as a model of simultaneous hexacarbon solvent and organophosphorus occupational intoxication. Arch Toxicol 59:311–8.

Pellin MC, Vilanova E, Barril J (1988). Low non-neuropathic tri-o-cresyl phosphate (TOCP) doses inhibit neuropathy target esterase near the neuropathic threshold in n-hexane pretreated hens. Toxicology 49:999–1005.

Peraica M, Capodicasa E, Moretto A, Lotti M (1993). Organophosphate polyneuropathy in chicks. Biochem Pharmacol 45:131–5.

Pleasure DE, Mishler KC, Engel WK (1969). Axonal transport of proteins in experimental neuropathies. Science 166:524–5.

Pope CN, Chapman ML, Tanaka D Jr, Padilla S (1992). Phenylmethylsulfonyl fluoride alters sensitivity to organophosphorus-induced delayed neurotoxicity in developing animals. Neurotoxicology 13:355–64.

Pope CN, Padilla S (1990). Potentiation of organophosphorus-induced delayed neurotoxicity by phenylmethylsulfonyl fluoride. J Toxicol Environ Health 31:261–73.

Prineas J (1969). The pathogenesis of dying-back polyneuropathies. Part I. An ultrastructural study of experimental tri-ortho-cresyl phosphate intoxication in the cat. J Neuropathol Exp Neurol 28:571–97.

Przedborski S, Wright M, Fahn S, Cadet JL (1989). Autoradiographic evidence of [^{3}H]neurotensin binding changes in discrete regions of brain in the rat model of persistent spasmodic dyskinesia induced by iminodipropionitrile. Neurosci Lett 107:335–40.

Przedborski S, Wright M, Fahn S, Cadet JL (1990). Quantitative autoradiographic changes in 5-[3H]HT-labeled 5-HT1 serotonin receptors in discrete regions of brain in the rat model of persistent dyskinesias induced by iminodipropionitrile (IDPN). Neurosci Lett 116:51–7.

Puglia CD, Loeb GA (1987). Influence of rat brain superoxide dismutase inhibition by diethyldithiocarbamate upon the rate of development of central nervous system oxygen toxicity. Toxicol Appl Pharmacol 75:258–64.

Pyle SJ, Amarnath V, Graham DG, Anthony DC (1992). The role of pyrrole formation in the alteration of neurofilament transport induced during exposure to 2,5-hexanedione. J Neuropathol Exp Neurol 51:451–8.

Rana RS, Hokin LE (1990). Role of phosphoinositides in transmembrane signalling. Physiol Rev 70:115–64.

Rasul AR, Howell JM (1973a). A comparison of the effect of sodium diethyldithiocarbamate on the central nervous system of young and adult domestic fowl. Acta Neuropathol (Berlin) 24:68–75.

Rasul AR, Howell JM (1973b). Further observations on the response of the peripheral and central nervous system of the rabbit to sodium diethyldithiocarbamate. Acta Neuropathol 24:161–73.

Rasul AR, Howell JM (1974). The toxicity of some dithiocarbamate compounds in young and adult domestic fowl. Toxicol Appl Pharmacol 30:63–78.

Ravindranath V, Pai KS (1991). The use of rat brain slices as an *in* vitro model for mechanistic evaluation of neurotoxicity-studies with acrylamide. Neurotoxicology 12:225–34.

Reagan KE, Wilmarth KR, Abou-Donia MB (1993). Acrylamide and glycidamide treatments increased calcium/calmodulin-dependent phosphorylation of cytoskeletal proteins in rat brain and spinal cord (abstr). Toxicolgist 13:128.

Reddy GR, Babu GRV, Reddana P, Chetty CS (1990). Effect *in* vitro of benthiocarb on rat brain succinate dehydrogenase. Biochem Int 20:771–4.

Reichert BL, Abou-Donia MB (1980). Inhibition of fast axoplasmic transport by delayed neurotoxic organophosphorus esters: a possible mode of action. Mol Pharmacol 17:56–60.

Rossi A, Manzo L, Orrenius S, Vahter M, Nicotera P (1991). Modifications of cell signalling in the cytotoxicity of metals. Pharmacol Toxicol 68:424–9.

Ruffer-Turner ME, Read DJ, Johnson MK (1992). Purification of neuropathy target esterase from avian brain after prelabelling with [^{3}H]diisopropyl phosphorofluoridate. J Neurochem 58:135–41.

Sabri MI (1984). Further observations on *in* vitro and *in* vivo effects of 2,5-hexanedione on glyceraldehyde-3-phosphate dehydrogenase. Arch Toxicol 55:191–4.

Sabri MI (1992). Effects of 2,5-hexanedione and 3,4-dimethyl-2,5-hexanedione on retrograde axonal transport in sciatic nerve. Neurochem Res 17:835–9.

Sabri MI, Spencer PS (1990). Acrylamide impairs fast and slow axonal transport in rat optic system. Neurochem Res 15:603–8.

Sager PR, Matheson DW (1988). Mechanisms of neurotoxicity related to selective disruption of microtubules and intermediate filaments. Toxicology 49:479–92.

Saitoh T, Masliah E, Jin L-W, Cole GM, Wieloch T, Shapiro IP (1991). Protein kinases and phosphorylation in neurologic disorders and cell death. Lab Invest 64:596–616.

Sakamoto J, Hashimoto K (1985). Effect of acrylamide and related compounds on glycolytic enzymes in rat sciatic nerve in vivo. Arch Toxicol 57:282–4.

Savolainen H, Lehtonen E, Vainio H (1977). CS$_2$ binding to rat spinal neurofilaments. Acta Neuropathol (Berlin) 37:219–23.

Savolainen H, Vainio H (1976). High binding of CS$_2$ sulphur in spinal cord axonal fraction. Acta Neuropathol (Berlin) 36:251–7.

Sayre LM, Autilio-Gambetti L, Gambetti P (1985). Pathogenesis of experimental giant neurofilamentous axonopathies: a united hypothesis based on chemical modification of neurofilaments. Brain Res Rev 10:69–83.

Schulze GE, Boysen BG (1991). A neurotoxicity screening battery for the use in safety evaluation: effects of arylamide and 3,3′-iminodipropionitrile. Fund Appl Toxicol 16:602–15.

Shafer TJ, Atchison WD (1989). Block of ^{45}Ca uptake into synaptosomes by methylmercury: Ca^{2+}- and Nc^{+}-dependence. J Pharmcol Expt Ther 248:696–702.

Shafer TJ, Atchison WD (1991). Transmitter, ion channel and receptor properties of pheochromocytoma (PC12) cells: a model for neurotoxicological studies. Neurotoxicology 12:473–92.

Shea TB, Balikian P, Beermann ML (1992). Aluminium inhibits neurofilament protein degradation by multiple cytoskeleton-associated proteases. FEBS Lett 307:195–8.

Sickles DW (1989a). Toxic neurofilamentous axonopathies and fast anterograde axonal transport: II. The effects of single doses of neurotoxic and non-neurotoxic diketones and β,β′-iminodipropionitrile (IDPN) on the rate and capacity of transport. Neurotoxicology 10:103–12.

Sickles DW (1989b). Toxic neurofilamentous axonopathies and fast anterograde axonal transport: the effect of single doses of acrylamide on the rate and capacity of transport. Neurotoxicology 10:91–102.

Sickles DW (1991). Toxic neurofilamentous axonopathies and fast anterograde axonal transport.

III. recovery from single injections and multiple dosing effects of acrylamide and 2,5-hexanedione. Toxicol Appl Pharmacol 108:390–6.

Sickles DW (1992). Toxic neurofilamentous axonopathies and fast anterograde axonal transport: IV. In vitro analysis of transport following acrylamide and 2,5-hexanedione. Toxicol Lett 61:199–204.

Sickles DW, Fowler SR, Testino AR (1990). Effects of neurofilamentous axonopathy–producing neurotoxicants on in vitro production of ATP by brain mitochondria. Brain Res 528:25–31.

Sickles DW, Goldstein BD (1986). Acrylamide produces a direct, dose-dependent and specific inhibition of oxidative metabolism in motoneurons. Neurotoxicology 7:187–95.

Simpson J, Yates CM, Whyler DK, Wilson H, Dewar AJ, Gordon A (1985). Biochemical studies on rabbits with aluminum-induced neurofilament accumulations. Neurochem Res 10:229–38.

Smith MI, Elvove E, Frazier WH (1930). The pharmacological action of certain phenol esters, with special reference to the etiology of so called ginger paralysis. Pub Health Rep 45:2509–72.

Smitt PAES, de Jong JMBV (1989). Animal models of amyotrophic lateral sclerosis and the spinal muscular atrophies. J Neurolog Sci 91:231–58.

Spencer PS, Schaumburg HH (1977). Ultrastructural studies of the dying-back process. III. The evolution of experimental peripheral giant axonal degeneration. J Neuropathol Exp Neurol 36:276–99.

Spencer PS, Schaumburg HH (1976). Central-peripheral distal axonopathy—the pathology of dying-back polyneuropathies. In Zimmerman H, ed. Progress in neuropathology. Vol. 3. New York: Grune and Stratton, 253–95.

Spencer PS, Schaumburg HH, Sabri MI, Veronesi B (1980). The enlarging view of hexacarbon neurotoxicity. CRC Crit Rev 7:279–356.

Srinivas PN, Reddy GR, Chetty CS (1989). Modulation of benthiocarb in vitro inhibited neonate rat (Wistar strain) brain Na^+K^+-ATPase by norepinephrine. Biochem Int 19:209–14.

Srivastava SP, Seth PK (1985). Effects of mixed-function oxidase modifiers on neurotoxicity of acrylamide in rats. Biochem Pharmacol 34:1099—102.

Srivastava SP, Sabri MI, Agrawal AK, Seth PK (1986). Effect of single and repeated doses of acrylamide and bis-acrylamide on glutathione-S-transferase and dopamine receptors in rat brain. Brain Res 371:319–23.

Srivastava SP, Seth PK, Das M, Mukhtar H (1989). Effects of mixed-function oxidase modifiers on neurotoxicity of acrylamide in rats. Biochem Pharmacol 34:1099–1102.

Srivastava SP, Srivastava SP, Seth PK (1984). Acid hydrolases in brain, spinal cord, and sciatic nerves of acrylamide-intoxicated rats. Toxicol Lett 22:211–5.

Sterman AB, Sposito N (1985). 2,5-Hexanedione and acrylamide produce reorganization of motoneuron perikarya. Neuropathol Appl Neurobiol 11:201–12.

Sumner SCJ, MacNeela JP, Fennell TR (1992). Characterization and quantitation of urinary metabolites of $[1,2,3-^{13}C]$acrylamide in rats and mice using ^{13}C nuclear magnetic resonance spectroscopy. Chem Res Toxicol 5:81–9.

Suwita E, Lapadula DM, Abou-Donia MB (1986a). Calcium and calmodulin-enhanced in vitro phosphorylation of hen brain cold-stable microtubules and spinal cord neurofilament triplet proteins following a single dose of tri-o-cresyl phosphate. Proc Natl Acad Sci USA 83:6174–8.

Suwita E, Lapadula DM, Abou-Donia MB (1986b). Calcium and calmodulin stimulated in vitro phosphorylation of rooster brain tubulin and MAP-2 following a single oral dose of tri-o-cresyl phosphate. Brain Res 374:199–203.

Suzuki K, Pfaff LD (1973). Acrylamide neuropathy in rats. An electron microscopic study of degeneration and regeneration. Acta Neuropathol (Berlin) 24:197–213.

Tanaka D Jr, Brusian SJ (1989). Degeneration patterns in the chicken central nervous system induced by ingestion of the organophosphorus delayed neurotoxin tri-*ortho*-tolyl phosphate. A silver impregnation study. Brain Res 484:240–56.

Tandrup T, Braendgaard H (1992). The number and mean volume of neurons in the cerebral cortex of rats intoxicated with acrylamide. Neuropathol Appl Neurobiol 18:250–8.

Tanii H, Hayashi M, Hashimoto K (1988). Neurofilament degradation in the nervous system of rats intoxicated with acrylamide, related compounds or 2,5-hexanedione. Arch Toxicol 62:70–5.

Tarkowski S, Cremer JE (1972). Metabolism of glucose and free amino acids in brain, studied with ^{14}C-labelled glucose and butyrate in rats intoxicated with carbon disulfide. J Neurochem 19:2631–40.

Tarkowski S, Sobczak H (1971). Oxidation and phosphorylation processes in brain mitochondria of rats exposed to carbon disulfide. J Neurochem 18:177–82.

Thomas PK, Bradley DJ, Bradley WA, Degen PH, Krinke G, Muddle J, Schaumburg HH, Skelton-Stroud PN, Thomann P, Tzebelikos E (1984). Correlated nerve conduction, somatosensory evoked potential and neuropathological studies in clioquinol and 2,5-hexanedione neurotoxicity in the baboon. J Neurol Sci 64:277–95.

Thorn GD, Ludwig RA (1962). The dithiocarbamates and related compounds. Amsterdam, New York: Elsevier.

Thuranszky K, Kiss I, Botos M, Szebeni A (1982). Effect of dithiocarbamate-type chemicals on the nervous system of rats. Arch Toxicol 5(suppl): 125–8.

Traxinger DL, Atchison WD (1987). Reversal of methylmercury-induced block of nerve-evoked release of acetylcholine at the neuromuscular junction. Toxicol Appl Pharmacol 90:23–33.

Troncoso JC, March JL, Haner M, Aebi U (1990). Effects of aluminum and other multivalent cations on neurofilaments in vitro: an electron microscopic study. J Struct Biol 103:2–12.

Troncoso JC, Sternberger NH, Sternberger LA, Hoffman PN, Price DL (1986). Immunocytochemical studies of neurofilament antigens in the neurofibrillary pathology induced by aluminium. Brain Res 364:295–300.

Valentine WM, Amarnath V, Graham DG, Anthony DC (1992). Covalent cross-linking of proteins by carbon disulfide. Chem Res Toxicol 5:254–62.

Van der Voet GB, Marani E, Tio S, de Wolff FA (1991). Aluminum neurotoxicity. Prog Histochem Cytochem 23:235–42.

Vasilescu C (1976). Sensory and motor conduction in chronic carbon disulfide poisoning. Eur Neurol 14:447–57.

Verity MA (1992). Neurotoxins and environmental poisons. Curr Opin Neurol Neurosurgery 5:401–5.

Veronesi B (1984). Effect of metabolic inhibition with piperonyl butoxide on rodent sensitivity to tri-o-cresyl phosphate. Exp Neurol 85:651–60.

Vyas I, Lowndes HE, Howland RD (1985). Inhibition of glyceraldehyde-3-phosphate dehydrogenase in tissues of the rat by acrylamide and related compounds. Neurotoxicology 6(3):123–32.

Watson DF, Fittro KP, Hoffman PN, Griffin JW (1991). Phosphorylation-related immunoreactivity and the rate of transport of neurofilaments in chronic 2,5-hexanedione intoxication. Brain Res 539:103–9.

Watson DF, Griffin JW, Fittro KP, Hoffman PN (1989). Phosphorylation-dependent immunoreactivity of neurofilaments increases during axonal maturation and β,β′-iminodipropionitrile intoxication. J Neurochem 53:1818–29.

Wilmarth KR, Viana ME, Abou-Donia MB (1993). Carbon disulfide (CS₂) inhalation increased CA^{2+}/calmodulin-dependent phosphorylation of cytoskeletal proteins in the rat central nervous system (abstr.) Toxicologist 13:127.

Xintaras C, Burg JR (1980). Screening and prevention of human neurotoxic outbreaks: issues and problems. In: Spencer PS, Schaumburg HH, eds. Clinical and experimental neurotoxicology. Baltimore: Williams and Wilkins.

Xintaras C, Burg JR, Tanaka S, Lee ST, Johnson BL, Cottrill CA, Bender J (1978). NIOSH health survey of velsicol pesticides workers: occupation exposure to leptophos and other chemicals. U.S. Government Printing Office, Washington, D.C., pp. 663–74.

Yamada H, Yasunobu KT (1962). Monoamine oxidase. II. Copper. One of the prosthetic group of plasma monoamine oxidase. J Biol Chem 237:3077–82.

Yates CM, Simpson J, Russell D, Gordon A (1980). Cholinergic enzymes in neurofibrillary degeneration produced by aluminium. Brain Res 197:269–74.

8

Toxicant-Induced Demyelinating Neuropathy

Thomas W. Bouldin and Jeffry F. Goodrum
University of North Carolina at Chapel Hill
Chapel Hill, North Carolina

DEFINITION AND CLASSIFICATION OF NEUROPATHIES

The term "neuropathy" refers to a disease process that involves the peripheral nervous system (PNS). Neuropathy may be evidenced by weakness or atrophy of muscle, alteration or loss of sensation, abnormal functioning of the autonomic nervous system, or various combinations of motor, sensory, and autonomic abnormalities. Comprehensive discussions of the clinical, electrophysiological, and pathological features of neuropathy are available (Dyck et al., 1984b; Schaumburg et al., 1992).

Many different types of disease process, including many toxicant-induced diseases, are associated with neuropathy. These neuropathies may be classified by etiology, morphological features, electrophysiological abnormalities, or clinical presentation. A classification of neuropathy based on etiology is presented in Table 1. Although classification by etiology is preferable, many neuropathies are idiopathic and therefore must be classified by their morphological, electrophysiological, or clinical features. Even when the etiology of a neuropathy is known, morphological classification remains useful, because an understanding of the specific cell-type involved in the neuropathic process may give clues to the pathogenic mechanism by which the particular etiological agent causes neuropathy. An understanding of pathogenesis is, in turn, important for developing appropriate strategies of therapy.

Because neurons and Schwann cells are the principal cell types in the PNS, virtually all neuropathies affect neurons or Schwann cells. This has led to a simplified morphological classification in which neuropathies may be categorized into those preferentially involving the neuron, those preferentially involving the Schwann cell, and those that have a "mixed pathology" with significant involvement of both the neuron and the Schwann cell (Griffin, 1983). Neuropathies preferentially involving the neuron (neuronopathy) or its axon (axonopathy) are usually characterized morphologically in the PNS by degeneration and

Table 1 Classification of Peripheral Neuropathy

1. Exposure to toxicants
   a. Lead neuropathy, tellurium neuropathy, etc.
2. Systemic metabolic abnormalities
   a. Diabetic neuropathy, uremic neuropathy, etc.
3. Nutritional deficiencies
   a. Alcoholic neuropathy, beriberi neuropathy, etc.
4. Inherited neuropathies
   a. Charcot-Marie-Tooth disease, Friedreich's ataxia, etc.
5. Autoimmune mechanisms
   a. Acute inflammatory demyelinating neuropathy, etc.
6. Neuropathy as a remote effect of cancer (paraneoplastic neuropathy)
7. Neuropathy associated with amyloidosis (amyloid neuropathy)
8. Neuropathy associated with paraproteinemias
9. Hypoxia-ischemia of nerve
   a. Vasculitic neuropathy, diabetic polyneuropathy, etc.
10. Neuropathy associated with infections
    a. Herpes zoster, leprosy, human immunodeficiency virus (HIV), etc.
11. Neuropathy associated with sarcoidosis (sarcoid neuropathy)
12. Neuropathy associated with radiation (radiation neuropathy)
13. Neuropathy associated with trauma (traumatic neuropathy)
14. Neuropathy of unknown cause (cryptogenic neuropathy)

loss of axons and are classified as axonal neuropathies. Neuropathies involving the Schwann cell or its myelin sheath are usually characterized morphologically in the PNS by degeneration and loss of myelin, and are classified as demyelinating neuropathies. This simplified morphological classification scheme correlates well with the electrophysiological abnormalities found in these neuropathies—axonal neuropathies often have little or no loss of nerve conduction velocity, and demyelinating neuropathies have a significant decrease in nerve conduction velocity.

Neuropathies with a mixed pathology typically show both axonal degeneration and demyelination. In these neuropathies, the demyelination may be due to direct Schwann cell injury or to underlying axonal abnormalities. The term "secondary demyelination" is used to describe the demyelination that occurs as a response of the Schwann cell to axonal perturbations (Dyck et al., 1984a). The interactions of the axon and the Schwann cell are complex (see below, "Alterations in the Interactions Between Axon and Schwann Cell"), and it is not surprising that a variety of toxicant-induced axonal neuropathies also show evidence of secondary demyelination (Shimono et al., 1978; Bouldin and Cavanagh, 1979; Griffin and Price, 1981). Just as toxicant-induced axonal neuropathies may show a degree of secondary demyelination, toxicant-induced demyelinating neuropathies frequently show occasional degenerating axons. The cause of the axonal degeneration associated with demyelinating neuropathy is poorly understood (Said et al., 1981a).

Most toxic neuropathies are classified as axonal neuropathies. Among the toxicant-induced neuropathies classified as demyelinating neuropathies are those associated with inorganic lead salts, tellurium, hexachlorophene, triethyltin sulfate, buckthorn toxin, diphtheria toxin, lysolecithin, local anesthetics and acetyl ethyl tetramethyl tetralin (AETT). Some of these toxicants (e.g., triethyltin sulfate, local anesthetic agents) associated with "demyelinating" neuropathy clearly target the Schwann cell/myelin sheath but cause little demyelination. In the case of triethyltin, the Schwann cell/myelin injury results primarily in intramyelinic edema rather than actual breakdown and loss of the myelin sheath (demyelination) (Graham and Gonatas, 1973). In the case of local anesthetic agents, the Schwann cell injury results primarily in lysis of unmyelinating Schwann cells and the formation of lipid droplets in myelinating Schwann cells (Powell et al., 1988). It may be argued that a morphological category other than "demyelinating neuropathy" would be more appropriate to encompass the morphological range of toxic neuropathies in which the primary target is the Schwann cell or myelin sheath.

Other, more elaborate classification schemes have been devised for toxic neuropathies. One such scheme is that proposed by Spencer and Schaumburg (1980). In this scheme, the terminology is centered on the putative site of the toxic injury and distinguishes the cell's soma (neuron or Schwann cell) from its processes (axon or myelin sheath) (Table 2). This classification scheme offers considerable benefits in the conceptualization of disease processes and in the formation of hypotheses concerning the pathogenetic mechanisms of cellular injury. However, unlike classification schemes that simply describe the observed morphological changes associated with a particular toxicant, this scheme requires that an initial assumption be made about the site of the cellular injury. The subjectivity involved in assigning the site of cellular injury is highlighted by tellurium neuropathy. Tellurium intoxication results biochemically in an enzymatic block in cholesterol metabolism in the nerve and morphologically in a demyelinating neuropathy. Because of cholesterol's importance in myelin synthesis, it has been hypothesized that the tellurium-induced block in cholesterol synthesis causes the demyelination (Harry et al., 1989). Assuming that this hypothesis is correct, does the block in cholesterol synthesis in Schwann cells mark tellurium neuropathy as a schwannopathy or a myelinopathy?

PATHOLOGY OF DEMYELINATING NEUROPATHY

Morphological Changes

One of the earliest descriptions of demyelinating neuropathy is that provided by Gombault, who recorded the pathological changes in the nerves of guinea pigs intoxicated with inorganic lead salts (1880–81). Using the teased-fiber technique to isolate single myelinated nerve fibers, he found that affected fibers showed segments of myelin loss. Subsequent studies in a variety of animal models of neuropathy, as well as in acquired (e.g., Guillain-Barré type of inflammatory demyelinating neuropathy) and hereditary neuropathies (e.g., Charcot-Marie-Tooth disease) in humans, have confirmed that segmental

Table 2 Classification of Peripheral Neuropathy Based on Putative Cellular Target Site

1. Neuron
   a. Disease of the cell's soma—neuronopathy
   b. Disease of the cell's processes (axons)—axonopathy
      Proximal axon—proximal axonopathy
      Distal axon—distal axonopathy
2. Schwann cell
   a. Disease of the cell's soma—schwannopathy (myelin gliopathy)
   b. Disease of the cell's processes (myelin)—myelinopathy

Source: Adapted from Spencer and Schaumburg, 1980.

demyelination is a common manifestation of disease in peripheral nerve fibers. Other morphological changes accompanying the segmental myelin loss in demyelinating neuropathy are subcellular alterations in Schwann cells, proliferation of Schwann cells, infiltration of the nerve by macrophages to phagocytose the myelin debris, breakdown of the blood-nerve barrier, and remyelination. The temporal course of some of these changes in tellurium neuropathy is presented schematically in Fig. 1. The following general description of the pathology of demyelinating neuropathy is based on our experience with inorganic-lead neuropathy and tellurium neuropathy, which are two prototypical toxicant-induced demyelinating neuropathies.

Abnormalities of the Myelin Sheath

Normal myelinated fibers in teased-fiber preparations show multiple segments of myelin covering the axon (Fig. 2A). Each segment, or internode, represents the territory myelinated by a single Schwann cell. Between each internode and the next is a short gap, the node of Ranvier. The earliest evidence of demyelination in teased-fiber preparations is usually paranodal or internodal demyelination. Paranodal demyelination is evidenced by widening of the gap at the node of Ranvier and by loss of a variable amount of the paranodal myelin sheath (Fig. 2B). Ultrastructural studies of paranodal demyelination in diphtheritic neuropathy reveal that the nodal widening is due in part to retraction of the outer loops of myelin from the nodal area (Allt et al., 1969). The converse of paranodal demyelination—one or more focal areas of demyelination limited to the perinuclear region of the internode and not involving the paranodal regions—has not been described.

Internodal demyelination is characterized by the complete loss of one or more entire internodes of myelin (Fig. 2C). It is usual to find in demyelinating neuropathy that some internodes show paranodal demyelination while others show internodal demyelination. In her detailed analysis of teased-fiber preparations from diphtheritic neuropathy in the rat, Jacobs (1967) found that paranodal and internodal demyelination were dose-dependent, with paranodal demyelination predominating at lower doses and internodal demyelination predominating at higher doses.

Another teased-fiber abnormality found in some toxicant-induced demyelinating neuropathies is the presence of localized vacuolation (bubbling) of the myelin sheath. These

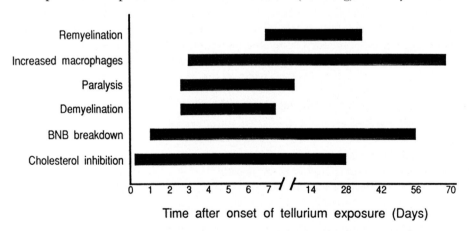

Figure 1 Approximate time intervals for some of the pathological and clinical findings in tellurium-induced demyelinating neuropathy. The observations are from a model in which a 1% tellurium diet is given to 20-day-old rats for 7 days. BNB = blood-nerve barrier.

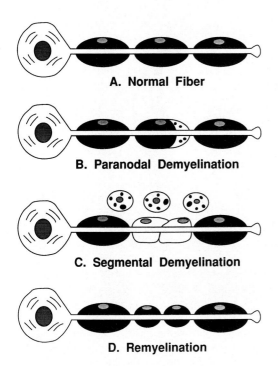

A. Normal Fiber

B. Paranodal Demyelination

C. Segmental Demyelination

D. Remyelination

Figure 2 Diagram of a neuron and its myelinated peripheral axon. Some of the morphological abnormalities found in demyelinating neuropathy are illustrated. The cells adjacent to the demyelinated segment (C) are macrophages.

internodal varicosities, which are due to intramyelinic edema, are commonly observed in tellurium neuropathy and are even more pronounced in AETT neuropathy and hexachlorophene neuropathy (Maxwell and Le Quesne, 1979; Spencer et al., 1979; Said and Duckett, 1981). The varicosities in AETT neuropathy and hexachlorophene neuropathy are due to splitting of the myelin sheath at the intraperiod line (Spencer et al., 1979; Towfighi, 1980).

Ultrastructural studies of the myelin sheath during the process of toxicant-induced demyelination typically reveal nonspecific degenerative changes in the myelin (Lampert and Schochet, 1968; Lampert and Garrett, 1971). Breakdown of myelin is evidenced by splitting and disorganization of the myelin lamellae (Fig. 3). The degenerating myelin may form a "honeycomb" pattern (vesicular degeneration of myelin) in which there are numerous contiguous membranous rings within the degenerating myelin sheath. Fluid sometimes accumulates between the myelin lamellae (intramyelinic edema), giving rise to the myelin bubbles visible in teased-fiber preparations. The degenerating myelin sheath is quickly and completely removed from the intact axon (Fig. 4). The demyelinated axon remains completed surrounded by Schwann cell cytoplasm, except in those uncommon toxicant-induced demyelinating neuropathies characterized by necrosis of Schwann cells and inhibition of Schwann cell proliferation (England et al., 1988).

Abnormalities of the Schwann Cell

A variety of ultrastructural abnormalities have been described in the cytoplasm of Schwann cells before and during the onset of myelin breakdown in demyelinating neuropathy. In

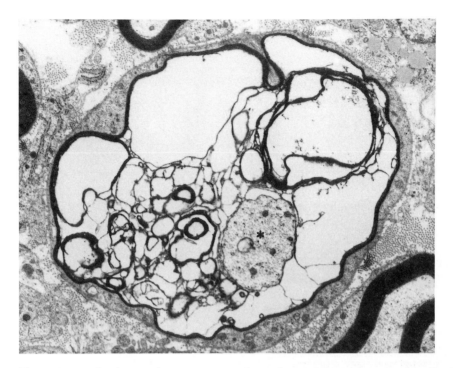

Figure 3 Myelin degeneration is present within 3 days in tellurium neuropathy. The degeneration is evidenced by vacuolation and disorganization of the myelin sheath. The underlying axon (asterisk) is intact. Portions of three intact myelin sheaths are visible at the edges of the figure.

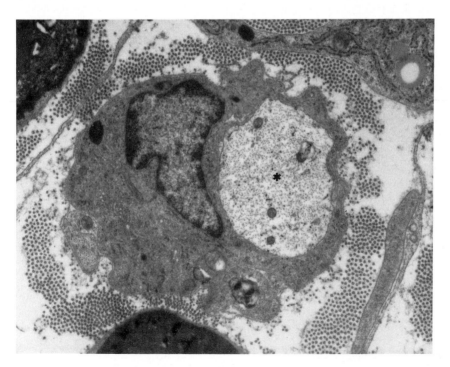

Figure 4 Numerous demyelinated axons are present in the rat sciatic nerve during the first week after beginning tellurium intoxication. This demyelinated axon (asterisk) is surrounded by Schwann cell cytoplasm. One of the Schwann cells is sectioned at the level of its nucleus.

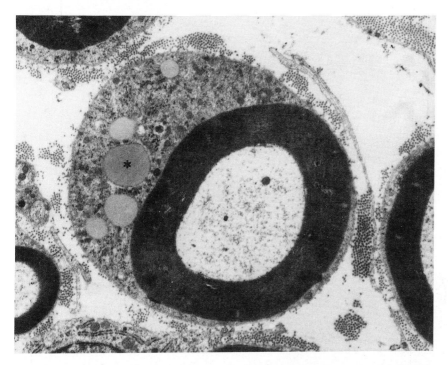

Figure 5 Subcellular, ultrastructural abnormalities are common in Schwann cells before the onset of myelin breakdown in tellurium neuropathy in the rat. This Schwann cell shows five intracytoplasmic lipid droplets (one marked with an asterisk) and an intact myelin sheath. These droplets are present within 24 h of starting the tellurium intoxication and are due to accumulation of squalene, an intermediary in the biosynthesis of cholesterol. Lipid droplets may also be due to lipid accumulation as a result of myelin breakdown. Lipid droplets are found in many demyelinating and axonal neuropathies.

general, these subcellular changes are nonspecific, with various combinations of abnormalities being reported in different neuropathies. Among the variety of changes described in Schwann cells are hypertrophy and mushroom-like excrescences of the Schwann cell cytoplasm, intracytoplasmic lipid droplets, increased numbers of pi bodies, dense bodies, myelin figures, membrane-bound vacuoles, subplasmalemmal caveolae, accumulations of intermediate filaments, and cytoplasmic edema (Fig. 5, 6) (Lampert and Schochet, 1968; Lampert and Garrett, 1971; Coria et al., 1986; Coria and Montón, 1988; Bouldin et al., 1989; Forcier et al., 1991). Inclusions within Schwann cell nuclei are a distinctive finding in inorganic lead neuropathy (Myers et al., 1980). Degeneration of Schwann cells, as evidenced by severe intracytoplasmic edema or accumulations of degenerating organelles, has been found in a variety of toxicant-induced demyelinating neuropathies (Fig. 7) (e.g., Lampert and Schochet, 1968; Lampert and Garrett, 1971). Profiles of necrotic Schwann cells may also occasionally be found in demyelinating neuropathies (Powell et al., 1982; Bouldin et al., 1989).

Intracytoplasmic lipid droplets (Figs. 5, 6) within Schwann cells are frequently found during the evolution of a demyelinating neuropathy or wallerian-type axonal degeneration and are considered nonspecific (Griffin et al., 1990). The lipid is usually considered to

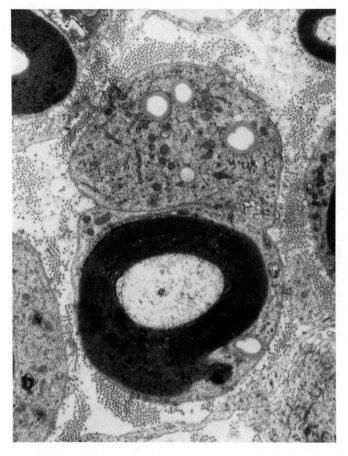

Figure 6 An ultrastructural abnormality occasionally found in Schwann cells before the onset of myelin breakdown is "capping" or "girdling" of the Schwann cell cytoplasm to form a mushroom-like cytoplasmic excrescence. Note the waist-like constriction of the Schwann cell cytoplasm just above the myelin sheath in this rat with tellurium neuropathy. This abnormality is reported in a variety of other demyelinating and axonal neuropathies. Intracytoplasmic lipid droplets are also present in the Schwann cell.

result from the catabolism of degenerating myelin, although the possibility of a direct toxic effect on the metabolism of the Schwann cell has also been raised (Kalichman et al., 1988). Recent studies in tellurium-induced demyelinating neuropathy indicate that both of these mechanisms are operative in tellurium neuropathy. Autoradiographic studies reveal that the lipid droplets forming in Schwann cells during the first 24 h after tellurium exposure, which is before the onset of myelin breakdown, are a consequence of the tellurium-induced block in cholesterol synthesis. These early lipid droplets represent intracytoplasmic storage of squalene due to tellurium's inhibition of squalene epoxidase, and thus they are derived from a toxicant-induced alteration in the Schwann cell's lipid metabolism (Goodrum et al., 1990). The lipid droplets that form later in Schwann cells after the onset of the tellurium-induced demyelination represent the cytoplasmic storage of lipid from the catabolism of myelin.

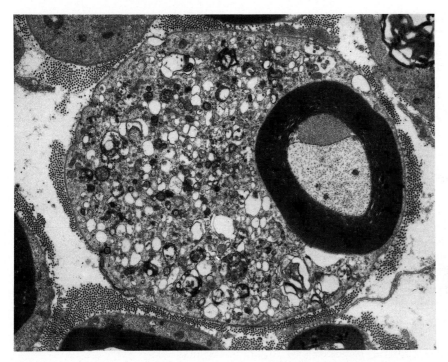

Figure 7 Degeneration of the Schwann cell cytoplasm has been described in several toxicant-induced demyelinating neuropathies. In this fiber from a rat intoxicated with tellurium, the Schwann cell cytoplasm is filled with degenerating organelles. The myelin sheath is intact.

Mushroom-like ("fungiform") excrescences of the Schwann cell cytoplasm (Fig. 6) are another common, nonspecific morphological alteration found in a variety of toxicant-induced demyelinating neuropathies (Lampert and Garrett, 1971; Coria et al., 1986; Bouldin et al., 1989; Griffin et al., 1990; Forcier et al., 1991). This alteration in the Schwann cell, which has been described as a "retraction," "capping," "girdling," or "stalk formation" of the Schwann cell cytoplasm, has also been observed in toxicant-induced axonal neuropathies with secondary demyelination and in wallerian-type axonal degeneration (Griffin et al., 1987). The significance of these excrescences is not clear. They are observed in tellurium neuropathy within 24 h of the beginning of intoxication and precede the onset of demyelination (Bouldin et al., 1989), suggesting that they may be an early morphological marker of Schwann cell perturbation.

Proliferation of Schwann Cells

Proliferation of Schwann cells is another early, stereotypic response of peripheral nerve to internodal demyelination. The Schwann cell proliferation in demyelinating neuropathy is similar in magnitude and timing to the Schwann cell proliferation found during wallerian-type axonal degeneration (Hall and Gregson, 1975; Said et al., 1981a; Saida and Saida, 1986). Hall and Gregson (1975) found an increase in Schwann cells at 48–72 hr after the onset of lysolecithin-induced demyelination in the mouse sciatic nerve. Said et al. (1981a) found in tellurium neuropathy in the rat that DNA synthesis in Schwann cells, as evidenced by ^{3}H-thymidine incorporation, began 4 days after starting the tellurium diet (demyelination was present in their model 2 days after starting the diet), reached a maximum at 7 days, and ended before 20 days. Many of these proliferated Schwann cells are superfluous; Said et al. (1981a) estimated that only one of four to six Schwann cells present at day 12 in the demyelinating nerve would be involved in the process of remyelination. In toxicant-induced demyelinating neuropathies characterized by repeated episodes of demyelination and remyelination, these superfluous Schwann cells may form concentric lamallae around the demyelinating/remyelinating axon ("onion-bulb" formation) (Lampert and Schochet, 1968; Powell et al., 1982).

The source of these daughter Schwann cells has been of considerable interest. Two recent studies of demyelination in toxic neuropathy by Griffin and associates (1987, 1990) suggest that the population of Schwann cells associated with unmyelinated fibers may be a major source of Schwann cells for the process of remyelination. Other identified sources of daughter Schwann cells were the newly formed, supernumerary Schwann cells in the endoneurial space and the Schwann cells associated with myelinated fibers. It is noteworthy that the proliferating Schwann cells associated with myelinated fibers usually showed morphological abnormalities of the Schwann cell or myelin sheath, suggesting that these Schwann cells were injured and would probably also undergo demyelination (Griffin et al., 1990). There was no strong evidence from these studies that Schwann cells can divide and continue to support a myelin sheath. Griffin et al. (1990) also found that the area of demyelination in their lysolecithin model was surrounded by a zone of Schwann-cell proliferation, and suggested that this "proliferative surround" was due to a diffusible mitogenic factor, possibly of macrophage origin.

Invasion of the Nerve by Macrophages

Macrophages invade peripheral nerves within 4 days and remain for several weeks after the onset of toxicant-induced demyelination (Gelman et al., 1987, 1991). A similar influx and persistence of macrophages in nerves is also found after wallerian-type axonal degeneration (Gibson, 1979). Gelman et al. (1991) found in their model of tellurium neuropathy, in which the demyelination is essentially limited to the first week after onset of tellurium exposure, that the peak density of macrophages in sciatic nerve occurs between days 4 and 10; the density of macrophages decreases toward control values thereafter. In contrast, they found in inorganic-lead neuropathy, in which demyelination continues to occur over the course of the intoxication, that the density of macrophages is related to the severity of the demyelination (Gelman et al., 1991). Most of these macrophages come from the blood (Beuche and Friede, 1986), although a small number appear to be derived from an indigenous population of endoneurial macrophages that are analogous to the microglia of the central nervous system (CNS) (Goodrum and Novicki, 1988). These macrophages are involved in the phagocytosis and catabolism of degenerating myelin (Fig. 8). There has been considerable controversy about the relative role played by the Schwann cell and the macrophage in the catabolism of degenerating myelin during neuropathy. Recent studies by Beuche and Friede (1984) and Crang and Blakemore (1986) suggest that it is invading macrophages rather than resident Schwann cells that are primarily responsible for the myelin degradation that occurs in nerves undergoing wallerian-type axonal degeneration. Interestingly, these studies also found that Schwann cells do not proliferate during Wallerian degeneration if macrophages are not present. Furthermore, as discussed below ("Role of Lipoproteins in Degeneration and Regeneration"), the role of invading macrophages in myelin metabolism appears to be considerably greater than simply functioning as phagocytes for the clearing of myelin debris after demyelination or wallerian-type axonal

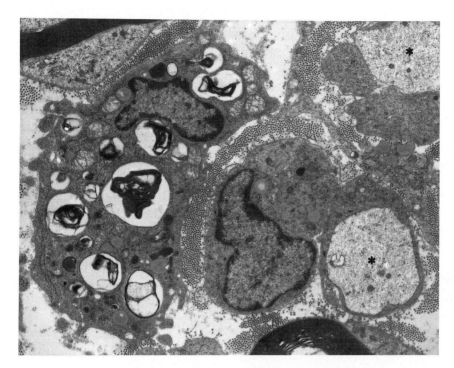

Figure 8 Infiltration of nerve by hematogenously derived macrophages occurs early in the course of demyelinating neuropathy. In this section of sciatic nerve from a rat with tellurium neuropathy, a crescent-shaped macrophage is adjacent to two demyelinated axons (asterisk). The phagocytic macrophage contains multiple clear vacuoles filled with myelin debris.

degeneration. It has also been speculated that macrophages release factors that contribute to the increased permeability of the blood-nerve barrier (BNB) found in most neuropathies (Olsson, 1984; Latker et al., 1991).

Remyelination

Before discussing the process of remyelination that occurs in toxicant-induced demyelinating neuropathy, it may be helpful to recall that the term "demyelination" refers to the loss of myelin from an intact axon and that the term "remyelination" refers to the myelination of an axon that was previously demyelinated. Demylination and remyelination are thus distinguished from the myelin degeneration that occurs following axonal degeneration and the myelin regeneration (with formation of new internodes) that occurs following axonal regeneration. In the remyelination that follows demyelination, the intact, demyelinated axons are surrounded by proliferating (daughter) Schwann cells and then myelinated by these cells. In the myelin regeneration that follows wallerian-type axonal degeneration and regeneration, the regenerating axons of the proximal nerve stump grow into the distal stump, establish contact with the proliferated Schwann cells in the denervated Schwann cell columns (bands of Büngner) of the distal nerve stump, and are then myelinated by these cells.

Remyelination of peripheral axons quickly follows demyelination in most toxicant-induced demyelinating neuropathies. This is in contrast to the CNS, where there is little remyelination of demyelinated central axons. Exceptions to this quick response of remyelination appear limited to those toxicant-induced demyelinating neuropathies in which proliferation of Schwann cells is inhibited (Hall and Gregson, 1975; England et al., 1988). The rapidity of the remyelinating process is illustrated by our model of tellurium neuropathy, in which demyelinated axons are present within 3 days of starting the intoxication and remyelinating axons are present by electron microscopy within 7 days. The remyelinating axons are characterized initially by a myelin sheath that is inappropriately thin for the diameter of the underlying axon (Fig. 9). Over a period of a few weeks, the new myelin sheaths quickly thicken so that it becomes difficult to distinguish remyelinated axons from unaffected myelinated axons in the nerve (Harry et al., 1989).

A characteristic feature of remyelinated internodes, regardless of the cause of the demyelination, is a short internodal length. These short internodal lengths permit easy recognition of remyelinated fibers in teased-fiber preparations (Fig. 2D). Jacobs and Cavanagh (1969) have evaluated quantitatively the internodal lengths of remyelinating internodes after diphtheria toxin–induced demyelination and of new internodes on myelinated fibers regenerating after nerve crush. In the rat, they found that the

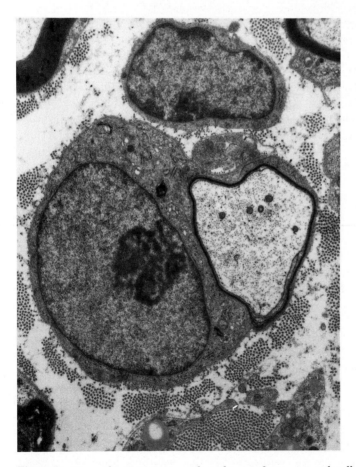

Figure 9   Remyelinating axons, such as this one from a rat with tellurium neuropathy, can be found quickly after the onset of the demyelinating process. Note the thinness of the myelin sheath compared with the diameter of the underlying axon. The Schwann cell has been sectioned at the level of its nucleus.

remyelinating internodes averaged 300 μm in internodal length, whereas internodal lengths are normally directly proportional to the diameter of the axon and vary between 300 and 1000 μm. The lengths of the new internodes on the regenerating axons after nerve crush were similar to the internodal lengths of the remyelinating internodes. This "unit length" of the remyelinating internodes and of the new internodes on the regenerating fibers was independent of the diameter of the remyelinating or regenerating axons. Unit-length remyelinating internodes are not found in all species, however. In the chicken, Jacobs and Cavanagh (1969) found that the internodal length of remyelinating internodes in diphtheritic neuropathy and of new internodes on regenerating axons is directly associated with axonal diameter.

Alterations of the Blood-Nerve Barrier in Demyelinating Neuropathy

Breakdown of the BNB has been documented in both axonal and demyelinating neuropathies (Olsson, 1984). In models of wallerian-type axonal degeneration in the rat, endoneurial fluid pressure is significantly increased by 90 min after nerve crush (Powell et al., 1979), and endoneurial edema is present by 24 h after nerve transection (Pettersson and Tengvar, 1986). Barrier breakdown may also occur early in the course of demyelinating neuropathy. In tellurium-induced demyelinating neuropathy, BNB breakdown is present within 24 h of beginning the tellurium exposure (Bouldin et al., 1989). Not all intoxications associated with demyelinating neuropathy have such a rapid onset of BNB breakdown after commencing the intoxication. Breakdown of the BNB is not present in inorganic-lead neuropathy in the rat until after several weeks of exposure (Myers et al., 1980; Poduslo et al., 1982).

The BNB may remain abnormally permeable or be restored over the course of a neuropathy (Bouldin et al., 1991). In tellurium neuropathy, where onset of demyelination is primarily restricted to the first week and remyelination is well under way by the second week, restoration of the BNB occurs between 3 and 14 weeks after onset of intoxication (Bouldin et al., 1991).

Selective Vulnerability in Demyelinating Neuropathy

"Selective vulnerability" refers to the phenomenon in which specific populations of cells show increased vulnerability to a disease process (Meyer, 1958). This selective targeting of specific cell populations is illustrated in the CNS by a variety of neurotoxic agents that with relative selectivity destroy only neurons or glia. This selective targeting is even more dramatically illustrated by neurotoxicants that with relative selectivity destroy only certain populations of neurons. Although myelinating Schwann cells may appear to be a rather homogeneous population of cells when compared with the diversity found among different populations of neurons, there is now considerable evidence that the phenomenon of selective vulnerability occurs in some toxicant-induced demyelinating neuropathies.

Several studies indicate that the size of the internode may determine in part its vulnerability to toxicant-induced demyelination. In tellurium neuropathy, the vulnerability of myelinating Schwann cells to demyelinate is directly related to the internodal length of the Schwann cell. Schwann cells with internodal lengths below 500 μm infrequently show demyelination, while those fibers with internodal lengths above 800 μm usually show one or more demyelinated internodes (Bouldin et al., 1988). Increased vulnerability of the longer internodes has also been found in AETT neuropathy (Spencer et al., 1979). That Schwann cells with longer internodes are more likely to demyelinate after exposure to certain toxicants may be related to the fact that these cells are maintaining larger volumes of myelin than Schwann cells with shorter internodes (Smith et al., 1982; Bouldin et al., 1988). This greater vulnerability of the longest, largest internodes in several toxicant-induced demyelinating neuropathies appears analogous to the greater vulnerability of the longest, largest axons in many toxicant-induced axonal neuropathies.

Not all toxicant-induced demyelinating neuropathies show a greater vulnerability of the longer internodes. The relationship is reversed in diphtheritic neuropathy in the chicken, in which the small-diameter myelinated fibers (which have proportionally shorter internodes) are the first to show demyelination (Cavanagh and Jacobs, 1964).

Given that different peripheral nerves vary in their proportions of fibers with long and short internodes, this differential vulnerability of longer and shorter internodes may explain why certain neuropathies appear to selectively involve some peripheral nerves more than others (Friede, 1983; Bouldin et al., 1985 and 1988). Such is the case in tellurium neuropathy in the rat, where the frequency of demyelination is greater in the sciatic nerve, a mixed motor and sensory nerve, than in the sural nerve, a sensory nerve (Bouldin et al., 1988). Analysis of teased fibers from the sciatic and sural nerves of rats reveals that this preferential involvement of the sciatic nerve is explained by its greater proportion of fibers with longer internodes (Bouldin et al., 1988). The frequency of demyelination is also greater in the sciatic nerve than in the sural nerve in inorganic-lead neuropathy in the rat (Bouldin et al., 1985). Presumably, this greater vulnerability of the sciatic nerve in lead neuropathy is also due to the increased vulnerability of longer internodes to lead-induced demyelination.

A curious and unexplained observation in demyelinating neuropathies is that along an individual fiber showing segmental demyelination, it is usual to find that not all internodes on the fiber have been affected. Dyck et al. (1977) found that the involvement of internodes along a fiber was random in inorganic-lead neuropathy, and they concluded that this random involvement argues against the demyelination's being secondary to underlying axonal abnormalities. No explanation has been put forward to explain why some Schwann cells are affected and others are not on the same fiber, even though all internodes along the fiber have comparable internodal lengths.

While the distal axon shows increased vulnerability to degeneration in many toxicant-induced axonal neuropathies ("distal axonopathies"), no proximodistal gradient of demyelination has been found in lead-induced demyelinating neuropathy (Ohnishi et al., 1977; Bouldin et al., 1985). A proximodistal gradient of demyelination has been found, however, in toxic neuropathies in which the demyelination is secondary to underlying axonal abnormalities (Shimono et al., 1978; Griffin and Price, 1981). The intramyelinic edema found in hexachlorophene neuropathy and triethyltin neuropathy also shows a proximodistal gradient of severity (Graham et al., 1976; Towfighi, 1980).

Vulnerability of the PNS to toxicant-induced demyelination may also be associated with age. Weanling rats between 15 and 25 days of age are very vulnerable to tellurium-induced demyelination, yet adult rats show only little demyelination, even after long-term exposure to tellurium (Lampert et al., 1970; Lampert and Garrett, 1971; Said and Duckett, 1981). Diphtheria toxin and 6-aminonicotinamide are other Schwann cell toxicants with which the age of the animal influences the expression of the nerve injury (Thomas, 1980).

BIOCHEMISTRY OF DEMYELINATING NEUROPATHY

Evolution of the Biochemical Changes

To put the biochemical events of demyelinating neuropathy in perspective, this section begins with a description of the major biochemical changes in peripheral nerves during wallerian-type axonal degeneration and the subsequent myelination of regenerating axons. By comparing the limited data on toxicant-induced demyelinating neuropathies with the data on wallerian degeneration we will see that, although the biochemical events of demyelination/remyelination and myelin degeneration/regeneration are likely to be the same regardless of etiology, study of neurotoxicant-induced neuropathies can provide insights into basic neurobiological questions. Schematic flow charts of the major morphological and biochemical changes occurring during wallerian-type axonal degeneration and tellurium-induced demyelination are presented in Figs. 10 and 11.

Biochemical Changes Following Wallerian-Type Axonal Degeneration

Schwann cells associated with myelinated axons respond extremely rapidly to axonal injury. Within hours of nerve crush or transection, total lipid synthesis within the nerve is reduced by 50%, with synthesis preferentially decreased in myelin-enriched lipids such as

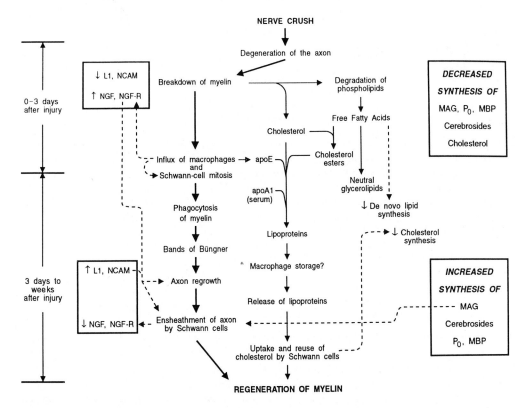

Figure 10   Flow chart of some of the major morphological and biochemical events occurring during wallerian-type axonal degeneration following nerve crush. The temporal sequence of the major morphological events is indicated by thick arrows, the metabolic pathways of myelin lipid metabolism are indicated by medium arrows, and known and presumed "trophic" influences are indicated by dashed arrows. The time scale on the left is provided to indicate the time frame within which the described events are initiated. Changes in expression of myelin-specific components are designated in the right-hand boxes, and changes in expression of growth factors and cell adhesion molecules are indicated in the left-hand boxes. MAG = myelin associated glycoprotein; MBP = myelin basic protein; NCAM = neural cell adhesion molecule; NGF = nerve growth factor; NGF-R = NGF receptor.

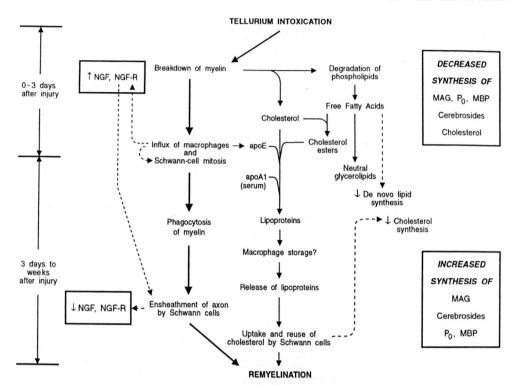

Figure 11   Flow chart of some of the major morphological and biochemical events occurring during the demyelinating neuropathy caused by tellurium intoxication. The temporal sequence of the major morphological events is indicated by thick arrows, the metabolic pathways of myelin lipid metabolism are indicated by medium arrows, and known and presumed "trophic" influences are indicated by dashed arrows. The time scale on the left is provided to indicate the time frame within which the described events are initiated. Changes in expression of myelin-specific components are designated in the right-hand boxes, and changes in expression of growth factors and cell adhesion molecules are indicated in the left-hand boxes. MAG = myelin-associated glycoprotein; MBP = myelin basic protein; NGF = nerve growth factor; NGF-R = NGF receptor.

cerebrosides and cholesterol (Rawlins and Smith, 1971; Yao and Cannon, 1983, White et al., 1989; Goodrum, 1990). By 3 days after injury, synthesis of cholesterol and cerebroside is near zero. Cholesterol synthesis is rapidly down-regulated at the key regulatory step, 3-hydroxy-3-methylglutaryl-coenzyme A (HMG-CoA) reductase (Goodrum, 1990). Enzyme activities associated with the synthesis of other myelin lipids are also down-regulated rapidly (e.g., Constantino-Ceccarini and Poduslo, 1989). While the synthesis of most lipids decreases, the synthesis of cholesteryl esters and neutral glycerolipids within the nerve increases 1–3 days following injury (Yao and Cannon, 1983; White et al., 1989; Goodrum, 1990). The increased synthesis of glycerolipids represents the removal of potentially toxic fatty acids produced from the degradation of phospholipids (Fig. 10). Cholesteryl esters are also formed from these fatty acids by esterification of preexisting cholesterol.

Synthesis of myelin proteins is also rapidly down-regulated following nerve crush or transection. Steady-state levels of mRNA for the myelin proteins P_0, myelin basic protein (MBP), and myelin-associated glycoprotein (MAG) appear to be decreased to 10–40% of control levels by 1 day after injury and to be near zero by 4 days (Gupta et al., 1988; Trapp et al., 1988; Tacke and Martini, 1990). These parallel changes in the synthesis of myelin lipids and myelin proteins suggest that the Schwann cell's program of myelin production is coordinately down-regulated.

The steady-state mRNA levels of a variety of proteins not associated with meylin synthesis also change very rapidly following injury. For example, message levels for the cell adhesion molecules L1 and neural cell adhesion molecule (NCAM), which are thought to be involved in the interaction between Schwann cell and axon, decrease by 50% within 2 days, while the expression of nerve growth factor (NGF) and NGF receptor, which are also thought to be involved in Schwann cell–axonal interactions, increase dramatically within the first 3 days following injury (Heumann et al., 1987; Tacke and Martini, 1990).

These data demonstrate that myelinating Schwann cells respond very rapidly to wallerian-type axonal degeneration by halting synthesis of myelin and other proteins of the differentiated phenotype and by up-regulating the expression of proteins of the precursor Schwann cell phenotype (see Jessen and Mirsky, 1991). These changes occur within the first 48 hr following onset of wallerian-type axonal degeneration, a time when blood-derived macrophages have yet to infiltrate the degenerating nerve and little structural breakdown of myelin has occurred. Infiltration of nerve by macrophages occurs by 3 days following injury and is coincident with the peak proliferation of Schwann cells.

The first detectable loss of myelin proteins from nerves undergoing nerve crush–induced wallerian-type axonal degeneration is around 4 days after injury, but significant losses of myelin proteins and lipids are not evident until a week after injury (Johnson et al., 1949; Manell, 1952; Wood and Dawson, 1974; McDermott and Wisniewski, 1977). By 2–3 weeks after injury there is little myelin-specific protein or lipid remaining in the injured nerve. Cholesterol is the exception. The total (free plus esterified) cholesterol content of the nerve changes little if at all following injury (Johnson et al., 1949; Manell, 1952; Wood and Dawson, 1974; Belin and Smith, 1976; Yao et al., 1980). Cholesterol cannot be metabolized by mammalian cells, and it has been presumed that phagocytic macrophages eventually carry away the unmetabolized myelin debris. However, Rawlins et al. (1970, 1972) have reported that previously labeled myelin cholesterol could be found in newly synthesized myelin following a nerve crush and subsequent axonal regeneration, suggesting that at least some degenerating myelin cholesterol could be retained and reutilized during the myelination of regenerating axons. The postulated mechanism for such reutilization is discussed below ("Role of Lipoproteins in Degeneration and Regeneration").

Most of the biochemical events associated with axonal regeneration and myelin regeneration in peripheral nerves comprise the reversal of the events described above. By 2–4 weeks after crush injury the levels of mRNA for myelin proteins have returned to or exceeded control levels, and lipid synthesis has recovered (Rawlins and Smith, 1971; Yao and Cannon, 1983; LeBlanc et al., 1987; Gupta et al., 1988; Trapp et al., 1988; White et al., 1989; Goodrum, 1990; Tacke and Martini, 1990). The expression of L1 and NCAM rebounds to a level several times higher than control, and that of NGF and its receptor falls to control levels. One of the most striking biochemical events during the period of myelin regeneration is that cholesterol synthesis remains at extremely low levels despite the rapid synthesis of new myelin (Goodrum, 1990). While the other metabolic changes described above have all returned to control values by 6 weeks after injury, cholesterol synthesis is only 50% of that in control nerve and does not reach control levels until 15 weeks after injury. This observation is consistent with the hypothesis that cholesterol from degenerated myelin is reutilized by Schwann cells to make new myelin (see below, "Role of Lipoproteins in Degeneration and Regeneration").

Biochemical Events During Toxicant-Induced Demyelination

The only toxicant-induced demyelinating neuropathy that has been studied biochemically in any detail is tellurium neuropathy. Therefore, this section details the biochemical events of tellurium-induced demyelinating neuropathy. (For additional information on the biochemistry of other toxicant-induced myelinopathies, including those of the CNS, see Chapter 21.)

Within 1 day of initiating exposure of weanling rats to 1% tellurium in the diet, total lipid synthesis in the sciatic nerve is decreased 15–30%; at 5 days, the peak of the demyelinating phase of the neuropathy, lipid synthesis is decreased 50–80% (Bouldin et al., 1989, Harry et al., 1989, personal observations). As in wallerian degeneration, this decrease in lipid synthesis in tellurium neuropathy is preferentially localized to the myelin-enriched lipids. Synthesis rates for nonspecific lipids such as phosphatidylcholine remain unchanged. Cholesteryl esters appear within 3 days of the start of dosing. In contrast to the large changes in general lipid synthesis, which approximate those found in wallerian degeneration, the levels of synthesis of the cholesteryl esters are only about 30% of the levels found in wallerian degeneration.

Cholesterol synthesis is inhibited rapidly and drastically following tellurium exposure. Synthesis is depressed by over 80% within hours of initiating exposure and is decreased to nearly zero by 3–5 days (Wagner-Recio et al., 1991). This block in cholesterol synthesis is due to two separate events. First, tellurium specifically blocks cholesterol synthesis at the squalene epoxidase step (Harry et al., 1989; Wagner-Recio et al., 1991). The initial effect of this metabolic block is the accumulation of the intermediary metabolite squalene and the concomitant decrease in the production of cholesterol. This enzymatic block and resultant accumulation of squalene is not limited to peripheral nerves, but occurs in all tissues. The second event, which may be specific to nerves, is that cholesterol synthesis is rapidly down-regulated at the level of HMG-CoA reductase, so that by 5 days activity of this enzyme is at very low levels (Toews et al., 1991a). As in wallerian degeneration, cholesterol synthesis remains at low levels during the remyelination phase of tellurium neuropathy, while the synthesis of other lipids rapidly returns to normal.

Along with the decreases in synthesis rate for myelin lipids following exposure to tellurium, there is a dramatic drop in the production of myelin proteins. The steady-state levels of mRNA for P_0, MBP, and MAG in sciatic nerve decrease after 1 day of dosing and are reduced to 20–50% of control levels by 5 days of dosing, a time course similar to that following a nerve crush (Toews et al., 1990, 1991b). The large decreases in P_0 mRNA expression have been shown by in situ hybridization studies to take place not only in demyelinating Schwann cells but also in Schwann cells that do not demyelinate (Toews et al., 1992; personal observations). This observation supports the hypothesis that myelin synthesis is a coordinately regulated process. That is, the decreased synthesis of cholesterol that occurs in all Schwann cells leads to a coordinate decrease in the synthesis of myelin proteins in all Schwann cells.

Changes in expression of other proteins in tellurium neuropathy are also similar to those found following a nerve crush. For example, NGF receptor mRNA is rapidly up-regulated in tellurium neuropathy (Toews et al., 1991b). Expression of the NGF receptor appears to peak during the period of initial remyelination and to be restricted to Schwann cells associated with demyelinated internodes (Fan and Gelman, 1992; Toews et al., 1992).

Several conclusions can be drawn from these studies of tellurium-induced demyelinating neuropathy. Many of the biochemical events taking place during toxicant-induced demyelination appear to be the same as those occurring during myelin degeneration secondary to axonal degeneration and may represent nonspecific reactive responses of the Schwann cell. This overall similarity in biochemical changes in Schwann cells following nerve crush or tellurium intoxication also indicates that physical loss of axonal contact is not necessary to initiate these events. Furthermore, it appears from the magnitude of the biochemical changes in tellurium neuropathy that Schwann cells can severely down-regulate their myelin synthesis for more than a week without demyelinating. Thus, most of the metabolic changes measured in the studies reported above could not be used to establish unequivocally the presence of demyelination. The best biochemical indicator of demyelination within a nerve may be the formation of cholesteryl esters.

Role of Lipoproteins in Degeneration and Regeneration

As discussed above, cholesterol from degenerating myelin appears to be retained within the nerve, and at least some part seems to be reutilized for new myelin synthesis. Although this observation was first made in 1970, it was generally ignored until 1986, when a protein whose synthesis is greatly increased in degenerating nerve was identified as apolipoprotein E (apoE) (Ignatius et al., 1986, Snipes et al., 1986). Apolipoprotein E, as a component of serum lipoproteins, plays a key role in "reverse cholesterol transport," i.e., the transport of cholesterol from extrahepatic tissues to the liver (see Weisgraber, 1986). In analogy to this function, it was hypothesized that during nerve degeneration endoneurial apoE served to salvage myelin cholesterol in the form of lipoprotein particles and to supply this lipoprotein-bound cholesterol to the Schwann cell during myelination of regenerated axons (see Mahley, 1988). Macrophages within the degenerating nerve are the source of endoneurial apoE (Boyles et al., 1989; Goodrum and Novicki, 1988) and may serve as a temporary storage depot for the salvaged cholesterol.

    If such a lipoprotein-mediated salvage and reutilization process occurs in nerves, then one would predict 1.) that following a nerve crush degenerating myelin cholesterol would become associated with apoE-containing lipoproteins, 2.) that Schwann cells would express the low-density lipoprotein (LDL) receptor necessary for uptake of such lipoproteins, and 3.) that as a result of such lipoprotein uptake, de novo synthesis of cholesterol in Schwann cells would be down-regulated at the HMG-CoA reductase step during regeneration. Evidence in support of each of these predictions has been reported (Boyles et al., 1989; Goodrum, 1990, 1991).

    Evidence is now accumulating that this same process of myelin cholesterol salvage and reutilization occurs in toxicant-induced demyelinating neuropathies. Gelman et al. (1987, 1991) documented the endoneurial synthesis and secretion of apoE in the demyelinating neuropathies caused by lead or tellurium. Furthermore, as stated earlier, cholesterol synthesis in the tellurium neuropathy is down-regulated during the remyelination period.

PATHOGENESIS OF DEMYELINATING NEUROPATHIES

Alterations in the Metabolism of Schwann Cells and Myelin

There are several specialized aspects of the Schwann cell and its metabolism that may make it especially vulnerable to injury by toxicants. First, the Schwann cell supports a peripheral structure, the myelin sheath, that has a membrane surface area many orders of magnitude larger than that of the perikaryon. It is presumed that specialized processes are involved in supporting such a large and distant structure, and that interference with these processes could lead to demyelination. Second, myelin is a highly ordered structure with a specialized protein and lipid composition. Alterations in this specialized composition could lead to instability of the myelin and demyelination. Third, the majority of PNS myelin is rapidly synthesized over a relatively short period during the maturation of the nervous system. Schwann cells are particularly vulnerable to certain toxicants during this time period of rapid myelin synthesis. Fourth, mature myelin is not metabolically inert, as was once thought. The lipids and proteins of myelin do turn over, though not as rapidly as those in the Schwann cell plasma membrane or in membranes of other cells. Furthermore, certain components of PNS myelin, such as the polyphosphoinositides and phosphate groups on P_0, actually turn over very rapidly (e.g., Toews et al., 1987; Day, 1991). Because the Schwann cell must continuously maintain its myelin sheath, perturbations of Schwann cell metabolism may lead to demyelination long after the cell has synthesized the myelin sheath. Fifth, it appears that there are active transport systems in myelin membranes (Lees and Saperstein, 1983; Norton and Cammer, 1984). Alterations in these transport systems within myelin might also lead to intramyelinic edema or myelin degeneration.

Alterations in the Interactions Between Axon and Schwann Cell

There is a large body of literature from both in vivo and in vitro studies indicating that during development of peripheral nerves, as well as during regeneration of nerves, the up-regulation of myelin-specific macromolecules, the formation of myelin, and the down-regulation of macromolecules such as NGF receptor, cell adhesion molecules, and glial fibrillary acidic protein involve membrane-to-membrane interactions between axons and Schwann cells (see Jessen and Mirsky, 1991). The loss of axonal contact following wallerian-type axonal degeneration is also generally assumed to provide the signal for the degeneration of myelin and the associated changes in Schwann cell expression of macromolecules that occur in wallerian degeneration. However, the nature of the signal(s) involved is unknown, and the necessity of axonal contact for maintenance of normal myelin is not absolute (Kidd and Heath, 1991). There are now several neuropathies in which the demyelination is considered a consequence of underlying axonal abnormalities interfering with the normal axon–Schwann cell interaction (Dyck et al., 1984a).

Role of the Blood-Nerve Barrier in Neuropathy

The BNB tightly regulates the extracellular environment of the endoneurial space in peripheral nerves (Rechthand and Rapoport, 1987). This barrier is located at the level of the endoneurial-capillary endothelium and the perineurium. Breakdown of the BNB occurs in many, and perhaps all, neuropathies in which there is axonal degeneration or demyelination (Olsson, 1984). Barrier breakdown has been documented in a variety of morphologic types of toxic neuropathy, including demyelinating neuropathy, neuronopathy, and axonopathy (Olsson, 1984; Bouldin et al., 1989, 1990). Breakdown of the BNB permits passage of osmotically active molecules into the endoneurial space, which in turn leads to an efflux of water from the blood to the endoneurial space and the formation of endoneurial edema (Olsson, 1984; Low, 1984). The mechanism for this increased barrier permeability in neuropathy and the mediators of this increased permeability are not known. It has been speculated that the BNB breakdown may be due to direct injury of the endothelium of the endoneurial capillaries or to release of vasoactive factors from degenerating or regenerating axons, Schwann cells, endoneurial mast cells, or macrophages (Olsson, 1984). At least in wallerian degeneration, the increased barrier permeability is a nonspecific, reactive response of the BNB to nerve-fiber injury rather than a response to direct injury of the capillary endothelium or perineurium (Latker et al., 1991).

Because breakdown of the BNB occurs in most neuropathies (Olsson, 1984, 1990; Low, 1984), it has long been suspected of playing a role in the pathogenesis of nerve fiber injury (Jacobs, 1980; Olsson, 1984; Low, 1984). Evidence of the potential importance of the BNB in the pathogenesis of neuropathy is found in models of diphtheritic neuropathy in which the demyelination is largely limited to dorsal root ganglia—structures without a well-developed BNB (Waksman, 1961). There is now a growing body of evidence supporting the hypothesis that BNB breakdown and its consequence, endoneurial edema, may cause nerve-fiber damage (Mizisin et al., 1990). Endoneurial edema has been associated with increased endoneurial fluid pressure (Low, 1984), decreased nerve blood flow (Myers et al., 1982; Myers and Powell, 1984; McManis et al., 1986), endoneurial hypoxia (Low et al., 1985), demyelination (Powell and Myers, 1983; Myers and Powell, 1984), axonal atrophy (Nukada et al., 1986) and axonal degeneration (Low et al., 1982). However, the precise role of BNB breakdown in the pathogenesis of toxicant-induced neuropathy remains to be determined.

ACKNOWLEDGMENT

The authors' work was supported by NIH grant ES01104.

REFERENCES

Allt G (1972). An ultrastructural analysis of remyelination following segmental demyelination. Acta Neuropathol 22:333–44.

Allt G, Cavanagh JB (1969). Ultrastructural changes in the region of the node of Ranvier in the rat caused by diphtheria toxin. Brain 92:459–68.

Belin J, Smith AD (1976). Wallerian degeneration of rat sciatic nerve. Changes in cholesteryl ester content and fatty acid composition. J Neurochem 27:969–70.

Beuche W, Friede RL (1984). The role of non-resident cells in wallerian degeneration. J Neurocytol 13:767–96.

Beuche W, Friede RL (1986). Myelin phagocytosis in wallerian degeneration of peripheral nerves depends on silica-sensitive, bg/bg-negative and fc-positive monocytes. Brain Res 378:97–106.

Bouldin TW, Earnhardt TS, Goines ND, Goodrum J (1989). Temporal relationship of blood-nerve barrier breakdown to the metabolic and morphologic alterations of tellurium neuropathy. Neurotoxicology 10:79–90.

Bouldin TW, Cavanagh JB (1979). Organophosphorous neuropathy. I. A teased-fiber study of the spatio-temporal spread of axonal degeneration. Am J Pathol 94:241–52.

Bouldin TW, Earnhardt TS, Goines ND (1990). Sequential changes in the permeability of the blood-nerve barrier over the course of ricin neuronopathy in the rat. Neurotoxicology 11:23–34.

Bouldin TW, Earnhardt TS, Goines ND (1991). Restoration of blood-nerve barrier in neuropathy is associated with axonal regeneration and remyelination. J Neuropathol Exp Neurol 50:719–28.

Bouldin TW, Meighan ME, Gaynor JJ, Goines ND, Mushak P, Krigman MR (1985). Differential vulnerability of mixed and cutaneous nerves in lead neuropathy. J Neuropathol Exp Neurol 44:384–96.

Bouldin TW, Samsa G, Earnhardt TS, Krigman MR (1988). Schwann-cell vulnerability to demyelination is associated with internodal length in tellurium neuropathy. J Neuropathol Exp Neurol 47:41–7.

Boyles JK, Zoellner CD, Anderson AJ, Kosik LM, Pitas RE, Weisgraber KH, Hui DY, Mahley RW, Gebicke-Harter PJ, Ignatius MJ, Shooter EM (1989). A role for apolipoprotein E, apolipoprotein A-1, and low density lipoprotein receptors in cholesterol transport during regeneration and remyelination of rat sciatic nerve. J Clin Invest 83:1015–31.

Cavanagh JB, Jacobs JM (1964). Some quantitative aspects of diphtheritic neuropathy. Br J Exp Pathol 45:309–22.

Constantino-Ceccarini E, Poduslo JF (1989). Regulation of UDP-galactose:ceramide galactosyl-transferase and UDP-glucose:ceramide glucosyltransferase after crush and transection nerve injury. J Neurochem 53:205–11.

Coria F, Montón F (1988). Recovery of the early cellular changes induced by lead in rat peripheral nerves after withdrawal of the toxin. J Neuropathol Exp Neurol 47:282–90.

Coria F, Montón F, Silos I, Fernandez R, Lafarga M (1986). Laminated cytoplasmic bodies in Schwann cells and phagocytes: an ultrastructural and cytochemical study in the normal and lead-damaged peripheral nervous system of the rat. J Submicrosc Cytol 18:153–9.

Crang AJ, Blakemore WF (1986). Observations on wallerian degeneration in explant cultures of cat sciatic nerve. J Neurocytol 15:471–82.

Day NS, Berti-Mattera LN, Eichberg J (1991). Muscarinic cholinergic receptor–mediated phospho-inositol metabolism in peripheral nerve. J Neurochem 56:1905–13.

Duckett S, Said G, Streletz LG, White RG, Galle P (1979). Tellurium-induced neuropathy: correlative physiological, morphological and electron microprobe studies. Neuropathol Appl Neurobiol 5:265–78.

Dyck PJ, O'Brien PC, Ohnishi A (1977). Lead neuropathy. 2. Random distribution of segmental demyelination among "old internodes" of myelinated fibers. J Neuropathol Exp Neurol 36:570–5.

Dyck PJ, Nukada H, Lais AC, and Karnes JL (1984a). Permanent axotomy: a model of chronic neuronal degeneration preceded by axonal atrophy, myelin remodeling, and degeneration. In: Dyck PJ, Thomas PK, Lambert, EH, Bunge R, eds. Peripheral neuropathy. 2nd ed. Vol. 1. Philadelphia: W. B. Saunders, 666–90.

Dyck PJ, Thomas PK, Lambert EH, Bunge RP, eds. (1984b). Peripheral neuropathy. 2nd ed. Philadelphia: W. B. Saunders.

England JD, Rhee EK, Said G, Summer AJ (1988). Schwann cell degeneration induced by doxorubicin (Adriamycin). Brain Res 111:901–13.

Fan X, Gelman BB (1992). Schwann cell nerve growth factor receptor expression during initiation of remyelination. J Neurosci Res 31:58–67.

Forcier NJ, Mizisin AP, Rimmer MA, Powell HC (1991). Cellular pathology of the nerve microenvironment in galactose intoxication. J Neuropathol Exp Neurol 50:235–55.

Friede RL (1983). Variance in relative internode length (l/d) in the rat and its presumed significance for the safety factor and neuropathy. J Neurol Sci 60:89–104.

Gelman BB, Goodrum JF, Bouldin TW (1991). Macrophage apolipoprotein synthesis and endoneurial distribution as a response to segmental demyelination. J Neuropathol Exp Neurol 50:383–407.

Gelman BB, Rifai N, Goodrum JF, Bouldin TW, Krigman MR (1987). Apolipoprotein E is released by rat sciatic nerve during segmental demyelination and remyelination. J Neuropathol Exp Neurol 46:644–52.

Gibson JD (1979). The origin of the neural macrophage: a quantitative ultrastructural study of the cell population changes during wallerian degeneration. J Anat 129:1–19.

Gombault A (1880–81). Contribution à l'étude anatomique de la névrite parenchymateuse subaiguë et chronique: névritre segmentaire périaxile. Arch Neurol (Paris) 1:11–38,177–90.

Goodrum JF (1990). Cholesterol synthesis is down-regulated during regeneration of peripheral nerve. J Neurochem 54:1709–15.

Goodrum JF (1991). Cholesterol from degenerating nerve myelin becomes associated with lipo-proteins containing apolipoprotein E. J Neurochem 56:2082–6.

Goodrum JF, Earnhardt TS, Goines ND, Bouldin TW (1990). Lipid droplets in Schwann cells during tellurium neuropathy are derived from newly synthesized lipid. J Neurochem 55:1928–32.

Goodrum JF, Novicki DL (1988). Macrophage-like cells from explant cultures of rat sciatic nerve produce apolipoprotein E. J Neurosci Res 20:457–62.

Graham DI, Gonatas NK (1973). Triethyltin sulfate–induced splitting of peripheral myelin in rats. Lab Invest 29:628–32.

Graham DI, De Jesus PV, Pleasure DE, Gonatas NK (1976). Triethyltin sulfate–induced neuropathy in rats: electrophysiologic morphologic and biochemical studies. Arch Neurol 33:40–8.

Griffin JW (1983). Diseases of the peripheral nervous system. In: Rosenberg RN, ed. Clinical neurosciences. Vol. 1. New York: Churchill Livingstone, 529–568.

Griffin JW, Drucker N, Gold BG, Rosenfield J, Benzaquen M, Charnas LR, Fahnstock KE, Stocks A (1987). Schwann cell proliferation and migration during paranodal demyelination. J Neurosci 7:682–99.

Griffin JW, Stocks EA, Fahnstock K, Van Praagh A, Trapp BD (1990). Schwann cell proliferation following lysolecithin-induced demyelination. J Neurocytol 19:367–84.

Griffin JW, Price DL (1981). Demyelination in experimental β, β′-iminodipropionitrile and hexacarbon neuropathies. Evidence for an axonal influence. Lab Invest 45:130–41.

Gupta SK, Poduslo JF, Mezie C (1988). Temporal changes in P$_0$ and MBP gene expression after crush-injury of the adult peripheral nerve. Mol Brain Res 4:133–41.

Hall SM, Gregson NA (1975). The effects of mitomycin C on the process of remyelination in the mammalian peripheral nervous system. Neuropathol Appl Neurobiol 1:149–70.

Harry GJ, Goodrum JF, Bouldin TW, Wagner-Recio M, Toews AD, Morell P (1989). Tellurium-induced neuropathy: metabolic alternations associated with demyelination and remyelination in rat sciatic nerve. J Neurochem 52:938–45.

Heumann R, Lindholm D, Bandtlow C, Meyer M, Rawdeke MJ, Misko TP, Shooter E, Thoenen H (1987). Differential regulation of mRNA encoding nerve growth factor and its receptor in rat sciatic nerve during development, degeneration and regeneration: role of macrophages. Proc Natl Acad Sci USA 84:8735–9.

Ignatius MJ, Gebicke-Haerter PJ, Skene JH, Schilling JW, Weisgraber KH, Mahley RW, Shooter EM (1986). Expression of apolipoprotein E during degeneration and regeneration. Proc Natl Acad Sci USA 83:1125–9.

Jacobs JM (1967). Experimental diphtheritic neuropathy in the rat. Br J Exp Pathol 48:204–16.

Jacobs JM (1980). Vascular permeability and neural injury. In: Spencer PS, Schaumburg, HH, eds. Experimental and clinical neurotoxicology Baltimore: Williams and Wilkins, 102–17.

Jacobs JM, Cavanagh JB (1969). Species differences in internode formation following two types of peripheral nerve injury. J Anat 105:295–306.

Jessen KR, Mirsky R (1991). Schwann cell precursors and their development. Glia 4:185–94.

Johnson AC, McNabb AR, Rossiter RJ (1949). Chemical studies of peripheral nerve during wallerian degeneration. I. Lipids. Biochem J 45:500–8.

Kalichman MW, Powell HC, Myers RR (1988). Pathology of local anesthetic–induced nerve injury. Acta Neuropathol 75:583–9.

Kidd GJ, Heath JW (1991). Myelin sheath survival following axonal degeneration in doubly myelinated nerve fibers. J Neurosci 11:4003–14.

Lampert PW, Garrett RS (1971). Mechanism of demyelination in tellurium neuropathy. Electron microscopic observations. Lab Invest 25:380–8.

Lampert PW, Schochet SS (1968). Demyelination and remyelination in lead neuropathy: electron microscopic study. J Neuropathol Exp Neurol 27:527–45.

Lampert PW, Garro F, Pentschew A (1970). Tellurium neuropathy. Acta Neuropathol (Berlin) 15:308–17.

Latker CH, Wadhwani KC, Balbo A, Rapoport SI (1991). Blood-nerve barrier in the frog during wallerian degeneration: are axons necessary for maintenance of barrier function? J Comp Neurol 309:650–64.

LeBlanc AC, Poduslo JF, Mezie C (1987). Gene expression in the presence or absence of myelin assembly. Mol Brain Res 2:57–67.

Lees MB, Saperstein VS (1983). Myelin-associated enzymes. In: Lajtha A, ed. Handbook of Neurochemistry. 2nd ed. Vol. 4. New York: Plenum Press, 435–60.

Low PA (1984). Endoneurial fluid pressure and microenvironment of nerve. In: Dyck PJ, Thomas PK, Lambert EH, Bunge R, eds. Peripheral Neuropathy 2nd ed. Vol. 1. Philadelphia: W. B. Saunders, 599–617.

Low PA, Dyck PJ, Schmelzer JD (1982). Chronic elevation of endoneurial pressure is associated with low-grade fiber pathology. Muscle Nerve 5:162–5.

Low PA, Nukada H, Schmelzer JD, Tuck RR, Dyck PJ (1985). Endoneurial oxygen tension and radial topography in nerve edema. Brain Res 341:147–54.

Mahley RW (1988). Apolipoprotein E: cholesterol transport protein with an expanding role in cell biology. Science 240:622–30.

Manell WA (1952). Wallerian degeneration in the rat. A chemical study. Can J Med Sci 30:173–9.

Maxwell IC, Le Quesne PM (1979). Conduction velocity in hexachlorophene neuropathy. Correlation between electrophysiological and histological findings. J Neurol Sci 43:95–110.

McDermott JR, Wisniewski HM (1977). Studies on the myelin protein changes and antigenic properties of rabbit sciatic nerves undergoing Wallerian degeneration. J Neurol Sci 33:81–94.

McManis PG, Low PA, Yao JK (1986). Relationship between nerve blood flow and intercapillary distance in peripheral nerve edema. Am J Physiol 251(Endocrinol Metab 14):E92–7.

Meyer A (1958). Anoxias, intoxications and metabolic disorders. In: Greenfield JG, Meyer A, Norman RM, McMenemey WH, Blackwood W, eds. Neuropathology. London: Edward Arnold, 230–99.

Mizisin AP, Kalichman MW, Myers RR, Powell HC (1990). Role of the blood-nerve barrier in experimental nerve edema. Toxicol Pathol 18:170–85.

Myers RR, Mizisin AP, Powell HC, Lampert PW (1982). Reduced nerve blood flow in hexachlorophene neuropathy. Relationship to elevated endoneurial fluid pressure. J Neuropathol Exp Neurol 41:391–9.

Myers RR, Powell HC (1984). Galactose neuropathy: impact of chronic endoneurial edema on nerve blood flow. Ann Neurol 16:587–94.

Myers RR, Powell HC, Shapiro HM, Costello ML, Lampert PW (1980). Changes in endoneurial fluid pressure, permeability, and peripheral nerve ultrastructure in experimental lead neuropathy. Ann Neurol 8:392–401.

Norton WT, Cammer W (1984). Isolation and characterization of myelin. In: Morell P, ed. Myelin. New York: Plenum Press, 147–80.

Nukada H, Dyck PJ, Low PA, Lais AC, Sparks MF (1986). Axonal caliber and neurofilaments are proportionately decreased in galactose neuropathy. J Neuropathol Exp Neurol 45:140–50.

Ohnishi A, Schilling K, Brimijoin WS, Lambert EH, Fairbanks VF, Dyck PJ (1977). Lead neuropathy. 1. Morphometry, nerve conduction, and choline acetyltransferase transport: new finding of endoneurial edema associated with segmental demyelination. J Neuropathol Exp Neurol 36:499–518.

Olsson Y (1984). Vascular permeability of the peripheral nervous system. In: Dyck PJ, Thomas PK, Lambert EH, Bunge R, eds. Peripheral neuropathy. 2nd ed. Vol. 1. Philadelphia: W. B. Saunders, 579–97.

Olsson Y (1990). Microenvironment of the peripheral nervous system under normal and pathological conditions. Crit Rev Neurobiol 5:265–311.

Pettersson CAV, Tengvar C (1986). Formation of oedema in transected rat sciatic nerve. A microgravimetric study. Acta Neuropathol (Berlin). 70:177–84.

Poduslo JF, Low PA, Windebank AJ, Dyck PJ, Berg CT, Schmelzer JD (1982). Altered blood-nerve barrier in experimental lead neuropathy assessed by changes in endoneurial albumin concentration. J Neurosci 2:1507–14.

Powell HC, Kalichman MW, Garrett RS, Myers RR (1988). Selective vulnerability of unmyelinated fiber Schwann cells in nerves exposed to local anesthetics. Lab Invest 59:271–80.

Powell HC, Myers RR (1983). Schwann cell changes and demyelination in chronic galactose neuropathy. Muscle Nerve 6:218–27.

Powell HC, Myers RR, Costello ML, Lampert PW (1979). Endoneurial fluid pressure in wallerian degeneration. Ann Neurol 5:550–7.

Powell HC, Myers RR, Lampert PW (1982). Changes in Schwann cells and vessels in lead neuropathy. Am J Pathol 109:193–205.

Rawlins FA, Smith ME (1971). Metabolism of sciatic nerve myelin in wallerian degeneration. Neurobiology 1:225–231.

Rawlins FA, Hedley-White ET, Villegas G, Uzman BG (1970). Reutilization of cholesterol-1,2-^{3}H in the regeneration of peripheral nerve. Lab Invest 22:237–40.

Rawlins FA, Villegas G, Hedley-White ET, Uzman BG (1972). Fine structural localization of cholesterol-1,2-^{3}H in degenerating and regenerating mouse sciatic nerve. J Cell Biol 52:615–25.

Rechthand E, Rapoport SI (1987). Regulation of the microenvironment of peripheral nerve: role of the blood-nerve barrier. Prog Neurobiol 28:303–43.

Said G, Duckett S (1981). Tellurium-induced myelinopathy in adult rats. Muscle Nerve 4:319–25.

Said G, Duckett S, Sauron B (1981a). Proliferation of Schwann cells in tellurium-induced demyelination in young rats. Acta Neuropathol 53:173–9.

Said G, Saida K, Saida T, Asbury AK (1981b). Axonal lesions in acute experimental demyelination: a sequential teased nerve fiber study. Neurology 31:413–21.

Saida K, Saida T (1986). Proliferation of Schwann cells in demyelinated rat sciatic nerve. Acta Neuropathol 71:251–8.

Schaumburg HH, Berger AR, Thomas PK (1992). Disorders of peripheral nerves, 2nd ed. Philadelphia: F. A. Davis.

Shimono M, Izumi K, Kuroiwa K (1978). 3,3'-Iminodipropionitrile induced centrifugal segmental demyelination and onion bulb formation. J Neuropathol Exp Neurol 37:375–386.

Smith KJ, Blakemore WF, Murray JA, Patterson RC (1982). Internodal myelin volume and axon surface area. A relationship determining myelin thickness? J Neurol Sci 55:231–46.

Snipes GJ, McGuire CB, Norden JJ, Freeman JA (1986). Nerve injury stimulates the secretion of apolipoprotein E by non-neuronal cells. Proc Natl Acad Sci USA 83:1130–4.

Spencer PS, Schaumburg HH (1980). Classification of neurotoxic disease. In: Spencer PS, Schaumburg HH, eds. Experimental and clinical neurotoxicology. Baltimore: Williams and Wilkins, 92–9.

Spencer PS, Sterman AB, Horoupian D, Bischoff M (1979). Neurotoxic changes in rats exposed to the fragrance compound acetyl ethyl tetramethyl tetralin. Neurotoxicology 1:221–37.

Tacke R, Martini R (1990). Changes in expression of mRNA specific for cell adhesion molecules (L1 and NCAM) in the transected peripheral nerve of the adult rat. Neurosci Lett 120:227–30.

Thomas PK (1980). The peripheral nervous system as a target for toxic substances. In: Spencer PS, Schaumburg HH, eds. Experimental and clinical neurotoxicology. Baltimore: Williams and Wilkins, 35–47.

Toews AD, Goodrum JF, Lee SY, Eckermann C, Morell P (1991a). Tellurium-induced alterations in 3-hydroxy-3-methylglutaryl-coA reductase gene expression and enzyme activity: differential effects in sciatic nerve and liver suggest tissue-specific regulation of cholesterol synthesis. J Neurochem 57:1902–6.

Toews AD, Eckermann CE, Roberson MD, Lee SY, Morell P. (1991b). Primary demyelination induced by exposure to tellurium alters mRNA levels for nerve growth factor receptor, SCIP, 2',3'-cyclic nucleotide 3'-phosphodiesterase, and myelin proteolipid in rat sciatic nerve. Mol Brain Res 11:321–5.

Toews AD, Lee SY, Popko B, Morell P (1990). Tellurium-induced neuropathy: a model for reversible reductions in myelin protein gene expression. J Neurosci Res 26:501–7.

Toews AD, Fischer HR, Goodrum JF, Windes S, Morell P (1987). Metabolism of phosphate and sulfate groups modifying the P$_0$ protein of peripheral nervous system myelin. J Neurochem 48:883–7.

Toews AD, Griffiths IR, Kyriakides E, Goodrum JF, Eckermann CE, Morell P, Thomson CE (1992). Primary demyelination induced by exposure to tellurium alters Schwann-cell gene expression. J Neurosci 12:3676–87.

Towfighi J (1980). Hexachlorophene. In: Spencer PS, Schaumburg HH, eds. Experimental and clinical neurotoxicology. Philadelphia: Williams and Wilkins, 440–55.

Trapp BD, Hauer P, Lemle G (1988). Axonal regulation of myelin protein mRNA levels in actively myelinating Schwann cells. J Neurosci 8:3515–21.

Wagner-Recio M, Toews AD, Morell P (1991). Tellurium blocks cholesterol synthesis by inhibiting squalene metabolism: preferential vulnerability to this metabolic block leads to peripheral nervous system demyelination. J Neurochem 57:1891–1901.

Waksman BH (1961). Experimental study of diphtheritic polyneuritis in the rabbit and guinea pig. III. The blood-nerve barrier in the rabbit. J Neuropathol Exp Neurol 20:35–77.

Weisgraber KH (1986). The role of apoE in cholesterol metabolism. In: Scanu AM, Spector AA, eds. Biochemistry and biology of plasma lipoproteins. New York: Marcel Dekker, 301–30.

White FV, Toews AD, Goodrum JF, Novicki DL, Bouldin TW, Morell P (1989). Lipid metabolism during early stages of Wallerian degeneration in the rat sciatic nerve. J Neurochem 52:1085–92.

Wood JG, Dawson RMC (1974). Lipid and protein changes in sciatic nerve during Wallerian degeneration. J Neurochem 22:631–5.

Yao JK, Cannon KP (1983). [14C]Acetate metabolism in the peripheral nervous system. Biochim Biophys Acta 752:331–8.

Yao JK, Natarajan V, Dyck PJ (1980). The sequential alterations of endoneurial cholesterol and fatty acid in Wallerian degeneration and regeneration. J Neurochem 35:933–40.

9

Schwann Cell–Axon Interactions: Implications for Neurotoxic Mechanisms

Richard M. LoPachin and Ellen J. Lehning
State University of New York at Stony Brook
Stony Brook, New York

INTRODUCTION

Neurotoxicologists traditionally have considered xenobiotic-induced nervous tissue dysfunction a consequence of altered neuron activity. In contrast, glial cell involvement has been regarded as either incidental or reactive. This predisposition is based in part on the historical view of glia as passive support cells that respond appropriately to the needs of the neuron. However, research over the past two decades has revised this subservient perception of glial function. It is now well established that a complex reciprocal relationship exists between glial cells and neurons in the peripheral and central nervous systems, and that this association is vital for development and function of each cell type (Fedoroff and Vernadakis, 1986a,b,c; Vernadakis, 1988; Abbott, 1991). Because of this relationship, perturbation of glial-neuronal interactions has deleterious consequences for both the developing and the mature nervous system (Kimelberg and Norenberg, 1989). It is therefore possible that nerve damage induced by chemicals or neuropathic disease processes involves disruption of glial-neuronal interactions.

The purpose of this chapter is to discuss the Schwann cell–axon relationship and its possible relevance to neurotoxicity. Schwann cells are the major glial component of the peripheral nervous system (PNS) and are remarkable and highly versatile cells. During the early stages of neuroembryogenesis, they establish an intricate relationship with axons. As will be demonstrated, this relationship has extensive reciprocal influences on the form and function of each constituent. The Schwann cell–axon association is vigorously maintained throughout life and has been shown to be vital for continued peripheral nerve function. In developing the concept of the Schwann cell–axon relationship and its importance to neurotoxicity, we will first provide a brief description of general Schwann cell physiology and morphology. Numerous Schwann cell reviews have been published to which the reader is referred for more detailed information (Landon and Hall, 1976;

Berthold, 1978; H..ll, 1978; Gould et al., 1982; Thomas and Ochoa, 1984; Webster and Favilla, 1984). We will then discuss the influence of the Schwann cell–axon partnership on peripheral nerve development, regeneration, and function. On the basis of the aforementioned reciprocity and obvious mutual dependency, we will then consider the Schwann cell–axon relationship as a basic unit of function in the PNS. The multifaceted nature of this intercellular relationship provides numerous potential sites of disruption for neurotoxic chemicals and diseases that have heretofore gone unrecognized or unappreci-ated. Therefore, the final goal of this chapter is to use previously described Schwann cell–axon interactions as a basis for predicting several sites of neurotoxicant action. Where available, relevant examples from the neurotoxicology literature will be presented. It should be noted, however, that a compendium of Schwann cell toxicants will not be provided. The reader is referred to Cammer (1980) and Anthony and Graham (1991) for information about specific Schwann cell toxicants.

PRINCIPLES OF SCHWANN CELL PHYSIOLOGY AND MORPHOLOGY

In the PNS, a single myelinated axon is enclosed by a longitudinal series of Schwann cells. Each Schwann cell of this series surrounds a segment of axon (500–1500 mm in length) in a spiral of plasma membrane. During the development of the Schwann cell–axon association, compaction of the multilayered spiral occurs. The resulting structure is myelin, which exhibits both lipid- and protein-dependent birefringence and has a characteristic x-ray diffraction pattern, biochemical composition, and water content (see below). The length of myelinated axon encompassed by a single Schwann cell is termed the internodal segment (Fig. 1). The length of this segment and the corresponding myelin thickness were thought to be determined by axon caliber, but it now appears that multiple factors including Schwann cell determinants affect these parameters (Griffin et al., 1988). The region

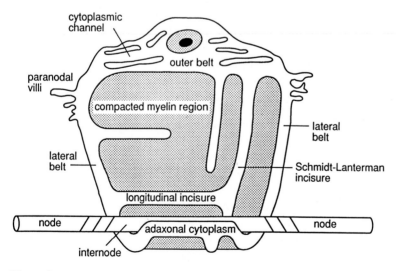

Figure 1   Diagrammatic representation of a Schwann cell and associated axon. The Schwann cell is shown unwrapped to depict the myelin and the various cytoplasmic regions. Schwann cell cytoplasm is present in the perinuclear region, as a belt around the perimeter of the cell and in longitudinal and Schmidt-Lanterman incisures within the compacted myelin.

between two adjacent Schwann cells is termed the node of Ranvier (Fig. 1). The amyelinated nodal area contains kinetically slow K^+ channels and a high concentration of Na^+ channels. In contrast, the internodal region expresses both fast and slow K^+ channels (Waxman and Ritchie, 1985; Black et al., 1990). It is the high-resistance, low-capacitance nature of myelin in conjunction with the localized concentration of nodal Na^+ channels that promotes impulse propagation in a rapid saltatory fashion (i.e., jumping from one non-myelinated nodal region to the next). As will be discussed, Schwann cells appear to play a significant role in restricting the nodal distribution of Na^+ channels and regulating channel turnover.

The unrolled myelinating Schwann cell can best be described as a flattened, trapezoid-shaped cell (Fig. 1). The Schwann cell nucleus contains clumped peripheral chromatin and is elongated in shape. The paranuclear cytoplasm contains the usual profusion of organelles (e.g., rough endoplasmic reticulum, mitochondria, Golgi membranes) and also contains two unique inclusion bodies: Reich granules and Elzholz bodies. In the unrolled state (Fig. 1), the innermost portion of the Schwann cell, which is in direct contact with the axon, is termed the adaxonal cytoplasmic margin; the outer margin surrounding the external aspects of the myelin sheath is the abaxonal cytoplasm. The margins of the abaxonal region are invaginated and form the paranodal villi. Not only does Schwann cell cytoplasm connect the perinuclear and paranodal regions, but a thin border of cytoplasm also circumscribes and invades the compact myelin. The role of these cytoplasmic invasions or Schmidt-Lanterman incisures is uncertain, although it has been suggested that they permit axonal elongation during stretch (Friede and Samorajski, 1970) or participate in the passage of metabolites along myelin (Krishnam & Singer, 1973).

Compact myelin (Fig. 1) is devoid of cytoplasm, and thus, wrapping of the plasmallema to form myelin results in a unique ultrastructure and x-ray diffraction pattern. When viewed by electron microscopy, myelin appears as a series of alternating dark and less dark lines (protein layers) separated by unstained zones (hydrophobic hydrocarbon chains). The less dark zones represent the intraperiod line, which is formed by the abutment of the outer faces of Schwann cell membranes. The dark or major period line results from fusion of the proteinaceous inner faces of the Schwann cell membranes (see Morell et al., 1989). The biochemical composition of myelin is well documented (see Morell et al., 1989) and is characterized by a high lipid-to-protein ratio. The high lipid content excludes water and water-soluble constituents such as Na^+ and K^+. This is evidenced by the relatively low content of these elements and water (33–40%) in rat sciatic nerve myelin as determined by electron probe x-ray microanalysis (LoPachin et al., 1988, 1992b). The high lipid content and low concentrations of diffusible ions contribute to the insulating role of myelin.

Unmyelinated fibers in the PNS also form close physical associations with Schwann cells. In contrast to myelinated axons, which form a 1:1 relationship with respective Schwann cells, groups of unmyelinated fibers (5–20/Schwann cell) become enclosed in individual furrows of glial membranes. The Schwann cells form branching and anastomosing cords of cells that provide continuous envelopment along the proximodistal length of the axons. Individual Schwann cells are difficult to differentiate in unmyelinated fibers, since the membranes interdigitate. Whether a Schwann cell myelinates a given axon appears to depend on axon caliber and other appropriate axonal signals (see below).

It should be clear that regardless of phenotype (i.e., myelinating vs. nonmyelinating), Schwann cells encircle nearly all peripheral nerve axons and, therefore, form a physical and, as we will see, a functional unit. All Schwann cell–axon units are enclosed by a sleeve of basal lamina that probably performs several functions: it limits the access of macromolecules to the unit, it provides an adhesive substratum for the unit, and it offers a binding site for trophic factors and signals (Bunge et al., 1986). Furthermore, synthesis of the basal lamina is a necessary step for continued Schwann cell differentiation and myelination (Eldridge et al., 1987, 1989). Axonal signals initiate Schwann cell expression of basal lamina components (e.g., type I, III, IV and V collagens, laminin, entactin, and heparin sulfate proteoglycan) and subsequent assembly (see below). The identity of these signals remains to be determined.

Patch-clamp studies of freshly isolated mammalian Schwann cell membranes have demonstrated the presence of voltage-gated sodium and potassium channels. This is a rather unexpected membrane property, especially since Schwann cells are nonexcitable and the channel types found were kinetically similar to those of axons. Specifically, only one type of sodium channel is present, but multiple types of potassium channels have been identified (Jonas et al., 1989; Howe and Ritchie, 1990). Anion channels (e.g., chloride currents) have also been reported for Schwann cell membranes (Howe and Ritchie, 1988; Quasthoff et al., 1992).

A specific ion channel phenotype for nonmyelinating and myelinating Schwann cells has been identified (Chiu, 1987). Nonmyelinating cells express voltage-gated sodium channels and outward rectifying potassium currents only in the cell body region. The low surface density of sodium channels probably accounts for the inability of these Schwann cells to generate action potentials (Chiu, 1987). In contrast, cell bodies of the myelinating phenotype do not normally exhibit ion channel currents. Chiu (1987) has proposed that ion channel expression in the cell body region is down-regulated as a function of differentiation and myelination. Paranodal Schwann cell membranes in adult myelinated peripheral nerves, however, do contain functional voltage-gated potassium channels that are similar to those found in the cell body region of nonmyelinating Schwann cells (Wilson and Chiu, 1990a,b). This resemblance suggests either developmental migration of channels to the paranodal area or differential temporal regulation of cell body channel expression vs. that of the paranode. Sodium channels were not detected in paranodal areas (Wilson and Chiu, 1990a). It is possible that such paranodal channels exist but are physically inaccessible to patch clamp analysis. This would appear to be the case, since antibodies to the α subunit of sodium channels label Schwann cell cytoplasm (Ritchie et al., 1990). Preliminary evidence suggests that unidentified axon signals regulate expression of the ion channel phenotype in myelinating and nonmyelinating Schwann cells (Chiu, 1988; Howe and Ritchie, 1990).

The functional relevance of ion channels in Schwann cell membranes is not understood. One possible role of membrane potassium channels is regulation of cell proliferation and differentiation. Pharmacological blockade of potassium channels (e.g., with 4-aminopyridine[4-AP], tetraethylammonium [TEA]) has been shown to cause dose-dependent inhibition of Schwann cell proliferation following wallerian degeneration in vitro (Chiu and Wilson, 1989). Additional in vitro studies suggest that potassium channels play a role in the early phases of Schwann cell proliferation during PNS development (Konishi, 1989). How changes in mitosis might be brought about by potassium currents is unknown, but the process could involve membrane hyperpolarization that initiates second messenger signals or fast induction of c-*fos* gene expression, both of which had been implicated in altering cell status (Morgan and Curran, 1986; Chiu and Wilson, 1989). As will be discussed later in this chapter, Schwann cell ion channels also appear to participate in regulation of the extracellular ion microenvironment and may represent a localized, transferable source for renewal of axolemmal ion channels.

A major precept of this chapter is that Schwann cells and axons establish a very close reciprocal relationship that has pervasive influence on nervous tissue form and function. The extent of this cell-cell association necessitates a complex communication system to coordinate the multiple levels of interaction. Indeed, Schwann cell membranes exhibit several types of transmitter receptor presumably directed toward receiving extracellular signals. For example, Schwann cells from squid giant nerve fiber express specific receptors for acetylcholine (ACh), octopamine, glutamate, and a number of endogenous peptides (e.g., vasoactive intestinal polypeptide [VIP], substance P) (Villegas et al., 1988). Many of these receptors are linked to classical second messenger systems such as cyclic adenosine monophosphate (cAMP) and inositol phosphate (Evans et al., 1985, 1986; Reale et al., 1986). Studies of Schwann cells in denervated amphibian neuromuscular junctions suggested release of acetylcholine (Dennis and Miledi, 1974). Efflux was induced by electrical stimulation and did not occur via classical release processes (i.e., calcium-dependent quantal release). That the presence of ACh in Schwann cells is the product of a specific synthetic process rather than uptake is indicated by the presence of choline acetyltransferase, the major synthetic enzyme for ACh (Tucek et al., 1978). Release and uptake of γ-aminobutyric acid (GABA) have also been demonstrated in Schwann cells of in vitro dorsal root ganglion preparations (Minchin and Iversen, 1974). Although there is clear evidence for release of neuroactive compounds from Schwann cells and central nervous system (CNS) neurologlia, the mechanism of release (i.e., vesicular, reversal of membrane transport, tension-controlled release) is poorly understood (Martin, 1992).

SCHWANN CELL–AXON INTERACTIONS: INFLUENCE ON PERIPHERAL NERVE DEVELOPMENT AND REGENERATION

Axonal Influence on Schwann Cell Development

Development of Schwann cells is a multistep process that involves the following: proliferation and migration of precursor cells on neurite extensions, cessation of division and association of axons with Schwann cell processes, synthesis of the basal lamina, and final differentiation into a myelinating or nonmyelinating Schwann cell (Landon and Hall, 1976; Webster and Favilla, 1984). The factors that regulate the process of Schwann cell development are not understood completely, but they probably include intrinsic (programmed) as well as extrinsic (environmental) components (Anderson, 1989). It is clear, however, that most stages of Schwann cell development depend, at least in part, on extrinsic influences (e.g., soluble factors, cell-cell contact) provided by axons.

The neural crest is a transient embryonic population of multipotential precursor cells that migrate into the periphery and differentiate into a multitude of cell types including Schwann cells (Le Douarin, 1982; Le Douarin et al., 1991). The mechanisms by which a multipotential neural crest cell becomes progressively restricted to the Schwann cell developmental pathway are not well understood, but it appears that axons play a significant role in the early stages of this process. Smith-Thomas et al. (1990) examined the effect of embryonic retinal axons on rat trunk neural crest cell differentiation in culture. They found that although retinal axons did not affect the number of neural crest cells that expressed the earliest Schwann cell markers (217c and nerve growth factor [NGF] receptor), their presence did increase the number of crest cells that progressed to the next stage of Schwann cell development. Cells that reached this stage, characterized by bipolar morphology and S-100 expression, were close to (e.g., 200 mm) but not necessarily in direct physical contact with an axon. The results suggest that before axon contact, a diffusible axon-derived factor causes Schwann cell precursors to continue along the Schwann cell developmental pathway.

The newly inducted Schwann cells eventually associate with axons. This initiates proliferation and differentiation into myelinating and nonmyelinating forms. The molecular signal or signals responsible for this induction have not been completely identified, although several lines of in vivo and in vitro evidence suggest that these processes are under axonal control (see reviews by Pleasure et al., 1985; Lemke, 1990; Mirsky and Jessen, 1990; Eccleston, 1992). For example, purified Schwann cell cultures divide very slowly when grown in standard serum (10% fetal calf)–containing medium. However, rapid proliferation can be initiated by coculture with peripheral neurons (sensory or sympathetic), where Schwann cells become associated with neurite extensions (Wood and Bunge, 1975). That this induction is specific for axon contact is suggested by a lack of division following exposure of purified Schwann cell cultures to neuron-conditioned medium or when Schwann cells and neurons are cocultured but separated by a permeable membrane (Salzer and Bunge, 1980; Salzer et al., 1980a,b). Studies with cell fractions from in vivo and in vitro neural preparations (e.g., brain, PC12 cell line) suggest that the mitogenic factor is associated with the axolemma and is possibly a positively charged polypeptide bound to a negatively charged axonal heparin sulfate proteoglycan (Salzer et al., 1980b; Sobue and Pleasure, 1985; DeCoster and DeVries, 1989). The proteoglycan composition of this membrane mitogen receptor was identified by studies employing pharmacological blockade of membrane glycoprotein and proteoglycan synthesis. For example, castanospermine, which interferes with asparagine-linked oligosaccharide metabolism in neurons, did not affect Schwann cell proliferation in vitro (Ratner et al., 1986). In contrast, β-D-xylosides, which are antimetabolites that specifically inhibit surface glycosaminoglycan chain extension, block Schwann cell proliferation initiated by coculture with treated neurons (Ratner et al., 1985).

Axonal membrane binding of mitogen probably ensures immobilization and might account for the requirement of Schwann cell–axon contact. The intracellular mechanism by which mitogen binding induces proliferation is not understood. However, a series of in vitro studies by Saunders and DeVries (1988a) suggested that Schwann cell binding of mitogen stimulated an increase in polyphosphoinositide phospholipid metabolism. Additional research indicated that subsequent production of diacylglycerol and activation of protein kinase C stimulated activity of the membrane Na^+/H^+ pump. It was hypothesized that cytoplasmic alkalinization may be important for promoting the protein synthesis and maximal activity of DNA polymerases necessary for cell division (Saunders and DeVries, 1988b; Saunders et al., 1989).

In addition to an axolemma-bound mitogen, Schwann cells also respond to soluble growth factors such as glial growth factor (GGF), platelet-derived growth factor (PDGF), transforming growth factor-β (TGF-β) and fibroblast growth factor (FGF) (Ridley et al., 1989; Davis and Stroobant, 1990; Eccleston et al., 1990). The physiological role of these soluble factors has not been fully elucidated, but it is probable that they contribute to proliferation of Schwann cells during nerve development and regeneration (Baichwal and DeVries, 1989; Ridley et al., 1989; Lemke, 1990; Davis and Stroobant, 1990). It is also not clear whether one or more of these growth factors is involved in Schwann cell stimulation. Moreover, the cellular source of soluble mitogen is unknown. An obvious site of origin is the neuron (Ayer-LeLivre et al., 1988), although some evidence points to the possibility of a modified autocrine mechanism whereby the neuron induces Schwann cell expression of growth factors (see reviews by Lemke, 1990; Mirsky and Jessen, 1990; Eccleston, 1992).

As with axonally initiated proliferation, our understanding of the intracellular mechanism of soluble growth factor–induced Schwann cell mitosis is limited. Several lines of evidence suggest that elevation of cAMP is a component in this process. For example, increasing intracellular cAMP by a variety of factors (e.g., forskolin, cholera toxin) has been shown to stimulate proliferation when Schwann cells are cultured in the presence of serum (Porter et al., 1986; Sobue et al., 1986; Raff et al., 1989). Increased intracellular cAMP has a synergistic effect on Schwann cell mitogenic responses to several growth factors (e.g., GGF, PDGF, TGF-β) and also up-regulates PDGF receptor expression by Schwann cells (Davis and Stroobant, 1990; Weinmaster and Lemke, 1990; Stewart et al., 1991). On the basis of these and other in vitro studies, cAMP appears to mediate Schwann cell differentiation, expression of myelin phenotype, and final maturation of non-myelin-form-ing Schwann cells. Both mitogenesis and effects of cAMP on differentiation are thought to be a specific product of growth factor receptor modulation on Schwann cell membranes, rather than stimulation of an independent intracellular mitogenic pathway. It is evident that Schwann cells respond to both bound and soluble mitogens and that cell division is induced by different signal transduction pathways (i.e., inositol phosphates and cAMP, respectively). However, the level of participation of each during development and regeneration is unknown, as is how the mitogenic processes might interact. Nevertheless, it is clear that Schwann cell proliferation and differentiation are strongly influenced by axonal directives.

The neuron, via axonal influences, also modulates Schwann cell production of basal lamina and myelin. Under direction of associated neurons, Schwann cells secrete several collagens, glycoproteins (e.g., fibronectin, laminin), and proteoglycans (e.g., heparin sulfate proteoglycan) that are major constituents of the basal lamina (see reviews by Bunge et al., 1986; Reichardt and Tomaselli, 1991; Eccleston, 1992). Formation of this extracellular matrix, which completely surrounds the Schwann cell–axon unit, is a necessary, but not an absolute, requirement for both myelin formation and the maturation of unmyelinated fibers (Aguayo et al., 1976a,b; Eldridge et al., 1987, 1989; Brunden et al., 1990). The basal lamina produced by Schwann cells probably serves as an immobilization site for growth factors (Klagsbrun, 1990) and as a substrate for cell-matrix adhesive interactions (see below). It should also be noted that many basal lamina constituents (e.g., fibronectin, laminin) promote division of cultured Schwann cells (Baron-Van Evercooren et al., 1982; McGarvey et al., 1984). Thus, the mature, quiescent Schwann cell is in contact with possibly two mitogenic factors; basal lamina and axon. The mechanism by which Schwann cell division is held in check in the normal mature nerve is unknown but may involve both glial and neuronal release of growth inhibition factors (e.g., gliostatin, glial maturation factor-β) (Lim et al., 1989; Asai et al., 1992; also see review by Eccleston, 1992).

In addition to possible basal lamina influences, axonal input appears necessary for induction of myelination by Schwann cells. This has been demonstrated using the cervical sympathetic trunk (CST), a nerve containing approximately 99% unmyelinated fibers. In studies by Aguayo et al. (1976a,b) and Weinberg and Spencer (1976), CST Schwann cells were shown to be capable of producing myelin when cross-anastomosed with a myelinating peripheral nerve. These results suggest that CST Schwann cells are not intrinsically different from those of myelinating nerves and that the decision to myelinate is primarily axon-based. The molecular identity of the axon stimulus for myelination has not been determined. However, two suggestions are prominent in the literature; axon caliber and the interaction of Schwann cells with specific axolemmal signaling molecules (Friede, 1972; Griffin et al., 1988). The signal to myelinate may (Sobue et al., 1986; Lemke and Chao,

1988) or may not (Mirsky et al., 1990) involve activation of Schwann cell adenylate cyclase. In any case, the axonal signal induces the myelin-forming phenotype, which is characterized by expression of major and minor myelin protein genes such as P_0, myelin basic protein (MBP), myelin-associated glycoprotein (MAG), proteolipid protein (PLP), and P_2 (Table 1) (Trapp et al., 1984; Eccleston et al., 1987; Hahn et al., 1987; Brunden et al., 1990). Nonmyelinating Schwann cells also express a characteristic molecular phenotype that includes expression of the genes for GFAP, nerve growth factor receptor, Ran-2, and the adhesion molecules NCAM (neural cell adhesion molecule) and L1 (Table 1) (Mirsky et al., 1986; Jessen et al., 1990).

   Axons may also govern differentiation of non-myelin-forming Schwann cells. Jessen et al. (1987) used immunohistochemical methods to examine expression of galactocerebroside (GalC), which is a marker for differentiated nonmyelinating Schwann cells, in the cervical sympathetic trunk. Ninety-nine percent of the Schwann cells in this nerve are of the nonmyelinating type. The percentage of GalC-positive Schwann cells declined to basal levels after nerve crush or transection and returned to control values when the nerve regenerated. Since parallel in vitro studies indicated that extracellular matrix components (laminin, collagen) did not affect GalC expression in non-myelin-forming Schwann cells, the results suggest that axonal influences (e.g., soluble factors, cell-cell contact) mediate differentiation of this type of Schwann cell. The nature of this axonal influence and the mechanism by which it might promote differentiation of non-myelin-forming Schwann cells are unknown.

Schwann Cell Influence on Axonal Differentiation

As the previous section indicates, peripheral axons modulate Schwann cell differentiation, proliferation, and myelin formation (see additional references: Wood and Bunge, 1975; Weinberg and Spencer, 1976). In contrast, Schwann cell modulation of nerve cell structural differentiation has been considered to be limited. However, as reviewed below, a growing body of evidence challenges these precepts, and it now appears that the effects of Schwann cells on neuronal characteristics are far more extensive and meaningful than previously expected (Griffin et al., 1988).

   Accumulating evidence suggests that glial cell influences have a significant impact on determining the characteristic morphology of nerve cells and axons. For example, in vitro studies have revealed a remarkable influence of Schwann cells on morphological differenti-

Table 1   Protein Markers of Schwann Cells

Myelin-forming Schwann cells	Non-myelin-forming Schwann cells	Common markers
P_0	NCAM	S100
P_2	GFAP	Vimentin
Myelin basic protein	NGF receptor	Laminin
CNPase	L1	Galactocerebroside
Proteolipid protein	A5E3	Seminolipid
Myelin-associated glycoprotein	Ran-2	04

NCAM = neural cell adhesion molecule; GFAP = GFAP = glial fibrillary acidic proteinNGF = nerve growth factor; CNPase = CNPase = 2':3'-cyclic nucleotide 3'-phosphodiesterase

ation of neurons (Mudge, 1984). Purified cultures of dorsal root ganglion sensory neurons exhibit an immature bipolar morphology. However, when cocultured with Schwann cells, sensory neurons undergo morphological differentiation to the mature pseudo-unipolar phenotype (see also Vernadakis, 1988). Influencing structural phenotype does not appear to be a distinguishing characteristic of Schwann cells, since astrocytes have been shown to modify gross morphological features (e.g., neurite extension, branching, and varicosities) and expression of cytoskeletal components in cocultured mesencephalic neurons (Denis-Donini et al., 1984; Chamack et al., 1987). Provided these in vitro studies of central and peripheral cells systems reflect the in vivo situation, glial cells in general appear to have a significant and reciprocal influence on morphological differentiation of neurons.

Axon caliber is a hallmark morphological feature of nerve cells that has functional implications related to electrophysiological properties, energy metabolism, elemental composition, and water content (see reviews by LoPachin et al., 1991, 1992a). The final diameter attained by an axon at maturity is directly related to cross-sectional neurofilament number. This parameter is controlled by gene expression in the cell body and by subsequent slow axonal transport (Friede and Samorajski, 1970; Lasek et al., 1983). However, it is now clear that adult axon size is determined not only by cell body influences but also by local glial effects as well. The best evidence for the impact of glia on axon morphology is provided by research using the *Trembler* mutant mouse. The *Trembler* mouse expresses a dominant mutation characterized by a dysfunctional axon–Schwann cell relationship. Manifestations of this dysfunctional association are hypomyelination and reduced axon caliber (see Aguayo and Bray, 1984). Aguayo and colleagues (1977) used cross-transplantation of peripheral nerve grafts into mutant and normal mice and found that axon caliber was specifically modulated by local Schwann cell–axonal interaction. This finding is supported by other studies indicating that attainment of mature axon size is dependent on the extent of myelination (Windebank et al., 1985; Parhad et al., 1987; Pannese et al., 1988).

How local glial cell–axon interactions might modify axon caliber is not known, although results from recent studies with the *Trembler* mutant provide some insight. DeWaegh and colleagues have found that the hypomyelination which characterizes mutant mouse peripheral nerve is associated with decreases in both slow axonal transport and phosphorylation of neurofilaments (deWaegh and Brady, 1990, 1991; deWaegh et al., 1992). An increase in neurofilament packing density is also observed that may be directly related to the decrease in phosphorylation (deWaegh et al., 1992). On the basis of their observations the authors suggest the following heuristic model: the process of myelination is associated with a heterophilic Schwann cell–axon adhesion molecule interaction possibly involving MAG and an unknown axonal counterpart. Via respective cytoplasmic domains (see above), binding of the axonal adhesion molecule modulates net activity of an axonal kinase-phosphatase pair so that kinase activity predominates. Elevated kinase activity results in increased phosphorylation of neurofilaments (and probably other substrates), which increases sidearm surface charge and subsequently interneurofilament repulsion. This enlarges neurofilament spatial occupation and thereby axon caliber. In contrast, hypomyelination would be associated with reduced intercellular adhesion molecule binding and a corresponding predominance of phosphatase activity. Increased enzymatic dephosphorylation would result in decreased neurofilament side arm phosphorylation and axonal diameter. Clearly, this fascinating model has potential implications for neurotoxic mechanisms (see below). Moreover, the studies discussed above provide evidence that local glial influences represent a regulatory step in determining axon caliber.

In addition to influencing neuronal morphology and axon diameter, glial contact also appears to affect molecular organization and differentiation of the axon membrane. Several investigators have used freeze-fracture techniques to study the distribution of large intramembranous particles (IMPs) in myelinated central and peripheral nerve axons (see reviews by Rosenbluth, 1989; Waxman, 1989). Large IMPs are presumed to be the structural correlates of voltage-sensitive Na^+ channels (Rosenbluth, 1983). Results show that in premyelinated axolemma, large IMPs loosely cluster at nodal precursor sites. Maturation of nodal regions is characterized by IMP condensation at nodal sites. This region is sharply bracketed by paranodal areas where particles are sparse under terminal loops of myelin but are present in axolemma between loop indentations. In juxtaparanodal internode portions, IMPs are present, but their concentrations decline rapidly as a function of lateral distance from the node. This spatial organization of axolemmal particles is presumed to be a product of glial cell contact and myelination. On the basis of corresponding studies (Joe and Angelides, 1992), it has been proposed that axon myelination maintains regional clustering of Na^+ channels and thereby defines the nodal domain. It should be noted, however, that other research indicates that clustering of voltage-dependent sodium channels at nodes may occur independently of glial cell contact (Ellisman, 1979; LeBeau et al., 1987; England et al., 1990, 1991). It has also been suggested (although recently disputed, see Barres et al., 1990) that astrocytes and Schwann cells actively participate in nodal function by regulating the turnover of ion channels (see review by Waxman and Ritchie, 1985). If nodal IMPs actually represent Na^+ channels, these studies indicate that development of electrogenic mechanisms is not entirely an intrinsic product of the axon but is instead due to complex glial-neuronal interactions that modify axolemmal structure and macromolecular distribution.

In contrast to the supposed unidirectional influence of axons on Schwann cell structure, the research discussed in this section provides evidence that glial cell contact significantly affects the morphological and functional differentiation of nerve cells and axons. This demonstrates that ample reciprocity exists between neurons and glial cells and suggests that corresponding adult morphological and neurophysiological attributes are a product of this cell-cell interaction.

Schwann Cell–Axon Interactions During Regeneration in the Peripheral Nervous System

Although Schwann cells are similar in many respects to their CNS counterparts (astrocytes and oligodendrocytes), they differ markedly in their ability to support axonal regeneration. Previously it was believed that CNS neurons were inherently incapable of regeneration. Over the past decade this notion has been questioned, and it now appears that the CNS neuroglial environment may be the major obstacle to axon sprouting. In fact, evidence suggests that oligodendrocytes produce factors that inhibit neurite outgrowth (see reviews by Bunge and Hopkins, 1990; Fawcett and Keynes, 1990; Schwab, 1990). In contrast, Schwann cells act as a nurturing substrate for regenerating axons by providing stabilization, guidance signals, and trophic factors (see below). This nurturing role is clearly evident when a peripheral nerve is transected or otherwise severely damaged. Both distal axons and myelin break down according to a process known as Wallerian degeneration. The bulky cell detritus is phagocytosed by Schwann cells (oligodendroglia in the CNS) and macrophages (Gray, 1970; Spencer and Thomas, 1974; see review by Cavanagh et al., 1990). Schwann cells in the degenerating nerve reenter the cell cycle and proliferate within the basal lamina. Schwann cell mitosis appears to be stimulated by components of the basal lamina (see above) and a number of other factors involved in axon degeneration, e.g., axonal and myelin debris (Salzer and Bunge, 1980), and factors released by macrophages that have phagocytosed myelin (Baichwal et al., 1988). Dividing Schwann cells form the bands of Büngner through which regenerating axons will grow. The regenerating axons or neurite extensions emanate from proximal nodes of Ranvier and, throughout elongation, are in constant physical contact with both basal lamina and Schwann cell membranes (Haftek and Thomas, 1968). However, research indicates that it is Schwann cells, and not basal lamina or fibroblasts, that are of primary importance to axon regeneration. For example, even though intact basal lamina is present, axons will not regenerate through peripheral nerve grafts in which Schwann cells have been selectively eliminated (Hall, 1986). Axons will regenerate through acellular nerve grafts only if accompanied by Schwann cells that originate in the host proximal stump (Gulati, 1988; Nadim et al., 1990).

Schwann Cell–Axon Contact Is Mediated by Membrane Adhesion Molecules

It is evident from the above discussion that peripheral nerve regeneration depends on physical contact between Schwann cell and axonal growth cone surfaces. As we have also discussed, developmental processes such as myelination and Schwann cell proliferation and differentiation exhibit a similar dependency on glial cell–axon contact. The molecular nature of these cell-cell interactions has not been fully defined, although it appears that such contact is mediated by a number of adhesive or recognition molecules that are expressed by both neurons and glial cells. For example, neurite outgrowth along glial surfaces (i.e., astrocytes, Schwann cells) and the extracellular matrix is characterized by a specific spatiotemporal elaboration of several adhesive molecules including L1, NCAM, N-cadherin, and integrin-class extracellular matrix receptors (Bixby et al., 1988; Martini and Schachner, 1988; Seilheimer and Schachner, 1988; Smith et al., 1990). Intercellular adhesive molecule binding is described as either homophilic (e.g., L1-L1 binding) or heterophilic (e.g., integrin-laminin binding). Regardless of the type of binding, adhesive interactions stabilize cell-cell contact (e.g., NCAM 180) and facilitate neurite motility (e.g., L1) (Table 2) (Pollerberg et al., 1985, 1987; Martini and Schachner, 1988). Moreover, adhesion molecule binding mediates a number of additional processes that are also critical for development and regeneration (Table 2): nerve fiber fasciculation (e.g., fasciclins, cadherins), pathway cues for guidance and target connectivity (e.g., L2/HNK-1 carbohy-

Table 2 Developmental Processes Mediated by Adhesion Molecules

Cell-cell stabilization (NCAM 180)
Neuronal cell body migration (NCAM, astrotactin, L1)
Glial cell proliferation and differentiation (L1)
Myelination (MAG)
Neurite outgrowth (L1, NCAM, N-cadherin, integrin)
Guidance and target connectivity (L2/HNK-1 epitope)
Nerve target adhesion (NCAM)
Topographic demarcation (J1 antiadhesion molecules)
Regulation of ionic milieu (AMOG)
Peripheral nerve regeneration (L1, N-CAM)

NCAM = neural cell adhesion molecule; MAG = myelin-associated glycoprotein;
AMOG = adhesion molecule on glia.

drate epitope), demarcation of topographic boundaries (e.g., J1 antiadhesion molecules), glial differentiation (e.g., L1), regulation of intra- and extracellular ion composition (i.e., adhesion molecule on glia, AMOG) and nerve-target adhesion (e.g., NCAM) (Kruse et al., 1985; Seilheimer et al., 1989; Gloor et al., 1990; Schachner, 1991).

Thus, adhesion molecule interactions promote growth cone motility along Schwann cell surfaces and also provide the neurite with directional cues and other information regarding the extracellular environment (e.g., boundaries). Processing of this information requires signal transduction and intracellular integration. How this occurs is not currently known, although it has been shown that the cytoplasmic domains of certain adhesion molecules (e.g., integrins, NCAM 180, L1) are linked (via spectrin?) to various cytoskeletal elements (e.g., actin bundles) (Chen et al., 1985; Chamak et al., 1987; Hirano et al., 1987; Pollerberg et al., 1987). Specific binding-induced changes in these membrane-cytoskeleton linkage complexes might be responsible for alterations in cytoskeletal components that are the basis of cell-cell stabilization and growth cone extension (Bixby et al., 1988; Chuong, 1990). In addition, in vitro evidence suggests that adhesion molecule binding influences second messenger turnover (i.e., inositol phosphates, Ca^{2+}), which might mediate appropriate and necessary changes in neurite metabolism and membrane ion channel function (Acheson and Thoenen, 1983; Acheson and Rutishauser, 1988; Schuch et al., 1989; Sontheimer et al., 1990).

The Trophic Role of Schwann Cells in Development and Regeneration

Neurite outgrowth during development and regeneration not only is dependent on Schwann cells for stabilization and guidance, but also requires glia-derived neurotrophic support. For example, during peripheral nerve regeneration (e.g., following nerve transection), Schwann cells produce and release NGF and express corresponding low-affinity (type II) plasmalemmal receptors. Released NGF subsequently binds to these type II glial receptors (Heumann et al., 1987a; Taniuchi et al., 1988). Nerve growth factor–responsive sympathetic and sensory fiber growth cones have high-affinity (type I) axolemmal NGF receptors (Taniuchi et al, 1988; Verge et al., 1989), and it is thought that Schwann cell receptors release dimeric NGF to these neurite receptors. In this way, growth cones are guided to their targets via Schwann cell membranes that act as a trophic factor–ladened substratum and chemotactic pathway. In regenerating peripheral nerves, glia-derived trophic factor transiently substitutes for target-derived trophic support. Reestablishment of axonal contact suppresses Schwann cell synthesis of the NGF protein and receptor (Heumann et al., 1987b; Taniuchi et al., 1988). In many respects, these regenerative glial-axonal interactions recapitulate those occurring during development (see Bixby et al., 1988). Johnson and others (see reviews by Johnson et al., 1988; Uzman et al., 1989) have offered the aforementioned scenario as a generic model in which Schwann cells express and bind a variety of neurotrophic factors derived from non-neuronal sources. This includes those factors that participate in the regeneration and development of non-NGF-sensitive fibers (e.g., motor and preganglionic autonomic fibers).

Schwann Cell–Axon Interactions During Peripheral Nerve Development and Regeneration: Conclusions

Schwann cell–axon interactions are important determinants of PNS development and regeneration. Axonal signals stimulate Schwann cell proliferation and eventual differentiation into myelinating and nonmyelinating phenotypes. On the other hand, Schwann cells provide a pathway for stabilization and guidance of nerve cell migration and neurite outgrowth. Schwann cells also offer neurotrophic support and additional haptotactic guidance that ensures proper end-target connection. These functional interactions require physical contact between the glial cells and axons. Such contact is mediated by intercellular binding of different membrane adhesion molecules expressed by each cell type. Homophilic and heterophilic binding events appear to stimulate neurite second messenger systems, with subsequent appropriate intracellular changes in physiological processes and cytoskeletal status.

SCHWANN CELL–AXON INTERACTIONS: INFLUENCE ON PERIPHERAL NERVE FUNCTION

The primary role of nervous tissue is transmission and integration of information. Schwann cells are not excitable and do not appear capable of vesicular neurotransmitter release, and therefore they do not participate directly in information processing. Nevertheless, research has shown that Schwann cell input significantly affects neuronal activity and that this influence is indispensable for proper operation of nervous tissue. In this section, we will discuss several glial-mediated processes that support and preserve nerve cell function; i.e., potassium buffering, intercellular communication, and Schwann cell–axon transfer of macromolecules and substrates. Although some of these functional influences have been better characterized in CNS neuroglia, it is likely that continued research will lead to identification of similar processes in Schwann cells.

Potassium Buffering

Repetitive firing of action potentials results in significant increases in extracellular concentrations of K^+ ($[K^+]_O$). Increased $[K^+]_O$ can cause depolarization blockade of action potentials and interfere with continued neuronal signaling (see reviews by Sykova, 1983; Waltz and Hertz, 1983). Therefore, in order to preserve neuronal activity, a method must exist by which excess $[K^+]_O$ is buffered. Evidence has been provided that this task is mediated by glial cells in both the CNS and the PNS (for reviews see Walz, 1989; Barres et al., 1990; Chiu, 1991). In the PNS, the mechanism by which extracellular K^+ is buffered is different for unmyelinated and myelinated axons. Konishi (1990) has shown that nonmyelinating Schwann cells exhibit dye-coupling that suggests formation of a glial syncytium. Consequently, high $[K^+]_O$ might be handled by a "spatial buffering" mechanism whereby activity-related localized increases in $[K^+]_O$ promote transmembrane K^+ movement into nonmyelinating Schwann cells through ion channels (Chiu, 1991). Intracellularly, entering K^+ would move across gap junctions into lower-K^+ environments of glial cells not exposed to high extracellular ion (Orkand et al., 1966). This proposed mechanism is applicable to nonmyelinating Schwann cells only, since myelinating cells do not exhibit dye-coupling (Konishi, 1990).

The suggested mechanism for clearance of extracellular K^+ in myelinated fibers may involve Schwann cells in paranodal, but not nodal, regions (Chiu, 1991). For example, theoretical calculations of activity-dependent potassium accumulation in nodal regions indicate that rapid ion clearance can be achieved by diffusion alone (Chiu, 1991). Thus, nodes of Ranvier might function normally in the absence of specific buffering mechanisms. Because myelin does not completely isolate the paranode from the node, the paranodal axolemma is believed to contribute to the electrogenesis of action potentials (Chiu and Ritchie, 1980; Mackenzie et al., 1984). On the basis of several lines of evidence it appears that high-frequency impulse activity can result in substantial paranodal K^+ accumulation that cannot be "buffered" by simple diffusion (Chiu, 1991). How such ion buildup might be redistributed is unknown, but it is possible that previously discussed inward rectifying potassium channels on paranodal Schwann cell processes might permit passive glial entry of axonally derived K^+ (Wilson and Chiu, 1990a). Regardless of the buffering mechanism, an important question remains unanswered; how is the acquired K^+ returned to the axon? In lieu of a specific method for reinvesting K^+, axons would rapidly become K^+-deficient, with corresponding functional perturbations.

Potassium buffering is clearly a necessity for proper function of myelinated and nonmyelinated axons. It appears that ion channels on Schwann cell membranes play a significant role in mediating extra-axonal K^+ homeostasis. However, it is important to note that, in contrast to CNS neuroglia (see Walz, 1989; Barres, 1991), changes in intracellular Schwann cell K^+ have not been demonstrated in association with axonal impulse activity. Moreover, both axons and Schwann cells have a number of additional mechanisms (e.g., membrane ion pump, ion exchangers) that could participate in K^+ homeostasis.

Intercellular Transfer of Macromolecules and Substrates

That glial cells might act as an energy source for neurons was proposed over 100 years ago by Golgi (see Kuffler et al., 1984). Neuroglia are well known to be glycogen-rich (Peters et al., 1991), and experimental evidence has been obtained in insects (honeybee) for transfer of glycogen from glia to neuron (Tsacopoulos et al., 1988). Although unequivocal data from vertebrate nervous systems is lacking, it seems possible that metabolic support for increased neuronal activity is derived from breakdown of astrocytic glycogen stores with subsequent intercellular transfer of substrate (Magistretti et al., 1986).

In addition to possible transfer of metabolic substrates, it appears that exchange of macromolecules routinely occurs between axons and Schwann cells (Lasek et al., 1983; Politis and Ingoglia, 1979; Byrne et al., 1988; Buchheit and Tytell, 1992). The functional significance and mechanisms of intercellular exchange are unknown. However, axon–to–Schwann cell transfer of material might alert glia to changes in intra-axonal status and thereby initiate appropriate supportive alterations in glial metabolism or macromolecule synthesis. In addition, metabolic waste products might be transferred to Schwann cells, where they may be handled more readily. Schwann cell–to–axon transfer has been studied extensively in invertebrate systems. Results indicate that transfer of material to the axon is mediated by either microphagocytosis of Schwann cell evaginations or vesicle external-ization and subsequent axon uptake (Buchheit and Tytell, 1992). In any case, a variety of protein and lipid macromolecules appear to be transferred, including constituents of the glial cytoskeleton (e.g., actin) and heat shock proteins (Tytell and Lasek, 1984; Tytell et al., 1986). Glia-to-axon transfer might serve several purposes, such as trophic factor export and rapid, localized replacement of high-turnover axonal constituents, e.g., enzymes, and ion channels; and finally, transferred material might protect the axon during metabolic or neurotoxic stress (Tytell et al., 1986; Grossfeld, 1991; Buchheit and Tytell, 1992). Regarding the last suggestion, local glial contribution of defensive factors represents an efficient and rapid means of responding to acute injury as opposed to relatively slow appearance of these molecules via cell body synthesis and axonal transport. It is important to note that much of the evidence for axon-glia exchange of macromolecules is based on studies using invertebrate or fish species. Thus, the relevance to mammalian systems is, as yet, unclear. In any case, direct or indirect retardation of glial expression of stress proteins or other transferred essential factors might significantly exacerbate the development of neurotoxicity (see below).

Intercellular Communication via Neuroactive Substances

As indicated earlier, Schwann cells exhibit the necessary neurotransmitter synthetic machinery, receptors, and membrane signal transduction mechanisms for sophisticated intercellular communication. Presumably, dialogue between axons and Schwann cells coordinates the intimate functional relationship that exists between these cells. Direct evidence for Schwann cell–axon signaling has been provided by studies using invertebrate nervous systems, e.g., the isolated Schwann cell–giant axon preparations of tropical squid and crayfish (see reviews by Villegas et al., 1988; Evans et al., 1991; Lieberman, 1991; Martin, 1992). Research involving these systems suggests the following communication scenario; high-frequency axonal stimulation promotes nonsynaptic (nonvesicular?) release of glutamate, which acts at quisqualate/kainate (non-NMDA) membrane receptors on surrounding Schwann cells. This receptor activation initiates an intracellular cascade of events culminating in the release of ACh from Schwann cells. Through autoreceptor interaction, ACh stimulates a Schwann cell cholinergic system that produces long-lasting hyperpolarization. The function of this hyperpolarization is unknown, but it is thought to facilitate K^+ regulation in the periaxonal space. It remains to be determined whether this communication scheme is representative of other "cross-talk" mechanisms that regulate functional glial-neuronal interactions. Preliminary indications from vertebrate studies suggest that chemical transmitter–mediated signaling between glial cells and axons is a common phenomenon.

Schwann Cell–Axon Interactions: Conclusions

For over 150 years neurobiologists have wondered about the role(s) of glial cells in nervous tissue physiology. Rudolph Virchow, in the mid-19th century, first used the word "glia" to reflect the perceived function of these cells as a nervous tissue glue or putty (Virchow, 1858). It is evident that the role of Schwann cells in neurophysiology extends well beyond passive structural support and sensitivity to axon commands. In fact, early in development, Schwann cells and axons establish a highly dynamic reciprocal relationship that influences subsequent nervous tissue growth, morphology, behavior and repair (Fig. 2). Considering the interdependence and diversity of influence, it is reasonable to suggest that the Schwann cell–axon association represents the functional unit of peripheral nervous tissue (Arenander and de Vellis, 1983).

SCHWANN CELL–AXON INTERACTIONS: FUTURE CONSIDERATIONS FOR NEUROTOXIC STUDIES

Neurotoxicologists have typically classified acquired and inherited neuropathies along morphological lines (see for example Spencer and Schaumburg, 1980). For example, tellurium and hexachlorophene have been classified as primary myelinotoxicants, whereas acrylamide and *n*-hexane have been considered to be axonopathic chemicals. The selective occurrence of structural changes in one cell compartment has been the rationale for

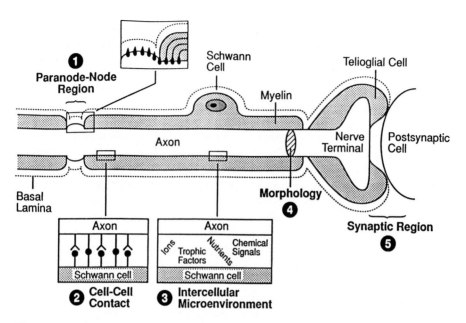

Figure 2 Schwann cell–axon interactions. Schematic representation of composite Schwann cell–axon interactions in the peripheral nervous system. Each number represents a site of probable influence. 1.) In the paranode-node region, Schwann cells appear to participate in Na^+ channel turnover and in delineating nodal ion channel domain. 2.) During development, intermolecular binding (homophilic or heterophilic) of membrane adhesion and recognition molecules directs migration of nerve cells and neurite projections. In the mature nervous system, adhesion molecule binding assures physical proximity and stabilizes cell-cell contact. This facilitates continued functional interactions between Schwann cells and axons. 3.) Both Schwann cells and axons condition the intercellular microenvironment through the uptake and release of effector chemicals, metabolic substrates, hormones, and ions. This environmental modulation affects development and function of each cell type. 4.) Schwann cells and axons influence the morphology and differentiation of each other. This is represented in the figure as the effect of the Schwann cell on axon caliber. 5.) Synaptic glial cells (i.e., telioglial cells) modulate neurotransmission by altering the synaptic ion concentration, by uptake of neurotransmitters, and by release of neuromodulatory chemicals. In addition, Schwann cells assist in removal of aged or defective nerve terminals.

implementation of this organizing scheme. However, morphological alterations are an insensitive index of dysfunction; biochemical lesions can occur in the absence of such alterations and/or structural changes can be temporally dissociated with respect to biochemically relevant perturbations (LoPachin and Saubermann, 1990; LoPachin et al., 1990,1992a). Therefore, a lack of morphological change in either the Schwann cell or the axon should not preclude considerations of functional deficits. Moreover, it is clear that the axon and Schwann cell are linked in a reciprocal and mutually dependent relationship and consequently function as a unit. Thus, it is ultimately the response pattern of this unit to injury that determines the magnitude and extent of neuropathic expression. Our current understanding of neurotoxic mechanisms has been influenced by inherent technical difficulties in the dissociation of neurotoxicant-induced functional changes in glia vs. axons. Technological advances in cell and molecular biology have provided the neurotoxicologist with several powerful new research tools; e.g., patch clamp, assays of glia- and neuron-specific proteins, tissue print, electron x-ray microanalysis, and in situ hybridization. These techniques offer means of detecting the impact of neurotoxicants on both cell types in the Schwann cell–axon unit. The next section of this chapter is devoted to developing the concept of neurotoxicant action within the Schwann cell–axon unit. Relevant examples will be provided from the neurotoxicology literature where available. The suggested mechanisms are for the most part speculative and are by no means inclusive; other possibilities are limited only by the reader's level of understanding and creativity.

Schwann Cell Injury with Axonal Consequences

It is possible that certain neurotoxic mechanisms in the PNS involve an effect on Schwann cell physiology that either causes secondary axonal injury or augments simultaneous axon damage. For example, many neurotoxicants, including tellurium, hexachlorophene, and lead, injure Schwann cells and interfere with their ability to maintain the insulating myelin sheath. The physiological consequences of this demyelination include slowing of action potential conduction and aberrant conduction of impulses (Anthony and Graham, 1991). The nerve damage induced by these neurotoxicants has been classified as a myelinopathy, since axons appear structurally intact. However, it is evident from our discussion of Schwann cell–axon relationships that many axonal properties necessary for normal impulse conduction (e.g., axon caliber, axonal transport, segregation and turnover of nodal sodium channels) depend on interactions of axons with the myelin sheath (Waxman and Ritchie, 1985; Joe and Angelides, 1992; deWaegh et al., 1992). Loss of this sheath would therefore be expected to alter normal axolemmal organization and axon function. Indeed, several lines of evidence suggest that demyelination perturbs fiber geometry, causes loss of regional differentiation of the axolemma, and modifies distribution of membrane sodium channels (Bostock and Sears, 1978; Quick and Waxman, 1978; Rasminsky, 1980). Thus deficits in impulse conduction that result from demyelination may be more complex than simple loss of insulation. Such deficits are likely also to involve perturbation of myelin-dependent electrogenic axonal characteristics.

   Glial cell swelling is a common morphological feature associated with several pathological conditions (e.g., hypoxia, trauma, diabetes) and exposure to certain neurotoxicants (lead, acrylamide, 2,5-hexanedione) in both the peripheral and central nervous systems (Powell et al., 1978; Norenberg, 1981; Philbert et al., 1987; Coria and Monton, 1988; LoPachin et al., 1992b). Glial swelling is often interpreted as an innocuous or reactive event in the course of neurotoxicity. However, regardless of whether a direct or indirect effect causes swelling, loss of cellular osmoregulation can have specific functional consequences that could impair the glial-neuronal relationship and ultimately neuron (axon) performance. Although the effects of swelling on cellular function have been best described in CNS tissues and cultures (Aschner and Kimelberg, 1991), the occurrence of Schwann cell swelling is likely to be a mechanistic issue in peripheral neurotoxicity. In general, cell swelling is associated with disruption of transmembrane ionic gradients and concomitant accumulation of cytoplasmic sodium ions and loss of potassium ions (Macknight, 1984). This impairs cellular processes such as energy metabolism, macromolecular synthesis, and extracellular K^+ buffering that depend on maintenance of transmembrane gradients (see reviews by Macknight, 1984, 1988; LoPachin and Saubermann, 1990; LoPachin et al., 1992a). Therefore, chemicals that produce swelling could compromise important homeostatic Schwann cell processes (e.g., ion buffering, metabolic support) that maintain axon integrity. In addition, modification of cell shape associated with swelling could alter the physical proximity of the Schwann cell and respective axon, which is important for maintenance of cell-cell contact, signaling mechanisms, and macromolecular transport.

Finally, as mentioned above, it is possible that the Schwann cell and axon are affected coincidentally by a neurotoxicant. In such an instance, the Schwann cell would be incapable of performing homeostatic functions that might modify the severity of axon injury (see below). For example, neurotoxic chemicals such as acrylamide and 2,5-hexanedione, which are traditionally considered to selectively injure axons, have been shown to alter several Schwann cell and astrocyte parameters (e.g., elemental content, cytoskeletal proteins, energy metabolism) (Powell et al., 1978; Ross et al., 1985; Karlsson et al., 1991; LoPachin et al., 1992b). These results may indicate that the attending glial cell is also injured by exposure to neurotoxicant. In any case, future investigations concerning neurotoxicant-induced nerve dysfunction should consider the possible involvement of Schwann cell injury or compromise as a factor contributing to the loss of axon structure and function.

Disruption of Schwann Cell–Axon Interactive Processes

The possibility exists that a neurotoxicant interferes with the unifying processes that physically and functionally bind the Schwann cell and axon. These processes include intercellular communication via neuroactive substances, adhesion molecule binding, and intercellular transfer of macromolecules. As indicated earlier, intercellular dialogue is a fundamental process for coordinating Schwann cell–axon interactions. Consequently, neurotoxicant disruption of communication will effectively sever the link between Schwann cell and axon and open the possibility of subsequent injury. However, to date this possibility remains unexplored.

Cell-cell contact mediated by membrane adhesion molecule binding regulates many Schwann cell–axon interactive processes (e.g., Schwann cell proliferation and differentiation, neurite outgrowth, myelination) and maintains Schwann cells and axons in the close physical proximity required for intercellular communication and transfer of macromolecules. Any neurotoxic agent that interferes with adhesion molecule binding or genetic expression might, therefore, be expected to "uncouple" Schwann cell–axon contact. As indicated elsewhere, this could have extensive impact on the form and function of each cell type. Cell-cell contact as a putative site of neurotoxicant action is a relatively recent consideration and has been investigated only in the CNS (Reuhl and Lowndes, 1992; Verity, 1992). For example, low-level lead exposure of rat pups in utero altered NCAM sialylation, which presumably impairs the intermolecular binding process important for cell-cell stabilization (Cookman et al., 1987). In addition, Reuhl and Borgeson (1990) showed that in vitro exposure to methylmercury caused an alteration in membrane NCAM distribution and a parallel reduction in neuronal aggregation and neurite fasciculation. Such studies provide a basis for related investigation in the PNS involving neurotoxic agents.

Schwann Cell Modification of Neurotoxic Expression

Axons are thought to be selectively vulnerable to many chemical neurotoxicants (e.g., organophosphates, *n*-hexane, diethyldithiocarbamate, and carbon disulfide). By virtue of their previously described homeostatic or defensive actions (e.g., ion buffering, trophic factor release, phagocytosis), Schwann cells could conceivably delay and/or modify expression of the axonopathy produced by these chemicals. For example, Schwann cells might sequester and metabolize neurotoxicants. This would reduce the effective microenvironment concentration of toxicant to which target axons are exposed. Alternatively,

Schwann cells might transfer to the axon factors such as heat shock proteins, energy substrates, and trophic factors (see above) that impede neurotoxic expression or restore compromised function. Finally, it is well recognized that Schwann cells insert cytoplasmic processes into axonal cytoplasm to remove debris that results from toxicant-induced damage (phagocytosis) and are intimately involved in the regenerative process by which peripheral nerves are able to recover from neurotoxic insult (see above).

Schwann Cell Participation in Neurotoxic Mechanisms: Conclusions

Definitions of neurotoxicity are traditionally presented in terms of neuron (axon) injury. Consistent with this neuron-centric theme, Schwann cells have been relegated to a secondary role involving reactive or supportive responses. It is clear that Schwann cells and axons function as a unit, the integrity of which is of fundamental importance to nearly all aspects of nervous system operation and morphology. In this chapter we have suggested general ways in which the Schwann cell–axon unit might participate in neurotoxic mechanisms. These possibilities represent nontraditional sites of action for many neurotoxicants. The design of future research investigating neurotoxic mechanisms should take into account the possible involvement of Schwann cells in peripheral neurotoxicities and, where appropriate, should be directed toward defining that involvement as either primary, coincidental, reactive, or supportive.

ACKNOWLEDGMENT

Preparation of this manuscript and the authors' work described herein were supported in part by NIEHS grant 5R01ES03830-07.

REFERENCES

Abbott NJ, ed. (1991). Glial-neuronal interactions. New York: New York Academy of Sciences.

Acheson A, Thoenen H (1983). Cell contact–mediated regulation of tyrosine hydroxylase synthesis in cultured bovine adrenal chromaffin cells. J Cell Biol 97:925–8.

Acheson A, Rutishauser U (1988). Neural cell adhesion molecule regulates cell contact–mediated changes in choline acetyltransferase activity of embryonic chick sympathetic neurons. J Cell Biol 106:479–86.

Aguayo AJ, Bray GM (1984). Cell interaction studied in the peripheral nerves of experimental animals. In: Dyck PJ, Thomas PK, Lambert EH, Bunge R, eds: Peripheral neuropathy. Vol. 1. Philadelphia: W. B. Saunders, 360–77.

Aguayo AJ, Charron L, Bray GM (1976a). Potential of Schwann cells from unmyelinated nerve to produce myelin: a quantitative ultrastructural and radiographic study. Neurocytology 5:565–73.

Aguayo AJ, Epps J, Charron L, Bray GM (1976b). Multipotentiality of Schwann cells in cross-anastomosed and grafted myelinated and unmyelinated nerves: quantitative microscopy and radioautography. Brain Res 104:1–20.

Aguayo AJ, Attiwell M, Trecarten J, Perkins S, Bray GM (1977). Abnormal myelination in transplanted trembler mouse Schwann cells. Nature 265:73–6.

Anderson DJ (1989). The neural crest cell lineage problem: neuropoiesis? Neuron 3:1–12.

Anthony DC, Graham DG (1991). Toxic responses of the nervous system. In: Amdur MO, Doull J, Klaassen CD, eds. Casarett and Doull's toxicology: the basic science of poisons. 4th ed. New York: Pergamon Press, 407–29.

Arenander AT, de Vellis J (1983). Frontiers of glial physiology. In: Rosenberg R, ed. The clinical neurosciences. New York: Churchill Livingstone, 53–91.

Asai K, Hirano T, Kaneko S, Moriyama A, Nakanishi K, Isobe I, Eksioglu YZ, Kato T (1992). A novel glial growth inhibitory factor, gliostatin, derived from neurofibroma. J Neurochem 59:307–17.

Aschner M, Kimelberg HK (1991). The use of astrocytes in culture as model systems for evaluating neurotoxic-induced injury. Neurotoxicology 12:505–18.

Ayer-LeLivre D, Olson L, Ebendal T, Seiger A, Perrson H (1988). Expression of the β-nerve growth factor gene in hippocampal neurons. Science 240:1339–41.

Baichwal RR, DeVries GH (1989). A mitogen for Schwann cells is derived from myelin basic protein. Biochem Biophys Res Commun 164:883–8.

Baichwal RR, Bigbee JW, DeVries GH (1988). Macrophage-mediated myelin-related mitogenic factor for cultured Schwann cells. Proc Natl Acad Sci USA 85:1701–5.

Baron-Van Evercooren A, Kleinman HK, Seppa HEJ, Rentier B, Dubois-Dalcq M (1982). Fibronectin promotes rat Schwann cell growth and motility. J Cell Biol 93:211–6.

Barres BA (1991). New roles for glia. J Neurosci 11:3685–94.

Barres BA, Koroshetz WJ, Chun LLY, Corey DP (1990). Ion channel expression by white matter glia: the type-1 astrocyte. Neuron 5:527–44.

Berthold C-H (1978). Morphology of normal peripheral axons. In: Waxman SG, ed. Physiology and pathobiology of axons. New York: Raven Press, 3–63.

Bixby JL, Lilien J, Reichardt LF (1988). Identification of the major proteins that promote neuronal process outgrowth on Schwann cells in vitro J Cell Biol 107:353–61.

Black JA, Kocsis JD, Waxman SG (1990). Ion channel organization of the myelinated fiber. Trends Neurosci 13:48–54.

Bostock H, Sears TA (1978). The internodal axon membrane: electrical excitability and continuous conduction in segmental demyellination. J Physiol (London) 280:273–301.

Brunden KR, Windebank AJ, Poduslo JF (1990). Role of axons in the regulation of P_0 biosynthesis by Schwann cells. J Neurosci Res 26:135–143.

Buchheit TE, Tytell M (1992). Transfer of molecules from glia to axon in the squid may be mediated by glial vesicles. J Neurobiol 23:217–30.

Bunge RP, Hopkins JM (1990). The role of peripheral and central neuroglia in neural regeneration in vertebrates. Semin Neurosci 2:509–18.

Bunge RP, Bunge MB, Eldridge CF (1986). Linkage between axonal ensheathment and basal lamina production by Schwann cells. Annu Rev Neurosci 9:305–28.

Byrne MC, Farooq M, Sbaschnig-Agler M, Norton WT, Ledeen RW (1988). Ganglioside content of astroglia and neurons isolated from maturing rat brain: consideration of the source of astroglial gangliosides. Brain Res 461:87–97.

Cammer W (1980). Toxic demyelination: biochemical studies and hypothetical mechanisms. In: Spencer PS, Schaumburg HH, eds. Experimental and clinical neurotoxicology. Baltimore: Williams and Wilkins, 239–56.

Cavanagh JB, Nolan CC, Brown AW (1990). Glial cell intrusions actively remove detritus due to toxic chemicals from within nerve cells. Neurotoxicology 11:1–12.

Chamak B, Fellous A, Glowinski J, Prochiantz A (1987). MAP2 expression and neuritic outgrowth and branching are coregulated through region-specific neuro-astroglial interactions. J Neurosci 7:3163–70.

Chen W-T. Hasegawa E, Hasegawa T, Weinstock C, Yamada KM (1985). Development of cell surface linkage complexes in cultured fibroblasts. J Cell Biol 100:1103–14.

Chiu SY (1987). Sodium currents in axon-associated Schwann cells from adult rabbits. J Physiol (London) 386:181–203.

Chiu SY (1988). Changes in excitable membrane properties in Schwann cells of adult rabbit sciatic nerves following nerve transection. J Physiol (London) 396:173–88.

Chiu SY (1991). Functions and distributions of voltage-gated sodium and potassium channels in mammalian Schwann cells. Glia 4:541–58.

Chiu SY, Ritchie JM (1980). Potassium channels in nodal and internodal axonal membrane of mammalian myelinated fibre. Nature 284:170–171.

Chiu SY, Wilson GF (1989). The role of potassium channels in Schwann cell proliferation in Wallerian degeneration of explant rabbit sciatic nerves. J Physiol (London) 408:199–202.

Chuong CM (1990). Differential roles of multiple adhesion molecules in cell migration: granule cell migration in cerebellum. Experientia 46:892–9.

Cookman GR, King W, Regan CM (1987). Chronic low-level lead exposure impairs embryonic to adult conversion of the neural cell adhesion molecule. J Neurochem 49:399–403.

Coria F, Monton F (1988). Recovery of the early cellular changes induced by lead in rat peripheral nerves after withdrawal of the toxin. J Neuropathol Exp Neurol 47:282–90.

Davis JB, Stroobant P (1990). Platelet-derived growth factors and fibroblast growth factors are mitogens for rat Schwann cells. J Cell Biol 110:1353–60.

DeCoster MA, DeVries GH (1989). Evidence that the axolemmal mitogen for cultured Schwann cells is a positively-charged, heparin sulfate proteoglycan–bound, heparin-displaceable molecule. J Neurosci Res 22:283–88.

Denis-Donini S, Glowinski J, Prochiantz A (1984). Glial heterogeneity may define the three-dimensional shape of mouse mesencephalic dopaminergic neurons. Nature 307:641–3.

Dennis MJ, Miledi R (1974). Electrically induced release of acetylcholine from denervated Schwann cells. J Physiol 237:431–52.

DeWaegh S, Brady ST (1990). Altered slow axonal transport and regeneration in a myelin-deficient mutant mouse: the Trembler as an in vivo model for Schwann cell–axon interactions. J Neurosci 10:1855–65.

DeWaegh S, Brady ST (1991). Local control of axonal properties by Schwann cells: neurofilament and axonal transport in homologous and heterologous nerve grafts. J Neurosci Res 30:201–12.

DeWaegh S, Lee VM-Y, Brady ST (1992). Local modulation of neurofilament phosphorylation, axonal caliber, and slow axonal transport by myelinating Schwann cells. Cell 68:451–63.

Eccleston PA (1992). Regulation of Schwann cell proliferation: mechanisms involved in peripheral nerve development. Exp Cell Res 199:1–9.

Eccleston PA, Mirsky R, Jessen KR, Sommer I, Schachner M. (1987). Postnatal development of rat peripheral nerves: an immunohistochemical study of membrane lipids common to non-myelin forming Schwann cells, myelin forming Schwann cells and oligodendrocytes. Dev Brain Res 35:249–56.

Eccleston PA, Collarini E, Jessen KR, Mirsky R, Richardson WD (1990). Platelet derived growth factor stimulates Schwann cell DNA synthesis: a possible autocrine method of growth. Eur J Neurosci 2:985–92.

Eldridge CF, Bunge MB, Bunge RP, Wood PM (1987). Differentiation of axon-related Schwann cells in vitro. I. Ascorbic acid regulates basal lamina assembly and myelin formation. J Cell Biol 105:1023–34.

Eldridge CF, Bunge MB, Bunge RP (1989). Differentiation of axon-related Schwann cells in vitro. II. Control of myelin formation by basal lamina. J Neurosci 9:625–38.

Ellisman MH (1979). Molecular specialization of the axon membrane at nodes of Ranvier are not dependent on myelination. J Neurocytol 8:719–35.

England JD, Gamboni F, Levinson SR, Finger TE (1990). Changed distribution of sodium channels along demyelinated axons. Proc Natl Acad Sci USA 87:6777–80.

England JD, Gamboni F, Levinson SR (1991). Increased numbers of sodium channels form along demyelinated axons. Brain Res 548:334–7.

Evans PD, Reale V, Villegas J (1985). The role of cyclic nucleotides in modulation of the membrane potential of the Schwann cell squid giant nerve fibre. J Physiol (London) 363:151–67.

Evans PD, Reale V, Villegas J (1986). Peptidergic modulation of the membrane potential of the Schwann cell of the squid giant nerve fibre. J Physiol (London) 379:61–82.

Evans PD, Reale V, Merzon RM, Villegas J (1991). Mechanisms of axon–Schwann cell signaling in the squid nerve fiber. In: Abbott NJ, ed. Glial-neuronal interactions. New York: New York Academy of Sciences, 434–47.

Fawcett JW, Keynes RJ (1990). Peripheral nerve regeneration. Annu Rev Neurosci 13:43–60.

Fedoroff S, Vernadakis A, eds. (1986a). Astrocytes: development, morphology, and regional specialization. Vol. 1. New York: Academic Press.

Fedoroff S, Vernadakis A, eds. (1986b). Astrocytes: development, morphology, and regional specialization. Vol. 2. New York: Academic Press.

Fedoroff S, Vernadakis A, eds. (1986c). Astrocytes: development, morphology, and regional specialization. Vol. 3. New York: Academic Press.

Friede RG (1972). Control of myelin formation by axon caliber (with a model of the central mechanism). J Comp Neurol 144:233–52.

Friede RL, Samorajski T (1970). Axon caliber related to neurofilaments and microtubules in sciatic nerve fibers of rats and mice. Anat Rec 167:379–88.

Gloor S, Antonicek H, Sweadner KJ, Pagliusi S, Frank R, Moos M, Schachner M (1990). The adhesion molecule on glia (AMOG) is a homologue of the β subunit of the Na,K-ATPase. J Cell Biol 110:165–74.

Gould RM, Matsumoto D, Mattingly G (1982). The Schwann cell. In: Lajtha A, ed. The handbook of neurochemistry. New York: Plenum Press, 397–414.

Gray EG (1970). The fine structure of nerve. Comp Biol Chem Physiol 36:419–48.

Griffin JW, Rosenfeld J, Hoffman PN, Gold BG, Trapp BD (1988). The axonal cytoskeleton: influences on nerve fiber form and Schwann cell behavior. In: Lasek RJ, Black MM, eds. Intrinsic determinants of neuronal form and function. New York: Alan R. Liss, 403–39.

Grossfeld RM (1991). Axon-glial exchange of macromolecules. In: Abbott NJ, ed. Glial-neuronal interactions. New York: New York Academy of Sciences.

Gulati AK (1988). Evaluation of acellular and cellular nerve grafts in repair of rat peripheral nerve. J Neurosurg 68:117–23.

Haftek J, Thomas PK (1968). Electron microscope observations on the effects of localized crush injuries on the connective tissue of peripheral nerves. J Anat 103:233–43.

Hahn AF, Whitaker JN, Kachar B, Webster HF (1987). P_2, P_1, and P_0 myelin expression in developing rat sixth nerve: a quantitative immunocytochemical study. J Comp Neurol 260:501–12.

Hall SM (1978). The Schwann cell: a reappraisal of its role in the peripheral nervous system. Neuropathol Appl Neurobiol 4:165–76.

Hall SM (1986). Regeneration in cellular and acellular autografts in the peripheral nervous system. Neuropathol Appl Neurobiol 12:27–46.

Heumann R, Korsching S, Bandtlow C, Thoenen H (1987a). Changes of nerve growth factor synthesis in nonneuronal cells in response to sciatic nerve transection. J Cell Biol 104:1623–31.

Heumann R, Lindholm D, Bandtlow C, Meyer M, Radeke MJ, Misko TP, Shooter E, Thoenen H (1987b). Differential regulation of mRNA encoding nerve growth factor and its receptor in rat sciatic nerve during development, degeneration, and regeneration: role of macrophages. Proc Natl Acad Sci USA 84:8735–9.

Hirano S, Nose A, Hatta K, Kawakami A, Takeichi M (1987). Calcium-dependent cell-cell adhesion molecules (cadherins): subclass specificities and possible involvement of actin bundles. J Cell Biol 105:2501–10.

Howe JR, Ritchie JM (1988). Two types of potassium current in rabbit cultured Schwann cells. Proc R Soc Lond (Biol) 235:19–27.

Howe JR, Ritchie JM (1990). Sodium currents in Schwann cells from myelinated and non-myelinated nerves of neonatal and adult rabbits. J Physiol (London) 425:169–210.

Jessen KR, Mirsky R, Morgan L (1987). Axonal signals regulate the differentiation of non-myelin-forming Schwann cells: an immunohistochemical study of galactocerebroside in transected and regenerating nerves. J Neurosci 7:3362–9.

Jessen KR, Morgan L, Stewart HJS, Mirsky R (1990). Three markers of adult non-myelin-forming Schwann cells, 217c(Ran-1), A5E3 and GFAP; development and regulation by neuron-Schwann cell interactions. Development 109:91–103.

Joe E, Angelides K (1992). Clustering of voltage-dependent sodium channels on axons depends on Schwann cell contact. Nature 356:333–5.

Johnson EM, Taniuchi M, DiStefano PS (1988). Expression and possible function of nerve growth factor receptors on Schwann cells. Trends Neurosci 11:299–304.

Jonas P, Brau ME, Hermsteiner M, Vogel W (1989). Single-channel recording in myelinated nerve fibers reveals one type of Na channel but different K channels. Proc Natl Acad Sci USA 86:7238–42.

Karlsson J-E, Rosengren LE, Haglid KG (1991). Quantitative and qualitative alterations of neuronal and glial intermediate filaments in rat nervous system after exposure to 2,5-hexanedione. J Neurochem 57:1437–44.

Kimelberg HK, Norenberg MD (1989). Astrocytes. Sci Am 260:66–76.

Klagsbrun M (1990). The affinity of fibroblast growth factors (FGF) for heparin and FGF heparin sulfate. Curr Opin Cell Biol 2:857–63.

Konishi T (1989). Voltage-dependent potassium channels in cultured mammalian Schwann cells. Brain Res 499:273–80.

Konishi T (1990). Dye coupling between mouse Schwann cells. Brain Res 508:85–92.

Krishnam N, Singer M (1973). Penetration of peroxidase into peripheral nerve fibers. Am J Anat 136:1–7.

Kruse J, Keilhauer G, Faissner A, Timpl R, Schachner M. (1985). The J1 glycoprotein-a novel nervous system cell adhesion molecule of the L2/HNK-1 family. Nature 316:146–8.

Kuffler SW, Nicholls JG, Martin AR (1984). Physiology of neuroglial cells. In: Kuffler SW, Nicholls JG, Martin AR, eds. From neuron to brain: a cellular approach to the function of the nervous system 2nd ed. Sunderland, Massachusetts: Sinauer Associates.

Landon DN, Hall S (1976). The myelinated nerve fiber. In: Landon DN, ed. The peripheral nerve. New York: John Wiley & Sons, 1–105.

Lasek RJ, Gainer H, Barker JL (1977). Cell-to-cell transfer of glial proteins to the squid axon. J Cell Biol 74:501–30.

Lasek R, Oblinger M, Drake P (1983). Molecular biology of neuronal geometry: expression of neurofilament genes influences axonal diameter. Cold Spring Harbor Symp Quant Biol 18:731–44.

LeBeau JM, Powell HC, Ellisman MH (1987). Node of Ranvier formation along fibers regenerating through silicone tube implants: a freeze fracture and thin-section electron-microscopic study. J Neurocytol 16:347–58.

Le Douarin NM (1982). The neural crest. Cambridge, England: Cambridge University Press.

Le Douarin NM, Dulac C, Dupin E, Cameron-Curry P (1991). Glial cell lineages in the neural crest. Glia 4:175–84.

Lemke G (1990). Glial growth factors. Semin Neurosci 2:437–43.

Lemke G, Chao M (1988). Axons regulate Schwann cell expression of the major myelin and NGF receptor genes. Development 102:499–504.

Lieberman EM (1991). Role of glutamate in axon–Schwann cell signaling in the squid. In: Abbott NJ, ed. Glial-neuronal interactions. New York: New York Academy of Sciences.

Lim R, Miller JF, Zaheer A (1989). Purification and characterization of glia maturation factor β: a growth regulator for neurons and glia. Proc Natl Acad Sci USA 86:3901–5.

LoPachin RM, Saubermann AJ (1990). Disruption of cellular elements and water in neurotoxicity: studies using electron probe X-ray microanalysis. Toxicol Appl Pharmacol 106:355–74.

LoPachin RM, Lowery J, Eichberg J, Kirkpatrick JB, Cartwright J Jr, Saubermann AJ (1988). Distribution of elements in rat peripheral axons and nerve cell bodies determined by x-ray microprobe analysis. J Neurochem 51:764–75.

LoPachin RM, LoPachin VR, Saubermann AJ (1990). Effects of axotomy on distribution and concentration of elements in rat sciatic nerve. J Neurochem 54:320–32.

LoPachin RM, Castiglia CM, Saubermann AJ (1991). Elemental composition and water content of myelinated axons and glial cells in rat central nervous system. Brain Res 549:253–9.

LoPachin RM, Castiglia CM, Saubermann AJ (1992a). Perturbation of axonal elemental composition and water content: implication for neurotoxic mechanisms. Neurotoxicology 13:123–38.

LoPachin RM, Castiglia CM, Saubermann AJ (1992b). Acrylamide disrupts elemental composition and water content of rat tibial nerve. II. Schwann cells and myelin. Toxicol Appl Pharmacol 115:35–43.

Mackenzie ML, Ghabriel MN, Allt G (1984). Nodes of Ranvier and Schmidt-Lanterman incisures: an in vivo lanthanum tracer study. J Neurocytol 13:1043–55.

Macknight ADC (1984). Cellular response to injury. In: Staub NC, Taylor AE, eds. Edema. New York: Raven Press, 489–520.

Macknight ADC (1988). Principles of cell volume regulation. Renal Physiol Biochem 3–5, 114–141.

Magistretti PJ, Hof PR, Martin JL (1986). Adenosine stimulates glycogenolysis in mouse cerebral cortex: a possible coupling mechanism between neuronal activity and energy metabolism. J Neurosci 6:2558–62.

Martin DL (1992). Synthesis and release of neuroactive substances by glial cells. Glia 5:81–94.

Martini R, Schachner M (1988). Immunoelectron microscopic localization of neural cell adhesion molecules (L1, N-CAM, and myelin-associated glycoprotein) in regenerating adult mouse sciatic nerve. J Cell Biol 106:1735–46.

McGarvey ML, Baron-Van Evercooren A, Kleinman HK, Dubois-Dalcq M (1984). Synthesis and effects of basement membrane components in cultured rat Schwann cells. Dev Biol 105:18–28.

Minchin MCW, Iversen LL (1974). Release of [^{3}H]gamma-aminobutyric acid from glial cells in rat dorsal root ganglia. J Neurochem 23:535–40.

Mirsky R, Jessen KR (1990). Schwann cell development and the regulation of myelination. Semin Neurosci 2:423–35.

Mirsky R, Jessen KR, Schachner M, Goridis C (1986). Distribution of the adhesion molecules N-CAM and L1 on peripheral neurons and glia in adult rats. J Neurocytol 15:799–815.

Mirsky R, DuBois C, Morgan L, Jessen KR (1990) O4 and AO07-sulfatide antibodies bind to embryonic Schwann cells prior to the appearance of galactocerebroside; regulation of the antigen by axon–Schwann cell signals and cyclic AMP. Development 109:105–6.

Morell P, Quarles RH, Norton WT (1989). Formation, structure, and biochemistry of myelin. In:Siegel GJ, Agranoff BW, Albers RW, Molinoff PB, eds. Basic neurochemistry. New York: Raven Press, 109–36.

Morgan JI, Curran T (1986). Role of ion flux in the control of c-fos expression. Nature 322:552–5.

Mudge AW (1984). Schwann cells induce morphological transformation of sensory neurones in vitro. Nature 309:367–9.

Nadim W, Anderson PN, Turmaine M (1990). The role of Schwann cells and basal lamina tubes in the regeneration of axons through long lengths of freeze-killed nerve grafts. Neuropathol Appl Neurobiol 16:411–21.

Norenberg MD (1981). The astrocyte in liver disease. In: Fedoroff S, Hertz L, eds. Advances in cellular neurology. Vol 2. New York: Academic Press, 304–38.

Orkand RK, Nicholls JG, Kuffler SW (1966). Effect of nerve impulses on the membrane potential of glial cells in the central nervous system of amphibia. J Neurophysiol 29:788–806.

Pannese E, Ledda M, Matsuda S (1988). Nerve fibers with myelinated and unmyelinated portions in dorsal spinal roots. J Neurocytol 17:693–700.

Parhad IM, Clark AW, Griffin JW (1987). The effect of impairment of slow transport on axonal caliber. In: Bisby M, ed. Axonal transport. New York: Alan R. Liss, 263–77.

Peters A, Palay SL, Webster HF (1991). The fine structure of the nervous system. 3rd ed. New York: Oxford University Press.

Philbert MA, Nolan CC, Cremer JE, Tucker D, Brown AW (1987) 1,3-Dinitrobenzene–induced encephalopathy in rats. Neuropathol Appl Neurobiol 13:371–89.

Pleasure D, Kreider B, Shuman S, Sobue G (1985). Tissue culture studies of Schwann cell proliferation and differentiation. Dev Neurosci 7:364–73.

Politis MJ, Ingoglia NA (1979). Axonal transport of nucleosides, nucleotides and 4S RNA in the neonatal rat visual system. Brain Res 169:343–56.

Pollerberg GE, Sadoul R, Goridis C, Schachner M (1985). Selective expression of the 180-kD component of the neural cell adhesion molecule N-CAM during development. J Cell Biol 101:1921–9.

Pollerberg GE, Burridge K, Krebs KE, Goodman SR, Schachner M (1987). The 180-kD component of the neural cell adhesion molecule N-CAM is involved in cell-cell contacts and cytoskeleton-membrane interactions. Cell Tiss Res 250:227–36.

Porter S, Clark MB, Glaser L, Bunge RP (1986). Schwann cells stimulated to proliferate in the absence of neurons retain full functional capability. J Neurosci 6:3070–8.

Powell HC, Koch T, Garrett R, Lampert PW (1978). Schwann cell abnormalities in 2,5-hexanedione neuropathy. J Neurocytol 7:517–28.

Quasthoff S, Strupp M, Grafe P (1992). High conductance anion channels in Schwann cell vesicles from rat spinal roots. Glia 5:517–24.

Quick DC, Waxman SG (1978). Demyelination of Sternarchus electrocyte fibers by injection of diphtheria toxin. J Neurol Sci 35:235–41.

Raff MC, Hornby-Smith A, Brockes JP (1989). Cyclic AMP as a mitogenic signal for cultured rat Schwann cells. Nature 273:672–3.

Rasminsky M (1980). Physiological consequences of demyelination. In: Spencer PS, Schaumburg HH, eds. Experimental and clinical neurotoxicology. Baltimore: Williams and Wilkins, 257–71.

Ratner N, Bunge RP, Glaser L (1985). A neuronal cell surface heparin sulfate proteoglycan is required for dorsal root ganglion neuron stimulation of Schwann cell proliferation. J Cell Biol 101:744–54.

Ratner N, Elbein A, Bunge MB, Porter S, Bunge RP, Glaser L (1986). Specific asparagine-linked oligosaccharides are not required for certain neuron-neuron and neuron–Schwann cell interactions. J Cell Biol 103:159–70.

Reale V, Evans PD, Villegas J (1986). Octopaminergic modulation of the membrane potential of the Schwann cell of the squid giant nerve fibre. J Exp Biol 121:421–43.

Reichardt LF, Tomaselli KJ (1991). Extracellular matrix molecules and their receptors: functions in neural development. Annu Rev Neurosci 14:531–70.

Reuhl KR, Borgeson R (1990). Methylmercury, N-CAM expression and dysmorphogenesis (abstr). Toxicologist 10:136.

Reuhl KR, Lowndes HE (1992). Factors influencing morphological expression of neurotoxicity. In: Tilson H, Mitchell C, eds. Neurotoxicology New York: Raven Press, 67–81.

Ridley AJ, Davis JB, Stroobant P, Land H (1989). Transforming growth factors-β1 and β2 are mitogens for rat Schwann cells. J Cell Biol 109:3419–24.

Ritchie JM, Black JA, Waxman SG, Angelides KJ (1990). Sodium channels in the cytoplasm of Schwann cells. Proc Natl Acad Sci USA 87:9290–4.

Rosenbluth J (1983). Structure of the node of Ranvier. In: Chang CD, Tasaki I, Adelman WJ, Leuchtag HR, eds. Structure and function in excitable cells. New York: Plenum Press, 25–52.

Rosenbluth J (1989). Role of Schwann cells in differentiation of the axolemma: consequences of myelin deficiency in spinal roots of the dystrophic mouse mutant. In: Scarpini E, Fiori MG, Pleasure D, Scarlato G, eds Peripheral nerve development and regeneration: recent advances and clinical application. Fidia Research Series, Vol. 19. Padua, Italy: Liviana Press, 39–53.

Ross SM, Sabri MI, Spencer PS (1985). Action of acrylamide on selected enzymes of energy metabolism in denervated cat peripheral nerves. Brain Res 340:189–91.

Salzer JL, Bunge RP (1980). Studies of Schwann cell proliferation: I. An analysis in tissue culture of proliferation during development, wallerian degeneration, and direct injury. J Cell Biol 84:739–52.

Salzer JL, Williams AK, Glaser L, Bunge RP (1980a). Studies of Schwann cell proliferation: II. Characterization of the stimulation and specificity of the response to a neurite membrane fraction. J Cell Biol 84:753–66.

Salzer JL, Bunge RP, Glaser L (1980b). Studies of Schwann cell proliferation: III. Evidence for the surface localization of the neurite mitogen. J Cell Biol 84:767–78.

Saunders RD, DeVries GH (1988a). Schwann cell proliferation is accompanied by enhanced inositol phospholipid metabolism. J Neurochem 50:876–82.

Saunders RD, DeVries GH (1988b). 1-Oleoyl-2-acetylglycerol and A23187 potentiate axolemma- and myelin-induced Schwann cell proliferation. J Neurochem 51:876–82.

Saunders RD, Brandon YW, DeVries GH (1989). Role of intracellular pH in the axolemma- and myelin-induced proliferation of Schwann cells. J Neurochem 52:1760–4.

Schachner M (1991). Cell surface recognition and neuron-glia interactions. In: Abbott NJ, ed. Glial-neuronal interactions. New York: New York Academy of Sciences, 105–12.

Schuch U, Lohse MJ, Schachner M (1989). Neural cell adhesion molecules influence second messenger systems. Neuron 3:13–20.

Schwab ME (1990). Myelin-associated inhibitors of neurite growth and regeneration in the CNS. Trends Neurosci 13:452–6.

Seilheimer B, Schachner M (1988). Studies of adhesion molecules mediating interactions between cells of peripheral nervous system indicate a major role of L1 in mediating sensory neuron growth on Schwann cells in culture. J Cell Biol 107:341–51.

Seilheimer B, Persohn E, Schachner M (1989). Neural cell adhesion molecule expression is regulated by Schwann cell–neuron interactions in culture. J Cell Biol 108:1909–15.

Smith GM, Rutishauser U, Silver J, Miller RH (1990). Maturation of astrocytes in vitro alters the extent and molecular basis of neurite outgrowth. Dev Biol 138:377–90.

Smith-Thomas LC, Johnson AR, Fawcett JW (1990). The effects of embryonic retinal neurons on neural crest cell differentiation into Schwann cells. Development 109:925–34.

Sobue G, Pleasure D (1985). Adhesion of axolemmal fragments to Schwann cells: a signal- and target-specific process closely linked to axolemmal induction of Schwann cell mitosis. J Neurosci 5:379–87.

Sobue G, Shuman S, Pleasure D (1986). Schwann cell responses to cyclic AMP: proliferation, change in shape, and appearance of surface galactocerebrosides. Brain Res 362:23–32.

Sontheimer H, Kettenmann H, Schachner M, Trotter J (1990). The neural cell adhesion molecule (N-CAM) modulates K^+ channels in cultured glial precursor cells. Eur J Neurosci 3:230–6.

Spencer PS, Thomas PK (1974). Ultrastructural studies of the dying back process. II. The sequestration and removal by Schwann cells and oligodendrocytes of organelles from normal and diseased axons. J Neurocytol 3:763–83.

Spencer PS, Schaumburg HH (1980). Classification of neurotoxic disease: a morphological approach. In: Spencer PS, Schaumburg HH, eds. Experimental and clinical neurotoxicology. Baltimore: Williams and Wilkins, 92–9.

Stewart HJS, Eccleston PA, Jessen KR, Mirsky R (1991). Interaction between cAMP elevation, identified growth factors and serum components in regulating Schwann cell growth. J Neurosci Res 30:346–52.

Sykova E (1983). Extracellular K^+ accumulation in the central nervous system. Prog Biophys Mol Biol 42:135–89.

Taniuchi M, Clark HB, Schweitzer JB, Johnson EM (1988). Expression of nerve growth factor receptors by Schwann cells of axotomized peripheral nerves: ultrastructural location, suppression by axonal contact and binding properties. J Neurosci 8:664–81.

Thomas PK, Ochoa J (1984). Microscopic anatomy of peripheral nerve fibers. In: Dyck PJ, Thomas PK, Lambert EH, Bunge R, eds. Peripheral Neuropathy Vol. 1. Philadelphia: W.B. Saunders, 39–96.

Trapp BD, Dubois-Dalcq M, Quarles RH (1984). Ultrastructural localization of P2 protein in actively myelinating Schwann cells. J Neurochem 43:944–8.

Tsacopoulos M, Evequoz-Mercier V, Perrottet P, Buchner E (1988). Honeybee retinal cells transform glucose and supply the neurons with metabolic substrate. Proc Natl Acad Sci USA 85:8727–31.

Tucek S, Zelena J, Ge I, Vyskocil F (1978). Choline acetyltransferase in transected nerves, denervated muscles and Schwann cells of the frog: correlation of biochemical, electron microscopical and electrophysiological observations. Neuroscience 3:709–24.

Tytell M, Lasek RJ (1984). Glial polypeptides transferred into the squid giant axon. Brain Res 324: 223–32.

Tytell M, Greenburg SG, Lasek RJ (1986). Heat shock–like protein is transferred from glia to axon. Brain Res 363:161–4.

Uzman BG, Snyder DS, Villegas GM (1989). Status of peripheral nerve regeneration. In: Seil FJ, ed. Neural regeneration and transplantation. New York: Alan R. Liss, 15–28.

Verge VMK, Riopelle RJ, Richardson PM (1989). Nerve growth factor receptors on normal and injured sensory neurons. J Neurosci 9:914–22.

Verity MA (1992). Determination of neurotoxicity using molecular biological approaches. In: Tilson H, Mitchell C, eds. Neurotoxicology. New York: Raven Press, 1–20.

Vernadakis A (1988). Neuron-glia interrelations. Int Rev Neurobiol 30:149–211.

Villegas J, Evans PD, Reale V (1988). Electrophysiology of Schwann cell receptors. In: Kimelberg HK, ed. Glial Cell Receptors. New York: Raven Press, 141–57.

Virchow R (1858). Cellular pathology as based upon physiological and pathological histology. Translated by F. Chance from 2nd ed., 1859. New York: Dover, 1971.

Walz W (1989). Role of glial cells in the regulation of the brain ion microenvironment. Prog Neurobiol 33:309–33.

Walz W, Hertz L (1983). Functional interactions between neurons and astrocytes. II. Potassium homeostasis at the cellular level. Prog Neurobiol 20:133–83.

Waxman SG (1989). Axon-glial interactions in regeneration. In: Seil FJ, ed. Neural regeneration and transplantation. New York: Alan R. Liss, 43–66.

Waxman SG, Ritchie JM (1985). Organization of ion channels in the myelinated nerve fiber. Science 228:1502–7.

Webster HF, Favilla JT (1984). Development of peripheral nerve fibers. In: Dyck PJ, Thomas PK, Lambert EH, Bunge R, eds. Peripheral neuropathy. Philadelphia: W.B. Saunders, 329–59.

Weinberg HJ, Spencer PS (1976). Studies on the control of myelinogenesis. II. Evidence from neuronal regulation of myelin production. Brain Res 113:363–78.

Weinmaster G, Lemke G (1990). Cell-specific cyclic AMP–mediated induction of the PDGF receptor. EMBO J 9:915–20.

Wilson GF, Chiu SY (1990a). Ion channels in axon and Schwann cell membranes at paranodes of mammalian myelinated fibers studied with patch clamp. J Neurosci 10:3263–74.

Wilson GF, Chiu SY (1990b). Potassium channel regulation in Schwann cells during early developmental myelinogenesis. J Neurosci 10:1615–25.

Windebank AJ, Wood P, Bunge RP, Dyck PJ (1985). Myelination determines the caliber of dorsal root ganglion neurons in culture. J Neurosci 5:1563–9.

Wood PM, Bunge RP (1975). Evidence that sensory axons are mitogenic for Schwann cells. Nature 256:662–4.

10

The Neuromuscular Junction as a Target for Toxicity

William D. Atchison
Michigan State University
East Lansing, Michigan

John M. Spitsbergen
University of Virginia College of Medicine
Charlottesville, Virginia

INTRODUCTION

The junction of an axon terminal with an effector cell, whether it is another nerve cell or a muscle or glandular cell, is known as a synapse. In this chapter we will examine the neurotoxicity of a specific synapse, that made by motor axons on skeletal muscle, a synapse known as the neuromuscular junction. Because of the importance of skeletal muscle function to respiration as well as voluntary movement, it is not surprising that a number of naturally occurring toxins are directed at the neuromuscular junction. This fact was not lost on the South American Indian tribes who used curariform alkaloids to coat their arrows and thus paralyze their prey. In addition, however, the neuromuscular junction has been commonly studied not only as a specific target of toxins such as botulinum toxin or neurotoxicants such as cholinesterase inhibitors, but also as a model synapse to examine the actions of putative neurotoxicants or neurotoxins on synaptic function. This is due in large part to its well-characterized physiology, biochemistry, and microscopic anatomy.

Neurotoxicants that act at the neuromuscular junction can be divided into two classes: those that alter the presynaptic synthesis, storage, or release of acetylcholine (ACh) and those that disrupt the postsynaptic function of the effector cells, usually associated either with the recognition of ACh by its target receptor, activation of conductances through the receptor-associated ion channel, or impaired hydrolysis of ACh.

The neuromuscular junction possesses the typical morphological features of a chemical synapse. The presynaptic terminal contains the characteristic synaptic vesicles. A synaptic cleft separates the presynaptic nerve terminal from the postsynaptic muscle end plate membrane. Within this region, the membrane is highly invaginated. At this site are the nicotinic cholinergic receptors for ACh.

The physiology of normal neuromuscular transmission has been extensively detailed in a number of excellent reviews and chapters (see Martin, 1966; Hubbard, 1970, 1973; Silinsky, 1985). Therefore, only a brief synopsis will be given. The process of chemical neurotransmission can be simplified into two steps: 1.) those processes associated directly with the synthesis and release of neurotransmitter, which occur in the presynaptic nerve terminal (presynaptic processes), and 2.) those processes associated with the binding of transmitter to its receptor sites in the postsynaptic membrane, with subsequent opening of ionic conductance channels leading to the postsynaptic polarization (postsynaptic processes). Effects at either presynaptic or postsynaptic sites would be expected to alter neurotransmission and hence depress the final result, which at the neuromuscular junction is the muscle twitch. Consequently, to obtain further information about the nature of potential effects on neurotransmission, both processes must be studied independently.

Propagation of an action potential into the nonmyelinated terminal depolarizes the nonmyelinated terminal. This induces opening of voltage-dependent ion channels for Ca, which allow entry of Ca^{2+} from the extracellular fluid down its steep concentration gradient (Katz and Miledi, 1967a, 1969b). Influx of Ca^{2+} increases the probability of transmitter release by interacting with Ca^{2+} receptor molecules, a process whose exact details are only now being elucidated (see Südhoff and Jahn, 1991; Trimble et al., 1991). It is believed that the Ca^{2+} channels are closely apposed to the release sites (Robitaille et al., 1990; Cohen et al., 1991; Llinàs, et al., 1992). The identity of the pharmacological type of Ca^{2+} channels at the mammalian motor nerve terminal is still unclear, although the predominant form does not appear to be of the "L" (Atchison and O'Leary, 1987; Atchison, 1989b) or "N" subtype (Sano et al., 1987; Anderson and Harvey, 1987; Protti, et al., 1991). However, both L and N channels can contribute to mammalian neuromuscular transmission under certain circumstances (Atchison and O'Leary, 1987; Atchison, 1989b; Wessler et al., 1990). More recent studies using venom fractions from the spider *Agelenopsis aperta* suggest that at the mammalian neuromuscular junction Ca^{2+} channels of a different subtype known as "P" may play a predominate role in transmitter release (Uchitel et al., 1992). At the amphibian neuromuscular junction, N-type channels play a predominant role in transmitter release (Kerr and Yoshikami, 1984; Robitaille et al., 1990). Irrespective of the type of Ca^{2+} channel involved, this influx of Ca probably raises the local [Ca] around the release sites to very high levels, inducing the release of numerous packets or quanta of ACh into the synaptic cleft. The action of more than one Ca^{2+} ion is thought to be involved in each release event (Dodge and Rahamimoff, 1967). Each packet contains approximately 10,000–20,000 ACh molecules. Diffusion of the ACh across the synaptic cleft results in its ability to interact with receptor macromolecules located in the postjunctional muscle membrane (acetylcholine receptors {AChRs}). Receptors bound with ACh undergo a conformational change resulting in opening of a cation channel permeable normally to Na^+, K^+, and, to a lesser extent, Ca^{2+}. These ions move down their respective concentration gradients; permeability to sodium is higher than that to potassium; thus the net charge movement is inward, and the muscle end plate membrane depolarizes. The ACh is hydrolyzed quickly by acetylcholinesterase, yielding the inactive products choline and acetate. If the depolarization of the end plate reaches a threshold level, a muscle action potential propagates from the end plate region in both directions, leading ultimately to muscle contraction. Choline generated by the breakdown of ACh is taken up into the nerve terminal by high-affinity transport systems, Ca^{2+} that entered the terminal during the action potential is sequestered by intracellular binding proteins or organelles and slowly dissipated back to the extracellular fluid, and vesicles probably move from a reserve pool to release sites at the terminal membrane.

Quantal release of transmitter at chemical synapses occurs in two forms (see Katz, 1969). The first, in response to stimulation of the presynaptic neuron, is assumed to result in the synchronous discharge of multiple packets or quanta of transmitter and gives rise to a graded polarization of the postsynaptic cell—either a depolarization or a hyperpolarization, depending on the ionic conductances involved, known respectively as an excitatory postsynaptic potential or an inhibitory postsynaptic potential. The second form occurs spontaneously and presumably consists of random discharge of single quanta of transmitter, although this is still open to some debate. The postsynaptic responses to these random discharges are known as miniature postsynaptic potentials. Release of ACh at the neuromuscular junctions occurs in both quantal and nonquantal forms. The quantal form of release is generally, though not universally, considered to be associated with the vesicular pool of transmitter. Electrophysiologically, quantal release is observed in two forms: that which occurs in response to stimulation of the motor axon, and that which occurs spontaneously. Release in response to nerve stimulation is observed in electrophysiological recordings as a depolarizing response at the end plate membrane. This response is of variable amplitude, depending on the number of quanta of ACh released as well as the postsynaptic sensitivity, and is known as the end plate potential (EPP). Under normal in vivo conditions, the EPP is sufficiently large to trigger a regenerative action potential in the myofiber. Under normal conditions, the EPP cannot be measured, because 1.) the upstroke of the action potential obscures the decay phase of the EPP, and 2.) the resulting muscle twitch dislodges the electrode from its recording site.

As shown by the work of Katz and colleagues (Fatt and Katz, 1951; Del Castillo and Katz, 1954b), the EPP is made up of multiple quanta released in synchrony in response to entry of calcium during the depolarization induced by the action potential. This process was shown to be probabilistic in nature and, under normal conditions, to behave according to binomial statistics (Del Castillo and Katz, 1954b; Boyd and Martin, 1956b). Normally, several hundred quanta are released from a terminal and contribute to the EPP. Under conditions in which the likelihood that any quantum will be released is low, the EPP fluctuates in amplitude. The fluctuations correspond to multiples of the amplitude of the basic quantum. Under these conditions, in which the probability of release of an individual quantum is very low, EPPs of unitary amplitude can be observed. The amplitude of these smallest EPPs is virtually identical to that of the second form of release, known as the miniature end plate potential (MEPP) (Fatt and Katz, 1952; Boyd and Martin 1956a). Miniature end plate potentials occur in the absence of nerve stimulation (i.e., spontaneously). They are generally held to represent the postsynaptic response to release of a single quantum of ACh, although this view is not held universally. Unlike the EPP, whose function is obvious, the function of MEPPs in normal synaptic physiology is less clear. It has been suggested that the occurrence of MEPPs may play a trophic role in maintaining normal synaptic structure, since during synapse degeneration, normal MEPPs do not occur (Miledi and Slater, 1968; Colmeus et al., 1982; Muniak et al., 1982). The occurrence of MEPPs implies both that the release apparatus is functional and that the sensitivity of the postsynaptic membrane to transmitter is intact. Factors that change the sensitivity of the postsynaptic AChRs, such as receptor-blocking agents, will decrease the amplitude of the MEPP, whereas agents that facilitate flow of ions through the receptor-activated channel or agents that prolong the duration of action of ACh, such as inhibitors of acetylcholinesterase, will increase the amplitude of the MEPP. Presynaptically, chemicals that impair the synthesis or storage of ACh in synaptic vesicles will similarly alter the amplitude of MEPPs. For example, hemicholinium-3, which blocks high-affinity transport of choline into the cholinergic axon terminal, and vesamicol (AH 5183) (Marshall, 1970), which impairs active uptake of ACh by the cholinergic vesicle, both reduce the amplitude of MEPPs.

Minature end plate potentials occur randomly. Under normal conditions, their frequency of occurrence is approximately 0.5–2 MEPPs/s (Hz). While MEPPs are not induced by nerve stimulation, their frequency of occurrence is nevertheless increased by factors that increase the Ca^{2+} concentration within the nerve terminal cytosol (Del Castillo and Katz, 1954b; Hubbard et al., 1968). Thus agents that either increase the entry of Ca^{2+} (Kita and Van der Kloot, 1976; Kita et al., 1981) or release Ca^{2+} from internal bound stores (Baker and Crawford, 1975; Alnaes and Rahamimoff, 1975) can increase the frequency of occurrence of MEPPs. Consequently, following a train of high-frequency stimuli delivered to the nerve (tetanus), there is a subsequent transient increase in MEPP frequency (Liley, 1956b). This effect is known generically as post-tetanic potentiation, but detailed studies of the process and its dependence on divalent cations have revealed several kinetically unique components of this response (Magleby and Zengel, 1975; Zengel and Magleby, 1977, 1981, 1982). Study of the effects of chemicals on these processes has provided clues to the ways in which chemicals can disrupt presynaptic processes associated with mobilization of transmitter (Atchison, 1989a) as well as maintenance of Ca^{2+} homeostasis within the axon terminal (Traxinger and Atchison, 1987a).

Two abnormal forms of quantal release also occur. These are the so-called giant MEPPs as well as abnormally small MEPPs known as sub-MEPPs. The "sub-MEPPs" represent a class of very small MEPPS that are found in certain preparations and that give rise to a separate distribution of amplitudes (Kriebel et al., 1982). It has been proposed that this class of small MEPPs represents subunits of the basic quanta, with the typical MEPP being composed of an integral number of subunits. While this hypothesis has not been disproved, evidence has been obtained that at least partially refutes the hypothesis (Magleby and Miller, 1981). No other adequate hypothesis to explain the presence of "sub-MEPPs" has been proposed, although incompletely filled vesicles or quanta released from release sites not adjacent to active zones are superficially possible.

The other form of MEPP observed is known as a "giant MEPP" (Liley, 1956a). These responses, which are observed at a variable rate at normal neuromuscular junctions and occur in a modified form more frequently at junctions during certain poisoning conditions (botulinum toxin, dithiobiuret) (Thesleff et al., 1983; Alkadhi, 1989; Atchison, 1989a), differ in several important respects from the more typical MEPP. The frequency of occurrence of these giant MEPPs is typically unaffected by modification of the intracellular $[Ca^{2+}]$, as by depolarization, release of bound Ca stores, etc. (Molenarr et al., 1987).

In addition to quantal release of ACh, electrophysiological (Katz and Miledi, 1972, 1973) and biochemical studies indicate that motor nerve terminals can release ACh in a nonquantal form. The source of this nonquantal release is presumed to be the cytoplasmic stores of ACh. However, both nerve and muscle can leak ACh. Electrophysiologically, this nonquantal release of ACh is observed as a hyperpolarization produced by application of d-tubocurarine to neuromuscular junctions treated with an irreversible inhibitor of acetylcholinesterase. This form of release is somewhat Ca^{2+}-dependent and is also increased somewhat by K^+-induced depolarization. The hyperpolarization is absent in denervated muscle, suggesting that muscle is not the source of the nonquantal ACh. In neurochemical experiments, over 95% of the ACh release measured from the nerve terminal at rest is nonquantal and not associated with MEPPs.

The nicotinic AChR to which ACh binds following its release is an integral membrane protein consisting of five subunits. These are two α subunits and one each of β, γ or ϵ, and δ. The γ and ε subunits replace one another during different stages of development. The γ subunit is expressed in developing or denervated muscle, while the ε subunit is expressed in adult muscle (Mishina et al., 1986). The names of the subunits were chosen from the distance that they migrated on SDS polyacrylamide gels, with α having the highest mobility and δ the lowest (Steinbach and Ifune, 1989). The five subunits combine in such a manner as to form a transmembrane pore, through which the transmitter-activated conductance change occurs. In addition to forming the transmembrane pore, the subunits also contain the binding sites for ACh. These sites are located on the α subunits; thus each receptor-channel complex contains two binding sites for ACh.

Three types of nicotinic AChR exist. They include 1.) those on muscle and electric organ, which function as ACh-gated cation channels; 2.) neuronal receptors, which in ganglia have a role similar to that of the muscle receptors, but in the brain may act to modulate the presynaptic release of transmitter; and 3.) neuronal α-bungarotoxin (α-BGT) binding proteins, which do not appear to act as ligand-gated ion channels (these have been localized to extrasynaptic sites), and whose function is as yet unknown (Halvorsen and Berg, 1987). Neuronal AChRs are similar in size to muscle AChRs but consist of only two different subunit types. The 75- to 79-kDa subunit binds agonist and is similar to the muscle α subunit. The 49- to 51-kDa subunit is similar to the muscle β subunit (Berg and Halvorsen, 1988; Berg et al., 1989). A number of different α and β subunits have been identified in a variety of different neuronal tissues, including α2–5,7 and β2–4 (Lukas and Bencherif, 1992). Although most neuronal AChRs appear to consist of combinations of α and β subunits, recent studies indicate that the α7 subunit can form a homo-oligomeric channel that is blocked by α-BGT (Couturier et al., 1990a,b). Recent studies investigating the function of the α-BGT–binding component present on ciliary ganglion neurons have demonstrated that activation of these receptors by ACh increases intracellular calcium (Vijayaraghavan et al., 1992).

Binding of ACh to the receptors leads to the opening of receptor-associated ion channels. These channels open for several milliseconds and allow cations (primarily Na^+ into the muscle cell and K^+ out) to flow through them. A variety of other positively charged molecules have been found to pass through the channel but do not appear to contribute to the current under physiological conditions (Adams et al., 1980; Dwyer et al., 1980). At a normal resting membrane potential of approximately –90 mV, the predominantly inward cationic current leads to depolarization of the end plate region, or EPP. Under conditions in which the current flowing across the membrane, but not the voltage, is under control (current clamp), the EPP is observed as a rapid 1- to 3-ms depolarization followed by a slower (5 or more ms) exponential repolarization phase. By holding the membrane potential steady (voltage clamp) during action of transmitter, the end plate current (EPC) underlying the change in membrane potential can be studied. End plate currents recorded in this way have a rapid rise of 1 ms or less and a slower exponential decay of several milliseconds. Perhaps the most powerful tool for studying AChR channel behavior is patch voltage clamp. With this method, current flowing through single AChR channels can be studied.

Following binding of two ACh molecules to an AChR, the channel undergoes a burst of activity, during which time it opens and closes several times. Figure 1 displays a schematic model that describes binding of agonist and opening of channels for AChR channels (Jackson et al., 1983; Colquhoun and Sakmann, 1985a,b). Two agonist molecules (A_2) bind to the receptor (R), and the channel opens for a short time (A_2R^* represents the doubly liganded open channel) proportional to the rate constant α. Upon channel closing, one or both agonist molecules dissociate from the receptor, and the cycle can repeat. When

$$2A + R \quad \rightleftharpoons \quad AR + A \quad \rightleftharpoons \quad A_2R \quad \rightleftharpoons \quad A_2R^*$$

$$\downarrow$$

$$AR^*$$

Figure 1 Acetylcholine (ACh) binding scheme. A = agonist (ACh); R = ACh receptor; AR* = singly liganded open channel; A_2R^* = doubly liganded open channel.

single channel currents are examined with very-high-resolution data-analysis systems, most openings appear as a burst of channel openings separated by brief closures. It appears as though each burst of openings represented an oscillation between the closed A_2R state and the open A_2R^* state, in which the channel opens, closes, and reopens before the agonist molecule can dissociate. The results of Colquhoun and Sakmann (1985a) indicate that, on average, each long-duration opening observed contains two rapid closures when ACh is the agonist and four rapid closures when suberyldicholine (SCh_2) is the agonist. This model also can account for openings associated with the singly liganded AChR channel (AR*). These are normally observed at a low frequency because of the positive cooperativity of binding of agonist to the AChR. The AChR has a greater affinity (up to $100\times$) for binding of the second agonist molecule once one molecule is bound (Sine et al., 1990). If the distribution of channel openings is examined it is found to be described by the sum of two exponentials. The fast component represents brief channel openings, predominantly singly liganded complexes, while the slower component describes the open time for the doubly liganded channels. The open time for channels can also be determined from the exponential decay phase of EPCs.

Presynaptic Nicotinic Acetylcholine Receptors

In early studies in which the effects of curare on transmission were examined, changes in transmission were observed that appeared to represent presynaptic effects of curare on transmitter release. These early studies indicated that ACh appeared to act presynaptically to mobilize transmitter stores (feed-forward mechanism) and that curare blocked this effect, causing a decline in transmitter release during repetitive stimulation (Hubbard and Wilson, 1973; Glavinovic, 1979). Recently, more evidence has been provided that both nicotinic and muscarinic receptors are present presynaptically at the neuromuscular junction and that these receptors play a role in the modulation of transmitter release (Wessler, 1989; Bowman et al., 1990). There is still debate whether these receptors, if present, exert positive or negative feedback control over transmitter release (Storella and Bierkamper, 1990).

TOXIC AGENTS AFFECTING NEUROMUSCULAR FUNCTION BY PREDOMINANTLY PREJUNCTIONAL EFFECTS

Effects of Biological Toxins on Presynaptic Neuromuscular Function

Botulinum Toxin

"Botulinum toxin" is a generic term applied to a group of toxins produced by the bacterium *Clostridium botulinum.* Currently, eight different botulinum toxins have been identified:

types A, B, C_1, C_2, D, E, F, and G. The molecular pharmacology and biochemistry of botulinum toxins have been the subject of a number of excellent reviews (Simpson, 1981, 1986; Howard and Gundersen, 1980; Sakaguchi, 1983), and readers are referred to these for more detailed information.

One of the unique features of the botulinum toxins is their exquisite potency as blockers of neuromuscular transmission. Block is relatively rapid in onset, and if death does not occur, paralysis is long-lived. This has been examined best in hind limb preparations from rats in which botulinum toxin is administered locally to the hind limb. The reestablishment of normal transmission occurs because of reinnervation due to nerve sprouting (Duchen and Strich, 1968; Duchen, 1971).

The neuromuscular blocking effects have been studied most for botulinum toxin A (Simpson, 1978). Slight differences, especially in potency, have been reported for other serotypes of botulinum toxin, most notably type B (Sellin et al., 1983b). Specifically, botulinum toxin type B was reported to have a shorter duration of action than type A, and to be less effectively antagonized by potassium channel blockers than type A. Botulinum toxins type D and E were similarly reported to be less potent than type A (Harris and Miledi, 1971; Simpson and DasGupta, 1983; Sellin et al., 1983a).

The neurotoxicity of botulinum toxin is directed at neuromuscular function and is not apparent in the central nervous system (CNS). However, the size of the native toxin (~150 kDa) precludes its entry into the CNS through the blood-brain barrier. A number of studies have used isolated nerve endings from the brain (synaptosomes) to study the actions of botulinum toxin on central cholinergic nerve terminals. In these systems, the toxin has similar actions and affinities. Thus the action of botulinum toxin is directed at cholinergic nerve endings in general, but by virtue of its size, it is precluded from inducing central cholinergic dysfunction during intoxication.

The actions of botulinum toxin are directed at ACh secretion. The characteristic effects of the toxins are to reduce evoked release of ACh to virtually complete block. Thus, EPPs recorded at botulinum toxin–poisoned junctions are subthreshold and usually of very small amplitude. The effects of botulinum toxin on nonquantal release of ACh are more controversial. Spontaneous "leakage" of ACh from hind limb muscles or diaphragms of rats intoxicated with botulinum toxin A was reportedly reduced in concert with evoked release (Polak et al., 1981; Dolezal et al., 1983; Gundersen and Jenden, 1983). On the other hand, Stanley and Drachman (1981) reported that spontaneous nonquantal release of ACh from mouse diaphragm was unaffected by botulinum toxin.

Several investigators have reported that during the early stages of poisoning with botulinum toxins, small-amplitude MEPPs (sub-MEPPs) occur, resulting in a shift of amplitude histograms to the left (Harris and Miledi, 1971; Boroff et al., 1974; Kriebel and Gross, 1974). In addition, after several days of poisoning, a different class of MEPPs appear. These MEPPs have an amplitude that is frequently much higher than the mean "bell MEPPs" and occasionally approach amplitudes of up to 10 mV (Sellin and Thesleff, 1981; Thesleff et al., 1983; Kim et al., 1984). A more characteristic feature of these MEPPs was their slow rise time compared with MEPPs at unpoisoned junctions. The incidence of slow MEPPs increased 6–10 days after intoxication with botulinum toxin A and was different for soleus and extensor digitorum longus muscles (Kim et al., 1984).

Because of the ability of raising extracellular Ca^{2+} ($[Ca^{2+}]_e$) to overcome the reduction of quantal content induced by botulinum toxin (Gundersen et al., 1982), and because of the critical role that voltage-dependent Ca^{2+} channels play in the release process, a natural hypothesis was that botulinum toxin blocked Ca^{2+} influx through these channels. This hypothesis was disproved, however, by measurements of effects of botulinum toxin A on presynaptic membrane currents at mouse motor nerve terminals (Dreyer et al., 1983). In the presence of potassium channel blockers, currents associated with nerve terminal Ca^{2+} channels could be observed. Botulinum toxin A did not reduce the amplitude of these currents.

A three-step process has been proposed as underlying the actions of botulinum toxins on ACh release (Simpson, 1981). The three steps involved are binding of the toxin to a membrane receptor, internalization of the toxin, and interaction with a component in the release process.

The distinction between the binding of botulinum toxin and its paralytic action was first observed indirectly by Burgen et al. (1949) and Hughes and Whaler (1962). Burgen et al. (1949) noted that botulinum toxin became bound to rat diaphragm preparations before onset of paralysis, suggesting that binding of the toxin to a membrane receptor did not in and of itself induce toxicity. Hughes and Whaler (1962), in turn, observed that the onset of paralysis with botulinum toxin was influenced by nerve activity. That is, for a given concentration of toxin, onset of paralysis was more rapid when the nerve was stimulated frequently. Conversely, paralysis occurred after much longer latencies when the nerve was not stimulated. Subsequent studies that contributed to the notion of separateness of binding from toxicity showed that botulinum antitoxin could not antagonize paralysis induced by the toxin, but could prevent paralysis when present during the initial binding stages (Simpson, 1974). Thus, toxin still bound to the membrane surface would be exposed to the antitoxin, while toxin internalized would be refractory to the action of antitoxin.

Perhaps because it is only an initial step in the process, binding has not been studied as extensively as other components of the toxic process. Botulinum toxin exists as an active dichain molecule containing an intramolecular disulfide bond. The two chains are referred to as light and heavy. Evidence suggests that the heavy chain of the toxin molecule is responsible for the binding step. Addition of the heavy chain itself to a nerve-muscle preparation does not paralyze the preparation but does protect the preparation from paralysis due to the intact toxin molecule (Simpson, 1986). Thus, apparently, the heavy chain binds to the receptor and can occlude it from the native toxin. Although the specific binding site has not yet been identified with certainty, botulinum toxin has been shown to bind to gangliosides (Simpson and Rapport, 1971). Specifically, ganglioside G_{T1b} is most effective in inactivating the toxin (Kitamura et al., 1980), although this effect is somewhat dependent on the toxin serotype (Kozaki et al., 1984).

The second step in the process of botulinum toxin–induced neuromuscular dysfunction is internalization of the toxin molecule. The proposal that the toxin underwent an internalization step before inducing block was based on the observation that there was a marked difference in sensitivity of neuromuscular transmission to botulinum toxin depending on the temperature. Specifically, incubation of diaphragm preparations with toxin at 4°C resulted in the toxin's remaining accessible to a neutralizing antibody. On the other hand, if incubation occurred at more physiological temperatures, the toxin rapidly disappeared from accessibility to neutralizing antibody. Studies in isolated lipid membranes suggest that the heavy chain of botulinum toxin forms a pore through which a peptide such as the light chain may pass.

The third step in the poisoning process is the intracellular step. The extraordinary sensitivity of neuromuscular transmission to block by botulinum toxin implies a unique and long-lasting action. An enzymatic action has been proposed by Simpson (1981), although the exact nature of this proposed action was unclear. More recently, it has been suggested that botulinum toxin A acts in an adenosine triphosphate (ATP)-dependent manner on the release process at a step proximal to the actual Ca^{2+} trigger step in release. Since the botulinum toxins A–E light chains contain a binding site for Zn^{2+} (Binz et al., 1990a,b; Whelen et al., 1992; Hauser et al., 1990; Poulet et al., 1992), and since blocking activity of proteases slows the onset of activity of the toxin, a Zn^{2+} protease site on a component of the release apparatus has been proposed. Synaptobrevin I/II has been implicated as a potential substrate, since botulinum toxin B and tetanus toxin have both been shown to cleave synaptobrevin (Schiavo et al., 1992a,b; Link et al., 1992), and this cleavage was prevented by chelation of zinc. Synaptobrevin has been implicated in formation of a fusion pore between the synaptic vesicle and plasma membrane at the active zone.

Tetanus Toxin

Tetanus toxin is another highly potent toxin produced by a clostridial bacterium (*Clostridium tetani*). Like botulinum toxin, tetanus toxin binds to the presynaptic motor nerve terminal and disrupts the release of ACh (Duchen and Tonge, 1973; Habermann et al., 1980). Specifically, the frequency of MEPPs is reduced, and nerve-evoked release of ACh is blocked (Dreyer and Schmitt, 1983; Dreyer et al., 1984). However, there the similarity ends. No effect of tetanus toxin on nonquantal release of ACh has been reported, nor does it induce appearance of the large-amplitude, slow-rise-time MEPPs. Tetanus toxin is apparently transported retrogradely to the CNS, where it exerts its primary action, namely to block release of the inhibitory amino acid transmitters γ-aminobutyric acid and glycine, leading ultimately to a spastic form of paralysis.

The general pattern of effects of tetanus toxin action on the neuromuscular junction resembles that of botulinum toxin (Dreyer et al., 1984). For both toxins, the paralytic process involves the three-step sequence of binding, internalization, and block. Like botulinum toxin, tetanus toxin is believed to bind to gangliosides of the 1b group (VanHeyningen, 1974; Simpson, 1984a,b). Again like botulinum toxin, tetanus toxin does not block nerve terminal Ca^{2+} channels (Dreyer et al., 1983). Even though the two toxins are reported to block neuromuscular transmission by different paths (Gansel et al., 1987), tetanus toxin has been shown to interact with synaptobrevin in what appears to be a zinc-dependent manner, just as is the case for botulinum toxins (Schiavo et al., 1992a; Link et al., 1992).

Snake Venom Toxins

A number of snake venoms display neurotoxic effects. These are obviously most commonly expressed at the neuromuscular junction, as envenomation is almost always by the intramuscular route. The actions of these venom toxins can be divided into those occurring at presynaptic and at postsynaptic loci. The postsynaptically acting toxins characterized by the snake alpha toxins (α-BGT) will be considered below ("Effects of Toxins and Neurotoxicants That Act Through Predominantly Postjunctional Mechanisms"). These toxins have proved to be vital tools in characterizing, identifying, and isolating the nicotinic receptor for ACh.

Neurotoxins that block neuromuscular transmission by presynaptic actions are found in crude venom of many of the same species of snakes whose venom contains postsynaptic toxins (Datyner and Gage, 1973; Chang and Lee, 1977). The best known of these, and the first to be described, was β-bungarotoxin (β-BGT), from the snake *Bungarus multicinctus*. This toxin was shown to block neuromuscular transmission irreversibly by reducing ACh release (Chang and Lee, 1963; Chang et al., 1973). Other neurotoxins with similar presynaptic actions are notexin from the Australian tiger snake (*Notechis scutatus*) (Halpert and Eaker, 1975; Halpert et al., 1976), taipoxin from the Australian taipan (*Oxyuranus scutellatus*) (Oberg and Kelly, 1976; Fohlman et al., 1976), and a myotoxin from the Asian sea snake *Enhydrina schistosa* (Fohlman and Eaker, 1977). β-Bungarotoxin has a triphasic pattern of effects on ACh release. Initially, release is decreased. This is followed by a transient increase in release, with a subsequent progressive inhibition leading to block (Abe et al., 1976, 1977). Actions of β-BGT are not limited to the neuromuscular junction, but have also been demonstrated in the CNS (Halliwell and Dolly, 1982). However, much higher concentrations of the toxin are needed to alter transmitter release in the brain. Nevertheless, its actions in the peripheral nervous system are proposed as being specific for cholinergic neurons (Chapell and Rosenberg, 1992). Peripheral adrenergic terminals are unaffected by β-BGT (Kato et al., 1977; Miura et al., 1981).

The precise mechanisms underlying the various actions of β-BGT are not yet completely understood. Several snake venoms contain toxins with phospholipase A_2 activity. These include notexin, β-BGT, and taipoxin. There is considerable sequence homology among amino acids for β-BGT and other snake venom phospholipase A_2 enzymes (Verheij, 1981). It is proposed that snake venom phospholipase A_2 neurotoxins act by hydrolyzing membrane phospholipids (Strong, et al., 1976, 1977; Abe et al., 1977). However, a number of studies suggest that the phospholipase A_2 activity in itself does not explain the toxin's effects (Caratsch et al., 1981, 1985). For example, a potassium channel blocking action has also been reported for β-bungarotoxin (Dreyer and Penner, 1987). This effect occurs independently of the phospholipase activity and has been proposed as being responsible for the transient increase in ACh release. However, it is unclear how this action could be specific for peripheral cholinergic terminals, since potassium channels would be found on other terminals as well. The cause of the ultimate block of release of ACh by β-BGT and other phospholipase A_2–type neurotoxins is unknown. Several of the suggested mechanisms include inhibition of oxidative phosphorylation (Wernicke et al., 1975), inhibition of cytoskeletal phosphorylation (Ueno and Rosenberg, 1990), and cytoskeleton disruption (Sen et al., 1976). However, a recent report suggests that β-BGT inhibits phosphorylation of synapsin I in rat brain synaptosomes (Ueno and Rosenberg, 1992). Synapsin I, a neuronal phosphoprotein associated with synaptic vesicles (Huttner et al., 1983), has been implicated in moving vesicles from a reserve to a releasable pool near the active zones (Llinás et al., 1985).

α-*Latrotoxin*

The venom of the black widow spider (*Latrodectus mactans*) also causes profound effects on vertebrate neuromuscular transmission (Clark et al., 1970, 1972; Ceccarelli et al., 1979). The syndrome is characterized by excessive cholinergic activity and is now known to be due to presynaptic effects of the venom, especially on the peripheral motor and autonomic nerve terminals. Inasmuch as these are markedly different from those caused by any other known group of toxins, the venom and its constituents have been a major tool in studying the dynamics of ACh release, as well as its origin (Gorio et al., 1978a).

α-Latrotoxin is the main protein component of the venom of the black widow spider (Frontali et al., 1976). The protein has a molecular weight of approximately 130 kDa and is thought to be responsible for all the major effects caused by the venom on the neuromuscular junction. The potency of the peptide is very high; effects are observed at isolated synapses in the 10^{-10} M range. The actions are not limited to the neuromuscular junction and are generalizable to all synapses thus far tested. Effects are also observed in the secretory cell pheochromocytoma cell line PC12 (Grasso et al., 1980). When the purified toxin or crude venom is applied to the neuromuscular junction, it induces a dramatic increase in MEPP frequency that eventually progresses to complete block of junctional transmission and depletion of synaptic vesicles (Clark et al., 1970, 1972). Thus, α-latrotoxin acts by greatly increasing the probability of vesicle fusion with the presynaptic membrane yet simultaneously appears to inhibit recycling of synaptic vesicles. The actions of the toxin are focused at the active zones, those sites at which transmitter release is thought to occur specifically; vesicle fusions do not occur randomly throughout the presynaptic terminal. The ultrastructure (Ceccarelli et al., 1979), resting membrane potential (Longenecker et al., 1970; Kawai et al., 1972), and sensitivity of postsynaptic membrane to neurotransmitter (Okamoto et al., 1971) are not significantly affected by black widow spider venom.

The effects of α-latrotoxin are temperature-dependent. When it is applied to mouse diaphragm bathed in solutions lacking divalent cations, no increase in MEPP frequency was observed at room temperature (presumably 22–25°C), whereas increasing the temperature to 35°C caused a normal toxin-induced increase in MEPP frequency to occur (Gorio and Mauro, 1978).

A peculiar aspect of the action of α-latrotoxin is that its effect is not blocked by high-potency clostridial toxins (botulinum, tetanus), which block ACh release (Cull-Candy et al., 1976; Figliomeni and Grasso, 1985). Thus the clostridial neurotoxins and α-latrotoxin have unique receptors, and the α-latrotoxin receptor appears to be "downstream" from the site of action of botulinum and tetanus toxin.

The actions of the venom are not reversed by prolonged washing of the preparation with toxin-free solution (Gorio and Mauro, 1978) but are prevented by preincubation of neuromuscular preparations with antivenin. Moreover, application of antivenin at the time of peak increase in MEPP frequency returns the frequency to control levels even 1 hour after treatment (Longenecker et al., 1970).

It has been suggested that α-latrotoxin acts in a dual manner to increase vesicular release of ACh at the neuromuscular junction, increasing cation permeability as well as directly bypassing the Ca^{2+}-dependent step (Gorio et al., 1978b).

The actions of black widow spider venom are not limited to peripheral motor nerve terminals, or even to cholinergic neurons. Since application of α-latrotoxin to isolated lipid membranes causes a pronounced increase in membrane cationic conductance (Finkelstein et al., 1976), early suggestions were made that α-latrotoxin increases MEPP frequency by increasing entry of Na^+ or Ca^{2+} into the nerve terminal. However, the venom stimulates MEPP frequency, blocks neuromuscular transmission, and depletes synaptic vesicles even in solutions deficient in Na^+ and Ca^{2+} (Gorio and Mauro, 1978; Gorio et al., 1978b). An observation that is consistent with an increase in cation permeability within the nerve terminal is swelling of some nerve terminals. Increased surface area of the terminal membrane was explained as being due to incorporation of vesicle membrane into the plasma membrane; however, increased terminal volume could not be explained in this way. In the absence of sodium in the extracellular medium, nerve terminal swelling in response to α-latrotoxin was not pronounced, suggesting that an increase in permeability to Na^+ was responsible for the nerve terminal swelling. More recently, the possibility that α-latrotoxin alters membrane cation permeability has been explored in more detail in isolated cells with patch voltage clamp techniques. α-Latrotoxin activates inward currents that cannot be blocked with tetrodotoxin, a potent blocker of voltage-gated Na^+ channels, or verapamil, which blocks a variety of different types of Ca^{2+} channel (Wanke et al.,

1986). The channels appear not to discriminate between Na^+ and K^+. A specific binding receptor for α-latrotoxin has been demonstrated in frog motor nerve terminals with immunofluorescence (Valtorta et al., 1984). Isolated nerve terminals from the brain (synaptosomes) also contain the α-latrotoxin receptor (Scheer and Meldolesi, 1985). Affinity of the toxin for this receptor is in the same range as the potency of the toxin in blocking neuromuscular transmission. Furthermore, reconstitution of α-latrotoxin receptors into liposomes causes Ca^{2+} transport in the presence of the toxin, whereas the toxin alone does not induce transport in receptor-deficient liposomes (Scheer et al., 1986). Taken together, these results are consistent with the hypothesis that the α-latrotoxin receptor is not only a binding site for the toxin, but actually participates in part of the toxin-mediated response. In this respect the action of α-latrotoxin differs from that of the clostridial neurotoxins.

Recent studies have characterized an α-latrotoxin–binding protein that is the putative receptor in the brain (Petrenko et al., 1990, 1991). The receptor appears to belong to a family of neuronal cell surface proteins known as the neurexins (Ushkaryov et al., 1992). It has been suggested that one of these proteins, neurexin Iα, is localized specifically to synapses, and in particular to the presynaptic membrane (Ushkaryov et al., 1992), and this localization is the same as that of the putative α-latrotoxin receptor (Valtorta et al., 1984). This receptor has been shown to interact with synaptotagmin, an integral membrane protein of synaptic vesicles thought to play a role in exocytotic fusion of the vesicle with the membrane (Brose et al., 1992). This has led to the proposal that perhaps α-latrotoxin causes transmitter release by a direct interaction with synaptotagmin, bypassing the normal Ca^{2+}-dependence (Petrenko et al., 1991; Hata et al., 1993).

In summary, it is believed that α-latrotoxin blocks neuromuscular transmission by two effects. One effect involves an ionophoric-like action to increase cationic conductances, while the other is independent of $[Ca^{2+}]_e$ and remains undefined, but may involve interactions with synaptic vesicle–specific proteins involved in the secretory process.

Miscellaneous Toxins

Because of the dependence of the EPP on functional conduction of normal nerve action potentials, any chemical that prevents or impairs excitation of the nerve terminal will impair neuromuscular function. Thus a number of toxins that alter invasion of the action potential into the nerve terminal by actions on sodium or potassium channels, or agents that prevent Ca entry by action on calcium channels, will disrupt neuromuscular transmission.

Several natural toxins that interact specifically with Ca^{2+} channels have been isolated from venom preparations. A family of polypeptide toxins with Ca^{2+}-channel activity has been isolated from venom of marine snails of the genus *Conus* (Olivera et al., 1987). ω-Conotoxin GVIA, isolated from the venom of *Conus geographus* (Olivera et al., 1985), is a potent inhibitor of nonmammalian Ca^{2+} channels, binding irreversibly in subpicomolar concentrations (Cruz and Olivera, 1986) and inhibiting neuromuscular transmission in the frog (Kerr and Yoshikami, 1984; Sano et al., 1987). In mammalian preparations, the actions of ω-conotoxin GVIA are less clear. This peptide does not block normal neurotransmitter release at the neuromuscular junction (Anderson and Harvey, 1987; Sano et al., 1987; Protti et al., 1991), suggesting that there may be differences in the Ca^{2+} channels at different terminal types or that the peptide may not gain access to certain nerve endings. In conotoxin-sensitive preparations, differential effects of ω-conotoxin were noted for the "N" and "L" types of Ca^{2+} channel (Nowycky et al., 1985). The L-type current was insensitive to ω-conotoxin, while the N current was resolved into a component blocked irreversibly by conotoxin and one blocked reversibly (Abe et al., 1986; McCleskey et al., 1987; Fox et al., 1987; Sano et al., 1987). More recently, other components of *Conus* toxins have been isolated. A fraction from the venom of *Conus magnus* known as conotoxin MVII-C is reported to inhibit the conotoxin GVIA-insensitive fraction of Ca channels present in mammalian synaptosomes and Purkinje cells (Hillyard et al., 1992). If the channel types present in these preparations are similar to those found at the mammalian neuromuscular junction, one would predict that this peptide might block mammalian neuromuscular transmission by virtue of its ability to block the Ca^{2+} channels responsible for transmitter release. Maitotoxin, which is produced by the marine dinoflagellate *Gambierdiscus toxicus*, activates Ca^{2+} channels in cultured neuronal cells (Takahashi et al., 1982, 1983) and therefore would be expected to increase evoked release of ACh at the neuromuscular junction. Spider venoms also contain peptides and polyamines that block Ca^{2+} channels. The ω-agatoxins have been isolated from the venom of the funnel-web spider (*Agelenopsis aperta*) and are potent blockers of Ca^{2+} channels (Adams et al., 1990; Mintz et al., 1992) and perhaps of mammalian neuromuscular transmission, although this apparently has not been tested directly. A polyamine toxin (FTX) that blocks Ca^{2+} channels has been purified from the venom of funnel-web spiders (Llinàs et al., 1989). Several synthetic compounds with similar activities although markedly reduced potency have been synthesized. Synthetic FTX and native venom from *Agelenopsis aperta* both block mammalian neuromuscular transmission (Uchitel et al., 1992). ω-Agatoxin and FTX have been shown to bind to the P class of Ca^{2+} channels, which are insensitive to both dihydropyridine-type blockers and ω-CgTx (Llinàs et al., 1989; Mintz et al., 1992).

Similarly, toxins that interact with voltage-gated sodium or potassium channels will also affect neuromuscular transmission. The classic sodium channel blockers tetrodotoxin and saxitoxin both block nerve evoked release of ACh and hence junctional transmission by blocking depolarization of the terminal subsequent to entry of sodium. However, as shown in the elegant work of Katz and Miledi (1967b, 1969a), this is the only effect that blocking Na entry has on junctional transmission, since focally induced depolarization of the terminal, *even in the absence of a regenerative action potential invasion*, still can elicit a normal EPP. Thus the basic process of ACh release is not dependent per se on Na entry. From this, it stands to reason that toxins such as tetrodotoxin and saxitoxin would have no prominent effect on resting MEPP amplitude or frequency. This is the case, although a slight reduction in MEPP frequency may be observed. The converse effect, activation of sodium channels by toxins such as batrachotoxin (Albuquerque et al., 1971; Albuquerque and Warnick, 1972), *Veratrum* alkaloids such as veratridine, or certain *Gymnodinium* (red tide) (Atchison et al., 1986b) or scorpion venoms, will have prominent effects on both resting and evoked release of ACh. Because these compounds prolong the open state of the Na^+ channel, they increase the duration of depolarization at the nerve terminal. This has the subsequent effect of keeping the voltage-gated Ca^{2+} channels in the terminal open for a longer time, which enhances Ca entry. Consequently, MEPP frequency is increased dramatically.

Several snake, insect, and arthropod venoms contain additional toxins that can block voltage-gated potassium channels. Included in this category is dendrotoxin, a component of the venom of *Dendroaspis angusticeps* (Harvey and Gage, 1981; Harvey and Karlsson, 1982; Halliwell et al., 1986) and charybdotoxin, from *Leiurus quinquestriatus* (Miller et al., 1985). As mentioned previously, at least one component of the action of β-BGT also consists of K^+ channel block. By virtue of their ability to block potassium efflux during the repolarization phase of the action potential, these toxins prolong the duration of depolarization and thus increase Ca^{2+} entry. This results in an increased EPP amplitude due to increased release of transmitter.

Antibiotics.   Neuromuscular block is a well-documented result of the use of antibiotics of the aminoglycoside, tetracycline, lincosamide, and polymyxin classes (for review see Pittinger and Adamson, 1972; Sander and Sanders, 1979; Sokoll and Gergis, 1981). Block is observed in both clinical and experimental situations (Caputy et al., 1981; Dunkley et al., 1973; Durant and Lambert, 1981; Farley et al., 1982; Fiekers, 1981, 1983a,b; Fiekers et al., 1983; Lee et al., 1977; Singh et al., 1978, 1979, 1982; Uchiyama et al., 1981; Vital-Brazil and Prado-Franceschi, 1969a,b; Wright and Collier, 1976a,b, 1977). This effect has been characterized in most detail for the aminoglycosides, but other antibiotics such as clindamycin, lincomycin, and polymyxin B have also been investigated. Despite the myriad studies describing antibiotic-induced neuromuscular block, the precise mechanisms by which block occurs are poorly understood. Antibiotics are reported to have both presynaptic and postsynaptic actions (Pittinger and Adamson, 1972; Sander and Sanders, 1979). Mechanisms proposed as being involved in antibiotic-induced block include 1.) diminished release of ACh from the motor nerve terminal in response to motor nerve stimulation, 2.) decreased sensitivity of the postjunctional ACh receptor due to competitive block, and 3.) decreased conductance through the ACh receptor–activated ionic channel due to block of the channel. Each of these factors alone would theoretically be sufficient to reduce the amplitude of the postsynaptic depolarization, the EPP, below the threshold necessary to evoke a muscle action potential. Hence, the contraction of the skeletal muscle would be blocked. For a particular antibiotic, neuromuscular block may involve any or all of these mechanisms. For some antibiotics (neomycin, streptomycin, and clindamycin), the prejunctional block appears to predominate at low doses while postjunctional block occurs at high doses (Fiekers, 1983a,b; Fiekers et al., 1983). For others (lincomycin and perhaps polymyxin B), postjunctional block is thought to be more dominant (Fiekers, 1981; Fiekers et al., 1983). Several thorough studies have examined the relative contribution of presynaptic and postsynaptic effects of neomycin, streptomycin (Farley et al., 1982; Fiekers, 1983a,b), and the lincosamides as a function of concentration (Fiekers et al., 1983), but for the most part, detailed studies of mechanisms responsible for the presynaptic effects of these and other antibiotics are lacking.

It is proposed that the predominant mechanism of neuromuscular block by amino-glycosides in general and neomycin in particular is presynaptic decrease in release of ACh due to competitive block of Ca^{2+} entry into the presynaptic nerve terminal during nerve stimulation (for review see Sander and Sanders, 1979). Diminished ACh release into the bath fluid has been demonstrated in tissue bath studies using isolated hemidiaphragms (Vital-Brazil and Prado-Franceschi, 1969a,b). Voltage clamp studies using transected muscle fibers of garter snake showed that neomycin and streptomycin caused a concentration-dependent reduction in EPC amplitude at concentrations that did not reduce miniature end plate current (MEPC) amplitude (Fieckers, 1983a,b). Neomycin was approximately ten times as potent as streptomycin in reducing evoked quantal release of ACh. This marked reduction in quantal content (m) was relieved in a competitive fashion by increasing the bath $[Ca^{2+}]$.

Blocking concentrations of polymyxin B also reduce m (Durant and Lambert, 1981) but not to as great an extent as do the aminoglycosides. The slope of the log Ca^{2+} concentration vs. log m relationship was similar for polymyxin B, magnesium, and aminoglycosides (Singh et al., 1979). It was suggested that this observation supports the notion that polymyxin B also competes prejunctionally with Ca^{2+} for entry into the nerve terminal through ionic channels.

In studies of the binding of ^{125}I-labeled ω-conotoxin GVIA, a putative blocker of N-type Ca^{2+} channels in some species (Dooley et al., 1987; Olivera et al., 1985, 1987; Reynolds et al., 1986), in the absence and presence of various antibiotics, aminoglycosides and polymyxin B were able to inhibit binding of the toxin to brain membrane fragments with IC_{50}s in the low-micromolar range (<25 μM) (Knaus et al., 1987). Other antibiotics tested, for which no measurable neuromuscular blocking capability has been reported, were ineffective at inhibiting conotoxin GVIA binding at concentrations up to 1 mM. With the exception of polymyxin B, which partially inhibited binding of labeled dihydro-pyridine-like drugs to putative L-type Ca^{2+} channel binding sites, none of the other antibiotics, including the aminoglycosides, affected binding at these sites or those labeled by desmethoxyverapamil (Knaus et al., 1987). These antibiotics also block the depolar-ization-dependent uptake of $^{45}Ca^{2+}$ into isolated nerve terminals from the brain (synap-tosomes) via pathways associated with voltage-dependent Ca^{2+} channels (Atchison et al., 1988). This effect occurs at concentrations that block transmitter release at the neuro-muscular junction.

Effects of Heavy Metals on Neuromuscular Transmission

Mercury and Methylmercury

Mechanistic studies designed to examine early effects of methylmercury have focused on effects of methylmercury on synaptic transmission. In part because of its well-characterized physiology, microscopic anatomy, and biochemistry, and in part because of the reported increased incidence of neuromuscular weakness in the Iraqi poisoning episode (Rustam et al., 1975), a number of studies have focused on the effects of inorganic and organic mercurials on the vertebrate neuromuscular junction. In isolated nerve-skeletal muscle preparations, acute bath application of mercuric chloride and methylmercuric chloride caused a time-dependent block of twitches evoked by electrical stimulation of the motor nerve (Von Burg and Landry, 1976; Juang, 1976a). Responses evoked by direct stimulation of the muscle were less affected, or unaffected. Thus these mercurials acted either to impair conduction of the nerve action potential or to disrupt synaptic transmission directly, or both. Muscle contractility measured in situ from the gastrocnemius of rats treated acutely (10 mg/kg/day s.c., 7 days) or subchronically (2 mg/kg/day, s.c., 5 days/week for 3–4 weeks) with methylmercury was diminished in comparison with pair-fed controls (Somjen et al., 1973). Both tension of individual twitches and tetanic tension were reduced. Twitches in response to direct electrical stimulation of the gastrocnemius-soleus were not measured, so it is impossible to determine whether the observed reductions were due to direct effects of methylmercury on skeletal muscle or effects on the motor nerve impulse or neuromus-cular junction. However, these results signify that effects of methylmercury on skeletal muscle contractility occur not only with direct bath application, but also at periods of 2–10 days following systemic application of the toxicant. These studies have provided the basis for further experimentation on effects of mercurials on synaptic transmission.

More recent studies using conventional intracellular microelectrode recording tech-niques have clarified the effects of mercurials on neuromuscular transmission. In the frog sartorius muscle (Manalis and Cooper, 1975; Juang, 1976b; Cooper and Manalis, 1983) and rat (Atchison and Narahashi, 1982; Atchison et al., 1984a) and mouse diaphragm (Atchison et al., 1984a) the primary effect of both divalent inorganic mercury and methylmercury is to decrease nerve-evoked release of ACh and increase, then decrease, spontaneous quantal release.

At the time of EPP block, MEPPs of normal amplitude and duration still occur (Atchison and Narahashi, 1982). In every instance in which it was tested, block of nerve-evoked transmitter release by inorganic or organic mercury could not be reversed by washing the preparation with mercury-free solutions (Atchison and Narahashi, 1982; Traxinger and Atchison, 1987b).

Effects of inorganic mercury and methylmercury on nerve-evoked transmitter release are time-dependent although not strictly concentration-dependent. Higher concentrations reduce the time required to produce an effect. At low concentrations of mercurials (0.1–10 μM) complete block of the EPP was not seen for 60 min or more (Manalis and Cooper, 1975; Juang, 1976b); concentrations of 20–100 μM methylmercury virtually completely blocked nerve-evoked postsynaptic responses between 5 and 30 min (Atchison and Narahashi, 1982; Atchison et al., 1986a; Traxinger and Atchison, 1987b). The decline in EPP amplitude was progressive with time, proceeding to complete block. Thus, block of the EPP does not attain a steady state short of complete block. For this reason, a strict concentration-dependence does not occur. There appears to be a lower threshold concentration below which block of evoked release does not occur (Atchison and Narahashi, 1982), but this may simply reflect the fact that the latent period to produce block at these concentrations was longer than the period over which the measurements were made and that the effect was missed. Thus, it is not possible to state unequivocally that there is a threshold concentration of mercury needed to block evoked transmitter release.

A transient increase in EPP amplitude that precedes the block of the EPP has been reported for both inorganic mercury and methylmercury. This effect occurred after 10–20 min of exposure to the mercurial (Manalis and Cooper, 1975; Juang, 1976b; Binah et al., 1978; Cooper and Manalis, 1983) and lasted 10–35 min. For example, Manalis and Cooper (1975) reported that at the frog neuromuscular junction inorganic mercury (1–10 μM) first increased EPP amplitude to 50 times the control values before subsequently depressing it. Juang (1976b) reported a similar phenomenon with 10 μM methylmercury but did not observe any such effect with 10 μM HgCl$_2$. Atchison and Narahashi (1982) observed a slight though statistically insignificant stimulatory effect of 4 μM methylmercury on the EPP at the rat motor end plate but no stimulation at 20 or 100 μM. Similar stimulatory effects of methylmercury have been observed on transmission at autonomic ganglia (Juang and Yonemura, 1975) and in hippocampal slices (Yuan and Atchison, 1993). It may be that at these higher concentrations, transmission block occurs too rapidly to permit stimulation of evoked release to be observed.

A number of different investigators (Juang, 1976b; Binah et al., 1978; Atchison and Narahashi, 1982) have reported that the effects of methylmercury and HgCl$_2$ on mean EPP amplitude paralleled those on mean quantal content (m), indicating that a predominant component of mercurial-induced block of synaptic transmission was due to presynaptic effects. Further analysis of statistical parameters of neurotransmitter release indicated that the depression of m produced by methylmercury was due primarily to depression of the immediately available store of neurotransmitter (n) (Atchison and Narahashi, 1982), an index of an intracellular action of the metal on the release process. The probability of transmitter release (p) was actually increased by methylmercury (Atchison and Narahashi, 1982). Release parameters have not been examined in the presence of divalent inorganic mercury.

Block of the EPP by mercurials appears initially to be independent of external Ca^{2+}

concentration. Increasing the bath concentration of Ca^{2+} from 2 mM to 4 or 8 mM did not prolong the time to block of the EPP or decrease the degree of block produced by methylmercury (Atchison et al., 1986a). However, the effect is somewhat complicated by the fact that methylmercury impairs axonal conduction, albeit at high concentrations (Shrivastav et al., 1976; Traxinger and Atchison, 1987b; Shafer and Atchison, 1992). Nonetheless, once an increase in membrane excitability is induced, then raising the Ca^{2+}_e concentration *can* cause partial reversal of effects of methylmercury on EPP amplitude (Traxinger and Atchison, 1987b). This suggests that there are complex effects of at least methylmercury on both membrane excitability and Ca^{2+}-dependent ACh release. A Ca^{2+} channel blocking action of methylmercury was demonstrated by block of Ca^{2+} entry during K^+-induced depolarization of isolated nerve terminals (synaptosomes) derived from rat forebrain (Atchison et al., 1986a; Shafer and Atchison, 1989) and of voltage-dependent Ca^{2+} currents in PC12 cells (Shafer and Atchison, 1991).

The effects of mercurials on spontaneous transmitter release are biphasic with continued exposure. The time course for effects on MEPP frequency differs from that observed for effects on the EPP amplitude. Initially, MEPP frequency is increased from control values of 0.3–3.0/s to frequencies of 10–100/s in the frog, rat, and mouse (Barrett et al., 1974; Juang, 1976b; Atchison and Narahashi, 1982; Miyamoto, 1983; Atchison et al., 1984a). This effect usually occurred following a latency of 2–40 min, depending on the concentration of mercury employed. Binah et al. (1978) and Cooper and Manalis (1983) reported that $HgCl_2$ increased MEPP frequency immediately upon exposure, but this has not been reported by others. The latent period can be cut dramatically by depolarizing the preparation using elevated extracellular K^+ (15–20 mM) (Miyamoto, 1983; Atchison, 1986). The increase in spontaneous release does not appear to be concentration-dependent. That is, similar frequencies are produced by concentrations of 10–100 μM. Reports vary as to whether $HgCl_2$ is more or less potent than methylmercury; Miyamoto (1983) reported that $HgCl_2$ increased MEPP frequency at a threshold concentration of 3 μM compared with 100 μM for methylmercury, while Binah et al. (1978) reported that $HgCl_2$ was more potent than the organomercurial mersalyl. On the other hand, Juang (1976b) showed that $HgCl_2$ and methylmercury at 10 μM were approximately equally effective in increasing MEPP frequency at the frog end plate but that $HgCl_2$ was less effective than methylmercury in stimulating transmitter release at isolated guinea pig ganglia (Juang and Yonemura, 1975). In the latter case, increased spontaneous release of ACh was also seen when mercury was given systemically as opposed to by bath application (Juang and Yonemura, 1975).

With continued bath application of mercurials, spontaneous transmitter release declines until eventually no further MEPPs can be recorded. Block of spontaneous release by methylmercury is not due to depletion of vesicular neurotransmitter stores, because treatment of the preparation at the time that MEPPs disappeared with $LaCl_3$, which is a profound stimulator of spontaneous release (Heuser and Miledi, 1971), was able to induce high frequencies of MEPPs (Atchison, 1986). Moreover, since normal-appearing MEPPs were evoked by La^{3+}, and since ACh depolarizations were normal at the time that spontaneous release ceased (Atchison and Narahashi, 1982), diminished postsynaptic sensitivity to ACh does not seem to account for the block of spontaneous release.

The increased MEPP frequency associated with mercurials is not prevented either by blocking the axon membrane Na^+ channels with tetrodotoxin (Atchison and Narahashi, 1982; Miyamoto, 1983) or by blocking membrane Ca^{2+} channels with high concentrations of Mg^{2+} (Atchison and Narahashi, 1982) or Co^{2+} (Miyamoto, 1983). Simultaneous block of both Na^+ and Ca^{2+} channels prevents the increase in MEPP frequency associated with

HgCl$_2$ but not that associated with methylmercury (Miyamoto, 1983). The implication is that inorganic mercuric ions can enter the nerve terminal through both Na$^+$ and Ca^{2+} channels. Methylmercury, on the other hand, may enter the cell not only through the channels but also directly through the membrane because of its increased lipophilicity. The latent period preceding increased MEPP frequency can be shortened dramatically by facilitation of Ca^{2+} entry into the axon terminal (Atchison, 1986, 1987) or in the presence of increased [Ca^{2+}]$_e$ (Atchison, 1986) as well as prolonged when the preparation is deficient in Ca^{2+} (Atchison, 1986). However, the increase in spontaneous release is not dependent on [Ca^{2+}]$_e$, because increases in MEPP frequency still occur with methylmercury in the absence of Ca^{2+} or in Ca^{2+}-deficient solutions (Atchison, 1986). The shortened latency obtained with a Ca^{2+} ionophore, a Ca^{2+} channel agonist, and depolarization are consistent with the notion that the latency is related at the time required for methylmercury to enter the nerve terminal and elevate intracellular Ca^{2+} ([Ca^{2+}]$_i$) (Atchison, 1987). Results in Ca^{2+}-deficient and Ca-free solutions suggest that [Ca^{2+}]$_i$ stores may be the source of increased Ca^{2+} responsible for the increased MEPP frequency. The ability of mitochondria to release Ca^{2+} in respone to methylmercury has been implicated in the increase in MEPP frequency (Levesque and Atchison, 1987, 1988, 1990). However, whether this is the only contributor, or even a major contributor, remains to be seen.

An explanation compatible with both the decreased evoked release of transmitter and the increased spontaneous release of transmitter by methylmercury is nerve terminal depolarization. Depolarization decreases the effectiveness of the presynaptic action potential in eliciting transmitter release (Hubbard and Willis, 1968; Krnjevic and Miledi, 1959). Conversely, depolarization opens membrane Na$^+$ and Ca^{2+} channels, increasing cation influx and provoking large increases in spontaneous release (Liley, 1956b). Methylmercury depolarizes the plasma membrane of guinea pig (Kauppinen et al., 1989) and rat brain synaptosomes (Hare and Atchison, 1992), but whether this is the only mechanism or even a major contributor is unclear.

Theoretically, blocking effects of mercurials on stimulus-evoked release of ACh at the neuromuscular junction could be due to either presynaptic or postsynaptic effects, but the results of measurements of MEPP amplitudes taken at the time of depressed EPP amplitude have indicated in general no significant effect of mercurials (Atchison and Narahashi, 1982; Miyamoto, 1983; Atchison et al., 1984a). Juang (1976b) noted a slight decrease in mean MEPP amplitude with 40 μM HgCl$_2$ and a slight increase with 40 μM methylmercury, but the magnitude of these changes was small. In view of the fact that the postsynaptic processes responsible for both the MEPP and the EPP are identical (i.e., receptor-agonist binding, receptor activation, ionic channel opening with resulting postsynaptic conductance changes; see Hubbard et al., 1969; Katz, 1969), a lack of effect of mercury on MEPP amplitude suggests that there is no significant postsynaptic blocking effect of mercurials at the time the EPP is blocked. This, coupled with the measurements of statistical release parameters, implies that the block of synaptic transmission is primarily presynaptic.

Iontophoretic application of exogenous ACh to the motor end plate of mercurial-poisoned preparations was used to test unequivocally for direct effects of mercurials on the AChR (Manalis and Cooper, 1975; Atchison and Narahashi, 1982). End plate depolarizations due to ACh are not decreased in amplitude by concentrations of mercurials as high as 100 μM or for periods of exposure of up to 60 min, by which time MEPPs are no longer observed. Thus, at the motor end plate, mercurials appear to produce few postsynaptic effects. In contrast to this, other experiments have indicated that mercurials do affect the postsynaptic membrane. For example, iontophoretic application of the organomercurial p-chloromercuribenzoate depolarized the postsynaptic membrane of the electric ray *Torpedo electroplax* in a manner similar to ACh and carbachol (del Castillo et al., 1972). These findings contrast with several biochemical studies indicating that methylmercury decreases the binding of cholinergic agonists to nicotinic (Eldefrawi et al., 1977) receptors. The apparent lack of effect of mercurials on the postsynaptic membrane at the neuromuscular junction is puzzling given the well-known affinity of inorganic and organic mercurials for sulfhydryl groups. The ACh receptor is known to contain sulfhydryl groups, whose modification leads to decreased affinity of the receptor to cholinergic agonists (Karlin and Bartels, 1966). Presumably, methylmercury should interact with the sulfhydryl groups to modify the ACh receptor and decrease the postsynaptic response to ACh.

Lead

Because of the interest in lead as an environmental neurotoxicant, it was one of the first agents whose effects on synaptic function were examined, and it is one of the most widely studied of the heavy metals. Since the neurotoxic effects of lead are not directed specifically at the neuromuscular junction, this is a classic example of use of this synapse to study more generalized effects of toxicants on synaptic function.

The pivotal report in this area was that of Manalis and Cooper (1973), in which for the first time intracellular microelectrode recording techniques were brought to bear to examine the effects of a suspected environmental neurotoxicant on synaptic transmission at the frog neuromuscular junction. A pattern of effects of Pb^{2+} was observed that is now recognized as being similar to that of a number of toxic heavy metals. That is, Pb^{2+} first decreased the amplitude of the EPP and then increased the frequency of occurrence of MEPPs. Both effects occurred in a concentration-dependent manner and were observed in the micromolar range, and both could be reversed by washing out the Pb^{2+} from the bathing solution. Differences in the time course of the effects of Pb^{2+} on the EPP and MEPPs led to the conclusion that the effects were mediated by distinct actions. Iontophoretic application of ACh to the end plate in the presence of 100 μM Pb^{2+} induced normal depolarizing responses of amplitude similar to that of responses elicited in Pb^{2+}-free solutions, implying a lack of postjunctional effect on the muscle nicotinic receptors. Subsequent studies revealed that Pb^{2+} had a similar spectrum of effects on the mammalian neuromuscular junction (Pickett and Bornstein, 1984; Atchison and Narahashi, 1984a).

In more recent studies, Cooper and Manalis (1983, 1984a,b; Manalis et al., 1984) examined the Ca-dependence of the effect of Pb^{2+} on the EPP. Varying the Ca concentration caused the amplitude of the EPP to increase. Addition of 1 μM Pb^{2+} caused a parallel shift of the concentration-response curve to the right, indicating that Pb^{2+} was a competitive antagonist to Ca^{2+} in the release process. A similar competitive relationship was observed, though not examined in as rigorous a quantitative fashion, at the rat neuromuscular junction (Atchison and Narahashi, 1984). One major difference between the mammal and amphibian preparations was that much higher concentrations of lead were needed to block transmission at rat neuromuscular junctions. The rapid, reversible nature of the interaction between lead and Ca^{2+} led to the proposal that block of the EPP occurs because of a Ca^{2+} channel–blocking effect of lead. This hypothesis was strengthened by the observation that Pb^{2+} blocked uptake of ^{45}Ca into nerve terminals isolated from the CNS (synaptosomes) (Suszkiw et al., 1984) and more recently by the demonstration of block of Ca^{2+} channels in isolated neural cell somas by Pb^{2+} (Reuveny and Narahashi, 1991; Evans et al., 1991).

In contrast to the inhibitory effect of Pb^{2+} on the EPP, spontaneous release as measured by MEPP frequency was increased dramatically by Pb^{2+}. As was the case with methylmercury, the effects on the two forms of release differed dramatically in their time courses. Increase of MEPP frequency by Pb^{2+} occurred after a latent period that presumably reflected the time necessary for Pb^{2+} to enter the axon terminal. This hypothesis was tested in a set of studies in which the ability of Cd^{2+} to block the action of Pb^{2+} on MEPP frequency was examined (Cooper and Manalis, 1984b).

Extracellular Ca^{2+} is not necessary for Pb^{2+} to increase MEPP frequency (Atchison and Narahashi, 1984; Kolton and Yaari, 1982). This led to the speculation that Pb^{2+} releases Ca^{2+} from bound intracellular stores, thereby increasing the free $[Ca^{2+}]_i$. This hypothesis remained a major tenet until the recent startling observation that Pb^{2+} can substitute for Ca^{2+} as a secretagogue in isolated chromaffin cells (Shao and Suszkiw, 1991). Whether this also occurs at the neuromuscular junction is unknown, but there is no reason a priori to expect that it will not. This would have profound implications for the basic process of transmitter release, especially with regard to the Ca-dependent substrates.

Effects of Other Heavy Metals on Neuromuscular Transmission

Other polyvalent cations besides lead and mercury also affect neuromuscular transmission. The principal effect is to block evoked transmitter release. This effect has been described for magnesium (del Castillo and Engbaek, 1954; Jenkinson, 1957); manganese (Balnave and Gage, 1973); cobalt (Weakly, 1973; Kita and Van der Kloot, 1973); lanthanum (Kajimoto and Kirperkar, 1972); cadmium (Forshaw, 1977; Cooper and Manalis, 1984a); nickel (Kita and Van der Kloot, 1973); praseodymium (Alnaes and Rahamimoff, 1974); zinc (Benoit and Mambrini, 1970), thallium (Wiegand et al., 1984a), gadolinium (Molgó et al., 1991), triethyltin (Allen et al., 1980), and erbium (Metral et al., 1978). Strontium is an exception in that it supports evoked release, although it is much less effective than equimolar concentrations of Ca^{2+} in generating an EPP (Miledi, 1966; Dodge et al., 1969; Meiri and Rahamimoff, 1972). Barium has an unusual effect on evoked release; it cannot support normal phasic evoked release but instead produces an asynchronous discharge of quanta, detectable as MEPPs, following nerve stimulation (Silinsky, 1977a,b, 1978a,b). Despite inhibition of evoked release, spontaneous transmitter release is stimulated by all of these polyvalent cations; this is evidenced by an increase in MEPP frequency (Anwyl et al., 1982; Cooper et al., 1984; Cooper and Manalis, 1984a; Nishimura, et al., 1984; Wiegand, 1984; Wiegand et al., 1984a,b; Nishimura, 1988; Wang and Quastel, 1990). Thus these other cations affect the neuromuscular junction in a manner very similar to that of Pb^{2+} and methylmercury. The mechanisms responsible for the effects of these divalent and trivalent cations are assumed to be on two distinct sites: block of entry of Ca^{2+} through membrane Ca^{2+} channels and displacement of intracellular Ca^{2+} stores. The ability of several of these polyvalent cations to block influx of Ca^{2+} through voltage-dependent membrane Ca^{2+} channels has been demonstrated (Baker et al., 1971; Kostyuk and Krishtal, 1977; Nachshen, 1984; Fox et al., 1987; Evans et al., 1991). It is this effect that is thought to be responsible for block of nerve-evoked transmitter release. This block is thought to be competitive and can be antagonized by higher concentrations of Ca^{2+} (Balnave and Gage, 1973; Kober and Cooper, 1976; Atchison and Narahashi, 1982). However, for at least thallium, Ca^{2+} channel block *is not* thought to be the mechanism responsible for block of the EPP (Wiegand et al., 1990). The metal is then postulated to gain entry to the nerve terminal, presumably through the same Ca^{2+} channels, and act intraterminally to increase spontaneous release. This notion is supported by studies in which, following substitution of Ni^{2+}, Mn^{2+}, or Mg^{2+} for Ca^{2+}, increased spontaneous release is produced by these cations under conditions that facilitate entry of the cation into the nerve terminal, such as depolarization (Kita et al., 1981), use of Ca^{2+} ionophores (Kita and Van der Kloot, 1976), or repetitive stimulation (Hurlbut et al., 1971; Kita and Van der Kloot, 1973; Kita et al., 1981).

Other Agents Affecting Neuromuscular Transmission by Presynaptic Effects

Dithiobiuret

2,4-Dithiobiuret (DTB) is a substituted thiourea derivative that produces a delayed-onset, flaccid neuromuscular weakness in rats (Astwood et al., 1945; Atchison and Peterson, 1981; Atchison et al., 1981b). Exposure to DTB does not appear to be a common toxicological problem, as the chemical is not widely used. On the other hand, DTB appears to produce a purely motor-directed neurodysfunction; sensory systems do not appear to be significantly affected (Atchison and Peterson, 1981; Crofton et al., 1991). In this regard, DTB is uniquely different from other chemicals inducing delayed onset neurotoxicity, with the sole exception of botulinum toxin. Muscle weakness induced by DTB typically requires accumulation of a threshold toxic dose as well as a minimum time of exposure to cause manifestation of the syndrome (Atchison et al., 1981b). When treatment is stopped, rats can recover apparently normal motor function in 4–10 days. The time course and severity of DTB-induced paralysis can be altered chemically. Daily treatment of rats with the sulfur-containing chelators d-penicillamine (d-PEN), disulfiram, or diethyldithiocarbamate (DEDTC) can protect them from DTB-induced paralysis (Williams et al., 1986). Moreover, rats paralyzed by DTB recover in approximately 2–7 days if, on the first day of paralysis, DTB treatment is supplemented by treatment with d-PEN or DEDTC. The mechanism responsible for protection against and reversal of DTB-induced paralysis is not known, but it does not appear to entail altered distribution or bioavailability of DTB (Williams et al., 1986).

A neuromuscular deficit is thought to be responsible for this weakness, as twiches of skeletal muscles isolated from rats affected by DTB are reduced in amplitude or blocked when elicited by electrical stimulation of the motor nerve, but not when elicited by direct stimulation of the muscle itself (Atchison et al., 1981a). A host of non-neural side effects are associated with DTB-induced paralysis, including decreased food and water intake, body weight loss, diuresis, and chromodacryorrhea (periorbital secretion of porphyrin-containing pigments from the harderian gland) (Atchison and Peterson, 1981a). However, extensive studies of potentially causative non-neural actions in inducing the neuromuscular weakness caused by DTB have failed to provide evidence that non-neural effects of DTB, such as thyroid dysfunction, electrolyte imbalance, or hypoxia cause or modulate this effect (Williams et al., 1987). Furthermore, DTB-induced motor dysfunction is not due to peripheral neuropathy (Williams et al., 1987). No systematic studies have yet been undertaken to ascertain whether DTB also affects CNS function.

Pharmacological investigations of the reductions in twitch tension induced by DTB suggested a prejunctional locus of action (Atchison et al., 1982b). This possibility was later tested in more detail using more definitive methods. Results of intracellular microelectrode recording studies indicate that both nerve-evoked and spontaneous release of ACh from motor nerve terminals is depressed in muscles taken from rats affected by DTB (Weiler et al., 1986; Atchison, 1989a). End plate potentials and MEPPs were recorded from single junctions of extensor digitorum longus (EDL) muscles isolated from male rats treated for 6–7 days with 1mg/kg/day i.p. of DTB or with 0.9% NaCl (1 ml/kg/day) as control. Paresis induced by DTB was associated with a diminished quantal content (m) (Atchison, 1989a).

This effect was attributed to a reduction of the immediately available store and not of the probability of release. Since the magnitude of reduction was similar for all frequencies of stimulation employed, no frequency-dependent fatigue was evident in evoked quantal release in the DTB-intoxicated group. However, as the stimulus frequency was increased, preparations from DTB-treated rats were characterized by failures of nerve impulses to elicit an EPP. Increasing $[Ca^{2+}]_e$ improved transmission in the DTB-poisoned group, but did not restore quantal release to control levels (Atchison, 1989a). Similarly, when Ca^{2+} influx into the axon terminal was facilitated with 4-aminopyridine, m was again increased in both groups, but evoked release was not restored to control levels in the DTB-poisoned group. When MEPPs were evoked by elevating $[K^+]_e$, the mean peak frequency was lower for DTB-treated rats. Thus asynchronous evoked release was also disrupted at DTB-affected junction. In the absence of a depolarizing stimulus, mean MEPP frequency was reduced significantly for the DTB-treated rats compared with controls. The DTB-paralyzed preparations were characterized by the presence of very large MEPPs (giant MEPPs) with prolonged rise and decay (Atchison, 1989a). Thus, paralysis induced by chronic DTB treatment is associated with impairment of presynaptic processes resulting in a diminution of the number of quanta liberated spontaneously and in response to motor nerve stimulation.

Differential muscle sensitivity occurs in a number of neuromuscular diseases and presumably is due to regional differences in transmission at junctions of different striated muscles, including different numbers of ACh receptors and different amounts of ACh released following motor axon stimulation. Differential muscle sensitivity associated with neuromuscular depression caused by DTB was examined using both the EDL muscle and the hemidiaphragm of male rats treated for 7–8 days with DTB 1 mg/kg/day, i.p., or with 0.9% NaCl (1 ml/kg/day) as control (Atchison, 1990). Decreased EPP amplitude associated with decreased m was observed in EDLs at the time of observable muscle weakness in DTB-treated rats. Conversely, analysis of quantal content of the EPPs from hemi-diaphragms of these treated rats indicated no difference from control. In hemidiaphragm preparations that were exposed to solutions containing elevated Mg^{2+} and lowered Ca^{2+} concentrations, motor nerve stimulation in DTB-poisoned rats was associated with decreased quantal content as compared with similarly treated control preparations. A lower peak frequency of MEPPs was evoked by K^+-induced depolarization in Mg^{2+}-treated DTB diaphragms as compared with control. Both mean MEPP frequency and MEPP amplitude were altered in Mg^{2+}-treated diaphragms of the DTB-treated group. Regardless of whether low Ca^{2+}/high Mg^{2+} solutions were used, diaphragms from treated rats exhibited pro-longation of decay times of synaptic potentials. The DTB-paralyzed preparations were also frequently characterized by the presence of very large MEPPs with prolonged decay times. Thus, differential muscle sensitivity is associated with paralysis induced by chronic DTB treatment and appears to be associated with the safety factor for ACh release. This reflects an impairment of presynaptic processes resulting in a diminution of the number of quanta liberated after motor nerve stimulation.

Whereas paralysis is produced reliably following chronic administration of DTB, acute application of the compound at doses far in excess of those needed to cause paralysis when given chronically does not cause paralysis (Atchison and Peterson, 1981). On the other hand, acute administration of DTB at high concentrations in an isolated bath, or by acute injection in rats, causes alterations of both EPPs and MEPPs that mimic those observed in rats treated chronically with DTB (Spitsbergen and Atchison, 1990). When neuromus-cular transmission was examined in rat hemidiaphragms taken 1 h following exposure to a single large dose of DTB, EPP amplitude and MEPP frequency and amplitude were all decreased, and rise and decay rates for both MEPPs and EPPs were prolonged. By 4, 8, and 24 h after treatment, these values, with the exception of rise and decay rates, returned toward control levels. Bath application (either 200 μM or 1.85 mM) of DTB to diaphragms taken from previously untreated rats initially increased EPP amplitude, MEPP amplitude, and MEPP frequency, but with continued exposure EPP amplitude decreased to below control levels. Block of EPPs occurred after approximately 10 or 37 min of exposure to 1.85 mM or 200 μM DTB, respectively. Frequency of MEPPs also decreased with continued exposure to DTB yet remained above control levels for the duration of DTB exposure. Bath application of DTB also slowed rise and decay rates of MEPPs and EPPs. Thus, a single large dose of DTB initially induces neuromuscular effects similar to those observed in rats paralyzed following chronic treatment with DTB, but these effects tend to reverse by 24 h after exposure. Bath exposure to high concentrations of DTB causes early effects on transmission, some of which mimic those seen in the paralyzed rat. These results correlate well with the earlier studies demonstrating cumulative dose and latency thresholds for the onset of DTB-induced muscle weakness (Atchison et al., 1981b), possibly indicating that DTB levels must be maintained in the rat for a given period of time to allow the early effects to progress to a more generalized muscle weakness observed with chronic dosing.

A curious aspect of the neurotoxicity of DTB is the observation that at high daily doses apparent refractoriness to the paresis occurs (Williams et al., 1992). Thus, increasing the daily dose of DTB in rats from 0.5 to 1 and 5 mg/kg shortened from 7 to 5 and 3 days, respectively, the latency to onset of treadmill failure, associated flaccid muscle tone, and reductions in gastrocnemius muscle contractions elicited by nerve stimulation; however, rats given 12 mg/kg of DTB for 3 days did not exhibit treadmill failure, flaccid skeletal muscle tone, or tetanic fade. Additional treatment with this dose for 2–3 days was required to produce treadmill failure, which was not accompanied by flaccid muscle tone but appeared to be associated closely with the moribund state of the rats before their death, which generally ensued within 24 h. Refractoriness to development of toxicity with DTB was limited in its spectrum; other non-neural effects of DTB occurred in the absence of flaccid muscle tone. Disposition of DTB-derived [^{14}C] determined 3 h after injection of ^{14}C-DTB (12 mg/kg) was unaffected by prior treatment with unlabeled DTB (12 mg/kg/day × 2 days). Electrophysiological studies using end plates of EDL muscles indicated that increased amplitude and frequency of occurrence and prolonged decay of MEPPS and decreased quantal content occurred after 5mg/kg/day but not 12 mg/kg/day of DTB (Williams et al., 1992).

Pathological examination of motor nerves and end plates using zinc iodide–osmium staining technique reveals striking changes in end plate morphology before and during development of neuromuscular weakness with DTB (Jones, 1989). By 3 days after initiation of treatment with DTB, rat neuromuscular junctions are characterized by changes in overall shape of the nerve terminal ("clumped," "globular," "string of beads") and by sprouting (Kemplay, 1984). Ultrastructurally, the earliest detected changes (24 h) include a swelling of Schwann cell processes, a separation of their myelin lamellae, and distended elements of rough endoplasmic reticulum. On day 2 an increase in smooth endoplasmic reticulum is seen within the nerve terminal, and by the third day of treatment, some terminals have abnormal accumulations of synaptic vesicles, abnormal mitochondria, a flocculent material next to the presynaptic membrane, and tangled intermediate filaments. In the preterminal axons, tubulovesicular profiles concentrate at the nodes of Ranvier. By the fourth day of treatment, changes in size of synaptic vesicles are seen, with an increase in dense-cored and coated vesicles, and Schwann cell processes are interposed between the postsynaptic muscle and the presynaptic membrane. Localization of Ca^{2+} in DTB-treated terminals, as measured with oxalate-pyroantimonate precipitation, is decreased, suggesting that DTB reduces the cytoplasmic "free" Ca^{2+} pool (Jones, 1989). The structural changes occurring in the later phases of DTB treatment include many features that are similar to those seen in a variety of situations in which neuromuscular junctions are diseased or degenerating. In fact, some of the later changes may be secondary and in response to dysfunction: retraction of the terminal, interposition of Schwann cell processes into the cleft, clumping of vesicles, and sprout formation are associated with other forms of degeneration (Birks et al., 1960; Miledi and Slater, 1968). Swelling of Schwann cells and changes in the myelin layer may be the basis for the increased number of failures to evoke an EPP at high stimulus frequencies (Atchison, 1989a) in DTB-paralyzed rats if there is conduction failure in the preterminal axonal branches.

The earlier changes, the swelling of glial cell processes, the increase in profiles of smooth and rough endoplasmic reticulum, and the appearance of an electron-dense flocculent material adjacent to the presynaptic active zone may reflect more direct actions of DTB resulting in the immediate decrease in transmitter release seen after acute application.

Whereas DTB clearly affects prejunctional aspects of neuromuscular transmission, its potential to disrupt postjunctional aspects is less clear. Evidence suggests that DTB may have additional postjunctional effects, inasmuch as rise and decay rates for MEPPs and EPPs are slowed at the time of muscle weakness (Atchison, 1989a). To determine whether an effect of DTB on current flow at the neuromuscular junction is related to the muscle weakness observed following DTB treatment, end plate currents (EPCs) and miniature end plate currents (MEPCs) were recorded, using two-microelectrode voltage clamp, in hemidiaphragm preparations from rats paralyzed with DTB and from rats given a single, nonparalytic dose of DTB (Spitsbergen and Atchison, 1991). Amplitude of EPCs was decreased both in muscles from rats paralyzed following 7 days of DTB treatment and in muscles from rats 1 and 24 h following a single large dose of DTB. Associated with the decrease in EPC amplitude was a decrease in quantal content both in muscles removed 24 h following a single dose of DTB and in muscles from rats paralyzed with DTB. Mean MEPC amplitude was unaffected by DTB treatment, but the frequency of abnormally large slow MEPCs was increased in muscles from chronically treated rats and at both 1 and 24 h following a single large dose of DTB. The decay time constant (τ) for EPCs was actually decreased as compared with control 24 h following a single DTB dose. The decay time constant for MEPCs was greater in muscles from DTB-treated rats compared with controls, but if the abnormally large slow MEPCs are not included in the calculation of τ, then τ is smaller in treated muscles compared with controls. Thus, exposure to DTB affects current flow at the neuromuscular junction, but the observed prolongation of MEPP and EPP rise and decay times cannot be explained by these effects (Spitsbergen and Atchison, 1991).

Hexanedione

Several solvents including methyl *n*-butyl ketone (MBK) and *n*-hexane induce a peripheral neuropathy through the common metabolite 2,5-hexanedione (Spencer and Schaumburg, 1975; DiVincenzo et al., 1976). Potential neuromuscular toxicity during the early stages of intoxication with 2,5-hexanedione was examined following administration of the toxicant to rats for up to 34 days (Cangiano et al., 1980). A number of fibers from the treated rats lacked EPPs as a result of denervation. In the denervated myofibers, no change was observed in resting membrane potential until the end of the 34-day treatment regimen. At earlier periods (14 days), MEPP frequency and amplitude of both soleus (a "slow-twitch" muscle) and EDL (a "fast-twitch" muscle) were increased. Mean quantal content (m) was reduced significantly in EDL but not soleus muscles. Cangiano et al. suggested that inhibition of glycolytic enzymes was responsible for the differences in sensitivity of fast- and slow-twitch fibers, and that this inhibition ultimately led to depolarization of the myofibers and increased MEPP frequency.

EFFECTS OF TOXINS AND NEUROTOXICANTS THAT ACT THROUGH PREDOMINANTLY POSTJUNCTIONAL MECHANISMS

By studying how chemicals, toxins, and other agents alter EPPs, EPCs, or single channel currents, information can be obtained concerning the mechanism of action by which these chemicals affect the neuromuscular junction.

Agents that alter or prevent the action of ACh at its receptors can be classified into two broad categories. Agents in one category compete with ACh for binding sites on the receptor complex (competitive antagonists), while the other category includes agents that bind irreversibly to ACh-binding sites or act at different sites from ACh to alter its effectiveness as an agonist (noncompetitive antagonists). In addition, there are a variety of ways in which the behavior of the AChR channel complex can be altered by these agents. First, compounds can bind to the same sites on the receptor as ACh and prevent ACh from exerting its effects. Second, they can bind to regions other than those to which ACh binds and alter the receptor's affinity for ACh. Third, these agents can chemically modify the ACh receptor region, to alter the affinity of the receptor for ACh. Finally, agents can bind to the channel portion of the receptor channel complex and alter the ionic conductance without altering the binding of ACh to the receptor.

Competitive Inhibition

Curare (*d*-tubocurarine), a quaternary alkaloid found in several species of South American plants, is probably the best-known of the neuromuscular blocking agents. Curare acts as a nondepolarizing competitive antagonist at ACh receptors. It binds to nicotinic AChRs, preventing ACh from binding and activating the receptor channel complex (Taylor, 1985). At the whole-cell level curare acts to decrease the amplitude of EPPs or EPCs, while decreasing the frequency of single channel currents. Recent reports, however, indicate that curare also has effects on channel conductance and may activate ACh channels in some preparations (Jackson et al., 1982; Strecker and Jackson, 1989). In addition, there have been numerous reports indicating prejunctional effects of curare, presumably on presynaptic nicotinic receptors (Hubbard and Wilson, 1973; Bowman et al., 1990).

α-Bungarotoxin is a polypeptide toxin purified from venom of the snake *Bungarus multicinctus*. This toxin binds to postjunctional nicotinic AChRs, causing a nondepolarizing block that is essentially irreversible. Binding of α-BGT to AChRs is antagonized to some extent by treatment with cholinesterase inhibitors or nicotinic agonists. Block of neuromuscular transmission by α-BGT occurs on a slower time course than that of curare; however, block by curare is readily reversible, while that of α-BGT is not. α-Bungarotoxin blocks transmission at junctions from eel electric organ but does not act presynaptically or block ganglionic transmission. The fact that α-BGT binds irreversibly to the binding sites for ACh has made it an important tool for the characterization and isolation of neuromuscular-type nicotinic AChRs.

Toxin F, BGT 3.1, and κ-bungarotoxin are all the same molecole. This toxin binds to two sites on ganglionic neurons. One site, which is also recognized by α-BGT, is dispersed over the cell body. Binding to this site does not affect ACh response. The second toxin binding site is not recognized by α-BGT and is localized to regions of synaptic contact (Loring and Zigmond, 1987). Binding to synaptic sites blocks responsiveness to ACh. The concentration of AChR at synaptic regions appears to be 20 times lower on neurons than on muscle cells.

Noncompetitive Inhibition

A number of agents exert effects on AChR function by interacting with the AChR at sites different from those at which ACh binds. Several noncompetitive inhibitors, such as histrionicotoxin (HTX), phencyclidine, and the local anesthetics, bind to the channel portion of the AChR (Sine and Taylor, 1982; Papke and Oswald, 1989). Block by several of these compounds is more effective in the presence of agonist, indicating that they bind preferentially to the open channel. In addition to blocking the AChR-channel, HTX, phencyclidine, and the local anesthetics increase the affinity of the AChR for ACh, leading to an increase in the rate of desensitization.

Chemical Modification of the Nicotinic Receptor

Previous studies have demonstrated the presence within the receptor region of the AChR channel complex of disulfide bonds that are critical to normal function (Karlin and Winnik, 1968; Rang and Ritter, 1971). Reduction of disulfides present on the receptor, with the reducing agent dithiothreitol (DTT), decreases the responsiveness to ACh, while reoxidation, with the oxidizing agent 5,5′-dithio-bis (2-nitrobenzoate) (DTNB), reverses these effects when examined in *Torpedo electroplax* preparations (Karlin and Winnik, 1968) and chick muscle (Rang and Ritter, 1971). Walker et al. (1981) examined both agonist binding and ion flux in membrane-bound vesicles containing AChRs from *T. electroplax*. They observed that reduction of the receptors with DTT decreased the binding affinity of AChRs for carbamylcholine (CCh) and shifted the dose-response curve for CCh-induced increases in $^{22}Na^+$ permeability to higher CCh concentrations. Effects of thiol-group modification on ion flux activation and inactivation kinetics were examined further by Walker et al. (1984). In these studies, CCh binding and ^{86}Rb influx into vesicles with reconstituted AChR channels purified from *Torpedo californica* were measured before and after reduction with DTT. Results of these studies demonstrated that the main effect of DTT reduction was to shift the EC_{50} values for activation and slow inactivation to higher agonist concentrations. These findings are consistent with a decrease in binding affinity for CCh previously described by this group. More recently Berstein et al. (1988) examined the effects of DTT and DTNB on muscarinic AChRs purified from pig brain. They observed that in the presence of DTT the afinity for muscarinic ligands was decreased without alteration of the total number of binding sites. Electrophysiological studies performed on muscles exposed to DTT have demonstrated that following exposure to DTT the amplitude and decay times for EPPs and MEPPs were decreased (Ben-Haim et al., 1973; Terrar, 1978). Studies using fluctuation analysis demonstrated that following reduction of AChRs with DTT, the time for which single channels remain open and the conductance for these channels are decreased (Ben-Haim et al., 1975). Thus reduction of critical disulfide groups located on the AChR leads to a decrease in affinity of the receptor for agonist, and associated with reduction is a decrease in single-channel conductance and open time. Oxidation or sulfonation (Steinacker and Zuazaga, 1981, 1987) of the postjunctional nicotinic receptor also cause alterations of decay kinetics of the EPP or EPC.

Lophotoxin, a coral toxin, is an uncharged molecule that reacts covalently with the AChR to block the agonist-recognition site. Previous reduction of cysteine groups in the binding region followed by alkylation prevents the activity of this toxin (Abramson et al., 1988). Lophotoxin reduces the amplitude of nerve-evoked EPCs as well as spontaneously occurring MEPCs (Atchison et al., 1984b).

Chemicals That Induce Channel Block

Many compounds block the AChR channel following its opening. All of the agonist molecules tested thus far block the channel (Ogden and Colquhoun, 1985; Sine and Steinbach, 1984). Moreover, agents such as *d*-tubocurarine, thought of as classical receptor blockers, also block the ion channel (Colquhoun et al., 1979; Strecker and Jackson, 1989), although not necessarily at the same concentrations as those at which they induce receptor block. In addition, a variety of other charged and uncharged molecules (Neher and Steinbach, 1978; Ogden et al., 1981; Neher, 1983) also appear to block the channel physically. During open-channel block, effects on both macroscopic (i.e., EPCs and MEPCs) and single-channel currents can be observed that are very characteristic for this mechanism. In the presence of compounds that can block open channels, the single-channel currents exhibit very characteristic bursts of activity. These bursts represent a single channel opening and becoming blocked and unblocked in rapid succession, followed by channel closure. The effects on EPCs and MEPCs of open-channel block are observed as a biphasic decay of the current. In the presence of open-channel blockers, the normal number of ion channels open following release of transmitter into the synaptic cleft. Thus the initial amplitude of the current is normal. Soon after opening, a portion of the channels become blocked. This leads to a very rapid initial decay of the current. The prolonged phase results from channels' becoming unblocked over time and allowing current to flow through them before their final closure (Adams and Sakmann, 1978; Lambert et al., 1980).

The lincosamide antibiotics and their analogues also act to block open ACh channels. Clindamycin interacts to produce a fast, single exponential decay for EPCs, while lincomycin produces a double exponential decay. Clindamycin is the more lipophilic of these molecules and thus has a substantially slower unblocking rate, leading to the single exponential decay of currents. Both agents decrease EPC amplitude as a result of fast blockade of open channels, but clindamycin also acts presynaptically to reduce quantal content, an effect that is only weakly dependent on external calcium (Prior et al., 1990).

Cholinesterase Inhibition

Following its initial release and binding to receptors, further action of ACh is prevented by the presence of the enzyme acetylcholinesterase (AChE). This enzyme, which has an extremely high turnover rate for ACh, is also present in very high concentrations within the synaptic cleft (Cooper et al., 1982). This combination leads to the removal of presynaptically released ACh from the synaptic cleft within a few hundred microseconds. In most cases, transmitter is released from the nerve terminal, diffuses across the synaptic cleft, binds a single time to receptors on the postsynaptic membrane, leading to channel opening, and then upon unbinding from the receptor is broken down very rapidly by AChE. Inhibition of AChE, by a variety of agents, leads to an increase in the amplitude and a prolongation of rise and decay times of synaptic potentials (Eccles and MacFarlane, 1949; Katz and Miledi, 1975; Laskowski and Dettbarn, 1979). Cholinesterase inhibition also leads to pathological alterations in skeletal muscles that can be observed as early as 30 min following AChE exposure and progress to encompass up to 7% of muscles in the body with chronic drug administration (Gwilt and Wray, 1986). Following 30 min of exposure to paraoxon (an irreversible cholinesterase inhibitor), mitochondria located within end plate regions of muscle become dilated, sarcoplasmic reticulum is increased, subsynaptic folds become widened and fused, and there is an increase in coated cleft vesicles. Twenty-four hours following exposure to paraoxon, muscle fiber architecture displays a generalized disruption and there is an accompanying infiltration of phagocytes (Wecker et al., 1978).

Addition prejunctional effects have been described for some inhibitors of AChE. Within 30 min following paraoxon exposure, evoked release of transmitter is blocked, while MEPP frequency is increased and rise and decay times for MEPPs are prolonged (Laskowski and Dettbarn, 1975, 1979). Acetylcholinesterase from *T. electroplax* has been shown to contain on its catalytic subunit a single free sulfhydryl group that can react with a number of sulfhydryl reagents. Modification of this group by thiol reagents has been found to inactivate the enzyme (Steinberg et al., 1990).

ACKNOWLEDGMENTS

The authors' work was supported by NIH grant NS20683.

The authors gratefully acknowledge the secretarial assistance of Robyn Bruining, Lisa Byrd, and Amy Verleger.

REFERENCES

Abe T, Alema S, Miledi R (1977). Isolation and characterization of presynaptically acting neurotoxins from the venom of *Bungarus* snakes. Eur J Biochem 80:1–12.

Abe T, Koyano K, Saisu H, Nishiuchi Y, Sakakibara S (1986). Binding of ω-conotoxin to receptor sites associated with the voltage-sensitive calcium channel. Neurosci Lett 71:203–8.

Abe T, Limbrick AR, Miledi R (1976). Acute muscle denervation by β-bungarotoxin. Proc R Soc Lond (Biol) 194:545–53.

Abramson SN, Culver P, Kline T, Li Y, Guest P, Gutman L, Taylor P (1988). Lophotoxin and related coral toxins covalently label the α-subunit of the nicotinic acetylcholine receptor. J Biol Chem 263:18568–73.

Adams ME, Bindokas VP, Hasegawa L, Venema VJ (1990). ω-Agatoxins: novel calcium channel antagonists of two subtypes from funnel web spider toxin (*Agelenopsis aperta*) venom. J Biol Chem 265:861–7.

Adams DJ, Dwyer TM, Hille B (1980). The permeability of endplate channels to monovalent and divalent metal cations. J Gen Physiol 75:493–510.

Adams PR, Sakmann B (1978). Decamethonium both opens and blocks end-plate channels. Proc Natl Acad Sci USA 75:2994–8.

Albuquerque EX, Warnick JE, Sansone FM (1971). The pharmacology of batrachotoxin. II. Effect on electrical properties of the mammalian nerve and skeletal muscle membranes. J Pharmacol Exp Ther 176:511–28.

Albuquerque EX, Warnick JE (1972). The pharmacology of batrachotoxin. IV. Interaction with tetrodotoxin on innervated and chronically denervated rat skeletal muscle. J Pharmacol Exp Ther 180:683–97.

Alkadhi K (1989). Giant miniature end-plate potentials at the untreated and emetine-treated frog neuromuscular junction. J Physiol (London) 412:475–91.

Allen JE, Gage PW, Leaver DD, Leow ACT (1980). Triethyltin depresses evoked transmitter release at the mouse neuromuscular junction. Chem Biol Interact 31:227–31.

Alnaes E, Rahamimoff R (1974). Dual action of praseodymium (Pr^{3+}) on transmitter release at the frog neuromuscular synapse. Nature 247:478–9.

Alnaes E, Rahamimoff R (1975). On the role of mitochondria in transmitter release from motor nerve terminals. J Physiol (London) 248:285–306.

Anderson AJ, Harvey AM (1987). ω-Conotoxin does not block the verapamil-sensitive calcium channels at mouse motor nerve terminals. Neurosci Lett 82:177–80.

Anwyl R, Kelly T, Sweeney F (1982). Alterations of spontaneous quantal transmitter release at the mammalian neuromuscular junction induced by divalent and trivalent ions. Brain Res 246:127–32.

Astwood EB, Hughes AM, Lubin M, VanderLaan WP, Adams RD (1945). Reversible paralysis of motor function in rats from the chronic administration of dithiobiuret. Science 102:196–7.

Atchison WD (1986). Extracellular calcium dependent and independent effects of methylmercury on spontaneous and potassium-evoked release of acetylcholine at the neuromuscular junction. J Pharmacol Exp Ther 237:672–80.

Atchison WD (1987). Effects of activation of sodium and calcium entry on spontaneous release of acetylcholine induced by methylmercury. J Pharmacol Exp Ther 241:131–9.

Atchison WD (1989a). Alterations of spontaneous and evoked release of acetylcholine during dithiobiuret-induced neuromuscular weakness. J Pharmacol Exp Ther 249:735–42.

Atchison WD (1989b). Dihydropyridine-sensitive and -insensitive components of acetylcholine release from rat motor nerve terminals. J Pharmacol Exp Ther 251:672–8.

Atchison WD (1990). Reduced safety factor for neuromuscular transmission precedes onset of neuromuscular weakness with 2,4-dithiobiuret. Toxicol Appl Pharmacol 106:234–44.

Atchison WD, Adgate L, Beaman CM (1988). Effects of antibiotics on uptake of calcium into isolated nerve terminals. J Pharmacol Exp Ther 245:394–401.

Atchison WD, Clark AW, Narahashi T (1984a). Presynaptic effects of methylmercury at the mammalian neuromuscular junction. In: Narahashi T, ed. Cellular and molecular neurotoxicology. New York: Raven Press, 23–43.

Atchison WD, Joshi U, Thornburg JE (1986a). Irreversible suppression of calcium entry into nerve terminals by methylmercury. J Pharmacol Exp Ther 238:618–24.

Atchison WD, Lalley PM, Cassens RG, Peterson RE (1981a). Depression of neuromuscular function in the rat by chronic 2,4-dithiobiuret treatment. Neurotoxicology 2:329–46.

Atchison WD, Mellon WS, Lalley PM, Peterson RE (1982b). Dithiobiuret-induced muscle weakness in rats: evidence for a prejunctional effect. Neurotoxicology 3:44–54.

Atchison WD, Narahashi T (1982). Methylmercury-induced depression of neuromuscular transmission in the rat. Neurotoxicology 3:37–50.

Atchison WD, Narahashi T (1984a). Mechanism of action of lead on neuromuscular junctions. Neurotoxicology 5:267–82.

Atchison WD, Narahashi T, Vogel SM (1984b). Endplate blocking actions of lophotoxin. Br J Pharmacol 82:667–72.

Atchison WD, SM O'Leary (1987). BAY K 8644 increases release of acetylcholine at the murine neuromuscular junction. Brain Res 419:315–9.

Atchison WD, Peterson RE (1981). Potential neuromuscular toxicity of 2,4-dithiobiuret in the rat. Toxicol Appl Pharmacol 57:63–8.

Atchison WD, Scruggs-Luke V, Narahashi T, Vogel SM (1986b). Nerve membrane sodium channels as the target site of brevetoxins at neuromuscular junctions. Br J Pharmacol 89:731–8.

Atchison WD, Yang KH, Peterson RE (1981b). Dithiobiuret toxicity in the rat: evidence for latency and cumulative dose thresholds. Toxicol Appl Pharmacol 61:166–71.

Baker PF, Crawford AC (1975). A note on the mechanism by which inhibitors of the sodium pump accelerate spontaneous release of transmitter from motor nerve terminals. J Physiol (London) 247:209–26.

Baker PF, Hodgkin AL, Ridway EB (1971). Depolarization and calcium entry in squid giant axons. J Physiol (London) 218:709–55.

Balnave RJ, Gage PW (1973). The inhibitory effect of manganese on transmitter release at the neuromuscular junction of the toad. Br J Pharmacol 47:339–52.

Barrett J, Botz D, Chang DB (1974). Block of neuromuscular transmission by methylmercury. In: Xintaras C, Johnson BL, de Groot I, eds. Behavioral toxicology, early detection of occupational hazards. Washington, DC: U.S. Department of Health, Education and Welfare, 5:277–287.

Ben-Haim BD, Dreyer F, Peper K (1975). Acetylcholine receptor: modification of synaptic gating mechanism after treatment with a disulfide bond reducing agent. Pflügers Arch 355:19–26.

Ben-Haim D, Landau EM, Silman I (1973). The role of a reactive disulfide bond in the function of the acetylcholine receptor at the frog neuromuscular junction. J Physiol (London) 234:305–25.

Benoit PR, Mambrini J (1970). Modification of transmitter release by ions which prolong the presynaptic action potential. J Physiol (London) 210:681–95.

Berg DK, Boyd RT, Halvorsen SW, Higgins LS, Jacob MH, Margiotta JF (1989). Regulating the number and function of neuronal acetylcholine receptors. TINS 12(1):16–21.

Berg DK, Halvorsen SW (1988). Acetylcholine receptor. Genes encoding nicotinic receptor subtypes on neurons (news). Nature 334:384–5.

Berstein G, Haga K, Haga T, Ichiyama A (1988). Agonist and antagonist binding of muscarinic acetylcholine receptors purified from porcine brain: interconversion of high- and low-affinity sites by sulfhydryl reagents. J Neurochem 50:1687–94.

Binah O, Meiri U, Rahamimoff H (1978). The effects of $HgCl_2$ and mersalyl on mechanisms regulating intracellular calcium and transmitter release. Eur J Pharmacol 51:453–7.

Binz T, Kurazono H, Popoff MR, Eklund MW, Sakaguchi G, Kozaki S, Krieglstein K, Henschen A, Gill DM, Niemann H (1990a). Nucleotide sequence of the gene encoding Clostridium botulinum neurotoxin type D. Nucl Acids Res 18:5556.

Binz T, Kurazono H, Wille M, Frevert J, Wernars K, Niemann H (1990b). The complete sequence of botulinum neurotoxin type A and comparison with other clostridial neurotoxins. J Biol Chem 265:9153–8.

Birks R, Katz B, Miledi R (1960). Physiological and structural changes at the amphibian myoneuronal junction in the course of nerve degeneration. J Physiol (London) 150:145–68.

Boroff DA, Del Castillo J, Evoy JH, Steinhardt RA (1974). Observations on the action of type A botulinum toxin on frog neuromuscular junctions. J Physiol (London) 240:227–53.

Bowman WC, Prior C, Marshall IG (1990). Presynaptic receptors in the neuromuscular junction. Ann NY Acad Sci 604:69–81.

Boyd IA, Martin AR (1956a). Spontaneous subthreshold activity at mammalian neuromuscular junctions. J Physiol (London) 132:61–73.

Boyd IA, Martin AR (1956b). The end-plate potential in mammalian muscle. J Physiol (London) 132:74–91.

Brose N, Petrenko AG, Südhof TC, Jahn R (1992). Synaptotagmin, a Ca^{2+} sensor on the synaptic vesicle surface. Science 256:1021–5.

Burgen ASV, Dickens F, Zatman LJ (1949). The action of botulinum toxin on the neuromuscular junction. J Physiol (London) 109:10–24.

Cangiano A, Lutzemberger L, Rizzuto N, Simonati A, Rossi A, Toschi G. (1980). Neurotoxic effects of 2,5-hexanedione in rats: early morphological and functional changes in nerve fibers and neuromuscular juinctions. Neurotoxicology 2:25–32.

Caputy AJ, Kim YI, Sanders DB (1981). The neuromuscular blocking effects of therapeutic concentrations of various antibiotics on normal rat skeletal muscle: a quantitative comparison. J Pharmacol Exp Ther 217:369–78.

Caratsch CG, Maranda B, Miledi R, Strong PN (1981). A further study of the phospholipase-independent action of β-bungarotoxin at frog end-plates. J Physiol (London) 319:179–91.

Caratsch CG, Miledi R, Strong PN (1985). Influence of divalent cations on the phospholipase-independent action of beta-bungarotoxin at frog neuromuscular junctions. J Physiol (London) 363:169–79.

Ceccarelli B, Grohovaz F, Hurlbut WP (1979). Freeze-fracture studies of the frog neuromuscular junction during intense release of neurotransmitter: effects of black widow spider venom and Ca^{2+}-free solutions on the structure of the active zone. J Cell Biol 81:163–77.

Chang CC, Chen TF, Lee CY (1973). Studies of the presynaptic effect of β-bungarotoxin on neuromuscular transmission. J Pharmacol Exp Ther 184:339–45.

Chang CC, Lee CY (1963). Isolation of neurotoxins from the venom of *Bungarus multicinctus* and their modes of neuromuscular blocking agents. Arch Int Pharmacodyn 144:241–57.

Chang CC, Lee JD (1977). Crotoxin, the neurotoxin of South American rattlesnake venom, is a presynaptic toxin acting like beta-bungarotoxin. Naunyn-Schmiedebergs Arch Pharmacol 296:159–68.

Chapell R, Rosenberg P (1992). Specificity of action of β-bungarotoxin on neurotransmitter release and its inhibitory effects on acetylcholine release from synaptosomes. Toxicon 30:621–33.

Clark AW, Hurlbut WP, Mauro A (1972). Changes in the fine structure of the neuromuscular junction of the frog caused by black widow spider venom. J Cell Biol 52:1–14.

Clark AW, Mauro A, Longenecker HE, Hurlbut WP (1970). Effects of black widow spider venom on the frog neuromuscular junction. Nature 225:703–5.

Colmeus C, Gomez S, Molgó J, Thesleff S (1982). Discrepancies between spontaneous and evoked synaptic potentials at normal, regenerating and botulinum toxin poisoned mammalian neuromuscular junctions. Proc R Soc Lond (Biol) 215:63–74.

Cohen MW, Jones OT, Angelides KJ (1991). Distribution of Ca^{2+} channels in frog motor nerve terminals revealed by fluorescent ω-conotoxin. J Neurosci 11:1032–9.

Colquhoun D, Dreyer F, Sheridan RE (1979). The actions of tubocurarine at the frog neuromuscular junction. J Physiol (London) 293:247–84.

Colquhoun D, Sakmann B (1985a). Fast events in single-channel currents activated by acetylcholine and its analogues at the frog muscle end-plate. J Physiol (London) 369:501–57.

Colquhoun D, Sakmann B (1985b). Bursts of openings in transmitter-activated ion channels. In: Neher E, Sakmann B, eds. Single-channel recording. New York: Plenum Press, 345–64.

Cooper JR, Bloom FE, Roth RH (1982). Acetylcholine. In: The Biochemical basis of neuropharmacology. New York: Oxford University Press, 77–108.

Cooper GP, Manalis RS (1983). Influence of heavy metals on synaptic transmission: a review. Neurotoxicology. 4:69–84.

Cooper GP, Manalis RS (1984a). Cadmium: effects on transmitter release at the frog neuromuscular junction. Eur J Pharmacol 99:251–6.

Cooper GP, Manalis RS (1984b). Interactions of lead and cadmium on acetylcholine release at the frog neuromuscular junction. Toxicol Appl Pharmacol 74:411–6.

Cooper GP, Suszkiw JJ, Manalis RS (1984). Presynaptic effects of heavy metals. In: T. Narahashi, ed. Cellular and molecular neurotoxicology. New York: Raven Press, 1–21.

Couturier S, Erkman L, Valera S, Rungger D, Bertrand S, Boulter J, Ballivet M, Bertrand D (1990a). Alpha 5, alpha 3, and non-alpha 3. Three clustered avian genes encoding neuronal nicotinic acetylcholine receptor–related subunits. J Biol Chem 265:17560–7.

Couturier S, Bertrand D, Matter J, Hernandez M, Bertrand S, Millar N, Valera S, Barkas T, Ballivet M (1990b). A neuronal nicotinic acetylcholine receptor subunit (α7) is developmentally regulated and forms a homo-oligomeric channel blocked by α-BTX. Neuron 5:847–56.

Crofton KM, Dean KF, Hamrick RC, Boyes WK (1991). The effects of 2,4-dithiobiuret on sensory and motor function. Fund Appl Toxicol 16:469–81.

Cruz LJ, Olivera BM (1986). Calcium channel antagonists. ω-Conotoxin defines a new high affinity site. J Biol Chem 261:6230–3.

Cull-Candy SG, Lundh H, Thesleff S (1976). Effects of botulinum toxin on neuromuscular transmission in the rat. J Physiol (London) 260:177–203.

Datyner ME, Gage PW (1973). Presynaptic and postsynaptic effects of the venom of the Australian tiger snake at the neuromuscular junction. Br J Pharmacol 49:340–54.

Del Castillo JD, Bartels E, Sobrino JA (1972). Microelectrophoretic application of cholinergic compounds, protein oxidizing agents, and mercurials to the chemically excitable membrane of the electroplax. Proc Natl Acad Sci USA 8:2081–5.

Del Castillo J, Engbaek L (1954). The nature of the neuromuscular block producted by magnesium. J Physiol (London) 124:370–84.

Del Castillo J, Katz B (1954a). Quantal components of the end-plate potential. J Physiol (London) 124:560–73.

Del Castillo J, Katz B (1954b). Statistical factors involved in neuromuscular facilitation and depression. J Physiol (London) 124:574–85.

DiVincenzo G, Kaplan CJ, Dedinas J (1976). Characterization of the metabolites of methyl-n-butyl ketone, methyl isobutyl ketone and methyl ethyl ketone in guinea pig serum and their clearance. Toxicol Appl Pharmacol 36:511–9.

Dodge FA, Miledi R, Rahamimoff R (1969). Strontium and quantal release of transmitter at the neuromuscular junction. J Physiol (London) 200:267–83.

Dodge FA, Rahamimoff R (1967). Co-operative action of calcium ions in transmitter release at the neuromuscular junction. J Physiol (London) 193:419–32.

Dolezal V, Vyskocil F, Tucek S (1983). Decrease of the spontaneous non-quantal release of acetylcholine from the phrenic nerve in botulinum-poisoned rat diaphragm. Pflügers Arch 397:319–22.

Dooley DJ, Lupp A, Hertting G (1987). Inhibition of central neurotransmitter release by ω-conotoxin GVIA, a peptide modulator of the N-type voltage-sensitive calcium channel. Naunyn-Schmiedebergs Arch Pharmacol 336:467–70.

Dreyer F, Becker C, Bigalke H, Funk J, Penner R, Rosenberg F, Zigler M. (1984). Action of botulinum A toxin and tetanus toxin on synaptic transmission. J Physiol (London) 79:252–8.

Dreyer F, Mallart A, Brigant JL (1983). Botulinum A toxin and tetanus toxin do not affect presynaptic membrane currents in mammalian motor nerve endings. Brain Res 270:373–5.

Dreyer F, Schmitt A (1983). Transmitter release in tetanus and botulinum A toxin–poisoned mammalian motor endplates and its dependence on nerve stimulation and temperature Pflügers Arch 399:228–34.

Dreyer F, Penner R (1987). The actions of presynaptic snake toxins on membrane currents of mouse motor nerve terminals. J Physiol (London) 386:455–63.

Duchen LW (1971). An electron microscopic study of the changes induced by botulinum toxin in the motor end-plates of slow and fast skeketal muscle fibres of the mouse. J Neurol Sci 14:47–60.

Duchen LW, Strich SJ (1968). The effects of botulinum toxin on the pattern of innervation of skeletal muscles in the mouse. Quart J Exp Physiol 53:84–9.

Duchen LW, Tonge DA (1973). The effect of tetanus toxin on neuromuscular transmission and on the morphology of motor end-plates in slow and fast skeletal muscle of the mouse. J Physiol (London) 228:157–72.

Dunkley B, Sanghoi I, Goldstein G (1973). Characterization of neuromuscular block produced by streptomycin. Arch Int Pharmacodyn 201:213–23.

Durant NN, Lambert JJ (1981). The action of polymyxin B at the frog neuromuscular junction. Br J Pharmacol 72:41–7.

Dwyer TM, Adams DJ, Hille B (1980). The permeability of the endplate channel to organic cations in frog muscle. J Gen Physiol 75:469–92.

Eccles JC, MacFarlane WV (1949). Actions of anticholinesterases on end-plate potential of frog muscle. J Neurophysiol 12:59–80.

Eldefrawi ME, Mansour NA, Eldefrawi AT (1977). Interactions of acetylcholine receptors with organic mercury compounds. In Miller MW, Shammoo AE, eds. Membrane toxicity. New York: Plenum Press. pp. 449–463.

Evans ML, Büsselberg D, Carpenter DO (1991). Pb^{2+} blocks calcium currents of cultured dorsal root ganglion cells. Neurosci Lett 129:103–6.

Farley JM, Wu CH, Narahashi T (1982). Mechanism of neuromuscular block by streptomycin: a voltage clamp analysis. J Pharmacol Exp Ther 222:488–93.

Fatt P, Katz B (1951). An analysis of the end-plate potential recorded with an intracellular electrode. J Physiol (London) 115:320–31.

Fatt P, Katz B (1952). Spontaneous subthreshold activity at motor nerve endings. J Physiol (London) 117:109–28.

Fiekers JF (1981). Neuromuscular blockade produced by polymyxin B: interaction with end-plate channels. Eur J Pharmacol 70:77–81.

Fiekers JF (1983a). Effects of the aminoglycoside antibiotics, streptomycin and neomycin, on neuromuscular transmission. I. Presynaptic considerations. J Pharmacol Exp Ther 225:487–95.

Fiekers JF (1983b). Effects of the aminoglycoside antibiotics, streptomycin and neomycin, on neuromuscular transmission. II. Postsynaptic considerations. J Pharmacol Exp Ther 225:496–502.

Fiekers JF, Henderson F, Marshall G, Parsons RL (1983). Comparative effects of clindamycin and lincomycin on end-plate currents and quantal content at the neuromuscular junction. J Pharmacol Exp Ther 227:308–15.

Figliomeni B, Grasso A (1985). Tetanus toxin affects the K^+-stimulated release of catecholamines from nerve growth factor-treated PC12 cells. Biochem Biophys Res Commun 128:249–56.

Finkelstein A, Rubin LL, Tzeng MC (1976). Black widow spider venom: effect of purified toxin on lipid bilayer membranes. Science 193:1009–11.

Fohlman J, Eaker D, Karlsson E, Thesleff S. (1976). Taipoxin, an extremely potent presynaptic neurotoxin from the venom of the Australian snake taipan (*Oxyuranus s. scutellatus*). Isolation, characterization, guaternary structure and pharmacological properties. Eur J Biochem 68:457–69.

Fohlman J, Eaker D (1977). Isolation and characterization of a lethal myotoxic phospholipase A from the venom of the common sea snake *Enhydrina schistosa* causing myoglobiniuria in mice. Toxicon 15:385–93.

Forshaw PJ (1977). The inhibitory effect of cadmium on neuromuscular transmission in the rat. Eur J Pharmacol 42:371–7.

Fox AP, Nowycky MC, Tsien RW (1987). Kinetic and pharmacological properties distinguishing three types of calcium currents in chick sensory neurones. J Physiol (London) 394:149–72.

Frontali N, Ceccarelli B, Gorio A, Mauro A, Siekevitz P, Tzeng M, Hurlbut WP (1976). Purification from black widow spider venom of a protein factor causing the depletion of synaptic vesicles at neuromuscular junctions. J Cell Biol 68:462–79.

Gansel M, Penner R, Dreyer F (1987). Distinct sites of action of clostridial neurotoxins revealed by double-poisoning of mouse motor nerve terminals. Pflügers Arch 409:533–9.

Glavinovic ML (1979). Voltage clamping of unparalysed cut rat diaphragm for study of transmitter release. J Physiol (London) 290:467–80.

Gorio A, Hurlbut WP, Ceccarelli B (1978). Acetylcholine compartments in mouse diaphragm; comparison of the effects of black widow spider venom, electrical stimulation, and high concentration of potassium. J Cell Biol 78:716–33.

Gorio A, Mauro A (1978). Reversibility and mode of action of black widow spider venom on vertebrate neuromuscular junction. J Gen Physiol 73:245–63.

Gorio A, Rubin LL, Mauro A (1978b). Double action of black widow spider venom on frog neuromuscular junction. J Neurocytol 7:193–205.

Grasso A, Alema S, Rufini S, Senni I (1980). Black widow spider toxin–induced calcium fluxes and transmitter release in a neurosecretory cell line. Nature 283:774–6.

Gundersen CB, Jenden DJ (1983). Spontaneous output of acetylcholine from rat diaphragm preparations declines after treatment with botulinum toxin. J Pharmacol Exp Ther 224:265–8.

Gundersen CB, Katz B, Miledi R (1982). The antagonism between botulinum toxin and calcium in motor nerve terminals. Proc R Soc Lond (Biol) 216:369–76.

Gwilt M, Wray D (1986). The effect of chronic neostigmine treatment on channel properties at the rat skeletal neuromuscular junction. Br J Pharmacol 88:25–31.

Habermann E, Dreyer F, Bigalke H (1980). Tetanus toxin blocks the neuromuscular transmission in vitro like botulinum A toxin. Naunyn Schmiedebergs Arch Pharmacol 311:33–40.

Halliwell JV, Dolly JO (1982). Preferential action of β-BuTX at nerve terminal regions in the hippocampus. Neurosci Lett 30:321–7.

Halliwell JV, Othman IB, Pelchen-Matthews A, Dolly JO (1986). Central action of dendrotoxin: selective reduction of a transient K conductance in hippocampus and binding to localized acceptors. Proc Natl Acad Sci USA 83:493–7.

Halpert J, Eaker D (1975). Amino acid sequence of a presynaptic neurotoxin from the venom of *Notechis scutatus scutatus* (Australian tiger snake). J Biol Chem 250:6990–7.

Halpert J, Eaker D, Karlsson E (1976). The role of phospholipase activity in the action of a presynaptic neurotoxin from the venom of *Notechis scutatus scutatus* (Australian tiger snake). FEBS Lett 61:72–6.

Halvorsen SW, Berg DK (1987). Affinity labeling of neuronal acetylcholine receptor subunits with an α-neurotoxin that blocks receptor function. J Neurosci 7:2547–55.

Hare MF, Atchison WD (1992). Comparative action of methylmercury and divalent inorganic mercury on nerve terminal and intraterminal mitochondrial membrane potentials. J Pharmacol Exp Ther 261:166–72.

Harris AJ, Miledi R (1971). The effect of type D botulinum toxin on frog neuromuscular junctions. J Physiol (London) 217:497–515.

Harvey AL, Gage PW (1981). Increase of evoked release of acetylcholine at the neuromuscular junction by a fraction from the venom of the eastern green mamba snake (*Dendroaspis angusticeps*). Toxicon 19:373–81.

Harvey AL, Karlsson E (1982). Protease inhibitor homologs from mamba venoms: facilitation of acetylcholine release and interactions with prejunctional blocking toxins. Br J Pharmacacol 77:153–61.

Hata Y, Davletov B, Petrenko AG, Jahn R, Südhof TC (1993). Interaction of synaptotagmin with the cytoplasmic domains of neurexins. Neuron 10:307–15.

Hauser D, Eklund MW, Kurazono H, Binz T, Niemann H, Gill DM, Boquet P, Popoff MR (1990). Nucleotide sequence of *Clostridium botulinum* Cl neurotoxin. Nucl Acids Res 18:4924.

Heuser J, Miledi FRS (1971). Effect of lanthanum ions on function and structure of frog neuromuscular junctions. Proc R Soc Lond (Biol) 179:247–60.

Hillyard DR, Monje VD, Gaur S, Nadasdi L, Miljanich G, Ramachandran J, Olivera BM (1992). Novel conopeptide inhibitors of mammalian presynaptic Ca channels derived from cDNA cloning and peptide synthesis (abstr). Soc Neurosci Abstr 18:970.

Howard BD, Gundersen CB Jr (1980). Effects and mechanisms of polypeptide neurotoxins that act presynaptically. Annu Rev Pharmacol Toxicol 20:307–36.

Hubbard JI (1970). Mechanisms of transmitter release. Progr Biophys Mol Biol 21:33–124.

Hubbard JI (1973). Microphysiology of the vertebrate neuromuscular junction. Physiol Rev 53:674–723.

Hubbard JI, Jones SF, Landau EM (1968). On the mechanism by which calcium and magnesium affect the spontaneous release of transmitter from mammalian motor nerve terminals. J Physiol (London) 194:353–80.

Hubbard JI, Llinàs R, Quastel DMJ (1969). Investigation of presynaptic function. In: Electrophysiological analysis of synaptic transmission. Baltimore: Williams and Wilkins, 112–73.

Hubbard JI, Willis WD (1968). The effects of depolarization of motor nerve terminals upon release of transmitter by nerve impulses. J Physiol (London) 194:381–405.

Hubbard JI, Wilson DF (1973). Neuromuscular transmission in a mammalian preparation in the absence of blocking drugs and the effects of d-tubocurarine. J Physiol (London) 228:307–25.

Hughes R, Whaler BC (1962). Influence of nerve-ending activity and of drugs on the rate of paralysis of rat diaphragm preparations by Cl. botulinum type A toxin. J Physiol (London) 160:221–33.

Hurlbut WP, Longenecker HE, Mauro A (1971). Effects of calcium and magnesium on the frequency of miniature end plate potentials during prolonged tetanization. J Physiol (London) 219:17–38.

Huttner WB, Schiebler W, Greengard P, DeCamilli P (1983). Synapsin I (protein I), a nerve terminal–specific phosphoprotein. III. Its association with synaptic vesicles studied in a highly purified synaptic vesicle preparation. J Cell Biol 96:1374–88.

Jackson MB, Lecar H, Askanas V, Engel WK (1982). Single cholinergic receptor currents in cultured human muscle. J Neurosci 2:1465–73.

Jackson MB, Wong BS, Morris CE, Lecar H, Christian CN (1983). Successive openings of the same acetylcholine receptor channel are correlated in open time. Biophys J 42:109–14.

Jenkinson DH (1957). The nature of the antagonism between calcium and magnesium ions at the neuromuscular junction. J Physiol (London) 138:434–44.

Jones HB (1989). Dithiobiuret neurotoxicity: an ultrastructural investigation of the lesion in preterminal axons and motor endplates in the rat lumbrical muscle. Acta Neuropathol 78:72–85.

Juang MS, Yonemura K (1975). Increased spontaneous transmitter release from presynaptic nerve terminal by methylmercuric chloride. Nature 256:211–3.

Juang MS (1976a). Depression of frog muscle contraction by methylmercuric chloride and mercuric chloride. Toxicol Appl Pharmacol 35:183–5.

Juang MS (1976b). An electrophysiological study of the action of methylmercuric chloride and mercuric chloride on the sciatic nerve–sartorius muscle preparation of the frog. Toxicol Appl Pharmacol 37:339–48.

Kajimoto N, Kirpekar SM (1972). Effect of manganese and lanthanum on spontaneous release of acetylcholine at frog motor nerve terminals. Nature 235:29–30.

Karlin A, Bartels E (1966). Effects of blocking sulfhydryl groups and of reducing disulfide bonds on the acetylcholine-activated permeability system of the electroplax. Biochim Biophys Acta 126:525–35.

Karlin A, Winnik M (1968). Reduction and specific alkylation of the receptor for acetylcholine. Proc Natl Acad Sci USA 60:668–74.

Kato AC, Pinto JEB, Glavinovic M, Collier B (1977). Action of a β-bungarotoxin on autonomic ganglia and adrenergic neurotransmission. Can J Physiol Pharmacol 55:574–84.

Katz B (1969). The release of neural transmitter substances. In: The Sherrington Lectures. Vol. 10. Liverpool: Liverpool University Press.

Katz B, Miledi R (1967a). The timing of calcium action during neuromuscular transmission. J Physiol (London) 189:535–44.

Katz B, Miledi R (1967b). A study of synaptic transmission in the absence of nerve impulses. J Physiol (London) 192:407–36.

Katz B, Miledi R (1969a). Tetrodotoxin-resistant electrical activity in presynaptic terminals. J Physiol (London) 203:459–87.

Katz B, Miledi R (1969b). Spontaneous and evoked activity of motor nerve endings in calcium Ringer. J Physiol (London) 203:689–706.

Katz B, Miledi R (1972). The statistical nature of the acetylcholine potential and its molecular components. J Physiol (London) 224:665–99.

Katz B, Miledi R (1973). The characteristics of "end-plate noise" produced by different depolarizing drugs. J Physiol (London) 230:707–17.

Katz B, Miledi R (1975). The nature of the prolonged endplate depolarization in anti-esterase treated muscle. Proc R Soc Lond (Biol) 192:27–38.

Kauppinen RA, Komulainen H, Taipale H (1989). Cellular mechanisms underlying the increase in cytosolic free calcium concentration induced by methylmercury in cerebrocortical synaptosomes from guinea pig. J Pharmacol Exp Ther 248:1248–54.

Kawai N, Mauro A, Grundfest H (1972). Effect of black widow spider venom on the lobster neuromuscular junctions. J Gen Physiol 60:650–64.

Kemplay S (1984). Effects of dithiobiuret intoxication of motor endplates on sternocostalis and hindlimb muscles of female rats. Acta Neuropathol (Berlin) 65:77–84.

Kerr LM, Yoshikami D (1984). A venom peptide with a novel presynaptic blocking action. Nature 308:282–4.

Kim YI, Lomo T, Thesleff S (1984). Miniature end-plate potentials in rat skeletal muscle poisoned with botulinum toxin. J Physiol (London) 356:587–99.

Kita H, Narita K, Van Der Kloot W (1981). Tetanic stimulation increases the frequency of miniature end-plate potentials at the frog neuromuscular junction in Mn^{2+}-, Co^{2+}-, and Ni^{2+}-saline solutions. Brain Res 205:111–21.

Kita H, Van Der Kloot W (1973). Action of Co and Ni at the frog neuromuscular junction. Nature 245:52–3.

Kita H, Van Der Kloot W (1976). Effects of the ionophore x-537A on acetylcholine release at the frog neuromuscular junction. J Physiol (London) 259:177–98.

Kitamura M, Iwamori M, Nagai Y (1980). Interaction between *Clostridium botulinum* neurotoxin and gangliosides. Biochem. Biophys. Acta 628:328–35.

Knaus H-G, Striessnig J, Koza A, Glossmann H (1987). Neurotoxic aminoglycoside antibiotics are potent inhibitors of [^{125}I]-omega-conotoxin GVIA binding to guinea-pig cerebral cortex membranes. Naunyn Schmiedebergs Arch Pharmacol 336:583–6.

Kober TE, Cooper GP (1976). Lead competitively inhibits calcium-dependent synaptic transmission in the bullfrog sympathetic ganglion. Nature 262:704–5.

Kolton L, Yaari Y (1982). Sites of action of lead on spontaneous transmitter release from motor nerve terminals. Isr J Med Sci 18:165–70.

Kostyuk PG, Krishtal OA (1977). Separation of sodium and calcium currents in the somatic membrane of mollusc neurones. J Physiol (London) 270:545–68.

Kozaki S, Sakaguchi G, Nishimura M, Iwamori M, Nagai Y (1984). Inhibitory effect of ganglioside G_{TIB} on the activities of *Clostridium botulinum* toxins. FEMS Microbiol Lett 21:219–23.

Kriebel ME, Gross CE (1974). Multimodal distribution of frog miniature endplate potentials in adult, denervated and tadpole leg muscle. J Gen Physiol 64:85–103.

Kriebel ME, Llados F, Matteson DR (1982). Histograms of the unitary evoked potential of the mouse diaphragm show multiple peaks. J Physiol (London) 322:211–22.

Krnjevic K, Miledi R (1959). Presynaptic failure of neuromuscular propagation in rats. J Physiol (London) 149:1–22.

Lambert JJ, Durant NN, Reynolds LS, Volle RL, Henderson EG (1980). Characterization of end-plate conductance in transected frog muscle: modification by drugs. J Pharmacol Exp Ther 216:62–9.

Laskowski MB, Dettbarn WD (1975). Presynaptic effects of neuromuscular cholinesterase inhibition. J Pharmacol Exp Ther 194:351–61.

Laskowski MB, Dettbarn WD (1979). An electrophysiological analysis of the effects of paraoxon at the neuromuscular junction. J Pharmacol Exp Ther 210:269–74.

Lee C, Chen D, Katz RL (1977). Characteristics of nondepolarizing neuromuscular blocks: (I) Post-junctional block by alpha-bungarotoxin. Can Anaesth Soc J 24:212–9.

Levesque PC, Atchison WD (1987). Interactions of mitochondrial inhibitors with methylmercury on spontaneous quantal release of acetylcholine. Toxicol Appl Pharmacol 87:315–24.

Levesque PC, Atchison WD (1988). Effect of alteration of nerve terminal Ca^{2+} regulation on increased spontaneous quantal release of acetylcholine by methylmercury. Toxicol Appl Pharmacol 94:55–65.

Levesque PC, Atchison WD (1990). Disruption of brain mitochondrial calcium seqestration by methylmercury. J Pharmacol Exp Ther 256:236–42.

Liley AW (1956a). An investigation of spontaneous activity at the neuromuscular junction of the rat. J Physiol (London) 132:650–66.

Liley AW (1956b). The effects of presynaptic polarization on the spontaneous activity at the mammalian neuromuscular junction. J Physiol (London) 134:427–43.

Link E, Edelmann L, Chou JH, Binz T, Yamasaki S, Eisel U, Baumert M, Südhof TC, Niemann

H, Jahn R (1992). Tetanus toxin inhibition of neurotransmitter release linked to synaptobrevin proteolysis. Biochem Biophys Res Comm 189:1017–23.

Llinàs R, McGuinness TL, Leonard CS, Sugimori M, Greengard P (1985). Intraterminal injection of synapsin I or calcium/calmodulin-dependent protein kinase II alters neurotransmitter release at the squid giant synapse. Proc Natl Acad Sci USA 82:3035–9.

Llinàs R, Sugimori M, Lin J-W, Cherksey B (1989). Blocking and isolation of a calcium channel from neruons in mammals and cephalopods utilizing a toxin fraction (FTX) from funnel-web spider poison. Proc Natl Acad Sci (USA) 86:1689–93.

Llinàs R, Sugimori M, Silver RB (1992). Microdomains of high calcium concentration in a presynaptic terminal. Science 256:677–9.

Longenecker HB, Hurlbut WP, Mauro A, Clark AW (1970). Effects of black widow spider venom on the frog neuromuscular junction. Nature 225:701–3.

Loring RH, Zigmond RE (1987). Ultrastructural distribution of ^{125}I-toxin F binding sites on chick ciliary neurons: synaptic localization of a toxin that blocks ganglionic nicotinic receptors. J Neurosci 7:2153–62.

Lukas RJ, Bencherif M (1992). Heterogeneity and regulation of nicotinic acetylcholine receptors. Int Rev Neurobiol 34:25–131.

Magleby KL, Miller DC (1981). Is the quantum of transmitter release composed of subunits? A critical analysis in the mouse and frog. J Physiol (London) 311:267–87.

Magleby KL, Zengel JE (1975). A dual effect of repetitive stimulation on post-tetanic potentiation of transmitter release at the frog neuromuscular junction. J Physiol (London) 245: 163–82.

Manalis RS, Cooper GP (1973). Presynaptic and postsynaptic effects of lead at the frog neuromuscular junction. Nature 243:354–6.

Manalis RS, Cooper GP (1975). Evoked transmitter release increased by inorganic mercury at frog neuromuscular junction. Nature 257:690–1.

Manalis RS, Cooper GP, Pomeroy SL (1984). Effect of lead on neuromuscular transmission in the frog. Brain Res 294:95–109.

Marshall IG (1970). Studies on the blocking action of 2-(4-phenyl piperidino) cyclohexanol (AH5183). Br J Pharmacol 38:503–16.

Martin AR (1966). Quantal nature of synaptic transmission. Physiol Rev 46:51–66.

McCleskey EW, Fox AP, Feldman DH, Cruz LJ, Olivera BM, Tsien RW, Yoshikami D (1987). ω-Contoxin: direct and persistant blockade of specific types of calcium channels in neurons but not muscle. Proc Natl Acad Sci (USA) 84:4327–31.

Meiri U, Rahamimoff R (1972). Neuromuscular transmission: inhibition by manganese ions. Science 176:308–9.

Metral S, Bonneton C, Hort-Legrand C, Reynes J (1978). Dual action of erbium on transmitter release at the frog neuromuscular synapse. Nature 271:773–5.

Miledi R (1966). Stromtium as a substitute for calcium in the process of transmitter release at the neuromuscular junction. Nature 212:1233–4.

Miledi R, Slater CR (1968). Electrophysiology and electron microscopy of rat neuromuscular junction after nerve degeneration. Proc R Soc Lond (Biol) 169:289–306.

Miller C, Moczydlowski E, Latorre R, Phillips M (1985). Charybdotoxin, a protein inhibitor of single Ca^{2+}-activated K^+ channels from mammalian skeletal muscle. Nature 313:316–18.

Mintz IM, Venema VJ, Swiderek KM, Lee TD, Bean BP, Adams ME (1992). P-type calcium channels blocked by the spider toxin ω-Aga-IVA. Nature 355:827–9.

Mishina B, Takai T, Imoto K, Noda M, Takahashi T, Numa S, Methfessel C, Sakmann B (1986). Molecular distinction between fetal and adult forms of muscle acetylcholine receptor. Nature 321:406–11.

Miura A, Muramatsu I, Fuliwara M, Hayashi K, Lee C-Y (1981). Species and regional differences in cholinergic blocking actions of β-bungarotoxin. J Pharmacol Exp Ther 217:505–9.

Miyamato MD (1983). Hg^{2+} causes neurotoxicity at an intracellular site following entry through Na and Ca channels. Brain Res 267:375–9.

Molenarr PC, Oen BS, Polak RL (1987). Effect of chloride ions on giant miniature end-plate potentials at the frog neuromuscular junction. J Physiol (London) 383:143–52.

Molgó J, del Pozo E, Baños JE, Angaut-Petit D (1991). Changes of quantal transmitter release caused by gadolinium ions at the frog neuromuscular junction. Br J Pharmacol 104:133–8.

Muniak CG, Kriebel ME, Carlson CG (1982). Changes in MEPP and EPP amplitude distributions in the mouse diaphragm during synapse formation and degeneration. Dev Brain Res 5:123–38.

Nachshen DA (1984). Selectivity of the Ca binding site in synaptosome Ca channels. Inhibition of Ca influx by multivalent metal cations. J Gen Physiol 83:941–67.

Neher E (1983). The charge carried by single-channel currents of rat cultured muscle cells in the presence of local anaesthetics. J Physiol (London) 339:663–78.

Neher E, Steinbach JH (1978). Local anaesthetics transiently block currents through single acetylcholine-receptor channels. J Physiol (London) 277:153–76.

Nishimura M, Tsutsui I, Yagasaki O, Yanagiya I (1984). Transmitter release at the mouse neuromuscular junction stimulated by cadmium ions. Arch Int Pharmacodyn Ther 271:106–21.

Nishimura M (1988). Zn^{2+} stimulates spontaneous transmitter release at mouse neuromuscular junctions. Br J Pharmacol 93:430–6.

Nowycky MC, Fox AP, Tsien RW (1985). Three types of neuronal calcium channel with different calcium agonist sensitivity. Nature 316:440–3.

Oberg SG, Kelly RB (1976). The mechanism of β-bungarotoxin action. I. Modification of transmitter release at the neuromuscular junction. J Neurobiol 7:129–41.

Ogden DC, Colquhoun D (1985). Ion channel block by acetylcholine, carbachol and suberyldicholine at the frog neuromuscular junction. Proc R Soc Lond (Biol) 225:329–55.

Ogden DC, Siegelbaum SA, Colquhoun D (1981). Block of acetylcholine-activated ion channels by an uncharged local anaesthetic. Nature 289:596–8.

Okamoto M, Longenecker HE Jr, Riker WF Jr, Song SK (1971). Destruction of mammalian motor nerve terminals by black widow spider venom. Science 172:733–6.

Olivera BM, Gray WR, Zeikus R, McIntosh JM, Varga J, Rivier J, DeSantos V, Cruz LJ (1985). Peptide neurotoxins from fish-hunting cone snails. Science 230:1338–43.

Olivera BM, Cruz LJ, DeSantos V, Lecheminant GW, Griffin D, Zeikus R, McIntosh JM, Galyean R, Varga J, Gray WR, Rivier J (1987). Neuronal calcium channel antagonists. Discrimination between calcium channel subtypes using ω-conotoxin from *Conus magnus* venom. Biochemistry 26:2086–90.

Papke RL, Oswald RE (1989). Mechanisms of noncompetitive inhibition of acetylcholine-induced single-channel currents. J Gen Physiol 93:785–811.

Petrenko AG, Kovalenko VA, Shamotienko OG, Surkova IN, Tarasyuk TA, Ushkaryov YA, Grishin EV (1990). Isolation and properties of the α-latrotoxin receptor. EMBO J 9:2023–7.

Petrenko AG, Perrin MS, Davletov BA, Ushkaryov YA, Geppert M, Südhoff TC (1991). Binding of synaptotagmin to the α-latrotoxin receptor implicates both in synaptic vesicle exocytosis. Nature 353:65–8.

Pickett JB, Bornstein JC (1984). Some effects of lead at mammalian neuromuscular junction. Am J Physiol 246:C271–6.

Pittinger C, Adamson R (1972). Antibiotic blockade of neuromuscular function. Annu Rev Pharmacol 12:169–84.

Polak RL, Sellin LC, Thesleff S (1981). Acetylcholine content and release in denervated or botulinum poisoned rat skeletal muscle. J Physiol (London) 319:253–9.

Poulet S, Hauser D, Quanz M, Niemann H, Popoff MR (1992). Sequences of the botulinal neurotoxin E derived from *Clostridium botulinum* type E (strain Beluga) and *Clostridium butyricum* (strains ATCC 43181 and ATCC 43755). Biochem Biophys Res Comm 183:107–13.

Prior C, Fiekers JF, Henderson F, Dempster J, Marshall IG, Parsons RL (1990). End-plate ion channel block produced by lincosamide antibiotics and their chemical analogs. J Pharmacol Exp Ther 255:1170–6.

Protti DA, Szczupak L, Scornik FS, Uchitel OD (1991). Effect of ω-conotoxin GVIA on neurotransmitter release at the mouse neuromuscular junction. Brain Res 557:336–9.

Rang HP, Ritter JM (1971). The effect of disulfide bond reduction on the properties of cholinergic receptors in chick muscle. Mol Pharm 7:620–31.

Reuveny E, Narahashi T (1991). Potent blocking action of lead on voltage-activated calcium channels in human neuroblastoma cells SH-SY5Y. Brain Res 545:312–4.

Reynolds IJ, Wagner JA, Snyder SH, Thayer SA, Olivera BM, Miller RJ (1986). Brain voltage-sensitive calcium channel subtypes differentiated by ω-conotoxin fraction GVIA. Proc Natl Acad Sci USA 83:8804–7.

Robitaille R, Adler EM, Charlton MP (1990). Strategic location of calcium channels at transmitter release sites of frog neuromuscular synapses. Neuron 5:733–9.

Rustam H, Von Burg R, Amin-Zaki L, El Hassani S (1975). Evidence for a neuromuscular disorder in methylmercury poisoning. Clinical and electrophysiological findings in moderate to severe cases. Arch Environ Health 30:190–5.

Sakaguchi G (1983). *Clostridium botulinum* toxins. Pharmacol Ther 19:165–94.

Sander WE, Sanders CC (1979). Toxicity of antibacterial agents: mechanism of action on mammalian cells. Annu Rev Pharmacol Toxicol 19:53–83.

Sano K, Enomoto K, Maeno T (1987). Effects of synthetic ω-conotoxin, a new type of Ca^{2+} antagonist, on frog and mouse neuromuscular transmission. Eur J Pharmacol 141:235–41.

Scheer H, Meldolesi J (1985). Purification of the putative α-latrotoxin receptor from bovine synaptosomal membranes in an active binding form. EMBO J 4:323–7.

Scheer H, Prestipino G, Meldolesi J (1986). Reconstitution of the purified α-latrotoxin receptor in liposomes and planar lipid membranes. Clues to the mechanism of toxin action. EMBO J 5:2643–8.

Schiavo G, Benfenati F, Poulain B, Rossetto, O, Polverino de Laureto P, DasGupta BR, Montecucco C (1992a). Tetanus and botulinum-β neurotoxins block neurotransmitter release by proteolytic cleavage of synaptobrevin. Nature 359:832–5.

Schiavo G, Rossetto O, Santucci A, DasGupta BR, Montecucco C (1992b). Botulinum neurotoxins are zinc proteins. J Biol Chem 267:23479–83.

Sellin LC, Kauffman JA, DasGupta BR (1983a). Comparison of the effects of botulinum neurotoxin types A and E at the neuromuscular junction. Med Biol 61:120–5.

Sellin LC, Thesleff S (1981). Pre- and post-synaptic actions of botulinum toxin at the rat neuromuscular junctions. J Physiol (London) 317:487–95.

Sellin LC, Thesleff S, DasGupta BR (1983b). Different effects of types A and B botulinum toxin on transmitter release at the rat neuromuscular junction. Acta Physiol Scand 119:127–33.

Sen I, Grantham PA, Cooper JR (1976). Mechanism of action of β-bungarotoxin on synaptosomal preparations. Proc Natl Acad Sci USA 73:2664–8.

Shafer TJ, Atchison WD (1989). Block of ^{45}Ca uptake into synaptosomes by methylmercury: Ca^{++}- and Na^{+}-dependence. J Pharmacol Exp Ther 248:696–702.

Shafer TJ, Atchison WD (1991). Methylmercury blocks N- and L-type Ca^{++} channels in nerve growth factor–differentiated pheochromocytoma (PC12) cells. J Pharmacol Exp Ther 258:149–57.

Shafer TJ, Atchison WD (1992). Effects of methylmercury on perineurial Na^{+} and Ca^{2+}-dependent potentials at neuromuscular junctions of the mouse. Brain Res 595:215–9.

Shao Z, Suszkiw JB (1991). Ca^{2+}-surrogate action of Pb^{2+} on acetylcholine release from rat brain synaptosomes. J Neurochem 56:568–74.

Shrivastav B, Brodwick MS, Narahashi T (1976). Methylmercury: effects on electrical properties of squid axon membranes. Life Sci 18:1077–82.

Silinsky EM (1977a). Can barium support the release of acetylcholine by nerve impulses? Br J Pharmacol 59:215–7.

Silinsky EM (1977b). An estimate of the equilibrium dissociation constant for calcium as an antagonist of evoked acetylcholine release: implications for excitation-secretion coupling. Br J Pharmacol 61:691–3.

Silinsky EM (1978a). Enhancement by an antagonist of transmitter release from frog motor nerve terminals. Br J Pharmacol 63:485–93.

Silinsky EM (1978b). On the role of barium in supporting th asynchronous release of aectylcholine quanta by motor nerve impulses. J Physiol (London) 274:157–71.

Silinsky EM (1985). The biophysical pharmacology of calcium-dependent acetylcholine secretion. Pharmacol Rev 37:81–132.

Simpson LL (1974). Studies on the binding of botulinum toxin type A to the rat phrenic nerve–hemidiaphragm preparation. Neuropharmacology 13:683–91.

Simpson LL (1978). Pharmacological studies on the subcellular site of action of botulinum toxin type A. J Pharmacol Exp Ther 206:661–9.

Simpson LL (1981). The origin, structure, and pharmacological activity of botulinum toxin. Pharmacol Rev 33:155–88.

Simpson LL, DasGupta BR (1983). Botulinum neurotoxin type E: studies on mechanism of action and on structure-activity relationships. J Pharmacol Exp Ther 224:135–40.

Simpson LL (1984a). Botulinum toxin and tetanus toxin recognize similar membrane determinants. Brain Res 305:177–80.

Simpson LL (1984b). The binding fragment from tetanus toxin antagonizes the neuromuscular blocking actions of botulinum toxin. J Pharmacol Exp Ther 229:182–7.

Simpson LL (1986). Molecular pharmacology of botulinum toxin and tetanus toxin. Annu Rev Pharmacol Toxicol 26:427–53.

Simpson LL, Rapport MM (1971). The binding of botulinum toxin to membrane lipids: phospholipids and proteolipid. J Neurochem 18:1671–7.

Sine SM, Claudio T, Sigworth FJ (1990). Activation of *Torpedo* acetylcholine receptors expressed in mouse fibroblasts; single channel current kinetics reveal distinct agonist binding affinities. J Gen Physiol 96:395–437.

Sine SM, Steinbach JH (1984). Activation of a nicotinic acetylcholine receptor. Biophys J 45:175–85.

Sine SM, Taylor P (1982). Local anesthetics and histrionicotoxin are allosteric inhibitors of the acetylcholine receptor. J Biol Chem 257:8106–14.

Singh YN, Marshall IG, Harvey AL (1978). Reversal of antibiotic-induced muscle paralysis by 3,4-diaminopyridine. J Pharm Pharmacol 30:249–50.

Singh YN, Marshall IG, Harvey AL (1979). Depression of transmitter release and postjunctional sensitivity during neuromuscular block produced by antibiotics. Br J Anaesth 51:1027–33.

Singh YN, Marshall IG, Harvey AL (1982). Pre-and postjunctional blocking effects of aminoglycoside, polymyxin, tetracycline and lincosamide antibiotics. Br J Anaesth 54:1295–1305.

Sokoll MD, Gergis SD (1981). Antibiotics and neuromuscular function. Anesthesiology 55:148–59.

Somjen GG, Herman SP, Klein R (1973). Electrophysiology of methylmercury poisoning. J Pharmacol Exp Ther 186:579–92.

Spencer PS, Schaumburg HH (1975). Experimental neuropathy produced by 2,5-hexanedione, a major metabolite of the neurotoxic industrial solvent methyl-*n*-butyl ketone. J Neurol Neurosurg Psychiatry 38:771–82.

Spitsbergen JM, Atchison WD (1990). Acute alterations of neuromuscular transmission following exposure to a nonparalytic dose of dithiobiuret. Toxicol Appl Pharmacol 102:68–79.

Spitsbergen JM, Atchison WD (1991). Voltage clamp analysis reveals multiple populations of quanta released at neuromuscular junctions of rats treated with 2,4-dithiobiuret. J Pharmacol Exp Ther 256:159–63.

Stanley EF, Drachman DB (1981). Non-quantal ACh release in the mouse diaphragm: effects of botulinum toxin and denervation (abstr). Neurosci Abstr 7:440.

Steinacker A, Zuazaga C (1981). Changes in neuromuscular junction endplate current time constants produced by sulfhydryl reagents. Proc Natl Acad Sci USA 78:7806–9.

Steinacker A, Zuazaga C (1987). Further kinetic analysis of the chemically modified acetylcholine receptor. Pflügers Arch 409:555–60.

Steinbach JH, Ifune C (1989). How many kinds of nicotinic acetylcholine receptor are there? Trends Neurosci 12:3–6.

Steinberg N, Roth E, Silman I (1990). Torpedo acetylcholinesterase is inactivated by thiol reagents. Biochem Int 21:1043–50.

Storella RJ, Bierkamper GG (1990). Effects of nicotinic agonists and antagonists on acetylcholine release from the rat hemidiaphragm. Ann NY Acad Sci 604:569–71.

Strecker GJ, Jackson MB (1989). Curare binding and the curare-induced subconductance state of the acetylcholine receptor channel. Biophys J 56:795–806.

Strong PN, Goerke J, Oberg SG, Kelly RB (1976). β-Bungarotoxin, a presynaptic toxin with enzymatic activity. Proc Natl Acad Sci USA 73:178–82.

Strong PN, Kelly RB (1977). Membranes undergoing phase transitions are preferentially hydrolyzed by β-bungarotoxin. Biochim Biophys Acta 469:231–5.

Südhoff TC, Jahn R (1991). Proteins of synaptic vesicles involved in exocytosis and membrane recycling. Neuron 6:665–77.

Suszkiw J, Toth G, Murawsky M, Cooper GP (1984). Effects of Pb^{2+} and Cd^{2+} on acetylcholine release and Ca^{2+} movements in synaptosomes and subcellular fractions from rat brain and *Torpedo* electric organ. Brain Res 323:31–46.

Takahashi M, Ohizumi Y, Yasumoto T (1982). Maitotoxin, a Ca^{2+} channel activator candidate. J Biol Chem 257:7287–9.

Takahashi M, Tatsumi M, Ohizumi Y, Yasumoto T (1983). Ca^{2+} channel activating function of maitotoxin, the most potent marine toxin known, in clonal rat pheochromocytoma cells. J Biol Chem 258:10944–9.

Taylor P (1985). Neuromuscular blocking agents. In: Gilman A, Goodman LS, Rall TW, Murad F, eds. The pharmacological basis of therapeutics. New York: Macmillan, 222–35.

Terrar DA (1978). Effects of dithiothreitol on end-plate currents. J Physiol (London) 276:403–17.

Thesleff S, Molgó J, Lundh H (1983). Botulinum toxin and 4-aminoquinoline induce a similar abnormal type of spontaneous quantal transmitter release at the rat neuromuscular junction. Brain Res 264:89–97.

Tonge DA (1974). Chronic effects of botulinum toxin on neuromuscular transmission and sensitivity to acetylcholine in slow and fast skeletal muscle of the mouse. J Physiol (London) 241:127–39.

Traxinger DL, Atchison WD (1987a). Comparative effects of divalent cations on the methylmercury-induced alterations of acetylcholine release. J Pharmacol Exp Ther 240:451–9.

Traxinger DL, Atchison WD (1987b). Reveral of methylmercury-induced block of nerve-evoked release of acetylcholine at the neuromuscular junction. Toxicol Appl Pharmacol 90:23–33.

Trimble WF, Linial M, Scheller RH (1991). Cellular and molecular biology of the presynaptic nerve terminal. Annu Rev Neurosci 14:93–122.

Uchitel OD, Protti DA, Sanchez V, Cherksey BD, Sugimori M, Llinàs R (1992). P-type voltage-dependent calcium channel mediates presynaptic calcium influx and transmitter release in mammalian synapses. Proc Natl Acad Sci USA 89:3330–3.

Uchiyama T, Molgó J, Lemeignan M (1981). Presynaptic effects of bekanamycin at the frog neuromuscular junction. Reversibility by calcium and aminopyridines. Eur J Pharmacol 72:271–280.

Ueno E, Rosenberg P (1990). Inhibition of phosphorylation of rat synaptosomal proteins by snake venom phospholipase A2 neurotoxins (β-bungarotoxin, notexin) and enzymes (*Naja naja atra, Naja nigricollis*). Toxicon 28:1423–37.

Ueno E, Rosenberg P (1992). Inhibition of phosphorylation of synapsin I and other synaptosomal proteins by β-bungarotoxin, a phospholipase A2 neurotoxin. J Neurochem 59:2030–9.

Ushkaryov YA, Petrenko AG, Geppert M, Südhof TC (1992). Neurexins: synaptic cell surface proteins related to the α-latrotoxin receptor and laminin. Science 257:50–6.

Valtorta F, Madeddu L, Meldolesi J, Ceccarelli B (1984). Specific localization of the α-latrotoxin receptor in the nerve terminal plasma membrane. J Cell Biol 99:124–32.

VanHeyningen WE (1974). Gangliosides as membrane receptors for tetanus toxin, cholera toxin and serotonin. Nature 249:415–7.

Verheij HM, Slotboom AJ, DeHaas GH (1981). Structure and function of phospholipase A2. Rev Physiol Biochem Pharmacol 91:91–203.

Vijayaraghavan S, Pugh PC, Zhang Z, Rathouz MM, Berg DK (1992). Nicotinic receptors that bind α-bungarotoxin on neurons raise intracellular free Ca^{2+}. Neuron 8:353–62.

Vital-Brazil O, Prado-Franceschi J (1969a). The nature of neuromuscular block produced by neomycin and gentamicin. Arch Int Pharmacodyn 179:78–85.

Vital-Brazil O, Prado-Franceschi J (1969b). The neuromuscular blocking action of gentamicin. Arch Int Pharmacodyn 179:65–77.

Von Burg R, Landry T (1976). Methylmercury and the skeletal muscle receptor. J Pharm Pharmacol 28:548–51.

Walker JW, Lukas RJ, McNamee MG (1981). Effects of thio-group modifications on the ion permeability control and ligand binding properties of *Torpedo californica* acetylcholine receptor. Biochemistry 23:2191–9.

Walker JW, Richardson CA, McNamee MG (1984). Effects of thio-group modifications of *Torpedo californica* acetylcholine receptor on ion flux activation and inactivation kinetics. Biochemistry 23:2329–38.

Wang Y-X, Quastel DMJ (1990). Multiple actions of zinc on transmitter release at mouse end-plates. Pflügers Arch 415:582–7.

Wanke E, Ferroni A, Gattanini P, Meldolesi J (1986). α-Latrotoxin of the black widow spider venom opens a small, non-closing cation channel. Biochem Biophys Res Commun 134:320–5.

Weakly JN (1973). The action of cobalt ions on neuromuscular transmission in the frog. J Physiol (London) 234:597–612.

Wecker L, Laskowski MB, Dettbarn W (1978). Neuromuscular dysfunction induced by acetylcholinesterase inhibitor. Fed Proc 37:2818–22.

Weiler MH, Williams KD, Peterson RE (1986). Effects of 2,4-dithiobiuret treatment in rats on cholinergic function and metabolism of the extensor digitorum longus muscle. Toxicol Appl Pharmacol 84:220–31.

Wernicke JF, Vanker AD, Howard BD (1975). The mechanism of action of β-bungarotoxin. J Neurochem 25:483–96.

Wessler I (1989). Control of transmitter release from the motor nerve by presynaptic nicotinic and muscarinic autoreceptors. Trends Pharmacol Sci 10:110–4.

Wessler I, Dooley DJ, Osswald H, Schlemmer F (1990). Differential blockade by nifedipine and ω-conotoxin GVIA of alpha$_1$- and beta$_1$-adrenoceptor–controlled calcium channels on motor nerve terminals of the rat. Neurosci Lett 108:173–8.

Whelan SM, Elmore MJ, Bodsworth NJ, Brehm JK, Atkinson T (1992). Molecular cloning of the *Clostridium botulinum* structural gene encoding the type B neurotoxin and determination of its entire nucleotide sequence. Appl Environ Microbiol 58:2345–54.

Wiegand H (1984). The action of thallium acetate of spontaneous transmitter release in the rat neuromuscular junction. Toxicology 55:253–7.

Wiegand H, Csicsaky M, Kramer U (1984a). The action of thallium acetate on neuromuscular tranmission in the rat phrenic nerve–diaphragm preparation. Arch Toxicol 55:55–8.

Wiegand H, Papadopoulos R, Csicsaky M, Kramer U (1984b). The action of thallium acetate on spontaneous transmitter relase in the rat neuromuscular junction. Arch Toxicol 55:253–7.

Wiegand H, Uhlig S, Gotzsch U, Lohmann H (1990). The action of cobalt, cadmium and thallium on presynaptic currents in mouse motor nerve endings. Neurotoxicol Teratol 12:313–8.

Williams KD, Lopachin RM, Atchison WD, Peterson RE (1986). Antagonism of dithiobiuret toxicity in rats. Neurotoxicology 7:33–50.

Williams KD, Miller MS, Boysen BG, Peterson RE (1987). Temporal analysis of dithiobiuret neurotoxicity in rats and assessment of potential nonneural causes. Toxicol Appl Pharmacol 91:212–221.

Williams KD, Peterson RE, Atchison WD (1992). High dose refractoriness to the neuromuscular toxicity of dithiobiuret in rats. Neurotoxicology 13:331–46.

Wright JM, Collier B (1976a). Characterization of the neuromuscular block produced by clindamycin and lincomycin. Can J Physiol Pharmacol 54:937–44.

Wright JM, Collier B (1976b). The site of the neuromuscular block produced by polymixin B and rolitetracycline. Can J Physiol Pharmacol 54:926–36.

Wright JM, Collier B (1977). The effects of neomycin upon transmitter release and action. J Pharmacol Exp Ther 200:576–87.

Yuan Y, Atchison WD (1993). Disruption by methylmercury of membrane excitability and synaptic transmission in hippocampal slices of the rat. Toxicol Appl Pharmacol 120:203–15.

Zengel JE, Magleby KL (1977). Transmitter release during repetitive stimulation: selective changes produced by Sr^{2+} and Ba^{2+}. Science 197:67–9.

Zengel JE, Magleby KL (1981). Changes in miniature endplate potential frequency during repetitive nerve stimulation in the presence of Ca^{2+}, Ba^{2+}, and Sr^{2+} at the frog neuromuscular junction. J Gen Physiol 77:503–29.

Zengel JE, Magleby KL (1982). Augmentation and facilitation of transmitter release; a quantitative description at the frog neuromuscular junction. J Gen Physiol 80:583–611.

Part III
Behavioral Toxicology
Introductory Overview

Hugh A. Tilson
U.S. Environmental Protection Agency
Research Triangle Park, North Carolina

INTRODUCTION

Over the last 15 years, there have been several symposia and conferences devoted to the use of behavioral techniques in toxicological testing and research (Tilson, 1990). Many of these conferences have dealt with methodological advances and problems of evaluation and interpretation of data, while others have focused on the use of behavioral methods to identify and characterize effects of chemicals on the nervous system. In addition, behavioral measures play a prominent role in two recent publications on environmental neurotoxicology (Office of Technology Assessment [OTA], 1990; National Research Council [NRC], 1992). These documents contain overviews of all the disciplines within neurotoxicology, including principles of risk assessment, animal and human neurotoxicology, and techniques to assess chemical-induced changes in neurobehavioral, neurophysiological, neurochemical, and neuroanatomical end points. These two publications underscore the utility and application of behavioral techniques in integrated toxicological studies to determine chemical-induced alterations in the nervous system.

USE AND ADVANTAGES OF BEHAVIORAL TESTS

Several expert committees have recommended that behavioral end points, such as a functional observational battery, motor activity, and/or schedule-controlled behavior be used, in some cases with neuropathology, to screen chemicals for potential neurotoxicity (cf. Tilson, 1990). It has also been recommended that behavioral techniques be used in a tiered-testing approach (NRC, 1975). In such a schema, each phase of evaluation

This paper has been reviewed by the Health Effects Research Laboratory, U.S. Environmental Protection Agency, and approved for publication. Mention of trade names or commercial products does not constitute endorsement or recommendation for use.

incorporates decision points based on whether suitable information exists to conclude that a chemical is or is not neurotoxic. First-tier procedures address hazard-identification issues, i.e., the neurotoxic potential of a chemical, while second- or third-tier tests address questions concerning mechanism of action, the lowest observed (adverse) effect level, or benchmark dose determination.

The use of behavioral procedures in toxicological assessments has increased in recent years. Behavioral testing of animals to determine developmental neurotoxicity of new drugs is required in Great Britain and Japan (Kimmel, 1988). The Organization for Economic Cooperation and Development is currently considering several behavioral testing protocols for neurotoxicological assessment. The United States Environmental Protection Agency (US EPA) has published several testing guidelines for behavioral procedures, including a functional observational battery and tests for motor activity and schedule-controlled behavior (US EPA, 1991). The recently published EPA testing guidelines for developmental neurotoxicity include several behavioral testing protocols, including tests for motor activity, acoustic startle reflex, and learning/memory. Recently, the EPA indicated that a battery of behavioral tests and neuropathology studies will be required in rodents for the registration and reregistration of pesticides covered under the Federal Insecticide, Fungicide and Rodenticide Act (US EPA, 1991). The Food and Drug Administration requires a number of clinical observations in the routine testing of drugs (Tilson, 1990), and behavioral data have been used in setting threshold limit values for exposure to many chemicals in the workplace (Anger, 1984).

Neurotoxicity can be measured at multiple levels of neural organization, including chemical, anatomical, physiological, and behavioral. Behavioral tests are sometimes referred to as "apical tests" because they measure the net integrated output of the nervous system; chemical-induced change in behavior might be a relatively sensitive indicator of significant neurochemical or neurophysiological dysfunction or action at a neuroanatomical site mediating observable behavioral alterations (NRC, 1975). Weiss (1988) has pointed out that behavioral changes are frequently among the first to be detected following chemical exposure in humans and may precede more obvious signs of neurotoxicity. Under the appropriate testing conditions, it is clear that behavioral tests can be used to characterize specific neurological or behavioral deficits in sensory, motor, and cognitive function (Weiss and Laties, 1975; Cory-Slechta, 1989). Behavioral tests are also important in toxicological studies because they are generally noninvasive and can be used to determine functional alterations during the course of repeated exposure and following cessation of exposure.

BEHAVIOR DEFINED

Behavior has been defined as what an organism does (Cory-Slechta, 1989) and can be classified as being respondent or operant. Respondent behaviors are elicited by a known environmental stimulus that usually has a specific temporal relationship to the occurrence of the response (Tilson, 1987; Cory-Slechta, 1989). The frequency of respondent behaviors depends on the frequency of the eliciting stimulus. Examples of respondent behavior include kineses, taxes, reflexes, and specific action patterns. Operants behaviors are emitted or voluntary responses. The frequency of an operant response is controlled by the consequences of the response. Exploratory motor activity in a novel environment is an example of an operant response.

Behaviors can also be unconditioned or conditioned (learned). Respondent conditioning consists of the pairing of two stimulus events, an unconditioned stimulus that elicits an unconditioned response and a conditioned stimulus. With repeated pairing of the two stimuli, a new response, the conditioned response, is formed. An example of an unconditioned stimulus and response is the presentation of an aversive stimulus to an arm or leg and the withdrawal response that is elicited. If another stimulus that does not elicit a withdrawal response initially (e.g., a flashing light)—a conditioned stimulus—is paired repeatedly with the unconditioned stimulus, then the conditioned stimulus comes to elicit a conditioned withdrawal response.

In the case of operant conditioning, a behavioral response occurring with some frequency shows a change in probability of recurrence following presentation of a stimulus after the response is emitted. Unconditioned operant responding (e.g., pecking a lighted panel on the wall of a test cage) will increase in frequency if the response is followed by presentation of a food or liquid reward. An increase in the probability of panel-pecking is evidence of operant conditioning. If the probability of panel-pecking increases, then positive reinforcement has occurred, while decreases in the probability of panel-pecking indicate negative reinforcement. Operant responses are typically studied by means of defined relationships or schedules established between responses and reinforcement.

TYPES OF BEHAVIORAL TEST

The chapters contained in this section focus on methods commonly used to assess chemical-induced behavioral deficits in animals. Dr. Deborah Cory-Slechta describes the use of schedule-controlled operant responding to study neurotoxicant-induced alterations in behavior. Dr. Gordon Pryor reviews the literature concerning effects of neurotoxicants on auditory function, while Dr. Mary Jeanne Kallman describes methods used to assess motor dysfunction. Neurotoxicants are also known to affect cognitive functions such as learning and memory, and this literature is reviewed by Dr. Charles Mactutus. Finally, Drs. Hugh Evans and Stephen Daniel focus on naturalistic or unlearned behaviors to assess neurotoxicity. This is important because batteries of simple, unlearned behaviors are frequently used in the initial or first-tier stage of hazard identification.

REFERENCES

Anger WK (1984). Neurobehavioral testing of chemicals: impact on recommended standard. Neurobehav Toxicol Teratol 6:147–53.

Cory-Slechta DA (1989). Behavioral measures of neurotoxicity. Neurotoxicology 10:271–96.

Kimmel CA (1988). Current status of behavioral teratology: science and regulation. CRC Rev Toxicol 19:1–10.

National Research Council (1975). Principles for evaluating chemicals in the environment. Washington, D.C.: National Academy Press.

National Research Council (1992). Environmental neurotoxicology. Washington, D.C.: National Academy Press.

Office of Technology Assessment (1990). Neurotoxicity: identifying and controlling poisons of the nervouse system. Washington, D.C.: U.S. Government Printing Office.

Tilson HA (1987). Behavioral indices of neurotoxicity: what can be measured? Neurotoxicol Teratol 9:427–43.

Tilson HA (1990). Neurotoxicology in the 1990s. Neurotoxicol Teratol 12:293–300.

United States Environmental Protection Agency (1991). Neurotoxicity testing guidelines. Springfield, Virginia: National Technical Information Service.

Weiss B (1988). Quantitative perspectives on behavioral toxicology. Toxicol Lett 43:285–93.

Weiss B, Laties V (1975). Behavioral toxicology. New York: Plenum Press.

11

Neurotoxicant-Induced Changes in Schedule-Controlled Behavior

Deborah A. Cory-Slechta
University of Rochester School of Medicine and Dentistry
Rochester, New York

INTRODUCTION

Defining Schedules of Reinforcement and Schedule-Controlled Behavior

The fate of our learned operant behavior is determined by the consequences that follow it, i.e., by its reinforcement contingencies. These consequences are deemed reinforcing stimuli if they function to maintain or increase the frequency of an operant behavioral response when presented contingent on that response. In contrast, these stimuli are deemed punishing stimuli if their presentation contingent on the behavioral response produces a subsequent decline in the frequency of that response. It is important to note that the classification of a stimulus as a reinforcer or punisher is based on the change in behavior that its contingent presentation produces, not on a common-sense usage, since many factors can influence the efficacy and potency of such stimuli. Thus, while it might be assumed that food would always serve as a positive reinforcing stimulus, it may not do so in the event of an upset stomach, for example, or if given just after completion of a meal. Conversely, one might anticipate that the presentation of shock contingent on a particular response would always serve as a punisher, but given a behavioral history of shock-avoidance responding, shock presentation can actually serve as a reinforcing stimulus.

These reinforcing or punishing stimuli may not and need not necessarily follow every occurrence of the particular response; they may be presented only intermittently after the response or may be withheld completely after the response. A possible example of the former would be phone calls that are only intermittently reinforced by a voice at the other end; a typical example of the latter would include withholding attention after a child's tantrum. It is precisely these conditions under which reinforcing or punishing stimuli are presented, i.e., the schedule of reinforcement, that determine the rate (frequency) and pattern of responding in time. As might be expected, different methods of scheduling reinforcement availability may generate marked differences in the subsequent rate and pattern of responding, i.e., in schedule-controlled behavior. Typically, however, different reinforcement schedules generate very characteristic patterns of behavior that show pronounced similarities across a wide array of species (e.g., Kelleher and Morse, 1969), attesting to the generality of such behavioral processes.

Classification of Schedules of Reinforcement

Typically, reinforcement availability is scheduled either on the basis of time, as in what are designated interval schedules, or on the basis of a required number of responses, as in ratio schedules. Moreover, the time-interval or response-number requirement may either be fixed or may vary from one instance of reinforcement availability to the next. From these designations come four simple schedules of reinforcement, with the characteristic performance of each depicted in the left side of Fig. 1. The fixed-interval (FI) schedule of reinforcement stipulates that the first response emitted after a fixed interval or period of time has elapsed since delivery of the preceding reinforcer will result in reinforcement delivery; an FI 1-min schedule schedule would reinforce the first instance of the designated response occurring 1 min after the preceding reinforcer delivery. On a variable-interval (VI) schedule of reinforcement, this time interval between instances of reinforcement availability varies from interval to interval, with the mean value of those times as the indicated parameter value. Thus, on a VI 1-min schedule, the intervals separating reinforcement availability would vary, but would average 1 min. On interval schedules, responses occurring during the time interval itself have no programmed consequence; they are neither directly reinforced nor punished.

The fixed-ratio (FR) schedule of reinforcement dictates that a specified number of responses must occur to produce reinforcement delivery; FR 100 indicates that 100 occurrences of the designated response will result in reinforcement delivery. On a variable-ratio (VR) reinforcement schedule, the number of responses required varies from one reinforcement delivery to the next, and the average number is the indicated parameter value. On a VR 100 schedule, then, the number of required responses would vary between reinforcement deliveries, but the average of those response requirement values would be 100.

Schedules of reinforcement with greater complexity, such as might be more characteristic of the human behavioral environment, arise from various combinations of these four simple reinforcement schedules. For example, in a compound schedule, the availability of reinforcement is jointly determined by both interval and ratio requirements. In an interlocking fixed-ratio, fixed-interval schedule, reinforcement availability depends on the number of responses emitted, but this ratio requirement changes as a function of time since the last reinforcement. Perhaps most characteristic of the human environment are concurrent schedules of reinforcement, which offer two (or presumably more) independent simultaneously available reinforcement schedules, each of which may be a complex schedule itself and which require one to "make choices." Thus, the possibilities for invoking complex schedules of reinforcement are almost unlimited. In addition, it should be noted that these conditions or schedules of reinforcement may not be static, but will change as other conditions of the environment change. A simple example can be drawn from the behavior of a child learning to count. While the parent may initially reinforce each correct occurrence of counting, even those with almost unlimited patience will eventually shift their praise to a more intermittent schedule of presentation, or may even try to reinforce alternative behaviors.

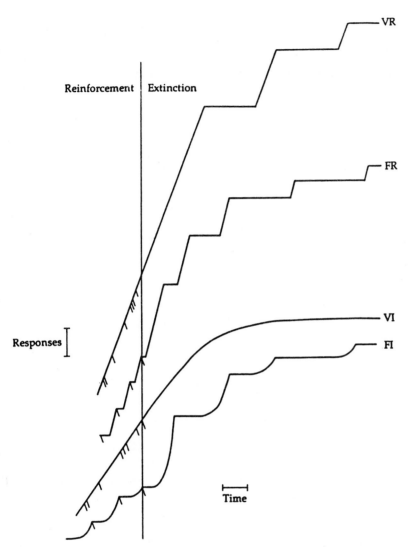

Figure 1   Typical patterns of responding on the four simple schedules following reinforcement (left) and during extinction. Responses cumulate vertically, and time is represented horizontally. The pip marks on the reinforcement side indicate reinforcement delivery. (From Reynolds, 1968.)

An additional classification basis for reinforcement schedules is derived from the presence or absence of environmental cues used to signal the currently operational reinforcement schedule and the availability of reinforcement. For example, in a multiple schedule of reinforcement, the operational reinforcement schedule alternates on the basis of time or number of reinforcements delivered, and each of the component schedules is signaled by a different external stimulus. On a multiple FI FR reinforcement schedule, then, the FI and FR components would alternate during the course of an experimental session, with different external stimuli signaling which of the two component schedules was currently in effect. In an experimental operant chamber, a red light might first appear, signaling that the FI schedule component was in effect. Following a specified period of time or number of reinforcement deliveries on the FI, the red light could change to blue, for example, signaling that the FR schedule component was now in effect. These two schedules could then continue to alternate during an experimental session. A mixed schedule of reinforcement operates identically to a multiple schedule but without the differential environmental stimuli to signal which component is in effect. Thus, on a mixed FI FR schedule, the component schedules would alternate, as they do in a multiple schedule, but without external stimuli to signal the transitions. Only the feedback to the behaver from its own behavior would signal that a transition had occurred. On a chained schedule of reinforcement, reinforcement follows the completion of a sequence of component schedules, with each component schedule being signaled by a different external environmental stimulus. A chained FI FR schedule of reinforcement would require completion of the FI component and then completion of the FR component for reinforcement delivery, with each of the component schedules signaled by a different external stimulus. A tandem schedule of reinforcement is similar to the chained schedule, with the difference that no external stimuli signal the completion of one component and the beginning of the next.

Standard-Dependent Variables

For all schedules, the most frequently measured aspect of schedule-maintained responding is overall response rate, which is simply calculated as the total number of responses emitted divided by the total time, and represents the most global measure of schedule-controlled performance. Both FI and FR schedules generate a characteristic pause following reinforcement delivery (see Fig. 1). This pause, known as the postreinforcement pause (PRP) time, is measured as the time from reinforcement delivery to the first response in the next interval (FI) or in the next ratio (FR) of the session. A measure of response rate calculated from the end of the PRP to the time of reinforcement delivery is known as running rate and provides a more direct or true estimate of response rate than does overall response rate, since running rate does not include the PRP time. The advent of computer technology permits a determination of the actual times between responses, known as interresponse times (IRTs). Interresponse times are generally presented as a frequency distribution plotting observed frequency of IRTs of various lengths.

As indicated in Fig. 1, the FI schedule generates what is referred to as a scalloped pattern of responding, which is the result of low rates of responding early in the interval followed by a gradually increasing rate of responding as the time of reinforcement availability approaches. One measure of the extent of scalloping in the interval is provided by a measure termed the index of curvature (IOC), devised by Fry et al. (1960), in which a value of zero indicates a constant rate of responding throughout the interval, while increasing positive values reflect increasing degrees of acceleration of responding. An alternative measure, the quarter-life, is defined as the percentage of the interval in which the first 25% of that interval's responses occur (Gollub, 1964). Another assessment frequently undertaken with FI performance is the rate-dependency analysis, in which the effects of the treatment are examined separately for the low response rates early in the interval and the higher response rates later in the interval, since many drugs have been shown to have rate-dependent effects increasing low response rates and decreasing higher rates.

Behavioral Mechanisms of Toxicant Effects on Schedule-Controlled Behavior

Three classes of variables control the rate, pattern, and form of operant behavior. The first of these is the nature of the consequences that follow behavior, in conjunction with the particular schedule of reinforcement according to which those consequences are presented, i.e., the consequence variables. Also important to our operant behavior are the current stimulus conditions, such as the external discriminative stimuli described above in multiple and chained reinforcement schedules that may signal reinforcement conditions, as well as the internal behaviorally generated stimuli operative in mixed and tandem schedules. In addition to the importance of consequence variables and current stimulus conditions to the control of operant behavior, antecedent variables, that is, the factors that influence the "motivational state" of the behaver, including the degree of deprivation or satiation relative to the reinforcing stimulus, are also critical. The efficacy of food as a reinforcing stimulus, for example, may be modulated by the time since the last meal consumed, our state of health, etc.

Characterizing the nature of toxicant-induced changes in schedule-controlled behavior, e.g., identifying the nature of the changes in rate or patterns of behavior (behavioral processes), must be distinguished from understanding the way in which these altered behavioral processes are produced, i.e., identifying the behavioral mechanisms of effect (Cory-Slechta, 1992). Toxicants may induce changes in schedule-controlled behavior by interacting with any or all of the variables that control behavior: the consequence variables, current stimulus conditions, or antecedent variables. For example, a toxicant may produce changes in the rate of schedule controlled-behavior by altering the efficacy of the reinforcing stimulus (consequence variable), or it may induce sensory changes that alter the perception of the current stimulus conditions, or it could change the motivational state of the behaver. Defining the behavioral mechanisms by which toxicants alter schedule-controlled behavior is critical for several reasons, including that it permits a prediction of the effects of the compound on other behavioral processes and may permit us to devise "behavioral therapeutics" to reverse or attenuate such behavioral changes.

An understanding of the behavioral mechanisms of toxicant action may derive from any or all of several sources. Some indications of behavioral mechanisms may be provided by the performance measures themselves. For example, changes in the temporal patterning of behavior on an FI schedule may suggest changes in temporal stimulus control and alterations in temporal discrimination capacity. Specific behavioral challenges designed to probe these possibilities may also be useful in elucidating behavioral mechanisms. If, for example, one suspected that exposure to a particular toxicant resulted in lack of attention to changes in stimuli signaling changed reinforcement contingencies, the stimuli could be made more salient in a probe session to determine whether the changes in schedule-controlled behavior were thereby attenuated. Another strategy designed to gain more information relating to behavioral mechanisms of toxicant action is the use of multiple schedules of reinforcement, with the multiple FI FR schedule perhaps the most frequently used. This multiple schedule format allows the evaluation of several aspects of behavior at one time, such as the importance of differential reinforcement contingencies (interval vs. ratio) and indices of stimulus control (the stimuli associated with component transitions), as well as the information from performance measures of each schedule per se.

As described above, particular schedules of reinforcement produce very characteristic patterns of behavior, as shown in Fig. 1, that tend to show considerable generality across species. Given these specific patterns, schedules of reinforcement can be used to study learning in the context of the acquisition of the characteristic response pattern, as, for example, the time (number of experimental sessions) required to attain this characteristic steady-state performance. One can further extend the use of schedules of reinforcement to study learning by imposing repeated transitions in schedule parameter values that then require changes in behavior. A simple example of such a strategy would be increasing the FI length each time stable performance is reached at the current FI value. Moreover, schedules of reinforcement can likewise be used in the context of "remembering", when the schedule value is returned to a previously imposed FI length to assess how long it takes for stable behavior to reemerge.

An additional variable that appears to modulate the effects of a wide variety of drugs at least on interval schedules, such as the FI, is the baseline rate of responding, a phenomenon known as rate-dependency. For reasons that are as yet unclear, low rates of responding, which tend to occur early in the interval during FI schedules, may be increased by drugs, whereas the higher response rates that tend to prevail as reinforcement availability approaches, i.e., as the interval approaches its end, are, instead, decreased by many drugs. The basis for rate-dependency is as yet unclear, but it is known to occur across a variety of drug classes, including amphetamine (e.g., Dews and Wenger, 1977), barbiturates (Dews, 1964; McMillan, 1973), scopolamine (McKim, 1973), and morphine (Stitzer, 1974). Thus, baseline rates of responding are an important determinant of drug effects, and rate-dependency may serve as a generalized basis of drug- and toxicant-induced changes.

Focus of the Review

This chapter focuses its review on the impact of four different classes of neurotoxicants on schedule-controlled behavior, including lead, organic, solvents, alkyl tins, and pesticides. These choices represent those classes of neurotoxicants for which the greatest amount of overall information was available and, also, for which contrasting information for interval-based and ratio-based schedules was reported. Since most of the relevant studies to date have focused on FI and FR schedules, effects on these schedules predominate in the review. However, comparative effects of other interval and ratio schedules are included where possible, particularly where they assist in differentiating generality from selectivity of an effect.

INORGANIC LEAD

Inorganic lead (Pb) has long been recognized as having neurotoxic properties, and early periods of development have been considered to be those of greatest vulnerability to the impact of Pb. However, studies of schedule-controlled behavior indicate effects that span developmental periods of exposure.

Interval Schedules

Lead exposure has been associated with very reliable and reproducible changes in FI schedule–controlled behavior, yielding a dose-effect curve for response rate that assumes an inverse U-shape (Rice, in press; Rice, 1988; Rice et al., 1979; Mele et al., 1984; Cory-Slechta and Weiss, 1989; Cory-Slechta, 1990; Cory-Slechta and Pokora, 1991; Cory-Slechta and Thompson, 1979; Cory-Slechta et al., 1983, 1985; Angell and Weiss, 1982; Van Gelder et al., 1973; Zenick et al., 1979; Barthalmus et al., 1977; Nation et al., 1989; reviewed by Cory-Slechta, 1984, 1985). Specifically, lower levels of lead exposure increase FI response rates, whereas higher levels of exposure appear, at least initially, to decrease rates of responding, as summarized in Fig. 2, which plots changes in response rate as a function of Pb exposure concentration derived from those studies reported to date. A similar function is produced when Pb-induced changes in FI response rates are plotted against the blood lead concentrations, in that low blood lead levels are associated

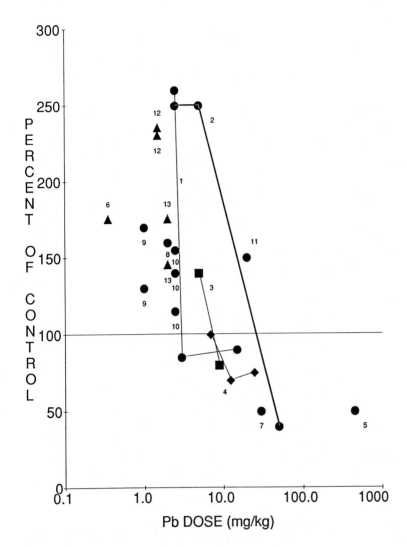

Figure 2 Dose-effect function for lead-induced changes in fixed-interval performance. The lead effect (response rate, interresponse time, or percentage of reinforcement) was plotted as a percentage of the control group value for sessions in which peak effects were observed. Different symbols represent different experimental species: circles, rats: triangles, monkeys: squares, sheep; diamonds, pigeons. Numbers next to curves or selected points represent data from the following studies: 1, Cory-Slechta et al., 1983; 2, Cory-Slechta and Thompson, 1979; 3, Van Gelder et al., 1973; 4, Barthalmus et al., 1977; 5, Zenick et al., 1979; 6, Rice et al., 1979; 7, Angell and Weiss, 1982; 8, Cory-Slechta and Pokora, 1991; 9, Cory-Slechta et al., 1985; 10, Cory-Slechta and Weiss, 1989; 11, Nation et al., 1989; 12, Rice, in press; 13, Rice, 1988. (Modified from Cory-Slechta, 1984.)

with increases in response rates, while relatively higher blood lead concentrations are associated with decreased response rates. However, it is important to note that blood lead concentration may actually serve as a surrogate in these studies for total lead body burden, or perhaps more precisely, total brain lead exposure. The importance of total lead burden as a determinant of the nature of the changes in FI response rates was demonstrated in a study examining changes following a 1-month exposure of rats to 50 ppm Pb acetate in drinking water as compared with an 8- to 11-month exposure to 50 ppm, both of which produced the same blood lead concentration (20–25 µg/dl) but would obviously produce very different total brain lead burdens. In that study, the 1-month 50-ppm exposure was associated with FI response rate increases, while the 8- to 11-month 50-ppm exposure resulted in the initial decreases in FI response rate typically associated with much higher exposure levels (Cory-Slechta, 1990).

While total lead burden appears to be an important determinant of the ensuing changes in FI response rate produced by Pb exposure, other variables seem to produce less of an impact on the shape of the dose-effect function. For example, the studies summarized by Fig. 2 include prenatal, postnatal, postweaning, and adult developmental periods of Pb exposure, but this does not appear to modify outcome patterns in any distinguishable way. In further support for the absence of a strong role for developmental exposure period, Rice (1992) found similar effects of Pb on FI performance in monkeys exposed to Pb continuously from birth, from birth to 400 days of age, or from 300 days of age onward. Moreover, the parameters of these FI schedules, including the length of the FI itself, are quite diverse across studies, ranging from 30 s to 8 min, again without any apparent effect on the dose-effect function. Finally, species differences do not appear to play any key role in this inverse U-shaped function, since comparisons across nonhuman primates (e.g., Rice, 1988; Rice, 1992; Rice et al., 1979) and rodents (Cory-Slechta and Thompson, 1979; Cory-Slechta et al., 1983, 1985; Cory-Slechta and Weiss, 1989; Cory-Slechta, 1990; Cory-Slechta and Pokora, 1991), which have included replications within species, generally yield similar functions.

Analyses of the components of FI responding reveal that Pb exposure generally does not change the temporal patterning of responses during the interval, since two measures that are related to temporal patterning, namely, PRP time (i.e., the time between reinforcement delivery and the first response in the next interval) and index of curvature, which stipulates the extent of scalloping during the interval (see above), are frequently reported to be unaffected in these studies. Instead, the primary impact of Pb is on local rates of responding, as manifest in the distribution of IRTs or the times between successive responses during the interval (Fig. 3). Low Pb exposure levels, which have stimulant effects on response rates, correspondingly shift the distribution of IRTs towards increasingly short values, whereas the higher exposure concentrations associated with depressions of response rate correspondingly shift the distribution towards longer IRTs.

The type of inverse U-shaped dose-effect curve relating Pb exposure level to FI response rate is actually not unusual. Other classes of drugs likewise produce inverse U-shaped dose-effect curves relating dose to FI response rate (e.g., Dews, 1955; Barrett, 1974). Frequently, these drug effects are also found to be rate-dependent, in that the compound increases the low rates of responding that predominate early in the interval whereas the much higher rates of responding that are characteristic later in the interval, as the time of reinforcement availability approaches, are decreased. In contrast, Pb exposure does not appear to produce rate-dependent effects. When response rates during each successive third of the FI were separately examined, it was found that the most pronounced increases in response rates as a result of Pb exposure occurred during the last third of the interval, when baseline response rates were already the highest (Cory-Slechta, unpublished data). The emergent picture, then, is that Pb-exposed organisms begin to respond at the same point during the interval as do normal subjects, but once responding begins, it occurs at a much higher rate than normal.

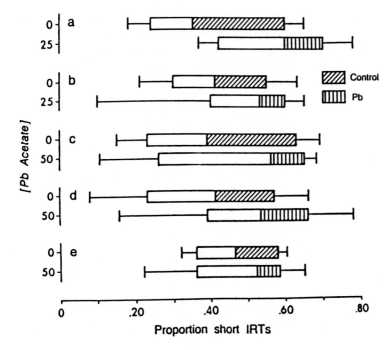

Figure 3 Stem and leaf plots summarizing low-level lead–induced changes in the frequency of short interresponse times (IRTs) (0.5 s or less), from Cory-Slechta and Weiss, 1989 (panels c, d, and e from experiments 1, 2, and 3, respectively), Cory-Slechta et al., 1985 (panel a), and Cory-Slechta, unpublished data (panel b). In each stem and leaf plot, the shaded area encompasses the 50–75th percentile of short IRT values, and the unshaded area represents the 25–50th percentile; thus the group median value is shown by the point where the shaded and unshaded areas meet. Error bars extend the data to the 10th (left side) and 90th (right side) percentiles. (From Cory-Slechta and Weiss, 1989.)

Several other characteristics effects of Pb on FI schedule–controlled behavior deserve mention not because they are unique to this behavioral enpoint or most likely to occur in response to Pb as a toxicant, but because they have simply been elaborated in some detail. The first is the observation of both "responders" and "nonresponders" to Pb treatment. Within a group of comparably Pb-exposed rats (e.g., Cory-Slechta et al., 1985) or monkeys (e.g., Rice, 1988), the majority of animals will exhibit deviate response rate or IRT values relative to controls, whereas the remaining animals within the Pb-treated group will show values well within the norm of the control group. This same phenomenon is noted in children with regard to the blood lead concentration at which acute lead encephalopathy is observed. While for some children, a blood lead level as low as 60–80 μg/dl may provoke acute encephalopathy, in others a level of 200 μg/dl may be attained with no evidence of encephalopathy. In cases where control performance is characterized by a wide range of values, one may frequently observe that the distribution of values within the Pb-exposed group is shifted toward the more extreme end or deviant values of controls. The fact that such effects occur repeatedly across studies (e.g., Fig. 3) and across laboratories speaks more to the biological significance of these findings than does any statistical evaluation.

An additional observation, again one not limited to schedule-controlled behavior as an end point, is that Pb exposure frequently not only changes rates of responding, but also increases the variability of performance from session to session. That is, the percent change in response rate or median IRT may change to a greater extent from session to session than occurs under normal conditions (e.g., Rice, 1988). Thus, behavior does not reach the same level of stability as is achieved by control animals, even in a situation in which reinforcement contingencies remain unchanged.

Also noted, at least in rodents exposed to Pb after weaning, is that the pattern of FI response rate changes produced by Pb exposure can change markedly over time, as shown in Fig. 4, modifying the shape of the concentration-effect function substantially. The bases

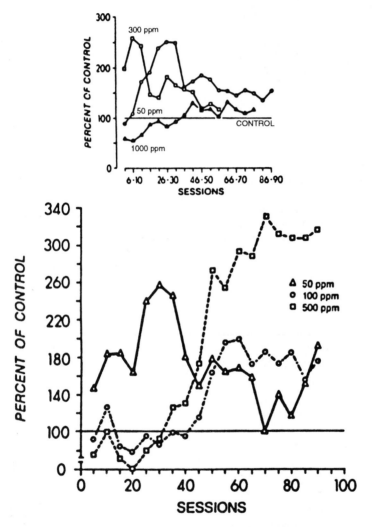

Figure 4   Median overall response rates (as percentage of corresponding control group) on a fixed-interval (FI) 30-s reinforcement schedule (inset: Cory-Slechta and Thompson, 1979) and FI 1-min schedule (Cory-Slechta et al., 1983). Each data point represents the median of the median rates over five sessions. In both studies, postweaning exposure to lower concentration(s) increased rates, which subsequently declined but remained above control levels. Exposure to higher concentration(s) initially decreased rates, after which rate increases were observed. (From Cory-Slechta, 1984.)

of these changing FI response rates across sessions is unclear; they may reflect changes in toxicokinetics or the incorporation of additional target organ effects as Pb body burden accumulates. Since most other studies have concentrated on Pb's effects on schedule-controlled behavior assessed more immediately (e.g., sessions 1 through 30), the extent to which this represents a phenomenon unique to rodents or to this particular developmental period of exposure, or to both, is not yet known.

Finally, studies by Rice (1992) and Cory-Slechta (1988) suggest that Pb-induced changes in FI schedule-maintained behavior may persist long after exposure ceases. Cory-Slechta (1988) described persistent FI rate increases in rats 3–4 months after termination of exposure to either 100 or 500 ppm Pb acetate in drinking water lasting for approximately 6 months, even though brain Pb concentrations had declined by 90% over this period. In the study by Rice (1992), monkeys whose Pb exposures ended at 400 days of age nevertheless exhibited changes in FI response rates at 7–8 years of age. Only Mele et al. (1984) failed to find long-term changes in FI performance in reponse to earlier Pb exposures of monkeys.

Ratio Schedules

Relative to its effects on FI schedules, Pb exposure appears to produce less marked and comparatively transient changes in behavior maintained by FR schedules of reinforcement. In a direct comparison in rodents, Cory-Slechta et al. (1985) reported effects of Pb on FI performance at an exposure concentration of 25 ppm Pb acetate, while Pb acetate exposure levels of 500 ppm were required to alter FR behavior in rats (Cory-Slechta, 1986). The dose-effect curve summarizing the results of the six studies that have examined FR responding following Pb exposure is shown in Fig. 5. It reveals little if any effect of Pb on FR performance at relatively low exposure levels. In fact, two additional studies employing

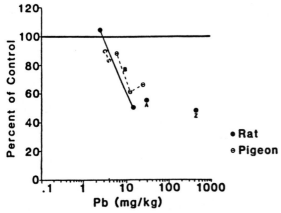

Figure 5 Dose-effect function for lead-induced changes in fixed-ratio (FR) performance. The lead effect (response rate) was plotted as a percentage of the control group value for the session(s) in which peak effects were observed. Different symbols represent different experimental species. The different letters represent the following studies: C-S, Cory-Slechta, 1986; A, Angell and Weiss, 1982; Z, Padich and Zenick, 1977; B, Barthalmus et al., 1977. Two additional studies (Rice, 1992; Rice, 1988) reported no effects of Pb on FR response rate and did not present any data, and thus they are not shown graphically. (From Cory-Slechta, 1984.)

low Pb exposure levels reported essentially negligible effects of Pb on FR performance at exposure concentrations of either 1.5 (Rice, 1992) or 2.0 mg/kg/day (Rice, 1988); thus they presented no absolute data and are not shown in Fig. 5. Exposure to higher Pb concentrations is associated with suppression of response rates, although, again, even these effects have sometimes been reported to be relatively transient (Cory-Slechta, 1986). Lead-induced decreases in response rates of pigeons were relatively short-lived in some birds but not in others.

Lead-induced changes that do occur in FR performance appear to derive primarily from changes in the distribution of responses, i.e., in a lengthening of IRTs, at least in rodents (Cory-Slechta, 1986; Padich and Zenick, 1977; Angell and Weiss, 1982). In nonhuman primates, a lengthening of the PRP time has been noted in addition to increased IRTs (Rice, 1988; Rice, 1992).

Some information on the role of developmental-period of Pb exposure in these effects can be gained from Angell and Weiss (1982) and Rice (1992). In both of those studies, changes in FR performance were noted primarily in groups with ongoing Pb exposure; prior cessation of Pb exposure resulted in negligible effects. In conjunction with those observations, the two Pb-exposed groups that did exhibit changes in FR response rates in Angell and Weiss (1982) were those exposed to Pb continuously from birth or continuously from 21 days of age and having brain Pb levels elevated relative to controls at the time of behavioral evaluation; the group exposed to Pb only during lactation did not have elevated brain Pb concentrations and also did not exhibit significant changes in FR response rate.

ORGANIC SOLVENTS

Organic solvents constitute a diverse chemical group that includes hydrocarbons, alcohols, ketones, esters, aliphatic nitrites, anesthetics, and propellants, many of which enjoy widespread industrial use and result in occupational exposure primarily via inhalation, although self-administration of these compounds is also a source of exposure for many people. This class of compounds was recently provided an excellent review by Glowa (1985).

Toluene

Interval Schedules

Because of its widespread industrial use and its association with a variety of behavioral impairments, toluene is the aromatic hydrocarbon that has been most intensively investigated with respect to changes in schedule-controlled behavior. Several different studies have examined changes in FI performance in response to toluene, using either a simple FI schedule or an FI schedule as one component of a multiple FI FR schedule, and these studies have generally reported quite similar results (Geller et al., 1979; Moser and Balster, 1986; Glowa, 1981; Glowa et al., 1983; Glowa and Dews, 1983; Glowa, 1987; reviewed by Glowa, 1985). Specifically, at lower levels of exposure, toluene is found to increase FI rates of responding, whereas at higher exposure concentrations, rates of FI responding are suppressed, resulting in an inverse U-shaped dose-effect function, as Fig. 6, summarizing several different studies, shows.

The toluene concentration at which the dose-effect curve begins to descend appears to depend on whether FI performance is assessed during toluene exposure, in which case response rate increases occur at lower exposure concentrations, or whether FI schedule–

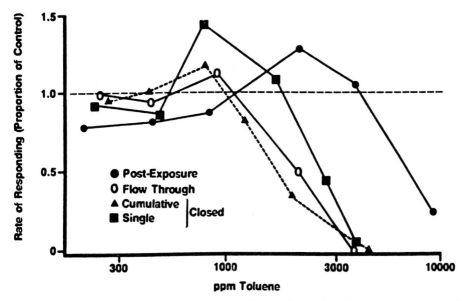

Figure 6 Concentration-effect functions for toluene obtained with mice responding under similar conditions. Abscissa: exposure concentration of toluene. Ordinate: effect, expressed as a proportion of average control rates of responding. Data were taken from the following studies: postexposure, Moser and Balster, 1981; flowthrough, Glowa and Dews, 1983; both cumulative and single, Glowa et al., 1983. (From Glowa, 1985.)

controlled responding is evaluated after exposure ends, in which case the curve is shifted to the right (Glowa, 1985). This rightward shift is related to the rapid clearance of toluene following cessation of exposure, so that the nominal exposure concentrations are higher than the actual toluene burden at the time of behavioral assessment. Moser and Balster (1986) demonstrated that complete recovery to the FI rate-suppressing effects of a 30-min exposure to 3200 ppm toluene occurred within 10 min after exposure ended. Thus, by averaging across this recovery period, postexposure assessments of the effects of toluene on schedule-controlled responding can markedly underestimate the magnitude of the behavioral change. Figure 6 also shows the relative unimportance of the method of toluene exposure (static vs. dynamic) as a determinant of the nature of these effects.

As the emphasis of these studies to date has largely been on characterizing the effects of toluene on FI schedule–controlled performance, little information is available with regard to the components of FI performance that are disrupted by toluene. Moser and Balster (1986) did report that the exposure concentrations of toluene associated with decreased FI response rates also decreased quarter-life values, indicating a less scalloped pattern of FI responding at high doses. However, while statistically significant, the magnitude of the change in quarter-life was quite small. Changes in IRT distributions, run rates, PRP time, or index of curvature have not been described, nor has any full evaluation of rate-dependency been reported. The absence of any information on the molecular basis of these changes in FI performance makes it difficult to compare the effects of toluene directly with those of other aromatic hydrocarbons, organic solvents, or drugs that likewise produce inverse U-shaped dose-effect curves relating dose to change in FI response rate.

A study by Glowa (1987) suggests the need to evaluate the effects of toluene on FI

performance under a wider array of experimental conditions. In that study, low concentrations of toluene increased rates of FI responding when a nose-poke was the required
response, but not when running in a wheel was the required response (Fig. 7), even though
the reinforcement schedule was the same. One possible explanation proposed by the author
for this difference related to the increased level of activity required for the running
response, with the possibility that it resulted in increased toluene uptake and thus higher
effective levels of the compound. Another possibility discussed derives from the rate-dependency hypothesis. As previously pointed out, that hypothesis holds that low rates of
responding, typically occurring early in the interval, are increased, while higher rates of
responding, which typically occur later in the interval, are decreased by an agent. With
respect to the differential effect of toluene on nose-poking and running, the argument
speculates that bringing a normally high-rate behavior such as locomotor activity (running)
under schedule control and maintaining an increase in rate makes it unlikely that a further
increase in rate could be produced. Glowa (1987) also pointed out that such an
interpretation is consistent with the fact that the high rates of responding maintained by
FR schedules are not increased by toluene (e.g., Moser and Balster, 1985), while the lower
rates of responding maintained under FI schedules are increased, as described above.

Interestingly, the effects of toluene on behavior maintained under a DRL (differential
reinforcement of low rates) schedule of reinforcement appear to be similar to those reported
for FI schedules. The DRL schedule is similar to the FI in that it too is a time-based

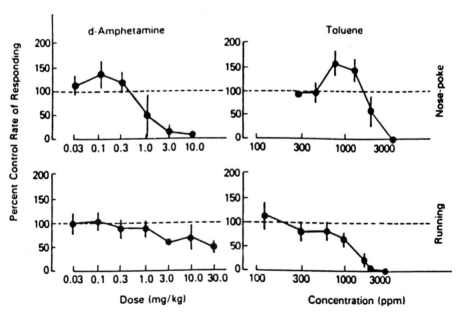

Figure 7   Dose-effect curves for acute exposure to incrementally increased concentrations of toluene
or *d*-amphetamine. The effect is expressed as the average percentage of the control rate of responding
for two separate determinations in each of four mice, i.e., the average effect of eight determinations
for each concentration of dose. Average control response rates (with the standard error of the mean
expressed as a percent of control) were 0.748 (21%) and 0.894 (18%) for nose-poke, and 0.332 (14%)
and 0.412 (5%) for running, for *d*-amphetamine and toluene, respectively. The abscissa shows
concentration (toluene) during the 30-min time out (TO) preceding, or the dose (*d*-amphetamine
given 5 min before responding was assessed). (From Glowa, 1987.)

schedule; it stipulates that responses must be separated by a specified interval of time in order to be reinforced. A report by Moser and Balster (1981) indicates that, as with FI schedules, rates of responding on the DRL schedule are increased at low toluene concentrations (800–3200 ppm) and decreased at higher exposure levels (6400 ppm). In conjunction with that report, concentrations of toluene ranging from approximately 575 to 2300 ppm likewise increased rates of responding on the DRL component of a multiple FR DRL schedule of reinforcement (Colotla et al., 1979).

Ratio Schedules

The impact of toluene on behavior maintained under FR reinforcement schedules has been less intensively investigated than under FI schedules, and the reported results are seemingly less consistent. Specifically, Geller et al. (1979) reported that short exposures (less than 2 h) to 150 ppm toluene increased FR response rates, while longer exposures (2–4 h) to 150 ppm decreased these rates, resulting, again, in an inverse U-shaped dose-effect function. Moser and Balster (1985) and Colotla et al. (1979), however, reported only exposure-related decrements in FR rate. This apparent inconsistency may relate to the fact that the lower exposure levels employed by Geller et al. (1979) were not examined by either Moser and Balster (1985), in whose study the range of toluene concentrations was 500–5000 ppm, or by Colotla et al. (1979), who used toluene levels ranging from 575 to 2300 ppm. Thus, it seems safe to conclude at this point that moderate to high toluene exposure concentrations result in suppression of FR performance, and that very low levels of toluene may stimulate FR response rates, but further studies to verify the latter conclusion, including the use of simple FR schedules and modifications of FR parameter values, are clearly warranted.

Trichloroethane

Interval Schedules

Chlorinated hydrocarbons such as trichloroethane (TCE) induce a variety of behavioral effects, including apparent changes in FI performance. While the evidence for FI response rate changes is currently based on a relatively limited data base, the reported findings are consistent with stimulation of FI response rates at low TCE concentrations and a suppression of FI responding at higher TCE exposure levels. Moser and Balster (1986) reported that TCE-1 exposure levels ranging from 1800 to 3600 ppm increased FI 60-s response rates of mice, while concentrations of 7200–10800 ppm depressed rates of responding. In a report focused on screening for behavioral toxicity, Dews (1978) presented a dose-effect curve for TCE-2 effects on FI performance that was suggestive of increased rates at lower concentrations and clearly demonstrative of suppression with increasing TCE-2 exposure levels, with a reported EC_{50} (50% effective concentration) of 4275 ppm. While these two reports raise the possibility that TCE affects responding maintained under FI schedules in a manner similar to toluene, it is obvious that additional investigative efforts are required to verify and elaborate this contention.

Ratio Schedules

Trichloroethane exposures have been consistently demonstrated to produce an exposure-related decline in rates of responding maintained under FR schedules of reinforcement (Balster and Borzelleca, 1982; Moser et al., 1985), with an EC_{50} in one case reported to be 2800 ppm (Balster and Borzelleca, 1982), with concentrations of 8000 ppm abolishing responding. In an extension of those findings, the study of Moser et al. (1985) also demonstrated that very little tolerance ever developed to the rate-suppressing properties of 6000 ppm TCE-1 on FR maintained behavior, as shown in Fig. 8.

Ketones

Interval Schedules

Ketones are organic solvents that are widely used in industrial operations and for which typical exposure is via inhalation. The effects of three such ketones, methyl *n*-amyl ketone (MAK), methyl *n*-butyl ketone (MBK), and acetone, have been investigated with respect to their effects on both FI and FR maintained behavior. Both MBK and MAK have been reported to produce exposure-related decreases in FI response rates, unlike the reported effects of toluene and of TCEs on this baseline. Using a multiple FR 5 FI 3-min schedule of reinforcement, Anger and Lynch (1977) demonstrated decrements in response rate following MBK exposures with an EC_{50} of 350 mg/kg orally, an effect they showed to include an increase in IRT length. Other measures of FI performance were not presented. They also noted that some tolerance to the rate-decreasing properties of MBK occurred over successive administrations. Johnson et al. (1977) examined the effects of prolonged inhalational exposures to MBK of either 100 or 1000 ppm for 6 h per day, 5 days per week for up to 10 months on the same multiple FR 5 FI 3-min schedule of reinforcement. While the lower MBK exposure concentration was without effect on FI performance, which was measured 2–3 h after termination of the daily exposure, the 1000-ppm exposure concentration induced decrements in response rate within 1–2 weeks of exposure, as shown in

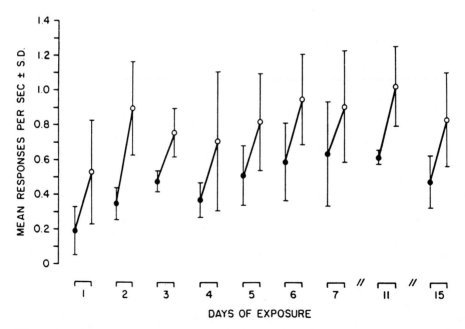

Figure 8   Mean response rates (± standard deviation [SD]) during the first 5 min (closed circles) and second 5 min (open circles) of recovery in various sessions of repeated exposure to 6000 ppm 1,1,1-trichloroethane. (From Moser et al., 1985.)

Fig. 9. As it also shows, within 6 weeks, there was some evidence for tolerance, at least in some rats.

Anger et al. (1979) investigated the effects of both injections and acute 6- or 8-h inhalational exposures to MAK on the multiple FR 5 FI 3-min schedule of reinforcement in a subsequent study. Both routes of exposure to MAK were again associated with response rate decreases on the FI schedule, with a dose of 37 mg/kg sufficient to decrease the rate by 30% and 175 mg/kg sufficient to abolish responding. For inhalational exposures, consistent declines in rate occurred only in response to concentrations of 1575–1900 ppm administered for 8 h, leading the authors to suggest that MAK was less potent than MBK with respect to changes in FI maintained responding. However, the 1575–1900 ppm exposure group was tested within 5–10 min following the termination of exposure, whereas at lower exposure concentrations, testing was not initiated until 40–50 min after exposure, leading to the possibility that recovery may already have occurred before behavioral evaluation at these lower exposure levels. Moreover, it is unclear from the study of Johnson et al. (1977) whether single exposures to 1000 ppm MBK were sufficient to induce response rate changes, since only weekly data were presented. Thus, a more systematic comparison of the two compounds is necessary before conclusions regarding potency differences can be finalized.

Geller et al. (1979) likewise used a multiple FI FR schedule to investigate the effects of acetone. In that experiment, short exposures (less than 2 h) to 150 ppm acetone increased FI response rates, whereas the longer exposure durations (2–4 h) at 150 ppm decreased rates of responding on the FI schedule. This report of increased rates at low levels of acetone exposure thus differs from the reports of only rate decreases on the FI schedule

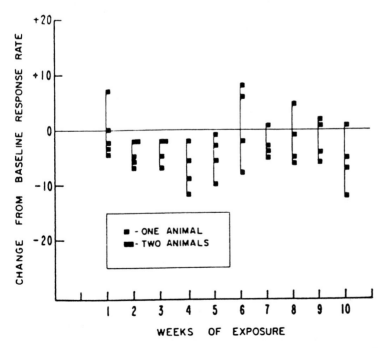

Figure 9   Effect of 1081 ppm methyl *n*-butyl ketone on response rate of rats performing a bar press task. (From Johnson et al., 1977.)

following MBK and MAK exposures. Again, however, additional investigations of these ketones at lower exposure levels will be required to clarify this issue.

Ratio Schedules

Even though virtually all of the studies looking at the effects of ketones on behavior have used a multiple schedule that included an FR component, only two of those studies presented any information on the extent to which the FR maintained behavior was altered by ketones. Anger and Lynch (1977) briefly pointed out that IRTs on the FR component of a multiple FI FR schedule were increased in length by MBK, which would be consistent with a decline in response rate. Unfortunately, neither the study of Johnson et al. (1977) examining protracted MBK exposures nor the study of Anger et al. (1979) investigating the impact of MAK reported the nature of any changes observed in the FR component of the multiple schedule. Geller et al. (1979) reported that the effects of acetone on responding under an FR schedule were identical to its effects on the FI schedule: short exposures (less than 2 h) to 150 ppm were associated with increased FR response rates, whereas more prolonged exposure (2–4 h) to 150 ppm acetone suppressed FR responding. Taken together, these studies of ketones suggest that such compounds may produce comparable effects on responding maintained under FI and FR reinforcement schedules. Together with the findings for the FI schedule that lower exposure levels may have stimulant properties, these lower exposure concentrations require more extensive experimental consideration with respect to the nature of change produced in FR performance as well.

ORGANIC TINS

The alkyl tins are used for industrial purposes, but experimental interest in these compounds also stems from early report that various alkyl tins induce central nervous system effects of interest because they may relate to neurodegenerative disorders and to hippocampal function.

Trimethyltin

Trimethyltin (TMT) has been reported to cause a variety of behavioral disturbances, including pronounced changes in learning and memory functions (e.g., Bushnell, 1988) and in both FI and FR schedule–controlled behavior (excellently reviewed by Wenger, 1985, and McMillan and Wenger, 1985).

Interval Schedules

Single injections of TMT produce relatively complex and, in some cases, contrasting patterns of FI response rate changes over time. It appears that the earliest effects of TMT on FI maintained behavior are either negligible or stimulatory, producing response rate increases. This, however, is followed by marked suppression of response rate that eventually recovers and may then even be followed by additional increases in FI response rate. Wenger et al. (1984) first demonstrated this pattern of results in two different strains of mice, as shown in Fig. 10. Following a single dose of 3 mg/kg TMT, FI response rates were substantially elevated in C57BL/6N mice within 3 h, while at 51 h, rates had declined below control levels. However, by day 5 after injection, increased rates of responding on the FI schedule reemerged, and these subsequently persisted over the 12-week period of the experiment. A corresponding pattern of effects was noted in BALB/c mice, except that the initial increase in response rate at 3 h after TMT adminisration was not observed. Some

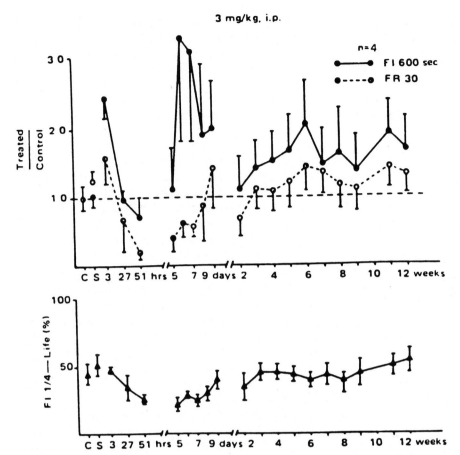

Figure 10 The effect of 3 mg/kg trimethyltin (TMT) on the rate of responding and fixed-interval (FI) quarter-life in C57BL/6N mice responding under the multiple fixed-ratio (FR) 30 FI 600-s schedule. Abscissa: time after TMT administration; ordinate (top): the rate of responding after TMT administration divided by the mean rate of responding before TMT administration; ordinate (bottom): FI quarter-life expressed as a percentage of the total 600-sec interval. Points above 3–51 h and above 5–9 days represent the mean of each daily test session for the four mice. Points above 2–12 weeks represent the weekly means of the four mice. Points above C and S represent noninjection control and saline injection (3 h), respectively. Mean control rates of responding were 0.20 and 1.33 responses per second for the FI and FR, respectively. Vertical bars indicate +/− standard error. (From Wenger et al., 1984.)

aspects of this time course of TMT-induced changes in FI response rate are exhibited by other species as well. Wenger (1985) noted that doses of 7.5 and 8.7 mg/kg TMT in rats both produce decreases in FI response rates that gradually recover over the subsequent 2-month period. McMillan et al. (1987) examined the impact of TMT in pigeons responding under a multiple FI FR schedule of reinforcement. At a dose of 1.75 mg/kg, rates of responding in the FI component were markedly suppressed, and in some birds there was evidence for behavioral recovery within about 6 weeks.

While the most consistent effect of TMT on FI maintained behavior appears to be a decline in rates of responding, increases in response rate on another temporally based schedule, the DRL schedule, have been reported. Both Wenger et al. (1985) and Mastropaolo et al. (1984) found that TMT administration increased rates of responding in rats under a DRL schedule of reinforcement. This increase in rate was apparently brought about by a shortening of IRTs (Wenger et al. 1985) which consequently produced a decline in the number of reinforcers earned. Thus, in the case of TMT, the differential reinforcement contingencies of the FI and DRL schedules appear to support effects of TMT that differ in direction.

Ratio Schedules

Interestingly, quite opposite effects of TMT or FR schedule–controlled responding have been reported across studies, as have differences in the permanence of such effects. Three reports suggest that TMT administration is associated with a decline in FR response rates. In a study using a multiple FR 30 FI 600-sec reinforcement schedule, Wenger et al. (1984) found that a 3 mg/kg dose of TMT produced declines in rates of responding on the FR schedule in both BALB/c and C57BL/6N mice that persisted for approximately 1 week, at which time response rates had recovered to control levels. However, while Wenger (1985) described a comparable decrease in FR response rates in rats exposed to 7.5 or 8.7 mg/kg TMT, there was no evidence of a recovery of such effects over the 2-month observation period, suggesting a permanent effect of TMT. A more mixed pattern of recovery of suppressed FR response rates after 1.75 mg/kg TMT was noted by McMillan et al. (1987) in pigeons, with some birds evidencing a subsequent recovery, while others continued to exhibit dramatically decreased response rates over the 8-week period of the experiment.

In contrast to the decrease in FR response rates reported in the three studies described above, Swartzwelder et al. (1981) found that a single injection of 7.0 mg/kg TMT produced a sustained increase in FR response rates, as can be seen in Fig. 11, which apparently represented a permanent effect of TMT on this baseline, since behavioral evaluation did not begin until 40 days after TMT administration. Moreover, even on a simple FR 1 schedule of reinforcement, McMillan et al. (1986) noted an initial decrease in response rate following an injection of 6.0 mg/kg TMT to rats that lasted for approximately 1 week, but this was followed by substantially elevated response rates for another week before response rates recovered to control levels. Thus, both increases and decreases in FR response rates have been reported following TMT injection. The one difference between those studies reporting decreases in FR response rates and those describing increased rates is that the former studied FR performance in the context of a multiple-schedule format, whereas the latter examined FR responding using a simple FR schedule. Differences in permanence of effect may reflect species differences, as permanent changes were not observed in mice but were found in both rats and pigeons. Further studies will certainly be required to resolve these apparent discrepancies.

Triethyltin

Like its counterpart, triethyltin (TET) has been reported to induce a wide variety of behavioral manifestations, although these effects appear to have a more rapid onset and, for the most part, a much shorter duration of action than those produced by TMT (Wenger, 1985; McMillan and Wenger, 1985).

Interval Schedules

The primary effect of TET on FI maintained behavior appears to be one of temporary rate suppression. Wenger et al. (1986) found that doses of 5–10 mg/kg TET given to mice pro-

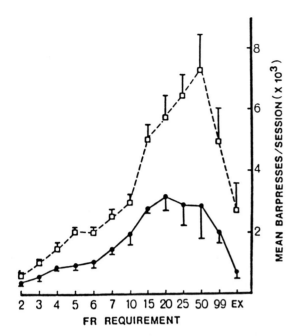

Figure 11   The effects of 7 mg/kg trimethyltin (TMT), administered 40 days before testing, on the total number of responses on the fixed-ratio (FR) schedule of reinforcement. Each data point represents the mean number of responses in a 3-h session. Points above EX represent data from an extinction session. Vertical bars indicate +/– standard error. Solid lines and filled points indicate data from control rats; dashed lines and open squares indicate data from TMT-treated rats. (From Swartzwelder et al., 1981.)

duced a decline in FI response rates for approximately 2 days, after which control rates of responding were resumed. Even repeated injections of 7.5 mg/kg produced only transient decreases in FI response rate that had disappeared within 24 h. Likewise, Rastogi et al. (1985) reported that administration of 3.0 mg/kg to rats under a multiple FR 30 FI 5-min schedule of reinforcement produced a short decrease in FI response rate that was gone within 24 h, with no residual effects noted over the next 6 weeks. In a study by DeHaven et al. (1982), doses of 1.0 and 1.5 mg/kg TET given to rats under a simple FI 1-min schedule resulted in transient decreases in response rates. McMillan et al. (1987) examined the effect of TET in pigeons under a multiple FR FI schedule of reinforcement and also found that response rates decreased within 3 h after injections of 1–5.6 mg/kg TET, with recovery noted afterward. In that study, however, some evidence for increased FI response rates emerging after several weeks was noted, although not consistently among animals.

As was the case with TMT, the effects of TET on another time-based schedule, the DRL schedule, appear to be the opposite of those described for FI schedules. Wenger et al. (1985) found that doses of TET increased rates of responding of rats on a DRL 10- to 14-s schedule by decreasing the IRTs. This increase in DRL response rate was associated with a decline in the number of reinforcers earned.

Ratio Schedules

Administration of TET likewise appears to result primarily in generally transient decreases in FR rates of responding. Wenger et al. (1986) reported that doses of 7.5–10 mg/kg TET given to mice decreased FR response rates, which then returned to baseline levels within 2 days. Even repeated injections of 7.5 mg/kg produced only transient suppression of FR responding. Rastogi et al. (1985) likewise reported a decline in response rate in the FR component of a multiple FI FR schedule in rats following 3 mg/kg TET, with recovery evident at 24 h. However, there was some evidence of rate increases over the next 2–6 weeks. In the study of DeHaven et al. (1982), doses of 1.5 mg/kg TET produced temporary decreases in response rates on a simple FR schedule. Transient decrements in FR response rates of pigeons under a multiple FR FI schedule were demonstrated by McMillan et al. (1987), although, as in the study of Rastogi et al. (1985), some evidence for a subsequent increase in rates over the next several weeks was observed. Even performance on a simple FR 1 schedule of reinforcement was suppressed by administration of 3.0–4.5 mg/kg TET to rats, although these effects appeared to be more prolonged, requiring 1–2 weeks to return to control levels of responding.

PESTICIDES

Pesticides are a broad and diverse class of chemicals that have been used on insects, fungi, nematodes, and rodents, among others. The extensive and widespread use of these compounds, with their well known central nervous system (CNS) effects, renders them an important environmental health problem. Only a few classes of pesticides have received sufficient experimental attention with respect to schedule-controlled responding to be included here, and an excellent review of the impact of these and some other classes of pesticides on schedule-controlled behavior was previously written by MacPhail (1985). His comments and conclusions are upheld by this review and are updated where additional information has been reported.

Organophosphates

The organophosphate compounds inhibit cholinesterases, and three members of the class, mevinphos, diisopropyl fluorophosphate (DFP), and parathion, have been studied most frequently.

Interval Schedules

Mertens and colleagues (Mertens et al., 1975, 1976; Lewis et al., 1973) have examined the effects of mevinphos on VI schedule–controlled responding in a variety of species, including gerbils, pigeons, and squirrel monkeys. While the effective dose differed by species, in all cases the organophosphate mevinphos produced only decreases in VI response rates and appeared to do so by increasing pausing, as can be seen in Fig. 12, which depicts the performance of a monkey responding after saline administration and after administration of mevinphos (Phosdrin). The same effect has been reported for FI maintained responding following administration of other organophosphates. For example, Ford and Rosenblum (1979) examined the effects of DFP in hens, pigeons, and rhesus monkeys under multiple FI FR schedules of reinforcement. Administration of DFP invariably resulted in a decrease in response rate in the absence of any changes in temporal patterning of behavior. McMillan and colleagues (1975) studied the effects of parathion on responding reinforced under a multiple FI 5-min FR 30 schedule of reinforcement in pigeons and likewise reported a decrement in FI response rates occurring in the absence of changes in temporal patterning. In their 1975 study, Mertens et al. also investigated

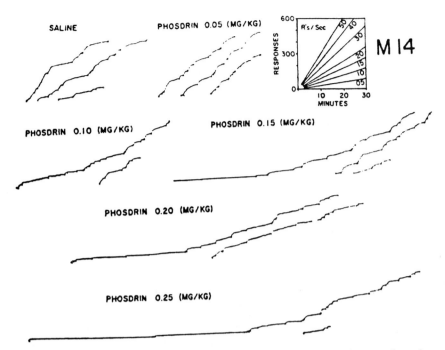

Figure 12 Cumulative records of responding for one particular monkey during the second presentation of the mevinphos (Phosdrin) dose series. Responses cumulate vertically, and time is represented horizontally. (From Lewis et al., 1973.)

the effects of mevinphos on another time-based reinforcement schedule, the DRL schedule, where a corresponding decrease in response rate accompanied by an increase in IRTs was observed. Thus, response rates on three different temporally based schedules are all suppressed by organophosphates, with such effects occuring across a wide variety of species.

Ratio Schedules

As with temporally based schedules, rates of responding on ratio-based schedules also appear to be suppressed by organophosphates across species. Fixed-ratio response rates of gerbils declined following mevinphos administration, again as a result of increased pausing (Mertens et al., 1975). Similarly, Ford and Rosenblum (1979) reported that DFP administration resulted in suppression of FR response rates in hens pigeons, and rhesus monkeys under a multiple FI FR schedule of reinforcement. Decreased FR response rates of pigeons exposed to parathion were reported by McMillan et al. (1975) in a study that used a multiple FI 5-min FR 30 schedule of reinforcement as a baseline. A study by Chambers and Chambers (1989) and another by Carr and Chambers (1991) demonstrated decreased FR 10 response rates of rats exposed to paraoxon at doses of 0.75 to 1.0 mg/kg.

Carbamates

Carbamates are a class of relatively reversible cholinesterase inhibitors and include agents such as carbaryl and aldicarb and compounds with nonpesticidal uses such as physostigmine and neostigmine.

Interval Schedules

Studies to date indicate that representative carbamate compounds produce only decreases in rates of responding maintained by temporally based schedules of reinforcement and do so primarily by generating long periods of pausing, as illustrated in the top panel of Fig. 13, which was also the case with the organophosphate mevinphos. Anger and Wilson (1980) reported a decline in VI response rates of rats following the administration of carbaryl. In 1964, Vaillant found a complete suppression of FI response rates in pigeons working under a multiple FR 30 FI 180-s or FR 30 FI 720-s schedule of reinforcement after injections of neostigmine. Vaillant (1964) describes this basically as an all-or-none phenomenon, in that prolonged periods of pausing were subsequently followed by the resumption of relatively normal responding patterns. In a study that included an evaluation of the effects of both physostigmine and neostigmine in mice, Wenger (1979) reported a decrement in rates of responding on the FI component of a multiple FR 30 FI 600-s schedule following administration of either compound.

Ratio Schedules

Performance maintained by ratio-based schedules of reinforcement is likewise suppressed by carbamates. Sideroff and Santolucito (1972) described a decrease in FR 25 response rates in rats produced by 10 mg/kg carbaryl administered once per week, an effect that persisted for weeks. This decrease in rates was at least partly attributable to increases in PRP length. A dose of 7.0 mg/kg carbaryl given to rats similarly decreased response rates during the VR component of a multiple VR 10 extinction schedule (Goldberg and Johnson, 1964). The nonpesticidal compounds neostigmine and physostigmine act similarly to their pesticidal counterparts. Both Vaillant (1964), using pigeons, and Wenger (1979), using mice, reported that physostigmine and neostigmine decreased the rates of responding on the FR component of multiple FI FR schedules.

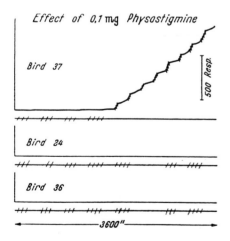

Figure 13 Cumulative records of performance on a multiple fixed-interval 180-s fixed-ratio 30 schedule for three pigeons starting 50 minutes after treatment with 0.1 mg physostigmine. Upper record demonstrates that bird 37 abruptly resumed a nearly normal pattern of behavior following a prolonged period of pausing. Hatches on the lower line of each record indicate programmed progression to the next schedule component with no occurrence of reinforcing stimuli. (From Vaillant, 1964.)

Pyrethroids

Pyrethroid insecticides have been considered to include two classes (type I and type II) based on some differences in the profiles of behavioral effects with which each is associated. Type I compounds include permethrin and cismethrin, while type II compounds include cypermethrin and deltamethrin.

Interval Schedules

Current evidence suggests that both type I and type II pyrethroids decrease response rates on interval schedules of reinforcement. Bloom et al. (1983) found a decrease in VI 20-s response rates in rats as a result of exposure to either permethrin or deltamethrin. A study by Leander and MacPhail (described by MacPhail, 1985) reported that deltamethrin administration decreased pigeons' response rates in the FI component of a multiple FI FR schedule but produced no changes in temporal patterning of behavior. Glowa (1986) studied the effects of deltamethrin exposure on the FI 60-s performance of mice. That study too reported a decrement in response rates with no evidence of tolerance following repeated injections over a 10-day period. MacPhail (1985) described a study of the impact of deltamethrin on response rates of rats whose behavior was maintained under an FI 180-s schedule of reinforcement in which declines in rates were likewise observed and changes in temporal patterning of behavior occurred only at the highest deltamethrin dose. In a later study, Peele and Crofton (1987) compared the effects of the type I compound permethrin and the type II compound cypermethrin on a multiple VI VI VI VI schedule of reinforcement. Both compounds decreased VI response rates, with cypermethrin, but not permethrin, producing rate-dependent effects.

Ratio Schedules

Pyrethroid compounds also appear to produce suppression of response rates on ratio-based reinforcement schedules. Decamethrin decreased FR 40 response rates in rats, at least in part by increasing periods of pausing (MacPhail et al., 1981). Corresponding effects of deltamethrin in pigeons were found in the FR component of a multiple FI FR schedule (Leander and MacPhail, cited in MacPhail, 1985). Stein et al. (1987) compared the effects in rats of permethrin, allethin, deltamethrin, and fenvalerate on a simple VR 25 schedule of reinforcement. As depicted in Fig. 14, all four compounds produced dose-related declines in response rates.

FUTURE RESEARCH NEEDS

As should be evident from the summaries provided here, our current understanding of the effects of exposures to inorganic lead, organic solvents, alkyl tins, and pesticides on schedule-controlled behavior is relatively restricted as a result of the rather limited data base from which pertinent information can as yet be derived. For all of the compounds reviewed here except inorganic lead, there are generally not more than four studies relating to effects on a given reinforcement schedule. Since this chapter has focused only on those compounds for which the greatest amount of information was available, that necessarily means that for numerous other neurotoxicants and for other classes of pesticides and solvents, almost nothing is known about their impact on schedule-controlled behavior. Given the critical role of schedules of reinforcement to all behavioral processes, this lack of understanding truly represents a major void in the area of behavioral toxicology.

In addition, most of the work to date examining the impact of neurotoxicants on schedule-controlled behavior has focused on characterizing the nature of the resulting effects, i.e., describing the direction and magnitude of the changes in response rates observed. This is of course appropriate and necessary in a scientific area of relative infancy, since any studies of behavioral mechanisms of action must certainly be based on reliable information about the change in schedule-controlled responding. As yet, however, few of the studies provide any in-depth information on indices of behavior other than overall response rate, by far the crudest measure of schedule-controlled behavior. Assessments of the other dependent variables related to schedule-controlled responding, such as PRP times, index of curvature or quarter-life, local response rates, IRT distributions, and rate-dependency, are seldom provided. Part of this failure to provide microanalyses of the behavior may relate to the absence of the necessary behavioral technology in some laboratories, so that collection of data required for these analyses is not possible.

Yet these measures are vital for two reasons. The first is that it is already obvious, as can be seen from the outcomes of the reviews provided here, that it will only be through the inclusion of such measures that full differentiation of the behavioral effects of various compounds will be achieved. For example, considering just the pesticides, all three classes of pesticides described, organophosphates, carbamates, and pyrethroids, decreased inter-val-based (FI and VI) response rates. However, it is very possible and highly likely, given the differences in structures of these agents, that these decreased rates were achieved through very different means. For example, IRTs can be lengthened in the absence of changes in PRP, or, alternatively, PRP may be lengthened in the absence of any local response rate changes. Both effects may result in declines measured in overall response rates. Thus it is possible that the three classes of pesticides do affect interval-based reinforcement schedules through very different behavioral processes with the same net effect on overall response rate.

Not only does the above argument apply to differentiation of subclasses of a compound (e.g., rate-dependent effects of the type II pyrethroid cypermethrin but not of the type I pyrethroid permethrin, even though both decreased VI response rates [Peele and Crofton, 1987]), it may also apply to differentiating agents within a class. A good example of this comes from a study by Moser and MacPhail (1986) examining the effects of three different formamidine pesticides (chlordimeform [CDM], amitraz [AMZ], and formetanate [FMT]) on a multiple FI 1-min FI 5-min schedule of reinforcement. In that study, all three compounds decreased rates of responding maintained by the FI 1-min schedule compo-nent, but only CDM altered index of curvature, i.e., the temporal patterning of behavior. Similarly, in the FI 5-min component, DCM did not affect overall response rate, but did decrease index of curvature values, AMZ decreased the rate of responding and altered the temporal patterning of behavior, and FMT suppressed response rates in the absence of any changes in the index of curvature. Thus, although all three formamidine compounds decreased FI response rates and thus produced ostensibly similar effects on behavior, a more refined analysis revealed a separate profile of activity for each.

The assessment of more fine-grained measures of schedule-controlled behavior is also critical to delineating the behavioral mechanism(s) of action of a compound. As previously pointed out, drugs or neurotoxicants can alter schedule-controlled behavior by interacting with the variables that control this behavior, as described above (see "Introduction"). These factors were also outlined by MacPhail (1990) as depicted in Table 1, indicating how neurotoxicants may affect schedule-controlled behavior through interactions with its controlling discriminative stimuli, the dynamics of the response, aspects of the reinforcing

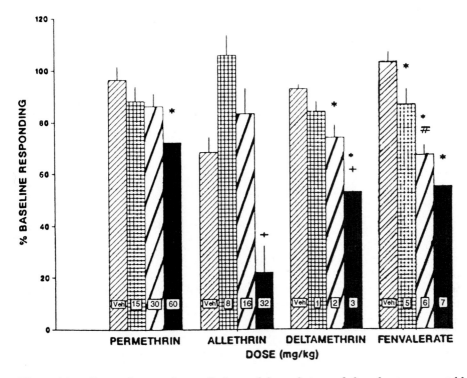

Figure 14 Effects of permethrin, allethrin, deltamethrin, and fenvalerate on variable-ratio 25 responding. Data (mean +/– standard error) are expressed as the percentage of the prior 4-day (less Monday) baseline response rate. Baseline (100%) response rates for each group of animals were permethrin 1440 +/– 135; allethrin: 4963 +/– 554; deltamethrin: 4055 +/– 233; fenvalerate: 3224 +/– 223. Rats were injected 20 min before the initiation of the 30-min test session except for allethrin, which was injected immediately before testing. Dose values are given. Numbers of subjects per group were as follows: permethrin, n = 12; allethrin, n = 7; deltamethrin, n = 12; fenvalerate, n = 11. *p .05 when compared with vehicle; ^{+}p .05 when compared with all other doses; $^{\#}p$ .05 when compared with the 5 mg/kg fenvalerate dose. (From Stein et al., 1987.)

stimuli, the nature of the schedule contingencies, the relationships between discriminative and reinforcing stimuli, and past or current behavioral history.

    With respect to the assessment of behavioral mechanisms of action, the additional use of probe sessions, i.e., intermittent sessions in which environmental manipulations are imposed, can be useful. For example, an occasional extinction session (during which no responses are reinforced) might be imposed during a long-term assessment of schedule-controlled responding. Changes in the persistence of responding under such conditions might be suggestive of alterations in motivational status, or, alternatively, in stimulus control (e.g., failure to attend to or detect changes in reinforcement density). The creative use of probe sessions should be encouraged to further the understanding of the behavioral mechanisms by which neurotoxicants alter schedule-controlled behavior.

    An additional need in this area is for studies that vary schedule parameter values and response parameters. The need for the first is underscored by findings such as those reported by Moser and MacPhail (1986) and described above, in which the formamidine pesticide chlordimeform was found to significantly suppress responding on the FI 1-min

Table 1 Operant Paradigm and the Variables Determining
Schedule-Controlled Behavior

---

1. Schedule-controlled behavior: operant paradigm[a]
    $S^D \times R \rightarrow S^R$
2. Controlling variables:
    A. S^D: Discrimintative stimuli
        1. Qualitative difference
        2. Quantitative difference
    B. R: Response effects
        1. Topography
        2. Ongoing rate
    C. S^R: Reinforcer effects
        1. Qualitative differences
        2. Quantitative differences
    D. $R \rightarrow S^R$: Schedule effects
        1. Differing schedules
        2. Differing parameters of the same schedule
    E. S^D: S^R effects
    F. Historical variables
        1. Long-term
        2. Short-term (context)

---

[a]Behavior (R) occurring in a stimulus environment ($S^D \times R$) produces
changes (right arrow) in that environment. Changes that maintain or
strengthen behavior are called reinforcers (S^R).
Source: MacPhail, 1990.

component but not on the FI 5-min component of the multiple schedule. The reasons for
these types of difference are not yet explored, but findings such as these emphasize that
the nature of a neurotoxicant's effects on behavior may be critically dependent on the
particular schedule parameter value chosen and the context in which it is examined.

The importance of evaluating different response parameters is illustrated by the
findings of Glowa (1987) that toluene exposure produced an inverse U-shaped dose-effect
function when the required response was a nose-poke, but instead produced a montonic
decline in responding on the same schedule when the required response was running in
a wheel (Fig. 7), even though the reinforcement schedule was the same. Again, such data
indicate that the nature of the effects of a given neurotoxicant may be highly dependent
on response parameters, and consequently efforts must be expended to consider diverse
response parameters.

A more complete understanding of the effects of neurotoxicants on schedule-controlled behavior will also require the evaluation of performance changes across a wider
array of reinforcement schedules. Currently, most investigators have focused their initial
efforts on FI or FR schedules, an initial strategy with the decided advantage of providing
a large data base for comparative purposes. An assessment of performance on additional
interval-based (e.g., VI, random interval, DRL) and other ratio-based (e.g., VR, random
ratio, differential reinforcement of high rates) schedules will permit a more precise
understanding of the degree of generality of any changes observed or indicate their
specificity with respect to particular contingencies. In the same vein, a broader evaluation
of the compounds within certain classes of neurotoxicants is required for determination of
structure-activity (response rate) relationships.

Finally, while the effects of several of the compounds discussed in this chapter have been examined across a relatively wide range of species, there is a continuing need to extend such efforts to include human subjects who have been inadvertently exposed to neurotoxicants. Such efforts will provide the final link bridging the issues of validation and cross-species extrapolation.

REFERENCES

Angell NF, Weiss B (1982). Operant behavior of rats exposed to lead before or after weaning. Toxicol Appl Pharmacol 63:62–71.

Anger WK, Lynch DW (1977). The effect of methyl *n*-butyl ketone on response rates of rats performing on a multiple schedule of reinforcement. Environ Res 14:204–11.

Anger WK, Wison SM (1980). Effects of carbaryl on variable interval response rates in rats. Neurobehav Toxicol 2:21–4.

Anger WK, Jordan MK, Lynch DW (1979). Effects of inhalation exposures and intraperitoneal injections of methyl *n*-amyl ketone on multiple fixed-ratio, fixed-interval response rates in rats. Toxicol Appl Pharmacol 49:407–16.

Balster RL, Borzelleca JF (1982). Behavioral toxicity of trihalomethane contaminants of drinking water in mice. Environ Health Perspec 46:127–36.

Barrett JE (1974). Conjunctive schedules of reinforcement I: Rate-dependent effects of pentobarbital and *d*-amphetamine. J Exp Anal Behav 22:561–73.

Barthalmus GT, Leander JD, McMillan DE, Mushak P, Krigman MR (1977). Chronic effects of lead on schedule-controlled pigeon behavior. Toxicol Appl Pharmacol 42:271–84.

Bloom AS, Staatz CG, Dieringer T (1983). Pyrethroid effects on operant responding and feeding. Neurobehav Toxicol Teratol 5:321–4.

Bushnell PJ (1988). Effects of delay, intertrial interval, delay behavior and trimethyltin on spatial delayed response in rats. Neurotoxicol Teratol 10:237–44.

Carr RL, Chambers JE (1991). Acute effects of the organophosphate paraoxon on schedule-controlled behavior and esterase activity in rats: dose-response relationships. Pharmacol Biochem Behav 40:929–36.

Chambers JE, Chambers HW (1989). Short-term effects of paraoxon and atropine on schedule-controlled behavior in rats. Neurotoxicol Teratol 11:427–32.

Colotla VA, Bautista S, Lorenzana-Jimenez M, Rodriguez R (1979). Effects of solvents on schedule-controlled behavior. Neurobehav Toxicol 1(suppl 1):113–8.

Cory-Slechta DA (1984). The behavioral toxicity of lead: problems and perspectives. In: Thompson T, Dews PB, Barrett JE, eds. Advances in behavioral pharmacology. Vol. 4. New York: Academic Press, 211–55.

Cory-Slechta DA (1985). Alterations in schedule-controlled behavior of rodents correlated with prolonged lead exposure. In: Seiden LS, Balster RL, eds. Behavioral pharmacology: the current status. New York: Alan R. Liss, 487–502.

Cory-Slechta DA (1986). Prolonged lead exposure and fixed ratio performance. Neurobehav Toxicol Teratol 8:237–44.

Cory-Slechta DA (1988). Chronic low-level lead exposure: behavioral consequences, biological exposure indices, and reversibility. Sci Total Environ 71:433–40.

Cory-Slechta DA (1990). Exposure duration modifies the effects of low level lead on fixed interval performance. Neuro toxicology 11:427–42.

Cory-Slechta DA (1992). Schedule-controlled behavior in neurotoxicology. In: Tilson H, Mitchell C, eds. Neurotoxicology. New York: Raven Press, 271–94.

Cory-Slechta DA, Pokora MJ (1991). Behavioral manifestations of prolonged lead exposure initiated at different stages of the life cycle: I. Schedule-controlled responding. Neurotoxicology 12:745–60.

Cory-Slechta DA, Thompson T (1979). Behavioral toxicity of chronic postweaning lead exposure in the rat. Toxicol Appl Pharmacol 47:151–9.

Cory-Slechta DA, Weiss B (1989). Efficacy of the chelating agent CaEDTA in reversing lead-induced changes in behavior. Neurotoxicology 10:685–98.

Cory-Slechta DA, Weiss B, Cox C (1983). Delayed behavioral toxicity of lead with increasing exposure concentration. Toxicol Appl Pharmacol 71:342–52.

Cory-Slechta DA, Weiss B, Cox C (1985). Performance and exposure indices of rats exposed to low concentrations of lead. Toxicol Appl Pharmacol 78:291–9.

DeHaven DL, Wayner MJ, Barone FC, Evans SM (1982). Effects of triethyltin on schedule dependent and schedule induced behaviors under different schedules of reinforcement. Neurobehav Toxicol Teratol 4:231–9.

Dews PB (1955). Studies on behavior. I. Differential sensitivity to pentobarbital of pecking performance in pigeons depending on the schedule of reward. J Pharmacol Exp Ther 113:393–401.

Dews PB (1964). A behavioral effect of amobarbital. Arch Exp Pathol Pharmakol 248:296–307.

Dews PB (1978). Epistemology of screening for behavioral toxicity. Environ Health Perspec 26:37–42.

Dews PB, Wenger GR (1977). Rate dependency of the behavioral effects of *d*-amphetamine. In: Thompson T, Dews PB, eds. Advances in behavioral pharmacology. Vol. 1. New York: Academic Press, 167–227.

Ford RD, Rosenblum I (1979). The acute behavioral effects of diisopropyl fluorophosphate in the chicken, pigeon and rhesus monkey. Ecotoxicol Environ Safety 3:428–38.

Fry W, Kelleher R, Cook L (1960). A mathematical index of performance on fixed-interval schedules of reinforcement. J Exp Anal Behav 3:193–9.

Geller I, Hartmann RJ, Randle SR, Gause EM (1979). Effects of acetone and toluene vapors on multiple schedule performance of rats. Pharmacol Biochem Behav 11:395–9.

Glowa JR (1981). Some effects of sub-acute exposure to toluene on schedule-controlled behavior. Neurobehav Toxicol Teratol 3:463–5.

Glowa JR (1985). Behavioral effects of volatile organic solvents. In: Seiden LS, Balster RL, eds. Behavioral pharmacology: the current status. New York: Alan R. Liss, 537–52.

Glowa JR (1986). Acute and sub-acute effects of deltamethrin and chlordimeform on schedule-controlled responding in the mouse. Neurobehav Toxicol Teratol 8:97–102.

Glowa JR (1987). Comparisons of some behavioral effects of *d*-amphetamine and toluene. Neurotoxicology 8:237–48.

Glowa JR, Dews PB (1983). Behavioral toxicology of volatile organic solvents. II. Comparison of results of toluene by flow-through and closed chamber procedures. J Am Coll Toxicol 2:319–23.

Glowa JR, DeWeese J, Natale ME, Holland JJ, Dews PB (1983). Behavioral toxicology of volatile organic solvents I. Methods: acute effects of toluene. J Am Coll Toxicol 2:175–85.

Goldberg ME, Johnson HE (1964). Behavioral effects of a cholinergic stimulant in combination with various psychotherapeutic agents. J Pharmacol Exp Ther 145:367–72.

Gollub LR (1964). The relations among measures of performance on fixed-interval schedules. J Exp Anal Behav 7:337–43.

Johnson BL, Setzer JV, Lewis TR, Anger WK (1977). Effects of methyl *n*-butyl ketone on behavior and the nervous system. Am Ind Hyg Assoc J 38:567–79.

Kelleher RT, Morse WH (1969). Determinants of the behavioral effects of drugs. In: Tedeschi DJ, Tedeschi RE, eds. Importance of fundamental principles in drug evaluation. New York: Raven Press, 383–405.

Lewis MF, Mertens HW, Steen JA (1973). Behavioral changes from chronic exposure to pesticides used in aerial application: effects of phosdrin on the performance of monkeys and pigeons on variable interval reinforcement schedules. Aerosp Med 44:290–3.

MacPhail RC (1985). Effects of pesticides on schedule-controlled behavior. In: Seiden LS, Balster RL, eds. Behavioral pharmacology: the current status. New York: Alan R. Liss, 519–35.

MacPhail RC (1990). Environmental modulation of neurobehavioral toxicity. In: Russel RW, Flattau PE, Pope AM, eds. Behavioral measures of neurotoxicity. Washington, D.C.: National Academy Press, 347–58.

MacPhail RC, Gordon WA, Johnston MA (1981). Behavioral effects of a synthetic pyrethroid insecticide (decamethrin). Fed Proc 40:678 (abstract).

McKim WA (1973). The effects of scopolamine on fixed-interval behaviour in the rat: a rate-dependency effect. Psychopharmacologia 32:255–64.

McMillan DE (1973). Drugs and punished responding I: Rate-dependent effects under multiple schedules. J Exp Anal Behav 19:133–45.

McMillan DE, Wenger GR (1985). Neurobehavioral toxicology of trialkyltins. Pharnmacol Rev 37:365–79.

McMillan DE, Leander JD, Lucot JB (1975). Some effects of parathion on the schedule-controlled behavior of the pigeon. Pharmacologist 17:204 (abstract).

McMillan DE, Chang LW, Idemudia SO, Wenger GR (1986). Effects of trimethyltin and triethyltin on lever pressing, water drinking and running in an activity wheel: associated neuropathology. Neurobehav Toxicol Teratol 8:499–507.

McMillan DE, Wenger GR, Brocco MJ, Idemudia SO, Chang LW (1987). Effects of trialkyltins on the schedule-controlled behavior of the pigeon. Neurotoxicol Teratol 9:67–74.

Mastropaolo JP, Decanay RJ, Luna BH, Tuck DL, Riley AL (1984). Effects of trimethyltin chloride on differential-reinforcement-of-low-rate responding. Neurobehav Toxicol Teratol 6:193–9.

Mele PC, Bushnell PJ, Bowman RE (1984). Prolonged behavioral effects of early postnatal lead exposure in rhesus monkeys: fixed-interval responding and interactions with scopolamine and pentobarbital. Neurobehav Toxicol Teratol 6:129–35.

Mertens HW, Steen JA, Lewis MA (1975). The effects of mevinphos on appetitive operant behavior in the gerbil. Psychopharmacology 41:47–52.

Mertens HW, Steen JA, Lewis MA (1976). Some behavioral effects of pesticides: the interaction of mevinphos and atropine in pigeons. Aviation Space Environ Med 47:137–41.

Moser VC, Balster RL (1981). The effect of acute and repeated toluene exposure on schedule-controlled responding in mice. Neurobehav Toxicol 3:471–5.

Moser VC, Balster RL (1985). Effects of toluene, halothane and ethanol vapor on fixed-ratio performance in mice. Pharmacol Biochem Behav 22:797–802.

Moser VC, Balster RL (1986). The effects of inhaled toluene, halothane, 1,1,1-trichloroethane, and ethanol on fixed-interval responding in mice. Neurobehav Toxicol Teratol 8:525–31.

Moser VC, MacPhail RC (1986). Differential effects of formamidine pesticides on fixed-interval behavior in rats. Toxicol Appl Pharmacol 84:315–24.

Moser VC, Scimeca JA, Balster RL (1985). Minimal tolerance to the effects of 1,1,1-trichloroethane on fixed-ratio responding in mice. Neurotoxicology 6:35–42.

Nation JR, Fry GD, Von Stultz J, Bratton GR (1989). Effects of combined lead and cadmium exposure: changes in schedule-controlled responding and in dopamine, serotonin, and their metabolites. Behav Neurosci 5:1108–14.

Padich R, Zenick H (1977). The effects of developmental and/or direct lead exposure on FR behavior in the rat. Pharmacol Biochem Behav 6:371–5.

Peele DB, Crofton KM (1987). Pyrethroid effects on schedule-controlled behavior: time and dosage relationships. Neurotoxicol Teratol 9:387–94.

Rastogi SK, McMillan DE, Wenger GR, Chang LW (1985). Effects of triethyltin and its interaction with *d*-amphetamine and chlorpromazine on responding under a multiple schedule of food presentation in rats. Neurobehav Toxicol Teratol 7:239–42.

Reynolds GS (1968). A primer of operant conditioning. Glenview, Illinois: Scott, Foresman and Company.

Rice DC (1988). Schedule-controlled behavior in infant and juvenile monkeys exposed to lead from birth. Neuro toxicology 9:75–88.

Rice DC (1992). Lead exposure during different developmental periods produces different effects on FI performance in monkeys tested as juveniles and adults. NeuroToxicol *13*:757–770.

Rice DC, Gilbert SG, Willes RF (1979). Neonatal low-level lead exposure in monkeys: locomotor activity, schedule-controlled behavior, and the effects of amphetamine. Toxicol Appl Pharmacol 51:503–13.

Sideroff SI, Santolucito JA (1972). Behavioral and physiological effects of the cholinesterase inhibitor carbaryl (1-naphthyl methylcarbamate). Physiol Behav 9:459–62.

Stein EA, Washburn M, Walczak C, Bloom AS (1987). Effects of pyrethroid insecticides on operant responding maintained by food. Neurotoxicol Teratol 9:27–31.

Stitzer M (1974). Comparison of morphine and chlorpromazine effects of moderately and severely suppressed punished responding in the pigeon. J Pharmacol Exp Ther 191:172–8.

Swartzwelder HS, Dyer RS, Holahan W, Myers RD (1981). Activity changes in rats following acute trimethyltin exposure. Neurotoxicology 2:589–93.

Vaillant GE (1964). Antagonism between physostigmine and atropine on the behavior of the pigeon. Naunyn-Schmiedebergs Arch Exp Pathol Pharmakol 248:406–16.

Van Gelder GA, Carson T, Smith RM, Buck WB (1973). Behavioral toxicologic assessment of the neurologic effect of lead in sheep. Clin Toxicol 6:405–18.

Wenger GR (1979). Effects of physostigmine, atropine and scopolamine on behavior maintained by a multiple schedule of food presentation in the mouse. J Pharmacol Exp Ther 209:137–43.

Wenger GR (1985). The effects of trialkyl tin compounds on schedule-controlled behavior. In: Seiden LS, Balster RL, eds. Behavioral pharmacology: the current status. New York: Alan R. Liss, 503–18.

Wenger GR, McMillan DE, Chang LW (1984). Behavioral effects of trimethyltin in two strains of mice. II. Multiple fixed ratio, fixed interval. Toxicol Appl Pharmacol 73:89–96.

Wenger GR, McMillan DE, Chang LW, Zitaglio T, Hardwick WC (1985). The effects of triethyltin and trimethyltin in rats responding under a DRL schedule of reinforcement. Toxicol Appl Pharmacol 78:248–58.

Wenger GR, McMillan DE, Chang LW (1986). Effects of triethyltin on responding of mice under a multiple schedule of reinforcement. Neurotoxicol Teratol 8:659–65.

Zenick H, Rodriquez W, Ward J, Elkington B (1979). Deficits in fixed-interval performance following prenatal and postnatal lead exposure. Dev Psychobiol 12:509–14.

12
Assessment of Auditory Dysfunction

Gordon T. Pryor
SRI International
Menlo Park, California

INTRODUCTION

Partial or complete deafness is a serious handicap for those afflicted. In the United States it was estimated in 1988 that some 21.9 million persons (about 9% of the population) suffer from some form of hearing impairment (U.S. Department of Commerce, 1991). Some 6 million also suffer from tinnitus to the extent of coming to the attention of medical personnel. The incidence of hearing loss increases progressively with age from about 2% among persons up to 18 years old to over 25% among persons 65 or older. The causes of various hearing disorders include genetic errors, congenital malformation or insults from various sources, various disease states and infections, auditory overstimulation, mechanical injury, exposure to drugs such as the aminoglycoside antibiotics, and apparently the aging process itself ("presbycusis") (Dublin, 1976; Hood and Berlin, 1986).

Another cause of auditory dysfunction that has come to be recognized as a potentially serious problem is exposure to certain industrial chemicals and environmental pollutants. The extent to which such exposures may have contributed to the large number of people suffering from some form of hearing disorder, especially in the older population, is unknown. However, this cause, regardless of the magnitude of its contribution to the problem, is potentially avoidable. When it is determined which chemicals or chemical classes are capable of causing hearing dysfunction, measures can be taken to reduce human exposure by establishing safe levels or eliminating them entirely from the ever-growing number of chemicals to which people are exposed.

At present only a handful of industrial chemicals have been proved to cause hearing impairment in animals. The number is even smaller for which convincing evidence is available for humans as well. In view of the expanding use of, and requirements for, neurotoxicity testing batteries that include tests of sensory function, this small number may imply that the concern about ototoxic chemicals is exaggerated. However, the tests for auditory dysfunction typically included in such batteries may be too insensitive to detect anything short of almost total deafness in rodents. Indeed, as researchers have begun to use tests that are designed specifically to detect and characterize auditory dysfunction in rodents and that can be administered to relatively large numbers of animals fairly rapidly, the number of known ototoxic chemicals has begun to grow.

The auditory system, especially the peripheral receptors, appears to be especially vulnerable, and sometimes specifically so, to certain classes of chemicals. The purpose of this chapter will be to examine the auditory system in this context (for more in-depth coverage of the topics covered, the reader is encouraged to consult the following sources: Dublin, 1976; Smith and Vernon, 1976; Altschuler et al., 1986; Jahn and Santos-Sacchi, 1988; Corwin and Warchol, 1991). First, the anatomy and electrophysiology of the acoustic apparatus, both of which have been extensively characterized, will be summarized to provide a basis and background for considering the auditory system as a target for toxic chemicals. Then, methods for assessing auditory dysfunction and its pathological basis will be briefly presented. Finally, a review of currently known agents and chemicals that cause temporary or permanent damage to the auditory system will be provided.

BASIC PRINCIPLES

Understanding of the anatomical and physiological basis of hearing is a relatively modern development, having been achieved mainly in the 20th century (see Hawkins, 1988, for a brief, but delightful, history of efforts to discover how we hear). Indeed, it was not until the 18th century that the doctrine of "implanted air" put forth by Aristotle was challenged seriously. Not until the 19th century was this unfounded speculation finally put to rest, and modern theories of hearing then began to emerge. Unraveling the mysteries of how vibrations in the air are translated into nerve impulses in the brain had to await technological advances that have became available only since the turn of the century. The initial slow progress in understanding cochlear function can be attributed mainly to the small size and inaccessibility of the auditory apparatus. However, once appropriate technologies became available, progress was rapid. The advent of scanning and transmission electron microscopes made possible the detailed description of the fine structure of the inner ear and its elegant geometry. Developments in biophysical and electrophysiological techniques provided the tools for recording and analyzing the earliest electrical events occurring in the transduction process and their subsequent journey through the 8th cranial nerve, the brain stem, the midbrain, and ultimately the cortex. Finally, modern biochemical methods are beginning to unravel the complex molecular substrate and functional components of the end organ.

By far the greatest number of agents known to cause auditory dysfunction do so in the cochlea. More specifically, the majority damage or destroy the receptor cells responsible for the final peripheral transduction, although the biochemical mechanisms involved are generally unknown at this time. The intricacy and high energy requirements of the elements involved in the transduction process appear to make this end organ especially vulnerable to damage, whether by acoustic overstimulation or by certain chemicals. This vulnerability makes the inner ear a potentially prime target for toxic insult by the myriad chemicals in our environment.

The purpose of this section is to provide a brief summary of the basic anatomy, physiology, and biochemistry of the auditory system. The reader is referred to several recent textbooks and reviews for more detailed information and to get a flavor of the rapid advances that are being made in our understanding of "how we hear" (e.g., Altschuler et al., 1986; Jahn and Santos-Sacchi, 1988).

Anatomy of the Auditory System

The cochlea is a complex spiral structure divided into three fluid-filled ducts, the scala tympani, the scala media, and the scala vestibuli (Fibs. 1 and 2) (Harrison and Hunter-Duvar, 1988). A duct at the apex of the cochlea connects the scala tympani with the scala vestibuli. The scala tympani ends at the round window, which serves to release the pressure changes within the cochlea. The lateral wall of the scala media is formed by the highly vascular stria vascularis (Axelsson and Ryan, 1988). The two outer ducts are filled with perilymph, and the middle duct, which bathes the auditory receptors, is filled with endolymph (Salt and Konishi, 1986). These ducts are also connected with other fluid-filled compartments of the skull and thus are continuous with comparable ducts within the vestibular apparatus and the cerebrospinal fluid.

The cochlear ducts are separated by Reissner's membrane and the basilar membrane,

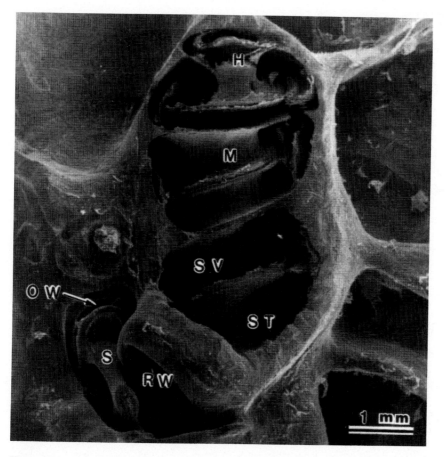

Figure 1 A scanning electron micrograph of the opened cochlea as seen from a lateral aspect. H = helicotrema; M = modiolus; OW = oval window; RW = round window; S = stapes; SV = scala vestibuli; ST = scala tympani. (From Harrison and Hunter-Duvar, 1988.)

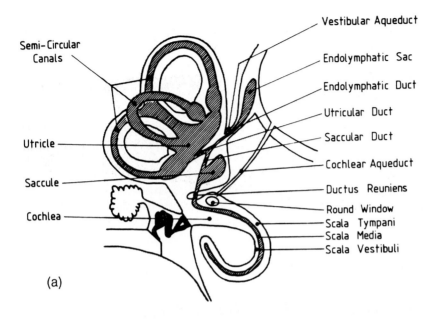

(a)

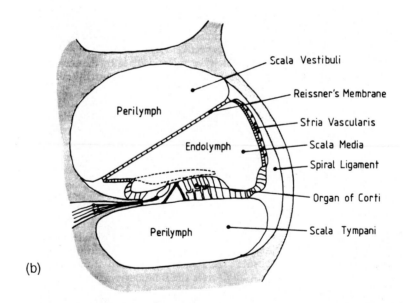

(b)

Figure 2 (a) Anatomy of the inner ear showing the major compartments and interconnecting ducts. Perilymph within the bony labyrinth is shown in white. The membranous structures, containing endolymph, are shaded with diagonal lines. (b) Diagrammatic cross-section through one turn of the cochlea. The tectorial membrane is represented by the dashed line. (From Salt and Konishi, 1986.)

the latter containing the organ of Corti. The organ of Corti is an elegant structure that contains the auditory receptors or hair cells (Santi, 1988). The hair cells are arranged in three rows of outer hair cells and one row of inner hair cells (Fig. 3). The stereocilia on each hair cell protrude into the endolymph of the scala media (Nielsen and Slepecky, 1986). They are cross-linked and attached to one another at their tips (Pickles et al., 1984). This cross-linking is important in the transduction process, because only the tallest row of stereocilia appears to be attached to the overlying tectorial membrane (Kimura, 1966).

Vibrations of the air are channeled through the auditory meatus of the external ear, where they strike the tympanic membrane or eardrum (Fig. 4). Vibrations of the tympanic membrane are modulated by the malleus, incus, and stapes. In turn, the mechanical motions of these three tiny bones of the middle ear, by attachment of the stapes to the oval window of the cochlea, set in motion the fluid in the cochlear ducts, vibrating the basilar membrane. The sensory epithelial cells on this membrane convert the mechanical energy to ionic fluxes, resulting in transmitter release to afferent nerve endings that synapse on the base of the hair cells (Santos-Sacchi, 1988). The afferent endings are dendrites of

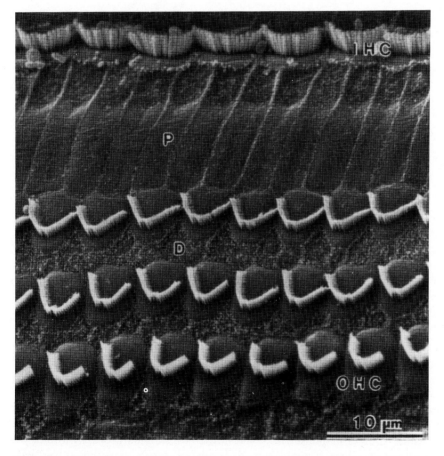

Figure 3   The sensory epithelium of the organ of Corti showing the stereocilia arising from the three rows of outer hair cells and one row of inner hair cells. D = Deiters' cells; IHC = inner hair cells; OHC = outer cells; P = pillar cells. (From Harrison and Hunter-Duvar, 1988.)

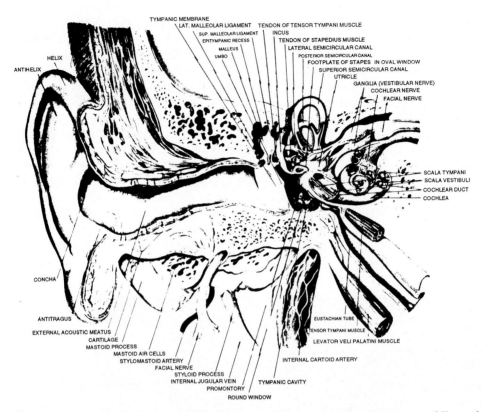

Figure 4   Drawing of the peripheral auditory-vestibular system showing outer, middle, and inner portions in relation to other anatomic features in this saggital section through the human head. (From Guth and Bobbin 1971.)

bipolar cells located in the spiral ganglion, the axons of which form a major portion of the 8th nerve (Spoendlin, 1988).

Because of the biophysics involved in the fluid-filled ducts of the cochlea, the hair cells are excited by sounds of increasing frequency from the apex to the base (Allen, 1988). The inner hair cells, with cell bodies in the spiral ganglion, synapse with about 90–95% of the myelinated afferent nerve endings contained in the 8th nerve (Spoendlin, 1988). The outer hair cells receive a rich supply of efferent input from cells in the superior olivary nucleus (Fig. 5).

Physiology of the Auditory System

The electrical responses of the elements of the auditory system have been studied extensively and are now fairly well understood (see Nauton, 1978; Allen, 1988; Santos-Sacchi, 1988; Harrison, 1988; Phillips, 1988). What follows is a brief description of the main characteristics of these responses from the initial transduction process through the activity of the 8th nerve, which terminates in the cochlear nuclear complex of the brain stem. The interactions that occur beyond the cochlear nuclear complex are intricate and are beyond the scope of this chapter (see Phillips, 1988). Nevertheless, pathways to the

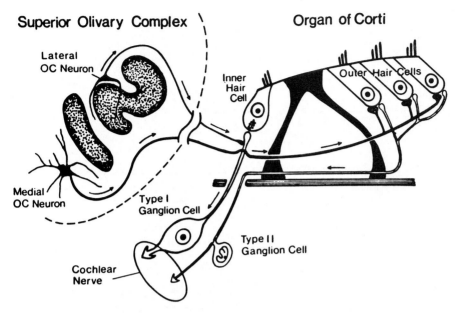

Figure 5 Schematic diagram showing the principal relations between the two afferent and the two efferent innervations of the organ of Corti. (From Warr et al., 1986.)

cortex will be outlined and a few prominent characteristics of their electrophysiology will be noted.

Displacement of the stereocilia on the hair cells results in an alternating current that faithfully follows the frequency of the sound stimulus, i.e., the cochlear microphonic (Weaver and Bray, 1930). The alternating current is generated by a differential ion flux between the extracellular (endolymph) and intracellular sides of the hair cell membrane (Santos-Sacchi, 1988). These currents are conditioned by direct-current potential between the endolymph of the scala media and the perilymph of the scala tympani, the resting, or endolymphatic, potential. This resting potential provides the electrical driving force for the movement of positively charged ions (Ca^+ and K^+) through the channels in the stereocilia of the hair cells (Russell, 1983).

Recordings made from various locations along the organ of Corti have clearly demonstrated that the hair cells generating the cochlear microphonic respond differentially as a function of the frequency of the acoustic stimulus (Fig. 6) (see Dallos, 1973; Santos-Sacchi, 1988). This frequency-specificity is related to the location of the hair cells along the basilar membrane, from low-frequency response at the apex to high-frequency response at the base. Because of the vibrational properties of the basilar membrane with respect to the fluid motion in the cochlear ducts, the location of the hair cells along the membrane is generally considered sufficient to account for their frequency-specificity (Khanna and Leonard, 1982; Sellick et al., 1982). However, this frequency-specificity is not absolute. At threshold stimulation with tones of varying frequency, the hair cells exhibit a tuning curve. The frequency at which the cell has the lowest threshold is that cell's best or characteristic frequency (CF). Frequencies on either side of the CF require higher intensities to produce a threshold response. The tails of the tuning curve are very asymmetrical for high-frequency tones, being shallow for frequencies below the CF and

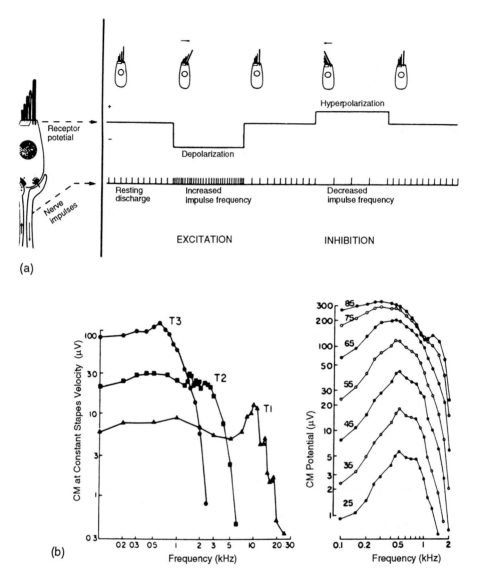

Figure 6   (a) Hair cell afferent nerve activity recorded during displacements of hair bundles in the lateral line organ showing the relations between direction of displacement, changes in polarization, and frequency of spike discharge. (b) Left: Recording of cochlear microphonic (CM) magnitude from turn 1 (T1), turn 2 (T2), and turn 3 (T3) along the cochlear duct of the guinea pig. A constant input stimulus was delivered to the ear at frequencies across the spectrum. The best frequency decreases from base to apex as indicated by the frequency at which the responses fall precipitously. Right: A family of curves illustrating CM magnitude versus frequency at several constant intensities. The sharpness of the tuning curve increases as the intensity decreases toward threshold. (From Santos-Sacchi, 1988.)

steep for those above it. This asymmetry decreases as the CF decreases (Santos-Sacchi, 1988).

The response of the inner hair cells is thought to be almost entirely responsible for the conversion of the cochlear microphonic to spike propagation in the 8th nerve. Over 90% of the fibers in the 8th nerve synapse one-on-one with the inner hair cells (Morrison et al., 1975). Most of the remainder, including efferents, synapse diffusely with the three rows of outer hair cells (Spoendlin, 1969; Perkins and Morest, 1975). Thus, activity recorded from single or massed unit fibers of the 8th nerve reflects the tuning characteristics of their respective associated hair cells (see Harrison, 1988). However, unlike the cochlear microphonic, the response of these fibers does not follow the stimulus frequency, except over a narrow range. Thus, frequency is coded spatially at the organ of Corti, and this tonotopic representation is remarkably preserved throughout the auditory pathways to the cortex (see Phillips, 1988).

The roles of the inner and outer hair cells in the hearing process are distinctly different. Whereas the inner hair cells transmit the primary information about the acoustic stimulus to the afferent fibers of the 8th nerve, the outer hair cells are believed to modulate the transduction process. The mechanism by which the outer hair cells may affect this modulation is truly remarkable and has only recently begun to be unraveled (Mountain, 1986; Yates et al., 1992; Pickles and Corey, 1992). The stereocilia of the outer hair cells have been observed to shorten or lengthen in response to appropriate stimulation (Brownell et al., 1985). This motion could alter the micro–fluid dynamics set in motion by the sound stimulus and thus alter the vibrational pattern of the basilar membrane. The result would be a modulation of the tuning characteristics of the basilar membrane and, consequently, the tuning curves for the inner hair cells on it.

Although coding for frequency can be satisfactorily accounted for by location of the hair cells along the organ of Corti, a universally accepted explanation for the coding of stimulus intensity (loudness) remains to be achieved. Hair cells and nerve fibers typically respond to an increase in stimulus intensity with an increase in firing rate up to some maximum (e.g., Evans, 1981; Palmer and Evans, 1982). The psychophysical dynamic range in humans (i.e., the range over which an increase in intensity can be perceived as an increase in loudness) is about 100 decibels (dB). However, the dynamic range for most fibers of the 8th nerve (substitute firing rate for loudness) is only about 40–50 dB. Therefore, other and/or additional mechanisms must be invoked to account for the dynamic range of perceived loudness. One possibility is that different neuron populations code smaller, overlapping segments of the dynamic range.

Several other characteristics of auditory signal processing should be mentioned. Adaptation, reflected by decreased spike rate in the 8th nerve, occurs exponentially with sustained sound stimulation (see Harrison, 1988). This phenomenon is associated with synaptic transmission between the hair cells and their afferent endings; such adaptation is not seen in the cochlear microphonic or the electrically stimulated fibers of the 8th nerve (Mulroy et al., 1974; Norris et al., 1977). When a sound stimulus is terminated, the spike rate decreases below the spontaneous discharge rate, the "off-response" (e.g., Harris and Dallos, 1979). These two phenomena may be related to the decreased response to the second of two acoustic stimuli. The reduction in response to the second stimulus is a function of the intensity of the first stimulus and the interval between the two stimuli. Other characteristics include masking, where the increase in response rate is conditioned by the presence of a simultaneously occurring tone or noise, and two-tone interactions (e.g., Evans, 1974; Arthur et al., 1971). These temporal and frequency-dependent characteristics of the responses to sound at the cochlea and 8th nerve clearly suggest that considerable signal processing of complex sounds, such as occur in speech and music, can occur at distal loci (see Harrison, 1988).

A brief tour through the central auditory system concludes this section (Fig. 7). The fibers from the cochlea make their first synapse in the cochlear nuclear complex of the brain stem. From here, ascending axons project ipsilaterally and contralaterally to the superior olivary complex and the inferior colliculi. Thus, it is at these levels that binaural interactions, critical in sound localization, can occur (see Phillips, 1988; Phillips and Brugge, 1985). Cells in the superior olivary complex that receive inputs from numerous sources, including the cochlea, also send efferents back to the hair cells of the cochlea. Ipsilateral and contralateral neurons from the cochlear nuclear complex and the superior olivary complex converge in the inferior colliculi and associated nuclei. From here they project ipsilaterally and contralaterally to the medial geniculate nuclei of the thalamus. The thalamocortical connections are exclusively ipsilateral and reciprocal. It is important to note that the tonotopic organization seen in the cochlea is preserved throughout the auditory pathway to the cortex. Equally important, however, is the modulatory influence of both ascending and descending neurons on this tonotopic organization. These interactions undoubtedly are intimately involved in the perception and decoding of complex sounds and the organism's response to them. The unraveling of this communications network remains a challenge for neuroscience.

Neurochemistry of the Peripheral Auditory System

The transduction process occurs as a result of the bending of the stereocilia in response to mechanical vibration of the basilar membrane. Deflection of the stereocilia opens ion channels in their tips (Hudspeth, 1982). The stereocilia are laterally cross-linked, which is thought to distribute the mechanical force throughout the stereocilia bundle (see Santi, 1988). The composition of these external linkages has not yet been determined, but they may consist of glycoproteins or proteoglycans (Lim, 1985; Santi and Anderson, 1987). Internally, the stereocilia contain axial microfilaments consisting of F-actin (Flock and Cheung, 1977) arranged in tightly packed arrays. These arrays are cross-linked by fimbrin to form rigid bundles that extend into the cuticular plate (Slepecky and Chamberlain, 1985).

Movement of the stereocilia in the direction of the tallest stereocilia causes depolarization of the hair cell, which opens voltage-sensitive Ca^{2+} channels in the basolateral membrane of the cell (Lewis and Hudspeth, 1983). Influx of Ca^{2+} is thought to promote release of the afferent neurotransmitter by fusion of vesicles with the presynaptic plasma membrane. The neurotransmitter interacts with a receptor on the postsynaptic membrane to cause depolarization and, if this is sufficient, initiation of an action potential.

The neurotransmitter between the hair cells and the afferent nerve endings has not been unequivocally identified (see Altschuler and Fex, 1986; Bledsoe et al., 1988). Indeed, multiple transmitters may be involved, depending on whether the synapses are on inner or outer hair cells and on the types of fibers being innervated.

At present the evidence strongly suggests an excitatory amino acid (EAA)-like substance as the endogenous afferent transmitter (see Bledsoe et al., 1988). Pharmacological evidence has shown that kainic acid (KA) and quisqualic acid (QA) receptors are present and functional in the cochlea and that they are probably postsynaptic to the hair cells

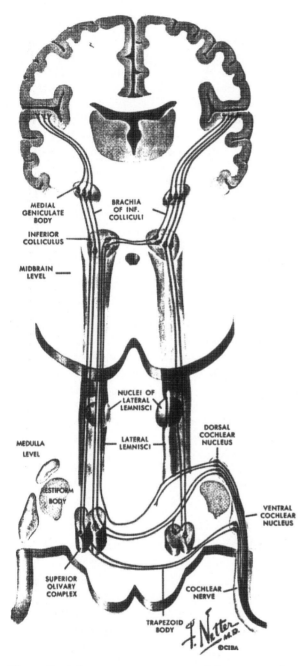

Figure 7 Schematic representation of the major pathways from the cochlea to the cortex. (From Netter, 1962.)

(Bledsoe et al., 1981; Jenison et al., 1986). In contrast, the *N*-methyl-D-aspartate (NMDA)-type EAA receptor does not appear to be present (Jenison et al., 1986). Thus, glutamate and aspartate, both of which are present presynaptically (Godfrey et al., 1976), or a structurally related analogue, are candidates. A number of substances that act as neurotransmitters in other parts of the nervous system have been virtually eliminated as the afferent transmitter in the hair cells—acetylcholine (ACh), 5-hydroxytryptamine, norepinephrine, dopamine, glycine, taurine, and substance P (reviewed by Bledsoe et al., 1982). Evidence also suggests that γ-amino-butyric acid (GABA) does not serve this function in the hair cells (also reviewed by Bledsoe et al., 1988) but may do so in the vestibular system (Felix and Ehrenberger, 1982) and possibly in the efferent innervation of the organ of Corti (reviewed by Altschuler and Fex, 1986).

The efferent transmitter is most likely ACh (reviewed by Altschuler and Fex, 1986; Bledsoe et al., 1988). Strong pharmacological evidence is provided by the finding that anticholinergic compounds such as atropine block the effects of efferent stimulation without affecting afferent transmission. The synthetic degradative enzymes for ACh, choline acetyltransferase (ChAT) and acetylcholinesterase (AChE), are present persynaptically, as demonstrated by transection experiments. Moreover, ACh-like activity has been demonstrated in the perilymph after electrical stimulation of the efferent system (Fex, 1968; Norris and Guth, 1974).

Finally, a number of substances have been identified as potential neuromodulators in the cochlea. Enkephalin-like immunoreactivity has been identified in efferent neurons of the cochlea (Fex and Altschuler, 1981), and a methionine-enkephalin-like component was elevated in the perilymph in response to noise (Drescher et al., 1983). Other candidates include adenosine triphosphate (ATP), calcitonin, gene-related peptide, taurine, aspartate, dopamine, and GABA (reviewed by Bledsoe et al., 1988).

Clearly, much more work is needed to identify the exact roles of these and other substances in the neurotransmission process in the peripheral auditory system. Nevertheless, it should be apparent that the potential for chemical interference or interaction with exogenous substances is substantial, and that any disturbances in the exquisitely tuned biochemical machinery of this organ could lead to reversible or irreversible auditory dysfunction.

METHODS FOR ASSESSING AUDITORY DYSFUNCTION IN ANIMALS

Behavioral Methods

A number of behavioral methods have been used to assess auditory dysfunction in a variety of animal species (Stebbins, 1970; Crofton, 1992). The choice of which method and species to use will depend largely on the precision needed and the resources available.

For screening purposes it may be sufficient to use a simple reflex procedure (the Preyer reflex). This reflex (observed as a twitch of the pinna) is elicited by a sharp-onset, brief click or tone of moderate intensity. Thus, in its simplest form (e.g., using a fingersnap or click stimulus) it is easily incorporated into a screening battery such as the functional observational battery (e.g., Moser et al., 1988). However, for more precise characterization of auditory dysfunction using this method, additional equipment is needed (appropriate sound-generation equipment and an acoustically neutral environment). Moreover, because it requires a human observer, it is very labor-intensive except in the screening mode, where it is probably the least sensitive. Thus, although many investigators have used this method successfully to characterize the temporary and permanent hearing losses associated with various drugs and noise (e.g., Parravicini et al., 1982), it has been largely abandoned in favor of more efficient methods.

For precise characterization of normal hearing and auditory dysfunction in various animal species, classical and operant conditioning procedures based on both positive and negative reinforcement have been the methods of choice (see Stebbins, 1970). These methods share the common characteristic that the animal subject is taught to report its perception of a stimulus by performing some act, such as pressing a lever, or, in the case of conditioned suppression, withholding some response. Thus, a simple communication system is established between the nonverbal subject and the experimenter or his or her surrogate computer. However, establishing this communication link can be very time-consuming and often requires weeks or months before actual testing can begin. Thus, these methods, in spite of their great precision and general usefulness, are not suited for testing large numbers of subjects.

Most of the operant procedures used in auditory research have employed positive reinforcement to motivate responding (e.g., food or water). However, negative reinforcement has also been used successfully in animal psychophysics. A shock-avoidance procedure has been used extensively to identify and characterize the hearing loss associated with inhalation exposure to a number of solvents (Pryor et al., 1983). The system developed to implement this procedure requires a relatively small investment in training time (5–10 days), because the subjects (rats) rapidly learn this task. Thus, fairly large numbers of subjects can be trained and tested efficiently. A shortcoming of this procedure is that it requires a motor response (climbing or pulling a pole suspended from the ceiling of the test chamber). Thus, agents that interfere with this motor response make auditory testing untenable.

A relatively recent addition to the behavioral methods for auditory assessment in animals is prepulse inhibition or reflex modification (see Crofton, 1992, for recent review). This method takes advantage of the discovery that a brief, low-intensity stimulus will attenuate the magnitude of the startle response elicited by a subsequent high-intensity stimulus (Ison, 1984; Young and Fechter, 1983; Fechter et al., 1988). Thus, no training is necessary, and, with the proper equipment (which is commercially available with computer automation for multiple test chambers), a fairly complete audiogram (intensity thresholds as several frequencies) can be obtained in a matter of days rather than the months required by traditional operant methods. Also, in contrast to the method just described, auditory function can be assessed in the presence of fairly severe motor disturbances (Fechter and Young, 1983; Crofton, 1992).

Electrophysiological Methods

A variety of methods have been used to examine the electrophysiological properties of the normal and damaged auditory system from the periphery to the cerebral cortex (Nauton and Fernández, 1978). The choice of methods will depend largely on the questions being asked and the time and resources available for their execution. For example, single-cell recordings from hair cells in the cochlea and individual fibers in the 8th nerve have provided us with much of the information we now have about the basic functioning and characteristics of the auditory system (see, e.g., Sellick and Russell, 1978; Antoli-Candela and Kiang, 1978). Similar methods have also been used to map the auditory system centrally (reviewed in Phillips, 1988). However, although such methods may be appropriate for uncovering the mechanisms by which ototoxic chemicals affect the auditory system, they are not generally suitable for identifying such chemicals. More efficient methods for this purpose include recording the cochlear microphonic (CM), the compound action potential (CAP) from the 8th nerve, and the brain stem auditory evoked response (BAER). Use of these methods, alone or in combination, can reveal damage throughout the auditory system and help identify the locus of such damage.

The CM, first recorded by Weaver and Bray in 1930, represents the electrical signal generated by the hair cells in response to acoustic stimulation. For accurate localization along the organ of Corti, a differential recording procedure between the scala tympani and the scala media is used (see Aran, 1981; Raslear, 1974). However, this procedure is tedious, technically difficult, and not practical for routine assessment of auditory dysfunction. The CM can also be recorded from an electrode on the round window, which is technically simpler (e.g., Saunders and Hirsch, 1976). However, this method does not permit accurate localization of the damaged hair cells along the cochlea. This restriction may be of little concern in most investigations of potentially ototoxic chemicals. The amplitude of the CM can be used for quantitation. However, many investigators have defined a threshold as the sound intensity required to generate a CM of 1 µV at each frequency tested (e.g., Saunders and Hirsch, 1976). These thresholds are then used to construct an isopotential intensity-frequency function. An increase in threshold indicates damage to the hair cells associated with the frequencies affected.

The CAP has been used extensively to investigate the effects of chemicals on peripheral auditory function. It is reliably recorded from an electrode on or near the round window (Aran, 1981; Norris et al., 1978). This evoked potential represents the integrated activity of all fibers in the 8th nerve. Intensity-frequency response thresholds or latencies can be rapidly generated using filtered clicks, tone pips, or tone bursts. The electrodes for recording the CAP can be chronically implanted for monitoring the onset and progression of any peripheral dysfunction caused by ototoxic agents (e.g., Aran, 1981). Further localization of the site of damage can be inferred by also observing the CM. Thus, a deterioration of the CAP in the presence of an intact CM would imply damage to fibers of the 8th nerve or their cell bodies in the spiral ganglia rather than to the hair cells.

The BAER is recorded from electrodes in the scalp or skull, either acutely or chronically implanted (see Rebert, 1983). It is a far-field potential evoked by discrete sound stimuli (usually clicks or tone pips). The shape of its waveform is informative of activity from the periphery through the auditory pathways of the brain stem. The first component of the BAER represents activity in the 8th nerve. Thus, changes in latency or amplitude of this component indicate peripheral dysfunction at the level of the hair cells or the 8th nerve itself. Disturbances in later components indicate dysfunction in the cochlear nuclear complex (wave II), the superior olivary nucleus (wave III), the lateral lemniscus (wave IV), and the inferior colliculi (wave V) (see Spehlman, 1985). Changes in the time intervals between the various components can be informative of possible damage to the structures associated with the components and fiber conduction velocity. The amplitude and latencies of the components of the BAER vary as a function of the intensity and frequency of the sound stimulus. Various methods have been used to quantitate the BAER, including peak-to-trough amplitude measurements, full-wave integrated amplitude, latencies of the various components and the intervals between them, and cross-correlation to evaluate changes in waveform. Threshold determinations have been based on visual definitions of a perceptible response and quantitative or qualitative assessment of intensity-response functions. In its present form and with modern equipment, this method for rapidly assessing auditory dysfunction is becoming the electrophysiological method of choice among various investigators charged with the task of evaluating the neurotoxic potential of large numbers of chemicals (cf. Mattsson et al., 1992).

Anatomical Methods

Histopathological methods for assessing lesions of the central auditory system are the same as those used to assess other regions of the central nervous system (CNS) and are not discussed. However, assessment of damage to the peripheral end organ is associated with special difficulties because of its small size, lack of ready accessibility, and unique geometry. The methods described below have evolved over several decades and have as one major goal a quantitative evaluation of the structural integrity of the hair cells along the entire length of the organ of Corti (surface preparations were described by Retzius in 1881).

The cochlea and its internal structures must be removed in a well-preserved condition. Then the cochlea is microdissected and/or decalcified and the structures of interest carefully removed and prepared for subsequent histological examination. The next step depends on the information sought. If a quantitative estimate of the number of damaged hair cells is needed, whole-mount surface preparations of sections of the organ of Corti are made. If the integrity of other structures is of interest, the preparation is sectioned in the desired orientation and processed in a manner similar to that used for other tissues. Both goals can be achieved by using one cochlea for surface preparation and the other for sectioning (e.g., see Fechter and Carlisle, 1990).

The specific methods used to prepare the tissues for examination differ somewhat among investigators, and the reader should consult the original references for details (e.g., Engström et al., 1966; Axelsson et al., 1975; Hawkins and Johnsson, 1976; Davies and Forge, 1987; Voelker et al., 1980). Examination of the surface preparations can be done readily by using differential interference contrast microscopy. A cochleogram (see Engström et al., 1966) can be constructed by counting the number of easily recognizable dead hair cells along the length of the basilar membrane. For more subtle effects, as might occur to the stereocilia before frank death of the cell, a scanning electron microscope (SEM) is needed to provide resolution and three-dimensional characteristics of these structures. Viewed through the SEM, damage can be seen as fused bundles of stereocilia with small cytoplasmic protrusions and stereocilia having a "floppy" appearance. If functional measures of auditory dysfunction are also available over a range of frequencies (i.e., an audiogram), the amount and range of damage to the hair cells can be compared and correlated with these functional measures.

In Vitro Tissue Cultures

Organotypic tissue cultures have been only sparingly used to study the effects of chemicals on the developing or relatively mature cochlea (e.g., Anniko et al., 1982; Richardson and Russell, 1991). These methods may offer considerable promise for screening chemicals for ototoxic effects and for examining their mechanisms of action without the various complications of an in vivo system. Possible differences between in vitro and in vivo systems in terms of such parameters as bioavailability and metabolism must always be kept in mind when drawing conclusions and making predictions. Nevertheless, most of the features associated with the ototoxic effects of neomycin have been elegantly demonstrated in such cultures of 1- or 2-day old mouse cochleas (Richardson and Russell, 1991), including differential sensitivity of inner and outer hair cells and their location along the basilar membrane.

AGENTS AFFECTING AUDITORY FUNCTION

Acoustic Overstimulation

Exposure to intense sounds can cause temporary or permanent hearing loss. These phenomena have been studied extensively in both humans and animals (see Henderson et al., 1976; Hamernick et al., 1982; Saunders et al., 1985; Henderson and Hamernick, 1986). The intensity, frequency composition, duration, and temporal patterns of the sound stimulus all interact in fairly systematic ways to determine the pattern of damage and its reversibility. As a sound stimulus of sufficient duration increases in intensity above some level (e.g., 80–90 dB, depending on other parameters), there is a temporary threshold shift (TTS). This TTS is reversible, as the term implies, and the rate of recovery (minutes, hours, or days) depends on the intensity, duration, and frequency composition of the eliciting stimulus. As the intensity or duration of the sound increases further, the shift in hearing thresholds becomes permanent, with little or no recovery. This permanent threshold shift (PTS) is associated with damage to or death of the hair cells on the organ of Corti (e.g., see Slepecky, 1986). The outer hair cells are more susceptible to acoustic overstimulation than the inner hair cells, and those at the basal end are more susceptible than those at the apical end. The damage, whether temporary or permanent, is dependent on the frequency composition of the stimulus. Thus, sounds composed mainly of high frequencies are more effective than those composed mainly of low frequencies (e.g., Henry, 1984). Also, the frequencies affected and the area of the cochlea damaged are related to the frequency composition of the sound stimulus. However, this relationship is not perfect because of the differential sensitivity of the hair cells along the basilar membrane. Thus, hearing loss typically occurs at frequencies higher than the dominant frequency of the eliciting stimulus. Pulsatile sound stimuli of sufficient intensity, such as might be generated by gunfire or even a toy cap pistol (Poche et al., 1969) can cause TTS and/or PTS. Again, the frequencies affected and the area of the organ of Corti damaged are related to the frequency composition of the pulsatile sound stimulus. Finally, it should be noted that there appears to be a period around the final maturation of the cochlea when it is most vulnerable to acoustic overstimulation (Bock and Saunders, 1977), and damage has been shown to result from in utero exposure in species in which nearly complete maturation occurs before birth (e.g., the guinea pig) (Cook et al., 1982). From this brief summary of the characteristics of sound-induced hearing loss, it is easy to speculate that this is a major cause of the marked age-related increase in human hearing disorders noted in the introduction.

Ototoxic Therapeutic Drugs

A number of drugs used therapeutically have been known for some time to cause auditory dysfunction and/or vestibular disturbances (see Hawkins, 1973; Matz et al., 1981; Govaerts et al., 1990; Walker et al., 1990; Rybak, 1986). These effects are often the limiting factor for the drugs' therapeutic usefulness, and efforts continue to find substitutes that retain their efficacy without such adverse effects. There are several classes of ototoxic drugs, including the aminoglycoside antibiotics, the loop diuretics, certain cancer chemotherapeutic agents, and salicylates.

Streptomycin, as the prototype aminoglycoside antibiotic, was found clinically to affect the inner ear in 1945 (Hinshaw and Feldman, 1945), and this finding was confirmed in animals shortly thereafter (Hawkins, 1950). Since then, a host of aminoglycoside antibiotics have been developed with the hope of discovering one free of this major side effect. Thus far, none has been found, although there are wide differences in potency among the various drugs in this class (e.g., Parravicini et al., 1982; Rybak, 1986). The ototoxic aminoglycoside antibiotics all appear to cause a similar pattern of damage to the cochlea. The outer hair cells of the basal end of the organ of Corti are damaged first, accompanied by a high-frequency hearing loss. With further treatment there is a loss of both outer and inner hair cells that progresses along the basilar membrane toward the apical end, accompanied by a loss of hearing at the lower frequencies. It should be noted that the hair cells on the organ of Corti are not the only target of the aminoglycosides. Some (e.g., streptomycin) are more selective for the hair cells of the vastibular system, whereas others (e.g. dihydrostreptomycin) are relatively selective for the auditory hair cells. It should also be noted that most, if not all, of the aminoglycosides are also nephrotoxic (Walker et al, 1990). As noted above for acoustic overstimulation, a period of enhanced vulnerability to the aminoglycosides also occurs around, or just preceding, full maturation of the peripheral auditory system. The mechanisms whereby the aminoglycoside antibiotics cause their effects are still under investigation. Their acute effect has been attributed to binding of the positively charged molecule to the negatively charged phospholipids in the hair cell membrane, which can be reversed by increasing calcium in the scala media (e.g., Takada and Schacht, 1982). Their irreversible effects are thought to occur intracellularly, perhaps by inhibition of an enzyme such as phosphatidylinositol phospholipase C, resulting in decreased degradation of phospholipids and altered membrane permeability (Schacht, 1986; Au et al., 1987).

Unlike the aminoglycoside antibiotics, the loop diuretics, exemplified by ethacrynic acid and furosemide, rarely cause irreversible hearing loss (see Rybak, 1986). Also, the loop diuretics affect a wide range of frequencies at effective doses. Finally, this class of compounds appears to act by interfering with ion transport at the stria vascularis rather than by a direct effect on the hair cells (Bosher, 1979; Pike and Bosher, 1980). Thus, the effect of the loop diuretics appears initially as a change in the endocochlear potential, with secondary reduction in the cochlear microphonics and the CAP of the 8th nerve.

A number of antineoplastic agents, such as *cis*-dichlorodiammine platinum (II) (cisplatin) and vincristine, cause temporary and/or permanent hearing loss (Fleischman et al., 1975; Stadnicki et al., 1975). The pattern of damage to the organ of Corti is similar in many respects to that of the aminoglycoside antibiotics. Accordingly, the progression of the hearing loss associated with these drugs also resembles that seen with the aminoglycoside antibiotics.

The salicylates, such as aspirin, can, in sufficiently high doses given over sufficient time, cause permanent hearing loss (Jarvis, 1966). However, such permanent effects are rare, and the hearing loss is generally reversible (reviewed in Guth and Bobbin, 1971). Moreover, tinnitus ("ringing in the ears") is more common than hearing loss with these drugs. It is unlikely that the mechanism of action is the same as that mediating the ototoxicity of acoustic overstimulation and the aminoglycoside antibiotics.

Nontherapeutic Chemicals

The potential for nontherapeutic chemicals to cause sensory dysfunction, including auditory dysfunction, was recognized early in the emergence of the field of neurotoxicology (see

Tilson and Cabe, 1978; Mitchell et al., 1982). However, neurotoxicologists have been slow to apply appropriate methodologies to the evaluation of potentially ototoxic industrial chemicals. As a result, only a handful of such chemicals have been adequately evaluated for their ototoxic potential.

Trimethyltin (TMT) has received considerable attention as a neurotoxic chemical (see Krigman and Cranmer, 1984). It causes neuronal loss and terminal degeneration in the hippocampus and entorhinal cortex, and scattered degeneration elsewhere in the CNS. Visual alterations accompanied by necrosis of retinal neurons have also been described. More recently, the effects of TMT on the auditory system have been described and characterized (Young and Fechter, 1986; Fechter et al., 1986; Eastman et al., 1987; Crofton et al., 1990; Hoeffding and Fechter, 1991). This compound appears to have two distinct effects on the auditory system, one reversible and the other irreversible. Initially there is a loss of hearing across a wide range of frequencies. With time, hearing at the lower frequencies recovers almost completely, leaving only a residual high-frequency deficit. The irreversible high-frequency hearing loss is associated with a loss of hair cells, especially the outer hair cells, in the basal turn of the cochlea. This effect appears to be similar to that caused by the aminoglycoside antibiotics. In addition, TMT causes marked changes in the stria vascularis, which may be responsible for the reversible wide-frequency-range hearing losses. Thus, these latter effects of TMT appear to be similar to the largely reversible effects of the loop diuretics. Interestingly, triethyltin, unlike TMT, does not appear to be ototoxic (Flechter and Young, 1983).

Iminodiproprionitrile (IDPN) has also recently received some experimental attention as an ototoxicant. In contrast to the aminoglycoside antibiotics and TMT, IDPN appears to cause an irreversible loss of sensitivity over a range of frequencies from 0.5 to 40 kHz in adult rats (Crofton et al., 1989). However, when rat pups were treated on postnatal days 4–7, only a high-frequency (40 kHz) loss was seen when they were tested as young adults (64–65 days of age) (Crofton et al., 1990). The mechanisms involved in these ototoxic effects of IDPN are currently unknown.

An interesting result with monosodium glutamate (MSG) also contrasts with the classic effects of other ototoxicants. Administered neonatally, MSG causes a selective high-frequency hearing loss in animals tested as adults (Crofton, 1990). However, the hearing loss appears to be associated with loss of neurons in the spiral ganglion rather than loss of hair cells (Janssen et al., 1991).

As a general class, the industrial solvents have been examined for their ototoxic potential to a greater extent than other nontherapeutic chemical classes. Toluene was first reported in 1983 to cause irreversible hearing loss in rats at frequencies from 8 to 20 kHz (Pryor et al., 1983; Rebert et al., 1983). This effect was found to be associated with damage to and loss of hair cells in the basal turn of the cochlea (the only section examined), and weanling rats were more sensitive than young adults (Pryor et al., 1984a). Since then, toluene and the closely related solvents mixed xylenes and styrene have been studied fairly extensively in this context (Pryor et al., 1984b; Pryor and Howd, 1986; Pryor et al., 1987), as has trichloroethylene (Pryor et al., 1991; Crofton and Zhao, 1992). A shortcoming of these studies has been a lack of cochlear histology to clearly identify the structural substrate for the hearing loss associated with these and other solvents. This mechanism has been documented only for toluene (Pryor et al., 1983; Sullivan et al., 1989) and styrene (Yano et al., 1992) thus far.

More recently, the author and his colleagues have been examining a wide range of solvents, with the goal of identifying the structural requirements for their ototoxic effects.

The strategy has been to expose rats to concentrations of each solvent ranging from those with no effect to nearly lethal concentrations for 8 h per day for 7 days in most experiments. This schedule of exposure is more than sufficient to cause a marked hearing loss for the prototype ototoxic solvent toluene (Pryor et al., 1984b). The rats are usually tested at 4, 8, and 16 kHz, using the BAER procedure (Rebert et al., 1983), although for some solvents they were tested behaviorally as well, using the shock-avoidance procedure described above (Pryor et al., 1983).

Table 1 summarizes the results for all of the solvents tested thus far as to whether hearing loss was observed. Where there was hearing loss, it was progressively greater from 4 to 20 kHz in all cases; frequencies higher than 20 kHz were not tested. Although considerable additional work is needed to establish a quantitative structure-activity relationship, several interesting and, in some cases, surprising observations can be made. First, there is clear evidence for structural specificity among the various solvents. Of the straight-chain solvents tested thus far, only carbon disulfide (Rebert and Becker, 1986) and trichloroethylene (Rebert et al., 1991) have caused hearing loss. No structural characteristics that might distinguish ototoxic from nonototoxic solvents in this series have yet emerged. However, the series of benzene ring structures is more interesting and provides some basis for speculation. Somewhat unexpectedly, benzene itself was inactive. Extending the side chain linearly from methyl (toluene) to *n*-propyl, including styrene and methoxybenzene, preserved the effect. However, activity was lost with the branched extension of isopropylbenzene. The dimethyl analogue (xylene) was tested initially as a mixture of the three isomers and was found to be potently ototoxic (Pryor et al., 1987). Therefore, it was somewhat unnerving when *o*-xylene and *m*-xylene (the major component of the

Table 1 Summary Effects of Solvents on Auditory Sensitivity

Solvent	Hearing loss
Benzene	No
Methylbenzene (toluene)	Yes
Ethylbenzene	Yes
n-Propylbenzene	Yes
Isopropylbenzene (cumene)	No
Methoxybenzene	Yes
Dimethylbenzenes (xylenes)	Yes
1,2-Dimethylbenzene (*o*-xylene)	No
1,3-Dimethylbenzene (*m*-xylene)	No
1,4-Dimethylbenzene (*p*-xylene)	Yes
Styrene	Yes
Monochlorobenzene	Yes
Carbon disulfide	Yes
Dichloromethane	No
Trichloroethane	No
Trichloroethylene	Yes
Tetrachloroethylene	No
2-Propanone (acetone)	No
Methylethylketone	No
Ethyl alcohol[a]	No
n-Hexane	No

[a]Administered in drinking water (6%).

mixture) were tested and both were found to be inactive. However, *p*-xylene was very active, accounting for the results with the mixed xylenes. Finally, activity was preserved by the substitution of chlorine for the methyl group (monochlorobenzene). From these results, a tentative hypothesis can be proposed. If these solvents interact specifically with some membrane structures (e.g., a receptor or ion channel), the geometry of this interaction may be quite restricted. The results for the dimethylbenzenes and the propylbenzenes suggest the possibility of a relatively narrow opening along the linear dimension of the molecule that is impeded by the presence of lateral groups. Moreover, a functional group must be present, as evidenced by the lack of effect of benzene itself. This hypothesis does not address the site of the interaction or the biochemical nature of the interaction. It only suggests a structural configuration whereby the solvent can gain access to the site of the interaction. Further tests of this hypothesis are in progress, which may also provide clues as to the mechanism involved.

Interactions Among Ototoxic Agents

The world is not simple, and people are exposed to a variety of agents simultaneously and sequentially—noise, drugs, industrial chemicals, pollutants, etc. Thus there is the possibility for a variety of adverse interactions that might not be predicted from the effect of single agents alone. The interactions that might occur among ototoxic agents have not, except in a few cases, received much experimental attention. However, there has been some work, which is summarized below (also see Rybak, 1986).

A potentiation between noise exposure and the aminoglycoside antibiotics has been known for some time (e.g., Brown et al., 1978, 1980; Jauhiainen et al., 1972; Marques et al., 1975). On the other hand, the combination of noise with the loop diuretics does not appear to result in such synergistic effects (Vernon and Brummett, 1977). Although the profound hearing loss associated with the loop diuretics is generally reversible (within hours, depending on dose), when loop diuretics are combined with the aminoglycoside antibiotics the irreversible damage associated with the latter when given alone is more severe and occurs sooner (e.g., Brummett et al., 1975, 1981). A possible explanation for this interaction is that the loop diuretics enhance the entry of the aminoglycoside antibiotics into the endolymph (Tran Ba Huy et al., 1983). Noise has also been reported to enhance the ototoxic effect of cisplatin when exposures are simultaneous (Boettcher et al., 1987) but not when the exposures are sequential (Laurell and Borg, 1986). On the other hand, no permanent damage was caused by the combination of noise and sodium salicylate, although they caused temporary threshold shifts (Woodford et al., 1978). Carbon monoxide alone causes reversible hearing losses. However, it has been reported to potentiate the cochlear damage induced by noise (Fechter et al., 1988; Young et al., 1987). There are suggestions that workers exposed to noise and various solvents may experience more severe hearing disorders than would be expected from exposure to either alone (e.g., Morata, 1991). This possibility has received some experimental support. Exposure to toluene preceding exposure to noise caused a hearing deficit in rats that was greater than expected from an additive model (Johnson et al., 1988). However, when the exposure sequence was reversed, only additive effects were observed (Johnson et al., 1990).

Potential interactions among various solvents have received some attention by the author and his colleagues (Pryor et al., 1985; Pryor and Rebert, 1990). Ototoxic solvents such as toluene, when combined with nonototoxic solvents such as dichloromethane, methylethylketone, and alcohol did not interact to enhance the effect of the ototoxic solvent alone. However, the combination of *n*-hexane, which is not ototoxic, and toluene resulted in a synergistic effect on the BAER, perhaps by independent effects on the auditory pathways and the cochlea, respectively (Pryor and Rebert, 1992). Combinations of solvents, both of which are ototoxic alone, have resulted thus far in effects that appear to be additive, suggesting a common mechanism (Pryor and Rebert, 1990; Rebert et al., 1992). Interestingly, induction of the metabolism of toluene (Pryor et al., 1991) and styrene (Pryor et al., 1992) by phenobarbital prevented the hearing loss associated with exposure to the solvents in uninduced rats, indicating that the solvents themselves, and not a metabolite, were the ototoxic agents.

EPILOGUE

The purpose of this chapter was to provide the neurotoxicologist with an introduction to the auditory system. It is hoped that this introduction will stimulate interest in the auditory system as a target for neurotoxicants, and that this interest will motivate further, more in-depth inquiry through the references cited herein. As noted in the introduction, hearing disorders are a major age-related problem in the United States. The extent to which exposure to various chemicals in our environment, either alone or in combination with other ototoxic agents such as noise, contributes to this problem is currently unknown. Nevertheless, a number of industrial chemicals are already known to be ototoxic, and this number can be expected to grow as more are examined with the sophisticated methods that are currently available. Thus, the neurotoxicologist who would presume to include sensory systems in his or her purview must make better use of such methods than has been common up to now.

ACKNOWLEDGMENTS

Work done by the author cited herein was supported by NIDA contract nos. 271-77-3402, 271-80-3712, 271-87-3132, and 371-90-7202.

REFERENCES

Allen JB (1988). Cochlear signal processing. In: Jahn A, Santos-Sacchi J, eds. Physiology of the ear. New York: Raven Press, 243–70.

Altschuler RA, Bobbin RP, Hoffman DW, eds. (1986). Neurobiology of hearing: the cochlea. New York: Raven Press.

Altschuler RA, Fex J (1986). Efferent neurotransmitters. In: Altschuler RA, Bobbin RP, Hoffman OW, eds. Neurobiology of hearing: the cochlea. New York: Raven Press, 383–96.

Anniko M, Takeda A, Schacht J (1982). Comparative ototoxicities of gentamicin and netilmicin in three model systems. Am J Otolaryngol 3:422–33.

Antoli-Candela F Jr, Kiang NYS (1978). Unit activity underlying the N_1 potential. In: Nauton RF, Fernández C, eds. Evoked electrical activity in the auditory system. New York: Academic Press, 165–91.

Aran J-M (1981). Electrophysiology of cochlear toxicity. In: Matz CJ, Lerner S, Hawkins JE Jr, eds. Aminoglycoside ototoxicity. Chicago: Little, Brown, 31–50.

Arthur RM, Pfeiffer RR, Suga N (1971). Properties of "two-tone inhibition" in primary auditory neurones. J Physiol 212:593–609.

Au S, Weiner ND, Schacht J (1987). Aminoglycoside antibiotics preferentially increase permeability in phosphoinositide-containing membranes: a study with carboxyfluorescein in liposomes. Biochem Biophys Acta 902:80–6.

Axelsson A, Miller J, Larsson B (1975). A modified "soft surface specimen technique" for examination of the inner ear. Acta Otolaryngol 80:362–74.

Axelsson A, Ryan AF (1988). Circulation of the inner ear: comparative study of the vascular anatomy in the mammalian cochlea. In: Jahn A, Santos-Sacchi J, eds. Physiology of the ear. New York: Raven Press, 295–315.

Bledsoe SC Jr, Bobbin RP, Chihal DM, (1981). Kainic acid: an evaluation of its action on cochlear potentials. Hearing Res 4:109–20.

Bledsoe SC Jr, Bobbin RP, Puel J-L (1988). Neurotransmission in the inner ear. In: Jahn A. Santos-Sacchi J, eds. Physiology of the ear. New York: Raven Press, 385–406.

Bock GR, Saunders JC (1977). A critical period for acoustic trauma and its relation to cochlear development. Science 197:396–8.

Boettcher FA, Henderson D, Gratton MA, Danielson RW, Byrne CD (1987). Synergistic interactions of noise and other ototraumatic agents. Ear Hearing 8:192–212.

Bosher SK (1979). The nature of the negative endocochlear potentials produced by anoxia and ethacrynic acid in the rat and guinea pig. J Physiol 293:329–245.

Brown JJ, Brummett RE, Fox KE, Bendrick TW (1980). Combined effects of noise and kanamycin. Cochlear pathology and pharmacology. Arch Otolaryngol 106:744–50.

Brown JJ, Brummett RE, Meikle MB, Vernon J (1978). Combined effects of noise and neomycin. Cochlear changes in the guinea pig. Acta Otolaryngol 83:394–400.

Brownell WE, Bader CR, Bertrand D, de Ribaupierre Y (1985). Evoked mechanical responses of isolated cochlear outer hair cells. Science 227:194–6.

Brummett RE, Bendrick T, Himes D (1981). Comparative ototoxicity of bumetanide and furosemide when used in combination with kanamycin. J Clin Pharmacol 21:628–36.

Brummett RE, Traynor J, Brown R, Himes DL (1975). Cochlear damage resulting from kanamycin and furosemide. Acta Otolaryngol 80:86–92.

Cook RO, Konishi T, Salt AN, Hamm CW, Lebetkin EH, Koo J (1982). Brainstem-evoked responses of guinea pigs exposed to high noise levels *in utero*. Dev Psychobiol 15:95–104.

Corwin JT, Warchol ME (1991). Auditory hair cells: structure, function, development, and degeneration. Annu Rev Neurosci 14:301–33.

Crofton KM (1990). Reflex modification and the detection of toxicant-induced auditory dysfunction. Neurotoxicol Teratol 12:461–8.

Crofton KM (1992). Reflex modification and the assessment of sensory dysfunction. In: Tilson H, Mitchell C, eds. Neurotoxicology. New York: Raven Press, 181–211.

Crofton KM, Dean KF, Menache MG, Janssen R (1990). Trimethyltin effects on auditory function and cochlear morphology. Toxicol Appl Pharmacol 105:123–32.

Crofton KM, Janssen R, Williams LD, Hamrick RC (1989). Effects of iminodipropionitrile on auditory function in the rat (abstr). Soc Neurosci Abstr 15:688.

Crofton KM, Stanton ME, Peele DB (1990). Developmental neurotoxicity following neonatal exposure to iminodipropionitrile in the rat (abstr). Toxicologist 10:305.

Crofton KM, Zhao X (1992). Frequency-dependent ototoxicity following inhalation exposure to trichloroethylene in the rat (abstr). Toxicologist 12:275.

Dallos P (1973). Cochlear potentials and cochlear mechanics. In: Moller AR, ed. Basic mechanisms in hearing. New York: Academic Press, 335–72.

Davies S, Forge A (1987). Preparation of the mammalian organ of Corti for scanning electron microscopy. J Microscopy 147:89–101.

Drescher MJ, Drescher DG, Medina JE (1983). Effects of sound stimulation at several levels on concentrations of primary amines, including neurotransmitter candidates in perilymph of the guinea pig inner ear. J Neurochem 41:309–20.

Dublin WB (1976). Fundamentals of sensorineural auditory pathology. Springfield, Illinois: C. C. Thomas.

Eastman CL, Young JS, Fechter LD (1987). Trimethyltin ototoxicity in albino rats. Neurotoxicol Teratol 9:329–32.

Engström H, Ades H, Anderson S (1966). Structural patterns of the organ of Corti. Baltimore: Williams & Wilkins.

Evans EF (1974). Auditory frequency selectivity and the cochlear nerve. In: Zwicker E, Terhardt E, eds. Facts and models in hearing. Berlin: Springer-Verlag, 118–29.

Evans EF (1981). The dynamic range problem: place and time coding at the level of the cochlear nerve and nucleus. In: Syka J, Aitkin L, eds. Neuronal mechanisms of hearing. New York: Plenum Press, 69–85.

Fechter LD, Carlisle L (1990). Auditory dysfunction and cochlear vascular injury following trimethyltin exposure in the guinea pig. Toxicol Appl Pharmacol 105:133–43.

Fechter LD, Sheppard L, Young JS, Zeger S (1988). Sensory threshold estimation from a continuously graded response produced by reflex modification audiometry. J Acoust Soc Am 84:179–85.

Fechter LD, Young JS (1983). Discrimination of auditory from nonauditory toxicity by reflex modification audiometry: effects of triethyltin. Toxicol Appl Pharmacol 70:216–27.

Fechter LD, Young JS, Nuttall AL (1986). Trimethyltin ototoxicity: evidence for a cochlear site of injury. Hearing Res 23:275–82.

Fechter LD, Young JS, Carlisle L (1988). Potentiation of noise-induced threshold shifts and hair cell loss by carbon monoxide. Hearing Res 34:39–48.

Felix D, Ehrenberger K (1982). The action of putative neurotransmitter substances in the cat labyrinth. Acta Otolaryngol 93:101–5.

Fex J (1968). Efferent inhibition in the cochlea by the olivocochlear bundle. In: De Reuck AVS, Knight J, eds. Ciba Foundation symposium on hearing mechanisms in vertebrates. Boston: Little, Brown, 169–81.

Fex J, Altschuler RA (1981). Enkephalin-like immunoreactivity of olivocochlear nerve fibers in cochlea of guinea pig and rat. Proc Natl Acad Sci USA 78:1255–59.

Fleischman RW, Stadnicki SW, Ethier MF, Schaeppi U (1975). Ototoxicity of *cis*-dichlorodiammine platinum (II) in the guinea pig. Toxicol Appl Pharmacol 33:320–32.

Flock Å, Cheung HC (1977). Actin filaments in sensory hairs of inner ear receptor cells. J Cell Biol 75:339–43.

Godfrey DA, Carter JA, Berger SJ, Matschinsky FM (1976). Levels of putative transmitter amino acids in the guinea pig cochlea. J Histochem Cytochem 24:468–72.

Govaerts PJ, Claes J, van der Heyning PH, Jorens PG, Marquet J, de Broe ME (1990). Aminoglycoside-induced ototoxicity. Toxicol Lett 52:227–51.

Guth PS, Bobbin RP (1971). The pharmacology of peripheral auditory processes: cochlear pharmacology. Adv Pharmacol Chemother 9:93–130.

Hamernik RP, Henderson D, Salvi R, eds. (1982). New perspectives on noise-induced hearing loss. New York: Raven Press.

Harris DM, Dallos P (1979). Forward masking of auditory nerve fiber response. J Neurophysiol 42:1083–1107.

Harrison RV (1988). The physiology of the cochlear nerve. In: Jahn A, Santos-Sacchi J, eds. Physiology of the ear. New York: Raven Press, 359–84.

Harrison RV, Hunter-Duvar IM (1988). An anatomical tour of the cochlea. In: Jahn A, Santos-Sacchi J, eds. Physiology of the ear. New York: Raven Press, 159–71.

Hawkins JE Jr (1950). Cochlear signs of streptomycin intoxication. J Pharmacol Exp Ther 100:38–44.

Hawkins JE Jr (1973). Comparative otopathology: aging, noise and ototoxic drugs. Adv Oto-Rhino-Laryngol 20:125–41.

Hawkins JE Jr (1988). Auditory physiological history: A surface view. In: Jahn A, Santos-Sacchi J, eds. Physiology of the ear. New York: Raven Press, 1–28.

Hawkins JE Jr, Johnsson L-G (1976). Microdissection and surface preparations of the inner ear. In: Smith CA, Vernon JA, eds. Handbook of auditory and vestibular research methods. Springfield, Illinois: C. C. Thomas, 5–52.

Henderson D, Hamernick RP (1986). Impulse noise: critical review. J Acoust Soc Am 80:569–84.

Henderson D, Hamernick RP, Dosanjh DS, Mills JH, eds. (1976). Effects of noise on hearing. New York: Raven Press.

Henry KR (1984). Cochlear damage resulting from exposure to four different octave bands of noise at three ages. Behav Neurosci 96:107–17.

Hinshaw HC, Feldman WH (1945). Streptomycin in the treatment of clinical tuberculosis: a preliminary report. Proc Mayo Clin 20:313.

Hoeffding V, Fechter LD (1991). Trimethyltin disrupts auditory function and cochlear morphology in pigmented rats. Neurotoxicol Teratol 13:135–45.

Hood JL, Berlin CI (1986). Contemporary applications of neurobiology in human hearing assessment. In: Altschuler RA, Bobbin RP, Hoffman DW, eds. Neurobiology of hearing: the cochlea. New York: Raven Press, 397–423.

Hudspeth AJ (1982). Extracellular current flow and the site of transduction by vertebrate hair cells. J Neurosci 2:1–10.

Ison JR (1984). Reflex modification as an objective test for sensory processing following toxicant exposure. Neurobehav Toxicol Teratol 6:437–45.

Jahn A, Santos-Sacchi J, eds. (1988). Physiology of the ear. New York: Raven Press.

Janssen R, Schweitzer L, Jensen KF (1991). Glutamate neurotoxicity in the developing rat cochlea: physiological and morphological approaches. Glutamate excitotoxicity in rat auditory system. Brain Res 522:255–64.

Jarvis JF (1966). A case of unilateral permanent deafness following acetyl salicylic acid. J Laryngol 80:318–20.

Jauhiainen T, Kohonen A, Jauhiainen M (1972). Combined effect of noise and neomycin on the cochlea. Acta Otolaryngol 73:387–90.

Jenison GL, Winbery S, Bobbin RP (1986). Comparative action of quisqualate and N-methyl-D-aspartate, excitatory amino acid agonists, on guinea pig cochlear potentials. Comp Biochem Physiol 84:385–9.

Johnson AC, Juntunan L, Nylen P, Borg E, Hoglund G (1988). Effect of interaction between noise and toluene on auditory function in the rat. Acta Otolaryngol 105:56–63.

Johnson AC, Nylen P, Borg E, Hoglund G (1990). Sequence of exposure to noise and toluene can determine loss of auditory sensitivity in the rat. Acta Otolaryngol 109:34–40.

Keidel WD, Neff WD, eds. (1974). Handbook of sensory physiology. Berlin: Springer-Verlag.

Khanna SM, Leonard DGB (1982). Basilar membrane tuning in the cat cochlea. Science 215:305–6.

Kimura RS (1966). Hairs of the cochlear sensory cells and their attachment to the tectorial membrane. Acta Otolaryngol 61:55–72.

Krigman MR, Cranmer JM, eds. (1984). Mechanisms and manifestations of tin neurotoxicity. Neurotoxicology 5:129–299.

Laurell G, Borg E (1986). Cis-platin in previously noise-exposed guinea pigs. Acta Otolaryngol 101:66–74.

Lewis RS, Hudspeth AJ (1983). Voltage- and ion-dependent conductance in solitary vertebrate hair cells. Nature 304:538–41.

Lim DJ (1985). Functional structure of the organ of Corti: a review. Hearing Res 22:117–46.

Marques DM, Clark CS, Hawkins JE Jr (1975). Potentiation of cochlear injury by noise and ototoxic antibiotics in guinea pigs. J Acoust Soc Am 57(suppl):560–9.

Mattsson JL, Boyes WK, Ross JF (1992). Incorporating evoked potentials into neurotoxicity test schemes. In: Tilson H, Mitchell C, eds. Neurotoxicology. New York: Raven Press, 125–45.

Matz CJ, Lerner S, Hawkins JE Jr (1981). Aminoglycoside ototoxicity. Chicago: Little, Brown.

Mitchell CL, Tilson HA, Cabe PA (1982). Screening for neurobehavioral toxicity: factors to consider. In: Mitchell CL, ed. Nervous system toxicology. New York: Raven Press, 237–45.

Morata EC, Dunn DE, Lemasters LW, Santos UP (1991). Effects of simultaneous exposure to noise and toluene on workers' hearing and balance. In: Fechter LD, ed. Proceedings of the Fourth International Conference on the Combined Environmental Factors. Baltimore: Johns Hopkins University Press, 81–6.

Morrison D, Schindler RA, Wersall J (1975). A quantitative analysis of the afferent innervation of the organ of Corti in guinea pig. Acta Otolatyngol 79:11–7.

Moser VC, McCormick JP, Creason JP, MacPhail RC (1988). Comparison of chlodimeform and carbaryl using a functional-observational battery. Fund Appl Toxicol 11:189–216.

Mountain DC (1986). Electromechanical properties of hair cells. In: Altschuler RA, Bobbin RP, Hoffman DW, eds. Neurobiology of hearing: the cochlea. New York: Raven Press, 77–90.

Mulroy MJ, Altmann DW, Weiss TF, Peak WT (1974). Intracellular electric responses to sound in a vertebrate cochlea. Nature 249:482–5.

Nauton RF, Fernández C, eds. (1978). Evoked electrical activity in the auditory nervous system. New York: Academic Press.

Netter FH (1962). The Ciba collection of medical illustrations. Vol. 1, nervous system. Summit, New Jersey: Ciba Corporation.

Nielsen DW, Slepecky N (1986). Stereocilia. In: Altschuler RA, Bobbin RP, Hoffman DW, eds. Neurobiology of hearing: the cochlea. New York: Raven Press, 23–46.

Norris CH, Garcia-Quiroga J, Guth PS (1978). A new and nondestructive technique for testing the cochlear toxicity of drugs. Toxicol Appl Pharmacol 43:317–26.

Norris CH, Guth PS (1974). The release of acetylcholine (ACH) by the crossed olivocochlear bundle (COCB). Acta Otolatyngol 77:318–26.

Norris CH, Guth PS, Daignault EA (1977). The site at which peripheral auditory adaptation occurs. Brain Res 123:176–9.

Palmer AR, Evans EF (1982). Intensity coding in the auditory periphery of the cat. Hearing Res 7:305–24.

Parravicini L, Arpini A, Bamonte F, Marzanatti M, Ongini E (1982). Comparative ototoxicity of amikacin, gentamicin, netilmicin, and tobramycin in guinea pigs. Toxicol Appl Pharmacol 65:222–30.

Perkins RE, Morest DK (1975). A study of cochlear innervation in cats and rats with Golgi methods and Nomarski optics. J Comp Neurol 163:129–58.

Phillips DP (1988). Introduction to anatomy and physiology of the central auditory system. In: Jahn A, Santos-Sacchi J, eds. Physiology of the ear. New York: Raven Press, 407–29.

Phillips DP, Brugge JF (1985). Progress in neurophysiology of sound localization. Annu Rev Psychol 36:245–74.

Pickles JO, Comis SD, Osborne MP (1984). Cross-links between stereocilia in the guinea-pig organ of Corti. Hearing Res 15:103–12.

Pickles JO, Corey DP (1992). Mechanoelectric transduction by hair cells. Trends Neurosci 15:254–9.

Pike D, Bosher SK (1980). The time course of the strial changes produced by intravenous furosemide. Hearing Res 3:79–89.

Poche LB Jr, Stockwell CW, Ades HW (1969). Cochlear hair-cell damage in guinea pigs after exposure to impulse noise. J Acoust Soc Am 4:947–51.

Pryor GT, Dickinson J, Feeney E, Rebert CS (1984a). Hearing loss in rats first exposed to toluene as weanlings or as young adults. Neurobehav Toxicol Teratol 6:111–9.

Pryor GT, Dickinson J, Howd RA, Rebert CS (1983). Transient cognitive deficits and high-frequency hearing loss in weanling rats exposed to toluene. Neurobehav Toxicol Teratol 5:53–7.

Pryor GT, Howd RA (1986). Toluene-induced ototoxicity by subcutaneous administration. Neurobehav Toxicol Teratol 8:103–4.

Pryor GT, Howd RA, Uyeno ET, Thurber AB (1985). Interactions between toluene and alcohol. Pharmacol Biochem Behav 23:401–10.

Pryor GT, Rebert CS (1990). Neurotoxicity of inhaled substances. Final report, NIDA contract 271-87-3132. Menlo Park, California: SRI International.

Pryor GT, Rebert CS (1992). Interactive effects of toluene and *n*-hexane on behavior and neurophysiologic responses in Fischer-344 rats. Neurotoxicology 13:225–34.

Pryor GT, Rebert CS, Dickinson J, Feeney EM (1984b). Factors affecting toluene-induced ototoxicity in rats. Neurobehav Toxicol Teratol 6:223–38.

Pryor GT, Rebert CS, Howd RA (1987). Hearing loss in rats caused by inhalation of mixed xylenes and styrene. J Appl Toxicol 7:55–61.

Pryor G, Rebert C, Kassay K, Kuiper H, Gordon R (1991). The hearing loss associated with exposure to toluene is not caused by a metabolite. Brain Res Bull 27:109–13.

Pryor G, Rebert C, Kassay K, Shinsky N, Gordon R (1992). Induction of styrene metabolism prevents styrene-induced hearing loss in rats (abstr.). Toxicologist 12:235.

Raslear TG (1974). The use of the cochlear microphonic response as an indicant of auditory sensitivity: a review and evaluation. Psychol Bull 81:791–803.

Rebert CS (1983). Multisensory evoked potentials in experimental and applied neurotoxicology. Neurobehav Toxicol Teratol 5:659–71.

Rebert CS, Becker E (1986). Effects of inhaled carbon disulfide on sensory-evoked potentials of Long-Evans rats. Neurobehav Toxicol Teratol 8:533–41.

Rebert CS, Boyes WK, Svendsgaard DJ, Pryor GT (1992). Interactive effects of solvents on the rat's auditory system (abstr.). Toxicologist 12:236.

Rebert CS, Day VL, Matteucci MJ, Pryor GT (1991). Sensory-evoked potentials in rats chronically exposed to trichloroethylene: predominant auditory dysfunction. Neurotoxicol Teratol 13:83–90.

Rebert CS, Sorensen SS, Howd RA, Pryor GT (1983). Toluene-induced hearing loss in rats evidenced by the brainstem auditory-evoked response. Neurobehav Toxicol Teratol 5:59–62.

Retzius G (1881). Das Gehörorgan der Wirbeltiere. Morphologisch-histologische Studien. I. Das Gehörorgan der Fische und Amphibien. Stockholm: Samson & Wallin.

Richardson GP, Russell IJ (1991). Cochlear cultures as a model system for studying aminoglycoside ototoxicity. Hearing Res 53:293–311.

Russell IJ (1983). Origin of the receptor potential in inner hair cells of the mammalian cochlea—evidence for Davis theory. Nature 301:334–6.

Rybak LP (1986). Ototoxic mechanisms. In: Altschuler RA, Bobbin RP, Hoffman DW, eds. Neurobiology of hearing. New York: Raven Press, 441–54.

Salt AN, Konishi T (1986). The cochlear fluids: perilymph and endolymph. In: Altschuler RA, Bobbin RP, Hoffman DW, eds. Neurobiology of hearing. New York: Raven Press, 109–22.

Santi PA (1988). Cochlear microanatomy and ultrastructure. In: Jahn A, Santos-Sacchi J, eds. Physiology of the ear. New York: Raven Press, 173–99.

Santi PA, Anderson CB (1987). A newly identified surface coat on cochlear hair cells. Hearing Res 27:47–65.

Santos-Sacchi J (1988). Cochlear physiology. In: Jahn A. Santos-Sacchi J, eds. Physiology of the ear. New York: Raven Press, 271–93.

Saunders JC, Dear SP, Schneider ME (1985). The anatomical consequences of acoustic injury: a review and tutorial. J Acoust Soc Am 78:833–50.

Saunders JC, Hirsch KA (1976). Changes in cochlear microphonic sensitivity after priming C57BL/6J mice at various ages for audiogenic seizures. J Comp Physiol Psychol 90:212–29.

Schacht J (1986). Molecular mechanisms of drug-induced hearing loss. Hearing Res 22:297–304.

Sellick PM, Patuzzi R, Johnstone BM (1982). Measurement of basilar membrane motion in guinea pig using the Mossbauer technique. J Acoust Soc Am 72:131–41.

Sellick PM, Russell IJ (1978). Intracellular studies of cochlear hair cells: filling the gap between basilar membrane mechanics and neural excitation. In: Nauton RF, Fernández C, eds. Evoked electrical activity in the auditory system. New York: Academic Press, 113–9.

Slepecky N (1986). Overview of mechanical damage to the inner ear: Noise as a tool to probe cochlear function. Hearing Res 22:307–21.

Slepecky N, Chamberlain SC (1985). Immunoelectron microscopic and immunofluorescent localization of cytoskeletal and muscle-like contractile proteins in inner ear sensory hair cells. Hearing Res 20:245–60.

Smith CA, Vernon JA, eds. (1976). Handbook of auditory and vestibular research methods. Springfield, Illinois: C. C. Thomas.

Spehlman R (1985). Evoked potential primer: visual, auditory, and somatosensory evoked potentials in clinical diagnosis. Boston: Butterworth.

Spoendlin H (1969). Innervation patterns in the organ of Corti of the cat. Acta Otolaryngol 67:239–54.

Spoendlin H (1988). Neural anatomy of the inner ear. In: Jahn A, Santos-Sacchi J, eds. Physiology of the ear. New York: Raven Press, 201–9.

Stadnicki SW, Fleischman RW, Schaeppi U, Merriam P (1975). *Cis*-dichlorodiammineplatinum (II) (NSC-119875): hearing loss and other toxic effects in rhesus monkeys. Cancer Chemother Rep 59:467–80.

Stebbins WC, ed. (1970). Animal psychophysics: the design and conduct of sensory experiments. New York: Appleton-Century-Crofts.

Sullivan MJ, Rarey KE, Conolly RB (1989). Ototoxicity of toluene in rats. Neurotoxicol Teratol 10:525–30.

Takada A, Schacht J (1982). Calcium antagonism and reversibility of gentamicin-induced loss of cochlear microphonics in the guinea pig. Hearing Res 8:179–86.

Tilson HA, Cabe PA (1978). A strategy for the assessment of neurobehavioral consequences of environmental factors. Environ Health Perspect 26:287–99.

Tran Ba Huy P, Manuel C, Meulemans A, Sterkers O, Wassef, M, Amiel C (1983). Ethacrynic acid facilitates gentamicin entry into endolymph of the rat. Hearing Res 11:191–202.

U.S. Department of Commerce (1991). Statistical Abstract of the United States 1991: The National Data Book. 111th Ed. p. 120.

Vernon J, Brummett RE (1977). Noise trauma in the presence of loop diuretics. Trans Am Acad Ophthalmol Otolaryngol 84:407–13.

Voelker FA, Henderson CM, Macklin AW, Tucker WE (1980). Evaluating the rat inner ear. A technique using scanning electron microscopy. Arch Otolaryngol 106:613–7.

Walker EM Jr, Fazekas-May MA, Bowen WR (1990). Nephrotoxic and ototoxic agents. Clin Lab Med 10:323–54.

Warr WB, Guinan JJ Jr, White JS (1986). Organization of the efferent fiber system: the lateral and medial olivocochlear systems. In: Altschuler RA, Bobbin RP, Hoffman DW, eds. Neurobiology of hearing New York: Raven Press, 333–48.

Weaver EG, Bray CW (1930). Auditory nerve impulses. Science 71:215.

Woodford CM, Henderson D, Hamernimk RP (1978). Effects of combinations of sodium salicylate and noise on the auditory threshold. Ann Otol Rhinol Laryngol 87:117–27.

Yano BL, Dittenber DA, Albee RR, Mattson JL (1992). Abnormal auditory brainstem response and cochlear pathology in rats induced by an exaggerated styrene exposure regimen. Toxicol Pathol 20:1–6.

Yates GK, Johnstone BM, Patuzzi RB (1992). Mechanical preprocessing in the mammalian cochlea. Trends Neurosci 15:57–61.

Young JS, Fechter LD (1983). Reflex inhibition procedures for animal audiometry: a technique for assessing ototoxicity. J Acoust Soc Am 73:1686–93.

Young JS, Fechter LD (1986). Trimethyltin exposure produces an unusual form of toxic auditory damage in rats. Toxicol Appl Pharmacol 82:87–93.

Young JS, Upchurch MB, Kaufman MJ, Fechter LD (1987). Carbon monoxide exposure potentiates high-frequency auditory threshold shifts induced by noise. Hearing Res 26:37–43.

13
Assessment of Chemically Induced Alterations in Motor Function

Mary Jeanne Kallman
Lilly Research Laboratories, A Division of Eli Lilly and Company
Greenfield, Indiana

Stephen C. Fowler
University of Mississippi at Oxford
University, Mississippi

INTRODUCTION

This chapter will 1.) provide a selective overview of the current approaches to motoric assessment, 2.) examine the development of promising new methods of motoric assessment in humans and animals, and 3.) where possible, interrelate the methods of human and animal assessment. A detailed and exhaustive evaluation of all methods that have been used in the past was not undertaken, and readers interested in more comprehensive reviews of procedures for assessment of motor function are referred to the excellent papers by Kulig and Lammers (1992), Rafales (1987), and Reiter and MacPhail (1982). This discussion will emphasize the state of the art in motoric assessment and novel techniques that provide exciting new dimensions to our current approaches to motoric evaluation in neurotoxicology.

MOTORIC ASSESSMENT IN HUMANS

The development of laboratory approaches to measuring chemically induced alterations in motor function has been only partially influenced by the methods used to assess humans. Nevertheless, an awareness of the procedures frequently used in monitoring human motoric response to neurotoxic compounds can provide some guidance in the selection of techniques that could be profitably applied to nonhuman testing. A brief discussion of the human data also provides anchors for the relevance of motoric assessment of nonhuman subjects in making generalizations to the human case.

Estimates suggest that approximately 750 chemicals, from a total of 53,000 to 100,000 that are in commercial use, produce direct or indirect central nervous system (CNS) damage, and roughly 40% of the chemicals identified as hazardous chemicals in the workplace by the National Institute for Occupational Safety and Health (NIOSH) produce

CNS effects (Anger and Johnson, 1985). Historically, the NIOSH has made decisions about toxicity that rely more on acute effects of chemical exposure than the decisions made by the Environmental Protection Agency (EPA) or the Food and Drug Administration (FDA), which have both depended more on irreversible effects of repeated low doses. One consideration in the definition of worker safety is that performance of on-job tasks cannot be impaired to an extent that reduces performance quality or safety. Statistics derived from this definition have led the NIOSH to list neurotoxic disorders as one of the ten leading occupational problems in the United States (Centers for Disease Control 1983, 1986) and have stimulated research on behavioral indicators of chemical exposure and a corresponding explosion of publications on the consequences of chemical exposure. Anger and Johnson (1985) reported a fivefold increase from the 1970s to the 1980s in the publication of human investigations on neurobehavioral effects of chemicals. The data reported in the approximately 50 papers published in the 1970s were generated with 250 different tests, while the increase in publications in the 1980s was also associated with an increase in the number of tests used for assessment. These observations reflect increased attention to neurotoxic indicators and continual evolution of the methodology for assessing performance as a reflection of nervous system function.

Within the broad arena of neurobehavioral assessment, measures of motor function have always occupied a prominent position. For instance, investigations of the behavioral effects of chemicals in humans have included observations of convulsions, weakness, tremor, twitching, ataxia, paralysis, incoordination, unsteadiness, clumsiness, reflex abnormalities, and activity changes, which represent roughly 35% of all reported behavioral effects (as computed from data presented in Anger and Johnson, 1985). Clearly, motoric assessment represents the single most frequently used measure of chemical effect. The emphasis on motor function has been caused in part by the fact that the two most extensively studied classes of chemical agents of the last 20 years are solvents and heavy metals (especially lead and mercury), and that these substances are reported to produce observable motoric effects.

In human neurobehavioral assessment, test batteries that assess multiple capabilities have been used more frequently than a single measure of effect. Two specific human test batteries are preferred by investigators, and both will probably be used extensively in the future because of the broad base of validation that is accumulating for them. The first of the two is the Neurobehavioral Evaluation System (NES) developed jointly in 1983 by the World Health Organization and the NIOSH; the second is the Neurobehavioral Core Test Battery (NCTB) developed in 1985 (Baker et al., 1985). For a more comprehensive discussion of approaches that have been used for human assessment of chemical exposure, see the reviews of Anger (1990, 1992). Both the NES and the NCTB have been used extensively with worldwide populations. The NES is a computerized set of tests that can be easily used in the field and is amenable to rapid computerized data reduction. Tests included as part of the battery fall into three domains: psychomotor, memory and learning, and cognitive. Five specific tests are included in the motoric domain. These tests are symbol-digit, hand-eye coordination, simple reaction time, continuous performance, and finger tapping. The NCTB includes a smaller number of core tests but includes several assessments that specifically reflect motoric capabilities, i.e., aiming and simple reaction time. Arcia and Otto (1992) have recently examined the reliability of these procedures, and they report test-retest reliabilities of about 85% for the motoric measures. Overall, these approaches to human assessment have emphasized fine motor movement more than gross movement, and motor function over "cognitive" function. But the test batteries do include some tasks requiring presumably cognitively mediated functions such as attention and short-term memory. Methods are available that were developed for the assessment of specific neurological (Potvin et al., 1981) and orthopedic (Goh et al., 1984) disorders, but these have not been aggressively applied to the assessment of human chemical exposures.

MOTORIC ASSESSMENT IN ANIMALS

The measurement of motor function in animals has included a broader range of test procedures than is commonly used in human assessment. The tests most typically used with animals can be grouped within three general categories. These involve measurement of locomotion, motoric coordination, and tremor. The latter two categories parallel the typical procedures used to evaluate chemical effects in humans, while locomotor measures are rarely used in human testing. These three categories of motoric assessment do not always yield identical results, since alterations in function reflected by one type of measurement may not correlate well with alterations in one or both of the other categories.

Spontaneous Locomotion

Descriptions of locomotor activity, primarily in rodents, have been a mainstay of behavioral pharmacology and toxicology since the inception of these scientific disciplines. Measurement of simple locomotion is probably the most common motoric and behavioral assessment made in toxicology evaluation today. Numerous technical approaches to the quantification of locomotion have been fashionable at different historical points. Procedures for measuring locomotion in less frequent use today include direct observation to determine degree or type of motion abnormality, running wheels, microswitch-operated tilt cages, jiggle platforms or stabilimeters, and ultrasonic devices that rely on the disruption of a field of ultrasonic waves by the animal to detect movement. Many of these procedures have been abandoned because of the significant sensory feedback, either kinesthetic or auditory, provided to the animal during movement by the measuring process itself. Moreover, scientists have accepted the idea that locomotion can be altered under these conditions in normal animals and that these techniques can produce complex interactions with specific drug and chemical treatments. Currently, the most common approach to locomotor assessment has followed the EPA guideline for motoric assessment (Sette, 1989). The most typical procedure is the measurement of movement in a confined environment with strategically located infrared (area of visual spectrum not visible to the rodent eye) photobeams that generate counts corresponding to the number of beam interruptions that have occurred within a fixed period. Both horizontal and vertical movement can be monitored with commercially available equipment. The duration of measurement sessions is usually 30 min, divided into three 10-min intervals so that intrasession adaptation can be evaluated. Normal rodents typically display a gradual reduction in locomotion both within and across sessions when multiple test sessions are conducted. Other laboratories have assessed locomotion in more complex maze environments, of which the one that has been most often used is the figure-eight maze (Crofton and Reiter, 1984, 1988; Crofton et al., 1989). Procedures for the automated measurement of rodent locomotion have aided the evolution of standardized procedures, thereby allowing quantitative comparisons from laboratory to laboratory.

One new technique for measuring locomotion, the contrast-sensitive video tracking system, has been described recently by Vorhees and colleagues at the University of

Cincinnati (Vorhees et al., 1992). They have applied this technique to the assessment of prenatal and neonatal toxicity of drugs and chemicals, but this procedure is also applicable to adult rodents, as demonstrated by work in Geyer's laboratory assessing psychoactive agents (Geyer, 1990). This system produces a two-dimensional tracing of the movement pattern of the subject as it moves within the recording arena, providing a description of locomotion more complete than a simple quantification of amount of locomotion. In addition to the tracings generated, this system records total distance traveled, number of transitions from one area to another of the arena, and total time spent in motion. Figure 1, from Vorhees's laboratory (Vorhees et al., 1992), illustrates the tracings for a normal rat (left column) that can be obtained for successive 10-min intervals in a 60-min session. Normal movement can be characterized as predominantly around the outside of the field and gradually decreasing across the session. In comparison, tracings taken from subjects treated with 200 mg/kg phenytoin prenatally (center and right panels) display a different pattern of movement. Clearly this new technique offers the potential for more complex assessment of locomotion with an automated procedure, and future efforts will probably generate profiles for specific toxins in adult animals.

Motor Coordination

Tests of motor coordination challenge the animal with gravity-related stimulation and the concurrent possibility of a negative consequence such as falling. Thus, motor-coordination assessment is thought to provide more information about the integrative functions of the neuromuscular system than simple locomotion on a horizontal surface. These coordination tasks are more similar to those used to assess human motor function, since the assessment of simple locomotion is almost never made in human evaluations of a substance's toxic potential. Normal performance on tests of motor coordination typically requires the whole-body coordination of motor functioning under specific response demands. Although these tests are more structured than observation of locomotor activity, most are simple and time-efficient. Deficits in motoric coordination do not always correlate with deficits in locomotion, and in some instances motoric coordination can be disrupted at levels of chemical exposure lower than those that disrupt locomotion.

Probably the single most commonly used test of motoric coordination is rotarod performance. This testing apparatus was initially developed to assess deficits induced in rodents by brain damage (Dunhan and Miya, 1957). Since its introduction, the rotarod has been used extensively to assess the effects of drugs and chemicals. Testing is conducted by placing the rodent on an elevated moving drum that rotates at a fixed or accelerating speed. Data are collected as the length of time that the animal can maintain locomotion on the moving surface. The texture of the moving surface can produce variability in control measures of performance when data collected with rotarods from different suppliers are compared. Practice before the actual chemical testing reduces the variability that is often observed for normal animals.

Swimming ability has also been used successfully to measure motor coordination. Swimming endurance in an open tank is the simplest measure of coordination, but some investigators have examined the intricacies of swimming style and pattern of performance in diversely designed mazes. Even though measures of swimming endurance and swimming coordination may be distinguishable physiologically and psychologically, investigators have typically treated these two dependent variables as if they were equivalent. Rodents are relatively good swimmers, even with no previous swimming history, and this can

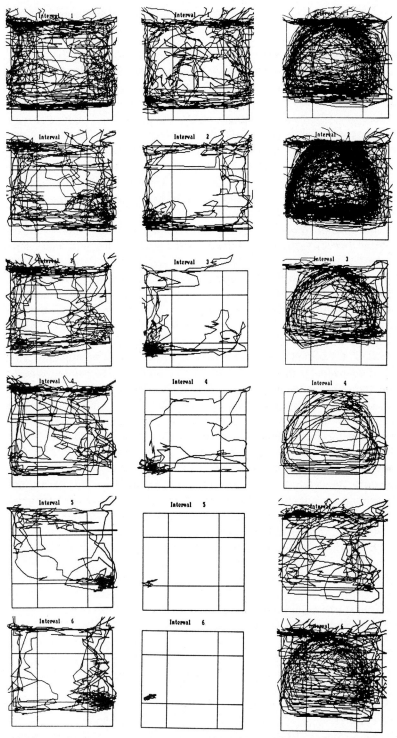

Figure 1 Video tracking activity patterns of one female rat from each treatment group/10-min intervals of a 60-min session. Panels on the left display the patterns of movement for controls, the center panels display the pattern for a phenytoin-exposed rat (200 mg/kg on prenatal days 7–18) that circled, and the right panel represents a phenytoin-exposed rat that did not circle. (From Vorhees et al., 1992.)

necessitate lengthy trials of observation to ascertain the limitations of ability. In our laboratory, two strategies have been used to standardize and shorten trials. First, task difficulty was increased by the addition of a "pack" or weight proportional to the body weight of the animal. As a second strategy, to increase the challenge of the test one can conduct trials in a cold-water (19°C) tank (Kallman et al., 1984). We have also observed that when repetitive tests of rodents are required, allowing the animal's coat to dry completely between trials leads to more consistent baseline scores. When the performance of control mice is compared across two swimming trials separated by a 30-min interval, there is no decrement in performance if the animals are permitted to dry completely between trials. If the mice are not permitted to dry, endurance measures on the second trial are reduced by about 10–20 s.

Another motor coordination procedure is the inverted-screen test, which was first used by Coughenour et al. (1977) to assess the effects of psychoactive drugs in mice. This test is conducted by placing a mouse on an elevated (e.g., 50 cm from the floor) wire mesh screen, inverting the screen 180°, and determining the mouse's speed in returning to an upright position on the side of the screen opposite to that on which it was placed initially. Occasionally, righting time has been used as the dependent measure for this task, but the more common dependent measure has been to determine whether an animal can right within a 60-s cut-off period. The quantal data based on the percent of mice succeeding on the task within the limited 60-s period can be used to compute ED_{50}s for comparison with other similarly obtained data sets for different doses or compounds. Table 1 is an example of such a comparison that was made in our lab. The table compares ED_{50}s from the inverted-screen test, which were computed at the time of peak effects, with LD_{50}s for the same halogenated hydrocarbons. The chemicals evaluated differed dramatically in the ratio between lethality and motor incoordination as measured by the screen test. The representative clinical anesthetic, chloral hydrate, has the largest ratio between effects. This test has been particularly sensitive to sedatives (Kallman et al., 1984) and solvents (Moser and Balster, 1985) that produce generalized reductions in motoric ability. Investigators should be attentive to the variability in mouse body weights, since we have observed that the task is more difficult for heavier animals, i.e., the percentage of animals not righting in 60 s will be larger for heavier animals. Another source of potentially confounding variance comes from practice effects that can occur with repetitive testing. In this laboratory, for

Table 1 Both ED_{50}s and LD_{50}s Determined in Male Mice Following Oral Exposure to Several Halogenated Hydrocarbons[a]

Chemical	Screen test ED_{50} (mg/kg)	LD_{50} (mg/kg)
Chloral	84.2	1442.0
Trichloroethylene	543.5	2402.0
Dichloroethylene	1172.0	2122.0
1,2-Trichloroethylene	128.0	378.0
1,2-Dichloroethylene	415.0	489.0

[a]ED_{50}s were determined by the assessment of inverted screen test performance. The tabled ED_{50} value was computed on data from the time point of peak effect. Screen test performance was recorded as the number of mice (10/exposure level) that righted in 60 s. LD_{50} values are determined across 14 days.

example, trial 2 righting speed will be 10–15 s faster than on trial 1 for body weight–matched nontreated controls.

Foot splay and gait in rodents have been used in behavioral toxicological assessment (Edwards and Parker, 1977; Parker and Clarke, 1990) as a measure of motor coordination. These methods derive from the assessment of abnormalities seen in human motor control that result from various neurological insults (for a review of these clinical methods, see Rosenbaum, 1991).

In the context of gait analysis as a reflection of motor coordination, Kulig has developed an interesting technique for assessing the adverse effects of a wide variety of chemical exposures (Kulig, 1987; Tanger et al., 1984). A transparent plastic drum (oriented vertically like the classical running wheel) is outfitted with equally spaced crosspieces or rungs attached to the floor of the apparatus, which rotates in one direction at 8 cm/s. The rat learns to walk by placing its feet on successive rungs as the wheel rotates, and the rat's performance is videotaped for scoring by observer or computer. This method has been used in Kulig's laboratory to measure neurobehavioral toxicity from acrylamide exposure (Kulig et al., 1985). Analyses have focused on the accuracy of the rat's hind-limb placement on the rungs. Data end points include duration of hind-paw placement on the rungs, durations of missteps, rung drops, and walking failures. A composite coordinated movement score can be computed from these separate measures. This approach has been used to examine both acute exposures (50 or 100 mg/kg) and repetitive 12-week exposures (14.4 mg/kg/day) to acrylamide, which is well known to produce peripheral neuropathies. Two disparate profiles were observed that were dependent on the course of acrylamide exposure. Acute exposures to acrylamide produced a decrease in the composite score that was predominantly due to failures of walking, while low-dose chronic exposure produced a different profile that was characterized by stepping deficits. Although the data-reduction component of this test procedure is complicated and quite sophisticated, the actual animal testing is rapid and easy to conduct. Moreover, this procedure has been found to be sensitive to known chemical alterations in motor function in rodents.

Tremor

Tremor phenomena (rhythmic or semirhythmic oscillations of a digit, a limb, or the whole body) have a prominent role in neurobehavioral toxicology, because several known neurological syndromes, whether idiopathic, iatrogenic, or induced by exposure to chemicals, have tremor as a prominent feature. Parkinson's disease (idiopathic or caused by 1-methyl-4-phenyl-1,2,3,6-tetrahydropyridine [MPTP] intoxication), multiple sclerosis, side effects of antipsychotic medications, and exposures to methylmercury, pesticides, organic solvents, or metals all produce tremors of some form. The application of tremor assessment to the workplace environment has direct utility for determining deviations in worker functioning that might reduce work capacity or safety on the job.

Methods for measuring both whole-body and finger or limb tremor have been devised. All of these methods transform mechanical movement via a transducer into an electrical signal that can in turn be quantized into computer-readable form by an analogue-to-digital converter. Four different types of transducer have been used to accomplish the energy transduction necessary for convenient electrical measurement. The four types are accelerometers, which quantify limb acceleration; force transducers, which quantify whole-body or limb force against a platform or other sensing surface; displacement potentiometers, which require very low force for their movement; and inductive or capacitive devices, which sense movement by magnetoelectric induction or by electric field variations. Accelerometers have been used most in human studies, and the force transducer has been most commonly used in animal investigations. An excellent review of problems and application details for each type of tremor assessment can be found in Newland's recent paper (Newland, 1988). Accelerometers detect alterations in position above about 4 Hz when subjects are evaluated in an unstructured test situation, while force transducers (Fowler, 1987; Gerhart et al., 1982, 1983; Herr et al., 1985) are more efficient for measuring both slow and fast frequencies when the subject is typically placed in a task-demand situation. These techniques require considerable expertise to implement, and one must be aware of the physical properties of the measurement system, especially resonance frequency, in order to avoid artifact contamination of the recordings. In the case of the use of force transducers for recording variations in forelimb force in rodents, system requirements for high-fidelity, artifact-free recordings have been described (Fowler, 1987).

Two examples of tremor assessment will be provided as illustrative of approaches that have been used to evaluate limb tremor in primates and in rodents. The first example is from Newland's research to evaluate the effects of chemical substances on squirrel monkey tremor as measured with a displacement transducer. The second example is from one of our laboratories, where rodent forelimb tremor was assessed with a force-transducer methodology.

Newland (1988) devised a test procedure in which a chaired squirrel monkey used one hand to position a lever within specific displacement limits and received sweetened fruit juice as a reinforcer (see Fig. 2) when correct performance was achieved. A rotary variable differential transformer, which required very low levels of force for its movement, was attached to the lever, and the direct output from the transformer was read by a computer via an analogue-to-digital converter. The low mass of the operandum was one of the key elements that made this measurement system so exquisitely sensitive to limb tremor. Newland reported little difficulty training monkeys to manipulate the lever in this situation. Data collected with this technique are displayed in Fig. 3, in which performance, with two doses (0.1 and 1.0 mg/kg) of the tremogenic agent oxotremorine (a muscarinic cholinergic agonist) was compared with control performance on the displacement lever. As can be seen in the figure, the two doses of oxotremorine that were tested produced different tremor characteristics. In the control tracing one sees normal, low-amplitude physiological tremor and a mean displacement falling within the 2-cm range. However, the low dose of oxotremorine produced an increase in the power at the higher frequencies, and this was accompanied by a large-amplitude drift in the animals' lever-manipulation behavior. At the higher dose, the displacement drift disappeared, and the power spectrum (bottom row of Fig. 3) showed that tremor had shifted to frequencies in the 6–10 Hz range, with the high-frequency oscillations returning to near control levels of power. Newland also compared ethanol (1 g/kg, P.O.) and oxotremorine with this same tremor-assessment procedure. Under these conditions ethanol flattens the power across the entire range of frequencies, a very different pattern from the one seen with oxotremorine. These examples suggest that tremor phenomena can be quite complex and that clearly distinguishable patterns of tremogenic responding can result from exposure to different types of CNS-active subtances.

Forelimb tremor measurement in rodents has been accomplished with an operant technique in which rats are required to exert pressure against a horizontal disk supported by the shaft of a force transducer (Fowler et al., 1990). Bouts of continuous force emission (downward force) are obtained by rewarding the rat with a dipperful of liquid reinforcement that remains accessible for licking only as long as the rat maintains the force above a specified

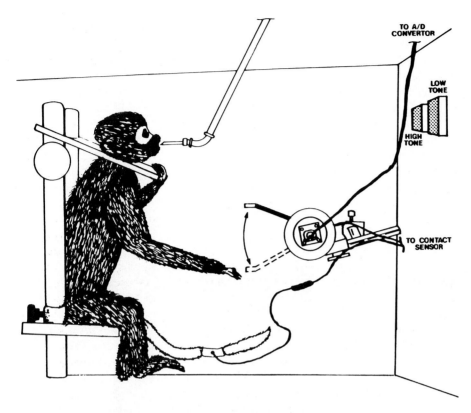

Figure 2   Lever-positioning task using a low-mass displacement transducer to quantify forelimb tremor. (From Newland, 1988.)

level. Thus, the rat licks the reward and makes its continuous holding response at the same time. To ensure that the force oscillations of the responding forelimb were not dampened by bracing of the forelimb or body against the cage, the operandum was located outside the operant chamber but was available through a rectangular opening positioned so that licking and forelimb bracing were not possible at the same time. Forelimb force of 20 g activated a solenoid that presented a reward dipper (filled with milk or water) to the rat as long as the force on the transducer was maintained above 6.7 g. After 3 weeks of training (mostly accomplished by the rat itself, as the manual shaping required only about 45 min), the typical performance consisted of 5- to 7-s bouts of continuous force emission while the rat licked the reward from the dipper. This press-while-you-lick methodology bears a resemblance to the discriminative motor control procedures introduced by Falk (1969) and pursued by Falk and colleagues (e.g., Samson and Falk, 1974; Lau et al., 1990), but the technique described here involves much less training time and higher-fidelity recordings as well. Once the dipper was emptied the rat released the pressure (usually entirely) for about a second, thereby allowing the dipper to drop and refill. Then the rat reapplied force to the operandum to gain access to the dipper contents. The oscillations in force during these bouts of holding (5 to 7 s) were recorded by computer at 100 samples/s, and the results were subjected to Fourier analysis to obtain power spectra of the tremor content. With this technique haloperidol was shown to dose-dependently increase the power in the 10–25 Hz region of the power spectrum

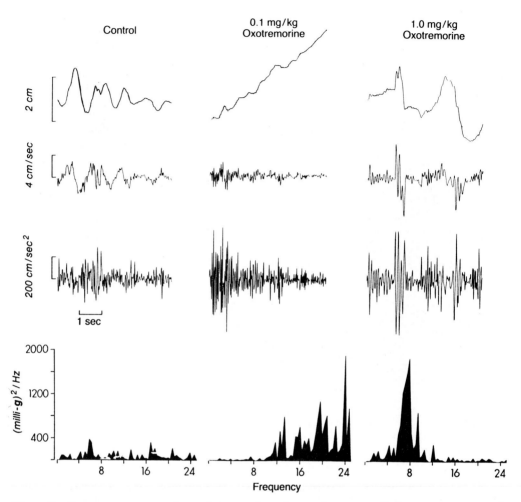

Figure 3   Representative recordings of a squirrel monkey performing on the lever-positioning task. Performance in the control condition and with 0.1 and 1.0 mg/kg oxotremorine is depicted. The first row of tracings shows displacment of the bar, the second row shows the derivative of row 1, the third row shows the second derivative of row 1 in units of acceleration, and the bottom row is the power spectrum of the acceleration signal in row 3. (From Newland, 1988.)

(Fowler et al., 1990). However, haloperidol did not appreciably affect the power of the dominant peak in the spectrum near 6–7 Hz.

In a heretofore unpublished replication of the haloperidol tremogenic effect, 12 rats were administered 0.04 mg/kg of haloperidol. The resulting power spectra for 10 of the rats are plotted in Fig. 4 as the functions represented by the heavy lines. Data for only 10 rats are shown because in the pentobartital phase described below, only 10 of the 12 rats provided sufficient responses for analysis. The power spectra of the force oscillations for these same rats after vehicle treatment are depicted by the lighter lines. Inspection of the spectra suggests that power was increased by haloperidol in the frequency range primarily above 10 Hz, and that the center frequency of the dominant peak at about 7 Hz was not affected by haloperidol treatment. Not all rats exhibited a noticeable effect (e.g.,

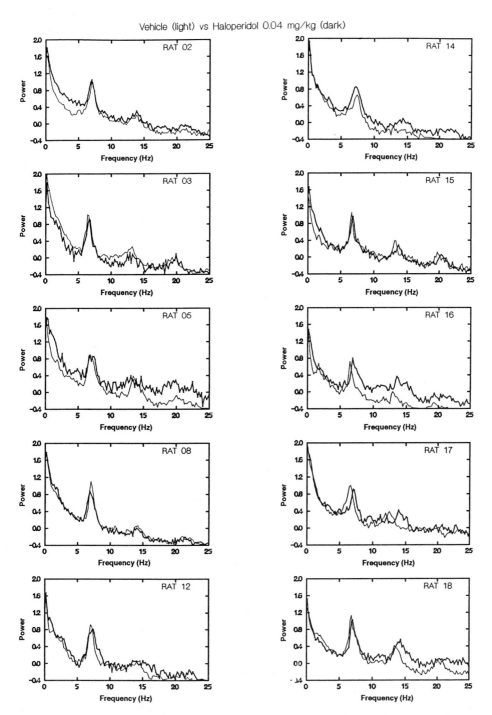

Figure 4   Power spectra of 10 rats' forelimb force oscillations after vehicle injection (light lines) or 45 min after treatment with 0.04 mg/kg of the neuroleptic haloperidol (dark lines). Rats were trained to use the right forelimb to press a force-sensing operandum, and while force remained above 20 g, a solenoid-operated dipper presented liquid reinforcer for the rat to lick. Voltage proportional to force was computer-sampled at 100 Hz, and 5.12-s segments of responding were subjected to fast Fourier analysis. For each rat several power spectra were computed and then ensemble-averaged to produce the functions shown. Under vehicle conditions each power spectrum is made up of an average of 32.75 separately estimated functions. In the drug conditions as shown by the dark lines, a mean of 24.8 separately estimated functions were averaged together for each rat.

rat 15, right column, second from the top, Fig. 4), illustrating that some individual differences in drug response are the biological rule. Quantitative group data given in Table 2 confirm that haloperidol significantly increased power in the 10–25 Hz frequency band. Inasmuch as few compounds have been evaluated with this paradigm, the rats were injected with 10.0 mg/kg pentobarbital in an attempt to demonstrate that the effects witnessed for haloperidol were not nonspecific sedative or motor-incoordination effects. The results for pentobarbital are shown in Fig. 5 (again, dark lines are drug and lighter lines are vehicle). These data differ from the haloperidol data in two ways: 1.) pentobarbital did not have a pronounced tendency to increase frequency in the 10–25 Hz band, and 2.) pentobarbital, unlike haloperidol, shifted the dominant peak near 6–7 Hz to demonstrably lower frequencies. Table 2 makes several statistical comparisons based on data averaged across the 12 rats responding after haloperidol treatment and the 10 rats that responded after pentobarbital treatment. These data show that both drugs were significantly effective in reducing the number of responses, but that only haloperidol significantly increased the high-frequency power. The graphic data show that only pentobarbital had a pronounced tendency to shift the 6–7 Hz peak to lower frequencies. Thus, in this paradigm, both haloperidol and pentobarbital disrupted performance, but each drug had distinctly different power spectra. In view of the fact that Fowler et al. (1990) reported that the centrally acting muscarinic anticholinergic agent atropine sulfate partially reversed the haloperidol-induced increase in power in the 10–25 Hz region, the tremogenic effect of haloperidol in the rat appears to be analogous, if not homologous, to neuroleptic-induced parkinsonism in human patients.

Assessment of Motor Function in Animal Test Batteries

Although many different test batteries have been described in the literature for assessing the toxic effects of chemicals, two batteries have been used most frequently for rodent screening. These test batteries are the National Toxicology Program (NTP) Battery (Tilson et al., 1979) and the functional observational battery (FOB) (Moser, 1989). Both of these batteries include the assessment of motor function as part of the more general behavioral measurement procedures.

Tilson's Animal Neurobehavioral Test Battery, which originated at the National Institute of Environmental Health Sciences (NIEHS), has been extensively used by the NTP to evaluate rats exposed to various chemicals. The battery includes 17 discrete tests that can be subdivided into five major categories of evaluation: sensory, motor, arousal, associative, and physiological-consummatory responses. The motor category includes the measurement of spontaneous motor activity, tremor, and forepaw/hind-limb strength. The methods for measuring locomotor activity and tremor are similar to those methods previously discussed, but testing of forepaw/hind-limb grip strength was a novel approach to evaluating neuromuscular strength, which had previously been evaluated with the inclined screen. Tilson's methods for forepaw/hind-limb grip strength assessment are time-efficient and more sensitive to mild neuromuscular dysfunction than the previously used inclined screen. The testing of forepaw/hind-limb grip strength has been used in many laboratories over the past 15 years to assess the motoric effects of chemicals.

Moser's more recent FOB (1989, 1990a,b) includes observations of rodents in three different conditions: home cage–open field, manipulative, and physiological. The FOB is typically used in conjunction with an automated measure of locomotor activity. This approach has been used in her laboratory to screen a wide array of pesticides and positive

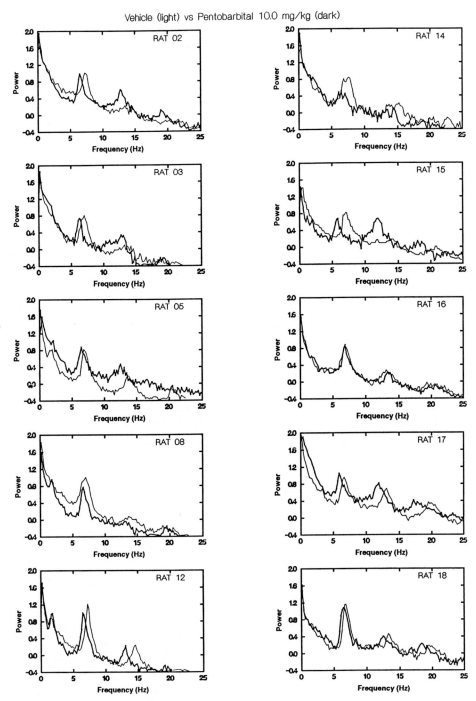

Figure 5   Power spectra for the same rats shown in Fig. 4, but in this case the effects of pentobarbital (10.0 mg/kg) are depicted. Computational methods were as described in the caption of Fig. 4, except that the mean number of functions combined for each rat under vehicle conditions was 28.45, and under drug conditions 23.5 functions were combined per rat.

Table 2 Statistical Data for the Performances Depicted for Haloperidol in Fig. 4 and for Pentobarbital in Fig. 5

Dependent variable	Haloperidol					Pentobarbital				
	Vehicle	Hal. (0.04 mg/kg)	t	df	p	Vehicle	Pent. (10.0 mg/kg)	t	df	p
Responses	43.42 (2.23)	30.17 (3.94)	3.478	11	0.005	45.82 (3.04)	37.00 (3.56)	2.617	9	0.028
Power in 10–20 Hz Band	58.69 (4.71)	74.49 (6.68)	2.889	10	0.016	62.85 (9.00)	77.15 (11.63)	1.516	9	NS
Peak Force (g)	35.03 (2.25)	36.34 (1.39)	0.573	11	NS	39.13 (2.47)	41.30 (3.62)	0.558	9	NS
Duration (s)	6.13 (0.35)	6.32 (0.32)	0.473	11	NS	5.64 (0.30)	5.84 (0.52)	0.224	9	NS

[a]Group means and standard errors of the mean, in parentheses, for the indicated behavioral measures and treatment conditions. A response was defined as force output above 6.67 g for 0.75 s or longer. Baseline differences in peak force and duration for haloperidol and pentobarbital may reflect the fact that the haloperidol data were collected with sweetened condensed milk as the reinforcer, whereas water was the reinforcer in the pentobarbital condition.

controls known to produce diverse neurotoxicity syndromes. In addition to the measure of locomotor activity, the FOB explores other aspects of motor functioning. In the home cage–open field situation, observations are made of posture, tremors, rearing, gait, and stereotypy. In a more structured test environment, righting reflex, landing foot splay, and fore-limb and hind-limb grip strength are measured. Many of the measurement techniques in the FOB are not unique to it, since all have been used in other laboratories, but the total FOB assessment is unique. Some toxicologists, who have failed to appreciate the diversity of motor functions, have suggested that a single measure of motor function might be sufficient. Data collected in Moser's laboratory (1989, 1992) on several pesticides clearly indicated that a single assessment procedure is not encompassing. Comparison of 90-day exposures to acrylamide (1–12 mg/kg), a compound that produces a known peripheral neuropathy, and 2-hydroxyethyl acrylate (HEA) (3–60 mg/kg), through six different assessments of neuromuscular functioning indicated that acrylamide and HEA produced distinctly different profiles. HEA produced no alteration of neuromuscular functioning, while acrylamide reduced functioning on all of the assessments except that of fore-limb grip strength, which remained normal under the exposure conditions. These data support the contention that multiple motoric measures or a battery approach to screening can provide a more complete evaluation of overall motor functioning than measurement of a single end point.

Even though primates have not been used as much as rodents to assess chemically induced neurobehavioral alterations, primate test batteries have been developed either for detecting side-effect liabilities of psychotherapeutic agents (O'Keeffe and Lifshitz, 1989) or for evaluating toxic effects of commonly abused drugs (Paule et al., 1988, 1990). A functional observational battery for primate assessment, similar to that used for rodents, has been developed by O'Keeffe and Lifshitz (1989) for evaluating the long-term effects of neuroleptic exposure in macaque monkeys. The O'Keeffe and Lifshitz FOB includes the observation of both nonsocial and social behaviors, since their monkeys are housed in group environments. A component of their FOB assesses motor function. In the nonsocial situation, observations of walking, climbing, lying and sleeping, and stereotyped pacing are made. In the social situation, chase and attack of other animals are scored. These procedures could be adapted directly or modified to evaluate a whole range of potential chemical toxicities.

Merle Paule and his colleagues at the National Center for Toxicological Research have designed an operant test battery for assessing the performance of rhesus monkeys subsequent to exposure to various chemicals and drugs (Paule et al., 1988, 1990). Their battery includes sequential testing on delayed matching-to-sample, conditioned position responding, progressive-ratio responding, temporal response differentiation, and incremental repeated acquisition responding. Most of these procedures are traditional operant tasks that have been used singly in the laboratory to examine various alterations in normal performance levels. One of these measures, the temporal response differentiation (TRD) task, is highly dependent on the animal's use of interoceptive cues to sustain the response for several seconds and is similar to some of the rodent procedures that have been found to be sensitive to tremogenic compounds. This procedure requires that responses on a conventional switch-closure lever must be between 10 and 14 s in duration for the delivery of reinforcement, which occurs upon response release. All other responses made, whether too long or too brief, are considered subcriterion. Although the TRD response is not an easy one to shape to criterion, primates do acquire the response. In the laboratory at NCTR the TRD has been found to be one of the most sensitive tasks in the operant test battery.

Δ-9-Tetrahydrocannabinol (THC), THC smoke, diazepam, amphetamine, morphine, and phencyclidine disrupted TRD performance at doses that did not affect the other tasks in the test battery. Only atropine sulfate disrupted performance in one of the other tasks, the incremental repeated acquisition task, at a dose that did not alter TRD responding (Schultze et al., 1988).

Interestingly, the NCTR laboratory has also applied this same test battery to human testing (Paule and Cranmer, 1990). Extensive cross-species validation, other than the examination of baseline performance for various age groups (4- to 8-year-olds), has not been conducted at this time, but future data bases will permit direct comparisons between laboratory primates and human populations.

INNOVATIVE APPROACHES TO THE MEASUREMENT OF CHEMICAL EFFECTS ON DISCRIMINATIVE MOTOR BEHAVIOR

The methods described in this section require subjects to respond appropriately to sensory cues, either internal or environmental. These techniques represent the most sophisticated approaches to assessing motor functioning; therefore, they are not intended as screening techniques (with the possible exception of the measurement of lick force described below) but rather are strategies for elucidating the intricacies of chemically induced alterations in motor behavior. Although relatively labor-intensive, these inventive techniques hold promise for identifying the neurobehavioral processes most sensitive to disruption by exposure to chemical substances.

Motor Function as Effort Expenditure

Newland and Weiss (1990) have developed a method for assessing primate effort expenditure in an operant procedure. This method for assessing effortful responding was originally developed in their laboratory to evaluate the effects of amphetamine and pentobarbital in cebus monkeys (*Cebus apella*). As is illustrated in Fig. 6, restrained monkeys were trained to perform a rowing motion, arm flexion coupled with leg extension, requiring a force of 39–41 newtons, and returning the manipulandum to the original resting position. Newland and Weiss failed to observe the expected generalized enhancement by

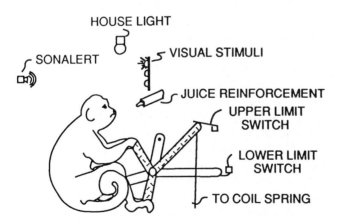

Figure 6   Rowing task to implement contingencies requiring varying amounts of work. (From Newland and Weiss, 1990.)

amphetamine or a generalized degradation of performance by pentobarbital at doses known to have effects in other behavioral paradigms.

More recently, Newland and Weiss (1992) have reported the effects of manganese on this unique laboratory measurement of required effort expenditure. Human manganese poisoning ensues in three distinct stages, as described by several authors (Catzios et al., 1968; Barbeau, 1984; Cawte, 1985). The first stage is characterized by mania, including the symptoms of hysterical laughter and crying, insomnia, and hypersexuality. The first stage is followed by a period of clumsiness, fatigue, and a mask-like facial expression. The final, irreversible stage is characterized by hyperflexion of the muscles and dystonia. The unique procedure used to quantify the rowing motion was applied to assess the effects of manganese in primates as a potential model of the second stage of the human syndrome. Newland and Weiss observed that the overall energy expentiture (i.e., work output, the distance integral of force) of the rowing response, but not the topography or motivational component of the response, degenerated across the period of repetitive exposure to a concentration that produced nigral and pallidal accumulation of manganese visualized by magnetic resonance imaging. The rowing motion assessed in this study has compelling face validity for describing manganese toxicity, since the observations made with monkeys correlate reasonably well with the human syndrome, which gradually worsens with extended exposure and the concomitant accumulation of manganese. This ingenious approach to assessing motoric responding is representative of the potential sophistication that can be applied to measuring chemically induced changes, but techniques like this one have not been used often.

Motor Function as Reflected by Variations in Response Force

Although operant methods usually emphasize the rate or probability of "simple" motor responses, it is possible to measure the amplitude and duration of these operant responses. This is accomplished by replacing the switch-closure lever with a force-sensing operandum that can measure the force of each individual response (Notterman and Mintz, 1965; Fowler, 1987). Under the latter circumstances new behavioral tasks and new measurements become available for the study of motor function. Two behavioral measurements of particular interest are the peak force of response (the maximum force amplitude attained during one strike of the operandum by some portion of the organism's body) and the duration of the response (the time the force remains above a specific force threshold that defines a response). In addition, the entire force-time waveform of these operant events can be used to characterize the disruptive effects of chemical agents. Because different portions of the musculoskeletal system are endowed with different muscle masses and force-generating capacities, it is usually important to restrict the response topography to forelimb(s), tongue, or nose. Otherwise, treatment-induced changes in response force would be difficult to interpret, because one could not know, without additional independent observations, whether large shifts in topography produced the force changes. For example, if the operandum were available to the jaws and teeth of a rodent as well as to forelimbs, a topographical shift from forelimb pressing to biting could produce a 10-fold increase in peak force. These considerations account for the location of the operandum outside the operant chamber, as illustrated in Fig. 7. With respect to the chemical agents studied with these methods, data have been collected mainly with psychotherapeutic drugs, especially neuroleptics, in an attempt to understand both their therapeutic effects and their side effects as these may be expressed in rats.

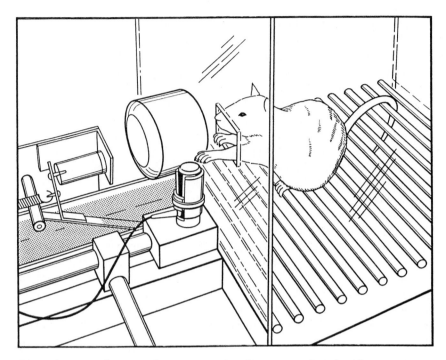

Figure 7 Line drawing of an operant chamber equipped with a force-sensing operandum and a solenoid-operated reinforcement dipper. This apparatus, or one similar to it, has been used to measure the motor effects of drugs on peak force and duration of operant responses (cf. Notterman and Mintz, 1965). This drawing was made through the support of National Science Foundation grant BNS-8510387 (Aaron Ettenberg, P.I.), while the second author (S.C.F.) was on sabbatical at the University of California, Santa Barbara, 1986.

In a representative study, Fowler et al. (1986) trained rats to reach and press a force operandum (see Fig. 7) and then examined the effects of haloperidol (0.04–0.16 mg/kg) on peak force, duration, and rate of response. In addition, individual force-time waveforms were recorded and analyzed for possible evidence of bradykinesia (retarded speed of forelimb withdrawal from the operandum) induced by this drug. Withdrawal time was defined as the time from attainment of peak force in a single response to the complete cessation of force on the operandum (this was called fall time). By computer methods, the rise and fall times were calculated for each response. The data indicated that haloperidol dose-dependently increased peak force of response, increased response duration, and decreased response rate. The rise-fall analysis of the force-time waveforms showed that the increase in duration of response was the result of increased fall time (i.e., was associated with sluggish forelimb withdrawal). Taken together, the results suggested that low doses (i.e., "subcataleptic") of haloperidol produced pseudoparkinsonism in rats, just as it engenders this prominent side effect in the clinic.

If the apparatus depicted in Fig. 7 has a photodetector added to the cylindrical recession giving access to the reinforcement dipper, one can measure the duration of the rat's head entry events along with the peak force, duration, and rate of response (Fowler et al., 1991). This technique provided useful information in an experiment in which the effects of haloperidol (0.04–0.16 mg/kg) were contrasted with those of nonparalytic doses

(0.2–0.8 mg/kg) of decamethonium bromide (a peripheral neuromuscular blocking agent). Because decamethonium bromide produces a relatively brief, reversible muscle weakness, it was thought the comparison with haloperidol would provide an additional anchor-point for understanding neuroleptics' effects on rats. Results indicated that "haloperidol increased peak force and duration of operant response, increased maximum head entry duration, and temporally dissociated forelimb and head entry behavior. Decamethonium decreased force and duration of operant response, did not appreciably affect maximum head entry duration, and did not influence the normal temporal coupling of forelimb and head entry responses" (Fowler et al., 1991). In addition to peak force of response, the maximum head entry duration (i.e., the duration of the longest photobeam break in a given operant session) discriminated quite consistently between the very different motor effects of these two drugs. Haloperidol produced "microcatalepsy," but decamethonium bromide did not. When used in combination, the multiple dependent variables in this study may serve as the basis for inferences about the contribution of CNS and peripheral factors to the disruption of motor function caused by chemical agents.

Falk and colleagues (Falk, 1969; Samson and Falk, 1974; Lau et al., 1990) and Fowler et al. (1984) trained rats in a discriminative motor control task in which the rat was required to hold force continuously for a few seconds within specified upper and lower force limits. While this task clearly requires a quite demanding (for a rat) level of discriminative motor behavior, it suffers from the disadvantage that the training time required is extensive. In a different force-discriminative task introduced by Notterman and Mintz (1962), the peak force band task, the animal is reinforced for brief, relatively ballistic responses having peak forces that fall within specified upper and lower limits. There is no time requirement. Nevertheless, the rats must make use of feedback from the response to guide further responding. Training rats to perform this task is comparatively rapid, but will depend on the width of the force band relative to the absolute force requirement of the band lower limit (i.e., Weber's law is true for rats). With the peak force band technique one can independently vary the discriminative requirement (band width) and the effort requirement (force level of the lower band limit) and thereby operationalize two separate dimensions of motor function in the same test preparation.

Figure 8 shows previously unpublished data gathered for diazepam with this force-band technique. Two groups of rats were first trained on relatively wide, low or high peak force bands (see legend of Fig. 8 for details). Under these conditions the rats' force emission becomes tightly controlled by the reinforcement contingencies, as is demonstrated by the separation of the mean peak force (upper left in Fig. 8) curves representing low- and high-force requirements and by the small standard error brackets for each group. As shown in the dose-effect functions in the left column of Fig. 8, diazepam dose-dependently increased peak force of response in both the low- and high-force-band groups. The data on the ratio of reinforced responses to total responses show that under vehicle conditions the two tasks were approximately equally difficult discriminatively. However, diazepam interfered with the performance of the low-band group more than it did with that of the high-band group, as is shown by the greater drug-related decline in the success ratio for the low-force group (see the middle left panel of Fig. 8). In neither group was response rate decreased by the doses of diazepam studied. Examination of force distributions showed that the disruptive effect of the drug was to produce overshooting of the force band in the low-band group. Mean peak force also increased significantly with increasing dose in the high-force-band group, but not enough to cause many responses to overshoot the upper band limit of 80 g.

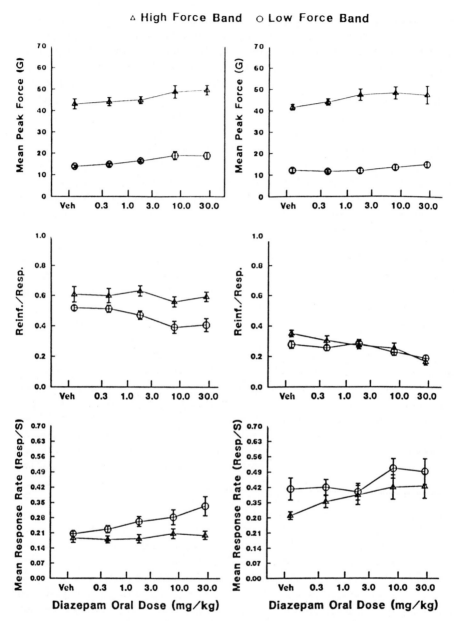

Figure 8 Effects of diazepam on rats' performance in an operant force-band task. In the wide-band condition (left panels), the peak force requirements were 8–16 g in the low-force group (n = 16) and 40–80 g in the high-force group (n = 16). For the narrow band (right panels), the low-force requirement was 10–12 g and the high-force requirement was 40–50 g. Responses with peak forces falling outside the force-band requirements had no scheduled consequences, whereas in-band responses were reinforced upon response termination. The ordinate label "Reinf./Resp." is an abbreviation for the number of reinforcers obtained divided by the total number of responses emitted; this success ratio is independent of the time rate of responding and provides information about the discriminative difficulty of the task. The brackets indicate ± 1 SEM.

After the collection of dose-effect information with the wide force band, the rats were given an additional 2 weeks of training with the force band narrowed considerably (i.e., the discriminative difficulty nearly doubled, as judged by the success ratio in the middle right panel of Fig. 8), but the effort level was kept approximately constant for each band group. Under these new, narrower peak-force-band conditions, dose-effect functions for diazepam were again obtained. The narrowing of the bands shifted the mean peak force output to levels lower than those emitted under the wider bands (compare left and right sets of axes in the top row of Fig. 8), but diazepam again produced an elevation in peak force in both groups. Likewise, for both groups, the ratio of reinforced responses to total responses emitted was lower in the narrower band condition, and the ratio declined significantly as dose increased for both groups. Average response rate was increased by diazepam, and, as is suggested by the data in the lower right panel of Fig. 8, the high-force group generally responded at a lower rate than the low-force group. The latter result suggests that the higher effort requirement may have had a suppressive effect on rate. Although much work needs to be done with these techniques before their relevance to neurobehavioral toxicology can be fully appreciated, these results with diazepam are instructive because they show that a drug with muscle-relaxing properties in human beings may lead to increased force output in rats even in a setting where force emission has been constrained to relatively narrow limits by operant-conditioning methods. Whether compounds with high neuromuscular toxicity, such as acrylamide, can be successfully evaluated with these new methods must await further experimentation.

From the perspective of investigators charged with the task of screening large numbers of doses or compounds for toxic effects, operant methods may be viewed as prohibitively labor-intensive and expensive. In this context it is important to note that the response force–recording methodology can be profitably applied to nonoperant as well as operant settings. For example, the effects of low doses of haloperidol (0.03–0.25 mg/kg) on rats' tongue forces during licking were characterized in a procedure that required only 2 min/day/rat and comparatively brief initial training in the lick task (Fowler and Mortell, 1992). Haloperidol was observed to decrease the peak force of tongue contacts against a metal disk from which water was licked by the rat. This lick-force impairment was in contrast to haloperidol-induced increases in forelimb force produced by the same dose range of this drug (Fowler et al., 1986, 1991). Thus, motor function disturbances produced by a toxic agent may be expressed differently by different neuromuscular subsystems in the same organism. Fourier methods applied to the tongue force-time waveforms were able to detect a significant but quite small slowing of the lick oscillator. For example, a haloperidol dose of 0.06 mg/kg slowed the burst rate of licking from 5.250 Hz to 5.096 Hz, $t(29)$, $p = .014$. In terms of the period (the reciprocal of the frequency) for a single lick, this slowing of frequency amounts to a lengthening of the period from 0.1905 s to 0.1962 s, or a prolongation of each lick averaging only 0.0057 s, or 5.7 ms per lick event. Results from this experiment suggest that conjoint assessment of tongue force and lick timing may provide an efficient and exquisitely sensitive procedure for detecting orobuccolingual motor impairments.

OVERVIEW

The interests of simplicity and efficiency have kept locomotor activity assessment the most frequently used technique for measuring motor function in contemporary pharmacology and toxicology. However, in the attempt to reduce neurobehavioral motor function to a single quantal value, much of the important complexity of neuromuscular function may be obscured, and correspondingly, disruptions of these functions by chemical substances may go undetected. A glimpse at the early work of Muybridge in the late 1800s describing equine movement through a series of time-lapse photographs (Rosenbaum, 1991) leads to astonishment at the complexity of motor behavior as expressed by a galloping horse. Newer techniques for examining specific complex aspects of motor function are available and probably will be applied by various laboratories to provide more intricate and revealing descriptions of specific chemical effects, such as those reported by Newland and Weiss (1992), Vorhees et al. (1992), and Fowler et al. (1990, 1991, 1992). To some extent, motoric assessment has been driven by the need to provide qualitative judgments about the toxicity of chemical exposure that can be applied to the broader needs of safety assessment rather than dwelling on the specific nature of those toxicities. The breadth of available techniques for examining the complexities of movement should generate more sophisticated descriptions of motoric toxicities and aid in delineating mechanisms responsible for those toxicities.

ACKNOWLEDGMENTS

Preparation of this chapter was supported in part by National Institute on Drug Abuse grant DA05253 and National Institute of Mental Health grant MH43429. We thank Scott Bowen for preparation of Fig. 8.

REFERENCES

Anger WK (1990). Worksite behavioral research: results, sensitive methods, test batteries and the transition from laboratory data to human health. Neurotoxicology 11:629–720.

Anger WK (1992). Assessment of neurotoxicity in humans. In: Tilson H, Mitchell C, eds. Neurotoxicology. New York: Raven Press, 363–86.

Anger WK, Johnson BL (1985). Chemicals affecting behavior. In: O'Donoghue J, ed. Neurotoxicity of industrial and commercial chemicals. Boca Raton, Florida: CRC Press, 51–148.

Arcia E, Otto DA (1992). Reliability of selected tests from the neurobehavioral evaluation system. Neurotoxicol Teratol 14:103–10.

Baker EL, Letz R, Fidler A (1985). A computer-administered neurobehavioral evaluation system for occupational and environmental epidemiology. Rationale, methodology, and pilot study results. J Occup Med 27:206–12.

Barbeau A (1984). Manganese and extrapyramidal disorders. Neurotoxicology 5:13–36.

Catzios GC, Horiuchi K, Fuenzalida S, Mena I (1968). Chronic manganese poisoning: clearance of tissue manganese concentrations with persistence of the neurological picture. Neurology 18:376–82.

Cawte J (1985). Psychiatric sequelae of manganese exposure in the adult, foetal and neonatal nervous systems. Aust NZ J Psychiatry 19:211–7.

Centers for Disease Control (1983). Leading work related diseases and injuries—United States. MMWR 32:24–6.

Centers for Disease Control (1986). Leading work related diseases and injuries—United States. Neurotoxic disorders. MMWR 35:113–6.

Coughenour LL, McClean JR, Parker RB (1977). A new device for the rapid measurement of impaired motor function in mice. Pharmacol Biochem Behav 6:351–3.

Crofton KM, Boncek VM, MacPhail RC (1989). Evidence for monoaminergic involvement in triadimefon-induced hyperactivity. Psychopharmacology 97:326–30.

Crofton KM, Reiter LW (1984). Effects of two pyrethroid insecticides on motor activity and the acoustic startle response in the rat. Toxicol Appl Pharmacol 75:318–28.

Crofton KM, Reiter LW (1984). Effects of two pyrethroid insecticides on motor activity and the acoustic startle response in the rat. Toxicol Appl Pharmacol 75:318–28.

Crofton KM, Reiter LW (1988). The effects of type I and II pyrethroids on motor activity and acoustic startle response in the rat. Fund Appl Toxicol 10:624–34.

Dunham NW, Miya TS (1957). A note on a simple apparatus for detecting neurological deficits in rats and mice. J Am Pharmacol Assoc 46:208–9.

Edwards PM, Parker VH (1977). A simple, sensitive, and objective method for early assessment of acrylamide neuropathy in rats. Toxicol Appl Pharmacol 40:589–91.

Falk J (1969). Drug effects on discriminative motor control. Physiol Behav 4:421–7.

Fowler SC (1987). Force and duration of operant response as dependent variables in behavioral pharmacology. In: Thompson T, Dews PB, Barrett JE, eds. Neurobehavioral pharmacology, advances in behavioral pharmacology, vol 6. Hillsdale, New Jersey: Erlbaum, 83:127.

Fowler SC, Ford KE, Gramling SE, Nail GL (1984). Acute and subchronic effects of neuroleptics on quantitative measures of discriminative motor control in rats. Psychopharmacology 84:368–73.

Fowler SC, LaCerra MM, Ettenberg A (1986). Effects of haloperidol on the biophysical characteristics of operant responding: implications for motor and reinforcement processes. Pharmacol Biochem Behav 25:791–6.

Fowler SC, Liao RM, Skjoldager PD (1990). A new rodent model for neuroleptic-induced pseudoparkinsonism: low doses of haloperidol increase forelimb tremor in the rat. Behav Neurosci 104:449–56.

Fowler SC, Mortell C (1992). Low doses of haloperidol interfere with rat tongue extensions during licking: a quantitative analysis. Behav Neurosci 106:386–95.

Fowler SC, Skjoldager PD, Liao R-M, Chase JM, Johnson JS (1991). Distinguishing between haloperidol's and decamethonium's disruptive effects on operant behavor in rats: use of measurements that complement response rate. J Exp Anal Behav 56:239–60.

Gerhart JM, Hong JS, Tilson HA (1983). Studies on the possible sites of chlordecone-induced tremor in rats. Toxicol Appl Pharmacol 70:382–9.

Gerhart JM, Hong JS, Uphouse LL, Tilson HA (1982). Chlordecone-induced tremor: quantification and pharmacological analysis. Toxicol Appl Pharmacol 66:234–43.

Geyer MA (1990). Approaches to the characterization of drug effects on locomotor activity in rodents. In: Adler MW, Cowan A, eds. Modern methods in pharmacology, vol. 6. Testing and evaluation of drugs of abuse. New York: Wiley-Liss, 81–99.

Goh JCH, Solomonidis SE, Spence WD, Paul JP (1984). Biomechanical evaluation of sach and uniaxial feet. Prosthet Orthot 8:147–54.

Herr DW, Hong JS, Tilson HA (1985). DDT-induced tremor in rats: effects of pharmacological agents. Psychopharmacology 86:426–31.

Kallman MJ, Balster RL, Kaempf G (1984). Behavioral toxicity of chloral in mice: an approach to evaluation. Neurobehav Toxicol Teratol 6:137–46.

Kulig BM (1987). An automated technique for the evaluation of coordinated movement deficits in rats. Zbl Bakt Hyg Biol 185:28–31.

Kulig BM, Lammers JHCM (1992). Assessment of neurotoxicant-induced effects of motor function. In: Tilson H, Mitchell C, eds. Neurotoxicology. New York: Raven Press, 147–79.

Kulig BM, Vanwersch RAP, Wolthuis OL (1985). The automated analysis of coordinated hindlimb movement in rats during acute and prolonged exposure to toxic agents. Toxicol Appl Pharmacol 80:1–10.

Lau CE, Falk JL, Tang M (1990). Motor performance decrement by midazolam: antagonism by Ro 15-1788 and CGS 8216. Pharmacol Biochem Behav 36:139–43.

Moser VC (1989). Screening approaches to neurotoxicity: a functional observational battery. J Am Coll Toxicol 8:85–93.

Moser VC (1990a). Approaches to assessing the validity of a functional observational battery. Neurotoxicol Teratol 12:483–8.

Moser VC (1990b). Application and assessment of neurobehavioral screening methods in rats. In:

Johnson BL, ed. Advances in neurobehavioral toxicology: applications in environmental and occupational health. Chelsea, Michigan: Lewis, 419–32.

Moser VC (1992). Applications of a neurobehavioral screening battery. J Am Coll Toxicol 6:661–9.

Moser VC, Balster RL (1985). Acute motor and lethal effects of inhaled toluene, 1,1,1-trichloroethane, halothane, and ethanol in mice: effects of exposure duration. Toxicol Appl Pharmacol 77:285–91.

Newland MC (1988). Quantification of motor function in toxicology. Toxicol Lett 43:295–319.

Newland MC, Weiss B (1990). Drug effects on an effortful operant: pentobarbital and amphetamine. Pharmacol Biochem Behav 36:381–7.

Newland MC, Weiss B (1992). Persistent effects of manganese on effortful responding and their relationship to manganese accumulation in the primate globus pallidus. Toxicol Appl Pharmacol 113:87–97.

Notterman JM, Mintz DE (1962). Exteroceptive cueing of response force. Science 135:1070–1.

Notterman JM, Mintz DE (1965). Dynamics of response. New York: Wiley.

O'Keeffe RT, Lifshitz K (1989). Nonhuman primates in neurotoxicity screening and neurobehavioral toxicity studies. J Am Coll Toxicol 8:127–40.

Parker AJ, Clarke KA (1990). Gait topography in rat locomotion. Physiol Behav 48:41–7.

Paule MG (1990). Use of NCTR operant test battery in nonhuman primates. Neurotoxicol Teratol 12:413–8.

Paule MG, Cranmer JM (1990). Complex brain function in children as measured in NCTR monkey operant test battery. In: Johnson BL, ed. Advances in neurobehavioral toxicology: applications in environmental and occupational health. Chelsea, Michigan: Lewis, 433–47.

Paule MG, Schulze GE, Slikker W Jr (1988). Complex brain function in monkeys as a baseline for studying the effects of exogenous compounds. Neurotoxicology 9:463–70.

Potvin AR, Tourtellotte WW, Syndulko K, Potvin J (1981). Quantitative methods in assessment of neurologic function. CRC Crit Rev Bioeng 10:177–224.

Rafales LS (1987). Assessment of locomotor activity. In: Annau Z, ed. Neurobehavioral toxicology. London: Edward Arnold, 54–68.

Reiter LW, MacPhail RC (1982). Factors influencing motor activity measurements in neurotoxicology. In: Mitchell CL, ed. Nervous system toxicology. New York: Raven Press, 45–65.

Rosenbaum DA (1991). Human motor control. New York: Academic Press.

Samson H, Falk J (1974). Ethanol and discriminative motor control: effects on normal and dependent animals. Pharmacol Biochem Behav 2:791–801.

Schultze GE, McMillan DE, Baily JR, Scallet A, Ali SF, Slikker W Jr, Paule MG (1988). Acute effects of delta-9-tetrahydrocannabinol in rhesus monkeys as measured by performance in a battery of complex operant tests. J Pharmacol Exp Ther 245:178–86.

Sette W (1989). Adoption of new guidelines and data requirements for more extensive neurotoxicity testing under FIFRA. Toxicol Indust Health 5:181–94.

Tanger HJ, Vanwersch RAP, Wolthuis OL (1984). Automated quantitative analysis of coordinated locomotor behaviour in rats. J Neurosci Meth 10:237–45.

Tilson HA, Mitchell CL, Cabe PA (1979). Screening for neurobehavioral toxicity: the need for examples of validation of testing procedures. Neurobehav Toxicol 1(suppl 1):137–48.

Vorhees CV, Acuff-Smith KD, Minck DR, and Butcher RE (1992). A method for measuring locomotor behavior in rodents: contrast-sensitive computer-controlled video tracking activity assessment in rats. Neurotoxicol Teratol 14:43–9.

14

Conceptual and Procedural Issues Concerning the Neurotoxicological Assessment of Learning and Memory Processes

Charles F. Mactutus
University of Kentucky
Lexington, Kentucky

INTRODUCTION

Memory is an extremely important cognitive process with capabilities that are simply astounding. Flexibility, redundancy, and apparently limitless capacity are among the inherent properties of our cognitive processes and their underlying neural mechanisms that permit us to function, rather flawlessly, day after day, year in, year out. Our memory provides the ability to recognize familiar faces in a crowd, recall the meanings of thousands of words, and reproduce many hard-earned motor skills in a brief instant. Indeed, it is not surprising that with but a moment's reflection one is acutely aware that impairments of memory can exert a profound effect on everyday life.

Dysfunctions of cognitive processes such as learning and memory have no unitary cause. The sustaining of an acute accident-related brain trauma warns us of the potential temporariness of our able-bodied state. The loss of cognitive function with advancing age documents a process that few will escape in their ripe old years. Affliction with a progressive neurodegenerative disease, for those less fortunate, precipitates an even more rapid loss of age-related cognitive abilities. Truly, the diversity of conditions that share some form of cognitive dysfunction attests to the formidable task that lies before us.

We are also now well aware that symptoms of memory impairment, such as those that have long been recognized as accompanying brain injury, disease states, and aging, are also often reported following neurotoxicant exposure. Untoward effects on the developing organism, potentially reflected as later learning disabilities and memory problems, illustrate the subtle manner in which such exposures may exert their influence. Exposure to certain environmental agents at any point in one's life, however, may produce frank memory disturbances, a fact attributable to the ability of such agents to cause irreversible central nervous system damage. Fortunately, milder or more transient forms of mental confusion and memory loss are the more commonly reported outcomes, although they may follow exposure to a broad variety of compounds such as carbon monoxide, organic solvents, and insecticides.

This introduction implicitly argues several points. First, animal models are extremely important in providing the rigorous experimental control necessary for the study of neurotoxicant-induced cognitive dysfunction. Second, the study of neurotoxicants, like the study of brain injury, disease states, and aging, may provide new tools and models through which to increase our understanding of normal cognitive and brain function. Third, information concerning cognitive dysfunction is valuable in making regulatory decisions about the manner in which and extent to which a suspected "neurotoxicant" ought to be used.

SCOPE

Goal and Aims

The challenge of identifying and discussing issues concerning the assessment of learning and memory in neurotoxicology is formidable. An explicit effort has been made to avoid another compilation of what has been done, with unresolved contradictory outcomes. Such an approach generally does little to serve the readership, to challenge our thoughts, or to stimulate progress in the field. Rather, in the interest of providing information useful to a broad audience with different goals, as a primary aim I have favored a more general approach identifying both conceptual and procedural issues that should be considered in developing any successful assay of cognitive function. It is my hope that this material may serve both as a guide and as a springboard for the development of more innovative and comprehensive assessments of neurotoxicant-induced cognitive dysfunction.

In pursuit of my stated goal, this chapter will be focused on four specific aims. The initial aim, by way of introduction, is to discuss conceptual definitions and issues inherent in any toxicological assessment of the psychological processes of learning and memory. This information is important in identifying the criteria for drawing inferences about learning and memory processes. The second aim is to provide a comprehensive survey of the toxicological literature as it pertains to assessing potential learning and memory dysfunction. I use the term "toxicological literature" to refer broadly to studies of adverse effects occurring as a function of agent exposure at any time during the life span of the animal; thus, both teratological and toxicological data of are interest. Third, within the context of this survey both the most commonly held assumptions and the most pressing procedural issues in the study of neurotoxicant-induced learning and memory dysfunction will be identified. Fourth, this chapter will provide a brief overview of the major procedures that are being used for cognitive evaluation, and will identify by way of the better exemplars in this literature what is being done.

Background: Prior Publications

Several relatively recent chapters are available on the topic of neurotoxicology and learning/memory processes. In particular, the chapters by Eckerman and colleagues (Cabe and Eckerman, 1982; Miller and Eckerman, 1986; Eckerman and Bushnell, 1992) are not only very readable as introductory material, but illustrate state-of-the-art research from psychological, toxicological, and pharmacological journals. Messing (1987) has a contemporary chapter on organometal neurotoxicity and memory. Brief reviews/chapters are also available for ontogenetic studies of potential learning and memory dysfunction (Mactutus, 1985); for a lesion analysis of the effects of neurotoxicants on brain function (Wenk and Olton, 1986; Levin et al., 1992); and for an animal model of mental retardation (Strupp and Levitsky, 1990). More general articles on behavior, with specific sections on learning and memory, have been written by Adams and Buelke-Sam (1981), Tilson and Mitchell (1984), and Adams (1986).

There are also a number of excellent chapters within the psychological literature that deserve further consideration, as they may address issues relevant to the field of neurotoxicology. Two edited volumes contain much provocative information on the ontogeny of learning and memory (Kail and Spear, 1984; Spear and Campbell, 1979). The modern birth of the "cognitive" approach to animal behavior may be traced through several volumes (Medin et al., 1976; Hulse et al., 1978; Spear, 1978; Roitblat et al., 1984). The recent "Annual Review of Psychology" chapter by Spear and his colleagues is an important paper that summarizes major advances culminating over the last two decades and presents a forceful argument for a basic reconceptualization of our thinking about the field of animal learning/memory (Spear et al., 1990). The recent book by Denny (1992) is an excellent text for nearly anyone interested in, or using, aversively motivated behavioral tasks. Finally, the upcoming book by Spear and Riccio (1994) on animal memory also promises to be an invaluable resource.

CONCEPTUAL DEFINITIONS

The terms "learning" and "memory" have no universally accepted definitions. This difficulty, although partly attributable to the fact that these terms have a number of different connotations to each of us, is not insurmountable. First, it should be emphasized that learning and memory are examples of cognitive processes; neither is synonymous with cognition. Second, it should be appreciated that although the terms "learning" and "memory" are both used to refer to theoretical processes reflecting associative or cognitive capabilities, and are mutually dependent, they reflect different processes and emphases.

Learning

Let us begin then with a look at several respected definitions of learning. A classic definition:

Learning refers to more or less permanent change in behavior [potentiality] which occurs as a result of [reinforced] practice (Kimble, 1961, p. 2).

A modern definition:

Learning is an inferred change in the organism's mental state which results from experience and which influences in a relatively permanent fashion the organism's potential for subsequent adaptive behavior (Tarpy and Mayer, 1978, p. 3).

More contemporary definitions:

Learning is an enduring change in the mechanisms of behavior that results from experience with environmental events (Domjan and Burkhard, 1986, p. 12).

Learning is a neurological process that arises from experience and is inferred from changes in the organism's behavior (Hall, 1989, p. 14).

Learning is reflected by a relatively permanent change in an organism's potential for responding that results from prior experience or practice (Gordon, 1989, p. 6).

Although a complete exposition of the implications of any one of these definitions is most appropriately obtained from the original source, for our purposes it is most important to note the consensus that exists among these experts.

Implicit or explicit in every one of these definitions are the following points: 1.) Learning is a process that occurs within the organism. 2.) Learning is not directly observable, but is inferred from behavior. 3.) Learning may occur without any detectable change in an organism's current behavior, but there is a change in the organism's potential behavior. 4.) Learning arises as a result of experience; experience with environmental events obviously includes, but is not limited to practice. 5.) Learning is relatively permanent, i.e., distinct from short-term changes in behavior reflecting muscle fatigue, sensory adaptation, illness, or drugs. Persistent changes in behavior also occur as a result of maturation, but not with the experience that satisfies the definition of learning.

Memory

Let us next turn our attention to a definition of memory. One major difficulty in providing a conceptual definition of memory is that the traditional emphasis in the study of changes in animal behavior has been on the process of learning or acquisition, with a concomitant resistance to the term "memory." The advent and acceptance of behaviorism is responsible for kindling and fueling this historical resistance to the concept of memory, replacing it with the concept of retention. The impact of historical resistance to the concept of memory remains readily illustrated in a contemporary definition of memory:

Most generally, memory has been used as a synonym for retention and has been defined as the persistence of learned responding, with a retention test being used to measure such persistence (Hall, 1989, p. 15–16).

If one accepts the consensus on the definition of learning as reflecting a relatively permanent change, then the traditional concept of memory (retention) is obviously redundant. As all instances of learning involve memory, a retention test (training trial conducted under the condition of extinction, i.e., nonreinforcement) is most parsimoniously interpreted as simply indicating that learning has occurred.

Fortunately, the rise of cognitive psychology has permitted the reacceptance and further development of the concept of memory in the study of animal learning. Although its reception has been limited, relative to its acceptance in studies of human learning, the issues of animal memory are finally beginning to be appreciated in texts on basic learning processes. The following are some contemporary definitions:

The existence of memory in animals is identified by the fact that their current behavior can be predicted from some aspect of their earlier experience (Domjan and Burkhard, 1986, p. 276).

Memory is an internal record or representation of some prior event or experience (Gordon, 1989, p. 9).

Memory is a multi-attribute representation of what is acquired by learning the relationships among a set of events grouped by a temporal window (Spear et al., 1990).

Implicit or explicit in these definitions of memory are many of the same points seen in the definition of learning: 1.) an internal process; 2.) an inference from behavior; 3.) a change in potential behavior; and 4.) a consequence of experience. The notable difference from the definition of learning is the omission of any reference to the permanence of the process. Obviously, the concept of memory cannot preclude short-lived influences on behavior by prior experiences.

The influence of cognitive psychology within the last 20 years of research on animal memory is also clearly shown in the importance of the concept of memory independent of that of learning. Indeed, the concept of memory is indispensable, in at least two major paradigms:

1. Working-memory studies provide clear instances in which information from prior events has only a short-lasting effect on the organism's actions, thus precluding a learning interpretation. Indeed, if the information in such studies is not shortly discarded it may interfere with performance on the next trial.
2. Studies have demonstrated the modification of memory for past events by procedures that do not produce learning in and of themselves. There are numerous ways in which memory may be facilitated or disrupted, without producing any new learning, including:
    a. the disruption of memory by retroactive or proactive interference, directed forgetting procedures, and neurophysiological sources;
    b. the facilitation of memory by reminder treatments; and
    c. the modulation of memory by contextual cues.
    It is important to recognize that each of these procedures demonstrate that the processes of learning and memory differ functionally, i.e., they alter retention quite independently of any effect on learning.

In sum, although memory and learning are intimately related, it should be clear that they reflect different processes and emphases. Moreover, despite the fact that all instances of learning involve memory, not all instances of memory involve learning.

CONCEPTUAL ISSUES

Learning vs. Memory

Operationally, it is generally accepted that investigators interested in the study of the learning process provide their subjects with multiple trials. Despite the conceptual fact that performance in multitrial experiments reflects the operation of both learning and memory processes (i.e., training trials function in part to provide retrieval practice; Miller, 1982), there is an implicit time-honored assumption that the incremental changes in performance over these trials reflect the learning process. In comparison, it is generally accepted that investigators interested in the study of memory processes provide their test subjects with a training session of one or multiple trials, followed by at least a brief time interval. Performance of the subject on a trial (or trials) subsequent to this time interval reflects memory of the original material. Thus, the general rule applied is that a measure of memory is provided whenever the interval since the last learning trial is greater than the previous intervals between trials. In other words, a retention interval is any duration longer than an intertrial interval, regardless of whether that interval is measured in minutes, hours, or even days.

One-Trial Learning

The use of a single-trial learning paradigm, e.g., passive avoidance, deserves a further statement, as it is an alternative strategy commonly used by investigators interested in the study of memory processes. A single-trial task provides the operational advantage of knowing precisely when "learning" occurs as well as the advantage of being able to conceptually distinguish learning from memory, i.e., there are no multiple training trials to provide retrieval practice.

Neurotoxicant Exposure and the Learning-Expression Distinction

The timing of neurotoxicant exposure of the animal is the major determinant of the design of any study proposed to assess potential learning and/or memory dysfunction. Figure 1 illustrates the possible timing of neurotoxicant exposure in a generic multitrial assessment of learning and memory processes. Note that for a generic single-trial learning task, the acquisition curve would simply be replaced by a step function. In teratology studies as well as in many developmental neurotoxicology investigations, the exposure to a drug or neurotoxicant agent occurs very early in life. This typically results in an exposure at a time before acquisition of the information to be remembered (T_1). This is obviously the case with all prenatal drug/toxicant exposures as well as with many neonatal treatments. Time T_1 also applies to those toxicology studies using adult animals that employ acute or chronic dosing regimens and subsequently examine the processes of learning and memory. Clearly, any experimental treatment imposed on an organism at T_1 may alter the acquisition of the appropriate task contingencies (an associative process) or may readily disrupt any of a number of other processes that do not reflect learning, such as motivation, attention, perception, sensory transduction, activity, reactivity, etc. The latter variables are collectively referred to as nonassociative factors. Thus, to argue convincingly that any toxicant-induced alteration in behavior reflects an effect on learning, one must demonstrate the functional integrity of these nonassociative processes. Moreover, if the acquisition of a task

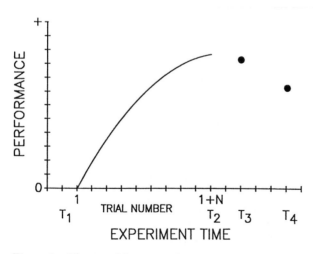

Figure 1   The possible timing (T_x) of neurotoxicant exposure is illustrated as a function of task performance in a generic multitrial learning-and-memory task. In a generic one-trial learning task, the negatively accelerating function would be replaced with a step function.

is altered, whether by associative or by nonassociative factors, a meaningful assessment of memory processes is a moot point, i.e., you can't remember what you did not learn. The accurate assessment of either learning or memory processes requires the use of procedures that permit the differentiation of associative alterations from changes in behavior attributable to nonassociative factors. This concern is absolutely critical to investigators studying basic cognitive processes and is at least as critical to those studying chemical- or toxin-induced learning and memory dysfunction.

The study of memory processes employs an experimental manipulation at some time after task acquisition, at time "T_2" (shortly after learning) or "T_3/T_4" (before a retention test). Although there is a substantial literature arguing whether a treatment at time T_2 reflects an effect on memory consolidation (initial storage) or memory retrieval processes (cf. Gold et al., 1973; Gold and King, 1974; Miller and Springer, 1973, 1974), it must be recognized that close temporal contiguity between an experimental treatment and the event to be remembered does not guarantee that the effect of that treatment is attributable to an effect on memory storage. The hypothetical construct of memory storage reflects a process that establishes a specific event or episode as a memory, whereas memory retrieval is a process that acts on the stored episode to distinguish it from others and promote its expression in behavior. The fact remains that one can never be certain that memory storage has been impaired, strengthened, or obliterated, as any such effect may be due to an effect on memory-retrieval processes (Spear, 1978). In sum, no currently available techniques permit the conclusion that the physiological representation of memory, once stored, has been altered. Accordingly, any toxicological exposure that impairs associative processes when administered at either T_2 or T_3/T_4 is most parsimoniously interpreted as reflecting a memory-retrieval failure.

In summary, what is of paramount importance to our goal of assessing cognitive dysfunction following neurotoxicant exposure is the conceptual fact that we do not and cannot measure learning or memory directly; they can only be inferred from the behavior of the animal. Although this distinction between learning and performance (Tolman, 1955) must be dealt with empirically, it reflects far more than a methodological issue. In recognition of 1.) the continuing shift in orientation from "learning" to "memory" in the field of animal learning and 2.) the evidence, from increasingly thorough measurement of behavior, that the processes responsible for the majority of variance in behavioral plasticity take place at the time of expression (retrieval) and not during the learning episode (encoding, attention, association), the distinction is more aptly drawn between learning and expression (Spear et al., 1990). Spear et al. (1990) provide an excellent summary of the recent discoveries that enable, if not force, such a bold and exciting reconceptualization.

Empirical Dissociations

The major purpose of any task designed to assess learning and memory processes is to demonstrate a selective change in overt behavior that, as indicated above, cannot be accounted for by nonassociative processes or factors. Three examples of empirical dissociation that are commonplace in the psychological literature on learning and memory processes are discussed below.

Comparison with Noncontingent Controls

Performance on a retention test presumably reflects prior learning. However, under some conditions an animal may perform the response required on a retention test, at above-chance levels, regardless of whether it has previously learned the task. Accordingly, it is of paramount importance to provide an explicit comparison between trained and untrained subjects if it is one's intention to make any definitive statements about learning and memory processes. This consideration then requires that half of any group of animals be trained as intended, whereas the other half experience all of the same stimuli but not in a paired, cue-predictive, or response-contingent fashion. It is only with this type of data that one has evidence to support the contention that an observed alteration in performance reflects an associative deficit.

Psychological "Dose-Response" Functions

The demonstration of a psychological "dose-response" function requires that a specific task dimension be manipulated to alter the importance or strength of the experience or episode; as the importance of the experience or episode is changed, behavior of the animal should be altered in a predictable, graded manner. For example, when assessment of memory processes is of particular interest, it is of great interpretive advantage to evaluate performance across multiple retention intervals while being careful to control for repeated testing effects. Clearly, a gradual loss of access to information would be expected with increasing length of the retention interval. Note that even for a "single-dose" study, two retention intervals are required. In other words, for a group of comparably trained subjects one would assess half of them after a very brief retention interval and the other half after an appreciably longer period. Evidence of intact memory-retrieval processes after short intervals would establish a baseline for the terminal degree of learning as well as establish the integrity of nonassociative processes. Further changes across time reflect the influence of the experimental treatment on memory processes. This consideration is very important, as it provides the basis for examining memory, as opposed to learning, processes (see above). The psychological literature has established numerous well-characterized dimensions that may serve to establish a "dose-response" function. For example, the factors of susceptibility to interference, similarily of training and test contexts, and length of interstimulus interval are of potential use as dimensions that can be quantitatively manipulated to assess memory processes.

Multiple Dependent Measures

Another strategy for partitioning the relative contribution of associative and nonassociative factors to task performance is to employ several response measures in the chosen procedure and thereby achieve their concurrent assessment. Within-task dissociations are readily provided by complex tasks such as a discriminated Y-maze. The measurement and recording of the number of avoidance responses, response latencies, and correct/incorrect discriminative choices should permit the differentiation of highly active animals from those that learn to which cue they should respond (e.g., Barrett et al., 1973). Unfortunately, implementation of this solution has been unnecessarily restricted to fairly complex tasks. Even with perhaps the "simplest," often misused, single-trial passive-avoidance task, there is no reason not to record a total preference measure as well as a response latency measure. Recording multiple indices of passive-avoidance behavior has been employed in the study of infantile amnesia (Mactutus and Wise, 1985) and amnesic effects of electroconvulsive shock (Adams and Calhoun, 1972; Sara et al., 1975) and hypothermia (e.g., Mactutus et al., 1982; Mactutus and Riccio, 1978), as well as in the evaluation of retention following exposure to pharmacological (Sara and Remacle, 1977) and toxicological agents (Flynn et al., 1979).

Besides the above rationale for using more than one dependent measure, it should be emphasized that any conclusions about learning and memory processes derived from tasks that employ a single dependent measure will be viewed skeptically. As a particularly convincing example, it is now well established that somatic and autonomic measures of classical conditioning are differentially sensitive to a variety of variables determinant to rate of acquisition (e.g., interstimulus interval) (Schneiderman, 1972) as well as differentially susceptible to sources of forgetting (Springer, 1975). Clearly, a reliance on only one measure of learning or memory in a neurotoxicological assessment would at this time appear questionable, if not foolhardy.

In sum, the use of multiple empirical dissociations is the key to assist one in drawing the learning-expression distinction in the assessment of learning and memory processes. Noncontingently trained control animals, psychological "dose-response" functions, and multiple dependent measures are among the tools that may be employed in this endeavor.

Task and Parameter Selection

The selection (or development) of a task and appropriate parameters must be considered with respect to at least three factors if they are to be successfully employed: validity, reliability, and sensitivity. Perhaps needless to say, the most sucessful tasks will be those that satisfy each of these requirements. Two important points are noteworthy about task selection (development). First, validity, reliability, and sensitivity are not intrinsic properties of a task per se; rather, they are a measure of performance of a particular group of subjects. Thus, proper design and careful execution of studies will have a marked influence on these factors. Second, despite the conceptual importance of distinguishing among the requirements of validity, reliability, and sensitivity, operationally it is often possible to assess them jointly. Among the most convincing ways to establish such requirements is to use empirical dissociations, as discussed directly above.

Validity

A valid task is one that measures what it is purported to measure. Neither great sensitivity nor high reliability insures validity. The demonstration of validity in a task of memory requires that animals, like humans, show learning and retention of experience. This brings us back to the principle that it is not enough to show a change in behavior to argue for a cognitive impairment. A valid task would be expected to reveal changes in performance that are not attributable to alterations in nonassociative processes. The reader is referred to Olton (1984) for further discussion of validity and animal memory models.

Reliability

"Reliability" refers to the reproducibility of the task outcome; i.e., to what extent the results will be replicated in the future by other investigators, with other species of animals, with females as well as males, etc. The validity of a test is limited by its reliability. In other words, a task that yields erratic scores will inherently lose validity. Perhaps the best way to determine reliability is through replication of the experiment, although statistical methods will provide a numerical estimate of the consistency of the data. In addition, assessments of reliability are also often useful in identifying boundary conditions and generality of observed effects. Any common statistical text will provide the necessary formula for computing reliability coefficients.

Sensitivity

The sensitivity of a task refers to its ability to detect alterations. The sensitivity of a task is often markedly affected by the specific procedure used. Training parameters, retention intervals, and contextual cues are among the many factors that can be manipulated to alter sensitivity. Ideally, mild impairments of associative processes should be readily detectable. Perusal of the exisiting literature will often provide a quite reasonable starting point for selecting parameters to evaluate.

TOXICOLOGY LITERATURE SURVEY

Rationale

The survey of primary publications concerning the assessment of learning and memory processes following exposure to a neurotoxicant was conducted for several reasons. The first reason was to directly assess exactly how much research was actually being conducted on the assessment of learning and memory processes following neurotoxicant exposure. Such an approach is not without precedent. Rodier (1978) conducted a survey of behavioral teratology studies covering the period from 1963 to 1978 through a page-by-page search of specific journals (Brain Research, Developmental Psychobiology, Journal of Comparative and Physiological Psychology, Radiation Research, and Teratology). Although the exact numerical data were not presented in reporting the survey, there were two remarkable findings: 1.) although some 30 to 40 different behaviors had been assessed, only three were used in more than a few studies, namely, open-field measures of activity, maze learning, and operant conditioning; and 2.) the vast majority of studies were based on evaluations of young adult animals. At approximately the same time, a questionnaire survey was conducted on general behavioral methods employed in teratogenic evaluations (Buelke-Sam and Kimmel, 1979); this survey included questions regarding the procedures commonly used to assess learning and memory processes. The responses of 69 (out of 110 polled) currently active investigators in the field of behavioral teratology in the late 1970s indicated that the major categories of learning and memory methods had a relative usage of 3% (classical conditioning) to 43% (maze behavior). The only more recent survey of which I am aware, covering the years 1978–1987, sought to identify any commonalities and distinctions between neurotoxicological research and the related fields of psychopharmacology and behavioral neuroscience in the procedures used to study learning and memory processes (Peele and Vincent, 1989). This survey found clear discipline-dependent biases in procedures employed (active avoidance and schedule-controlled behavior being the most commonly used in toxicology) and general reliance on a single test method (only 18% used more than one test of learning and memory function). Relative to this latter effort, the present survey sought a greater representation of teratology journals, an exclusive focus on toxicology/teratology journals (only 46% of the articles previously reviewed were from toxicology journals), and less restrictive criteria for including studies in the survey.

A second reason for conducting this survey was to trace explicitly the emergence of the assessment of learning and memory processes in toxicology. Thus, a broader time frame for the survey was sought. Coverage of the literature began with the year 1976, three years before the first issues of *Neurotoxicology and Teratology* (*Neurobehavioral Toxicology* in 1979) and *Neurotoxicology*, four years before the first issue of *Teratogenesis, Carcinogenesis, and Mutagenesis*, and five years before the first issue of *Fundamental and Applied Toxicology*. The main journals of the Society of Toxicology (*Toxicology and Applied Pharmacology*) and the Teratology Society (*Teratology*), however, had been firmly established years earlier. To render this chapter as current as possible the survey was extended through December 1991. Such extended sampling is necessary to determine the long-term trends that are present in research assessing neurotoxicant-induced cognitive dysfunction.

Search Strategy

I began with the rather ambitious goal of conducting a survey to identify all primary publications concerning the assessment of learning and memory in toxicology journals. Perhaps I was a little naive in hoping for a straightforward and comprehensive search via MEDLINE of 19 toxicology journals, covering the period 1976–1991. Using the subject headings of learning and memory only 67 articles were located; six of these articles were reviews and contained no new primary data. Despite my dismay with this minimal output, a closer examination revealed that several points were clear. First, much of the literature that dealt with the assessment of learning and memory (87%) was concentrated in four of the 19 journals (*Neurotoxicology and Teratology*, *Neurotoxicology*, *Toxicology and Applied Pharmacology*, and *Teratology*). Second, the small size of the output suggested 1.) that little such work had been conducted, 2.) the work was not published in toxicology journals, or 3.) that the search parameters "learning" and "memory" were poor choices for finding such papers. Accordingly, I redefined my approach by restricting the search to six journals that covered the major avenues of publication for the Society of Toxicology, the Behavioral Toxicology Society, the Neurobehavioral Teratology Society, and the Teratology Society. Table 1 summarizes the specifications on the journals from which the survey data were drawn. Second, I also increased the comprehensiveness of my search of all articles with a title and abstract search for key terms, employing the broadest term "behavior" for the toxicology and teratology (but not neuro-) journals. Third, recognizing that before 1983 MEDLINE does not include any abstracts, I conducted a manual title/abstract search of all six journals before that time. I also verified article count with the table of contents for each journal issue or volume and manually included any miskeyed or omitted articles in the title/abstract search.

Search Limitations

Although we were interested in generating as comprehensive a picture as possible, we did place a few restrictions on our search in order to keep the articles directly relevant to our goal of facilitating the development of experimental assessments of neurotoxicant-induced cognitive dysfunction. First, we considered only articles on nonhuman subjects. Second, original research contributions, whether full-length or short communications, were the basis of our survey material. Articles that used any of the behavioral techniques represented by the seven categories listed in Table 2 were included. Although we initially included

Table 1 Journals Surveyed[a]

Journal	Years (volumes) covered
Toxicology and Applied Pharmacology	1976 (35)–1991 (111)
Fundamental and Applied Toxicology	1981 (1)–1991 (17)
Neurotoxicology and Teratology	1988 (10)–1991 (13)
(*Neurobehavioral Toxicology and Teratology*)	1981 (3)–1987 (9)
(*Neurobehavioral Toxicology*)	1979 (1)–1980 (2)
Neurotoxicology	1979/1980 (1)–1991 (12)
Teratology	1976 (13)–1991 (44)
Teratogenesis, Carcinogenesis, and Mutagenesis	1980 (1)–1991 (11)

[a]A listing of the toxicology and teratology journals surveyed for articles that used learning and memory tasks. The inclusive years of the survey were 1976 through 1991.

Table 2 Learning/Memory Test Procedures[a]

Category	Task
Habituation/sensitization	Startle response Motor activity Head-dipping response Limb withdrawal Autonomic response
Classical conditioning	Taste aversion Odor aversion Conditioned suppression Nictitating membrane Autonomic conditioning Place preference

Instrumental conditioning, schedule-controlled	Simple schedules
	  Continuous
	  Partial
	    Fixed-ratio, variable-ratio, fixed-interval, variable-interval
	  Differential
	    Low rate, high rate
	Compound, complex, higher-order

Instrumental conditioning, discrete trials	Simple mazes
	  Straight alley maze, T-maze, Y-maze
	Complex mazes
	  Lashley III, Hebb-Williams, Beil water maze
	Complex "spatial" mazes
	  Radial arm maze, Morris water maze

Avoidance conditioning (classical and instrumental)	Passive (inhibitory) avoidance
	  Step-(down), -through
	Active avoidance
	  One-way, two-way, any-way, pole climb, Sidman (operant), T-, Y-maze (choice)

Working memory (short-term)	Non-maze
	  Delayed
	    Alternation, response, match-to-sample, match-to-position
	Maze
	  Simple, complex
	Spontaneous alternation
	  Simple, complex

Memory modification	Interference
	  Retroactive, proactive
	Reminder treatments
	  Prior cuing, reactivation
	Contextual cues

[a]A summary of categories of learning and memory tasks examined in the survey and the major tasks within each category. The task listing is representative and not exhaustive. Although the listed tasks were primarily mutually exclusive, this was not always the case. For example, Sidman avoidance was classified as both an avoidance and an operant task.

published papers that were the results of specific symposium presentations, any such articles that contained data previously published were not included in the survey. Review articles, teaching monographs, and editorials were also accordingly excluded. The data parameters that were incorporated into our survey were, at this time, restricted to those indicated in Table 3.

Search Results: Overview

An overview of the survey results is presented in this section, whereas discussion of the major assumptions and issues inherent within this literature is presented below. ("Procedural [Survey-Derived] Issues"). Of the 9316 articles surveyed, a total of 422 articles attempted at least some assessment of learning and memory processes. Figure 2 illustrates the number of journal articles that attempted to assess learning and memory processes as a function of the specific journals examined. Although the majority of learning/memory articles were published in Neurotoxicology and Teratology (65%), the journal Neurotoxicology contributed another 15%. The relative percentage of articles that included learning/memory assessment was between 0.5% and 2% for the remaining journals; nevertheless, these journals collectively contributed the final 20% of the total learning/memory observations. The cumulative growth of learning/memory assessments, as illustrated in Fig. 3, indicates a publication rate of 21 articles/year for Neurotoxicology and Teratology, 5 articles/year for Neurotoxicology, and 5 articles/year, collectively, for the remaining journals. The cumulative growth functions for articles that employed learning and memory tests, when separated as a function of those articles with a developmental (teratology) or adulthood (toxicology) focus (Fig. 3), suggested a comparable number of teratology (54%) and toxicology (46%) studies. This outcome confirmed our intention of providing a relatively balanced appraisal of potential long-term divergence in number of learning/memory articles as a function of teratology or toxicology research focus. Average publication rates of approximately 14 and 12 articles/year, respectively, were evident.

Table 3   Survey Data/Issues Encoded[a]

Parameter	Common variations
Neurotoxicology assessment strategy	General test battery, restricted test battery, and apical or stand-alone test
Exposure age	Developmental or adult
Number of learning/memory tasks	Single task, two tasks, or three or more tasks
Type of task/procedure	As specified
Motivational stimulus	Food deprivation/reward, water deprivation/reward, water escape, shock avoidance/escape, drug (toxin)-induced illness
Number of dependent variables	As specified
Gender	Male only, female only, male and female undifferentiated/unanalyzed, male and female explicity studied
Species	Avian, rodent, primate, other mammals, other species
Strain	As specified

[a]A summary of the data parameters and their common variations that were encoded in the survey data base. The terminology "as specified" was used when the possibilities defied a succinct description.

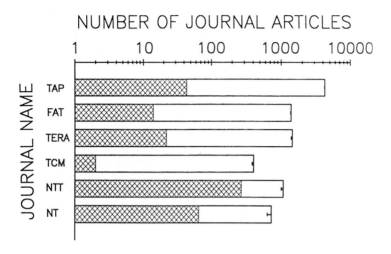

Figure 2   The number of journal articles that made some attempt to examine learning and memory processes is illustrated as a function of six journals representing the major avenues of publication for the Society of Toxicology, the Teratology Society, the Behavioral Toxicology Society, and the Neurobehavioral Teratology Society. The volume of material surveyed (9316 articles) dictated the use of a logarithmic scale. The open bars represent the total number of articles surveyed in the journal, whereas the crosshatched bars represent the number of articles within the journal that employed a learning/memory task. Also indicated are "error bars," which represent the number of journal articles published that were not indexed in MEDLINE; this represented 12% of the total for NT, 6% for NTT, 5% for TCM, 3.5% for TERA, and 1% or less for TAP and FAT. TAP = *Toxicology and Applied Pharmacology*; FAT = *Fundamental and Applied Toxicology*; TERA = *Teratology*; TCM = *Teratogenesis, Carcinogenesis, and Mutagenesis*; NTT = *Neurotoxicology and Teratology*; NT = *Neurotoxicology.*

PROCEDURAL (SURVEY-DERIVED) ISSUES

The assessment of learning and/or memory processes within neurotoxicology occurs in the context of a number of implicit assumptions. As indicated in Table 3, all studies incorporated in our data base were classified according to a series of parameters. Our approach was to examine the survey studies to tabulate the most common variations of each parameter as a window to the assumptions held by investigators. When implicit assumptions lead to near-universal selection of a particular variate, this outcome suggested the derivation of an important and pressing issue. Two measures of the study data are provided to examine these assumptions and issues. The first primary dependent measure was the number of articles that selected the individual variations of a parameter. A second

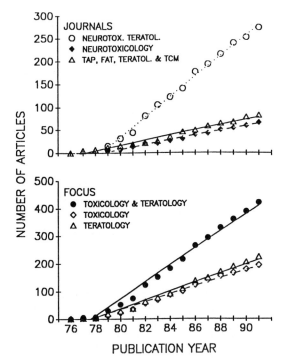

Figure 3 Top panel: The number of articles that utilized learning and memory assessments is shown as a function of publication year, from a time antecedent to the birth of four of the selected journals (Fundamental and Applied Toxicology; Teratogenesis, Carcinogenesis, and Mutagenesis; Neurotoxicology and Teratology; Neurotoxicology) to the present. Bottom panel: The composite cumulative growth function for articles that employed learning and memory tests is shown as are the cumulative growth functions separated into those articles with a developmental (teratology) or adulthood (toxicology) focus. TAP = *Toxicology and Applied Pharmacology*; FAT = *Fundamental and Applied Toxicology*; Teratol. = *Teratology*; TCM = *Teratogenesis, Carcinogenesis, and Mutagenesis*.

primary dependent measure was the rate of change in selection frequency across time, an index of a shift in the manner in which neurotoxicological assessments of learning and memory are conducted.

Between-Task vs. Within-Task Strategies

Background

The principal goal of any task designed to assess learning and memory processes must be to demonstrate a selective change in overt behavior that, as indicated above, is not attributable to alterations in nonassociative processes or factors (i.e., the learning-expression distinction). Accordingly, the major strategy for any such investigation must be to show behavioral dissociations, either between or within tasks, in which alternative explanations for behavioral change are in direct opposition through careful study design.

Between-task dissociations are epitomized by the test-battery approach. The strategy of a test-battery approach is to demonstrate that changes in a nonassociative process, such as motivation, are not produced by a neurotoxicant in a task sensitive to changes in motivation, while showing that changes in associative processes are produced by the neurotoxicant in a task sensitive to changes in learning or memory. This strategy relies on the implicit assumption that the nonassociative factor will influence behavior similarly in both tasks. At least for certain nonassociative factors, such as alterations in locomotor activity, this assumption is questionable. Locomotor activity is well known to be environmentally sensitive and task-sensitive. Therefore, the failure to find alterations in locomotion in a "nonlearning" task does not speak to the issue of potential differences in locomotion within the learning/memory task.

Within-task dissociations, the major alternative strategy, are illustrated by the use of a single complex task, i.e., a putative apical test. Accurate performance in an apical test requires the integration of motivational, sensory, motor, learning, and memory processes. From the screening perspective, that of detecting any form of toxicity, the value of performance in an apical test lies in its putative sensitivity in detecting a deficit in any of several subsystems (cf. Butcher, 1976; Grant, 1976). With respect to learning and memory assessment, the value of an apical test is that it permits the concurrent assessment in a particular test environment of the role of associative and nonassociative processes in any observed behavioral alterations. The most accurate interpretation of behavioral alterations in apical testing, however, not only requires the use of multiple dependent measures (an implicit assumption of employing a complex task), but also obligates the use of specific behavioral control groups and the determination of at least one psychological dose-response function. The discriminated Y-maze, previously mentioned under the topic of multiple dependent measures, is but one good example of an apical task.

A restricted test battery, reflecting a combined emphasis of the between- and within-task approach, might conceivably employ several tests of learning and memory processes. The several tests of associative processes would presumably use stimulus cues for different modalities (vision, audition, taction) and require different responses (inhibition vs. active responding). If both tasks were conducted in the same apparatus, differential alterations of activity per se would be precluded. If the neurotoxicant produced an increase in locomotion, inhibition would be expected to be impaired, but active responding would not. However, if the neurotoxicant produced a deficit in learning/memory processes, more rapid responding would be expected in the inhibitory task and less rapid responding would be expected in the response-requiring task.

As one final background comment, it should be emphasized that to the extent that one adheres to the use of the three empirical dissociations noted above (noncontingent controls, psychological dose-response functions, and multiple dependent measures), all tests of learning and memory are "apical."

There is extensive discussion in the neurotoxicological literature of the relative merits of battery (two-tier, three-tier) and apical testing approaches. It is not within the scope of this chapter to contribute to that discourse or to reiterate those positions (cf. Butcher, 1976; Buelke-Sam and Kimmel, 1979; Tilson and Mitchell, 1984). Rather, our aim was to define the respective approaches (see above) and subsequently to identify the use and apparent utility of each type of approach within the scientific literature as related to learning and memory assessment. As indicated in Table 3, all studies were classified according to whether they employed a general test battery, a restricted test battery, or a stand-alone, apical test.

Results

The assessment strategy for neurotoxicological research that included learning and memory testing is portrayed as a function of publication year (Fig. 4). The test battery approach

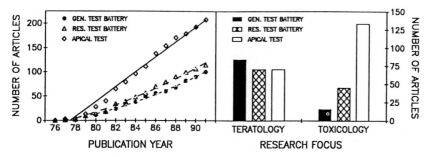

Figure 4   Left panel: The assessment strategy for neurotoxicological research that included learning and memory testing is portrayed as a function of publication year. Right panel: The assessment strategy for neurotoxicological research that included learning and memory testing is shown as a function of those articles with a developmental (teratology) or adulthood (toxicology) focus. Although the total number of articles is similar for those with a teratology focus and those with a toxicology focus, the toxicology studies clearly display a narrower focus. (Gen = general test battery; Res = restricted test battery).

was used markedly less often than an apical test. The use of restricted test batteries, where presumably some information is already known about the neurotoxicity of the compound in order to focus further study, appears to be showing a gradually increasing popularity, relative to a general test battery approach.

The assessment strategy for neurotoxicological research that included learning and memory testing is shown as function of those articles with a developmental (teratology) or adulthood (toxicology) focus (Fig. 4). Although the total number of articles with a teratology focus and with a toxicology focus is similar, the teratology studies conducted their learning/memory assessments nearly equally as part of a general test battery or a restricted test battery or as a single test. In marked contrast, learning/memory assessment within toxicology studies was routinely conducted as a single, presumably apical, test.

The profile demonstrated by the studies with a teratology focus is consistent with the use of increasingly selective tests as one learns more about a neurotoxicant. That is, at any point in time one would expect an approximately equal number of screening, replication, and mechanistic studies. Interpretation of the profile evidenced by the studies with a toxicology focus is much less definitive. One possibility is that a sufficient amount of background information is available on the majority of neurotoxicants studied in adult animals, and thus, specific mechanistic and hypothesis-driven studies are commonly performed using a single well-characterized "apical" task. Alternatively, no more may be known about most neurotoxicants in adulthood than in development, but the wealth of data recorded in an apical learning/memory task is more informative than a learning/memory task incorporated within a test battery. Whether one attributes the overall practice of employing apical tests in toxicology studies to knowledge about neurotoxicants or to an appreciation of the wealth of information generated by the apical approach, one might reasonably suppose that some change in the growth rate of both of these processes occurred across time as the science of neurotoxicology emerged. In this regard, subsequent analyses were conducted of the learning and memory studies with a toxicology focus. Interestingly, linear trends provided the best fit to the cumulative growth functions of apical testing, general test batteries, and restricted test batteries (rs > 0.97); i.e., all had constant rates of growth. Moreover, the initial incorporation of a learning/memory test within an adult restricted test battery or general test battery lagged 2 to 4 years behind the initial apical studies. Thus, from the inception of neurotoxicological assessments of learning and memory with adult animals it appears 1.) that the apical test approach has been used more frequently then either test battery approach, 2.) that all three strategies have displayed a constant rate of growth, and 3.) that the relative long-term publication rates averaged 8+, 3, and 1 article/year for the apical, restricted test battery, and general test battery approaches, respectively.

Number of Learning/Memory Tasks

Background

The number of tasks that assessed learning and memory processes within neurotoxicology provides an index of the investigators' perspective on the number of distinct learning and memory processes that exist. The number of options to which an assessment of learning and memory processes could be directed includes, at minimum, classical conditioning, operant or instrumental conditioning, avoidance conditioning, short-term or working memory, long-term memory, modifications of memory, and the nonassociative process of habituation. Perhaps an analogy to sensory systems is appropriate. Assessment of the integrity of the visual system following exposure to a neurotoxicant does not tell us anything about the integrity of olfaction, audition, gustation, taction, or pain. Clearly, one could not argue that a neurotoxicant had no detectable effect on sensory processing unless all sensory systems were evaluated. Similarly, with respect to learning and memory any one process may be preferentially affected. Thus, one cannot argue for a sparing of learning and memory processes unless multiple processes are investigated. The number of learning and memory tasks employed and the specific tasks chosen (see below, "Task Type") reflect the recognition and acceptance of this fact.

An examination of the number of learning and memory tasks employed per article should also provide an independent confirmation of the "apical" tendency noted within the overall neurotoxicology assessment strategy. As indicated in Table 3, all studies were classified according to the number of tasks employed to assess learning and/or memory, independent of the overall neurotoxicology assessment strategy. That is, one might have a test battery with one, two, three, or more learning and memory tasks. Obviously, however, use of an apical neurotoxicology assessment strategy would indicate not only that testing was restricted to one task (as examined above), but that this assessment was of a learning and/or memory process.

Results

The number of tasks that assessed learning and memory processes within each selected article is illustrated as a function of publication year in Fig. 5. These data could not more clearly indicate an early and sustained practice of relying on a single test of cognitive function. The relative use of one, two, and three or more distinct tests of learning and memory within an article was 71%, 18%, and 7%; the number of articles which examined the nonassociative process of habituation was 4%. All cumulative growth functions were primarily linear (rs > 0.96), suggesting a constant rate of growth in all cases.

The number of tasks that assessed learning and memory processes within each selected article is also shown as a function of those articles with a developmental (teratology) or adulthood (toxicology) focus (Fig. 5). Again observe that although the total number of articles with a teratology focus and with a toxicology focus is similar, the relative distribution of those studies with one, two, three, or more learning and memory tasks is notably

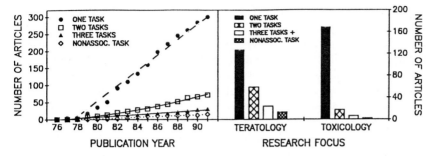

Figure 5 Left panel: The number of tasks that assessed learning and memory processes within each selected article is illustrated as a function of publication year. The prominent linear function indicates the stable growth in popularity of employing a single test of cognitive function. Right panel: The number of tasks that assessed learning and memory processes within each selected article is shown as a function of those articles with a developmental (teratology) or adulthood (toxicology) focus. Again note that although the total number of articles is similar for those with a teratology focus and those with a toxicology focus, the toxicology studies are greatly skewed toward a single task of learning and memory processes.

different. The relative distribution for the adult-focused studies was 87%, 9%, 3%, and 1%, respectively, whereas the parallel figures for developmentally focused research were 57%, 26%, 11%, and 6%.

Consistent with the data obtained from the overall neurotoxicology assessment strategy, the direct assessment of the number of learning and memory tasks employed confirmed that the majority of investigators depend on a single learning and memory task. This trend was present since the birth of the field of neurotoxicology and shows no evidence of changing. The measure of the number of learning and memory tasks employed as a function of major research area confirmed and extended the overall assessment strategy data. Specifically, those investigations focused on developmental, relative to adult, research displayed a marked reduction in reliance on only one learning and memory task, and a corresponding shift in using two, three, and four or more cognitive tasks. Although the explanation for this differential outcome is unclear, the use of multiple learning and memory tasks in the teratological studies is consistent with the recognition that multiple cognitive processes may be affected by a neurotoxicant.

Motivational Stimulus

Background

The motivational stimulus employed in the assessment of learning and memory processes has very important implications when assessing the influence of a neurotoxicant. For example, one common effect of neurotoxicant exposure is a loss of body weight. The loss of body weight could signify general malaise, a specific taste aversion, an effect on hormonal or neural feeding regulation, or even increased metabolism or physical activity. Obviously, a change in the level of motivation provided by a manipulation of food deprivation is conceivably attributable to any of these factors that precipitate a loss in body weight. A cursory examination suggests that this question is rarely addressed.

The use of a very different motivational stimulus, water escape, has some distinct advantages in this regard. The primary advantage is that one does not have to deprive the animal before training. Rodents are also very good swimmers, and procedures for assessing swimming ability and its development are readily available (mice, Rice and Milan, 1986; rats, Shapiro et al., 1970; Vorhees et al., 1984). However, the use of water escape as the motivational stimulus does not guarantee that neurotoxicant-exposed animals will respond comparably to nonexposed animals any more than does the use of food deprivation. If a toxicant affects thermoregulatory systems, metabolism, or fat disposition one must certainly consider that motivational factors, at any given level of water temperature, may be affected. Again, this situation appears to be at best unaddressed, at worst unrecognized.

There are at least three important issues to consider with respect to motivation. The first is whether investigators rely on any particular motivational stimulus, and if so, what it is. The second question is whether investigators employ more than a single motivational stimulus when performing more than one assessment of learning and memory. The third is whether for any given motivational stimulus, manipulations of the level of motivation are performed. The design of the survey data base can provide direct information concerning the first two questions. Data with respect to the third question come from a few studies that have shown some appreciation of the common effect of neurotoxicants on weight loss.

Results

The motivational stimuli employed in the assessment of learning and memory processes are illustrated as a function of publication year for both appetitive and nonappetitive classes of reinforcers (Fig. 6). Food deprivation/reward and shock avoidance show comparable use rates (37% vs. 40% of the reports). Food deprivation/reward overshadows water deprivation/reward (10%) by a factor of four. Shock avoidance similarly outranks drug- or toxin-induced illness (9.5%) and novelty (8%). Water escape represents the third most prominently employed motivational stimulus (13.5%).

With respect to cumulative growth functions, it is of particular note that the use of water escape is the only motivational stimulus that is increasing in relative use. This trend is attributable to two factors: 1.) the prolific laboratory of Vorhees and colleagues, with their use/development of the Biel/Cincinnati water maze (e.g., Vorhees, 1987a; Vorhees et al., 1991) and 2.) the adoption/adaptation of the Morris water maze from psychology (Morris, 1981) to the field of neurotoxicology (and behavioral neuroscience).

The number of articles that employed more than one motivational stimulus in their assessment of learning and memory function is plotted across publication year (Fig. 6). Of note is the increasing use of two different aversive motivational stimuli as well as the combination of aversive and appetitive motivational stimuli. In both instances this growth is attributable to the increasing use of water escape as a motivational stimulus, as discussed above. The use of two different appetitive stimuli as reinforcers has never been a very common choice.

Direct manipulation of motivational level is not typically performed in a neurotoxicological assessment of learning and memory processes. One notable exception examined complex spontaneous alternation under ad lib. and water-deprivation conditions in lead-exposed animals (Flynn et al., 1979). Although deprivation increased the mean difference between groups in number of arm entries, consistent with a lead-exposed increase, spontaneous alternation was not differentially affected. A second exception, although involving performance, and not acquisition, of a schedule-controlled behavior, is

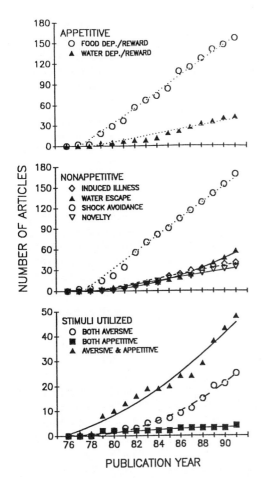

Figure 6 Top panel: The motivational stimulus employed in the assessment of learning and memory processes is illustrated for appetitive reinforcers. Middle panel: The motivational stimulus employed in the assessment of learning and memory processes is illustrated for nonappetitive reinforcers. Note the positively accelerating growth function for the use of water escape as a motivational stimulus. Bottom panel: The number of articles that employed more than one motivational stimulus in their assessment of learning and memory function is plotted across publication year. Note the increasing use of two different aversive motivational stimuli as well as the combination of aversive and appetitive motivational stimuli. These accelerating functions are attributable to the increasing use of water escape as a motivational stimulus.

also noted (DeHaven et al., 1982). The effects of triethyltin on stable fixed-ratio and fixed-interval responding were detectable sooner and at lower doses at recovered body weight than under conditions of reduced body weight.

Task Type

Background

The selection of tasks to assess learning and/or memory processes is a major issue because, as indicated above, the great majority of investigators rely primarily on only one task and only one motivational stimulus. In light of the commonly accepted position that neither learning nor memory reflects a unitary process, this situation places great importance on task selection. Clearly, the data thus far indicate that the question of task selection should be answered, if not posed, in the plural. Reference again to Table 2 will indicate the categories and individual tasks included in the current data base. The current information on task type should not be taken as an endorsement of any particular task. This statement is emphasized because, as stated previously, the specific task parameters selected have a primary role in determining the validity, reliability, and sensitivity of an assessment; a task per se has no such inherent properties.

Results

The relative use of the various types of tasks is illustrated as a function of publication year in Fig. 7. The major categories of learning and memory tasks used in any one article for assessing neurotoxicity included avoidance training (35%), free-operant, schedule-controlled behavior (32%), discrete-trial maze training (25%), classical conditioning (14%), and habituation (7%). The functions fitted to these cumulative growth curves (rs > 0.95) indicate constant growth rates for all major categories of tasks with the notable exception of an accelerating function for the use of maze tasks.

A closer examination of the major task categories was also conducted. When avoidance training was divided into two major categories, it was clear that active avoidance was more widely used (76%) than passive-avoidance procedures (44%). The preceding percentages do not sum to 100%, as approximately 20% of the investigations that employed avoidance procedures used both active and passive paradigms. Free-operant procedures to examine performance of acquired behavior (a well-learned "habit" not generally interpreted as reflecting either learning or memory) were used as frequently (48%) as procedures to examine acquisition of schedule-controlled behavior (52%). The relative use of mazes was 28% for the simple T-maze, 19% for the complex Biel/Cincinnati maze, 21% for the spatial

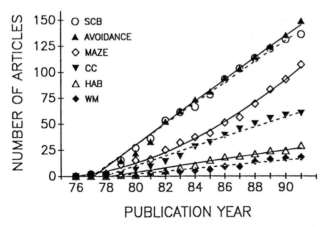

Figure 7   Use of the major categories of learning and memory tasks is plotted as a function of publication year. The accelerating function for the use of maze tasks reflects the increasing use of water maze tasks—the Biel/Cincinnati maze and the Morris water maze. SCB = schedule-controlled behavior (free operant); CC = classical or Pavlovian conditioning; HAB = habituation/sensitization; WM = working memory. There were no toxicological studies within the memory-modification category, as defined in the text, for inclusion in the survey.

radial-arm maze, and 20% for the spatial Morris water maze. The classical conditioning procedures used most frequently were conditioned taste aversion (63%) and conditioned suppression (12%). The nonassociative process of habituation was assessed with comparable frequency as a measure of motor activity (48%) and as the reflexive startle response (41%).

A summary of task use is detailed in Table 4, with a citation from the field of neurotoxicology of at least one exemplary article for each task/method. An article from the field of psychology is also cited for each task to provide an additional methodological/conceptual resource. Note that citation of an article as an exemplar should not be viewed as an uncritical acceptance of the methodology employed. Whenever possible the reference was selected for citation because the investigators attempted more than a comparison of the performance of vehicle- and neurotoxicant-exposed animals under one set of conditions. Consideration of the empirical dissociations explained at the beginning of this chapter (noncontingent controls, psychological dose-response functions, and multiple dependent measures) should illustrate the kinds of manipulation that would facilitate a less ambiguous interpretation of the majority of the neurotoxicological assessments and memory.

Number of Dependent Variables

Background

As discussed above ("Empirical Dissociations") and reiterated here for emphasis, any conclusion about learning and memory processes derived from tasks that employ a single dependent measure will be viewed skeptically. With that background already established, three major questions were considered. Given the widespread reliance on only a single task to assess the functional integrity of learning and memory processes, the first question posed was how many dependent measures are routinely used to assess an animal's behavior to assist in drawing inferences about cognitive processes. The second question was whether there has been a change in the number of behavioral measures used within learning and memory assessments with the evolution of the field of neurotoxicology. The third question derives from the difference between apical and test battery approaches in terms of the number of tasks assessed. It is presumed axiomatic that one gathers multiple measures of behavior in the single apical task relative to very few measures per task, perhaps even one, when using a battery. We sought to establish empirically the extent to which there was a difference in the number of dependent measures employed in a learning and memory task when it was used alone relative to incorporation within a restricted or general test battery.

Results

The number of dependent variables used within each learning and memory task (not article) is shown as a function of publication year (Fig. 8). The relative use of one to five dependent variables was 40%, 31%, 16%, 8%, and 5%, respectively. The cumulative growth functions suggested that linear functions were again prominent for all groups (rs > 0.96); however, note the progressively later initiation of increasing numbers of dependent variables. In light of the great majority of studies that employ only one learning and memory task, it was surprising to see that over 70% of all reported tasks used only one or two dependent measures.

Of great interest at this point was the comparison of the number of dependent measures used in learning and memory tasks as a function of neurotoxicology assessment strategy (Fig. 9). It is immediately obvious that whether the learning and memory task is

Table 4 Learning/Memory Task Exemplars[a]

Task	Neurotoxicology exemplar	Parametric resource
Habituation/sensitization		Groves and Thompson, '70; Peeke and Petrinovich, '84
Startle response	Geyer et al., '84; Foss and Riley, '91	Leaton et al., '85; Davis, '80
Motor activity	Shaywitz et al., '79; Booze and Mactutus, '90*	Reiter and MacPhail, '82
Heat-dipping response	Plonsky et al., '85; File, '86	File and Wardill, '75
Limb withdrawal	—	Stehouwer and Campbell, '78
Autonomic response	—	Haroutunian and Campbell, '81
Classical conditioning		Rescorla, 1978; Holland, 1984
Taste aversion	Peele et al., '87; Riley et al., '84	Riley and Tuck, '85
Odor aversion	Barron et al, '88; Stanton, '91	Kurcharski and Spear, '84; Hoffmann et al., 87
Conditioned suppression	Nation et al., '83; Vorhees et al., '90	Thomas and Riccio, '79; Coulter et al., '76
Nictitating membrane	Yokel, '83; Solomon et al., '88	Gormezano et al., '83
Autonomic conditioning	Caul et al, 83	Campbell and Ampuero, '85
Place preference	Heyser et al., '92	Bozarth, '87
Instrumental conditioning, schedule-controlled	Cory-Slechta, '92; Rice and Gilbert, '90; Laties, '82;	Ferster and Skinner, '57; Honig and Staddon, '77;
Simple schedules		
Partial		
Fixed-ratio,	Gentry and Middaugh, '88; Rice, '88	
Variable-ratio,	Sobotka et al., '81; Cory-Slechta et al., '85	
Fixed-interval,	Mele et al., '86; Lilienthal et al., '90	
Variable-interval	Glowa, '86; Cory-Slechta and Pokora, '91	
Differential		
Low rate	Driscoll et al., '80; Moser et al., '85	
High rate	Bornhausen et al., '80	
Compound, complex, or higher-order	Paule and McMillian, '86; Wenger et al., '86	

Instrumental conditioning, discrete trials		Domjan and Burkhard, '86; Hulse et al., '78
Simple mazes		
Straight alley maze,	Taylor et al., '82; Miller, '84	Amsel et al., '77
T-maze	Vorhees, '85; Lochry et al., '85	Kenny and Blass, '77
Y-maze	Anandam and Stern, '80; Adams et al., '82	
Complex mazes		
Lashley III,	Haddad et al., '79	Miller, '82
Hebb-Williams	Ryan and Pappas, '90; Swartzwelder et al., '82	Rabinovitch and Rosvold, '51; Davenport et al., '70
Beil water maze	Vorhees, '87a; Akaike et al., '88	Vorhees et al., '91
Complex "spatial" mazes		
Radial arm maze,	Rodier et al., '79; Walsh et al., '82;	Olton and Samuelson, '76; Olton et al., '77;
Morris water maze	Blanchard et al., '87b; Goodlett et al., '87*	Morris, '81; Rudy et al., '87
Avoidance conditioning (Classical and Instrumental)		Bolles, '70; Campbell and Church, '69; Brush, '71; Denny, '92
Passive avoidance		
Step-(down), -through	Flynn et al., '79; Mactutus et al., '82; Peele et al., '90	Mactutus and Wise, '85; Myslivecek and Hassmannova, '83; Stehouwer and Campbell, '80; Sara et al., '75
Active avoidance		
One-way,	Mactutus and Tilson, '84	
Two-way,	Mactutus and Fechter, '84	
Any-way,	Satinder and Sterling, '83	
Pole climb,	Pryor et al., '83a, '83b	Satinder, '76; Misanin et al., '80
Sidman (operant)	Riley et al., '82; Nation et al., '87	
T-maze	Lochry and Riley '80; Goldenring et al., '82	
Y-maze	Vorhees, '87b; Fernandez et al., '83	
Working memory		Nagy and Murphy, '74
Non-maze		Barrett et al., '73
Delayed		Honig, '78; Olton, '78
Alternation ("spatial" -position)	Milar et al., '81, Levin and Bowman, '86; Rice and Karpinski, '88	

Table 4 Continued

Task	Neurotoxicology exemplar	Parametric resource
Response		
Match-to-sample	McMillan, '81; Rice, '84	Pontecorvo, '85; Thomas et al., '91
Match-to-position	—	Zentall et al., '84; D'Amato & Colombo, '85
	Bushnell, '88	Dunnett et al., '88
Maze		
Simple	Stanton et al., '91	Olton, '83; Nonneman and Corwin, '81
Complex	McLamb et al., '88; De Boer et al., '89	Jarrard, '83; Bartus et al., '85
Spontaneous alternation		
Simple	Petit and LeBoutillier, '86; Smith et al., '89	Douglas, '66
Complex	Flynn et al., '79; Bushness and Levin, '83	
Memory modification		Balsam and Tomie, '85; Spear and Riccio, '93
Interference		
Retroactive,		Grant and Roberts, '76
Proactive	Bushnell, '88	Dunnett and Martel, '90; Pontecorvo, '85
Reminder treatments		
Prior cuing,	—	Gordon, '81
Reactivation	—	Miller et al., '90
Contextual cues	—	Hinderliter et al., '75; Richardson and Riccio, '86

[a]A listing of exemplar studies from the field of neurotoxicology that illustrates the use of each of the learning and memory tasks. The neurotoxicology references were selected from within the six surveyed journals, with but two exceptions (*). Tasks that were not found in the neurotoxicology literature but are commonly used in related fields are indicated by a dash (—). Articles from the field of psychology that may serve as general (task category) and specific (individual tasks) parametric resources are also provided. For those task categories with a voluminous literature, e.g., schedule-controlled behavior, no attempt was made to choose a specific parametric resource. For schedule-controlled behavior, an effort was made to select studies examining effects on acquisition, not on performance. (The latter studies are thoroughly reviewed by Cory-Slechta, 1992; also this volume). Note that inclusion of a study in this list does not imply an uncritical acceptance of its methodologies, and that exclusion from the list does not necessarily indicate that other comparable exemplars do not exist.

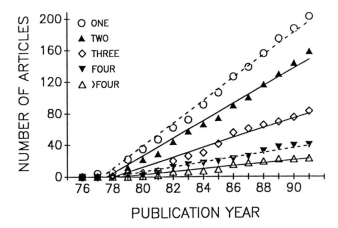

Figure 8 The number of dependent measures used for any given task in the assessment of learning and memory processes is depicted as a function of publication year.

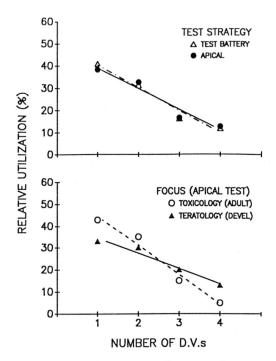

Figure 9 Top panel: The relative use of various numbers of dependent measures in the assessment of learning and memory processes is shown as a function of whether conducted as an apical task or as incorporated within a test battery (the average of general and restricted test batteries). Bottom panel: The relative use of various numbers of dependent measures in the assessment of learning and memory processes is shown as a function of major research focus, teratology vs. toxicology. Note that the conduct of an apical test in teratologically focused research shows a major shift toward using an increased number of dependent variables.

conducted as a single, apical test or as part of a test battery, there is no difference in the number of dependent measures employed. This outcome suggests that very little attempt is made to determine whether behavioral alterations observed in an apical task have anything to do with the associative processes of learning and memory. Paradoxically, that is the very rationale for conducting an apical test.

Recalling the difference in neurotoxicological assessment strategy as a function of major research focus, i.e., teratology (development) vs. toxicology (adult), and the parallel difference in number of learning and memory tasks employed as a function of major research focus, a comparison of the number of dependent variables recorded in an apical test was similarly examined as a function of major research focus. As may be readily observed (Fig. 9), there is a shift toward recording more dependent variables when apical tests are conducted within a developmental research focus than when they are conducted with a focus on adulthood. This outcome is consistent with the previous contention that in developmental studies there appears to be a progression from screening to mechanistic approaches, i.e., the apical tests are applied so as to collect a greater amount of information about the animals' behavior in the task. The immediately preceding outcome also suggests, contrary to prior speculation, that adult-focused studies are, relative to developmental studies, neither commonly hypothesis-driven nor appreciative of the wealth of data available in an apical test.

Gender-dependent Responses

Background

The rationale for using both males and females in the assessment of learning and memory processes within neurotoxicology is based on a number of observations. First and foremost, neurotoxicants have produced gender-dependent effects on learning and memory tasks. For example, gender-dependent alterations in performance have been reported following prenatal alcohol exposure for the Morris water maze (Blanchard et al., 1987b; Kelly et al., 1988) and the Lashley III maze (McGivern et al., 1984). It should be noted that gender differences in susceptibility to alcohol, administered prenatally, are not uncommon in other behaviors (Barron and Riley, 1985; Blanchard et al, 1987a), although the gender more affected varies as a function of the specific measure examined. As another example, gender-dependent responses to neonatal exposure to chlordecone, a compound with both inherent hormonal and hormonally inducing properties, have been noted in both passive-avoidance (Mactutus et al., 1982) and active-avoidance tasks (Mactutus and Tilson, 1984). Again, other nonassociative behaviors are also affected in a gender-dependent manner following neonatal chlordecone exposure (Mactutus and Tilson, 1985). Second, despite the unfortunate long-standing tradition within the psychological literature addressing learning and memory processes of relying on the study of male animals, it is known that gender differences do exist in learning/memory tasks commonly used in neurotoxicology, including avoidance (particularly two-way active) (Beatty and Beatty, 1970), complex mazes (e.g., Lashley III; Stewart et al., 1975; Barrett and Ray, 1970) and conditioned taste aversion (Chambers, 1976; Dacanay et al., 1984; Sengstake and Chambers, 1991). For each of these tasks, it is noteworthy that organizational influences of androgens have been shown to mediate the gender-dependent difference.

Given that learning and memory processes are presumably altered by neurotoxicants because they produce a structural or functional lesion in the brain circuitry necessary for the process under study, two additional sets of findings are relevant. Not only are gender differences in brain structure well documented in areas associated with reproduction, but brain regions less clearly related to reproductive function also show sexual dimorphism in neuronal structures (De Vries et al., 1984; Juraska, 1991). With respect to implications for the assessment of learning and memory processes, sexual dimorphism in neuronal structure has been found in the visual cortex (Juraska, 1984), corpus callosum (Juraska and Kopcik, 1988), and hippocampus (Wimer and Wimer, 1985; Loy, 1986). Gender differences in the last structure are noted in both granule (Juraska, 1990) and pyramidal neurons (Juraska et al., 1989). Second, gender-dependent responses have been demonstrated following lesions of specific, nonreproductive brain regions. For example, gender differences in the behavioral response to septal lesions have been noted (Bengelloun et al., 1976; Kondo and Lorens, 1971). Most notably, greater plasticity (as defined by axonal sprouting) has been found in females than in males following fimbria/fornix transection (Loy and Milner, 1980), an effect mimicked by castration of neonatal, but not adult, males (Milner and Loy, 1982). The effects of orbital-frontal lesions on delayed response, delayed alternation, and object reversal in rhesus monkeys are also gender-dependent (cf. Goldman et al., 1974); again, early androgen treatment markedly attenuates this difference.

In recognition of these clearly documented effects of early sex hormone milieu on the brain as well as on behavior in learning and memory tasks, the relative use of male and female animals in the assessment of learning and memory processes within neurotoxicology was of considerable interest. It would be regrettable if in the process of adopting/adapting techniques from psychology the field of neurotoxicology inherited the bias of relying on the study of male animals. Accordingly, the survey data were examined both for the relative use of males and females and for changes in the rate of use across time. If males and females were often studied with no differential effect, then we might expect to confirm a quadratic function reflecting a gradual decline in the use of both males and females across the extended period of our survey. On the other hand, it is quite possible that the majority studies have always focused on male animals (offspring) as test subjects and that the use of female subjects (offspring) has been neglected. Under the latter scenario, one would find a clear linear cumulative growth function for use of only males as subjects, i.e., a constant rate of growth since the beginning of the field.

Results

The gender of animals studied within learning and memory assessments is shown as a function of publication year (Fig. 10). The data clearly indicate that the majority of studies (57.8%) use only one gender, and of those studies 95.9% used males. Another 12.6% of all studies functionally employed only one gender, i.e., they either did not specify the gender of subject used or reported the use of both males and females but did not differentiate or analyze the data on the basis of gender. The remaining 29.6% of all studies employed both males and females and analyzed for potential gender-dependent effects.

With respect to the emergence of these trends in gender utilization, note that the best-fit function describing the use and analysis of both males and females indicates a cumulative growth function with a primary linear component, i.e., a constant rate of growth. The best-fit function for the growth in utilization of animals of one gender for assessment of learning and memory processes does display at least a minor quadratic component, but it reflects a minor acceleration in this long-term trend. Growth of the functionally single-gender studies was relatively constant, as indicated by a prominent linear trend in publication of articles that fail to specify or analyze for gender differences. When calculated on the basis of their primary linear components, average annual publication rates of 15.3, 3.3, and 7.8 were obtained for the single-gender, functionally single-gender, and both-gender studies, respectively.

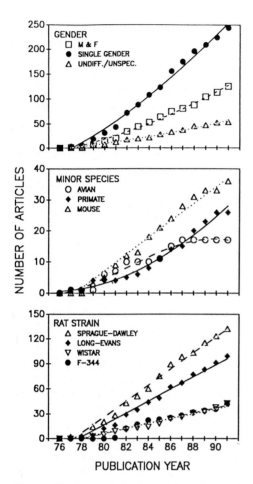

Figure 10 Top panel: The gender of animals studied within learning and memory assessments is shown as a function of publication year. It is particularly noteworthy that the majority of studies use only one gender, primarily males. Note that the best-fit function describing these data suggests at least a minor acceleration in this long-term trend. M & F = males and females studied and analyzed; Undiff./Unspec. = males and females undifferentiated and/or unanalyzed as well as gender unspecified. Middle panel: The minor species employed within learning and memory assessments are plotted as a function of publication year. In contrast to the sustained use of the mouse as a test subject, the use of avian species appears to have halted. The study of learning and memory in primates evidenced an early increase in use that has since been sustained. Bottom panel: The most prominent strains of rats employed in tests of learning and memory are shown as a function of publication year. The F-344 rat is the only inbred strain that has substantial use.

Consideration of the data on gender utilization with respect to area of major research focus indicated that of those studies that employed both genders, 90% had a teratological focus, whereas only 10% had an adult-toxicology focus. Conversely, of the single-gender studies, 73% had an adult-toxicology focus, with the remaining 27% displaying a teratological focus. The functionally single-gender studies were primarily teratological in focus (91%) and primarily reflected the typical use of relatively small numbers of male and female subjects in nonhuman primate studies as well as offspring of rodents not differentiated on the basis of gender.

In light of these observations indicating that the great majority of studies exclusively employ animals of a single gender, either purposefully or functionally, it is not surprising that there is little information available about gender-dependent responses. Quite simply, the question is not commonly asked! Perhaps the reliance on male animals (offspring) is a question of cost-effectiveness. Why should both males and females be studied if 1.) they provide the same response (data), or 2.) females, relative to males, display greater variability of response and thus for any given sample size would be less likely than males to be significantly affected by a neurotoxicant? The former view is obviously an assumption that has hindered the gathering of data to answer the question of whether we ought routinely to assess both males and females. The latter point, the greater variance among females attributable to estrus cycle, is also a questionable assumption, apparently based on the early discovery of estrus-linked changes in activity (cf. Wang, 1923). It is now clear, however, that estrus-related differences in motor activity are typically minimal or nondetectable, as long as the running wheel is not used as the measure of activity (Reiter and MacPhail, 1982). Moreover, when the question of the influence of ovarian hormones on learning and memory was directly examined, there was no evidence that internal hormonal state associated with estrus cycle or with pregnancy was capable of influencing retention (Kristal et al., 1978; Ebner et al., 1981; Riccio and Ebner, 1981). Under ovariectomized conditions, it was nevertheless possible to demonstrate that ovarian hormones would influence memory retrieval at short, but not long, retention intervals (Ebner et al., 1981). The latter conditions establish that the test procedures used were sensitive to detecting potential effects on memory retrieval and were similar to those used previously to demonstrate circadian fluctuations in memory retrieval (Holloway and Wansley, 1973).

In sum, it appears that the most parsimonious view at present is that the failure to find gender-dependent effects reported more commonly in the neurotoxicology literature may reflect, not their nonexistence, but rather that they are not often examined. Moreover, there appears to be little justification for excluding the female gender from neurotoxicological studies on learning and memory because of "estrus-related" differences.

Species (Strain) Generality/Extrapolation

Background

The significance of using multiple species (strains) in neurotoxicological investigations of learning and memory processes is multifold. Comparative studies represent the very foundation for toxicological investigations as they relate to the identification of adverse health effects and risk assessment. When scientific data are available from the study of multiple species for a given neurotoxic compound, the process of cross-species extrapolation is facilitated (e.g., McMillan, 1990). Conversely, sketchy or nonexistent information leads to the application of additional uncertainty factors in making regulatory decisions. In practice, although extrapolation from animals to humans is always difficult because of unknowns, the outcome one seeks to guard against by assessing multiple species is the failure to detect neurotoxicity because of species-specific toxicity (e.g., Stebbins and Moody, 1979). The ever-present difficulty in cross-species extrapolation is that of distinguishing homology from analogy (Atz, 1970); however, the problem is no less intractable with behavior than when considering anatomy or physiology. When considering functional domain as the basis (Stanton and Spear, 1990), recent reviews have argued for the comparability of human and animal neurotoxicity associated with methadone withdrawal (Hutchings, 1990) and with exposure to methylmercury (Burbacher et al., 1990), phenytoin (Adams et al., 1990), lead (Davis et al., 1990), ethanol (Driscoll et al., 1990), polychlorinated biphenyls (Tilson et al., 1990), and ionizing radiation (Schull et al., 1990). It should be clear that although there often will be procedural/operational differences in assessing the same functional domain across species (e.g., cognition), efforts focused on a specific process within a functional category (e.g., the assessment of short-term or working memory) represent a move toward the homology end of the continuum (Bitterman, 1976; Domjan, 1987b). The argument for homology may be bolstered via characterization by empirical dissociations to demonstrate that conceptually, the same process is under study across the species of interest.

Comparative data on learning and memory processes are another significant aspect of the issue of generality. As recently summarized by Galef (1987), depending on how one defines comparative psychology, that field may be held never to have existed (Lorenz, 1950), to be stillborn (Hodos and Campbell, 1969), to have died in its prime (Lockhard, 1971), to be alive but ailing (Adler et al., 1973), or to be in robust health (Dewsbury, 1984). If one asks the empirical question, however, there are numerous applications of the principles of learning, derived from animals, that are relevant to the human condition (cf. Domjan, 1987a), including such notable examples as Siegel's classical-conditioning model of drug addiction (1983), Seligman's research on learned helplessness and depression (1975), and Mineka's research on learned phobias (1987). Comparative studies have also greatly furthered our appreciation and understanding of basic conditioning through the area of research known as biological constraints. Stimulus salience, the animals' response repertoire, preparedness, and species-specific defensive reactions are all examples of biological influences and constraints on the learning situation (Domjan, 1983). The establishment of such influences and boundary conditions has helped to specify in greater detail the generalizability of instrumental conditioning (Domjan and Burkhard, 1986). Although biological constraints may be viewed as complicating the issue of cross-species extrapolation, it is not knowledge of them, but rather ignorance, that does so.

The question of species and strain generality of the neurotoxic effects of a given compound on learning and memory processes was the final, but hardly least important issue considered. Three major questions were addressed. First, is there a prominent species (strain) that is employed, and if so, what is it? Second, for the species (strains) used, have there been any changes in their use across time? Third, what evidence is there for current or prior use of cross-species (strain) research in neurotoxicological assessments of learning and memory processes?

Results

Rodents were employed in 87.9% of the neurotoxicological studies that used a learning/memory task. Of those studies, rats were used in 89.8%, mice in 9.7%, and guinea pigs in 0.5%. As an additional perspective, rats were the species used in 78.9% of all the neurotoxicological assessments of learning and memory.

The minor species employed within learning and memory assessments are plotted as a function of publication year (Fig. 10). Although the use of the mouse as a test subject began several years after the use of any avian species, the mouse has continued to be used at a reasonably constant rate (2.8 publications/year), whereas the use of any avian species has halted. Avian species (comprising pigeons, 70%; chicks, 18%; and quail, 12%) were used at a rate of approximately 1.5 publications/year up through 1987. The study of learning and memory in primates initially evidenced a low rate of use (< 1 publication/year) that has subsequently accelerated to a rather moderate rate (2.5 publications/year since 1984). The major primate species employed were Macaca fascicularis (50%) and M. mulatta (35%).

The most prominent strains of rats employed in tests of learning and memory are shown as a function of publication year (Fig. 10). The strains portrayed make up 94.9% of those used. Of those studies that used these prominent strains, the relative use was Sprague-Dawley, 41.8%; Long-Evans, 31.3%; Wistar, 13.6%; and F-344, 13.3%. Note that the F-344 rat is the only inbred strain that has substantial use. There is little, if any, evidence for any change in preference for rat strains across time (linear functions displayed rs > 0.97). Relative publication rate/year across the 16-year survey period, adjusted for year of initial use, was 8.8, 6.6, 3.1, and 3.8, respectively, as above.

To assess the extent to which comparative studies have been performed, the use of multiple species in learning/memory assessments within neurotoxicology was also assessed. We crossed each of the five categories of species present in the data base with the others; the outcome indicated only two investigations that used more than one species (Sandstead et al., 1977; Geller et al., 1979). A similar crossing of the five major strains of rats employed uncovered only seven articles that used two or more strains (Thomas et al., 1980; MacPhail and Leander, 1981; Commissaris et al., 1982; Walsh, Curley et al., 1982; Vorhees, 1983; Mokler et al., 1986; Crofton et al., 1991). The searching of all studies that employed mice found only two investigations that used multiple strains (MacPhail and Elsmore, 1980; Wenger et al., 1984). Note that the majority of these comparative papers were published over a decade ago, and only one was published within the last 5 years. Thus, it appears that the concurrent use of multiple species or strains was never very common and has all but halted. Perhaps it might be necessary to qualify this statement because of the tendency to publish less comprehensive bodies of data, i.e., authors who used multiple species or strains might simply publish their findings in different papers. Accordingly, we assessed the species- or strain-selection pattern of the more productive investigators (five who collectively contributed 21% of the data base). With respect to species use, two investigators restricted their animal use to rats; the third investigator employed primarily rats (96%), with one early publication using an avian species; the fourth investigator used rats (88%), mice (6%), and guinea pigs (6%); and the fifth investigator employed rats (79%), with early publications using mice (14%) or an avian species (7%). In only one of these publications was the issue of species generality explicitly addressed.

When considering strain use the following pattern was observed. Two investigators employed the same strain of rats through the 16-year period; one used three different strains, changing them sequentially during the period; and the remaining two investigators exclusively used a preferred strain 73–81% of the time. The use of nonpreferred strains by the last investigators was restricted to their interest in a particular neurotoxic compound, represented a sequential change of strain, or represented an explicit comparison study. It appears that the current work of Paule, Slikker, and colleagues is really the only contemporary "comparative" approach with respect to neurotoxicological assessment of learning and memory processes, with their application of operant procedures previously used in primates (Schulze et al., 1988) to human infants (Paule et al., 1988). Data collected on humans were outside the scope of this review.

In sum, despite the importance of comparative data for neurotoxicological assessment of learning and memory, the prominent trends are not comforting: an actual decrease in the number of species routinely used and the near-cessation of direct cross-species (strain) studies. These trends do not appear to be readily explained by the use of a comparative approach across, as opposed to within, publications.

CONCLUSIONS

The assessment of the cognitive processes of learning and memory following exposure to neurotoxicants poses a formidable challenge. The current chapter has pursued the goal of identifying both conceptual and procedural issues that should be considered in developing any successful assay of cognitive function. The conceptual background began with the presentation of a discussion of definitions for the terms "learning" and "memory." Subsequently, four major conceptual issues were discussed: the differences between learning and memory, the learning-expression distinction, three empirical dissociations, and task/parameter selection. Specific operational examples were cited to demonstrate the utility of these concepts in addressing otherwise common pitfalls in the assessment of learning and memory processes. With this conceptual guide, it is my hope that investigators are encouraged to take steps, where appropriate, to facilitate the interpretation of their research within the context of learning and memory processes. Single-task experiments demand a more accurate reflection of their apical nature. Clearly, their faithful interpretation cannot be made without supporting evidence. Conversely, investigators using a learning/memory task within a general test battery should not be compelled to interpret their findings as indexing learning and memory processes when there is no occasion to provide any empirical dissociations.

The primary body of the chapter was, however, devoted to procedural issues empirically derived from an exhausting, if not exhaustive, survey of the assessment of learning and memory processes in neurotoxicology. It is clear from the survey that an extensive amount of energy has been directed at the assessment of learning and memory processes within neurotoxicology. The major observations, reflecting both the current status and long-term trends, indicated 1.) a marked reliance on an apical neurotoxicological assessment strategy, 2.) the use of only one learning/memory task; 3.) the primary use of either foot shock or food deprivation/reward as the motivational stimulus; 4.) the most common use of the task categories of avoidance conditioning and schedule-controlled behavior; 5.) a primary reliance on using only one or two dependent measures/task; 6.) a pronounced bias for using animals of only one gender, primarily males, as the test subjects; and 7.) the prominent use of the rat in preference to other species, with Sprague-Dawley and Long-Evans rats being the most widely employed strains. The assessment of cumulative growth functions for each of these variables indicated that every one of these trends displayed a prominent linear component, i.e., a relatively stable growth rate. The picture of these major parameters that emerges thus reflects what previously was done, what is currently being done, and what will most likely continue to be done.

One most surprising outcome of the survey was that the research focus of teratology (developmental neurotoxicology) has a much broader base than that of adult neurotoxicology. This is true with respect not only to overall neurotoxicology assessment strategy, but also to the factors of number of learning and memory tasks per study, number of dependent variables per task, and gender utilization. More perplexing is the question of how these two focus areas have arrived at such different states since their common inception some 15 years ago (as shown empirically by the survey data), when there have been no differential rate changes in those four variables across time. These data force the conclusion that the distinction between research focus areas reflects an inherent, or perhaps inherited, bias with respect to breadth. It may very well be that the allied sciences of teratology and developmental biology display greater breadth than that of behavioral pharmacology and psychology. The adoption and adaptation of their methods may directly mirror that discipline-derived distinction.

The present data support much less speculation about the future of research on neurotoxicological assessment of learning and memory processes. Recognizing the constant growth rates of the primary variate of each parameter investigated, and the common observation that many of the secondary and higher variates also have stable, but relatively fractional growth rates, we are going to have to encourage ourselves to purposefully alter our course, if only to avoid becoming even more narrowly focused. We must ponder the wisdom of a narrow (and narrowing) focus as we grapple with the vexing number of potential neurotoxic compounds.

In sum, I hope that this chapter provides guidance in refining the application of established methodologies as well as in stimulating the development and application of new methodologies. Rather compelling evidence has been provided for an occasion to contemplate the breadth and direction of our research. I am optimistic that a future update of our data base will show that investigators have more than met the challenge of assessing the cognitive processes of learning and memory with superior analytical paradigms reflecting both greater precision and greater breadth.

ACKNOWLEDGEMENTS

The constructive comments of Dr. Rosemarie M. Booze, the literature data base assistance of Ms. Laura G. McIlwain, and the editorial assistance of Ms. Carol L. Smith are all gratefully appreciated. The present work was supported in part by grants from the National Institutes of Health, (ES 06259 and AG 10747), the Tobacco and Health Research Institute and the University of Kentucky Medical Center.

REFERENCES

Adams HE, Calhoun KS (1972). Indices of memory recovery following electroconvulsive shock. Physiol Behav 9:783–7.

Adams J (1986). Methods in behavioral teratology. In: Riley EP, Vorhees CV, eds. Handbook of behavioral teratology. New York: Plenum Press, 67–97.

Adams J, Buelke-Sam J (1981). Behavioral assessment of the postnatal animal: testing and methods development. In: Kimmel CA, Buelke-Sam J, eds. Developmental toxicology. New York: Raven Press, 233–58.

Adams J, Buelke-Sam J, Kimmel CA, LaBorde JB (1982). Behavioral alterations in rats prenatally exposed to low doses of *d*-amphetamine. Neurobehav Toxicol Teratol 4:63–70.

Adams J, Vorhees CV, Middaugh LD (1990). Developmental neurotoxicity of anticonvulsants: human and animal evidence on phenytoin. Neurotoxicol Teratol 12:203–14.

Adler HE, Adler LL, Tobach E (1973). Past, present and future of comparative psychology. Ann NY Acad Sci 223:184–92.

Akaike M, Tanaka K, Goto M, Sakaguchi T (1988). Impaired Biel and radial arm maze learning in rats with methylnitrosourea-induced microcephaly. Neurotoxicol Teratol 10:327–32.

Amsel A, Letz R, Burdette DR (1977). Appetitive learning and extinction in 11-day-old rat pups: effects of various reinforcement conditions. J Comp Physiol Psychol 91:1156–67.

Anandam N, Stern JM (1980). Alcohol in utero: effects on preweanling appetitive learning. Neurobehav Toxicol 2:199–205.

Atz JW (1970). The application of the idea of homology to behavior. In: Aronson LR, Jobach E,

Lehrman DS, Rosenblat JS, eds. Development and evolution of behavior: essays in memory of T.C. Schneirla. San Francisco: Freeman, 53–74.

Balsam PD, Tomie A eds. (1985). Context and learning. Hillsdale, New Jersey: Lawrence Erlbaum Associates.

Barrett RJ, Leith NJ, Ray OS (1973). A behavioral and pharmacological analysis of variables mediating active-avoidance behavior in rats. J Comp Physiol Psychol 82:489–500.

Barrett RJ, Ray OS (1970). Behavior in the open field, Lashley III maze, shuttle-box, and Sidman avoidance as a function of strain, sex, and age. Dev Psychol 3:73–7.

Barron S, Gagnon WA, Mattson SN, Kotch LE, Meyer LS, Riley EP (1988). The effects of prenatal alcohol exposure on odor associative learning in rats. Neurotoxicol Teratol 10:333–9.

Barron S, Riley EP (1985). Pup-induced maternal behavior in adult and juvenile rats exposed to alcohol prenatally. Alcohol Clin Exp Res 9:360–5.

Bartus RT, Dean RL, Pontecorvo MJ, Flicker C (1985). The cholinergic hypothesis: a historical overview, current perspective, and future directions. Ann NY Acad Sci. 444:332–58.

Beatty WW, Beatty PA (1970). Hormonal determinants of sex differences in avoidance behavior and reactivity to electric shock in the rat. J Comp Physiol Psychol 73:446–55.

Bengelloun WA, Nelson DJ, Zent HM, Beatty WW (1976). Behavior of male and female rats with septal lesions: influence of prior gonadectomy. Physiol Behav 16:317–30.

Bitterman ME (1976). Issues in the comparative psychology of learning. In: Masterton RB, Bitterman ME, Campbell CBG, Hotton N, eds. Evolution of brain and behavior in vertebrates. Hillsdale, New Jersey: Lawrence Erlbaum Associates, 217–25.

Blanchard BA, Hannigan JH, Riley EP (1987a). Amphetamine-induced activity after fetal alcohol exposure and undernutrition in rats. Neurotoxicol Teratol 9:113–9.

Blanchard BA, Riley EP, Hannigan JH (1987b). Deficits on a spatial navigation task following prenatal exposure to ethanol. Neurotoxicol Teratol 9:253–8.

Bolles RC (1970). Species-specific defense reactions and avoidance learning. Psychol Rev 71:32–48.

Booze RM, Mactutus CF (1990). Developmental exposure to organic lead causes permanent brain damage in Fischer-344 rats. Experientia 46:292–7.

Bornhausen M, Musch HR, Greim H (1980). Operant behavior performance changes in rats after prenatal methylmercury exposure. Toxicol Appl Pharmacol 56:305–10.

Bozarth MA (1987). Conditioned place preference: a parametric analysis using systemic heroin injections. In: Bozarth MA, ed. Methods of assessing the reinforcing properties of abused drugs. New York: Springer-Verlag, 241–74.

Brush FR, ed. (1971). Aversive conditioning and learning. New York: Academic Press.

Bulke-Sam J, Kimmel CA (1979). Development and standardization of screening methods for behavioral teratology. Teratology 20:17–29.

Burbacher TM, Rodier PM, Weiss B (1990). Methylmercury developmental neurotoxicity: a comparison of effects in humans and animals. Neurotoxicol Teratol 12:191–202.

Bushnell PJ (1988). Effects of delay, intertrial interval, delay behavior and trimethyltin on spatial delayed response in rats. Neurotoxicol Teratol 10:237–44.

Bushnell PJ, Levin ED (1983). Effects of zinc deficiency on lead toxicity in rats. Neurobehav Toxicol Teratol 5:283–8.

Butcher RE (1976). Behavioral testing as a method for assessing risk. Environ Health Perspect 18:75–8.

Cabe PA, Eckerman DA (1982). Assessment of learning and memory dysfunction in agent-exposed animals. In: Mitchell CL, ed. Nervous system toxicology. New York: Raven Press, 133–98.

Campbell BA, Ampuero MX (1985). Dissociation of autonomic and behavioral components of conditioned fear during development in the rat. Behav Neurosci 99:1089–1102.

Campbell BA, Church RM, eds (1969). Punishment and aversive behavior. Englewood Cliffs, New Jersey: Printice Hall.

Caul WF, Fernandez K, Michaelis RC (1983). Effects of prenatal ethanol exposure on heart rate, activity, and response suppression. Neurobehav Toxicol Teratol 5:461–4.

Chambers KC (1976). Hormonal influence on sexual dimorphism in rate of extinction of a conditioned taste aversion in rats. J Comp Physiol Psychol 90:851–6.

Commissaris RL, Cordon JJ, Sprague S, Keiser J, Mayor GH, Rech RH (1982). Behavioral changes in rats after chronic aluminum and parathyroid hormone administration. Neurobehav Toxicol Teratol 4:403–10.

Cory-Slechta DA (1992). Schedule-controlled behavior in neurotoxicology. In: Tilson HA, Mitchell CL, eds. Neurotoxicology. New York: Raven Press, 271–94.

Cory-Slechta DA, Pokora MJ (1991). Behavioral manifestations of prolonged lead exposure initiated at different stages of the life cycle: I. Schedule-controlled responding. Neurotoxicology 12:745–60.

Cory-Slechta DA, Weiss B, Cox C (1985). Performance and exposure indices of rats exposed to low concentrations of lead. Toxicol Appl Pharmacol 78:291–9.

Coulter X, Collier AC, Campbell BA (1976). Long-term retention of early Pavlovian fear conditioning in infant rats. J Exp Psychol Anim Behav Process 2:48–56.

Crofton KM, Howard JL, Moser VC, Gill MW, Reiter LK, Tilson HA, McPhail RC (1991). Interlaboratory comparison of motor activity experiments: implications for neurotoxicological assessments. Neurotoxicol Teratol 13:599–609.

D'Amato MR, Colombo M (1985). Auditory matching-to-sample in monkeys (Cebus apella). Anim Learn Behav 13:375–82.

Dacanay RJ, Mastropaolo JP, Olin DA, Riley AL (1984). Sex differences in taste aversion learning: an analysis of the minimal effective dose. Neurobehav Toxicol Teratol 6:9–11.

Davenport JW, Hagquist WW, Rankin JR (1970). The symmetrical maze: an automated closed-field intelligence test series for rats. Behav Res. Methods Instrumen 2:112–8.

Davis JM, Otto DA, Weil DE, Grant LD (1990). The comparative developmental neurotoxicity of lead in humans and animals. Neurotoxicol Teratol 12:215–29.

Davis MD (1980). Neurochemical modulation of sensory-motor reactivity: acoustic and tactile startle reflexes. Neurosci Biobehav Rev 4:241–63.

De Boer S, Mirmiran M, Van Haaren F, Louwerse A, van de Poll NE (1989). Neurobehavioral teratogenic effects of clomipramine and alpha-methyldopa. Neurotoxicol Teratol 11:77–84.

DeHaven DL, Wayner MF, Barone FC, Evans SM (1982). Effects of triethyltin on schedule dependent and schedule induced behaviors under different schedules of reinforcement. Neurobehav Toxicol Teratol 4:231–9.

De Vries GJ, De Briun JPC, Uylings HBM, Corner MAE, eds. (1984). Sex differences in the brain. Progress in brain research vol. 61. Amsterdam: Elsevier.

Denny MR, (1992). Fear, avoidance, and phobias. Hilsdale, New Jersey: Lawrence Erlbaum Associates.

Dewsbury DA (1984). Comparative psychology in the twentieth century. Stroudsburg, Pennsylvania: Hutchinson Ross.

Domjan M (1983). Biological constraints on instrumental and classical conditioning: implications for general process theory. In: Bower GH, ed. The psychology of learning and motivation. Vol. 17. New York: Academic Press, 215–77.

Domjan M (1987a). Animal learning comes of age. Am Psychol 42:556–64.

Domjan M (1987b). Comparative psychology and the study of animal learning. J Comp Psychol 101:237–41.

Domjan M, Burkhard B (1986). The principles of learning and behavior. Pacific Grove, California: Brooks/Cole.

Douglas RT (1966). Cues for spontaneous alternation. J Comp Physiol Psychol 62:171–83.

Driscoll CD, Chen JS, Riley EP (1980). Operant DRL performance in rats following prenatal alcohol exposure. Neurobehav Toxicol 2:207–11.

Driscoll CD, Streissguth AP, Riley EP (1990). Prenatal alcohol exposure: comparability of effects in humans and animal models. Neurotoxicol Teratol 12:231–7.

Dunnett SB, Badman F, Rogers DC, Evenden JL, Iversen SD (1988). Cholinergic grafts in the neocortex or hippocampus of aged rats: reduction of delay-dependent deficits in the delayed non-matching to position task. Exp Neurol 102:57–64.

Dunnett SB, Martel FL (1990). Proactive interference effects on short-term memory in rats: I. Basic parameters and drug effects. Behav Neurosci 104:655–65.

Ebner DL, Richardson R, Riccio DC (1981). Ovarian hormones and retention of learned fear in rats. Behav Neural Biol 33:45–58.

Eckerman DA, Bushnell PJ (1992). The neurotoxicology of cognition: attention, learning, and memory. In: Tilson HA, Mitchell CL, eds. Neurotoxicology. New York: Raven Press, 213–70.

Fernandez K, Caul WF, Osborne GL, Henderson GI (1983). Effects of chronic alcohol exposure on offspring activity in rats. Neurobehav Toxicol Teratol 5:135–7.

Ferster CB, Skinner BF (1957). Schedules of reinforcement. New York: Appleton-Century-Crofts.

File SE (1986). The effects of neonatal administration of clonazepam on passive avoidance and on social, aggressive and exploratory behavior of adolescent male rats. Neurobehav Toxicol Teratol 8:447–52.

File SE, Wardill AG (1975). Validation of head-dipping as a measure of exploration in a modified holeboard. Psychopharmacology 44:53–9.

Flynn JC, Flynn ER, Patton JH (1979). Effects of pre- and post-natal lead on affective behavior and learning in the rat. Neurobehav Toxicol 1(suppl):93–103.

Foss JA, Riley EP (1991). Elicitation and modification of the acoustic startle reflex in animals prenatally exposed to cocaine. Neurotoxicol Teratol 13:541–6.

Galef BG Jr (1987). Comparative psychology is dead! Long live comparative psychology. J Comp Psychol 101:259–61.

Geller I, Mendez V, Hamilton M, Hartmann RJ, Gause E (1979). Effects of carbon monoxide on operant behavior of laboratory rats and baboons. Neurobehav Toxicol 1:179–84.

Gentry GD, Middaugh LD (1988). Prenatal ethanol weakens the efficacy of reinforcers for adult mice. Teratology 37:135–44.

Geyer MA, Segal DS, Greenberg BD (1984). Increased startle responding in rats treated with phencyclidine. Neurobehav Toxicol Teratol 6:161–4.

Glowa JR (1986). Acute and sub-acute effects of deltamethrin and chlordimeform on schedule-controlled responding in the mouse. Neurobehav Toxicol Teratol 8:97–102.

Gold RA, King RD (1974). Retrograde amnesia: storage failure versus retrieval failure. Psychol Rev 81:465–9.

Gold RA, Marci J, McGaugh JL (1973). Retrograde amnesia effects: effects of direct cortical stimulation. Science 179:1343–5.

Goldenring JR, Batter DR, Shaywitz BA (1982). Sulfanilic acid: behavioral change related to azo food dyes in developing rats. Neurobehav Toxicol Teratol 4:43–9.

Goldman PS, Crawford HT, Stokes LP, Galkin TW, Rosvold HE (1974). Sex-dependent behavioral effects of cerebral cortical lesions in the developing rhesus monkey. Science 186:540–2.

Goodlett CR, Kelly SJ, West JR (1987). Early postnatal alcohol exposure that produces high blood alcohol levels impairs development of spatial navigation learning. Psychobiology 15:64–74.

Gordon WC (1981). Mechanisms of cue-induced retention enhancement. In: Spear NE, Miller RR, eds. Information processing in animals: memory mechanisms. Hillsdale, New Jersey: Lawrence Erlbaum, Associates, 319–39.

Gordon WC (1989). Learning and memory. Pacific Grove, California: Brooks/Cole.

Gormezano I, Kehoe EJ, Marshall BS (1983). Twenty years of classical conditioning research with the rabbit. In: Prague JM, Epstein AN, eds. Progress in psychobiology and physiological psychology. Vol. 10. New York: Academic Press, 197–275.

Grant DS, Roberts WA (1976). Sources of retroactive inhibition in pigeon short-term memory. J Exp Psychol Anim Behav Proc 2:1–16.

Grant LD (1976). Research strategies for behavioral teatology studies. Environ Health Perspec 18:85–94.

Groves PM, Thompson RF (1970). Habituation: a dual process theory. Psychol Rev 77:419–50.

Haddad R, Rabe A, Dumas R (1979). Neuroteratogenicity of methylazoxymethanol acetate: behavioral deficits of ferrets with transplacentally induced lissencephaly. Neurotoxicology 1:171–89.

Hall JF (1989). Learning and memory. Boston: Allyn and Bacon.

Haroutunian V, Campbell BA (1981). Development and habituation of the heart rate orienting response to auditory and visual stimuli in the rat. J Comp Physiol Psychol 95:166–74.

Heyser CJ, Miller JS, Spear NE, Spear LP (1992). Prenatal exposure to cocaine disrupts cocaine-induced conditioned place preference in rats. Neurotoxicol Teratol 14:57–64.

Hinderliter CF, Webster T, Riccio DC (1975). Amnesia induced by hypothermia as a function of treatment-test interval and recooling in rats. Anim Learn Behav 3:257–63.

Hodos W, Campbell CBG (1969). Scala naturae: why there is no theory in comparative psychology. Psychol Rev 76:337–50.

Hoffmann H, Molina JC, Kucharski D, Spear NE (1987). Further examination of ontogenetic limitations on conditioned taste aversion. Dev Psychobiol 20:455–63.

Holland PC (1984). Origins of behavior in Pavlovian conditioning. In: Bower G, ed. The psychology of learning and motivation. Vol. 18. New York: Academic Press, 129–174.

Holloway FA, Wansley RA (1973). Multiphasic retention deficits at periodic intervals after passive avoidance learning. Science 180:208–10.

Honig WK (1978). Studies of working memory in the pigeon. In: Hulse SH, Fowler H, Honig WK, eds. Cognitive processes in animal behavior. Hillsdale, New Jersey: Lawrence Erlbaum Associates, 211–48.

Honig WK, Staddon JER, eds (1977). Handbook of operant behavior. Englewood Cliffs, New Jersey: Prentice Hall.

Hulse SH, Fowler H, Honig WK, eds (1978). Cognitive processes in animal behavior. Hillsdale, New Jersey: Lawrence Erlbaum Associates.

Hutchings DE (1990). Issues of risk assessment: lessons from the use and abuse of drugs during pregnancy. Neurotoxicol Teratol 12:183–9.

Jarrard LE (1983). Selective hippocampal lesions and behavior: effects of kainic acid lesions on performance of place and cue tasks. Behav Neurosci 97:873–89.

Juraka JM (1984). Sex differences in dendritic response to differential experience in the rat visual cortex. Brain Res 295:27–34.

Juraska JM (1990). Gender differences in the dendritic tree of granule neurons in the hippocampal dentate gyrus of weaning age rats. Dev Brain Res 53:291–4.

Juraska JM (1991). Sex differences in "cognitive" regions of the rat brain. Psychoneuroendocrinology 16:105–9.

Juraska JM, Fitch JM, Washburne DL (1989). The dendritic morphology of pyramidal neurons in the rat hippocampal CA3 area: II. Effects of gender and the environment. Brain Res 479:115–9.

Juraska JM, Kopcik JR (1988). Sex and environmental influences on the size and untrastructure of the rat corpus callosum. Brain Res 450:1–8.

Kail R, Spear NE, eds (1984). Comparative perspectives on the development of memory. Hillsdale, New Jersey: Lawrence Erlbaum Associates.

Kelly SJ, Goodlett CR, Hulsether SA, West JR (1988). Impaired spatial navigation in adult female but not adult male rats exposed to alcohol during the brain growth spurt. Behav Brain Res 27:247–57.

Kenny JT, Blass EM (1977). Suckling as an incentive to instrumental learning in preweanling rats. Science 196:898–9.

Kimble G (1961). Hilgard and Marquis' conditioning and learning. New York: Appleton-Century-Crofts.

Kondo CY, Lorens SA (1971). Sex differences in the effects of septal lesions. Physiol Behav 6:481–5.

Kristal MB, Axlerod S, Noonan M (1978). Learning in escape/avoidance tasks in females rats does not vary with reproductive condition. Physiol Behav 21:251–6.

Kurcharski D, Spear NE (1984). Conditioning of aversion to an odor paired with peripheral shock in the developing rat. Dev Psychobiol 17:465–79.

Laties VG (1982). Contributions of operant conditioning to behavioral toxicology. In: Mitchell CL, ed. Nervous system toxicology. New York: Raven Press, 67–79.

Leaton RN, Cassella JV, Borszcz GS (1985). Short-term and long-term habituation of the acoustic startle response in chronic decerebrate rats. Behav Neurosci 99:901–12.

Levin ED, Bowman RE (1986). Long-term lead effects on the Hamilton search task and delayed alternation in monkeys. Neurobehav Toxicol Teratol 8:219–24.

Levin ED, Schantz SL, Bowman RE (1992). Use of the lesion model for examining toxicant effects on cognitive behavior. Neurotoxicol Teratol 14:131–41.

Lilienthal H, Neuf M, Munoz C, Winneke G (1990). Behavioral effects of pre- and postnatal exposure to a mixture of low chlorinated PCBs in rats. Fund Appl Toxicol 15:457–67.

Lochry EA, Hoberman AM, Christian MS (1985). Detection of prenatal effects on learning as a function of differential criteria. Neurobehav Toxicol Teratol 7:697–701.

Lochry EA, Riley EP (1980). Retention of passive avoidance and T-maze escape in rats exposed to alcohol prenatally. Neurobehav Toxicol 2:107–15.

Lockhard RB (1971). Reflections on the fall of comparative psychology: Is there a message for us all? Am Psychol 26:168–79.

Lorenz K (1950). The comparative method in studying innate behavior patterns. Symp Soc Exp Biol 4:221–68.

Loy R (1986). Sexual dimorphism in the septohippocampal system. In: Isaacson RL, Pribram KH, eds. The hippocampus. vol. 3. New York: Plenum Press, 301–21.

Loy R, Milner TA (1980). Sexual dimorphism in extent of axonal sprouting in rat hippocampus. Science 208:1281–4.

MacPhail RC, Elsmore TF (1980). Ethanol-induced flavor aversions in mice: a behavior-genetic analysis. Neurotoxicology 1:625–34.

MacPhail RC, Leander JD (1981). Chlordimeform effects on schedule-controlled behavior in rats. Neurobehav Toxicol Teratol 3:19–26.

Mactutus CF (1985). Conceptual and procedural considerations for developmental assessment of learning and memory (dys)function following neurotoxicant exposure. Neurobehav Toxicol Teratol 7:703–8.

Mactutus CF, Fechter LD (1984). Prenatal carbon monoxide exposure: learning and memory deficits. Science 223:409–11.

Mactutus CF, Riccio DC (1978). Hypothermia-induced retrograde amnesia: role of body temperature in memory retrieval. Physiol Psychol 6:18–22.

Mactutus CF, Tilson HA (1984). Neonatal chlordecone exposure impairs early learning and retention of active avoidance in the rat. Neurobehav Toxicol Teratol 6:75–83.

Mactutus CF, Tilson HA (1985). Evaluation of long-term consequences in behavioral and/or neural function following neonatal chlordecone exposure. Teratology 31:177–86.

Mactutus CF, Unger KL, Tilson HA (1982). Neonatal chlordecone exposure impairs early learning and memory in the rat on a multiple measure passive avoidance task. Neurotoxicology 3:27–44.

Mactutus CF, Wise NM (1985). The inaccessible, but intact, engram: a challenge for animal models of memory dysfunction. Ann NY Acad Sci 444:465–8.

McGivern RF, Clancy AN, Hill MA, Noble EP (1984). Prenatal alcohol exposure alters adult expression of sexually dimorphic behavior in the rat. Science 224:896–8.

McLamb RL, Mundy WR, Tilson HA (1988). Intradentate colchicine disrupts the acquisition and performance of a working memory task in the radial arm maze. Neurotoxicology 9:521–8.

McMillan DE (1981). Effects of chemicals on delayed matching behavior in pigeons I: acute effects of drugs. Neurotoxicology 2:485–98.

McMillan DE (1990). The pigeon as a model for comparative behavioral pharmacology and toxicology. Neurotoxicol Teratol 12:523–9.

Medin DL, Roberts WA, Davis RTE, eds (1976). Processes of animal memory. Hillsdale, New Jersey: Lawrence Erlbaum Associates.

Mele PC, Bowman RE, Levin ED (1986). Behavioral evaluation of perinatal PCB exposure in rhesus monkeys: fixed-interval performance and reinforcement-omission. Neurobehav Toxicol Teratol 8:131–8.

Messing RB (1987). Learning and memory dysfunction as selective neurotoxic effects. In: Tilson HA, Sparber SB, eds. Neurotoxicants and neurobiological function: effects of organoheavy metals. New York: Wiley-Interscience, 279–302.

Milar KS, Krigman MR, Grant LD (1981). Effects of neonatal lead exposure on memory in rats. Neurobehav Toxicol Teratol 3:369–73.

Miller DB (1984). Pre- and postweaning indices of neurotoxicity in rats: effects of triethyltin (TET), Toxicol Appl Pharmacol 72:557–65.

Miller DB, Eckerman DA (1986). Learning and memory measures. In: Annau Z, ed. Neurobehavioral toxicology. Baltimore: Johns Hopkins University Press, 94–149.

Miller JS, Jagielo JA, Spear NE (1990). Alleviation of short-term forgetting: effect of the CS and other conditioning elements in prior cueing or as context during test. *Learn Motiv 21*: 96–109.

Miller RR (1982). Effects of intertrial reinstatement of training stimuli on complex maze learning in rats: evidence that "acquisition" curves reflect more than acquisition. J Exp Psychol Anim Behav Proc 8:86–109.

Miller RR, Springer AD (1973). Amnesia, consolidation and retrieval. Psychol Rev 80:69–79.

Miller RR, Springer AD (1974). Implications of recovery from experimental amnesia. Psychol Rev 81:470–3.

Milner TA, Loy R (1982). Hormonal regulation of axonal sprouting in the hippocampus. Brain Res 243:180–5.

Mineka S (1987). A primate model of phobic fears. In: Eysenck H, Martin I, eds. Theoretical foundations of behavior therapy. New York: Plenum Press, 81–111.

Misanin JR, Brownback T, Shaughnessy LD, Hinderliter CF (1980). Acquisition and retention of multidirectional escape behavior in preweanling rats. Dev Psychobiol 13:85–93.

Mokler DJ, Robinson SE, Johnson JH, Hong JS, Rosecrans JA (1986). Effects of postweaning administration of delta-9-tetrahydrocannabinol (THC) on adult behavioral and neuroendocrine function in Sprague-Dawley and Fischer-344 rats. Neurobehav Toxicol Teratol 8:407–13.

Morris RGM (1981). Spatial localization does not require the presence of local cues. Learn Motiv 12:239–49.

Moser VC, Coggeshall EM, Balster RL (1985). Effects of xylene isomers on operant responding and motor performance in mice. Toxicol Appl Pharmacol 80:293–8.

Myslivecek J, Hassmannova J (1983). The development of inhibitory learning and memory in hooded and albino rats. Behav Brain Res 8:151–66.

Nagy ZM, Murphy JM (1974). Learning and retention of a discriminated escape response in infant mice. Dev Psychobiol 7:185–92.

Nation JR, Baker DM, Bratton GR, Fantasia MA, Andrews K, Womac C (1987). Ethanol self-administration in rats following exposure to dietary cadmium. Neurotoxicol Teratol 9:339–44.

Nation JR, Clark DE, Bourgeois AE, Baker DM (1983). The effects of chronic cadmium exposure on schedule controlled responding and conditioned suppression in the adult rat. Neurobehav Toxicol Teratol 5:275–82.

Nonneman AJ, Corwin JV (1981). Differential effects of prefrontal cortex ablation in neonatal, juvenile, and young adult rats. J Comp Physiol Psychol 95:588–602.

Olton DS (1978). Characteristics of spatial memory. In: Hulse SH, Fowler H, Honig WK, eds. Cognitive processes in animal behavior. Hillsdale, New Jersey: Lawrence Erlbaum Associates, 341–73.

Olton DS (1983). Memory functions and the hippocampus. In: Seifert W, ed. Neurobiology of the hippocampus. New York: Academic Press, 335–73.

Olton DS (1984). Animal models of human amnesia. In: Squire LR, Butters N, eds. Neuropsychology of memory. New York: Gilford Press, 367–73.

Olton DS, Collison C, Werz M (1977). Spatial memory and radial arm maze performance of rats. Learn Motiv 8:289–314.

Olton DS, Samuelson RJ (1976). Remembrances of places passed: spatial memory in rats. J Exp Psychol Anim Behav Proc 2:97–116.

Paule MG, Cranmer JM, Wilkins JD, Stern HP, McMillan DE (1988). Quantitation of complex brain function in children: preliminary evaluation using a nonhuman primate behavioral test battery. Neurotoxicology 9:367–78.

Paule MG, McMillan DE (1986). Effects of trimethyltin on incremental repeated acquisition (learning) in the rat. Neurobehav Toxicol Teratol 8:245–53.

Peeke HVS, Petrinovich L, eds (1984). Habituation, sensitization, and behavior. New York: Academic Press.

Peele DB, Allison SD, Crofton KM (1990). Learning and memory deficits in rats following exposure to 3,3'-iminodipropionitrile. Toxicol Appl Pharmacol 105:321–32.

Peele DB, Farmer JD, MacPhail RC (1987). Conditioned flavor aversions: applications in assessing the efficacy of chelators in the treatment of heavy-metal intoxication. Toxicol Appl Pharmacol 88:397–410.

Peele DB, Vincent A (1989). Strategies for assessing learning and memory, 1978–1987: a comparison of behavioral toxicology, psychopharmacology, and neurobiology. Neurosci Biobehav Rev 13:33–8.

Petit TL, LeBoutillier JC (1986). Zinc deficiency in the postnatal rat: implications for lead toxicity. Neurotoxicology 7:237–46.

Plonsky M, Riley EP, Lee MH, Haddad RK (1985). The effects of prenatal methylazoxymethanol acetate (MAM) on holeboard exploration and shuttle avoidance performance in rats. Neurobehav Toxicol Teratol 7:221–6.

Pontecorvo MJ (1985). Memory for a stimulus versus anticipation of a response: contrasting effects of proactive interference in two delayed comparison tasks. Anim Learn Behav 13:355–64.

Pryor GT, Dickinson J, Howd RA, Rebert CS (1983a). Transient cognitive deficits and high-frequency hearing loss in weanling rats exposed to toluene. Neurobehav Toxicol Teratol 5:53–7.

Pryor GT, Uyeno ET, Tilson HA, Mitchell CL (1983b). Assessment of chemicals using a battery of neurobehavioral tests: a comparative study. Neurobehav Toxicol Teratol 5:91–117.

Rabinovitch MS, Rosvold HE (1951). A closed-field intelligence test for rats. Can J Psychol 5:122–8.

Reiter LW, MacPhail RC (1982). Factors influencing motor activity measurements in neurotoxicology. In: Mitchell CL, ed. Nervous system toxicology. New York: Raven Press, 45–65.

Rescorla RA (1978). Some implications of a cognitive perspective on Pavlovian conditioning. In: Hulse SH, Fowler H, Honig WK, eds. Cognitive processes in animal behavior. Hillsdale, New Jersey: Lawrence Erlbaum Associates, 15–50.

Riccio DC, Ebner DL (1981). Postacquisition modifications of memory. In: Spear NE, Miller, RR, eds. Information processing in animals: memory mechanisms. New Jersey: Lawrence Erlbaum Associates, 291–317.

Rice DC (1984). Behavioral deficit (delayed matching to sample) in monkeys exposed from birth to low levels of lead. Toxicol Appl Pharmacol 75:337–45.

Rice DC (1988). Schedule-controlled behavior in infant and juvenile monkeys exposed to lead from birth. Neurotoxicology 9:75–87.

Rice DC, Gilbert SG (1990). Automated behavioral procedures for infant monkeys. Neurotoxicol Teratol 12:429–39.

Rice DC, Karpinski KF (1988). Lifetime low-level lead exposure produces deficits in delayed alternation in adult monkeys. Neurotoxicol Teratol 10:207–14.

Rice SA, Millan DP (1986). Validation of a developmental swimming test using Swiss Webster mice perinatally treated with methimazole. Neurobehav Toxicol Teratol 8:69–75.

Richardson R, Riccio DC (1986). An examination of a contextual component of memory following recovery from anterograde amnesia. Physiol Psychol 14:75–81.

Riley AL, Tuck DL (1985). Conditioned food aversions: a bibliography. Ann NY Acad Sci 443:381–437.

Riley EP, Barron S, Driscoll CD, Chen JS (1984). Taste aversion learning in preweanling rats exposed to alcohol prenatally. Teratology 29:325–31.

Riley EP, Plonsky M, Rosellini RA (1982). Acquisition of an unsignalled avoidance task in rats exposed to alcohol prenatally. Neurobehav Toxicol Teratol 4:525–30.

Rodier PM (1978). Behavioral teratology. In: Wilson JG, Fraser FC, eds. Handbook of teratology. Vol. 4. New York: Plenum Press, 397–428.

Rodier PM, Reynolds SS, Roberts WN (1979). Behavioral consequences of interference with CNS development in the early fetal period. Teratology 19:327–36.

Roitblat HL, Bever TG, Terrace HS, eds (1984). Animal cognition. Hillsdale, New Jersey: Lawrence Erlbaum Associates.

Rudy JW, Stadler-Morris S, Albert P (1987). Ontogeny of spatial navigation behaviors in the rat: dissociation of "proximal"- and "distal"-cue-based behaviors. Behav Neurosci 101:62–73.

Ryan CL, Pappas BA (1990). Prenatal exposure to antiadrenergic antihypertensive drugs: effects on neurobehavioral development and the behavioral consequences of enriched rearing. Neurotoxicol Teratol 12:359–66.

Sandstead HH, Fosmire GJ, Halas ES, Jacob RA, Strobel DA, Marks EO (1977). Zinc deficiency: effects of brain and behavior of rats and rhesus monkeys. Teratology 16:229–34.

Sara SJ, David-Remacle M, Lefevre D (1975). Passive avoidance behavior in rats after electroconvulsive shock: facilitative effects of response retardation. J Comp Physiol Psychol 89:489–97.

Sara SJ, Remacle J-F (1977). Strychnine-induced passive avoidance facilitation after electroconvulsive shock or undertraining: a retrieval effect. Behav Biol 19:565–75.

Satinder KP (1976). Sensory responsiveness and avoidance learning in rats. J Comp Physiol Psychol 90:946–57.

Satinder KP, Sterling JW (1983). Differential effects of pre- and/or post-natal *d*-amphetamine on avoidance response in genetically selected lines of rats. Neurobehav Toxicol Teratol 5:315–20.

Schneiderman N (1972). Response system divergencies in aversive classical conditioning. In: Black AH, Prokasy WF, eds. Classical conditioning II: current research and theory. New York: Appleton-Century-Crofts, 341–76.

Schull WJ, Norton S, Jensh RP (1990). Ionizing radiation and the developing brain. Neurotoxicol Teratol 12:249–60.

Schulze GE, McMillan DE, Bailey JR, Scallet AC, Ali SF, Slikker W Jr, Paule MG (1988). Acute effects of delta-9-tetrahydrocannabinol (THC) in rhesus monkeys as measured by performance in a battery of complex operant tests. J Pharmacol Exp Ther 245:178–86.

Seligman MEP (1975). Helplessness: on depression, development, and death. San Francisco: Freeman.

Sengstake CB, Chambers KC (1991). Sensitivity of male, female, and androgenized female rats to testosterone during extinction of a conditioned taste aversion. Behav Neurosci 105:120–5.

Shapiro S, Salas M, Vukovic K (1970). Hormonal effects on ontogeny of swimming ability in the rat: assessment of nervous system development. Science 168:147–51.

Shaywitz BA, Goldenring JR, Wool RS (1979). Effects of chronic administration of food colorings on activity levels and cognitive performance in developing rat pups treated with 6-hydroxy-dopamine. Neurobehav Toxicol 1:41–7.

Sigel S (1983). Classical conditioning, drug tolerance and drug dependence. In: Israel Y, Glaser FB, Kalant H, Popham RE, Schmidt W, Smart RG, eds. Research advances in alcohol and drug problems. vol 7. New York: Plenum Press, 207–246.

Smith RF, Mattran KM, Kurkjian MF, Kurtz SL (1989). Alterations in offspring behavior induced by chronic prenatal cocaine dosing. Neurotoxicol Teratol 11:35–8.

Sobotka TJ, Spaid SL, Brodie RE, Reed GF (1981). Neurobehavioral toxicity of ammoniated glycyrrhizin, a licorice component, in rats. Neurobehav Toxicol Teratol 3:37–44.

Solomon PR, Pingree TM, Baldwin D, Koota D, Perl DP, Pendlebury WW (1988). Disrupted retention of the classically conditioned nictitating membrane response in rabbits with aluminum-induced neurofibrillary degeneration. Neurotoxicology 9:209–21.

Spear NE (1978). The processing of memories: forgetting and retention. Hillsdale, New Jersey: Lawrence Erlbaum Associates.

Spear NE, Campbell BA, eds (1979). Ontogeny of learning and memory. Hillsdale, New Jersey: Lawrence Erlbaum Associates.

Spear NE, Miller JS, Jagielo JA (1990). Animal memory and learning. Annu Rev Psychol 41:169–211.

Spear NE, Riccio DC (1994). Memory: phenomena and principles. Boston: Allyn & Bacon.

Springer AD (1975). Vulnerability of skeletal and autonomic manifestation of memory in the rat to electroconvulsive shock. J Comp Physiol Psychol 88:890–903.

Stanton ME (1991). Neonatal exposure to triethyltin disrupts olfactory discrimination learning in preweanling rats. Neurotoxicol Teratol 13:515–24.

Stanton ME, Jensen KF, Pickens CV (1991). Neonatal exposure to trimethyltin disrupts spatial delayed alternation learning in preweanling rats. Neurotoxicol Teratol 13:525–30.

Stanton ME, Spear LP (1990). Workshop on the qualitative and quantitative comparability of human and animal developmental neurotoxicity, Work Group I report: comparability of measures of developmental neurotoxicity in humans and laboratory animals. Neurotoxicol Teratol 12:261–7.

Stebbins WC, Moody DB (1979). Comparative behavioral toxicology. Neurobehav Toxicol 1(suppl): 33–44.

Stehouwer DJ, Campbell BA (1978). Habituation of the forelimb-withdrawal response in neonatal rats. J Exp Psychol Anim Behav Proc 4:104–19.

Stehouwer DJ, Campbell BA (1980). Ontogeny of passive avoidance: role of task demands and development of species-typical behaviors. Dev Psychobiol 13:385–98.

Stewart J, Skvarenina A, Pottier J (1975). Effects of neonatal androgens on open-field and maze learning in the prepubescent and adult rat. Physiol Behav 14:291–5.

Strupp, BJ, Levitsky DA (1990). An animal model of retarded cognitive development. In: Rovee-Collier, C, Lipsett L eds. Advances in infancy research. Vol. 6 Norwood, New Jersey: Ablex, 149–85.

Swartzwelder HS, Hepler J, Holahan W, King SE, Leverenz HA, Miller PA, Myers RD (1982). Impaired maze performance in the rat caused by trimethyltin treatment: problem-solving deficits and perseveration. Neurobehav Toxicol Teratol 4:169–76.

Tarpy RM, Mayer RE (1978). Foundations of learning and memory. Glenview, Illinois: Scott, Foresman and Co.

Taylor DH, Noland EA, Brubaker CM, Crofton KM, Bull RJ (1982). Low level lead (Pb) exposure produces learning deficits in young rat pups. Neurobehav Toxicol Teratol 4:311–4.

Thomas DA, Riccio DC (1979). Forgetting of a CS attribute in a conditioned suppression paradigm. Anim Learn Behav 7:191–5.

Thomas JR, Ahlers ST, Schrot J (1991). Cold-induced impairment of delayed matching in rats. Behav Neural Biol 55:19–30.

Thomas JR, Schrot J, Banvard RA (1980). Behavioral effects of chlorpromazine and diazepam combined with low-level microwaves. Neurobehav Toxicol 2:131–5.

Tilson HA, Jacobson JL, Rogan WJ (1990). Polychlorinated biphenyls and the developing nervous system: cross-species comparisons. Neurotoxicol Teratol 12:239–48.

Tilson HA, Mitchell CL (1984). Neurobehavioral techniques to assess the effects of chemicals on the nervous system. Annu Rev Pharmacol Toxicol 24:425–50.

Tolman EC (1955). Principles of performance. Psychol Rev 62:315–25.

Vorhees CV (1983). Influence of early testing on postweaning performance in untreated F344 rats, with comparisons to Sprague-Dawley rats, using a standardized battery of tests for behavioral teratogenesis. Neurobehav Toxicol Teratol 5:587–91.

Vorhees CV (1985). Fetal anticonvulsant syndrome in rats: effects on postnatal behavior and brain amino acid content. Neurobehav Toxicol Teratol 7:471–82.

Vorhees CV (1987a). Maze learning in rats: a comparison of performance in two water mazes in progeny prenatally exposed to different doses of phenytoin. Neurotoxicol Teratol 9:235–41.

Vorhees CV (1987b). Fetal hydantoin syndrome in rats: dose-effect relationships of prenatal phenytoin on postnatal development and behavior. Teratology 35:287–303.

Vorhees CV, Butcher RE, Brunner RL, Wooten V (1984). Developmental toxicity and psychotoxicity of sodium nitrite in rats. Chem Toxicol 22:1–6.

Vorhees CV, Rindler JM, Minck DR (1990). Effects of exposure period and nutrition on the developmental neurotoxicity of anticonvulsants in rats: short and long-term effects. Neurotoxicology 11:273–83.

Vorhees CV, Weisenburger WP, Acuff-Smith KD, Minck DR (1991). An analysis of factors influencing complex water maze learning in rats: effects of task complexity, path order and escape assistance on performance following prenatal exposure to phenytoin. Neurotoxicol Teratol 13:213–22.

Walsh JM, Curley MD, Burch LS, Kurlansik L (1982). The behavioral toxicity of a tributyltin ester in the rat. Neurobehav Toxicol Teratol 4:241–6.

Walsh TJ, Miller DB, Dyer RS (1982). Trimethyltin, a selective limbic system neurotoxicant, impairs radial-arm maze performance, Neurobehav Toxicol Teratol 4:177–83.

Wang GH (1923). The relation between "spontaneous" activity and oestrous cycle in the white rat. Comp Psychol Monogr 2(6).

Wenger GR, McMillan DE, Chang LW (1984). Behavioral effects of trimethyltin in two strains of mice. II. Multiple fixed ratio, fixed interval. Toxicol Appl Pharmacol 73:89–96.

Wenger GR, McMillan DE, Chang LW (1986). Effects of triethyltin on responding of mice under a multiple schedule of reinforcement. Neurobehav Toxicol Teratol 8:659–65.

Wenk GL, Olton DS (1986). Lesion analysis. In: Annau Z, ed. Neurobehavioral toxicology. Baltimore: Johns Hopkins University Press, 268–76.

Wimer RE, Wimer C (1985). Three sexual dimorphisms in the granule cell layer of the hippocampus in house mice. Brain Res 328:105–9.

Yokel RA (1983). Repeated systemic aluminum exposure effects on classical conditioning of the rabbit. Neurobehav Toxicol Teratol 5:41–6.

Zentall TR, Hogan DE, Edwards CA (1984). Cognitive factors in conditional learning by pigeons. In: Roitblat HL, Bever TG, Terrace HS, eds. Animal cognition. Hillsdale, New Jersey: Lawrence Erlbaum Associates, 389–405.

15
Behavioral Toxicology: From the Lab to the Natural Environment

Hugh L. Evans
New York University Medical Center
Tuxedo, New York

Stephen A. Daniel
Mercy College
Dobbs Ferry, New York

DEFINITIONS AND PHILOSOPHICAL ISSUES

What Is Natural?

We occasionally are asked by nonspecialists whether behavioral data from lab animals can be extrapolated to the "real world" or whether we could create an experimental model that is more "natural." Similar questions are asked of studies of humans (Banaji and Crowder, 1991). We discourage thinking of a dichotomy between lab and field because to label some research as "natural" implies that other research is "unnatural." Such philosophizing starts one down a slippery slope in attempting to draw boundaries around the various research methods. Such thinking has been promulgated by antivivisectionists to bolster their claim that research with animals is irrelevant and to impede scientific research by provoking frivolous arguments among researchers. Our approach is integrative, searching for generalities, rather than exclusionary. The following paragraphs explain our approach to this paper.

Behavior Is Adaptable

Behavior is a major mechanism whereby animals adapt to changes in their environment, including the intrusion of toxic chemicals. Thus, the impact of environmental pollution should be gauged partly in terms of behavior. Adaptive behavior may indicate toxicity, or it may indicate successful coping. In either event, behavioral changes show that the environment, including chemicals, is impinging on the animal. When traveling through our coastal regions, one observes wild sea gulls at shopping malls many miles from the water. The gulls have been seen feeding on pizza crust and other products of modern, fast-food society. Certainly, pizza was not an important dietary staple during the thousands of years during which the feeding habits of gulls evolved through natural selection. Instead, the recent development of suburban malls with fast-food shops has triggered social learning,

443

a process much more rapid than genetic evolution. The feeding behavior of modern gulls has adapted to a new food source without training sessions provided by behavioral scientists! The gull's capability for rapid behavioral adaptation to changes in its environment accounts for its ability to thrive in many different ecological niches.

Changes in behavior may tell us something of the influence of chemical pollution on our natural environment. That is the theme of this chapter. As for gulls eating pizza, an apparent benefit to the survival of both the individual and species, what could more clearly illustrate the limited value of struggling to classify behavior as natural or unnatural? Who would propose that toxicant-induced impairment of feeding performance on a lab test means nothing about the chances that a similarly exposed animal will find ingest food in the wild? We conclude that the concept of the "natural" has been as overburdened in discourse about science as it has in attempts by the food and clothing industries to inflate the sense of a product's value.

Does Toxicity Include Adaptive Change?

Here, it is useful to recognize the adaptive character of behavior. A small change in the environment, or a very low dose of a chemical, may result in a behavioral change that is adaptive (i.e., a departure from the normal pattern of behavior may improve the animal's chances of survival without compromising its life span or the propagation of the species). Behavioral changes of this type might include the gull's adapting to suburban malls or an increase in locomotor behavior that increases chances of encountering food. Such behavioral changes are particularly sensitive and useful as *markers of exposure*. Such changes may provide valuable warning of a chemical's biological effects in advance of overt toxicity. Such advance warning provides time for remediation of the environmental contamination or protection of the exposed organism. The research reviewed here shows that many behaviors provide a marker of exposure.

In contrast to the adaptive change, a higher dose may produce a behavioral change that is clearly toxic, i.e., that indicates a compromised life span or the reduced propagation of the species. Such a change would be termed a *marker of toxicity*. Behavior can provide evidence of toxicity, or it can confirm health and well-being in the absence of toxicity (Evans et al., 1989).

It often is difficult to draw a clear line between adaptive change and behavior that manifests toxicity. The transition between the two types of change occurs at the low end of the dose-response curve, where change may appear only in the most sensitive individuals, and where changes are often small in magnitude. Thus, extensive effort is required to document a statistically significant effect at a near-threshold dose.

Do Laboratory Data Generalize to the "Real World"?

Research applied to concerns about the environment is sometimes questioned for its relevance or its "ecological realism" (Henry and Atchison, 1991). Can models with lab animals tell us anything relevant to the "real world"? Can models of animal behavior tell us anything about what animals do "naturally"? This question is as arbitrary and slippery as the one about "natural" behavior. The lack of consensus about the real world is easily illustrated by the ways in which politicians, ranging from conservative to liberal persuasion, define "natural" events in their view of the real world.

Sometimes the words "real world" are used to indicate complex social relationships, as in human or animal societies. Unfortunately, attempts to create large, complex social groups of animals in laboratories (Calhoun, 1963, 1973; Palmes and Del Pup, 1971; Del

Pup et al., 1978; Novak and Suomi, 1988) have yielded small dividends for toxicology and pharmacology compared with the substantial costs of establishing the group and of isolating and controlling variables that influence the experimental outcomes.

It often is desirable to select a simpler model, rather than a more complex one. A simpler model permits the scientist to concentrate on a few variables for intensive study. In toxicity testing, a simple model can collect evidence of changes in a wide variety of physiological processes. Apical tests (i.e., body weight, locomotor activity) are good as first-tier screens because they "cast a wide net." At the first tier, one need not try to decide among all alternative mechanisms that might explain the observed effect. Identification of mechanisms is the job for higher tiers of screening and for the research lab.

What Can Be Learned from Field Studies?

This chapter will review and, when possible, compare laboratory and field research findings. While the typical laboratory approaches and ethological approaches to behavioral toxicology are very different, it may be possible to build a bridge between these two divergent approaches. Ethology provides the primary methods of field study (Lehner, 1979; Dewsbury, 1978). A species is typically observed in its natural habitat to gain an accurate description of the species' normal ("species-typical") behavior. This observation and description of behavior includes objective operational definitions of behavior that can be recorded by well-trained observers (Silverman, 1987).

Henry and Atchison (1991) indicated the following desirable characteristics of behavioral end points for ethotoxicological studies: 1.) ease of observation in laboratory and field; 2.) sensitivity to chemicals being studied; 3.) being previously well described and well understood in the animal-behavior literature, in terms of their sequence, eliciting factors, etc. (Farr, 1980); 4.) being ecologically relevant to species survival; and 5.) integrating several sensory and motor modalities.

Ethology differs from laboratory approaches to the study of behavior in several important ways. The first of these is the habitat in which the animal is studied (lab or wild) and the complexity of the habitat (simple–complex). Behavioral toxicity is usually defined by ethologists in terms of obvious survival value to the species, such as escape from predators, social interactions, mating behavior, and feeding behavior. Another characteristic of the ethological approach is the study of the interactions between two or more animals. Lab studies usually observe a single animal or its interaction with a piece of equipment ranging in complexity from a running wheel to an operant-conditioning chamber. Critics of lab studies overlook the importance of an animal's interaction with inanimate objects (e.g., nest construction, tool use). Ethologists are more likely to study a broader range of species, which often include fish and birds. As related to the last two points, the results typically provide information about how toxicant-induced behavioral changes are detrimental to one or more species of animal, while lab studies yield results about one species. The sequences of species-specific behavior usually occur without experimenter-initiated learning. Observational methodology is more commonly employed in field studies, where it would be more difficult to use instrumentation for precise and automated measurement. Observational studies, whether in the field or in the lab, require time-sampling techniques, interobserver reliability, and blind scoring (e.g., Evans et al., 1981). Although field studies save on animal purchase and housing costs, lab studies save on costs of travel for staff and equipment.

An advantage of field studies over lab studies is access to animals that cannot easily be kept in the lab. One might refer to these as exotic species. The values of exotic or seldom-used animal species for neurotoxicology can be 1.) to test the generality of results from studies with common lab species; 2.) to model a response that is not readily available in other animal models; and 3.) to provide unusual sensitivity to some compounds. A disadvantage is the scarcity of background information for use in planning experiments or interpreting results with exotic species.

A limitation of field research is the sacrifice of control over many variables in order to gain the reality of the natural habitat. It is difficult to control variables such as temperature, predation, and health risks posed by factors unrelated to the toxicological question. One also sacrifices control over exposure to toxicants. Animals may be moving into and out of the area of contamination (Dinnel et al., 1979), raising the possibility that changes in behavior will be confounded with changes in exposure or with changes in the population at the test site. Such studies must employ the strategies of epidemiology. Even so, it is difficult to firmly establish cause and effect relationships and to extrapolate results from the unique field (habitat) in which a study was conducted to another habitat in which countless variables are different (Henry and Atchison, 1991). Finally, the quest for observation under "natural" conditions may increase the risk of anthropomorphism.

Few studies of animal behavior in the wild have appeared in toxicology. This reflects the bias of funding agencies toward human, rather than animal, epidemiology. The numerous environmental variables known to influence human behavioral traits (housing density, family size, socioeconomic status, etc.) would be difficult to model in animals, and identifying and controlling the many variables that combine to influence animal behavior in the wild presents great difficulty. Also, results with exotic species may be difficult to extrapolate to humans. Finally, it seems impossible to use animals in the wild to screen for toxicity of unknown compounds.

A more appropriate use of wild animals is as sentinels of environmental pollution (Moriarty, 1988; U.S. National Research Council, 1991). Field studies can make use of "natural experiments" to identify harmful effects of pollution. Fish may serve as sentinels of aquatic pollutants such as polychlorinated biphenyls (Evans et al., 1993; Baatrup, 1991). Birds have been proposed as sentinels of environmental health hazards (Fleming et al., 1991; Meydani and Post, 1979; Young et al., 1979). Most publications in this area report on the concentration of a toxicant in animal tissue, or on dose-response, with lethality as the most common end point. We shall review a few papers in which behavior was the end point.

Research Must Be Evaluated According to Its Purpose

Much of the debate about the appropriate role for behavioral studies in toxicology could be ended by recognizing that toxicological studies have divergent goals. Some are designed to document harm to the environment, others to predict health risks to humans posed by poorly understood chemicals; still others are designed to unravel the basic mechanisms of the nervous system's response to chemical injury. An experiment that is well designed for one purpose may not be well suited for the other purposes, but this does not render the scientific enterprise invalid. The above discussion suggests that the distinction between ethology and lab research in terms of "naturalness" is not as decisive as it at first seemed to be. There are advantages and disadvantages to each approach.

Instincts and "Unlearned" Behaviors

The most salient distinction between the different research strategies may be the use of instinctive behavior, i.e., predator attack or startle reflex, instead of learned behavior.

Animals can perform instinctive behavior without training or extensive advance preparation by the scientist. In contrast, behaviors such as schedule-controlled operant behavior (Chapter 11) are carefully created by the investigator in order to observe some aspect of behavior in greater detail or in greater quantity than can be observed without the researcher's intervention. Lab studies can create a behavioral sequence to provide the behavior desired for study, e.g, withhold food or increase palatability of food in order to study ingestive behavior, or "build" measurable sequences of instinctive behavior.

Other advantages of the study of instinctive, or reflexive, behavior are that little time is required to prepare animals before the start of the study, and that instinctive behavior usually relates directly to survival (e.g., mating or predation), while laboratory studies of an individual animal require extrapolation from the simplified test to the natural environment.

Home-Cage Behavior: An Amalgam of Lab and Naturalistic Approaches

The study of behavior in the home cage is an emerging trend enabled by technological advances in miniaturized electronics, and motivated by both economics and animal-care regulations that discourage transport of animals between housing room and laboratory. Advantages in studying behavior in the home cage have been discussed in detail (Evans et al., 1986; Evans, 1989). Advantages include minimal disruption of ongoing behavior (e.g., diurnal pattern of sleep); reduction of experimenter bias that occurs when an investigator must evaluate animals by handling them; reduction of injury and exchange of pathogens between animal and human; reduction of space and equipment requirements for the study; facilitation of collaboration with investigators—since animals have to be housed in cages regardless of the purpose of the study, one can easily add behavioral evaluation of animals being prepared for studies of end points other than those involving the nervous system; minimal time needed to prepare animals for study; use of standard animal cages instead of specialized test cages; automation; and greater statistical power because of the ability to evaluate large numbers of animals.

We have organized this review according to the various neurobehavioral functions, such as ingestion, reproduction, locomotion, aggression, and defense. Evaluation of each function has ranged, in various studies, from apical screens to more complex and detailed analyses. There is no clear dichotomy between simple and complex or between screening and research. Instead, one can perceive a continuum along which the investigator can position a study, depending on needs.

BEHAVIORAL FUNCTION OF THE INDIVIDUAL

Feeding and Drinking

Laboratory studies can be arranged so that the behavior being investigated is ecologically realistic. For example, feeding behavior in the wild is a complex set of behaviors that may include searching, selection, attack, capture, and handling of Prey. Laboratory models are available for the study of foraging or predation (Evans et al., 1989; Miczek et al., 1989; Morgan and Kiceniuk, 1990, 1991).

Body Weight

Body weight exemplifies what has come to be known as an "apical" index of toxicity, since it reflects changes in any of a wide variety of physiological and behavioral mechanisms (e.g., appetite or thirst, metabolism, digestive efficiency, sensory acuity, or motor coordination). Because of this, body weight is useful in screening for toxicity of unknown compounds, and also as a handy benchmark in evaluating data in research, where it is important to know whether changes in performance of positively rewarded learned behavior may be secondary to loss of appetite. Because of this, behavioral scientists are most interested in changes that occur in the absence of significant changes in body weight.

Amount of Food or Water Ingested

The daily quantity of food and water ingested can be measured easily by weighing the food or water containers; these data can reflect evidence of surgically induced pain (Flecknell and Liles, 1992) or toxicity (Dempster et al., 1984; Evans et al., 1986) when body weight does not. Boric acid increased consumption of both food and water by rats and mice. Trimethyltin increased consumption of water but not of food by rats (Bushnell and Evans, 1985).

Emesis

There is a surprisingly small literature on emesis in animal toxicology, perhaps because the rat, the dominant model, does not vomit. However, birds and mammals provide models of emesis (Carpenter et al., 1984, 1986; King and Landauer, 1990) that may be extrapolated to humans. Another reason emesis has seldom been reported in behavioral research is that the response is associated with inadequacy of dosing by the oral route or is irrelevant to the nervous system functions being studied in the experiment.

Birds provide sensitive models of several digestive disorders described in humans. For example, workers who inhale solvents while at work experience nausea. An early model was the observation that pigeons vomited during inhalation of carbon disulfide (T. Levine, personal communication, and Levine, 1976). Pigeons in our lab (M. J. Pontecorvo and H. L. Evans, unpublished) exhibited classical conditioning of regurgitation with repeated daily inhalation exposures to organic solvents. At first they regurgitated after an hour inside the inhalation exposure chamber; with more and more daily exposures, an increasing percentage of the birds began to regurgitate earlier in the exposure, until, after 1 week of daily exposures, the birds began to regurgitate when placed on a cart to transfer them from their living cages to the inhalation exposure chamber. Ducks exhibit conditioned aversion to aluminum (Sparling, 1990).

Pigeons develop crop stasis after oral exposure to lead (Cory-Slechta et al., 1980; Boyer et al., 1985). At the New York University laboratories, we found pigeons to regurgitate an aqueous solution of triethyltin shortly after oral gavage (P. J. Bushnell and H. L. Evans, unpublished); a similar solution was retained by rats (Bushnell and Evans, 1986). Macaque monkeys vomited within an hour after oral administration of trimethyltin; the effect was less pronounced if the animals were fasted and if the chemical was first absorbed into a food biscuit and then eaten (J. F. Graefe and H. L. Evans, unpublished).

Consumption of Unusual Substances

Several experiments have shown that exposure to toxicants can selectively increase ingestion of calorically rich substances. This phenomenon is comparable to stress-induced ingestion (Teal and Evans, 1982). It may reflect toxicant-induced changes in function of peripheral nerves that subserve taste. Mice will drink sweetened, condensed milk even when they have free access to a nutritionally complete diet. The ease with which this drinking can be established makes it practical for screening. Consumption of milk increased above control levels after exposure to benzene (Dempster et al., 1984; Evans et al., 1981) or to acrylamide (Teal and Evans, 1982). Rats exposed to lead (Pb) consumed more ethanol than controls (Nation et al., 1986).

Efficiency and Pattern of Ingestive Behavior

A greater sensitivity to low doses and information concerning potential mechanisms of toxicity can be obtained by a more detailed study of ingestive behavior. Simple measurements, while observing an animal pick up food, have been used to document toxicity. Decrements in efficiency of feeding have been described in minnows exposed to Pb (Weber et al., 1991), in pigeons exposed to acrylamide (Daniel et al., 1990; Evans, 1982), or methylmercury (Evans et al. 1982). In addition to the simplicity of implementation and minimal time needed for preparation of animals, food-retrieval tests provide the added advantage of clear relevance to health and have well-defined cellular and neurophysiological mechanisms (Kalaska and Cram- mond, 1992; Zeigler et al., 1975) to which toxic effects can be related.

Similar observational tests, based on visually guided reaching for food objects (Montoya et al., 1991; Evans et al., 1975; Maurissen et al., 1990), are about as sensitive to age-related decline in performance efficiency (Bachevalier et al., 1991) as are much more complex tests of learned behavior. Food-pickup tests were also sensitive in documenting changes in monkey's foraging efficiency related to test familiarity (Evans et al., 1989) or to exposure to methylmercury (Evans et al., 1975), toluene (Evans and Taylor, in preparation), or acrylamide (Maurissen et al., 1990). With all procedures, it is advisable to compare the total amount of food consumed in the test with the amount of standard diet consumed in the home cage. This prevents confounding changes in feeding efficiency with unrelated changes in motivation, motor coordination, or some other function.

Microcomputer technology has made possible the detailed, continuous examination of ingestion in the home cage (West et al., 1983; Evans et al., 1986). The diurnal pattern of ingestion can reveal subtle degrees of toxicity (Bushnell and Evans, 1985, 1986). Changes in diurnal pattern cannot always be deduced from changes in total daily amount of consumption (Evans, 1989). Low-level exposure to trimethyltin selectively impaired food pellet retrieval and mastication of rats without affecting drinking (Bushnell and Evans, 1985). Even more detailed analyses reveal that licking can vary more in response to chemical parameters of the test solution (Davis and Smith, 1992) or to drug toxicity (Fowler and Mortell, 1992) than had previously been thought.

In summary, toxicants, like other stimuli that stress nervous system function, can increase ingestion of specific substances. Toxicants also can increase consumption of food or water, but most commonly are reported to suppress intake of water and food. When a toxicant alters ingestion or body weight, it may be necessary to study a group of pair-fed and pair-deprived animals so as to control for changes that are secondary to wasting and loss of energy.

Locomotion

The total amount of locomotor behavior provides an apical index, in that it can result from changes in any of a variety of physiological processes. Some have questioned the confidence with which the nervous system can be identified as the primary target organ responsible for changes in locomotor activity (Maurissen and Mattsson, 1989), and attempts to define pain and analgesia in terms of locomotor behavior are not particularly convincing (Flecknell and Liles, 1992). Despite these limitations, spontaneous locomotor activity is meaningful in toxicology because it reflects a function that is important to survival of the individual and the species in the wild—e.g., the mobility needed to search for food or mate, or to elude predators. It is not necessary for researchers to bring the predators into the laboratory in order to make this point.

The evidence overwhelmingly indicates an important role for measures of locomotion in toxicological research (Crofton et al., 1991). Publications have become too numerous to be described here; Table 1 provides a sample. As we found to be true for ingestive behavior, the information content and mechanistic implications of studies in this area increase with the amount of effort expended by the experimenter in documenting detailed data.

The Home Cage

Many systems for automated measurement of an animal's locomotor behavior in the home cage have been employed since the New York University system was reported (Evans et al., 1986; Evans, 1988, 1989). Most measure the frequency with which a rodent's movements cause an interruption of an infrared photobeam (Evans et al., 1986; Flecknell and Liles, 1992; Fitzgerald et al., 1988; Crofton et al., 1991). Similar systems can be used with primates; both ultrasonic motion detectors (Holtzman and Young, 1991) and infrared photobeams (Evans, et al., 1989) have been used with similar results. An alternative technology records infrared energy emitted by an animal (Foss and Lochry, 1991; Tamborini et al., 1989). This passive infrared detector has an advantage in not requiring the precise alignment of a photobeam, but the specificity and meaning of the infrared analogue signal is not yet fully understood.

The ethological approach also has documented toxicant-induced changes in locomotion. Meydani and Post (1979) measured the dose effects of malathion on the ability of

Table 1 Compounds Affecting Locomotion

Compound	References
Acetanilide	Tamborini et al., 1989
Acrylamide	Kulig and Lammers, 1992; Schulze, 1990; Schulze and Boysen, 1991
Arecoline	Ferguson and Bowman, 1992
Carbaryl	Crofton et al., 1991
Chlorobiphenyl	Eriksson et al., 1991
IDPN	Shulze and Boysen, 1991
Isopropanol	Burleigh-Flayer et al., 1992
Lead	Lilienthal et al., 1986; Burdette and Goldstein, 1986; Ferguson and Bowman, 1992
Manganese	Komura and Sakamoto, 1991
Mercurials	Kulig and Lammers, 1992; Tamborini et al., 1989
Organophosphates	Meydani and Post, 1979; Dam and Gopal, 1991
Pyrethroids	Crofton and Reiter, 1988; Eriksson and Fredriksson, 1991; Crofton et al., 1991
Toluene	Forkman et al., 1991
Tin, organic	Bushnell and Evans, 1985, 1986; Ema et al., 1991; Kernan et al., 1991
Triadimefon	Crofton et al., 1991

IDPN = 3',3'-iminodipropionitrile.

Japanese quail to regain their feet after being placed on their backs on a table ("flap" test); this test is analogous to the "righting reflex" test used with rodents. The number of times birds were able to regain their feet decreased in a dose-dependent manner after exposure, then recovered by 20 days after malathion administration. There was a linear correlation between the results of the "flap" test and brain acetylcholinesterase activity. The authors conclude that sublethal concentrations of malathion can reduce an animal's ability to right itself from a sitting position, and thus impair escape from predation or searching for food and water.

Whitworth et al. (1991) measured the effects of boron and arsenic on time allocation of various behaviors in developing mallard ducklings. The high dose of arsenic increased time spent resting. Both arsenic and boron decreased time in alert posture and time in the water trough. Boron resulted in increased feeding and preening time. The overall picture of arsenic and boron intoxication is of an organism that is sedentary, less alert, and seeking supplemental heat. While these animals were able to survive in a latoratory setting, it is likely that these behavioral effects could compromise survival in the wild.

Fenitrothion increased surfacing, erratic movements, jumping, convulsions, and opercular movements and decreased distance traveled in *Channa punctatus*, a freshwater fish (Dam and Gopal, 1991). These behavioral changes were accompanied by changes in monoamine in several brain areas. Exposure generally resulted in a decrease in stamina and an apparent increase in stimulus-related behaviors. These neurobehavioral changes would have consequences for survival through effects on orientation and locomotor patterns such as decreased predator avoidance, decreased ability to focus on prey detection and capture, and decreased ability to engage in courtship displays and other reproductive behaviors. These authors, more than most, were willing to interpret changes in motor activity in terms of health and survival of the individual. This illustrates how lab studies of locomotor behavior can be intelligently applied to questions of health risk.

Analyses of the temporal *pattern* of locomotion can reveal evidence of change not seen in measures of the *total amount* of locomotion. Rats exposed to Pb exhibited normal amounts of locomotion in the residential maze but also had dampened cyclicity in the nocturnal phase (Reiter and MacPhail, 1982). Effects of trimethyltin were similar in rats and macaques, with an enhancement of the diurnal rhythm in locomotion, i.e., a selective increase of activity during the time of day, when animals were normally active (Evans, 1989). Tributyltin (Fig. 1) (Ema et al., 1991) produced an effect in rats that could be described as a dampening of the diurnal rhythm, different from that of trimethyltin in that the increased activity occurred in the light, when activity was normally low, while nocturnal activity, which is usually high, was decreased.

The Open Field

The open field is a quasistandardized arena for observation of behavior. Modern instrumentation permits automated measurement in the dark, an important capability if one is interested in rodents or other nocturnal species that normally display very little behavior in the light. The behavior of most species, ranging from humans (Bell, 1968; Colburn et al., 1976; Eaton et al., 1988; Muller et al., 1979; Saudino and Eaton, 1990) and nonhuman primates (Ferguson and Bowman, 1990; Rice et al., 1979) to the fruit fly (Akins et al., 1992), has been studied with open-field procedures. Locomotion of nonhuman primates exposed to lead was higher than that of control animals in the open field (Ferguson and Bowman, 1992). Locomotion of humans in the open field was used to evaluate pharmacotherapy for

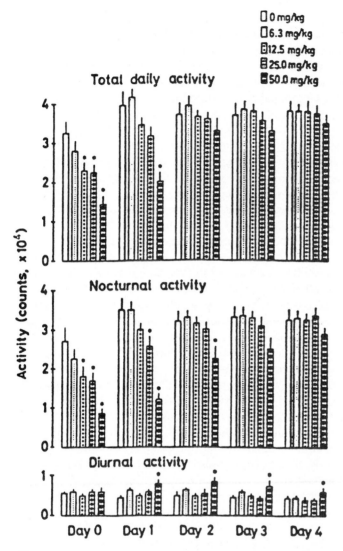

Figure 1   Changes in home-cage locomotor activity of rats after acute oral exposure to tributyltin. Separate evaluation of nocturnal activity (middle graph) and diurnal activity (lower graph) helped to indicate effects that were not apparent in total daily activity (top graph). (From Ema et al., 1991.)

hyperactivity disorders (Anderson et al., 1989). Locomotor behavior of humans has not been studied in toxicology. Reports of the effects of toxicants on open-field behavior of rodents are too numerous to review here; recent references are summarized in Table 1.

Computer-controlled video tracking of rodent locomotor behavior, the newest technology to be applied, is of interest to those who believe that one of the many different behavioral topographies (Maier et al., 1988) may provide information about toxicity that otherwise would be missed by apical tests of total activity (Voorhees et al., 1992; Mullenix et al., 1990). As with any new technique, data are needed to document the practical application of this technology to routine toxicity screening of large numbers of animals and the method's relative sensitivity in comparison with other methods. The technique proved to be as sensitive in documenting effects of acute triethyltin (Kernan et al., 1991) as the photocell method of Bushnell and Evans (1986), but the technique's cost is substantially higher than that of current photocell methods. Imaging techniques currently require that the animal be removed from its home cage for observation, and the complexity of instrumentation and software for data reduction limits the number of animals that can be observed simultaneously. A healthy skepticism might suggest that drugs and toxicants seldom respect the boundaries between different categories and classifications of behavior devised by human observers of an animal's behavior.

Habituation is a higher-order aspect of locomotor behavior in which the animal displays evidence of previously having been in the test situation. In one study (Eriksson and Frediksson, 1991), toxicant-exposed rats were indistinguishable from control rats during initial measurement of locomotion in an open field, but exposed rats failed to habituate as observation time continued (Fig. 2). Another study found Pb-exposed rats to exhibit less habituation in an open field (Burdette and Goldstein, 1986).

Gait Analyses

Behavioral assessment provides the standard evidence of gait disorders (e.g., Parkinson's disease) in humans (e.g., Blin et al., 1991; Pedersen et al., 1991). Behavior also provides clear evidence of other motor disabilities related to aging or toxicant exposure (Schaumburg and Spencer, 1979). These signs are readily modeled in animals. Models of gait are needed to evaluate therapeutic intervention (Van Der Zee et al., 19?9) as well as mechanisms of toxicity. A number of methods, ranging from simple to detailed, have been published for use with rats (Hruska et al., 1979; Lowden et al., 1988; De Medinaceli et al., 1982, 1984; Parker and Clarke, 1990) and chicks (Newby-Schmidt and Norton, 1980). Kulig and Lammers (1992) recently reviewed additional aspects of this topic.

Positive control substances and conditions (ethanol, thyroid deficiency, acrylamide) were used to develop models of toxicant-induced gait disturbances in the rat (Jolicoeur et al., 1979) and chick (Newby-Schmidt and Norton, 1980). Ethanol continues to be a major focus of investigations with rats (Clarke and Steadman, 1989; Hannigan and Riley, 1988; Meyer and Riley, 1990). However, avian models predominate in studies of organophosphate-induced delayed neuropathy, because the earliest and least ambiguous sign of neurotoxicity is hind-limb weakness in the hen.

Quadrupeds can be used to document behavioral deficits ensuing from exposure to pesticides nearly as well as bipeds. A semiobjective rating scale for gait of rats could document effects of chlordimeform or carbaryl (Moser et al., 1988) as well as 2-hydroxyethyl acrylate or acrylamide (Moser et al., 1992; Shell et al., 1992). A similar approach was used to document gait and other motor dysfunctions in pigeons exposed to methylmercury (Evans et al., 1982) and to investigate whether this type of motor impairment could be confounded with decrements in cognitive function (Laties and Evans, 1980).

Stride length (Fig. 3) and landing foot spread (Edwards et al., 1991; Teal and Evans, 1982) are readily quantified and provide unambiguous evidence of acrylamide's toxicity. As with acrylamide, a number of pesticides cause a reduction in stride length of chickens (Sheets et al., 1987; Farage-Elawar, 1988, 1989; Farage-Elawar and Francis, 1988; Farage-Elawar et al., 1989). It is useful to note that behavioral evidence of carbamate-induced motor dysfunction was a more sensitive end point than neurochemical evidence, e.g., neurotoxic esterase and acetylcholinesterase (Farage-Elawar, 1988; Farage-Elawar and Francis, 1988).

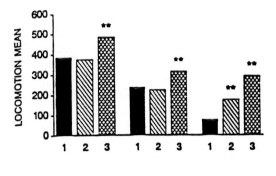

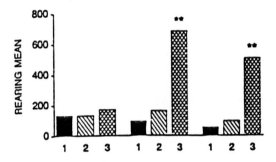

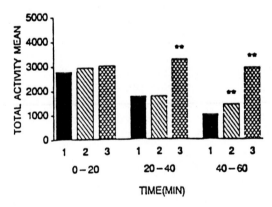

Figure 2   Habituation, shown by decline in amount of locomotor activity of control mice (solid bars, group 1) during a 60-min test in an open field. Mice previously exposed to pyrethroids (hatched bars, groups 2 and 3) did not habituate. This behavioral effect could not have been documented with a brief test, e.g., 20 min. (From Eriksson and Fredriksson, 1991.)

Swimming

Aquatic species have been used to assess preference and aversion for contaminated water. Henry and Atchison (1991) reviewed findings that various metals cause a variety of fish species to avoid contaminated streams. Copper, zinc, or arsenic in the water resulted in avoidance of the area of contamination. Many of the species studied tend to return to the streams in which they were born (natal streams). However, these streams may be avoided

17 Days of H₂O 　　　 17 Days of ACR 45 mg/kg

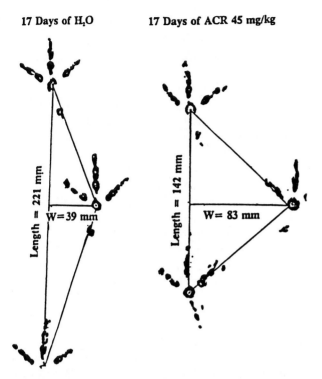

Figure 3 Change in a pigeon's gait following repeated oral exposure to 45 mg/kg acrylamide (right) compared with gait of a pigeon given sham treatment (left). Acrylamide exposure resulted in reduced stride length and increased stride width. (From Daniel et al., 1990).

if polluted with certain chemicals. Disruption of the fish's migration can lead to decreased reproduction (Geckler et al., 1986). However, other studies show that fish may spend more time in contaminated water than in clean water. These contradictory findings make it difficult to generalize from the data. Since rodents do not have to be trained to swim or be prepared in advance to be motivated to escape from water, swimming is convenient for studies of place learning and performance, e.g., with the Morris water maze (McNaughton and Morris, 1987). Observation of swimming helped to reveal methyl-mercury-induced incoordination (Spyker et al., 1972) and has been used in toxicology since then (Vorhees, 1987). As an endurance test, simply counting time a rodent spends swimming may not be a sensitive index, because animals often adapt a floating posture instead of swimming. The naturalistic character of swimming is sacrificed in attempts to overcome this by using extreme water temperatures or by attaching weights to the animal.

Tremor and Postural Sway

Tremor can be measured most effectively with behavioral tests (Roels, et al., 1989). Procedures reviewed have been used with humans. The measurement is of the finger, hand, or arm while the subject is performing a task that resembles a workplace action. Exposure to elemental mercury or vapors containing mercurial compounds has long been known to cause tremor (Wood et al., 1973; Evans et al., 1975). This technique was used to track humans exposed to carbon disulfide (Chapman et al., 1991). Whole-body tremor (Gerhart et al., 1982, 1983) and whole-body measurement of the startle reflex (Crofton, 1992) can indicate toxic effects with rodents. Additional information can be found in recent reviews (Kulig and Lammers, 1992; Newland, 1988).

Postural sway can be used to gauge normal growth and development of children (Ashmead and McCarty, 1991) or effects of toxicants. Systems for measuring sway employ detectors of light-emitting diodes worn by the subject (Ashmead and McCarty, 1991) or a force-transducing platform on which the subject stands (Bhattacharya et al., 1988; Ledin et al., 1989; Linz et al., 1992). Body sway of children aged 6 years was positively correlated with the maximal blood Pb level recorded at 2 years of age (Bhattacharya et al., 1988) and was selectively increased when the test was conducted without visual or proprioceptive cues (Bhattacharya et al., 1990; Bhattacharya and Linz, 1991). Sway-test performance improved with chelation therapy in an adult who had subacute Pb intoxication (Linz et al., 1992). Increased body sway was found in workers following long-term exposure to solvents (Ledin et al., 1989). The literature concerning solvents is particularly interesting because sway apparently can be "improved" by low-level exposure to organic solvents, but worsened by higher-level exposures (see review of Arlien-Soberg, 1992).

Functional Observational Battery

A battery of end points may be more likely to detect an effect than any single test. The functional observational battery (FOB) required by the U.S. Environmental Protection Agency (1985) is a neurological examination for rodents adapted from pharmaceutical screening. A number of studies have indicated that the FOB is capable of differentiating between toxicants of different chemical classes and that a number of labs can develop proficiency in the procedure (Moser et al., 1988, 1992; Tilson and Moser, 1992; Shell et al., 1992). The FOB has proved roughly equal to schedule-controlled behavior in sensitivity to several toxic agents. The FOB may be less sensitive than locomotor activity (Burleigh-Flayer et al., 1992), which is a more quantitative and less time-consuming procedure. Current work is exploring ways to abbreviate the FOB. Additional problems with the technique include potential for experimenter bias due to the semiquantitative nature of the technique, and health hazards to animal and investigator because the evaluation requires extensive handling of the animal. An advantage of the FOB is that it resembles the clinical neurological examination used by physicians for quick evaluation of humans.

Naturalistic Behavior in Humans

The value of observing human behavior in the natural environment was pointed out by Barocas and Weiss (1974) and by Robins (1981). Several techniques can be used as alternatives to paper-and-pencil tests or clinical examinations of the type described by Anger (1992). For example, prenatal alcohol exposure causes behavioral changes in children (Streissguth et al., 1984). Until recently, there have been few techniques that could be used with extremely young children. The key to successful testing of young children is to define and measure a response that infants are capable of producing, e.g., direction of gaze while looking at a target (Diamond, 1990). We expect to see more research with human infants by the time our next review is completed. Of the behavioral effects reviewed in this chapter, gait, tremor, and postural sway have been used most often with human subjects in toxicology and occupational medicine.

ETHOTOXICOLOGY: BEHAVIORAL INTERACTIONS BETWEEN INDIVIDUALS

Unfortunately, behavioral changes are seldom included in environmental assessments. Chemical analyses of water or air are typically monitored, but biological effects are less commonly used in environmental assessments. Very few studies have focused on behavior in nature (Little and Henry, 1990). Most studies of higher animals occur in lab settings; the distinguishing feature of this part of the scientific literature is the focus on two or more animals. We will review progress since the reviews of Davis (1982).

Predator-Prey Interactions

Predator-prey interactions focus on events that are critical to survival. The win-lose aspect of this interaction makes these studies of obvious relevance. The behaviors in question may result in either acquisition of food for the predator or survival for the prey. These behaviors are highly complex sequences of behaviors. For the predator, these behaviors may include prey seeking and stalking, prey capture and manipulation, and prey ingestion. For the prey species, predator avoidance may involve freezing, activity, or social behaviors.

Predation

Fenitrothion, an organophosphate pesticide, interferes with predation by decreasing distance of reaction to brine shrimp prey in adult (Morgan and Kiceniuk, 1991) and juvenile (Morgan and Kiceniuk, 1990) Atlantic salmon. After pesticide exposure, the prey had to be closer to elicit the salmon's attack response. Exposed salmon also captured fewer shrimp per attempt.

Weber et al. (1991) found that waterborne lead increased number of miscues and feeding time in juvenile fathead minnows preying on *Daphnia magna*. There also was an interaction between lead dose and prey size affecting feeding efficiency, in that lead effects were greater with larger prey. Therefore, lead decreased feeding efficiency by increasing the number of errors an intoxicated subject made in predatory behavior, by increasing the feeding time and by decreasing the distance at which the predator reacted to the prey. The authors interpret this as a lead-induced change in motor behavior rather than an effect on appetite, since the intoxicated minows attempted to consume all that was offered to them.

Hahn et al. (1991) found that lead acetate in the drinking water resulted in a tendency for male mice to attack cricket prey more quickly and increased the likelihood that female mice would attack the rear legs of the crickets first. This toxicant-induced change in attack strategy reduced the mouse's feeding efficiency, because the cricket's rear legs are readily detached from its body, permitting the cricket to escape.

Sandheinrich and Atchison (1989) investigated the effects of copper on the bluegill's foraging for five different prey types. They found that copper decreased the capture and consumption of zooplankton by bluegills and increased the amount of time spent investigating and manipulating prey (handling time), with no effects on the distance from the prey before the bluegills responded (reaction distance). The increase in handling time was greater for small prey than for large prey. Prey handling was the component of the foraging sequence most sensitive to copper intoxication. These findings indicate that copper increases the energy cost of certain components of foraging, such as the amount of time devoted to handling the prey, and therefore decreases the net energy gain for the predator by increasing the handling and decreasing the consumption of the prey.

The overall finding of this body of literature is that predators exposed to toxicants are less efficient in their pursuit and capture of prey. They seem to employ less optimal feeding strategies, are less reactive to the prey, and make more errors that allow the prey to escape. In addition, capture and consumption of larger prey were more affected than those of smaller prey.

Predation as a Route of Exposure

Species-typical feeding behavior is an important determinant of exposure to environmental toxicants. Frank and Braun (1990) analyzed organochloride residues in dead birds collected over a 16-year period. The lowest levels of brain residues were found in seed-eating birds, with higher residues in aquatic birds, e.g., loons and herons. Raptors had levels equivalent to those found in the aquatic birds, but with a much higher variability. The highest levels of organochloride residues were in gulls and terns, which may reflect the type of food eaten and the particular ecosystem in which each species lives.

Predator-Avoidance Behavior

Bildstein and Forsyth (1979) measured the effects of 10 ppm of dieldrin on the reaction of mice to a hawk predator flying overhead, in a laboratory setting. Dieldrin treatment resulted in increased locomotor activity, such as increased excitability during handling and increased somersaulting. In addition, during hawk reaction trials, the treated mice showed less reaction to the hawk and decreased freezing. Since the normal antipredator reaction of mice is to freeze, thereby making themselves a less salient stimulus for the visually oriented hawk, increased activity rendered the treated mice much more vulnerable to predation by the hawk. This increased vulnerability of the toxicant-exposed prey means that the predator's diet will have higher levels of toxicant. This is compatible with evidence that raptors tend to be sensitive to the effects of pesticides and tend to bioconcentrate the chemicals (Frank and Braun, 1990; Young et al., 1979).

Buerger et al. (1991) found that a high dose of methyl parathion decreased survival in wild Northern bobwhites. According to evidence obtained from postmortem inspections, this decreased survival was due to increased predation, not overt toxicity from the parathion. A possible reason for increased predation may be separation of the intoxicated bird from its covey, i.e., a group of quail. The covey is a behavioral defense mechanism that facilitates communication when a predator is detected. Behavioral toxicity thus weakens the rigid social network required for the covey to function effectively.

Reduced behavioral activity levels after exposure to a high dose (8 mg/kg) of methyl parathion increased the susceptibility of bobwhite quail to predation by domestic cats (Galindo et al., 1985). Treated quail spent less time walking and more time standing still, both before and after exposure to a predator cat in a lab setting. Exposed quail were more likely to be captured if they spent significantly more time standing still and less time walking before introduction of the cat. Toxicant-induced reduction in acetylcholinesterase activity was correlated with the quails' maladaptive behavior and with capture by the cat.

Hatfield and Anderson (1972) reported that fenitrothion or DDT reduced the ability of Atlantic salmon yearlings to escape predation by brook trout. Exposed salmon were less active and thus less able to escape predation by outswimming the trout. The effects of the pesticides also may involve specific antipredator strategies by the salmon yearlings, but this was not assessed.

Brown et al. (1985) measured the effects of pentachlorophenol on predator-avoidance behavior in juvenile guppies. These authors found that this toxicant did not consistently affect habitat use or the general behavior of the guppies. However, in the presence of bass predators, the guppies were more often alone, motionless, and in a different area of the habitat. In addition, the increased capture success of the predator species was due in large part to the decreased ability of intoxicated guppies to escape predation. These changes were reflected in decreased ability of guppies to accelerate and maintain acceleration in response to predator exposure.

In general, the consequences for survival of a toxicant-induced change in locomotor activity depend on the normal response to predation. In some instances, decreases in prey's activity may make it less detectable to predators; conversely, *increased* activity levels may result in greater predation (Bildstein and Forsyth, 1979). In other instances, those animals with decreased activity are *more* likely to be captured. These different outcomes emphasize the importance of understanding the predator as well as the prey. A visually oriented predator relies on the prey's movement, while other predators rely on their ability to outrun their prey. Quail and fish usually try to outrun their predators. Toxicants that compromise this ability also compromise survival (Brown et al., 1985; Hatfield and Anderson, 1972). Finally, the behavior of a group (quail in coveys or fish in schools) often aids in predator detection and antipredator activity. However, if an intoxicated member of the covey or school has decreased stamina and endurance and is unable to keep up with other members of the group, it is more likely that the intoxicated animal will be caught (e.g., Myllyvirta and Vuorinen, 1989).

Territoriality and Social and Aggressive Behavior

Drug-modified aggressive behavior is studied primarily in laboratory models with rodents (Miczek et al., 1989; Garmendia et al., 1992). Environmental toxicants have been studied with a wider variety of models, mostly in lab settings. Insecticides can increase aggressive behavior of chickens (Farage-Elawar and Francis, 1988). Fish have been the subject of several studies. Fenitrothion affects territorial defense in young Atlantic salmon, resulting in dose-dependent decreases in the number of salmon defending territories, especially in those subjects that were territorial before removal for control or insecticide treatment (Symons, 1973). Some treated fish showed decreases in feeding and swimming ability that lasted for 24–48 h after dosing. In addition, some subjects that had been dominant became completely subordinate and did not regain their territories for 2–3 weeks after treatment.

Bull and McInerney (1974) investigated the dose-dependent effects of fenitrothion on agonistic, feeding, and comfort behaviors in nuvenile Coho salmon. Fenitrothion resulted in dose-dependent decreases in several agonistic behaviors, including displays, flights, and vacating. Decreases in feeding, chewing, and yawns and increases in coughs, thrusts, and flicks were seen. The low-dose increases in comfort behaviors were interpreted as an irritant response, since there were no effects on locomotor behavior. At higher doses, there were effects on locomotor behavior that resulted in decreases in comfort behaviors and the inability of fish to maintain their position in the current. Decreases in agonistic behaviors and changes in territoriality are ecologically important in this species.

Exposure to metals frequently is reported to increase several aspects of aggressive behavior. Hyperaggressive behavior has been observed in laboratory rats exposed to trimethyltin and mercury (Evans et al., 1975). This is interpreted as resulting from damage to limbic structures known to regulate emotion. Burright et al. (1989) investigated the effects of lead on postpartum aggression in female mice toward intruder males. The results showed an increase in the duration and frequency of fighting with intruders. The increases in aggression were accompanied by decreased prolactin levels. Hahn et al. (1991) investigated the effects of lead on food competition and social contact in mice. They found that lead resulted in increased food possession time and increased social contacts. This increase in social contacts was not due to an increase in agonistic behavior; in fact, there was a nonsignificant decrease in agonistic behavior among the lead-treated animals.

In most territorial species, dominant animals reproduce most often, and their offspring probably have increased chances of survival. By affecting territoriality, environmental contaminants alter the survival of the contaminated animals. Agonistic and territorial behavior help insure adequate feeding areas for the competing animals. Disruption of stable social structure should lead to poorer food utilization and distribution.

Reproductive and Parental Behaviors: Offspring Development

As with predator-prey relationships, reproductive behaviors are a highly complex sequence involving two animals. Reproductive behaviors include courtship, mating, and parental behavior. These behaviors are often species-specific, vary little between individuals of the same species, occur with little or no learning involved, and are instinctual (hard-wired). Some references are summarized in Table 2.

Reproductive Displays

Schroder and Peters (1988a,b) measured the effects of lindane and waste water on reproductive displays in male guppies. Both treatments caused a decrease in the frequency and duration of courtship displays and an increase in thrusting toward a female. These

Table 2 Compounds Affecting Predator/Prey, Reproductive, or Social Behaviors

Compound	Species	Reference
Effects on predator behavior		
Fenitrothion	Fish	Morgan and Kiceniuk, 1990, 1991
Copper	Fish	Sandheinrich and Atchison, 1989
Lead	Mice	Hahn et al., 1991
Lead	Fish	Weber et al., 1991
Effects on predator-avoidance behavior		
Dieldrin	Mice	Bildstein and Forsyth, 1979
Methyl parathion	Birds	Buerger et al., 1991
		Galindo et al., 1985
Fenitrothion	Fish	Hatfield and Anderson, 1972
Pentachlorophenol	Fish	Brown et al., 1985
Lead	Birds	Burger and Gochfeld, 1993
Effects on territorial and social behavior		
Fenitrothion	Fish	Symons, 1973
		Bull and McInerney, 1974
Lead	Mice	Burright et al., 1989
		Hahn et al., 1991
Effects on reproductive and parental behavior		
Lindane and waste water	Fish	Schroder and Peters, 1988a,b
Methyl parathion	Birds	Bennett et al., 1991
		Meyers et al., 1990
Dictrophos	Birds	Grue et al., 1982
Carbofuran	Ducks	Martin et al., 1991

changes tend to decrease the probability of reproduction, since more active males have a greater chance of encountering receptive females and are preferred by females (i.e., courtship displays are a primary determinant of reproductive success). The male's sexual behavior (gonopodial thrusting) occurs more often when a female is not in the receptive cycle.

Egg Laying and Incubation

Methyl parathion has been studied in several species. The number of eggs laid by exposed mallard hens was significantly decreased (Bennett et al., 1991). These hens either stopped laying eggs and started incubating soon after treatment, or returned to their original clutch or abandoned their own clutch and initiated a new clutch. Hens treated during incubation were more likely to abandon their nest. Treatments early in incubation resulted in greater effect than treatments later in incubation. In addition, there were more signs of acute organophosphate poisoning during incubation than during egg laying. Gulls also decrease incubation time after exposure to parathion (White et al., 1983).

Red-winged blackbirds exposed to methyl parathion exhibited overt signs of toxicity and required a longer time to return to the nest after dosing (Meyers et al., 1990). Since the parents spent less time on the nest, eggs or nestlings would have been left unprotected and exposed to predators. While parathion resulted in some short-term effects on reproductive behavior, there were no long-term treatment effects on percent hatched and percent fledged.

Grue et al. (1982) measured the effects of dicrotophos, an organophosphate pesticide, on the care of nestlings by female starlings. They found that toxicant-treated females made fewer trips to feed their young and spent significantly more time away from the nest boxes than control females.

In general, parathion resulted in the production of fewer offspring, as a result of either decreased egg laying, increased nest abandonment, or increased time off the nest during incubation. Laboratory studies may underestimate the effect of returning to the nest in the wild, since in the laboratory the visual stimulus of the brood is much more salient, and the brood would be unprotected from predators in the wild. Greater toxicity during incubation may have resulted from the depletion of lipid reserves that commonly occurs during incubation.

These studies show that pesticides degrade the reproductive and parental behavior of animals by decreasing the amount of attention a parent pays to its young. Exposed parents spend more time away from the nest and less time laying eggs and incubating the eggs. These behaviors by the parent lead to increased exposure of the eggs or young to the elements or predators and decrease the likelihood of survival of the offspring.

Imprinting

Martin et al. (1991) studied the effects of carbofuran, a carbamate insecticide, on imprinting-induced activity in mallard ducklings. The ducklings were released in an area 60–90 min after carbofuran had been applied by air in one of three concentrations when the vegetation was dry. They were exposed in these three areas and allowed to walk three different distances. The behavioral testing involved the approach response toward an attractive stimulus: a group of similarly aged ducklings and a tape recording of the previous vocalization used to imprint these ducklings. Latency to approaching the stimuli was increased by two aspects of dosage: the concentration (spray rate) and the distance the duckling was allowed to travel in the exposure area. In addition, there was an interaction between these two factors; i.e., the longer distances traveled with the high dose of carbofuran resulted in slower approach times than the longer distances with the lower or control concentrations. Within the higher-dose group, ducklings exposed to the longer-distance treatments had slower approach rates than ducklings that walked shorter distances.

Slower approaches of intoxicated ducklings to imprinting stimuli probably decrease survival in the wild. Nonintoxicated ducklings maintain close contact with their mother and the rest of the brood. This maintenance of brood integrity probably allows rapid movement through the environment; rapid movement protects the ducklings from predators because they can hide more easily as a cohesive group. However, when intoxicated ducklings are slow to approach the rest of the brood or the hen, the hen and the unaffected brood remain near the slow or intoxicated duckling, apparently in response to distress vocalizations. Thus, a single intoxicated duckling may slow the entire brood, causing the brood to hide less effectively. Therefore, the entire brood would be more susceptible to predation as a result of intoxication of one or a few ducklings, since they would be traveling at a slower rate and might be more exposed to predators in unprotected areas.

GENERAL CONCLUSIONS

Can Behavior Provide Definitive Evidence of Neurotoxicity?

Evidence of target-organ specificity comes from the comparison of dose-response curves for several different organ systems. If indices of nervous system function are affected at doses below those that alter function of other organ systems, one may presume that the nervous system is the target organ. Morphological change has been the traditional "gold standard" for neurotoxicity. Histopathology can point to the anatomical structures and the cell population that are most prominently affected but can seldom define the functional consequence of the lesion. In contrast, the apical screens of behavior and other nervous system functions seldom identify a specific cell population.

As pointed out by Tilson and Moser (1992), many tests are sensitive (i.e. reliably indicate the effects of low doses), but few seem to have been demonstrated to be specific (i.e., to reflect specific damage to the nervous system rather than to some other organ system). Funding has seldom been directed toward the study of the negative control substances that are needed to demonstrate specificity (Weissman, 1990).

Behavioral results of the type illustrated in this chapter can suggest second-tier studies that illuminate mechanisms of toxicity. We cannot demand that a brief first-tier test provide all the data needed to decide among alternative hypotheses concerning target organ. Tests are more useful in screening if they can document secondary as well as primary effects, because data of either type can be used to protect the worker or consumer, even before details of the primary or secondary site of toxic action become known. Thus, locomotor behavior is valuable as an apical screen because of its well-documented ability to mark impairment at any of several levels in the nervous system or in other systems.

How Does Behavior Compare with Other End Points?

It is difficult to conclude, because behavior has seldom been compared directly with other end points. Neurotoxicity testing has almost never afforded behavioral studies equality to pathology studies, in terms of budget for equipment and manpower. Without a level playing field, comparisons are impossible.

Naturalistic Behavior Is as Sensitive as Other Types of Behavior

Although the various techniques for documenting behavioral toxicology seldom have been compared directly, our review suggests that differences in dose-response functions are small in the perspective of toxicity screening (i.e., most end points change within one half log unit, and few exceed one log unit). Drugs and toxicants affect a wide variety of behaviors at similar doses (within one half to one log unit). Toxicants show little respect for the labels and schemes of classifying behavior (learned vs. unlearned; higher order vs. reflexive; natural vs. artificial). Efficiency is an advantage of reflexes and unlearned behavior.

What Are the Trade-offs in Study of Exotic Species Instead of Common Lab Animals?

Have we discovered something with an exotic species that could not have been learned with a commonly available lab animal? Certainly, the understanding of emesis required an alternative to the rat. Most of the other topics reviewed here (foraging, reproductive and parental behaviors, predation, gait) can be studied with the common lab animals.

Can "Apical" Tests Provide Sufficient Information for First-Tier Screening?

An apical test is one that reflects change at any of the many integrated centers within the nervous system. Body weight and spontaneous locomotor behavior are perhaps the two most prevalent examples. Most behavioral tests (tremor, food consumption, visual discrimination) are capable of indicating changes in any of several anatomical sites. Despite seemingly valid philosophical objections, data continue to accumulate in support of the conclusion that the rodent's motor activity is a sufficiently sensitive and very practical test of toxicity.

What Are the Trade-offs Between Longer and Shorter Test Batteries?

Our review suggests that it may be time to reconsider the reliance on large test batteries for toxicity screening. Of course, batteries were never popular in mechanistic research. Most scientists have endorsed the rationale that more is better, or in the words of Confucius, "let a thousand flowers bloom." Thus, considerable effort has been devoted to assembling test batteries with multiple end points in the hope that one end point will prove to be much more sensitive than the others, or that it will detect a toxic effect that would have escaped detection by other battery items. Our review suggests that many items of behavior are highly correlated with each other, i.e., are redundant. If this is true, testing could be streamlined with little loss of sensitivity, but with a valuable gain in efficiency, much to the benefit of a society with too little funds to evaluate all chemicals.

In reviewing work with the FOB and with computerized image analyses, we find examples of the prevailing assumption that increasing the number of end points will increase the odds of detecting a toxic effect. Batteries with large numbers of end points create new statistical issues, such as intercorrelation and correcting for experiment-wise alpha inflation (Tilson and Moser, 1992). Just to be contrary, we might assert that the various items of rodent locomotion (stepping, rearing, walking, grooming) are partly correlated and that any single behavioral end point would provide a satisfactory dose-response determination in screening for neurotoxicity. Statistical methods are available to test our assertion. Multiple regression analyses can quantify the increment in detection or sensitivity gained by the addition of each endpoint to the battery. The identification of "domains" of effects on the FOB is a step in this direction (Tilson and Moser, 1992). The value of multiple end points may be greater for basic research, where studying a variety of end points may help to identify the underlying mechanisms of toxicity.

Promising New Methods

New methods have transformed all of neurobiology by providing more sensitive or convenient assays. New in vitro methods may help to screen for drug- and transmitter-binding sites but have not yet replaced live animals in providing evidence of nervous system function, e.g., hunger, learning, and libido. Methods derived from ethology have helped the researcher to understand chemically induced changes in the behavior of a group of animals in an ecologically relevant setting. This information is important, both for basic knowledge of group functions and because group interactions represent an often-overlooked aspect of environmental assessment. However, experiments with groups cannot achieve a practical advantage for screening, since the group counts statistically only as N = 1 (Evans, 1989).

Controversies Requiring Further Research

Is habitat complexity important to behavioral toxicity? Obviously, one cannot conclude much about the effects of toxicants on predation unless one gets a predator and prey together for a test. However, results of simple feeding tests convey significant information about appetite for food and motor coordination in obtaining food. Performance of an individual animal on such a test may predict toxic effects on animals in a more complex environment, as when pursuing prey. There has been very little research on extrapolation from simple to complex tests.

ACKNOWLEDGMENTS

Supported in part by a Center Grant (ES-00260) and a Program Project Grant (ES-04895) at New York University Medical Center and by an award from the Faculty Development Committee at Mercy College. We thank Hassan El-Fawal for contributions to the section on gait and postural sway.

REFERENCES

Akins JM, Schroeder JA, Brower DL, Aposhian HV (1992). Evaluation of drosophila-melanogaster as an alternative animal for studying the neurotoxicity of heavy metals. Biol Metals 5:111–20.
Anderson LT, Campbell M, Adams P, Small AM, Pery R, Shell J (1989). The effects of haloperidol on discrimination learning and behavioral symptoms in autistic children. J Autism Dev Disord 19:227–39.
Anger WK (1992). Assessment of neurotoxicity in humans. In: Tilson HA, Mitchell CL, eds. Neurotoxicology. New York: Raven Press, 363–86.
Arlien-Soborg P (1992). Solvent neurotoxicity. Boca Raton, Florida: CRC Press.
Ashmead DH, McCarty ME (1991). Postural sway of human infants while standing in light and dark. Child Dev 62:1276–87.

Baatrup E (1991). Structural and functional effects of heavy metals on the nervous system, including sense organs, of fish. Comp Biochem Physiol 100C:253–257.

Bachevalier J, Landis LS, Walker LC, Brickson M, Mishkin M, Price DL, Cork LC (1991). Aged monkeys exhibit behavioral deficits indicative of widespread cerebral dysfunction. Neurobiol Aging 12:99–111.

Banaji MR, Crowder RG (1991). Some everyday thoughts on ecologically valid methods. Am Psychologist 46:78–9.

Barocas R, Weiss B (1974). Behavioral assessment of lead intoxication in children. Environ Health Perspect 7:47–52.

Bell RQ (1968). Adaptation of small wrist watches for mechanical recording of activity in infants and children. J Exp Child Psychol 6:302–5.

Bennett RS, Williams BA, Schmedding DW, Bennett JK (1991). Effect of dietary exposure to methyl parathion on egg laying and incubation in mallards. Environ Toxicol Chem 10:501–6.

Bhattacharya A, Shukla R, Bornschein RL, Dietrich KN, Keith R (1990). Lead effects on postural balance of children. Environ Health Perspect 89:35–42.

Bhattacharya A, Linz DH (1991). Postural sway analysis of a teenager with childhood lead intoxication: a case study. Clin Pediatr 30:543–8.

Bhattacharya A, Shukla R, Bornschein RL, Dietrich KN, Kopke JE (1988). Postural disequilibrium quantification in children with chronic lead exposure: a pilot study. Neurotoxicology 9:327–40.

Bildstein KL, Forsyth DJ (1979). Effects of dietary dieldrin on behavior of white-footed mice (Peromyscus leucopus) towards an avian predator. Bull Environ Contam Toxicol 21:93–7.

Blackburn TP, Cox B, Heapy G, Lee TF (1982). Possible mechanism of 5-methoxy-N,N-dimethyltryptamine–induced turning behavior in DRN lesioned rats. Pharmacol Biochem Behav 16:7–11.

Blin O, Ferrandez AM, Pailhous J, Serratrice G (1991). Dopa-sensitive and dopa-resistent gait parameters in Parkinson's disease. J Neurol Sci 103:51–4.

Boyer IJ, Cory-Slechta DA, DiStefano V (1985). Lead induction of crop dysfunction in pigeons through a direct action on neural or smooth muscle components of crop tissue. J Pharmacol Exp Ther 234:607–15.

Brown JA, Johansen PH, Colgan PW, Mathers RA (1985). Changes in the predator-avoidance behavior of juvenile guppies (Poecilia reticulata) exposed to pentachlorophenol. Can J Zool 63:2001–5.

Buerger TT, Kendall RJ, Mueller BS, DeVos T, Williams BA (1991). Effects of methyl parathion on northern bobwhite survivability. Environ Toxicol Chem 10:527–32.

Bull CJ, McInerney JE (1974). Behavior of juvenile Coho salmon (Oncorhychus kisutch) exposed to Sumithion (fenitrothion), an organophosphate insecticide. J Fish Res Board Can 31:1867–72.

Burdette LJ, Goldstein R (1986). Long-term behavioral and electrophysiological changes associated with lead exposure at different stages of brain development in the rat. Dev Brain Res 29:101–10.

Burleigh-Flayer HD, Gill MW, Marino DJ, Masten LW, McKee RH, Tyler TR (1992). Isopropanol 14-week vapor inhalation study in rats and mice with neurotoxicity evaluation in rats. Toxicologist 12:277 (Abstract).

Burright RG, Engellenner WJ, Donovick PJ (1989). Postpartum aggression and plasma prolactin levels in mice exposed to lead. Physiol Behav 46:889–93.

Bushnell PJ, Evans HL (1985). Effects of trimethyltin on patterns of homecage behavior in rats. Toxicol Appl Pharmacol 79:134–42.

Bushnell PJ, Evans HL (1986). Diurnal patterns in homecage behavior of rats after acute exposure to triethyltin. Toxicol Appl Pharmacol 85:346–54.

Calhoun JB (1963). The social use of space. In: Mayer LW, Van Gelder R, eds. Physiological mammalogy. New York: Academic Press, 2–187.

Calhoun JB (1973). Death squared: the explosive growth and demise of a mouse population. Proc R Soc Med 66:80–8.

Carpenter DO, Briggs DB, Knox AP, Strominger NL (1986). Radiation-induced emesis in the dog: effects of lesions and drugs. Radiation Res 108:307–16.

Carpenter DO, Briggs DB, Strominger N (1984). Behavioral and electrophysiological studies of peptide-induced emesis in dogs. Fed Proc 43:2952–4.

Chapman LJ, Sauter SL, Henning RA, Levine RL, Matthews CG, Peters HA (1991). Finger tremor after carbon disulfide–based pesticide exposures. Arch Neurol 48:866–70.

Clarke KA, Steadman P (1989). Abnormal locomotion in the rat after administration of a TRH analogue. Neuropeptides 14:65–70.

Colburn TR, Smith BM, Guarini JJ, Simmons NN (1976). An ambulatory activity monitor with solid state memory. ISA Transactions 5:149–54.

Cory-Slechta DA, Garman RH, Seidman D (1980). Lead-induced crop dysfunction in the pigeon. Toxicol Appl Pharmacol 52:462–7.

Crofton KM (1992). Reflex modification and the assessment of sensory dysfunction. In: Tilson H, Mitchell C, eds. Neurotoxicology. New York: Raven Press, 181–211.

Crofton KM, Howard JL, Moser VC, Gill MW, Reiter LW, Tilson HA, MacPhail RC (1991). Interlaboratory comparison of motor activity experiments: implications for neurotoxicological assessments. Neurotoxicol Teratol 13:599–609.

Crofton KM, Reiter LW (1988). The effects of type I and type II pyrethroids on motor activity and the acoustic startle response in the rat. Toxicol Appl Pharmacol 10:624–34.

Dam MD, Gopal K (1991). Neurobehavioral changes in freshwater fish (Channa punctatus) exposed to fenitrothion. Bull Environ Contam Toxicol 47:455–8.

Daniel SA, El-Fawal HAN, Moon FR, Evans HL (1990). Effects of acrylamide on neurobehavioral function in the pigeon. Pharmacol Biochem Behav 36:436 (Abstract).

Davis JD, Smith GP (1992). Analysis of the microstructure of the rhythmic tongue movements of rats ingesting maltose and sucrose solutions. Behav Neurosci 106:217–28.

Davis JM (1982). Ethological approaches to behavioral toxicology. In: Mitchell C, ed. Nervous system toxicology. New York: Raven Press, 29–44.

De Medinaceli L, Freed WJ, Wyatt RJ (1982). An index of the functional condition of rat sciatic nerve based on measurements made from walking tracks. Exp Neurol 77:634–43.

De Medinaceli L, DeRenzo E, Wyatt RJ (1984). Rat sciatic functional index data management system with digitized input. Comput Biomed Res 17:185–92.

Del Pup JA, Pasternack BS, Harley NH, Kane PB, Palmes ED (1978). Effects of DDT on stable laboratory mouse populations. J Toxicol Environ Health 4:671–87.

Dempster AM, Evans HL, Snyder CA (1984). The temporal relationship between behavioral and hematological effects of inhaled benzene. Toxicol Appl Pharmacol 76:195–203.

Dewsbury D (1978). Comparative animal behavior. New York: McGraw-Hill.

Diamond A (1990). The development and neural bases of memory functions as indexed by the AB and delayed response tasks in human infants and infant monkeys. Ann NY Acad Sci 608:267–316.

Dinnel PA, Stober QJ, DiJulio DH (1979). Behavioral responses of shiner perch to chlorinated primary sewage effluent. Bull Environ Contam Toxicol 22:708–14.

Eaton WO, McKeen NA, Lam C-S (1988). Instrumented motor activity measurement of the young infant in the home: validity and reliability. Infant Behav Dev 11:375–8.

Edwards PM, Sporel-Ozakat RE, Gispen WH (1991). Peripheral pain fiber function is relatively insensitive to the neurotoxic actions of acrylamide in the rat. Toxicol Appl Pharmacol 111:43–8.

Ema M, Itami T, Kawasaki H (1991). Behavioral effects of acute exposure to tributyltin chloride in rats. Neurotoxicol Teratol 13:489–93.

Eriksson P, Fredriksson A (1991). Neurotoxic effects of two different pyrethroids, bioallethrin and deltamethrin, on immature and adult mice: changes in behavioral and muscarinic receptor variables. Toxicol Appl Pharmacol 108:78–85.

Eriksson P, Lundkvist U, Fredriksson A (1991). Neonatal exposure to 3,3′,4,4′-tetrachlorobiphenyl: changes in spontaneous behavior and cholinergic muscarinic receptors in the adult mouse. Toxicology 69:27–34.

Evans HL (1982). Assessment of vision in toxicology. In: Mitchell CL, ed. Nervous system toxicology. New York: Raven Press, 81-107.

Evans HL (1988). Quantitation of naturalistic behaviors. Toxicol Lett 43:345–59.

Evans HL (1989). Behaviors in the home cage reveal toxicity: recent findings and proposals for the future. J Am Coll Toxicol 8:35–52.

Evans HL, Bushnell PJ, Taylor JD, Monico A, Teal JJ, Pontecorvo M (1986). A system for assessing toxicity of chemicals by continuous monitoring of homecage behaviors. Fund Appl Toxicol 6:721–32.

Evans HL, Dempster AM, Snyder CA (1981). Behavioral changes in mice following benzene inhalation. Neurobehav Toxicol Teratol 3:481–5.

Evans HL, Garman RH, Laties VG (1982). Neurotoxicity of methylmercury in the pigeon. Neurotoxicology 3:21–36.

Evans HL, Laties VG, Weiss B (1975). Behavioral effects of mercury and methylmercury. Fed Proc 34:1858–67.

Evans HL, Little A, Gong ZL, Duffy JS, Wirgin I, El-Fawal HAN (1993). Glial fibrillary acidic protein (GFAP) indicates in vivo exposure to environmental contaminants: PCB in the Atlantic Tomcod. Ann NY Acad Sci 679:402–406.

Evans HL, Taylor JD (in preparation) Pharmacological and behavioral manipulation of visual vigilance in the primate.

Evans HL, Taylor JD, Ernst J, Graefe J (1989). Methods to evaluate the wellbeing of laboratory primates: comparisons of macaques and tamarins. Lab Animal Sci 39:318–23.

Farage-Elawar M (1988). Toxicity of aldicarb in young chicks. Neurotoxicol Teratol 10:549–54.

Farage-Elawar M (1989). Enzyme and behavioral changes in young chicks as a result of carbaryl treatment. J Toxicol Environ Health 26:119–31.

Farage-Elawar M, Duggy JS, Francis BM (1989). Developmental toxicity of desbromoleptophos in chicks: enzyme inhibition, malformations and functional deficits. Neurotoxicol Teratol 13:91–7.

Farage-Elawar M, Francis BM (1988). Effects of fenthion, fenitrothion and desbromoleptophos on gait, acetylcholinesterase, and neurotoxic esterase in young chicks after in ovo exposure. Toxicology 49:253–61.

Farr JA (1980). Social behavior patterns as determinants of reproductive success in the guppy (poecilia reticulata)—an experimental study of the effects of intermale competition, female choice, and sexual selection. Behavior 74:38–91.

Ferguson SA, Bowman RE (1990). A nonhuman primate version of the open field test for use in behavioral toxicology and teratology. Neurotoxicol Teratol 12:477–81.

Ferguson SA, Bowman RE (1992). Effects of arecoline and scopolamine on open field behavior of adult monkeys treated with lead during the first year postpartum. Neurotoxicol Teratol 14:73–80.

Fitzgerald RE, Berres M, Schaeppi U (1988). Validation of a photobeam system for assessment of motor activity in rats. Toxicology 49:433–9.

Flecknell PA, Liles JH (1992). Evaluation of locomotor activity and food and water consumption as a method of assessing postoperative pain in rodents. In: Short CE, Van Poznak A, eds. Animal pain. New York: Churchill Livingstone, 482–505.

Fleming WJ, Hill EF, Momot JJ, Pang VF (1991). Toxicity of trimethyltin and triethyltin to mallard ducklings. Environ Toxicol Chem 10:255–60.

Forkman BA, Ljungberg T, Johnson AC, Nylen P, Stahle L, Hoglund G, Ungerstedt U (1991). Long-term effects of toluene inhalation on rat behavior. Neurotoxicol Teratol 13:475–81.

Foss JA, Lochry EA (1991). The assessment of motor activity in neonatal and adult rodents using passive infrared sensors. Presentation at American College of Toxicology annual meeting. Savannah, GA.

Fowler SC, Mortell C (1992). Low doses of haloperidol interfere with rat tongue extensions during licking: a quantitative analysis. Behav Neurosci 106:386–95.

Frank R, Braun HE (1990). Organochlorine residues in bird species collected dead in Ontario 1972–1988. Bull Environ Contam Toxicol 44:932–9.

Galindo JC, Kendall RJ, Driver CJ, Lacher TE Jr (1985). The effect of methyl parathion on susceptibility of bobwhite quail (Colinus virginianus) to domestic cat predation. Behav Neural Biol 43:21–36.

Garmendia L, Sanchez JR, Azpiroz A, Brain PF, Simon VM (1992). Clozapine: strong antiaggressive effects with minimal motor impairment. Physiol Behav 51:51–4.

Geckler JR, Horning WB, Neiheisel QH, Robinson EL, Stephen CE (1986). Validity of laboratory tests for predicting copper toxicity in streams. Washington, D.C: U.S. Environmental Protection Agency Ecological Resource Service. EPA-600/3-76-116.

Gerhart JM, Hong JS, Uphouse JL, Tilson HA (1982). Chlordecone-induced tremor in rats. Toxicol Appl Pharmacol 66:234–43.

Gerhart JM, Hong JS, Tilson HA (1983). Studies on the possible sites of chlordecone-induced tremor in rats. Toxicol Appl Pharmacol 70:382–9.

Grue CE, Powell GVN, McChesney MJ (1982). Care of nestlings by wild female starlings exposed to an organophosphate pesticide. J Appl Ecol 19:327–35.

Hahn ME, Burright RG, Donovick PJ (1991). Lead effects on food competition and predatory aggression in Binghamton HET mice. Physiol Behav 50:757–64.

Hannigan JH, Riley EP (1988). Prenatal ethanol alters gait in rats. Alcohol 5:451–4.

Hatfield CT, Anderson JM (1972). Effects of two insecticides on the vulnerability of Atlantic salmon (Salmo salar) parr to brook trout (Salvelinos fontinalis) predation. J Fish Res Board Can 29:27–9.

Henry MG, Atchison GJ (1991). Metal effects on fish behavior—advances in determining the ecological significance of responses. In: Newman MC, McIntosh AW, eds. Metal ecotoxicology, concepts and applications. Chelsea, Michigan: Lewis, 131–43.

Holtzman SG, Young CW (1991). Motor activity of squirrel monkeys measured with an ultrasonic motion sensor. Pharmacol Biochem Behav 38:633–7.

Hruska RE, Kennedy S, Silbergeld EK (1979). Quantitative aspects of normal locomotion in rats. Life Sci 25:171–80.

Jolicoeur FB, Rondeau DB, Barbeau A (1979). Comparison of neurobehavioral effects induced by various experimental models of ataxia in the rat. Neurobehav Toxicol 1:175–8.

Kalaska JF, Crammond DJ (1992). Cerebral cortical mechanisms of reaching movements. Science 255:1517–24.

Kernan WJ, Hopper DL, Bowes MP (1991). Computer pattern recognition: spontaneous motor activity studies in rats following acute exposure to triethyltin. J Am Coll Toxicol 10:705–18.

King GL, Landauer MR (1990). Effects of zacopride and BMY25801 (batanopride) on radiation-induced emesis and locomotor behavior in the ferret. J Pharmacol Exp Ther 253:1026–33.

King KA, White DH, Mitchell CA (1984). Nest defense behavior and reproductive success of laughing gulls sublethally dosed with parathion. Bull Environ Contam Toxicol 33:499–504.

Komura J, Sakamoto M (1991). Short-term oral administration of several manganese compounds in mice: physiological and behavioral alterations caused by different forms of manganese. Bull Environ Contam Toxicol 46:921–8.

Kulig BM, Lammers JHCM (1992). Assessment of neurotoxicant induced effects on motor function. In: Tilson H, Mitchell C, eds. Neurotoxicology. New York: Raven Press, 147–79.

Laties VG, Evans HL (1980). Methylmercury-induced changes in an operant discrimination in the pigeon. J Pharmacol Exp Ther 214:620–8.

Ledin T, Odkvist LM, Moller C (1989). Posturography findings in workers exposed to industrial solvents. Acta Otolaryngol 107:357–61.

Lehner PN (1979). Handbook of ethological methods. New York: Garland STPM Press.

Levine TE (1976). Effects of carbon disulfide and FLA-63 on operant behavior in pigeons. J Pharmacol Exp Ther 199:669–78.

Lilienthal H, Winneke G, Brockhaus A, Molik B (1986). Pre- and postnatal lead-exposure in monkeys: effects on activity and learning set formation. Neurobehav Toxicol Teratol 8:265–72.

Linz DH, Barrett ET, Pflaumer JE, Keith RE (1992). Neuropsychological and postural sway improvement after Ca^{++}-EDTA chelation for mild lead intoxication. J Med 34:638–41.

Little EE, Henry MG (1990). Symposium on behavioral toxicology. Environ Toxicol Chem 9:1–120.

Lowdon IMR, Seaber AV, Urbaniak JR (1988). An improved method of recording rat tracks for measurement of the sciatic functional index of de Medinaceli. J Neurosci Meth 24:279–80.

Maier SE, Vandenhoff P, Crowne DP (1988). Multivariate analysis of putative measures of activity, exploration, emotionality, and spatial behavior in the hooded rat (Rattus norvegicus). J Comp Psychol 102:378–87.

Martin PA, Solomon KR, Forsyth DJ, Boermans HJ, Westcott ND (1991). Effects of exposure to carbofuran-srayed vegetation on the behavior, cholinesterase activity and growth of mallard ducklings (Anas platyrhynchos). Environ Toxicol Chem 10:901–9.

Maurissen JPJ, Mattsson JL (1989). Critical assessment of motor activity as a screen for neurotoxicity. Toxicol Indust Health 5:195–202.

Maurissen JPJ, Weiss B, Cox C (1990). Vibration sensitivity recovery after a second course of acrylamide intoxication. Fund Appl Toxicol 15:93–8.

McNaughton N, Morris RG (1987). Chlordiazepoxide, an anxiolytic benzodiazepine, impairs place navigation in rats. Behav Brain Res 24:39–46.

Meydani M, Post G (1979). Effect of sublethal concentrations of malathion on Coturnix quail. Bull Environ Contam Toxicol 21:661–7.

Meyer LS, Riley EP (1990). Alterations in gait following ethanol exposure during the brain growth spurt in rats. Alcoholism 14:23–7.

Meyers SM, Cummings JL, Bennett RS (1990). Effects of methyl parathion on red-winged blackbird (Agelaius phoeniceus) incubation behavior and nesting success. Environ Toxicol Chem 9:807–15.

Miczek KA, Haney M, Tidey J, Vatne T, Weerts E, DeBold JF (1989). Temporal and sequential patterns of agonistic behavior: effects of alcohol, anxiolytics and psychomotor stimulants. Psychopharmacology 97:149–51.

Montoya CP, Campbell-Hope LJ, Pemberton KD, Dunnett SB (1991). The "staircase test": a measure of independent forelimb reaching and grasping abilities in rats. J Neurosci Meth 36:219–28.

Morgan MJ, Kiceniuk JW (1990). Effect of fenitrothion on the foraging behavior of juvenile atlantic salmon. Environ Toxicol Chem 9:489–95.

Morgan MJ, Kiceniuk JW (1991). Recovery of foraging behavior of atlantic salmon exposed to a simulated commercial application of fenitrothion. Environ Toxicol Chem 10:961–5.

Moriarty F (1988). Ecotoxicology. Hum Toxicol 7:437–41.

Moser V, McCormich JP, Creson JP, MacPhail RC (1988). Comparison of chlordimeform and carbaryl using a functional observational battery. Fund Appl Toxicol 11:189–206.

Moser V, Anthony DC, Sette WF, MacPhail RC (1992). Comparison of subchronic neurotoxicity of 2-hydroxyethyl acrylate and acrylamide in rats. Fund Appl Toxicol 18:343–52.

Mullenix PJ, Kernan WJ, Tassinari MS, Schunior A, Waber DP, Howes A, Tarbell NJ (1990). An animal model to study toxicity of central nervous system therapy for childhood acute lymphoblastic leukemia: effects on behavior. Cancer Res 50:6461–5.

Muller PG, Crow RE, Cheney CD (1979). Schedule-induced locomotor activity in humans. J Exp Anal Behav 31:83–90.

Myllyvirta TP, Vuorinen PJ (1989). Effects of bleached kraft mill effluent (BKME) on the schooling behavior of vendace. Bull Environ Contam Toxicol 42:262–9.

Nation J, Baker DM, Taylor B, Clark DE (1986). Dietary lead increases ethanol consumption in the rat. Behav Neurosci 10:525–30.

Newby-Schmidt MB, Norton S (1980). Detection of subtle effects on the locomotor ability of the chicken. Neurobehav Toxicol Teratol 3:45–8.

Newland MC (1988). Quantification of motor function in toxicology. Toxicol Lett 43:295–319.

Novak MA, Suomi SJ (1988). Psychological well-being of primates in captivity. Am Psychologist 43:765–73.

Palmes ED, Del Pup J (1971). Procedure for the maintenance of stable laboratory mouse populations. Lab Animal Sci 21:932–6.

Parker AJ, Clarke KA (1990). Gait topography in rat locomotion. Physiol Behav 48:41–7.

Pedersen SW, Eriksson T, Oberg B (1991). Effects of withdrawal of antiparkinson medication on gait and clinical score in the parkinson patient. Acta Neurol Scand 84:7–13.

Reiter LW, MacPhail RC (1982). Factors influencing motor activity measurements in neurotoxicology. In: Mitchell CL, ed. Nervous system toxicology. New York: Raven Press, 45–66.

Rice DC, Gilbert SG, Willes RF (1979). Neonatal low-level exposure in monkeys: locomotor activity, schedule-controlled behavior, and the effects of amphetamine. Toxicol Appl Pharmacol 51:503–13.

Robins LN (1981). Epidemiological approaches to natural history research. J Am Acad Child Psychiatry 20:556–80.

Roels H, Abdeladim S, Braun M, Malchaire J, Lauwerys R (1989). Detection of hand tremor in workers exposed to mercury vapor: a comparative study of three methods. Environ Res 49:152–65.

Sandheinrich MB, Atchison GJ (1989). Sublethal copper effects on bluegill, lepomis macrochirus, foraging behavior. Can J Fish Acquat Sci 46:1977–85.

Saudino KJ, Eaton WO (1991). Infant temperament and genetics: an objective twin study of motor activity level. Child Dev 62:1167–74.

Schaumburg HH, Spencer PS (1979). Clinical and experimental studies of distal axonopathy—a frequent form of brain and nerve damage produced by environmental chemical hazards. Ann NY Acad Sci 329:14–29.

Schroder JH, Peters K (1988a). Differential courtship activity of competing guppy males (Poecilia reticulata Peters; Pisces; Poeciliidae) as an indicator for low concentrations of aquatic pollutants. Bull Environ Contam Toxicol 40:396–404.

Schroder JH, Peters K (1988b). Differential courtship activity of competing guppy males (Poecilia reticulata Peters; Pisces; Poeciliidae) as an indicator for low concentrations of aquatic pollutants. Bull Environ Contam Toxicol 41:385–90.

Schulze GE (1990). Large scale assessment of motor activity in rodents: procedures for routine use in toxicity studies. J Am Coll Toxicol 9:455–63.

Schulze GE, Boysen BG (1991). A neurotoxicity screening battery for use in safety evaluation: effects of acrylamide and 3′,3′-iminodipropionitrile. Fundam Appl Toxicol 16:602–15.

Sheets L, Hassanein RS, Norton S (1987). Gait analysis of chicks following treatment with tri-ortho-cresyl phosphate in ovo. J Toxicol Environ Health 21:445–53.

Shell L, Rozum M, Jortner BS, Ehrich M (1992). Neurotoxicity of acrylamide and 2,5-hexanedione in rats evaluated using a functional observational battery and pathological examination. Neurotoxicol Teratol 14:275–83.

Silverman PA (1987). An ethologist's approach to behavioral toxicology. Neurotoxicol Teratol 10:85–92.

Sparling DW (1990). Conditioned aversion of aluminum sulfate in black ducks. Environ Toxicol Chem 9:479–81.

Spyker JM, Sparber SB, Goldberg AM (1972). Subtle consequences of methylmercury exposure: behavioral deviations in offspring of treated mothers. Science 177:621–3.

Streissguth AP, Martin DC, Barr HM, MacGregor Sandman B (1984). Intrauterine alcohol and nicotine exposure: attention and reaction time in 4-year old children. Dev Psychol 4:533–41.

Symons PEK (1973). Behavior of young atlantic salmon (Salmo salar) exposed to or force-fed fenitrothion, an organophosphate insecticide. J Fish Res Board Can 30:651–5.

Tamborini P, Sigg H, Zbinden G (1989). Quantitative analysis of rat activity in the home cage by infrared monitoring: application to the acute toxicity testing of aetanildide and phenylmercuric acetate. Arch Toxicol 63:85–96.

Teal JJ, Evans HL (1982). Behavioral effects of acrylamide in the mouse. Toxicol Appl Pharmacol 63:470–80.

Tilson HA, Moser VC (1992). Comparison of screening approaches. Neurotoxicology 13:1–14.

U.S. Environmental Protection Agency (1985). Toxic substances control act testing guidelines. 40 CFR Part 798, subpart G, Section 798.6050. Fed Reg 50(188):39, 458–60.

U.S. National Research Council (1991). Animals as sentinels of environmental health hazards. Washington, D.C.: National Academy Press.

Van Der Zee CEEM, Schuurman ZT, Van Der Hoop, RG, Traber J, Gispen WH (1990). Beneficial effect of nimodipine on peripheral nerve function in aged rats. Neurobiol Aging 11:451–6.

Vorhees CV (1987). Reliability, sensitivity and validity of behavioral indices of neurotoxicity. Neurotoxicol Teratol 9:445–64.

Vorhees CV, Acuff-Smith KD, Minck DR, Butcher RE (1992). A method for measuring locomotor behavior in rodents: contrast-sensitive computer-controlled video tracking activity assessment in rats. Neurotoxicol Teratol 14:43–9.

Weber DN, Russo A, Seale DB, Spieler RE (1991). Waterborne lead affects feeding abilities and neurotransmitter levels of juvenile fathead minnows (pimephales promelas). Aquatic Toxicol 21:71–80.

Weissman A (1990). What it takes to validate behavioral toxicology tests: a belated commentary on the collaborative behavioral teratology study. Neurotoxicol Teratol 12:497–501.

West DB, Tengan C, Smith WS, Samson HH (1983). A microcomputer-based data acquisition system for continuous recording of feeding and drinking by rats. Physiol Behav 31:125–32.

White DH, Mitchell CA, Hill EF (1983). Parathion alters incubation behavior of laughing gulls. Bull Environ Contam Toxicol 31:93–7.

Whitworth MR, Pendleton GW, Hoffman DJ, Camardes MG (1991). Effects of dietary boron and arsenic on the behavior of mallard ducklings. Environ Toxicol Chem 10:911–6.

Wood RW, Weiss AB, Weiss B (1973). Hand tremor induced by industrial exposure to inorganic mercury. Arch Environ Health 26:249–52.

Young DR, Heesen TC, Esra GN, Howard EB (1979). DDE contaminated fish off Los Angeles are suspected cause in deaths of captive marine birds. Bull Environ Contam Toxicol 21:584–90.

Zeigler HP, Miller M, Levine RR (1975). Trigeminal nerve and eating in the pigeon (Columba livia): neurosensory control of the consummatory responses. J Comp Physiol Psychol 83:845–58.

Part IV
Biochemical and Molecular Neurotoxicology
Introductory Overview

Stephen C. Bondy
University of California
Irvine, California

This section of the handbook is directed toward delineation of the metabolic basis of neurotoxic injury. Two major concepts, which are examined from several perspectives, underlie this series of chapters.

The first of these is that there are many common features characterizing neurotoxic effects caused by apparently unrelated toxicants. This may reflect the existence of especially susceptible metabolic events within the brain. The existence of such "weak points" may also account for the resemblance between the effects of several neurotoxic agents and various neurological diseases. One chapter is specifically addressed to the use of toxic chemicals in the modeling of common neurological disorders. Some chapters deal with commonly occurring states, such as excitotoxicity or excess generation of free radicals, that may follow ineffective maintenance of cellular energy reserves. The unique structure of myelin also presents a significant and vulnerable target to toxicants. In addition to the distinctive properties of a given neurotoxic agent, some general properties may underlie the toxicity of a variety of chemicals: namely, the ability to effect nonspecific stress and to impair normal anabolic events. These unifying hazards lead to consideration of possible "final common pathways" that may recur following both neurotoxic exposures and other neurological dysfunctions not known to relate to chemical toxicity. Derangement of cell responses to endocrine or neural signals is a major issue that is discussed in a chapter on receptors and channels on the plasma membrane, and also in a chapter on intracellular signaling.

The second element unifying this section of the handbook is an emphasis on recent methodological advances. Toxicological studies have often been somewhat tardy in the exploitation of novel technological advances in biology, and thus this component of the handbook may be timely. This element is particularly important in the area of molecular biology, where great strides in understanding of neural mechanisms have been made. Neurotoxicologists as a whole have been slow to take advantage of the possibilities offered

473

by this field, which offers dynamic new concepts as well as methods. New procedures and conceptual perspectives are especially valuable in that they can be readily transferred between studies on a wide range of diverse neurotoxic chemicals.

Experiments that involve reversal or mitigation of the effects of neurotoxicants are also prevalent in these chapters. Such an approach has value both in the mechanistic understanding of toxic effects and in the potential development of new treatments for neurological disorders, whether of toxic or other origin. The potential of chronic low-level neurotoxic exposures to interact with normal aging processes either additively or synergistically is also a key issue that is addressed in several chapters. Such interactions potentially move neurotoxicology toward becoming a discipline relevant to a major proportion of the population, rather than only involving small select groups experiencing unusual occupational or environmental exposures.

16
Cell Signaling and Neurotoxic Events

Lucio G. Costa
University of Washington
Seattle, Washington

INTRODUCTION

A number of neurotransmitters, hormones, and growth factors serve as "first messengers" to transfer information from one cell to another by binding to specific cell membrane receptors. This interaction results in activation or inhibition of specific enzymes and/or opening of ion channels, which lead to changes in intracellular metabolism and, in turn, to a variety of effects ranging from activation of other specific enzymes to expression of selected genes. Examples of such "second-messenger" systems are the cyclic nucleotides, the products of phosphoinositide metabolism, and calcium ions. One of the features of these systems is that the receptors act only to transfer information from the incoming ligand to another entity (e.g., acetylcholine or norepinephrine through M_1 muscarinic receptors and α_1 receptors, respectively, to phospholipase C). In spite of its high specificity for its receptor, one ligand may produce the same final "nonselective" effect(s) as another ligand acting through an entirely distinct specific receptor (Lichtstein and Rodbard, 1987). This apparent lack of specificity of postreceptor events has been seen as one of the conceptual obstacles that have hampered the pharmaceutical industry's attempts to develop drugs aimed at second-messenger targets (Corda et al., 1990). Yet recent developments in the biochemistry and molecular biology of receptors have provided preliminary evidence confirming the hypothesis (Lichtstein and Rodbard, 1987) that receptors are considerably more active functionally in the information transfer process than had been generally believed, and that signal specificity may be encoded in part in the primary structure of the receptor. For example, the concept is now slowly unfolding that different receptor subtypes may couple to different second-messenger systems, that these could change depending, for example, on the cell type, and that all this may be ascribed to the interaction of guanosine triphosphate (GTP)-binding protein with the receptor itself (Ashkenazi et al., 1989; Boege et al., 1991). Furthermore, second-messenger responses are more specific than initially thought. For example, molecular cloning has so far revealed the existence of at least seven isoforms of protein kinase C, five isoforms of phospholipase C, and five families of cyclic nucleotide phosphodiesterase (Corda et al., 1990). This is allowing the development of very specific drugs that may selectively affect a metabolic pathway and, therefore, have selective therapeutic effects (Garattini, 1992); an example of this strategy is offered by inhibitors of various types of phosphodiesterase (Beavo and Reifsnyder, 1990).

Investigations on the molecular mechanisms of neurotoxicity have also for the most part shied away from studying second-messenger systems as potential targets for neurotoxicants. Yet in recent years, rapid advances in basic knowledge about signal-transduction mechanisms have opened the way for new research in the area of cell signaling and neurotoxicity. In this chapter I will briefly review the principal receptor-activated second-messenger systems and their potential functional consequences, and will then describe a few examples of neurotoxicity that may involve interaction with such cell-signaling systems.

THE PHOSPHOINOSITIDE/PROTEIN KINASE C PATHWAY

Production of Inositol Phosphates

Though the first observation that agonists for several receptors can stimulate the metabolism of inositol phospholipids was made almost 40 years ago (Hokin and Hokin, 1955), it was only in 1975 that Michell suggested that stimulation of inositol phospholipid breakdown was associated with a rise in cytosolic Ca^{2+} ion concentration in the stimulated cell (Michell, 1975). The past 15 years have seen a rapid advancement of knowledge in this area, and these findings have been summarized in several recent reviews (Kikkawa et al., 1989; Rana and Hokin, 1990; Berridge and Irvine, 1989; Martin, 1991; Hughes and Putney, 1990; Housley, 1991). Phosphoinositide metabolism in the nervous system has received particular attention because of the presence of several receptor systems coupled to this response, in both nerve and glial cells, and because of the high concentrations of protein kinase C (PKC) present in the brain (Fisher and Agranoff, 1987; Kikkawa et al., 1988; Chuang, 1989; Costa, 1990; Fisher et al., 1991; Fowler and Tiger, 1991; Patel et al., 1991).

When an agonist interacts with the appropriate receptor (e.g., cholinergic muscarinic M_1 or M_3 receptors, α_1-adrenergic receptors, or metabotropic excitatory amino acid receptors), it activates a phosphoinositidase (phospholipase C) that hydrolyzes phosphoinositide 4,5-bisphosphate (PtdIns 4,5-P_2) to form inositol 1,4,5-trisphosphate (Ins 1,4,5-P_3) and 1,2-diacylglycerol (DG). A GTP-binding protein couples the receptor to phospholipase C. Although the exact nature of this protein has not been fully determined, mounting evidence suggests that more than one protein exists, depending on the receptor subtype and the cell type (Lo and Hughes, 1987; Fain et al., 1988; Ashkenazi et al., 1989). Recent evidence obtained in a reconstituted system suggests that the G protein $G_{q/11}$ couples the muscarinic M_1 receptor to phospholipase C-β1 (Bernstein et al., 1992).

Inositol 1,4,5-trisphosphate binds to specific and saturable receptor sites located in the endoplasmic reticulum and in a recently proposed organelle, the calciosome (Worley et al., 1989; Volpe et al., 1988) and causes the mobilization of calcium ions in the cytosol. By the action of phosphatases, Ins 1,4,5-P_3 is then dephosphorylated to Ins 1,4-P_2, Ins 1-P, and inositol (Majerus et al., 1988). The latter reaction, catalyzed by an Ins 1-P phosphatase, is inhibited by lithium ions (Drummond et al., 1987), suggesting that this effect may be involved in the antimanic action of this compound. Inositol 1,4,5-triphosphate can also be phosphorylated by a 3-kinase to form inositol 1,3,4,5-tetrakisphosphate (Ins 1,3,4,5-P_4), which may play a role in modulating the mobilization of intracellular Ca^{2+} by Ins 1,4,5-P_3 and in regulating Ca^{2+} entry from outside the cell (Hughes and Putney, 1990). Other inositol phosphates that have been identified include Ins 1,3,4-P_3, Ins 1,3,4,5,6-P_5, Ins P_6, and cyclic inositol 1-2,4,5-trisphosphate; although all have been shown to exert some cellular effect, their precise roles in the phosphoinositide pathway are still far from clear (Costa 1990; Fisher et al., 1991).

Mobilization of Intracellular Calcium

A main consequence of the activation of the phosphoinositide pathway is a change in the intracellular concentration of calcium deriving from Ins 1,4,5-P_3–sensitive stores or from Ca^{2+}- and/or Ins 1,3,4,5-P_4–sensitive stores, or entering the cell from receptor-operated calcium channels (Hughes and Putney, 1990; Henzi and MacDermott, 1992). Intracellular calcium can bind to two types of broadly defined receptor protein. One type (e.g., calmodulin) does not possess enzymatic activity, but after binding calcium is capable of activating various enzymes, such as the Ca^{2+}-calmodulin–activated protein kinases or the calcium adenosinetriphosphatase (ATPase) (Rasmussen et al., 1990). The second type of protein, represented for example by PKC, possesses intrinsic enzymatic activity that can be activated by calcium (Rasmussen et al., 1990). While a transient increase in intracellular calcium is necessary for the normal physiological functions of the cell, a sustained increase can produce toxicity. In particular, calcium can activate phospholipases, proteases, and endonucleases, leading to fragmentation of phospholipids, proteins, and DNA (Orrenius et al., 1988; Komulainen and Bondy, 1988).

Activation of Immediate Early Genes

Several receptors that directly (e.g., via the phosphoinositide pathway and/or direct opening of calcium channels) or indirectly (e.g., via phosphorylations that follow an initial activation of the adenylate cyclase pathway) cause an increase in intracellular calcium levels lead to activation of immediate early genes (Arenander et al., 1989; Sheng and Greenberg, 1990). Expression of immediate early genes (e.g., c-fos, c-jun) is very low in quiescent cells but is rapidly induced at the transcriptional level (Sheng and Greenberg, 1990). The mRNAs accumulate for 1–2 h in the cytoplasm, and the respective proteins (e.g., Fos and Jun) are translated and then translocated to the nucleus, where they form a heterodimeric protein complex that binds to the DNA regulatory element known as the AP-1 binding site (Morgan and Curran, 1989). The binding of the Fos-Jun complex to DNA causes the activation of target genes that may code for a variety of structural or other proteins (Sheng and Greenberg, 1990; Hall, 1990). The transient nature of the mRNAs and their proteins suggests that these may act as a signaling system, i.e., as a third-messenger system within an intracellular cascade linking extracellular stimuli to long-term adaptive processes (Morgan and Curran, 1989; Macara, 1989).

Activation of Protein Kinase C

1,2-Diacylglycerol, the other product of phosphoinositide hydrolysis, activates a protein kinase, PKC. Activation of PKC requires the presence of calcium and phospholipids, particularly phosphatidylserine, and involves its translocation from the inactive form in the cytosol to the membrane (Nishizuka, 1988). As with other enzymes of the phosphoinositide cycle, several isozymes of PKC exist: at least seven subspecies of PKC have been found in nervous tissue, and their structures, deduced by analysis of their DNA sequences, have been elucidated (Parker et al., 1986; Nishizuka, 1988; Kikkawa et al., 1988). These different PKCs differ in their specific activity in different brain areas, in their developmental profile, and in their activation requirements (Nishizuka, 1988; Kikkawa et al., 1988). Protein kinase C is the receptor for, and can be activated by, phorbol esters, a known class of tumor promoters (Kikkawa et al., 1983). The gamma form of PKC, which is expressed only in the brain and spinal cord, can also be activated by arachidonic acid and by other eicosanoids (Kikkawa et al., 1988). A large number of proteins can be phosphorylated by PKC, including receptors, ion channels, cytoskeletal proteins, and membrane enzymes (Nishizuka, 1986). Protein kinase C has been involved in the release of a variety of neurotransmitters, an effect strongly correlated with phosphorylation of a synaptic protein known as B-50 or GAP43 (Kikkawa and Nishizuka, 1986; Dekker et al., 1989). This action may be linked to the role of PKC in the maintenance of long-term potentiation, suggesting a role for this enzyme in the process of memory (Chiarugi et al., 1989). Another important role of PKC, and of the phosphoinositide pathway in general, is in cell proliferation (Whitman and Cantley, 1988; Murphy et al., 1987; Saunders and DeVries, 1988). In the nervous system, proliferation of astrocytes and Schwann cells has been shown to be associated with activation of the phosphoinositide/PKC system. Phorbol esters have been shown also to enhance the differentiation of astrocytes and oligodendrocytes in culture (Honegger, 1986).

NEUROTOXICANTS AND PHOSPHOINOSITIDE METABOLISM

Metals

A limited number of studies exist on the interactions of neurotoxic chemicals with the phosphoinositide/PKC system (Costa, 1990). Several metals have been shown to interact with PKC or other elements of the phosphoinositide pathway. Inorganic mercury and various forms of organic mercury have been shown to inhibit PKC activity and the binding of ^{3}H-phorbol 12,13-dibutyrate at low micromolar concentrations (Inoue et al., 1988). This is not surprising, since PKC differs from other kinases because of its rich cysteine content, and mercurials are known to have a high affinity for sulfhydryl groups, which are present in the catalytic and regulatory domains of PKC. Although this interaction may be of interest and related to mercury neurotoxicity, the known ability of mercury compounds to affect a large number of biochemical and physiological processes (Costa, 1988) calls for caution in evaluating the relative contribution of each effect to its overall neurotoxicity. Additionally, inhibition of phorbol ester binding in brain regions was not observed following acute or repeated exposure of mice to methylmercury (Katsuyama et al., 1989). Inorganic mercury has also been shown to potentiate nerve growth factor (NGF)-induced DG production in neuroadrenergic PC12 cells and to have an effect on its own at submicromolar concentrations (Rossi et al., 1992). It appears that in these cells, the effect of NGF on cellular differentiation is mediated by stimulation of glycosylphosphatidylinositol hydrolysis, which generates inositol glycan and DG. In cultured cerebellar granule neurons methylmercury, but not mercury chloride, has been shown to increase inositol phosphates and free intracellular calcium levels, and it has been suggested that these actions are associated with the mechanism of neurotoxic injury of this compound (Sarafian and Verity, 1992). Increases in free cytosolic calcium by methylmercury have also been observed in synaptosomal preparations (Komulainen and Bondy, 1987a; Hare et al., 1991) and have been ascribed to either membrane or intracellular actions.

Lead is known to alter calcium-mediated processes and may also mimic calcium's effects (Pounds, 1984; Bressler and Goldstein, 1991). For example, lead has a higher affinity than calcium for calmodulin and can activate some calmodulin-dependent processes (Habermann et al., 1983). Lead can also substitute for calcium in stimulating PKC activity (Markovac and Goldstein, 1988a,b). In isolated immature rat microvessels, lead caused activation of PKC in a concentration range of 0.1–10 μM and also caused translocation of PKC from the cytosol to the particulate fraction. More surprisingly, lead has been shown to activate PKC, partially purified from rat brain, at concentrations as low as 10^{-15} M, being several orders of magnitude more potent than calcium itself (Markovac and Goldstein, 1988b). The reason for the apparent discrepancy between the potency of lead in the brain and in isolated microvessels is not clear, but it may be linked to the relative distribution of subspecies of PKC. It should be noted, however, that an inhibitory effect of lead on PKC activity has also been reported (Feng et al., 1990). As long-term potentiation, a possible functional equivalent of memory storage, is blocked by inhibitors of PKC, a lead-induced decrease in PKC activity (via inhibition or down-regulation due to sustained stimulation) may relate to learning and memory deficits caused by this compound. Potential interactions of lead with the calcium-releasing ability of Ins 1,4,5-P_3 could also be of interest. At micromolar concentrations, lead has been shown to enhance the binding of $[^3H]$-Ins 1,4,5-P_3 and $[^3H]$-Ins 1,3,4,5-P_4 to cerebellar membranes, and the effect is antagonized by adenosine triphosphate (ATP) (Vig and Desaiah, 1992).

Another neurotoxic metal, aluminum, can activate phosphoinositide metabolism where present alone or complexed with fluoride to form AlF^{4-} (Candura et al., 1991). The effect is believed to be due to an interaction with the G protein(s), but its possible physiological or pathological (e.g., in Alzheimer's disease) implications are far from clear. Aluminum has also been shown to inhibit rat brain PKC activity in vitro at micromolar concentrations (Cochran et al., 1990). Other metals (e.g., cadmium, manganese, organotins) have also been shown to activate or inhibit PKC in vitro at micromolar concentrations (see references in Costa, 1990; Speizer et al., 1989; Trottman et al., 1991). Vanadate has been shown to prevent the hydrolysis of Ins 1,4,5-P_3 to Ins 1,4-P_2 and of Ins 1,3,4,5-P_4 to Ins 1,3,4-P_3, thereby potentiating the basal and stimulated accumulation of inositol phosphates (Bencherif and Lukas, 1992). These effects of vanadium may be involved in the alleged role played by this metal in the etiology of some forms of depression and bipolar disorder (Bencherif and Lukas, 1992).

Pesticides

A number of studies have investigated the interactions of pesticides, particularly organophosphates, with the metabolism of phosphoinositides. Repeated exposures to organophosphates causes a decrease in carbachol-stimulated phosphoinositide metabolism in the rat cerebral cortex, which parallels a decrease in the density of muscarinic receptors (Costa et al., 1986; Pintor et al., 1992; Mundy et al., 1992). A series of studies by Savolainen et al. (Savolainen et al., 1988; Hirvonen et al., 1990; Savolainen et al., 1991) have investigated the involvement of phosphoinositides and calcium in the convulsing effect of organophosphates. An increase in cerebral Ins 1-P was observed in convulsing rats but was not present (or occurred only transiently) in nonconvulsing animals. Increased levels of calcium and morphological changes were also observed, and all effects, including convulsions, were potentiated by lithium, suggesting that the phosphoinositide signaling pathway may be involved in convulsions and, through elevation of intracellular calcium, contribute to neuronal injury. Potentiation of other direct (pilocarpine) or indirect (physostigmine) cholinergic agonists by lithium has also been reported (Honchar et al., 1983; Terry et al., 1990), confirming a role for the phosphoinositide pathway in cholinergic-induced seizures and brain damage.

Pyrethroids, of both type I and type II, can stimulate phosphoinositide breakdown in guinea pig synaptosomes; for type II compounds this effect is due to activation of sodium channels, while type I compounds may act through a different, still unknown, mechanism (Gusovsky et al., 1989). Several chlorinated hydrocarbons (e.g. chlordane, lindane) stimulate PKC from rat brain, an effect that may be related to the hepatic tumor-promoting action of some of these neurotoxic organochlorines (Moser and Smart, 1989).

Ethanol

A number of studies have been carried out in the past few years investigating the potential interaction of ethanol with phosphoinositide metabolism (Hoek and Rubin, 1990). Most of these studies have been conducted in adult animals and were aimed at defining a possible role for phosphoinositides in the process of ethanol tolerance and dependence or other specific organ effects (e.g. hepatotoxicity) (Costa et al., 1992; Hoek et al., 1992). In rat brain slices, ethanol has differential inhibitory effects on agonist-induced inositol metabolism, depending on the nature of the agonist and the regions examined (Gonzales et al., 1986). Chronic treatment with ethanol, however, did not modify stimulation of phosphoinositide metabolism in the cerebral cortex or cerebellum by glutamate, norepinephrine, or carbachol (Gonzales and Crews, 1988; Balduini and Costa, 1989), but it reduced the binding of Ins 1,4,5-P_3 to mouse cerebellar membranes (Smith, 1987). In astrocytes, ethanol has been found to potentiate the effect of serotonin and norepinephrine on phosphoinositide metabolism (Ritchie et al., 1988). In PC12 cells, ethanol (100 mM) has also been shown to inhibit muscarine-stimulated calcium mobilization, while having no effect on its own at this concentration (Rabe and Weight, 1988). Thus, ethanol seems to have differential effects on receptor-stimulated phosphoinositide metabolism depending on the tissue, the neurotransmitter, and the mode of exposure (e.g., acute vs. chronic).

Another aspect of the interaction of ethanol with phosphoinositides is the formation of phosphatidylethanol by the action of phospholipase D (Gustavsson and Alling, 1987). Phosphatidylethanol can activate PKC, particularly the gamma subtypes (Asaoka et al., 1988), and may contribute to the down-regulation of PKC observed following chronic in vivo exposure to ethanol (Battaini et al., 1989), since ethanol per se does not appear to activate PKC (Machu et al., 1991).

Recent studies have suggested the hypothesis that phosphoinositide metabolism stimulated by activation of cholinergic muscarinic receptors in the developing rat brain may represent a relevant target for the developmental neurotoxicity of ethanol (Balduini and Costa, 1989, 1990; Candura et al., 1992; Costa et al., 1992). The hypothesis stemmed from the observation that the developmental profile of muscarinic receptor–stimulated phosphoinositide metabolism in the rat has a striking resemblance to that of the brain growth spurt (Dobbing and Sands, 1979), suggesting a role for this system in the regulation of neurocytomorphogenesis, synaptogenesis, and glial cell proliferation (Balduini et al., 1987). The age-, brain region–, and receptor-specific inhibitory effects of ethanol on this system are intriguing and may relate to some of the effects found in the fetal alcohol syndrome (e.g., microencephaly). Inhibition of muscarinic receptor–induced increases in intracellular free calcium by ethanol in rat primary cortical neuronal cultures has also been found (K. Kovacs and L. G. Costa, unpublished observation).

Excitatory Amino Acids

Interactions with phosphoinositide metabolism may also be involved in the neurotoxicity of excitatory amino acids (Costa, 1990). In hippocampal slices, quisqualate- and glutamate-stimulated phosphoinositide breakdown is more pronounced in the neonatal than in the adult rat (Nicoletti et al., 1986; Balduini et al., 1991). This is of interest, since quisqualic acid is particularly toxic to the immature brain (Silverstein et al., 1986). L-Cysteine, which exerts profound neurotoxic effects in the immature rat (Olney et al., 1991), is also a potent activator of phosphoinositide metabolism in the immature rat brain (W. Balduini, L. G. Costa, and F. Cattabeni, unpublished observations). Excessive and prolonged translocation of PKC from the cytosol to the neuronal membrane and destabilization of calcium homeostatis have been suggested as important elements in the neurotoxicity of glutamate in cerebellar granule cells (Manev et al., 1990; Choi, 1990; Guidotti et al., 1991). A link between excitatory amino acid receptors, phosphoinositide metabolism, and neurotoxicity has been proposed. For example, hypoxia-ischemia causes a specific increase in quisqualate-stimulated phosphoinositide metabolism in hippocampal and striatal slices of the neonatal rat (Chen et al., 1988). This enhanced phosphoinositide hydrolysis may contribute to several potentially detrimental steps, including an increased availability of arachidonic acid, an important substrate for free radical formation, and a metabolic derangement due to the increased metabolic cost of phosphoinositide breakdown and resynthesis (Chen et al., 1988). On the other hand, it has also been reported that activation of the metabotropic glutamate receptor attenuates the neurotoxicity caused by N-methyl-D-aspartate in murine cortical cultures (Koh et al., 1991). Furthermore, recent studies with ibotenic acid have shown that stimulation of phosphoinositide metabolism was neither necessary nor sufficient for neurotoxicity in cortical neurons (Zinkand et al., 1992). Some apparently contradictory results may be explained by activation of different subtypes of excitatory amino acid receptors by different compounds. This has been recently shown by Nicoletti et al. (1992), who reported that activation of the metabotropic glutamate receptors 1 and 5 leads to activation of phosphoinositide hydrolysis as well as neurotoxicity, while other metabotropic glutamate receptors, negatively linked to adenylate cyclase, may exert neuroprotective effects. Of interest is that gangliosides appear to be capable of antagonizing intracellular events associated with glutamate receptor "abuse" (e.g., delayed PKC translocation and neural death) without affecting its physiological response (e.g., activation of phospholipase C) (Favaron et al., 1990; Guidotti et al., 1991).

Colchicine

A series of studies by Tilson and coworkers (Tandon et al., 1989a,b, 1991) have shown that direct intradentate administration of colchicine, a neurotoxicant known to block mitosis and axoplasmic transport, results in an alteration of carbachol-mediated phosphoinositide hydrolysis in the hippocampus. This change occurred between 3 and 12 weeks after infusion of colchicine and was present up to 1 year later. This increased sensitivity is believed to be a compensatory change associated with a loss of muscarinic receptors due to the destruction of granule cells and mossy fibers. Similar changes in ibotenate- and glutamate-induced phosphoinositide hydrolysis have also been reported following colchicine administration (Nicoletti et al., 1987).

CALCIUM AND NEUROTOXICITY

There is a strong evidence that the neurotoxicity of excitatory amino acids involves calcium ions, since removal of extracellular calcium or chelation of intracellular calcium prevents their neurotoxicity (Choi, 1985; Garthwaite and Garthwaite, 1986; Siesjo, 1990; Scharfman and Schwartzkroin, 1989). Indeed, increasing evidence is suggesting that calcium ions may be involved in the neurotoxicity of several compounds (Komulainen and Bondy, 1988; Bondy, 1989; Pounds and Rosen, 1988; Verity, 1992; Nicotera et al., 1990). Neurotoxic compounds may lead to a disruption of calcium-dependent mechanisms and to a sustained increase in intracellular calcium levels. While a transient increase in free Ca^{2+} within the cells is essential for normal cell function, a prolonged increase may lead to activation of proteases, phospholipases, and endonucleases, leading to protein, phospholipid, and DNA damage (Orrenius et al., 1988). Furthermore, prolonged elevation of free intracellular Ca^{2+} may activate compensatory mechanisms that require energy, thus leading to depletion of energy- related reserves (Komulainen and Bondy, 1988). Several neurotoxic chemicals are known to increase intracellular calcium levels. In addition to the excitatory amino acids, these include mercury and methylmercury (Rossi et al., 1991; Levesque and Atchison, 1991; Sarafian and Verity, 1992), other organometals such as triethyllead and trimethyltin (Komulainen and Bondy, 1987a), organochlorine insecticides such as chlordecone and lindane (Komulainen and Bondy, 1987b; Bondy and Halsall, 1988), and cyanide (Johnson et al., 1987). Several mechanisms may be involved in the increase of free calcium levels induced by neurotoxicants (Komulainen and Bondy, 1988; Levesque and Atchison, 1991). At the level of the plasma membrane these include inhibition of Na^+/K^+-ATPase or of Ca^{2+}-ATPase, prevention of Na^+-Ca^{2+} exchange, nonspecific membrane damage, receptor activation, and membrane depolarization. In the mitochondria, neurotoxic chemicals may cause membrane damage, inhibit the Ca^{2+} uniporter, inhibit respiration, or uncouple oxidative phosphorylation (Komulainen and Bondy, 1988; Levesque and Atchison, 1991). Any interference with the action of inositol phosphates in the endoplasmic reticulum will also lead to alteration in calcium homeostasis. An additional calcium-regulating mechanism that has been receiving much attention is represented by calmodulin. Calmodulin is a multifunctional regulatory protein that binds Ca^{2+} and can activate a number of enzymes involved in several physiological process (Stoclet et al., 1987). One of these targets, which has received much attention in neurotoxicology, is calmodulin-activated calcium ATPase, which has been shown to be inhibited by various heavy metals (Desaiah, 1988).

Increases in intracellular free calcium also result in the rapid, transient induction of immediate early genes, such as *c-fos* and *c-myc* (Morgan and Curran, 1988), possibly through a calmodulin-dependent pathway (Morgan and Curran, 1986). Expression of the immediate early gene *c-fos* has been suggested as a potential marker of neurotoxicity (Vendrell et al., 1991). The organochlorine insecticide lindane induces *c-fos* expression in the cerebral cortex and hippocampus in a dose-dependent manner (Vendrell et al., 1992). Two nonconvulsant isomers of lindane were not able to induce expression of *c-fos*, suggesting that expression of this proto-oncogene is linked to lindane-induced convulsions. Indeed, seizure activity is known to induce *c-fos* in a transient manner (Morgan et al., 1987). The exact molecular mechanism of this action of lindane is not known, but it may be linked to an increase in intracellular calcium (Bondy and Halsall, 1988; Vendrell et al., 1992), which is known to modulate the immediate early gene cascade in neurons (Morgan and Curran, 1988). An increase in *c-fos* and *c-jun* expression in the rat brain was observed also after exposure to acrylamide (Kittur et al., 1991).

REGULATION OF CYCLIC NUCLEOTIDE METABOLISM

Cyclic Adenosine Monophosphate

The role of cyclic adenosine monophosphate (AMP) as a mediator of several physiological processes has been established for more than two decades (Robison et al., 1971). Activation of a number of receptors (e.g., β-adrenoceptors), coupled through the GTP-binding protein Gs to the enzyme adenylate cyclase, causes the conversion of ATP to cyclic AMP. Before being inactivated by phosphodiesterases (Beavo and Reifsnyder, 1990), cyclic AMP can activate a cyclic AMP–dependent protein kinase that in turn can phosphorylate a number of cellular substrates, including proteins involved in neurotransmitter release, receptors, ion channels, cytoskeletal proteins, and other enzymes (Krebs, 1989; Walaas and Greengard, 1991). One of the substrates of this kinase is a protein known as CREB (cAMP response element binding protein) (Sheng et al., 1990). Interestingly, CREB can also be phosphorylated by calcium-calmodulin protein kinase, making it a common link between the cyclic AMP and the calcium-signaling pathways. Among the genes regulated by CREB are those coding for the neuropeptide somatostatin and the immediate early genes, including the proto-oncogenes *c-fos* and c-*myc*, which are believed to play a fundamental role in directing growth and differentiation of nerve cells.

Activation of certain receptors (e.g. muscarinic M_2, A_1-adenosine) can also cause inhibition of adenylate cyclase, leading to a decrease in the intracellular levels of cyclic AMP (Kendall-Harden, 1989). This "negative coupling" to adenylate cyclase is mediated by a G protein known as Gi.

Cyclic Guanosine Monophosphate

Activation of other receptors (e.g. glutamate, muscarinic M_1 or M_3) causes elevation in intracellular cyclic guanosine monophosphate (GMP) levels. The effect has been considered to be indirect, involving an additional second messenger, since receptor agonists, differently from compounds such as sodium nitroprusside, cannot activate guanylate cyclase (the soluble enzyme that converts GTP to cyclic GMP) in broken cell preparations. Two likely candidates for this role are calcium ions and a metabolite of arachidonic acid. A role for calcium is suggested by experiments showing that extracellular calcium ions are necessary for receptor stimulation of cyclic GMP and that calcium channel antagonists block this effect (El-Fakahany and Richelson, 1983). An involvement of a metabolite of arachidonic acid is suggested by the finding that inhibitors of lipoxygenase (but not cyclo-oxygenase) block the cyclic GMP response (McKinney and Richelson, 1989). The role of nitric oxide in the activation of guanylate cyclase is discussed below.

NEUROTOXICANTS AND CYCLIC NUCLEOTIDES

Despite the great importance of cyclic nucleotides in a large number of cell functions, there has been only a limited number of studies investigating the effects of neurotoxicants on these systems. Several pesticides (the organophosphates soman, tabun, and sarin; certain pyrethroids and DDT) have been shown to increase levels of cyclic GMP, while other pesticides (e.g., organochlorines) may enhance the brain cyclic AMP content (Bodnaryk, 1982; Costa, 1992a). Lead, on the other hand, has been shown to inhibit adenylate cyclase (Nathanson and Bloom, 1975). A large number of studies (summarized by Pennington, 1992) exist on the interaction of ethanol with the adenylate cyclase/cyclic AMP system.

Chronic alcohol exposure results in a decrease in effector-stimulated adenylate cyclase. This is believed to be due to a selective interaction of ethanol with Gs (Hoffman and Tabakoff, 1990). Ethanol was also shown to inhibit glutamate-induced cyclic GMP formation in primary cultures of cerebellar granule cells (Hoffman et al., 1989).

Nitric Oxide

The cyclic GMP pathway has recently received strong new attention, since it has been discovered that nitric oxide (NO) synthesized from L-arginine by NO synthase binds to a heme moiety that is attached to guanylate cyclase and stimulates the accumulation of cyclic GMP (Ignarro, 1991; Moncada et al., 1991; Bredt and Snyder, 1992). Nitric oxide is a free radical gas, formed in neurons and in glial cells by action of NO synthase, a calcium-calmodulin–dependent enzyme, which was recently cloned (Bredt et al., 1991), and which resembles cytochrome P-450 reductase. Nitric oxide diffuses from the cell where it is formed and activates guanylate cyclase in adjacent cells (Bredt and Snyder, 1992). This had been simply and elegantly shown by experiments with hemogobin, an NO-binding molecule that remains extracellular (Southan and Garthwaite, 1991), which is a potent inhibitor of glutamate-induced increase in cyclic GMP in cerebellar slices. Glutamate-stimulated cyclic GMP formation (East and Garthwaite, 1990) and neurotoxicity (Dawson et al., 1991) are believed to be mediated by NO, since analogues of arginine such as L-N^G-nitroarginine, which inhibit NO synthase, antagonize both effects. Additional evidence for a role of NO in mediating glutamate neurotoxicity is that toxicity is prevented in an arginine-free medium and is antagonized by hemoglobin (Dawson et al., 1991). The effect of glutamate through the NO pathway appears to be mediated by the NMDA receptors (Izumi et al., 1992), which may also be involved in the neurotoxicity of cyanide. Indeed, in primary neuronal cultures the toxicity of cyanide is antagonized by specific NMDA antagonists (Isom et al., 1992); additionally, cyanide-induced convulsions are inhibited by N^G-nitro-L-arginine (Yamamoto, 1992). Thus, cyanide-induced toxicity may involve, at least in part, release of glutamate that activates the NO–cyclic GMP pathway through NMDA receptors.

Recent attention has also been directed to the mechanism(s) by which NO causes cellular toxicity. The reaction between superoxide (O_2^-) and NO can result in the generation of a potent oxidant, the peroxynitrile ($DNOO^-$) radical, that can diffuse to other cells (Garthwaite, 1991; McCall and Vallance, 1992). Furthermore, NO can cause nitrosylation of nucleic acids and break DNA strands (McCall and Vallance, 1992). Judging from the recent developments and discoveries, it is apparent that the study of the role of NO in neurotoxicity is fertile terrain for further investigations.

PROTEIN PHOSPHORYLATION

Protein phosphorylation is a major additional step in the second-messenger cascade, and its importance in neuronal function is increasingly recognized (Walaas and Greengard, 1991). In addition to the aforementioned calcium/phospholipid-dependent protein kinase (PKC) and the cyclic AMP–dependent protein kinase, other well-characterized kinases are the cyclic GMP–dependent protein kinase and the Ca^{2+}-calmodulin–dependent protein kinases (I, II, and III) (Walaas and Greengard, 1991). A protein kinase phosphorylates a substrate protein by transferring a terminal phosphate from ATP; the so-formed phospho-protein changes its function, presumably by changing its structure, and is then reversed through removal of the phosphate group by phosphatases. A large number of proteins are regulated by phosphorylation, including enzymes involved in neurotransmitter synthesis, ion channels, receptors, cytoskeletal proteins, and proteins involved in regulation of transcription and translation. A number of protein kinases also exist in brain tissue that can phosphorylate endogenous proteins on serine and threonine residues and do not appear to be regulated by any known second-messenger system, but may be of neurotoxicological significance. For example, casein kinase II can phosphorylate DARPP-32, a region- and cell-specific phosphoprotein; glycogen synthase kinase 3 can catalyze the in vitro phosphorylation of the neuronal cell adhesion molecule N-CAM; several neurofilament protein kinases can phosphorylate the three neurofilament proteins (Walaas and Greengard, 1991). An additional class of protein kinases is represented by the tyrosine-specific protein kinases, which include proto-oncogene products (e.g., pp60$^{c\text{-}src}$, the gene product of *c-src*) as well as growth factor receptors (e.g, the insulin-like growth factor I) (Druker et al., 1989; Walaas and Greengard, 1991).

Surprisingly, while phosphorylation of proteins by protein kinases has been long recognized as a primary dynamic regulatory process for post-translational modifications in the nervous system, its possible role in neurotoxicity has received only limited attention. A role for endogenous protein phosphorylation in the delayed polyneuropathy induced by certain organophosphorus compounds was suggested some years ago (Abou-Donia et al., 1984). Triethyltin increases the phosphorylation of synapsin I, possibly by activation of cyclic AMP–dependent protein kinases (Neuman and Taketa, 1987). Alterations of phosphorylation have been found in various clinical disorders (e.g., diabetes, cystic fibrosis) and may also be relevant in Alzheimer's disease (Walaas and Greengard, 1991). Administration of the antimitotic agent methylazoxymethanol to rats at day 15 of gestation has been shown to reduce phosphorylation of the neuronal phosphoprotein B50 (GAP43) without altering the relative amount of the protein or the levels of mRNA (Di Luca et al., 1991). Several neuron- and glia-specific phosphoproteins are also being used as markers for neurotoxic damage (O'Callaghan, 1992).

METABOLISM OF ARACHIDONIC ACID

Another intracellular pathway whose importance is increasingly recognized, but which has received little or no attention in a neurotoxicology context, is the metabolism of arachidonic acid (AA). Arachidonic acid is liberated from membrane phospholipids by two pathways: a Ca^{2+}-activated phospholipase A_2 generates AA and lysophospholipid, while phospholipase C generates DG, which is then converted to AA and glycerol by lipases. Free AA can diffuse out of the cells, can be reincorporated into phospholipids, or can undergo intracellular metabolism. The three metabolic pathways of AA are initially catalyzed by cyclo-oxygenase, lypoxygenase, and cytochrome P-450 (Shimizu and Wolfe, 1990). The cyclo-oxygenase pathway leads to the formation of prostaglandins, thromboxanes, and prostacyclin, and is inhibited by anti-inflammatory drugs such as aspirin or indomethacin. Cytochrome P-450 catalyzes the conversion of AA into epoxyeicosatrienoic acids. Lipoxygenase metabolizes AA to hydroxyperoxyeicosatetraenoic acids (HPETE), which are then converted to leukotrienes.

Various neurotransmitters (e.g., glutamate via NMDA receptors, acetylcholine via muscarinic receptors) cause the formation of lipoxygenase metabolites in nervous tissue (Simmet and Peskar, 1990). Increases in lipoxygenase products occur as a consequence of ischemic insult and epilectic seizures (Simmet and Peskar, 1990). In certain systems (e.g.,

N1E-115 murine neuroblastoma cells), lipoxygenase products may also mediate the stimulation of cyclic GMP synthesis (McKinney and Richelson, 1989). Inhibition of neurotransmitter release by 12-HPETE (formed from AA by the action of a 12-lipoxygenase) has been documented. A cytochrome P-450–generated metabolite of 12-HPETE can activate K^+ channels, leading to decreased calcium entry and decreased neurotransmitter release. 12-HPETE can also inhibit calmodulin-dependent protein kinase II and thus reduce phosphorylation of synapsin I and neurotransmitter release (Piomelli and Greengard, 1990). Arachidonic acid itself may also have a role in long-term potentiation (Piomelli and Greengard, 1990). As knowledge of the functional role(s) of AA and its several metabolites in nerve tissue increases, their potential involvement in neurotoxic events will become more apparent.

CONCLUSION

The study of second- and third-messenger events linked to activation of membrane receptors is one of the most actively investigated fields of today's neurobiology. Yet the possible involvement of cell signaling in neurotoxic events has been considered only recently, and evidence of a direct causal relationship between alterations of signal transduction systems and neurotoxicity is still limited. This brief review was meant to summarize some of the principal signal-transduction mechanisms and to offer some examples of their interactions with neurotoxicants. As identification of molecular mechanisms of neurotoxicity remains a primary objective of neurotoxicological research, it is hoped that cell-signaling events will receive increasing attention in this regard. Furthermore, investigations of the possible consequences for signal transduction that may arise from other well-characterized toxicological effects (e.g., oxidative stress and cellular defense mechanisms, disruption of mitochondrial functions or role of xenobiotic metabolizing enzymes; Costa, 1992b) have the promise of providing valuable new information for neurotoxicology as well as basic neuroscience.

ACKNOWLEDGMENTS

Work by the author was supported by National Institute of Environmental Health Sciences (NIEHS) grant ES-04696, National Institute of Alcoholism and Alcohol Abuse (NIAAA) grant AA-08154, and grants from the Alcohol and Drug Abuse Institute, the University of Washington, and the Fondazione Clinica del Lavoro, Pavia, Italy. Ms. Chris Sievanen provided valuable secretarial assistance.

REFERENCES

Abou-Donia MB, Patton SE, Lapadula DM (1984). Possible role of endogenous protein phosphorylation in organophosphorous compound–induced delayed neurotoxicity. In: Narahashi T, ed. Cellular and molecular neurotoxicology. New York: Raven Press, 265–83.

Arenander AT, de Vellis J, Herschman HR (1989). Induction of *c-fos* and TIS genes in cultured rat astrocytes by neurotransmitters. J Neurosci Res 24:107–14.

Asaoka Y, Kikkawa U, Segiguchi K, et al. (1988). Activation of brain-specific protein kinase C subspecies in the presence of phosphatidylethanol. FEBS Lett 321:221–4.

Ashkenazi A, Peralta EG, Winslow JW, Rawachendran J, Capon DJ (1989). Functionally distinct G proteins selectively couple different receptors to PI hydrolysis in the same cell. Cell 56:487–93.

Balduini W, Costa LG (1989). Effects of ethanol on muscarinic receptor–stimulated phosphoinositide metabolism during brain development. J Pharmacol Exp Ther 250:541–7.

Balduini W, Costa LG (1990). Developmental neurotoxicity of ethanol: in vitro inhibition of muscarinic receptor–stimulated phosphoinositide metabolism in brain from neonatal but not adult rats. Brain Res 512:248–52.

Balduini W, Candura SM, Costa LG (1991). Regional development of carbachol-, glutamate-, norepinephrine-, and serotonin-stimulated phosphoinositide metabolism in rat brain. Dev Brain Res 62:115–20.

Balduini W, Murphy SD, Costa LG (1987). Developmental changes in muscarinic receptor–stimulated phosphoinositide metabolism in rat brain. J Pharmacol Exp Ther 241:421–7.

Battaini F, Del Vesco R, Govoni S, Trabucchi M (1989). Chronic alcohol intake modifies phorbol ester binding in selected rat brain areas. Alcohol 6:169–72.

Beavo JA, Reifsnyder DH (1990). Primary sequence of cyclic nucleotide phosphodiesterase isozymes and the design of selective inhibitors. Trends Pharmacol Sci 11:150–5.

Bencherif M, Lukas RJ (1992). Vanadate amplifies receptor-mediated accumulation of inositol trisphosphates and inhibits inositol tris- and tetrakis-phosphatase activities. Neurosci Lett 134:157–60.

Bernstein G, Blank JL, Smrcka AV, Higashijima T, Sternweis PC, Exton JH, Ross EM (1992). Reconstitution of agonist-stimulated phosphatidylinositol 4,5-biphosphate hydrolysis using purified m1 muscarinic receptor, G$_{9/11}$ and phospholipase C-β1. J Biol Chem 267:8081–8.

Berridge MJ, Irvine RJ (1989). Inositol phosphates and cell signalling. Nature 341:197–205.

Bodnaryk RP (1982). The effects of pesticides and related compounds on cyclic nucleotide metabolism. Insect Biochem 12:589–97.

Boege F, Neuman E, Helmreich EJM (1991). Structural heterogeneity of membrane receptors and GTP-binding proteins and its functional consequences for signal transduction. Eur J Biochem 199:1–15.

Bondy SC (1989). Intracellular calcium and neurotoxic events. Neurotoxicol Teratol 11:527–31.

Bondy SC, Halsall L (1988). Lindane-induced modulation of calcium levels within synaptosomes. Neurotoxicology 9:645–52.

Bredt DS, Snyder SH (1992). Nitric oxide, a novel neuronal messenger. Neuron 8:3–11.

Bredt DS, Hwang PM, Glatl CE, Lowenstein C, Reed RR, Snyder SH (1991). Cloned and expressed nitric oxide synthase structurally resembles cytochrome P-450 reductase. Nature 351:714–8.

Bressler JP, Goldstein GW (1991). Mechanisms of lead neurotoxicity. Biochem Pharmacol 41:479–84.

Candura SM, Castoldi AF, Manzo L, Costa LG (1991). Interaction of aluminum ions with phosphoinositide metabolism in rat cerebral cortical membranes. Life Sci 49:1245–52.

Candura SM, Manzo L, Costa LG (1992). Inhibition of muscarinic receptor– and G-protein–dependent phosphoinositide metabolism in cerebrocortical membranes from neonatal rats by ethanol. Neurotoxicology 13:281–8.

Chen CK, Silverstein FS, Fisher SK, Statman D, Johnston MV (1988). Perinatal hypoxic-ischemic brain injury enhances quisqualic acid–stimulated phosphoinositide turnover. J Neurochem 51:353–9.

Chiarugi VP, Ruggiero M, Corradetti R (1989). Oncogenes, protein kinase C, neuronal differentiation and memory. Neurochem Int 14:1–9.

Choi DW (1985). Glutamate neurotoxicity in cortical cell cultures is calcium dependent. Neurosci Lett 58:293–7.

Choi DW (1990). Glutamate neurotoxicity: a three-stage process. In: Guidotti A, ed. Neurotoxicity of excitatory amino acids. New York: Raven Press, 235–42.

Chuang DM (1989). Neurotransmitter receptors and phosphoinositide turnover. Annu Rev Pharmacol Toxicol 29:71–110.

Cochran M, Elliott DC, Brennan P, Chantur V (1990). Inhibition of protein kinase C activation by low concentrations of aluminium. Clin Chim Acta 194:167–72.

Corda D, Luini A, Garattini S (1990). Selectivity of action can be achieved with compounds acting at second messenger targets. Trends Pharmacol Sci 11:471–3.

Costa LG (1988). Interaction of neurotoxicants with neurotransmitter systems. Toxicology 49:359–66.

Costa LG (1990). The phosphoinositide/protein kinase C system as a potential target for neurotoxicity. Pharmacol Res 221:393–408.

Costa LG (1992a). Role of second-messenger systems in response to organophosphorous compounds. In: Chambers JE, Levi PE, eds. Organophosphates: chemistry, fate and effects. New York: Academic Press, 271–84.

Costa LG (1992b). Effect of neurotoxicants on brain neurochemistry. In: Tilson HA, Mitchell CL, eds. Neurotoxicology. New York: Raven Press, 101–23.

Costa LG, Balduini W, Candura SM, Castoldi AF, Manzo L (1992). Neurochemical effects of alcohol: the interaction of ethanol with the metabolism of inositol phospholipids. In: Manzo L, Imbriani M, Costa LG, eds. Current issues in alcoholism. Pavia, Italy: La Goliardica Pavese, 7–17.

Costa LG, Kaylor G, Murphy SD (1986). Carbachol- and norepinephrine-stimulated phosphoinositide metabolism in rat brain: effect of chronic cholinesterase inhibition. J Pharmacol Exp Ther 239:32–7.

Dawson VL, Dawson TM, London ED, Bredt DS, Snyder SH (1991). Nitric oxide mediates glutamate neurotoxicity in primary cortical cultures. Proc Natl Acad Sci USA 88:6368–71.

Dekker LV, De Graan PNE, Versteeg DHG, Oestreicher AB, Gispen WH (1989). Phosphorylation of B-50 (GAP 43) is correlated with neurotransmitter release in rat hippocampal slices. J Neurochem 52:24–30.

Desaiah D (1988). Action of metals on calmodulin-regulated calcium pump activity in brain. In: Foulkes EC, ed. Biological effects of heavy metals. Boca Raton, Florida: CRC Press, 59–67.

Di Luca M, Cimino M, De Graan PNE, Oestreicher AB, Gispen WH, Cattabeni F (1991). Microencephaly reduces the phosphorylation of the PKC substrate B50/GAP43 in rat cortex and hippocampus. Brain Res 538:95–101.

Dobbins J, Sands J (1979). Comparative aspects of the brain growth spurt. Early Hum Dev 3:79–83.

Downes CP, MacPhee CH (1990). Myo-inositol metabolites as cellular signals. Eur J Biochem 193:1–18.

Druker BJ, Mamon HJ, Roberts TM (1989). Oncogenes, growth factors and signal transduction. N Engl J Med 321:1382–91.

Drummond AH, Joels LA, Hughes PJ (1987). The interaction of lithium ions with inositol lipid signalling systems. Biochem Soc Trans 15:32–5.

East SJ, Garthwaite J (1990). Nanomolar N^G-nitroarginin inhibits NMDA-induced cyclic GMP formation in rat cerebellum. Eur J Pharmacol 184:311–3.

El-Fakahany E, Richelson E (1983). Effect of some calcium antagonists on muscarinic receptor–mediated cyclic GMP formation. J Neurochem 40:705–10.

Fain JN, Wallace MA, Wojcikiewicz RJH (1988). Evidence for involvement of guanine nucleotide–binding regulatory proteins in the activtion of phospholipases by hormones. FASEB J 2:2569–74.

Favaron M, Manev H, Vicini S, Guidotti A, Costa E (1990). Prevention of excitatory amino acid–induced neurotoxicity by natural and semisynthetic sphingoglycolipids. In: Guidotti A, ed., Neurotoxicity of excitatory amino acids. New York: Raven Press, 243–58.

Feng GP, Chen SG, Murakami K (1990). Lead inhibits purified protein kinase C subtypes from rat brain (abstr). Soc Neurosci Abst 16:1116.

Fisher SK, Agranoff BW (1987). Receptor activation and inositol lipid hydrolysis in neural tissue. J Neurochem 48:999–1017.

Fisher SK, Heacock AM, Agranoff BW (1991). Inositol lipids and signal transduction in the nervous system: an update. J Neurochem 58:18–38.

Fowler CJ, Tiger G (1991). Modulation of receptor-mediated inositol phospholipid breakdown in the brain. Neurochem Int 19:171–206.

Garattini S (1992). Pharmacology of second messengers: a critical appraisal. Drug Metab Rev 24:125–94.

Garthwaite G, Garthwaite J (1986). Aminoacid neurotoxicity: intracellular sites of calcium accumulation associated with the onset of irreversible damage to rat cerebellum neurons in vitro. Neurosci Lett 71:53–8.

Garthwaite J (1991). Glutamate, nitric oxide and cell-cell signalling in the nervous system. Trends Neurosci 14:60–7.

Gonzales RA, Crews FT (1988). Effects of ethanol *in vivo* and *in vitro* on stimulated phosphoinositide metabolism in rat cortex and cerebellum. Alcoholism Clin Exp Res 12:94–8.

Gonzales RA, Theiss C, Crews FT (1986). Effects of ethanol on stimulated inositol phospholipid hydrolysis in rat brain. J Pharmacol Exp Ther 237:92–8.

Guidotti A, de Erausquin G, Brooker G, Favaron M, Manev H, Costa E (1991). Receptor-abuse-dependent antagonism. A new strategy in drug targeting for excitatory aminoacid–induced neurotoxicity. In: Meldrum BS, Moroni F, Simon RP, Woods JH, eds. Excitatory amino acids. New York: Raven Press, 635–46.

Gusovsky F, Secunda SF, Daly JW (1989). Pyrethroids: involvement of sodium channels in effects on inositol phosphate formation in guinea pig synaptoneurosomes. Brain Res 492:72–8.

Gustavsson L, Alling C (1987). Formation of phosphatidylethanol in rat brain by phospholipase D. Biochem Biophys Res Commun 142:958–63.

Habermann E, Crowell K, Janicki P (1983). Lead and other metals can substitute for Ca^{2+} in calmodulin. Arch Toxicol 54:61–70.

Hall A (1990). Oncogene products involved in signal transduction. In: Naccache PH, ed. G-Proteins and calcium signaling. Boca Raton, Florida: CRC Press, 29–43.

Hare MF, Denny MF, Atchison WD (1991). Organic and inorganic mercury alter synaptosomal calcium concentrations (abstr). Soc Neurosci Abst 17:578.15.

Henzi V, MacDermott AB (1992). Characteristics and function of Ca^{2+} and inositol 1,4,5-trisphosphate–releasable stores of Ca^{2+} in neurons. Neuroscience 46:251–73.

Hirvonen MR, Paljarvi L, Nankarinen A, Komulainen H, Savolainen KM (1990). Potentiation of malaoxon-induced convulsions by lithium: early neuronal injury, phosphoinositide signaling and calcium. Toxicol Appl Pharmacol 104:276–89.

Hoek JB, Rubin E (1990). Alcohol and membrane-associated signal transduction. Alcohol Alcoholism 25:143–56.

Hoek JB, Thomas AP, Rooney TA, Higashi K, Rubin E (1992). Ethanol and signal transduction in the liver. FASEB J 6:2386–96.

Hoffman PL, Tabakoff B (1990). Ethanol and guanine nucleotide binding proteins: a selective interaction. FASEB J 4:2612–22.

Hoffman PL, Moses F, Tabakoff B (1989). Selective inhibition by ethanol of glutamate-stimulated cyclic GMP production in primary cultures of cerebellar granule cells. Neuropharmacology 28:1239–43.

Hokin LE, Hokin MR (1955). Effects of acetylcholine on the turnover of phosphonyl units in individual phospholipids of pancreas slices and brain cortex slices. Biochim Biophys Acta 18:102–10.

Honchar MP, Olney JW, Sherman WR (1983). Systemic cholinergic agents induce seizures and brain damage in lithium-treated rats. Science 200:323–5.

Honegger P (1986). Protein kinase C–activating promoters enhance the differentiation of astrocytes in aggregating fetal brain cell cultures. 46:1561–6.

Housley MD (1991). "Crosstalk": a pivotal role for protein kinase C in modulating relationships between signal transduction pathways. Eur J Biochem 195:9–27.

Hughes AR, Putney JW (1990). Inositol phosphate formation and its relationship to calcium signaling. Environ Health Perspect 84:141–7.

Ignarro LJ (1991). Signal transduction mechanisms involving nitric oxide. Biochem Pharmacol 41:485–90.

Inoue Y, Saijoh K, Sumino K (1988). Action of mercurials on activity of partially purified soluble protein kinase C from mice brain. Pharmacol Toxicol 62:278–81.

Isom GE, Yim GKW, Patel MN (1992). The role of NMDA receptor activation in cyanide neurotoxicity in primary hippocampal cultures. Toxicologist 12:293.

Izumi Y, Benz AM, Clifford DB, Zorumski CF (1992). Nitric oxide inhibitors attenuate *N*-methyl-D-aspartate excitotoxicity in rat hippocampal slices. Neurosci Lett 135:227–30.

Johnson JD, Conroy WG, Isom GE (1987). Alteration of cytosolic calcium levels in PC12 cells by potassium cyanide. Toxicol Appl Pharmacol 88:217–24.

Katsuyama H, Saijoh K, Inoue Y, Sumino K (1989). ^{3}H-PDBu binding after administration of methylmercury to mice. Bull Environ Contam Toxicol 43:886–92.

Kendall-Harden T (1989). Muscarinic cholinergic receptor–mediated regulation of cyclic AMP metabolism. In: Brown JH, ed. muscarinic receptors. Clifton, New Jersey: Humana Press, 221–58.

Kikkawa U, Nishizuka Y (1986). The role of protein kinase C in transmembrane signalling. Annu Rev Cell Biol 2:149–78.

Kikkawa U, Kishinoto A, Nishizuka Y (1989). The protein kinase C family: heterogeneity and its implications. Annu Rev Biochem 58:31–44.

Kikkawa U, Ogita K, Shearman MS, et al. (1988). The heterogeneity and differential expression of protein kinase C in nervous tissue. Phil Trans R Soc Lond (Biol) 320:313–24.

Kikkawa U, Takai Y, Tamaka Y, Miyake R, Nishizuka Y (1983). Protein kinase C as a possible receptor protein of tumor promoting phorbol esters. J Biol Chem 258:11442–5.

Kittur S, Endo H, Higgins GA, Sabri M, Spencer PL, Stephens JM, Pekala PH (1991). Immediate early gene expression in acrylamide neurotoxicity (abstr). Soc Neurosci Abst 17:96.

Koh JY, Palmer E, Cotman CW (1991). Activation of the metabotropic glutamate receptor attenuates *N*-methyl-D-aspartate neurotoxicity in cortical cultures. Proc Natl Acad Sci USA 88:9431–5.

Komulainen H, Bondy SC (1987a). Increased free intrasynaptosomal Ca^{2+} by neurotoxic organometals: distinctive mechanisms. Toxicol Appl Pharmacol 88:77–86.

Komulainen H, Bondy SC (1987b). Modulation of levels of free calcium within synaptosomes by organochlorine insecticides. J Pharmacol Exp Ther 241:575–81.

Komulainen H, Bondy SC (1988). Increased free intracellular Ca^{2+} by toxic agents: an index of potential neurotoxicity? Trends Pharmacol Sci 9:154–6.

Krebs EG (1989). Role of the cyclic AMP–dependent protein kinase in signal transduction. JAMA 262:1815–8.

Levesque PC, Atchison WD (1991). Disruption of brain mitochondrial calcium sequestration by methylmercury. J Pharmacol Exp Ther 256:236–42.

Lichtstein D, Rodbard D (1987). A second look at the second messenger hypothesis. Life Sci 40:2041–51.

Lo WWY, Hughes J (1987). Receptor–phosphoinositidase C coupling. Multiple G proteins? FEBS Lett 224:1–3.

Macara IG (1989). The role of oncogene and proto-oncogene products in signal transduction. In: Michell RH, Drummond AH, Downes CP, eds. Inositol lipids in cell signaling. New York: Academic Press, 501–19.

Machu TK, Olsen RW, Browning MD (1991). Ethanol has no effect on cAMP-dependent protein kinase–, protein kinase C–, or Ca^{2+}-calmodulin–dependent protein kinase II–stimulated phosphorylation of highly purified substrates *in vitro*. Alcoholism: Clin Exp Res 15:1040–4.

Majerus PW, Connolly TM, Bansall VS, Inhorn RC, Ross TS, Lips DL (1988). Inositol phosphates: synthesis and degradation. J Biol Chem 263:3051–4.

Manev H, Favaron M, Bertolino M, Brooker G, Guidotti A, Costa E (1990). Importance of sustained protein kinase C translocation and destabilization of Ca^{2+} homeostasis in glutamate-induced neuronal death. In: Guidotti A, ed, Neurotoxicity of excitatory amino acids. New York: Raven Press, 63–78.

Markovac J, Goldstein GW (1988a). Lead activates protein kinase C in immature rat brain microvessels. Toxicol Appl Pharmacol 96:14–23.

Markovac J, Goldstein GW (1988b). Picomolar concentrations of lead stimulate brain protein kinase C. Nature 334:71–3.

Martin TFJ (1991). Receptor regulation of phosphoinositidase C. Pharmacol Rev 49:329–45.

McCall T, Vallance P (1992). Nitric oxide takes centre-stage with newly defined roles. Trends Pharmacol Sci 13:1–6.

McKinney M, Richelson E (1989). Muscarinic receptor regulation of cyclic GMP and eicosanoid production. In: Brown JH, ed. The muscarinic receptors. Clifton, New Jersey: Humana Press, 309–40.

Michell RH (1975). Inositol phospholipids and cell surface receptor function. Biochem Biophys Acta 415:81–147.

Moncada S, Palmer RMJ, Higgs EA (1991). Nitric oxide: physiology, pathophysiology and pharmacology. Pharmacol Rev 43:109–42.

Morgan JI, Curran T (1986). Role of ion flux in the control of *c-fos* expression. Nature 322:552–5.

Morgan JI, Curran T (1988). Calcium as a modulator of the immediate-early gene cascade in neurons. Cell Calcium 9:303–11.

Morgan JI, Curran T (1989). Stimulus-transcription coupling in neurons: role of immediate-early genes. Trends Neurosci 12:459–62.

Morgan JI, Cohen DR, Hempstead JI, Curran T (1987). Mapping patterns of *c-fos* expression in the central nervous system after seizure. Science 237:192–7.

Moser GI, Smart RC (1989). Hepatic tumor promoting chlorinated hydrocarbons stimulate protein kinase C activity. Toxicologist 9:125.

Mundy WR, Ward TR, Forbis V, Tilson HA (1992). Effect of repeated organophosphate administration on carbachol-stimulated phosphoinositide metabolism in rat brain. Toxicologist 12:318.

Murphy S, McCabe N, Morrow C, Pearce B (1987). Phorbol ester stimulates proliferation of astrocytes in primary culture. Dev Brain Res 31:133–5.

Nathanson JA, Bloom FE (1975). Lead-induced inhibition of brain adenyl cyclase. Nature 255:419–20.

Neumann PE, Taketa F (1987). Effects of triethyltin bromide on protein phosphorylation in subcellular fractions from rat and rabbit brain. Mol Brain Res 2:83–7.

Nicoletti F, Jadarola MJ, Wroblewski JT, Costa E (1986). Excitatory aminoacid recognition sites coupled with inositol phospholipid metabolism: developmental changes and interactions with alpha$_1$-adrenoceptors. Proc Natl Acad Sci USA 83:1931–5.

Nicoletti F, Wroblewski JT, Alho H, Eva C, Fadda E, Costa E (1987). Lesions of putative glutamatergic pathways potentiate the increase of inositol phospholipid hydrolysis elicited by excitatory amino acids. Brain Res 436:103–12.

Nicoletti F, Aleppo G, Bruno V, Scapegnini U (1992). Metabotropic glutamate receptors: neurotoxic or neuroprotective? Toxicol Lett (suppl 1): 79–80.

Nicotera P, Bellomo G, Orrenius S (1990). The role of Ca^{2+} in cell killing. Chem Res Toxicol 3:484–94.

Nishizuka Y (1986). Studies and perspectives of protein kinase C. Science 233:305–12.

Nishizuka Y (1988). The molecular heterogeneity of protein kinase C and its implication for cellular regulation. Nature 334:661–5.

O'Callaghan JP (1992). Assessment of neurotoxicity using assays of neuron- and glia-localized proteins: chronology and critique. In: Tilson HA, Mitchell CL, eds. Neurotoxicology. New York: Raven Press, 88–100.

Olney JW, Zorumski C, Price MT, Labruyere J (1991). L-Cysteine, a bicarbonate-sensitive endogenous excitotoxin. Science 248:596–8.

Orrenius S, McConney DJ, Jones DP, Nicotera P (1988). Ca^{2+}-Activated mechanisms in toxicity and programmed cell death. ISI Atlas of Science/Pharmacology pp. 319–324.

Parker PJ, Coussens L, Totty N, et al. (1986). The complete primary structure of protein kinase C, the major phorbol ester receptor. Science 233:853–66.

Patel J, Keith RA, Salama AI, Moore WE (1991). Role of calcium in regulation of phosphoinositide signaling pathway. J Mol Neurosci 3:19–27.

Pennington SN (1992). Ethanol-induced teratology and second messenger signal transduction. In:

Miller MW, ed. Development of the central nervous system: effects of alcohol and opiates. New York: Wiley-Liss, 189–207.

Pintor A, Fortuna S, Nalepa I, Michalek H (1992). Effects of diisopropylfluorophosphate on muscarinic M_1-receptors and on receptor mediated responsiveness of the phosphatidylinositol system in the cerebral cortex of rats. Neurotoxicology 13:289–94.

Piomelli D, Greengard P (1990). Lipoxygenase metabolites of arachidonic acid in neuronal trans-membrane signalling. Trends Pharmacol Sci 11:367–73.

Pounds JG (1984). Effect of lead intoxication on calcium homeostasis and calcium mediated cell function: a review. Neurotoxicology 5:295–331.

Pounds JG, Rosen JF (1988). Cellular Ca^{2+} homeostasis and Ca^{2+}-mediated processes as critical targets for toxicant action: conceptual and methodological pitfalls. Toxicol Appl Pharmacol 94:331–41.

Rabe CS, Weight FF (1988). Effects of ethanol on neurotransmitter release and intracellular free calcium in PC12 cells. J Pharmacol Exp Ther 244:417–22.

Rana RS, Hokin LE (1990). Role of phosphoinositides in transmembrane signaling. Physiol Rev 70:115–64.

Rasmussen H, Barrett P, Smallwood J, Bollag W, Isales C (1990). Calcium ion as intracellular messenger and cellular toxin. Environ Health Perspect 84:17–25.

Ritchie T, Kim HS, Cole R, De Vellis J, Noble EP (1988). Alcohol-induced alterations of phosphoinositide hydrolysis in astrocytes. Alcohol 5:183–7.

Robison GA, Butcher RW, Sutherland EW (1971). Cyclic AMP. New York: Academic Press, 316.

Rossi A, Manzo L, Orrenius S, Vahter M, Nicotera P (1991). Modifications of cell signalling in the cytotoxicity of metals. Pharmacol Toxicol 68:424–9.

Rossi AD, Manzo L, Vanter M, Larsson O, Bergreen PO, Orrenius S, Nicotera P (1992). Interaction of inorganic mercury with cell signalling systems in PC12 cells. Toxicologist 12:314.

Sarafian TA, Verity MA (1992). Methylmercury specifically increases intracellular Ca^{2+} and inositol phosphate levels in cultured granule neurons. J Neurochem (in press).

Saunders RD, DeVries GH (1988). Schwann cell proliferation is accompanied by enhanced inositol phospholipid metabolism. J Neurochem 50:876–82.

Savolainen KM, Muona O, Nelson SR, Samson FE, Pazdernik TL (1991). Lithium modifies convulsions and brain phosphoinositide turnover induced by organophosphates. Pharmacol Toxicol 68:1–9.

Savolainen KM, Nelson SR, Samson FE, Pazdernik TL (1988). Soman-induced convulsions affect the inositol lipid signaling system: potentiation by lithium; attenuation by atropine and diazepam. Toxicol Appl Pharmacol 96:305–14.

Scharfman HE, Schwartzkroin PA (1989). Protection of dentate hilar cells from prolonged stimulation by intracellular calcium chelation. Science 246:257–60.

Sheng M, Greenberg ME (1990). The regulation and function of *c-fos* and other immediate early genes in the nervous system. Neuron 4:477–85.

Sheng M, McFadden G, Greenberg ME (1990). Membrane depolarization and calcium induced *c-fos* transcription via phosphorylation of transcription factor CREB. Neuron 4:571–82.

Shimizu T, Wolfe LS (1990). Arachidonic acid cascade and signal transduction. J Neurochem 55:1–15.

Siesjo BK (1990). Calcium, excitotoxins and brain damage. NIPS 5:120–5.

Silverstein FS, Chen R, Johnston MV (1986). The glutamate analogue quisqualic acid is neurotoxic in striatum and hippocampus of immature rat brain. Neurosci Lett 71:13–18.

Simmet T, Peskar BA (1990). Lipoxygenase products of polyunsaturated fatty acid metabolism in the central nervous system: biosynthesis and putative functions. Pharmacol Rev 22:667–82.

Smith TL (1987). Chronic ethanol consumption reduces ^{3}H-inositol (1,4,5)-trisphosphate specific binding in mouse cerebellar membrane fragments. Life Sci 41:2863–8.

Southam E, Garthwaite J (1991). Intercellular action of nitric oxide in adult rat cerebellar slices. NeuroReport 2:658–60.

Speizer LA, Watson MJ, Kanter JR, Brunton LL (1989). Inhibition of phorbol ester binding and protein kinase C activity by heavy metals. J Biol Chem 264:5581–5.

Stoclet JC, Gererd D, Kilhoffer MC, Lugvier C, Miller R, Schaeffer P (1987). Calmodulin and its role in intracellular calcium regulation. Prog Neurobiol 29:321–64.

Tandon P, Ali SF, Bonner M, Tilson HA (1989a). Characterization of receptor-coupled phosphoinsoitide hydrolysis in the rat hippocampus after intradentate colchicine. J Neurochem 53:117–25.

Tandon P, Barone S, Drust EG, Tilson HA (1991). Long-term behavioral and neurochemical effects of intradentrate administration of colchicine in rats. Neurotoxicology 12:67–78.

Tandon P, Harry G, Tilson HA (1989b). Colchicine-induced alterations in receptor-stimulated phosphoinositide hydrolysis in the rat hippocampus. Brain Res 477;308–13.

Terry JB, Pazdernik TL, Nelson SR (1990). Effect of LiCl pretreatment on cholinomimetic-induced seizures and seizure-induced brain edema in rats. Neurosci Lett 114:123–7.

Trottman CH, Pentyala SN, Sekhon BS, Desaiah D (1991). In vitro effect of triorganotins on protein kinase C activity in rat brain. Toxicologist 11:310.

Vendrell M, Tusell JM, Serratosa J (1992). Effect of γ-hexachlorocyclohexane and its isomers on protooncogene *c-fos* expression in brain. Neurotoxicology 13:301–8.

Vendrell M, Zawia NH, Serratosa J, Bondy SC (1991). *c-fos* and ornithine decarboxylase gene expression in brain as early markers of neurotoxicity. Brain Res 544:291–6.

Verity MA (1992). Ca^{2+}-dependent processes as mediators of neurotoxicity. Neurotoxicology 13:139–48.

Vig PJS, Desaiah D (1992). ATP inhibits lead-mediated increase in inositol 1,4,5-trisphosphate and 1,3,4,5-tetrakisphosphate receptor binding in rat cerebellum. Toxicologist 12:316.

Volpe P, Krause KH, Hashimoto S, Zorzato F, Pozzan T, Meldolesi J, Leiw DP (1988). "Calciosome," a cytoplasmic organelle: the inositol 1,4,5-triphosphate–sensitive Ca^{2+} store of nonmuscle cells? Proc Natl Acad Sci USA 85:1091–5.

Walaas SI, Greengard P (1991). Protein phosphorylation and neuronal function. Pharmacol Rev 43:299–349.

Whitman M, Cantley L (1988). Phosphoinositide metabolism in the control of cell proliferation. Biochim Biophys Acta 948:327–44.

Worley PF, Baraban JM, Snyder SH (1989). Inositol 1,4,5-trisphosphate receptor binding: autoradiographic localization in rat brain. J Neurosci 9:339–46.

Yamamoto HA (1992). Protective effect of N^G-nitro-L-arginine (N^5[imino (nitroamino) methyl]-L-ornithine) against cyanide-induced convulsions in mice. Toxicology 71:277–83.

Zinkand WC, Moore WG, Thompson C, Salama AI, Patel J (1992). Ibotenic acid mediates neurotoxicity and phosphoinositide hydrolysis by independent receptor mechanisms. Mol Chem Neuropathol 16:1–10.

17
Excitotoxicity

John W. Olney
Washington University Medical School
St. Louis, Missouri

INTRODUCTION

In recent years, glutamate (Glu) and aspartate (Asp) have become recognized as the Jekyll/Hyde molecules of the central nervous system (CNS). These common acidic amino acids, which are naturally present in higher concentrations than any other amino acids in the CNS, serve vitally important metabolic, neurotrophic, and neurotransmitter roles, but also harbor treacherous neurotoxic potential. Significant progress has been made recently in understanding the neurotoxic (excitotoxic) properties of Glu and related excitatory amino acids (EAAs). Three classes of EAA receptor that mediate excitotoxicity have been identified, drugs with antiexcitotoxic actions have been discovered, and evidence for the complicity of both exogenous and endogenous excitotoxins in neurodegenerative disorders has begun to unfold. There now is substantial evidence for the involvement of each EAA receptor subtype in one or more human neurodegenerative syndromes, and recent findings suggest that EAA receptors are sensitive mediators of excitotoxicity at both ends of the age spectrum.

Historical Perspective

Three decades ago, Curtis and Watkins (1963), using newly developed microelectrophoretic techniques to examine the membrane-depolarizing properties of Glu and related compounds, characterized the structural requirements for molecular interaction with an apparent EAA receptor. However, the myriad metabolic involvements of Glu, its ability to excite neurons throughout the CNS, and the lack of any known mechanism for terminating its excitatory action led neuroscientists of the 1960s and 1970s to reject Glu as a transmitter candidate. In the 1980s and 1990s, the pendulum has swung steadily in the opposite direction, and this common acidic amino acid is now widely accepted as the substance that most likely mediates fast neurotransmission at the majority of excitatory synapses in the mammalian CNS.

Thirty-six years ago, Lucas and Newhouse (1957) reported that subcutaneous administration of Glu to infant mice destroys neurons in the developing retina. This remarkable observation was largely ignored until it was found a decade later that either oral (Olney and Ho, 1970) or subcutaneous (Olney, 1969a,b, 1971) administration of Glu to immature animals of various species, including primates (Olney et al., 1972a), destroys neurons not only in the retina but in several regions of the brain. The brain lesions were localized to circumventricular organ (CVO) regions that lack blood-brain barriers. This suggested that Glu might be able to destroy neurons in any brain region to which it had free access, and it delineated CVO brain regions as a valuable in vivo testing ground for elucidating the neurotoxic properties of Glu. Ultrastructural examination of the retinal and CVO lesions (Olney 1969b, 1971; Olney et al., 1972a) localized the apparent site of toxic action to postsynaptic dendrosomal membranes where Glu excitatory synaptic receptors were presumed to be located. More definitive insight into the mechanism was provided by molecular-specificity studies (Olney et al., 1971) showing that specific Glu analogues that mimic the neuroexcitatory properties of Glu also mimic its CVO neurotoxic effects, that these analogues have a parallel order of potencies for their excitatory and toxic actions, and that analogues lacking excitatory activity also lack neurotoxicity. These and related observations gave rise to the excitotoxicity concept (Olney et al., 1971, 1975; Olney, 1974) that Glu destroys neurons by excessive activation of excitatory receptors on their dendrosomal surfaces.

The identification of EAA receptor subtypes differentially sensitive to specific agonists (N-methyl-D-aspartate [NMDA], quisqualic acid [Quis], and kainic acid [KA]), and the discovery of antagonists that block the excitatory actions of EAA agonists at such receptors (Watkins, 1978; Watkins and Evans, 1981), permitted the excitotoxic hypothesis to be rigorously tested. Shortly after the first EAA antagonists were identified electrophysiologically (e.g., α-amino adipate, D-2-amino-5-phosphonovalerate), it was shown that they protect neurons in the in vivo mouse hypothalamus against the neurotoxic actions of Glu or its more potent analogue, NMDA (Olney et al., 1979, 1981). By in vitro methods (Rothman, 1984; Olney et al., 1986b, 1987a,b; Choi et al., 1988), many EAA antagonist candidates were subsequently screened systematically and found to have antiexcitotoxic activities corresponding in potency and receptor specificity to their known antiexcitatory activities.

Special Features of NMDA Receptors

Of the three types of EAA receptor (NMDA, Quis, KA) that are capable of mediating excitotoxic events, the NMDA receptor has received the most attention (Fig. 1). Several features of the NMDA receptor distinguish it from other subtypes of EAA receptor. This receptor is linked to a cation channel that has a much higher Ca^{2+} conductance than ion channels associated with other EAA receptor subtypes (Dingledine 1983; MacDermott et al., 1986; but see Hume et al., 1991), and the NMDA ion channel is subject to a voltage-dependent Mg^{2+} blockade (Mayer et al., 1984). The NMDA receptor is closely associated with a strychnine-insensitive glycine receptor (Johnson and Ascher, 1987) and with a polyamine receptor (Ransom and Stec, 1988; Reynolds and Miller, 1989; Romano et al., 1991). When the former is activated by glycine and the latter by spermine or spermidine, this facilitates opening of the NMDA ion channel. Phencyclidine (PCP) receptors (Lodge et al., 1982, 1987) are positioned witin the NMDA ion channel, permitting PCP agonists to perform an open channel block (MacDonald et al., 1987). In addition, there is evidence that Zn^{2+}, acting at a separate site near the mouth of the NMDA ion channel, acts as an inhibitory modulator of channel function (Westbrook and Mayer, 1987). Thus, as Fig. 1 illustrates, the NMDA receptor system is a remarkably complex entity, the normal function of which depends on a dynamic equilibrium among multiple facilitative and inhibitory factors. It follows that any pathological process abnormally increasing any of the facilitative forces or decreasing inhibitory forces might create an imbalance rendering the system prone to an expression of excitotoxicity.

Other Excitatory Amino Acid Receptors

In addition to the NMDA receptor, two other EAA receptors linked to ion channels (ionotropic receptors) were initially described. These are the Quis and KA receptors, which are often referred to collectively as non-NMDA receptors because in electrophysiological studies it has been difficult to determine whether the non-NMDA receptor is two different receptors or merely one receptor that responds differently to Quis and KA. The bulk of evidence suggests that non-NMDA ionotrophic receptors are associated with Na^+/K^+ ion channels that, unlike the NMDA ion channel, have a low conductance for Ca^{2+}. However, recent site-directed mutagenesis experiments pertaining to newly cloned non-NMDA receptor subunits have resulted in the surprising finding that the presence or absence of a single amino acid in one transmembrane domain of these subunits determines whether

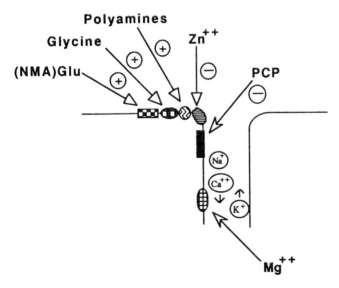

Figure 1 A schematic depiction of the various components of the *N*-methyl-D-aspatate (NMDA) receptor–ionophore complex. Recent evidence suggests that endogenous transmitter (presumably glutamate [Glu]) released from presynaptic axon terminals activates NMDA receptors on postsynaptic dendrosomal membranes, resulting in opening of a cation channel. Coupled with the NMDA receptor are recognition sites through which glycine and certain polyamines (spermine or spermidine) facilitate opening of the NMDA ion channel, whereas phencyclidine (PCP), Zn^{2+}, and Mg^{2+}, each acting at a separate site, are antagonists of channel function.

they will be permeable to Ca^{2+} (Hollmann et al., 1991; Verdoorn et al., 1991; Hume et al., 1991).

A Glu receptor that is differentially responsive to 2-amino-4-phosphonobutyrate (AP4) has been described in the retina (Miller and Slaughter, 1986) and dentate hippocampal gyrus (Koerner and Cotman, 1981). Relatively little is understood about this receptor, although in the hippocampus it appears to be on presynaptic axon terminals and may regulate the release of Glu, whereas in the retina it is presumably postsynaptic and mediates the natural action of Glu at the photoreceptor synapse with "on" bipolar cells.

Initially the Quis receptor was characterized as an ionotrophic receptor, but more recently it has been recognized that Quis activates two separate receptors, one being the above-mentioned non-NMDA ionotropic receptor and the other being a metabotropic receptor that is coupled by a G protein to phosphoinositide hydrolysis (Sladeczek et al., 1985; Sugiyama et al., 1987). The Quis ionotropic receptor has been renamed after AMPA (amino-3-hydroxy-5-methylisoxazole-4-propionic acid), an agonist that acts selectively at this receptor without activity at the Quis metabotropic receptor. Recently, trans-ACPD (aminocyclopentane dicarboxyic acid) was identified (Palmer et al., 1989) as an agonist that selectively activates the Quis metabotropic but not ionotropic receptor. Schoepp and colleagues (1989, 1990) have identified AP3 (2-amino-3-phosphonopropionic acid) as an apparent antagonist of the Quis metabotropic receptor in that it inhibits ACPD-stimulated phosphoinositide hydrolysis.

Recent Explosion in Excitatory Transmitter Receptor Cloning

Although I have referred above to EAA receptors identified by pharmacological and electrophysiological methods as if they were single invariant entities, molecular biology techniques have very recently transformed this scene (Fig. 2). Gene cloning has resulted recently in the identification of one NMDA receptor that appears to have most if not all biological properties of the NMDA receptor channel complex (Moriyoshi et al., 1991), and more recently in the description of four additional NMDA receptor subunits (Monyer et al., 1992; Meguro et al., 1992; Yamazaki et al., 1992). Over the past few years, four receptor subunits that are differentially sensitive to AMPA (Boulter et al., 1990; Keinanen et al., 1990), five that are differentially sensitive to KA (Bettler et al., 1990; Egebjerg et al., 1991; Werner et al., 1991), and five Glu metabotropic receptor subunits (Masu et al, 1991; Houamed et al., 1991; Watson and Abbot, 1990; Abe et al., 1992) have been described. It remains to be determined how these various subunits are combined into assemblies that constitute functional receptors in the mammalian CNS, and how many different assemblies are expressed and/or are functionally active in any given CNS region at any given time in ontogenesis. However, it is already evident that various EAA receptor subunits can form heteromeric receptors in which the specific combination of subunits present is a critical determinant of the functional properties of the receptor (Hollmann et al., 1991; Verdoorn et al, 1991; Hume et al., 1991; Monyer et al., 1992).

Excitotoxin Antagonists

Evidence implicating excitotoxins in neurodegenerative disorders (see below) stimulated interest in the possibility that EAA antagonists might prove valuable as neuroprotective agents in clinical neurology. In Table 1, the results of several in vitro EAA agonist/antagonist studies are summarized. The first generation of EAA antagonists identified were competitive NMDA antagonists that compete with NMDA agonists for binding at NMDA

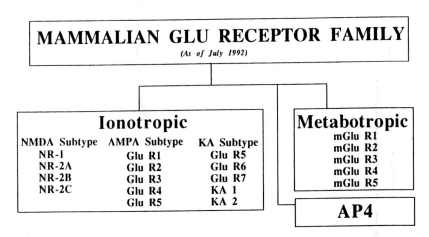

Figure 2   Over the past few years, molecular cloning experiments have resulted in the identification of 14 receptor subunits in the ionotropic subfamily and five in the metabotropic subfamily. Within the ionotropic subfamily, four receptor subunits show differential sensitivity to N-methyl-D-aspartate (NMDA), five to amino-3-hydroxy-5-methylisoxazole-4-propionic acid (AMPA), and five to kainic acid (KA). Within the metabotropic subfamily, five metabotropic receptor subunits have been cloned, all of which mediate signal transduction through G protein pathways that are still being characterized. No receptor subunits have been cloned in the α-amino-4-phosphonobutyrate (AP4) category.

receptors. The most powerful antiexcitotoxic drugs identified thus far are noncompetitive NMDA antagonists that act at PCP receptors to block both the excitatory and the toxic actions of NMDA. MK-801, a drug developed by Merck, Sharp and Dohme, is the most potent known compound in this category (Olney et al., 1987a). Certain currently marketed drugs, including dextromethorphan (Goldberg et al., 1987) and several antiparkinsonian agents (Olney et al., 1987b), are moderately potent noncompetitive NMDA antagonists. Mixed antagonists, such as kynurenic acid and 7-chloro-kynurenic acid, block the excitotoxic effects of both NMDA and non-MNDA agonists, but block the former more effectively than the latter. These compounds are of particular interest for their ability to block the excitotoxic effects of NMDA noncompetitively by an action at the strychnine-insensitive glycine site (Kemp et al., 1988). Ifenprodil is a recently described noncompetitive NMDA antagonist that blocks NMDA receptor function by an action at the polyamine site (Carter et al., 1988). The quinoxalinediones, CNQX, DNQX, and NBQX, have the important distinction of being the first agents found to block the excitatory (Honore et al., 1988; Sheardown et al., 1990) and excitotoxic (Mosinger et al., 1991) actions of non-NMDA agonists more powerfully than they block those of NMDA. GYKI 52466 is the first noncompetitive antagonist of non-NMDA receptors and the only agent that selectively blocks KA and Quis receptors without any blocking activity at NMDA receptors (Olney et al., 1992; Zorumski et al., 1992).

EXCITOTOXINS AND NEURODEGENERATIVE DISORDERS

Given the abundance of excitotoxins in the environment, the high concentration of these agents in the CNS, their intrinsic neurotoxic potential, and the several mechanisms by which such potential might be expressed, excitotoxins are logical candidates for complicity

Table 1 Potencies of Antagonists in Blocking N-Methyl-D-Aspartate (NMDA), Kainic Acid (KA), or Quisqualic Acid (QUIS) Toxicity[a]

Antagonists	vs. NMDA (μM)	vs. KA (μM)	vs. Quis (μM)
Competitive vs. NMDA			
CPP	10	—	—
D-AP5	25	—	—
Noncompetitive vs. NMDA			
PCP site			
MK-801	0.1	—	—
Phencyclidine	0.5	—	—
Unknown Site			
Procyclidine (Kemadrin)	15	—	—
Dextromethorphan	25	—	—
Polyamine Site			
Ifenprodil	50	—	—
Glycine Site			
Kynurenic acid	300	750	1000
7-Cl-Kynurenic acid	50	250	400
Competitive vs. non-NMDA			
CNQX	200	50	15
DNQX	100	50	15
Noncompetitive vs. non-NMDA			
GYKI 52466	>250	75	25

[a]Compounds were rated according to the minimal concentration (μM) required to provide total protection against the neurotoxic effects of NMDA (120 μM), KA (25 μM), or Quis (15 μM) in the isolated chick embryo retina. Antagonists were tested over a range of concentrations from 1000 μM downward until a minimal effective concentration was established. No blocking action at 1000 μM is indicated by a dash.

in neurodegenerative conditions. Over the past decade, evidence has begun to accumulate for the involvement of EAAs and an excitotoxic mechanism in the pathophysiology of a wide variety of neurological disorders, some involving exogenous excitotoxins, some endogenous ones, and some perhaps both.

Disorders Involving Exogenous (Environmental) Excitotoxins

Glutamate and Neuroendocrinopathies

Glutamate, in the form of its sodium salt (monosodium glutamate [MSG]), is one of the world's most widely and heavily used food additives. Currently, as in the past, food-regulatory authorities place no restrictions on the food-additive use of MSG, despite evidence that doses (mg/kg body weight) in the range that human young are exposed to in foods destroy CNS neurons when administered orally to immature animals (Olney, 1984). The immature brain is much more sensitive to MSG neurotoxicity than is the adult brain. Neurons most vulnerable to destruction by orally administered MSG are those lying in certain brain regions that lack blood-brain barriers, e.g., neurons in the arcuate nucleus of the hypothalamus that regulate neuroendocrine function. Since destruction of hypothalamic neurons in immature animals results in a complex delayed-onset neuroendocrine deficiency syndrome, the question arises whether ingestion of MSG by human young contributes to the occurrence of neuroendocrinopathies in later life (for recent reviews of this issue, see Olney, 1984, 1987).

Even if it could be proved that Glu ingestion by immature humans does not destroy neurons in the developing brain, there is basis for concern that Glu may disrupt normal growth and development by interacting erratically with neuroendocrine regulatory systems. It was demonstrated in the mid-1970s (Olney et al., 1976) that subcutaneous administration of a subtoxic dose of Glu to a young adult rat induces a rapid elevation of luteinizing hormone (LH) in the blood. It was also demonstrated (Price et al., 1978) that various EAA analogues of Glu elicit the same LH response, and it was determined that NMDA was particularly potent and reliable as a tool for exploring this phenomenon. In a series of subsequent studies (Olney and Price, 1980; Cicero et al., 1988) it was demonstrated that Glu and related EAAs exert their effects on the LH axis by entering the endocrine hypothalamus and activating neurons that secrete gonadotrophin-releasing hormone (GnRH) into the portal blood, which delivers GnRH to the pituitary, where it stimulates the release of LH into the systemic circulation. Wilson and Knobil (1982) then demonstrated that NMDA elicits an abrupt release of LH when administered to the female rhesus monkey. Plant and colleagues (1989, 1990) more recently showed that NMDA administration to the prepubescent male rhesus monkey causes premature onset of puberty. In addition, they have shown that administration of Glu or Asp to the prepubescent monkey causes an acute elevation of plasma LH, prolactin, and growth hormone (Medhamurthy et al., 1990). Others have corroborated these findings in other species (Urbanski and Ojeda, 1987, 1990; Urbanski, 1990). It is quite clear from these findings that administration of Glu or its excitatory analogues in doses substantially lower than those required to destroy hypothalamic neurons can stimulate neuroendocrine regulatory systems to cause an abrupt outpouring of hormones that regulate growth and development, including hormones that regulate reproductive cycling and onset of puberty. Thus, it is not unreasonable to suggest that frequent exposure of young children to Glu during critical periods of development might result in hormonal perturbations that could have an influence on growth and development.

L-Cysteine Neurotoxicity

Following systemic administration to infant or pregnant rodents, Glu and L-cysteine (Cys) induce a similar type of brain damage, but Glu damages only brain regions that lack blood-brain barriers and Cys induces a more generalized pattern of damage throughout the infant or fetal brain (Olney et al., 1972b). Interestingly, the pattern of damage induced by systemic Cys and that resulting from direct injection of NMDA into the immature rat brain are very similar, both preferentially involving the frontoparietal neocortex, hippocampus, septum, caudate nucleus, and thalamus (which is the same pattern of damage induced in immature rodent brain by hypoxia/ischemia) (Ikonomidou et al., 1989a,b). This suggests that Cys and NMDA neurotoxicity in the immature brain have something in common with each other and with hypoxic/ischemic brain damage—all three may be NMDA receptor–mediated phenomena. Consistent with this hypothesis, we have administered the NMDA antagonist MK-801 (1 mg/kg subcutaneously) to Cys-treated infant rats and found that it totally protects all regions of the immature brain against Cys neurotoxicity (Olney et al., 1990a).

Exploring the mechanism of Cys neurotoxicity further, we have found (Olney et al., 1990a) in the isolated chick embryo retina that Cys and NMDA have identical cytopathological effects, and that NMDA antagonists, including those acting at the NMDA, glycine, zinc, PCP, or Mg^{2+} sites, block Cys toxicity with potencies directly proportional to their potencies in blocking NMDA toxicity. We have also found that the excitotoxicity of Cys is bicarbonate-sensitive, i.e., in the absence of bicarbonate, Cys is a relatively weak excitotoxin, but in the presence of physiological concentrations of bicarbonate, it becomes a powerful excitotoxin. In addition, we have presented evidence that chelation of Zn^{2+} by Cys may play a role in Cys neurotoxicity (removal of the inhibitory influence Zn^{2+} on NMDA ion channel function increases the chances that NMDA receptor stimulation will have excitotoxic consequences). Since Cys is naturally present in both the brain and the environment, it qualifies as an agent that might contribute, as either an exogenous or an endogenous excitotoxin, to neurodegenerative diseases. Moreover, since it penetrates both blood-brain and placental barriers, it is a valuable systemic tool for probing, in the in vivo animal, the vulnerability of developing CNS neurons to NMDA receptor–mediated excitotoxic processes. While the mechanisms underlyng Cys excitotoxicity require further elucidation, it is already possible to point to three potentially important contributory factors—the Zn^{2+}-chelating properties of Cys, the potentiating effect conferred by the bicarbonate ion, and the hyperreactivity of the NMDA receptor–ion channel complex during development. Although Cys acts most potently at the NMDA receptor, it also triggers neuronal degeneration through quisqualate receptors (Olney et al., 1990a); this may be important for understanding its potential role in adult neurodegenerative processes (see below).

It is not clear what relevance this new information pertaining to Cys neurotoxicity may have in a food-safety context. Since it requires that a large oral dose of Cys (approximately 0.6–1 g/kg) be fed to the pregnant dam or the neonatal rodent in order to trigger the brain damage syndrome, it seems unlikely that this syndrome would ever occur in human populations solely as a result of dietary intake of Cys. However, it is of interest that the pattern of brain damage induced by Cys in the developing brain is similar to that associated with hypoxia/ischemia and with the clinical syndrome known as cerebral palsy. Since it is possible to induce a similar pattern of brain damage by direct injection of NMDA into the developing rodent brain, it seems likely that abnormal NMDA receptor activation is a common denominator of these neurodegenerative reactions. This raises the question whether some combination of factors, such as developmental hypersensitivity of NMDA receptors, mildly increased levels of exposure to Cys, and mild asphyxia or zinc deficiency, might conspire to produce a neurotoxic syndrome in which Cys, although not the sole cause, is an important contributory factor. Also to be considered is the possibility that some individuals may be genetically prone to metabolize sulfur amino acids differently and that this might result in exposure of hypersensive NMDA receptors in the developing human brain to abnormally high concentrations of Cys. If there were such a metabolic defect, the neurodegenerative consequences would be made worse by ingestion of Cys, even in normal dietary amounts. Although currently there is no evidence for expression of such a metabolic defect during development, recent evidence for expression of a heretofore unsuspected defect in cysteine metabolism in adulthood (Heafield et al., 1990; see below) lends credibility to the possibility that such a defect might exist on an occult basis during development.

β-*N*-Methylamino-L-Alanine and the Amyotrophic Lateral Sclerosis/Parkinsonism/Dementia Complex

Spencer and colleagues (1987) have postulated that a neurological disease endemic to certain South Sea islands, especially Guam, having combined features of amyotrophic lateral sclerosis, parkinsonism, and dementia may be caused by exposure to the seeds of a cycad plant that contain high concentrations of an excitotoxin, β-*N*-methylamino-L-alanine

(BMAA). It has been proposed that the gradual decrease in incidence of this disease in recent years can be attributed to a change in eating habits that has reduced the islanders' intake of BMAA (Spencer et al., 1987). Although it was first suggested on the basis of in vitro studies that BMAA may act primarily at NMDA receptors, more recent evidence depicts it as a mixed agonist that acts equipotently at NMDA and quisqualate receptors (Koh et al., 1990; Stewart et al. 1990). There are interesting parallels between BMAA and Cys in that both molecules lack the ω acidic group that characterizes all other straight-chain excitotoxic molecules, which probably facilitates their penetration of blood-brain barriers, and the excitotoxicity of both molecules is markedly enhanced in the presence of physiological concentrations of bicarbonate (Weiss and Choi, 1988; Olney et al., 1990a). Moreover, it was recently found that patients in England with motor neuron disease, parkinsonism, or Alzheimer's disease have an apparent metabolic disturbance in Cys pathways resulting in an abnormally high ratio of Cys to sulfate concentrations in the blood (Heafield et al., 1990). Inter alia, this raises the possibility, which remains to be explored, that Guamanian victims who suffer from mixed manifestations of all three of these diseases might have a Cys-metabolic disturbance plus BMAA exposure to account for their peculiar susceptibility to this devastating disease triad.

Since the Guamanian disease complex comprises features of three different neurodegenerative disease entities that occur independently of one another throughout many parts of the world, continued research into the potential role of BMAA and/or Cys in the pathophysiology of this disease syndrome could eventually lead to new insights into mechanisms underlying any or all of the three components of the disease triad. For example, if a link between either BMAA or Cys (or both) and the Guamanian disease complex is confirmed, this would suggest that excitotoxic molecules possessing mixed receptor specificity for the NMDA and quisqualate receptors may have uniquely versatile properties that can give rise to chronic neurodegenerative diseases with delayed onset and with varied modes of expression depending perhaps on the relative degree of involvement of each receptor type or the extent to which both receptors are simultaneously activated pathologically.

β-*N*-Oxalylamino-L-*Alanine and Neurolathyrism*

Neurolathyrism is a crippling neurological disorder that occurs endemically in certain parts of the world where the legume Lathyrus sativus is ingested in excess during periods of famine. The poisonous ingredient in Lathyrus sativus is believed to be β-*N*-oxalylamino-L-alanine (BOAA, also sometimes abbreviated ODAP), an acidic amino acid with powerful excitotoxic properties (Olney et al., 1976; Spencer et al., 1984, 1986; Zeevalk et al., 1988). Spencer and co-workers (1986) have recently demonstrated that the paralytic symptoms of neurolathyrism can be reproduced in monkeys maintained chronically on a diet enriched in BOAA. In the chick embryo retina, BOAA causes an excitotoxic lesion that conforms to the pattern of a quisqualate lesion (distinctly different from a KA lesion pattern). In this preparation, the neurotoxicity of BOAA is not blocked by NMDA antagonists but is blocked by CNQX introduced at low concentrations that are known to block the neurotoxicity of quisqualate but not that of kainic acid or NMDA. In other in vitro preparations, BOAA displays excitotoxicity that is blocked by non-NMDA antagonists but not by NMDA antagonists (Ross et al., 1987; Zeevalk et al., 1988). Therefore, the evidence strongly implicates a specific excitotoxin, BOAA, and a specific receptor, the quisqualate receptor, in the pathophysiology of neurolathyrism, a semichronic motor neuron disease that is moderately slow in onset and not progressive unless the victim continues to have exposure to BOAA.

It will be important to continue studying the potential role of BOAA in the pathophysiology of neurolathyrism, as such studies can provide valuable clues into the type of disease process that can be expected to occur in humans when the offending excitotoxin acts exclusively at the quisqualate receptor. Moreover, if neurolathyrism research can solve the puzzle of how food-borne agents can cause degeneration of neurons in parts of the CNS that are thought to be inaccessible to such agents, we will be in a better position to evaluate the possibility that other exogenous excitotoxins, including those used as food additives, might contribute (in concert with endogenous excitotoxins) to a variety of chronic neurodegenerative conditions.

Domoic Acid (Seafood) Poisoning

In 1987 there was an outbreak of food poisoning in Canada that affected more than 100 people, some of whom died and were found at autopsy to have disseminated acute lesions in the CNS (Teitelbaum et al., 1990; Perl et al., 1990). Some of the survivors apparently sustained permanent brain damage, as they continued to show signs of cognitive deficits, primarily memory impairment (anterograde amnesia), when retested by neuropsychologists several months after the poisoning (Teitelbaum et al., 1990). All of the afflicted persons had eaten mussels from Prince Edward Island, near Newfoundland, that were found to have exceedingly high concentrations of domoic acid, an excitotoxic analogue of Glu that interacts selectively and powerfully with the KA receptor (Biscoe et al., 1976; Debonnel et al., 1989; Stewart et al., 1990). It is well established that KA, when administered systemically to adult rats, induces persistent seizures and a seizure-mediated brain damage syndrome (Olney et al., 1986a). Recent studies have documented that domoic acid is approximately five times more powerful than KA in reproducing the same seizure–brain damage syndrome in adult rats (Stewart et al., 1990; Tryphonas and Iverson, 1990; Tryphonas et al., 1990). Persistent seizure activity (status epilepticus) was a prominent feature of the clinical symptomatology observed in the Canadian poisoning incident (Teitelbaum et al., 1990). As is discussed further below, a disproportionately high percentage of severely affected persons were elderly (Perl et al., 1990), which suggests that the KA receptor is a potentially sensitive mediator of excitotoxic neuropathology in the aged human brain.

Disorders Involving Endogenous Excitotoxins

Sulfite Oxidase Deficiency

The first human neurodegenerative condition to receive specific attention as a possible excitotoxin-mediated phenomenon was sulfite oxidase deficiency (Olney et al., 1975). This is a rare inherited disease in which an abnormal metabolite, cysteine-S-sulfate, accumulates in body tissues (Mudd et al., 1967) and disseminated degeneration of CNS neurons occurs over a relatively brief time course, resulting in blindness, spastic quadriplegia, and death in early infancy. Since cysteine-S-sulfate is a close structural analogue of Glu and mimics the excitatory action of Glu (Watkins, 1978), we synthesized a small batch of the compound and studied its neurotoxic properties. When administered systemically to infant rats or microinjected directly into the adult rat brain, it proved quite powerful in acutely destroying CNS neurons (Olney et al., 1975). This is consistent with the hypothesis that cysteine-S-Sulfate, acting by an excitotoxic mechanism, could be responsible for neuronal degeneration in sulfite oxidase deficiency.

Hypoxia/Ischemia

In 1984, Rothman (1984) demonstrated in an in vitro hippocampal cell culture preparation that EAA antagonists can prevent anoxic neuronal degeneration, and Simon et al. (1984) showed that injection of a competitive NMDA antagonist into the hippocampus protects CA-1 hippocampal neurons from degenerating in an adult rat model of cerebral ischemia. In the same year, Benveniste et al. (1984) demonstrated that cerebral ischemia causes a marked elevation in the extracellular concentration of the endogenous excitotoxins Glu and Asp in the rat hippocampus. Rothman's findings were readily confirmed in vitro (Weiss et al., 1986; Olney, 1988a), and considerable evidence suggesting that NMDA antagonists can protect against hypoxic/ischemic brain damage in vivo has now been generated (Gill et al., 1987; McDonald et al., 1987; Park et al., 1987; Olney et al., 1989; Kochhar et al., 1988). Studies from the author's laboratory have addressed this issue with respect to both the immature and the mature CNS, with the results supporting the conclusion that NMDA receptors are the primary mediators of ischemic neuropathology in the developing CNS (Ikonomidou et al., 1989a,b; Olney et al., 1989), whereas both NMDA and non-NMDA receptors are critically involved in ischemic neuropathology in the adult (Mosinger and Olney, 1989; Mosinger et al., 1991).

Epilepsy

Sustained limbic seizures induced in experimental animals by any of a number of methods result in brain damage that resembles Glu cytopathology and is distributed in a pattern similar to that seen at autopsy in patients with intractable epilepsy (for a review of seizure-related brain damage, see Olney et al., 1986a). When sustained seizure activity is induced in specific pathways believed to use Glu as transmitter, it results in acute Glu-like cytopathology in dendrosomal neural elements postsynaptic to such pathways (Collins and Olney, 1982; Sloviter, 1983; Olney et al., 1983). It is possible to prevent seizure-related brain damage by systemic administration of noncompetitive NMDA antagonists, including MK-801, PCP, and ketamine (Labruyere et al., 1986; Clifford et al., 1989, 1990). Curiously, however, the seizure activity, as recorded from depth electrodes in vulnerable brain regions, is not substantially suppressed by these agents (Clifford et al., 1989, 1990). Thus, we tentatively propose that these agents block only one component of seizure activity (the component mediated through NMDA receptors, which we postulate is the component responsible for seizure-related brain damage), while permitting seizure activity mediated through other pathways to continue relatively unabated.

Hypoglycemia

In humans, severe hypoglycemia results in brain damage, and it has been shown in the rat that hypoglycemic brain damage is associated with an increase in the release of endogenous excitotoxins (Asp > Glu) (Sandberg et al., 1986) and can be prevented by transection of Glu/Asp axonal inputs to vulnerable brain regions (Wieloch et al, 1985) or by administration of NMDA antagonists (Wieloch, 1985). Moreover, it has been shown (Auer, 1985; Auer et al., 1985) that hypoglycemic brain damage in the rat is indistinguishable, by either light- or electron-microscopic pathomorphological criteria, from Glu-induced brain damage. Thus, there is ample basis for concluding that endogenous excitotoxins play an important role in hypoglycemic brain damage.

Central Nervous System Trauma

It has been shown that CNS tissue injury entails an outpouring of endogenous excitotoxins from the intra- to the extracellular compartment (Katayama et al., 1988; Faden et al.,

1989), much as occurs under anoxic/ischemic conditions. Thus, edematous swelling or other brain tissue pathology associated with trauma may be due, at least in part, to an excitotoxic action of endogenous EAA. Consistent with this interpretation is evidence that neurological dysfunction associated with head trauma (Hayes et al., 1987; Faden et al., 1989) or spinal cord injury (Faden and Simon, 1987) is reduced by timely treatment with NMDA antagonists such as PCP and MK-801.

Dementia Pugilistica

Dementia pugilistica is a dementing illness associated with the sport of boxing (Corsellis, 1978). Since concussive brain injury in the rat is associated with elevated extracellular hippocampal concentrations of endogenous excitotoxins (Katayama et al., 1988, Faden et al., 1989), it is reasonable to propose that concussive blows delivered to the human head in a boxing contest might cause a similar intra- to extracellular translocation of excitotoxins. Conceivably, the initial concussive injury and associated excitotoxin outpourings might sensitize hippocampal or other CNS neurons to an excitotoxic process, rendering them hypervulnerable to eventual degeneration as subsequent concussive blows reexpose EAA receptors to abnormal concentrations of endogenous excitotoxins. It is noteworthy that neurofibrillary tangles (aggregates of paired helical filaments), which are prominently present in the brain in Alzheimer's disease, are found in great abundance in the brains of victims of dementia pugilistica (Corsellis, 1978). This establishes an interesting association between neurofibrillary tangles and repetitive exposure of EAA receptors to abnormal concentrations of endogenous excitotoxins. Reinforcing this association is the finding of De Boni and McLachlan (1985) that cultured human fetal spinal neurons develop paired helical filaments of the Alzheimer type when exposed in vitro to Glu or Asp. Also noteworthy is recent evidence that β-amyloid protein is present in abnormal concentrations in the brains of victims of dementia pugilistica (Roberts et al., 1990) and that the excitotoxic activity of Glu and related analogues in cerebrocortical cell cultures is increased by the presence of β-amyloid protein in the incubation medium (Koh et al., 1990).

Olivopontocerebellar Degeneration

It has been shown (Plaitakis et al., 1980, 1982, 1984) that patients with the adult-onset neurodegenerative disease olivopontocerebellar degeneration (OPCD), have a deficiency of glutamic dehydrogenase enzyme activity that impairs their ability to metabolize Glu. Ingestion of Glu by such patients causes abnormally high levels of the amino acid in the blood. On the basis of these findings, Plaitakis et al. (1982) have postulated a defect in CNS catabolism of Glu that may cause an excitotoxic build up of Glu at EAA receptors, with consequent slow degeneration of CNS neurons.

Amyotrophic Lateral Sclerosis

Amyotrophic lateral sclerosis (ALS), sometimes referred to as Lou Gehrig's disease, is a motor neuron disease that entails spontaneous degeneration of upper and/or lower motor neurons resulting in spasticity, muscle wasting, and paralysis. The disease is encountered sporadically throughout the world and occurs endemically in Guam and related islands, where it is one component of the ALS/parkinsonism/dementia complex. Although persons with ALS do not have a demonstrable deficiency of glutamic dehydrogenase, Plaitakis and Caroscio (1987) have shown that they resemble OPCD patients (see above) in developing abnormally high blood Glu levels following oral intake of Glu. Thus, a build-up of Glu at CNS synapses on the basis of an unknown metabolic defect has been postulated to account for the degeneration of motor neurons in this disease. (Plaitakis, 1991). More recently, Rothstein et al. (1990, 1991) have reported elevated cerebrospinal fluid levels of Glu and Asp in patients with ALS and have attributed this to a defect in transmitter Glu transport in both the brain and the spinal cord of ALS patients (Rothstein and Kuncl, 1991; Rothstein et al., 1992). In another recent study, abnormally high Cys-to-sulfate ratios were measured in the blood of patients with motor neuron disease (Heafield et al., 1990) suggesting that Cys may play a role in the degeneration of motor neurons in ALS. It should be noted that a metabolic impairment in the catabolism of Cys could easily have neurodegenerative consequences, since not only would the Cys generated in metabolic pathways tend to accumulate in the CNS, but Cys ingested in foods would enter the CNS and add to the abnormal accumulation.

Parkinson's Disease

It was not until very recently that evidence began to appear suggesting a possible link between an excitotoxic mechanism and neuronal degeneration in Parkinson's disease (PD). The first such evidence was presented by Sonsalla et al. (1989), who showed that the neurotoxic action of methamphetamine against dopaminergic nigrostriatal neurons (a dopamine-dependent form of neurotoxicity that may entail oxidative stress and associated metabolic impairment) is blocked by the NMDA antagonist MK-801. More recently, Turski and colleagues (1991) reported that MK-801 also protects against degeneration of nigrostriatal neurons in another animal model of PD, the MPTP (1-methyl-4-phenyl-1,2,3,6-tetrahydropyridine) model. In MPTP neurotoxicity, the pyridinium free radical MPP^+ is generated and is selectively taken up by dopaminergic neurons and accumulated by mitochondria, within which it inhibits complex I of the electron transport chain (Singer and Ramsay, 1990; Ramsay et al., 1990). It is postulated that this serves as a source of metabolic impairment interfering with the ability of nigral neurons to maintain a normal membrane potential, thus leading to partial membrane depolarization that removes the Mg^{2+} blockade that ordinarily impedes ion flow through the NMDA receptor channel. This predisposes the nigral neuron to NMDA receptor–mediated excitotoxic cell death, which can be prevented by MK-801. Thus, there is evidence from two animal models of PD supporting a bioenergetic-deficit hypothesis to explain neuronal degeneration on an excitotoxic basis in PD. Consistent with this, evidence for a mitochondrial complex I deficiency has been reported in PD (Parker et al., 1989; Schapira et al., 1990; Shoffner et al., 1991). The concept that metabolic impairment, by relieving the Mg^{2+} blockage of the NMDA receptor, might predispose neurons to excitotoxic degeneration, even in the absence of abnormally elevated concentrations of Glu at excitatory receptors, was first advanced by Henneberry et al. (1989) and currently is being entertained as a viable hypothesis to explain the pathophysiology of several neurodegenerative disorders (for example, see below, "Huntington's disease").

Also of interest is the observation (Corsellis, 1978) that PD symptoms and spontaneous degeneration of nigrostriatal neurons are features of the neuropathology in dementia pugilistica. Thus, it is possible that nigrostriatal neurons are sensitive to a pathological sequence in which either physical trauma or some toxic agent induces oxidative stress that unleashes the excitotoxic potential of endogenous EAA against these dopaminergic cells.

Very recently, evidence supporting an alternate excitotoxic hypothesis to explain neuronal degeneration in PD has been reported. In the chick embryo retina it has been shown that L-dopa, or its orthohydroxylated derivative 6-OH-dopa, destroys neurons by an excitotoxic mechanism involving non-NMDA receptors (quisqualate at low concentrations and possibly both quisqualate and kainate receptors at higher concentrations) (Olney et al., 1990b). The excitotoxic properties of 6-OH-dopa have also been demonstrated in cultured neurons (Aizenman et al., 1989). It is reasonable, therefore, to postulate an excitotoxic process mediated by L-dopa or an excitotoxic analogue with non-NMDA receptor specificity in the pathophysiology of either Huntington's disease (discussed below) or PD. In the case of PD, the hypothesis assumes a build-up of L-dopa or an excitotoxic derivative in the cell bodies of substantia nigra dopaminergic neurons, perhaps because of a defect preventing anterograde transport of the molecule from the nigral cell body to the axon terminal in the striatum. If the accumulated excitotoxin were to leak out of the nigral cell body to come in contact with quisqualate receptors on its dendrosomal surfaces, this could cause degeneration of the nigrostriatal tract, with the degenerative process originating at the level of the substantia nigra dopaminergic neuron. This hypothesis would explain why the neurodegenerative process in PD tends to be selective for substantia nigra dopaminergic neurons. It was recently shown that NMDA receptors are present in the pars compacta of the substantia nigra, presumably on dopaminergic cell bodies or their dendritic processes, and that such receptors are diminished in the brains of PD patients. Therefore, a compound mechanism might be entertained whereby L-dopa or an excitotoxic derivative would persistently stimulate quisqualate receptors, thereby holding the neuron at a reduced membrane potential, with consequent relief of the Mg^{2+} blockade, which might cause the physiological action of endogenous Glu at NMDA receptors to become pathological.

Finally, yet another excitotoxic mechanism that might explain degeneration of dopaminergic neurons in PD is suggested by two recent findings: 1.) that Cys, in the presence of bicarbonate ion, is a potent excitotoxin (Olney et al., 1990b), and 2.) that PD patients have an apparent metabolic disturbance interfering with the catabolism of Cys that is manifested by fivefold increases in Cys-to-sulfate ratios in the blood (Heafield et al., 1990). Since Cys exerts its excitotoxic activity through both NMDA and quisqualate receptors, the hypothesis advanced above relating L-dopa excitotoxicity to neuronal degeneration in PD would be equally applicable to Cys, i.e., instead of L-dopa or its derivatives accumulating extracellularly and stimulating quisqualate receptors on the dendrosomal surface of nigral neurons, Cys would accumulate extracellularly and join endogenous Glu in stimulating both quisqualate and NMDA receptors on these neurons.

Alzheimer's Disease

The first evidence providing a fundamental basis for suspecting that EAAs may play a role in Alzheimer's disease (AD) was developed approximately one decade ago. In AD, several types of neuron degenerate, including those of the cholinergic, noradrenergic, and somatostatinergic systems. Loss of basal forebrain cholinergic neurons that project to the cerebral cortex and limbic brain regions is a particularly striking feature of the neuropathology of AD that can be reproduced in experimental animals by injecting an excitotoxin into the basal forebrain region where these cells are located (Coyle et al., 1983). This has provided a useful animal model for studying the role of cholinergic neurons in the cognitive deficits associated with AD, and the fact that excitotoxins are effective in destroying cholinergic neurons and somatostatinergic neurons (Wozniak et al., 1991) implies that these neurons have EAA receptors through which either exogenous or endogenous excitotoxins could act pathologically to destroy them. Since EAA receptors are present on many types of CNS neuron, an excitotoxic process could probably explain the death of most, if not all, neurons that degenerate in AD.

Procter and colleagues (1988) have presented evidence suggesting a possible defect occurring in early stages of AD involving loss of Glu uptake sites; this might be interpreted as loss of glutamatergic axon terminals or as a loss of uptake binding sites without loss of the terminals. In the latter case, Glu would still be released by these terminals and, in the absence of adequate uptake capacity, might accumulate in excitotoxic concentrations extracellularly. Consistent with this possibility, Pomara et al. (1992) recently reported that Glu and Asp concentrations are significantly higher than normal in the cerebrospinal fluid of AD patients early in the course of the illness. They postulated that a Glu/Asp uptake defect might be reflected as an elevation of Glu and Asp cerebrospinal fluid concentrations early in the disease and as a reduction late in the disease due to loss of Glu-containing neurons as the disease progresses. Such a defect early in the disease might eventually cause neurons innervated by glutamatergic axons to undergo excitotoxic degeneration, which would be reflected as loss of Glu receptors in late stages of the disease (because the degenerating neurons have Glu receptors on their surfaces). Greenamyre et al. (1987) have described a striking loss of Glu receptors in the cerebral cortex and hippocampus of AD brains, a finding that apparently is associated only with the late stages of the disease (Cowburn et al., 1988).

While it is difficult to pinpoint the specific mechanism that is responsible for pathological changes in either dementia pugilistica or AD, it is remarkable that in both conditions the victims have widespread loss of neurons, become demented, and have abundant β-amyloid protein (Roberts et al., 1990) and neurofibrillary tangles (Corsellis, 1978) in their brains. Therefore, it is of interest to compare these two conditions in search of a common factor that might explain the similar mental and neuropathological changes. Since all victims of dementia pugilistica have in common a history of repeated brain trauma, whereas AD victims do not, brain trauma per se is not the answer. However, some factor associated with brain trauma might be worth considering. For example, brain trauma of the type encountered in dementia pugilistica is associated with an outpouring of endogenous excitotoxins (Glu and Asp) from the intra- to the extracellular compartment of the brain. As mentioned above, there is suggestive evidence for a similar extracellular accumulation of endogenous excitotoxins in the early stages of AD. A causal link between abnormal extracellular Glu/Asp concentrations and neurofibrillary tangles may be proposed on the basis of the observation that exposure of cultured human spinal neurons to abnormal concentrations of extracellular Glu and Asp causes these neurons to develop paired helical filaments of the Alzheimer type (De Boni and McLachlan, 1985). The presence of β-amyloid protein in the brains of victims of dementia pugilistica raises the possibility that periodic flooding of the extracellular compartment of the brain with abnormal concentrations of Glu and Asp could serve to trigger mechanisms underlying the generation of this protein. Moreover, if it could be established that the abnormal concentrations of Glu and Asp were present in the brain affected by dementia pugilistica at the same time that β-amyloid protein began to accumulate, this would have special significance in view of the recent finding that cultured neurons in vitro become more sensitive to the excitotoxic action of EAA agonists if β-amyloid protein is present in the incubation medium (Koh et al., 1990).

Until very recently, evidence implicating a specific excitotoxin (other than endogenous Glu) in AD has been lacking. However, recent reports describing Cys as a potent excitotoxin (Olney et al., 1990a) and revealing an apparent metabolic disturbance causing a fivefold increase in Cys-to-sulfate ratios in the blood of patients with AD (Heafield et al., 1990) identify Cys as an agent that warrants careful evaluation for its potential complicity in the pathophysiology of AD. Since Cys has dual receptor specificity (NMDA and quisqualate), an extacellular accumulation of Cys in the CNS coupled with an impairment in Glu reuptake (Procter et al., 1988) would create a situation in which both Cys and Glu might accumulate at and interact pathologically with both NMDA and quisqualate receptors.

Huntington's Disease

The demonstration that injection of excitotoxins, such as KA and ibotenic acid, into the rat corpus striatum results in biochemical and pathomorphological changes resembling those in Huntington's disease (HD) (Coyle et al., 1978) provided a useful animal model for studying this neurodegenerative disease. More recent evidence that quinolinic acid, an excitotoxin found naturally in the brain, is more potent in destroying striatal than other CNS neurons (Schwarcz and Kohler, 1983; Beal et al., 1986) but selectively spares a population of aspiny striatal neurons (Martin et al., 1987) that are also spared in HD (Ferrante et al., 1985) has raised hopes that the pathophysiology of neuronal degeneration in HD might be traced to quinolinic acid or a similarly selective endogenous excitotoxin. Although a role for quinolinic acid itself seems doubtful in view of the recent observation that quinolinic acid concentrations in the striatum of persons with HD is not elevated (Reynolds et al., 1988), this does not rule out the involvement of some other excitotoxic molecule with selective properties similar to those of quinolinic acid. It is thought that quinolinic acid acts predominantly at NMDA receptors, and it was recently shown (Young et al., 1988) that receptor loss in the striatum in HD is disproportionately greater for NMDA than for any other type of transmitter receptor.

As mentioned above in discussing PD, a modified excitotoxicity concept has been proposed in which the basic defect pertains to the maintenance of cellular energy (Henneberry et al., 1989). It is proposed that a bioenergetics defect would lead to failure of the Na^+/K^+-ATPase system that maintains polarity of neural membranes, and that this would cause partial membrane depolarization that would compromise the Mg^{2+} blockade of the NMDA receptor (a physiological neuroprotective mechanism), thereby leaving the neuron hypervulnerable to NMDA receptor–mediated excitotoxic cell death. While bioenergy impairment would be the basic defect that initiates the pathological process, excitotoxicity would be the proximal mechanism responsible for neuronal cell death. Since a wide variety of mechanisms might lead to an impairment in energy matabolism and such mechanisms might be expressed with various patterns of regional selectivity, the bioenergetic-deficiency hypothesis is versatile in its capacity to explain, on the basis of an excitotoxic mechanism, regionally selective neuronal degeneration such as occurs in HD. Beal and colleagues (1991) have recently presented evidence supporting the bioenergetic-deficiency hypothesis as a potential explanation for regionally selective neuronal degeneration in HD, inasmuch as they found that intrastriatal administration of amino-oxyacetic acid, which impairs mitochondrial energy metabolism, caused acute degeneration of striatal neurons by a mechanism involving NMDA receptors, since NMDA receptor antagonists protect against the neurotoxic process, but amino-oxyacetic acid does not directly bind to or activate NMDA receptors. Parker et al. (1990) have reported evidence for a mitochondrial complex I energy defect in HD.

Recent evidence (Olney et al., 1990b) that L-dopa, the natural precursor to dopamine in the brain, displays excitotoxicity in vitro (see above, "Parkinson's Disease") has given rise to the hypothesis that L-dopa, or an aberrant excitotoxic derivative of this compound (Aizenman et al., 1989), may play a role in HD. There is evidence that the dopaminergic nigrostriatal tract, which diffusely innervates the striatum, may give off branches that form presynaptic contacts with incoming axons of the glutamatergic corticostriatal tract (Rowlands and Roberts, 1980), the function of such branches being to tonically inhibit Glu release (Maura et al., 1990). A defect in the conversion of L-dopa to dopamine at the level of the nigrostriatal axon terminal would result in a build-up of L-dopa and a shortage of dopamine in the microenvironment of the striatal neuron. The shortage of dopamine would result in disinhibition of Glu release, with an excessive amount of Glu being released at striatal neuronal receptors. If L-dopa or an L-dopa derivative accumulating in the nigrostriatal axon terminal were to leak out, this would expose receptors on striatal neurons simultaneously to two excitotoxins (endogenous Glu and L-dopa or a derivative) that might act in concert to destroy these neurons. An attractive feature of this hypothesis is that it could readily explain the regional selectivity of the neurodegenerative process in HD. A potential problem with this hypothesis, as applied to HD, is that the neurodestructive action of L-dopa appears to be mediated by quisqualate receptors, whereas the most striking receptor losses in HD reportedly involve the NMDA receptor (Young et al., 1988). This problem can be resolved by assuming that the Glu released excessively by corticostriatal terminals acts predominately at NMDA receptors and perhaps is augmented in this action by the simultaneous depolarizing action of L-dopa at quisqualate receptors, which may be present on the same neurons. A high density of NMDA receptors and lower density of quisqualate receptors on the neurons that eventually degenerate might explain the greater loss of NMDA receptors in HD.

Wernicke-Korsakoff Syndrome

In both alcoholism and nutritional deficiency syndromes, especially thiamine deficiency, neuronal degeneration has been described in several regions of the brain, including periventricular and periaqueductal regions, the thalamus, the hypothalamus, and the mammillary bodies. Persons with this type of brain damage manifest the clinical syndrome known as the Wernicke-Korsakoff syndrome, which includes severe deficits in memory and cognitive functions. Langlais and Mair (1990) recently demonstrated that in a rat model of thiamine deficiency, which entails disseminated brain damage distributed in a Wernicke-Korsakoff pattern, the brain damage can be markedly attenuated by pretreatment with MK-801. Thus, it is possible that NMDA receptors may play a role in the mediation of brain damage associated with alcoholism and nutritional deficiency syndromes.

Infectious Disorders of the Central Nervous System

In Creutzfeldt-Jakob disease (CJD), a spongiform neurodegenerative disorder that is thought to be caused by a virus or viromimetic "prion" protein, neurons undergo a degenerative reaction in which the dendrites and cell bodies become grossly edematous and swollen, rupturing of the plasma membrane occurs, and the nucleus displays pyknotic changes (Lampert et al., 1972; Masters et al., 1976). Since these are precisely the classical signs of Glu-induced neuronal degeneration (Olney, 1971), it is an intriguing possibility that viral or related infectious agents can induce changes in neuronal homeostasis that permit an unleashing of the excitotoxic potential of Glu and Asp. In other words, endogenous excitotoxins might mediate the cell death process even though it is etiologically induced by an infectious agent. The hypothesis linking an excitotoxic mechanism to spongiform disorders is strengthened by recent evidence that β-amyloid protein, which accumulates in the CNS in CJD, sensitizes CNS neurons in vitro to the neurotoxic actions of NMDA (Koh et al., 1990). If a combined infectious/excitotoxic mechanism does underlie neuronal degeneration in CJD, it is conceivable that a similar combination might underlie other neurodegenerative diseases in which an infectious agent plays a role.

Recently, Heyes (1990) has demonstrated abnormally high concentrations of the excitotoxic agonist quinolinic acid in the cerebrospinal fluid of patients with CNS human immunodeficiency virus (HIV) infection. A high percentage of patients with CNS HIV infection display symptoms of dementia, but the underlying mechanism is poorly understood. Although it is known that HIV can gain access to the CNS, and although various neuropathological changes have been reported in this condition—some of which pertain to opportunistic CNS infections—spontaneous degeneration of neurons, as would be expected from an excitotoxic process, is not a typical feature of the disease. Reportedly, patients showing amelioration of CNS symptoms as a result of zidovudine therapy also show a lowering of cerebrospinal fluid concentrations of quinolinic acid (Heyes, 1990). Thus, there is an associational basis for postulating a role for quinolinic acid in the pathogenesis of symptoms in CNS HIV infection; however, specific evidence for a causal link between quinolinic acid and the neuropsychopathology of CNS HIV infection remains to be established. A further potential link between an excitotoxic mechanism and AIDS dementia complex is that proteins associated with HIV infection cause degeneration of cultured neurons that can be prevented by anatagonists of the NMDA receptor (Giulian et al., 1990).

Excitotoxicity and the Developing Central Nervous System

Hypersensitivity of the Immature NMDA Receptor

McDonald and colleagues (1988) have demonstrated that the immature rat brain at 7 days of age is much more sensitive to the neurotoxic action of NMDA than is the adult rat brain. In contrast, it has been known for years that KA, which is extremely powerful in destroying neurons when injected into the adult rat brain, is much less potent as a neurotoxin in the infant rat brain (Campochiaro and Coyle, 1978). While the status of the quisqualate receptor in the developing CNS is less clear, it apparently does not reach peak sensitivity until a slightly later stage of development in comparison with the NMDA receptor (McDonald et al., 1991). Ikonomidou et al (1989b) confirmed that NMDA, when injected directly into the brain (corpus striatum), is much more powerful in destroying neurons in the immature than in the mature rat brain. Moreover, they were impressed that the acute neurotoxic changes associated with injection of a small dose of NMDA (5 nmol) into the infant rat caudate nucleus spread widely throughout the forebrain and seemed to mimic, in both type of cytopathology and distribution pattern, changes associated with hypoxia/ischemia in the immature rat brain; by contrast, in the adult rat brain, doses of NMDA 10 times larger produced only a small focal lesion. These findings suggest that during development the NMDA receptor may be hypersensitive to excitatory stimulation and, therefore, excessively prone to express excitotoxicity.

Observations that lend credibility to the NMDA-receptor-hypersensitivity hypothesis include the following: 1.) The immature hypothalamus is much more sensitive to Glu neurotoxicity than is the adult hypothalamus, despite absence of blood-brain barriers in this hypothalamic zone at either age (Olney, 1984); the neurodestructive action of Glu in the immature mouse hypothalamus is mediated almost exclusively by NMDA receptors, since specific NMDA antagonists protect against such damage (Wang et al., 1990). 2.) In sulfite oxidase deficiency, fulminating neuronal necrosis occurs widely throughout the immature human CNS and appears to be caused by the abnormal endogenous excitotoxic metabolite cysteine-S-sulfate, which is an agent that acts powerfully and specifically at NMDA receptors. 3.) In the immature rodent brain, subcutaneously administered Cys penetrates blood–brain barriers and induces a disseminated pattern of brain damage that, according to all available evidence, appears to be mediated by NMDA receptors (Olney et al., 1990a).

Parallel Changes in Sensitivity to NMDA Neurotoxicity and Hypoxic/Ischemic Brain Damage During Development

Ikonomidou et al. (1989b) subjected rats at various ages to an intracaudate injection of NMDA or to hypoxic/ischemic conditions in order to compare CNS sensitivity at each stage in development to these two conditions. Sensitivity to the two conditions changed in parallel, being relatively low at birth, then steadily increasing to a peak level on the 6th to 10th postnatal days, and thereafter gradually declining to lower levels characteristic of the adult CNS. McDonald et al (1988, 1991), having conducted similar experiments, estimated the sensitivity of the 7-day-old rat brain to NMDA neurotoxicity to be approximately 60 times greater than that of the adult rat brain. These studies suggest that there is a period spanning approximately the first 2 weeks of neonatal life in the rat during which NMDA receptors may be hypersensitive to EAA stimulation. The findings of Ikonomidou et al. (1989b) also suggested that within this 2-week interval, each neuronal group may be governed by its own specific timetable for onset and duration of its period of peak sensitivity. We propose that any given neuronal group, during the period when its NMDA receptors are at peak sensitivity, may be hypervulnerable to excitotoxic degeneration, i.e., only mild disturbances in NMDA receptor homeostasis may be sufficient to trigger neuronal degeneration.

Unitary Hypothesis Relating Excitotoxicity to Developmental Neuropathological Processes

Beginning with the premise that NMDA receptors are hypersensitive during a certain period in development and that the NMDA receptors on different neuronal populations reach their period of peak sensitivity at different points in developmental time, it follows that an NMDA receptor–mediated excitotoxic process might induce various patterns of brain damage, depending on the developmental stage in which the neurotoxic process is triggered. Assuming that in human ontogenesis there is also a period during which NMDA receptors are hypersensitive, it is likely that this period would span months rather than weeks and that the period of peak vulnerability might occur prenatally rather than (or in addition to) postnatally. Thus, any type of disturbance, originating either exogenously or endogenously, that shifts the balance of forces governing homeostasis of the NMDA receptor in a direction favoring an expression of excitotoxicity could trigger an acute brain damage syndrome that would vary in distribution depending on the stage in development when the pathological event occurred.

Hypoxia/Ischemia Equivalency Concept

It has long been assumed that hypoxia/ischemia may play an important role in developmental brain damage, but it has not been possible to establish a close correlation between the degree of parapartum asphyxia experienced in the birth process and the subsequent development of clinical syndromes such as cerebral palsy, nor has it been possible to identify specific prenatal ischemic mechanisms that might be responsible for cerebral palsy–like syndromes. Thus, a high index of suspicion continues to link these syndromes to a hypoxia/ischemia-like mechanism, but the majority of such cases encountered in pediatric medicine today can be attributed only to occult and yet-to-be deciphered mechanisms.

We propose that Cys excitotoxicity qualifies as an occult hypoxia/ischemia-like mechanism that may underlie several developmental neuropathology syndromes. Just as Heafield and colleagues (1990) recently found that patients with certain adult-onset neurological disorders (motor neuron, Parkinson's and Alzheimer's diseases) have a disturbance in Cys metabolism resulting in markedly elevated Cys-to-sulfate ratios in the blood, it is possible that an adult woman during pregnancy might have such a metabolic abnormality and, therefore, might expose the fetus in utero to blood levels of Cys high enough to cause subtle excitotoxic brain damage by interaction of Cys with NMDA receptors during a period of NMDA-receptor hypersensitivity. It is possible that both the mother and the fetus might have the abnormal trait, so that the fetus, being compromised in dealing with the excess Cys received from the maternal blood, would develop exceedingly high blood and brain levels of the toxin. The type of brain damage produced by Cys or a related metabolite would be the same type that would be induced by ischemia at that stage in development, since all available evidence suggests that the same mechanism—excessive activation of hypersensitive NMDA receptors—underlies both Cys- and ischemia-induced damage in the immature CNS. In other words, Cys excitotoxicity may be viewed as a hypoxia/ischemia equivalent. Given a Cys-metabolic disturbance, it is reasonable to assume that tolerance of the fetal brain to ischemia would be compromised; even minor degrees of ischemia causing only small increases in extracellular brain Glu and Asp concentrations might be sufficient to trigger fetal brain damage by combined interaction of these three excitotoxins with hypersensitive NMDA receptors. Under such circumstances, exogenous Cys ingested by the mother, even if not sufficient by itself to trigger such a process, might contribute significantly to the excitotoxic outcome.

The above scenario provides a plausible explanation not only for cerebral palsy but for certain psychiatric conditions such as hyperkinetic child syndrome, infantile autism, and schizoprenia. Since each of these conditions could result from subtle brain damage induced during a particular stage in development, and since hypoxia/ischemia or its equivalent (Cys excitotoxicity) might give rise to various patterns of brain damage depending on the developmental stage when the damage occurs, the Cys-hypoxia/ischemia hypothesis is quite promising for explaining such neuropsychopathological syndromes.

Excitotoxicity in Adulthood and Old Age

Neuronal Attrition with Age

It is believed that CNS neurons begin to die in mid-adult life and that there is a steady attrition of neurons from that point until death. Considering the several agonist and antagonist principles that constitute counterbalancing components of the NMDA/Gly/polyamine/PCP/Zn^{2+}/Mg^{2+} receptor–ionophore complex, and evidence that this receptor-ionophore complex is widely distributed throughout the forebrain, it is not unreasonable to postulate an age-linked shift in the dynamic equilibrium of this system such that the agonist driving mechanisms overwhelm the antagonist forces in the microenvironment of a given neuron, the result being excitotoxic death of that neuron. Such a process could account for the "normal" death of a large number of CNS neurons as a function of age.

Sensitivity of Excitatory Amino Acid Receptors in Old Age

Whereas NMDA receptors are characteristically hypersensitive in early life and non-NMDA receptors are relatively hyposensitive, this is not the case in adulthood. It is known, for example, that direct injection of KA into the rat brain causes a much more severe excitotoxic reaction in the adult than in the infant brain (Campochiaro and Coyle, 1978). Therefore, although we know less about non-NMDA receptors, it is reasonable to postulate that eventually they may prove at least as important as NMDA receptors in mediating neurodegenerative phenomena in the adult and aging brain (including the "normal" attrition of neurons with age).

Although much attention has been paid to the potential role of NMDA receptors in the mediation of long-term potentiation and memory, the implication being that these receptors are prime candidates for complicity in memory-impairment disorders, recent studies (Izumi et al., 1987; Davies et al., 1989) also implicate quisqualate receptors in long-term potentiation, and evidence that domoic acid poisoning results in profound memory deficits in aged humans (Perl et al., 1990) suggests that excitotoxic mechanisms operating through KA receptors can efficiently disrupt memory in this critical age group. However, the situation is further complicated by the possibility that NMDA receptors may play a prominent role in domoic acid neurotoxicity. This suggestion is based on evidence that domoic acid and KA are both powerful convulsants that damage the brain by the same mechanism(s), and that much of the brain damage induced by KA is seizure-mediated damage that can be prevented by pretreatment with an NMDA antagonist (Clifford et al., 1990). In other words, although the persistent seizure activity induced by either domoic or kainic acid is triggered by activation of KA receptors, excessive seizure-mediated release of an excitotoxic transmitter (presumably Glu) at NMDA receptors is apparently responsible for most of the brain damage that ensues, and this explains the ability of NMDA receptor antagonists to prevent such damage. In addition, it permits the tentative conclusion that both the KA and the NMDA subtypes of Glu receptor are potentially sensitive mediators of excitotoxic events in the aging human brain.

CONCLUSIONS

Here I have discussed the potential role of excitotoxins (glutamate and related excitatory neurotoxins) in a variety of human neuropsychiatric conditions. I have suggested that excitotoxic mechanisms may underly neuropathological processes at both ends of the age spectrum, with the NMDA receptor subtype being the most sensitive mediator of excitotoxic pathology during development and both NMDA and non-NMDA receptors mediating excitotoxic events in adulthood and old age. I have pointed to L-cysteine as a promising candidate for complicity in a wide range of both developmental and adult neuropsychiatric disorders. I have briefly described several classes of antiexcitotoxic agents that are currently under study for their ability to protect neurons against excitotoxin-mediated neuronal degeneration. While it is possible that such agents will prove useful in the clinical management of neurodegenerative disorders, neither their efficacy nor their safety has been adequately established at present. With the plethora of new information about the NMDA receptor–ionophore complex, one tends to forget that non-NMDA receptors, about which we know comparatively little, can also mediate excitotoxic events. As we learn more about the physiology and makeup of non-NMDA receptors, this will undoubtedly help clarify the role of excitotoxic mechanisms in neuropsychiatric disease processes.

ACKNOWLEDGMENTS

Supported in part by National Institute of Mental Health Research Scientist Award MH 38894 (JWO) and Department of Health and Human Services grants HD 24237, DA 05072, DA 06054, EY 08089, and AG 05681.

REFERENCES

Abe T, Sugihara H, Nawa H, Shigemnoto R, Mizuno N, Nakanishi S (1992). Molecular characterization of a novel metabotropic glutamate receptor mGlu R5 coupled to inositol phosphate/Ca++ signal transduction. J Biol Chem 267:13361–8.

Aizenman E, White WF, Loring RH, Rosenberg PA (1989). Dopamine-related substance acts as a glutamatergic agonist (abstr). Neurosci Abstr 15:768.

Arendash GW, Millard WJ, Dunn AJ, Meyer EM (1987). Long-term neuropathological and neurochemical effects of nucleus basalis lesions in the rat. Science 238:952–6.

Auer RN (1985). Hypoglycemic brain damage. An experimental neuropathologic study in the rat. Doctoral thesis, Studentlitteratur, University of Lund, Sweden.

Auer RN, Kalimo H, Olsson Y, Siesjo BK (1985). The temporal evolution of hypoglycemic brain damage: II. Light and electron microscopic findings in the rat hippocampus. Acta Neuropathol (Berlin) 67:25–36.

Beal MF, Kowall NW, Ellison DW, Mazurek MF, Swartz KJ, Martin JB (1986). Replication of the neurochemical characteristics of Huntington's disease by quinolinic acid. Nature 321:168–71.

Beal MF, Swartz KJ, Hyman BT, Storey E, Finn SF, Koroshetz W (1991). Amino-oxyacetic acid results in excitotoxin lesions by a novel indirect mechanism. J Neurochem 57:1068–73.

Benveniste H, Drejer J, Schousboe A, Diemer NM (1984). Elevation of the extracellular concentrations of glutamate and aspartate in rat hippocampus during transient cerebral ischemia monitored by intracerebral microdialysis. J Neurochem 43:1369–74.

Bettler B, Boulter J, Hermans-Borgmeyer I, O'Shea-Greenfield A, Deneris ES, Moll C, Borgmeyer U, Hollmann M, Heinemann S (1990). Cloning of a novel glutamate receptor subunit, GluR5: Expression in the nervous system during development. Neuron 5:583–95.

Biscoe TJ, Evans RH, Headley PM, Martin MR, Watkins JC (1976). Structure-activity relations of excitatory amino acids on frog and rat spinal neurones. Br J Pharmacol 58:373–82.

Boulter J, Hollmann M, O'Shea-Greenfield A, Hartley M, Deneris E, Maron C, Heinemann S (1990). Molecular cloning and functional expression of glutamate receptor subunit genes. Science: 249:1033–7.

Campochiaro P, Coyle JT (1978). Ontogenetic development of kainate neurotoxicity: Correlates with glutamatergic innervation. Proc Natl Acad Sci USA 75:2025–9.

Carter C, Benavides J, Legendre P, Vincent JD, Noel F, Thuret F, Lloyd KG, Arbilla S, Zivkovic B, MacKenzie ET, Scatton B, Langer SZ (1988). Ifenprodil and SL 82.0715 as cerebral anti-ischemic agents. II. Evidence for N-methyl-D-asparate receptor antagonist properties. J Pharmacol Exp Ther 247:1222–32.

Choi DW, Koh J, Peters S (1988). Pharmacology of glutamate neurotoxicity in cortical cell culture: Attenuation by NMDA antagonists. J Neurosci 8:185–96.

Cicero TJ, Meyer ER, Bell RD (1988). Characterization and possible opioid modulation of N-methyl-D-aspartic acid induced increases in serum luteinizing hormone levels in the developing male rat. Life Sci 42:1725–32.

Clifford DB, Zorumski CF, Olney JW (1989). Ketamine and MK-801 prevent degeneration of thalamic neurons induced by focal cortical seizures. Exp Neurol 105:272–9.

Clifford DB, Olney JW, Benz AM, Fuller TA, Zorumski CF (1990). Ketamine, phencyclidine and MK-801 protect against kainic acid induced seizure-related brain damage. Epilepsia 31:382–90.

Collins RC, Olney JW (1982). Focal cortical seizures cause distant thalamic lesions. Science 218:177–9.

Corsellis JAN (1978). Posttraumatic dementia. In Katzman R, Terry RD, Bick KL, eds. Alzheimer's disease: senile dementia and related disorders. New York: Raven Press, 125–33.

Cowburn R, Hardy J, Roberts P, Briggs R (1988). Presynaptic and postsynaptic glutamatergic function in Alzheimer's disease. Neurosci Lett 86:109–13.

Coyle JT, McGeer EF, McGeer PL, Schwarcz R (1978). Neostriatal injections: a model for Huntington's chorea. In: McGeer EG, Olney JW, McGeer PL, eds. Kainic acid as a tool in neurobiology. New York: Raven Press, 139–59.

Coyle JT, Price DL, De Long MA (1983). Alzheimer's disease: a disorder of cortical cholinergic innervation. Science 219:1184–90.

Curtis DR, Watkins JC (1963). Acidic amino acids with strong excitatory actions on mammalian neurons. J Physiol 166:1–14.

Davies SN, Lester RAI, Reyman KG, Collinridge GL (1989). Temporally distinct pre and post synaptic mechanisms maintain long term potentiation. Nature 338:500–503.

De Boni U, McLachlan DRC (1985). Controlled induction of paired helical filaments of the Alzheimer type in cultured human neurons by glutamate and aspartate. J Neurol Sci 68:105–18.

Debonnel GL, Beauchesne GL, DeMontigny C (1989). Domoic acid, the alleged "mussel toxin," might produce its neurotoxic effect through kainate receptor activation: an electrophysiological study in the rat dorsal hippocampus. Can J Physiol Pharmacol 67:29–33.

Dingledine R (1983). N-methylaspartate activates voltage-dependent calcium conductance in rat hippocampal pyramidal cells. J Physiol 343:385–405.

Egebjerg J, Bettler B, Hermans-Borgmeyer I, Heinemann S (1991). Cloning of a cDNA for a glutamate receptor subunit activated by kainate but not A_1PA. Nature 351:745–8.

Faden AI, Simon RP (1987). N-methyl-D-aspartate receptor antagonist MK-801 improves outcome following experimental spinal cord injury in rats (abstr). Neurosci Abstr 13:1031.

Faden AI, Demediuk S, Panter S, Vink R (1989). The role of excitatory amino acids and NMDA receptors in traumatic brain injury. Science 224:798–800.

Ferrante RJ, Kowall NW, Beal MF, Richardson EP Jr, Bird ED, Martin JB (1985). Selective sparing of a class of striatal neurons in Huntington's disease. Science 230:561–3.

Gill R, Foster AC, Woodruff GN (1987). Systemic administration of MK-801 protects against ischemia-induced hippocampal neurodegeneration in the gerbil. J Neurosci 7:3343–9.

Goldberg MP, Pham P, Choi DW (1987). Dextrorphan and dextromethorphan attenuate hypoxic injury in neuronal culture. Neurosci Lett 80:11–15.

Greenamyre TJ, Penny JB, D'Amato CJ, Young AB (1987). Dementia of the Alzheimer's type: changes in hippocampal L-[^{3}H] glutamate binding. J Neurochem 48:543–51.

Hayes RL, Chapouris R, Lyeth BG, Jenkins L, Robinson SE, Young HF, Marmarou A (1987). Pretreatment with phencyclidine (PCP) attenuates long-term behavioral deficts following concussive brain injury in the rat (abstr). Neurosci Abstr 13:1253.

Heafield MT, Fearn S, Steventon GB, Waring RH, Williams AD, Sturman SG (1990). Plasma cysteine and sulphate levels in patients with motor neurone, Parkinson's and Alzheimer's disease. Neurosci Lett 110:216–20.

Henneberry PL, Novelli A, Cox JA, Lysko PG (1989). Neurotoxicity at the N-methyl-D-aspartate receptor in energy-compromised neurons. An hypothesis for cell death in aging and disease. Ann NY Acad Sci 568:225–33.

Heyes MP (1990). Quinolinic acid and kynurenic acid: potential mediators of neuronal dysfunction in infectious disease (Abstr). Neurochem Int 16:9.

Hollmann M, Hartley M, Heinemann S (1991). Ca++ permeability of KA-AMPA-gated glutamate receptor channels depends on subunit composition. Science 252:851–3.

Honore T, Davies SN, Drejer J, Fletcher EJ, Jacobsen P, Lodge D, Nielsen FE (1988). Quinox-alinediones: potent competitive non-NMDA glutamate receptor antagonists. Science 241:701–3.

Houamed KM, Kuijper JL, Gilbert TL, Haldeman BA, O'Hara PJ, Mulvihill ER, Almers W, Hagen FS (1991). Cloning, expression, and gene structure of a G protein–coupled glutamate receptor from rat brain. Science 252:1318–21.

Hume RI, Dingledine R, Heinemann SF (1991). Identification of a site in glutamate receptor subunits that controls calcium permeability. Science 253:1028–31.

Ikonomidou C, Price MT, Mosinger JL, Frierdich G, Labruyere J, Shahid Salles K, Olney JW (1989a). Hypobaric-ischemic conditions produce glutamate-like cytopathology in infant rat brain. J Neurosci 9:1693–1700.

Ikonomidou C, Mosinger JL, Shahid Salles K, Labruyere J, Olney JW (1989b). Sensitivity of the developing rat brain to hypobaric/ischemic damage parallels sensitivity to N-methyl-aspartate neurotoxicity. J Neurosci 9:2809–18.

Izumi Y, Miyakawa H, Ito K, Kato H (1987). Quisqualate and N-methyl-D-aspartate receptors in induction of hippocampal long term facilitation using conditioning solution. Neurosci Lett 83:201–6.

Johnson JW, Ascher P (1987). Glycine potentiates the NMDA response in cultured mouse brain neurons. Nature 325:529–31.

Kemp JA, Foster AC, Wong EHF (1987). Non-competitive antagonists of excitatory amino acid receptors. Trends Neurosci 10:294–9.

Kemp JA, Foster AC, Leeson PD, Priestley T, Tridgett R, Iversen LL, Woodruff GN (1988). 7-Chlorokynurenic acid is a selective antagonist at the glycine modulatory site of the N-methyl-D-aspartate receptor complex. Proc Natl Acad Sci USA 85:6547–50.

Katayama Y, Cheung MK, Gorman L, Tamura T, Becker DP (1988). Increase in extracellular glutamate and associated massive ionic fluxes following concussive brain injury (abstr). Neurosci Abstr 14:1154.

Keinanen K, Wisden W, Sommer B, Werner P, Herb A, Verdoorn TA, Sakmann B, Seeburg PH (1990). A family of AMPA-selective glutamate receptors. Science 249:556–8.

Kochhar A, Zivin JA, Lyden PD, Mazzarella V (1988). Glutamate antagonist therapy reduces neurologic deficits produced by focal central nervous system ischemia. Arch Neurol 45:148–53.

Koerner JF, Cotman CW (1981). Micromolar L-2-amino-4-phosphonobutyric acid selectively inhibits perforant path synapses from lateral entorhinal cortex. Brain Res 216:192–8.

Koh J-Y, Goldberg MP, Hartley DM, Choi DW (1990). Non-NMDA receptor-mediated neurotoxicity in cortical culture. J Neurosci 10:693–705.

Koh J, Yang LL, Cotman CW (1990). Beta-amyloid protein increases the vulnerability of cultured cortical neurons to excitotoxin damage. Brain Res 533:315–20.

Labruyere J, Fuller TA, Olney JW, Price MT, Zorumski C, Clifford D (1986). Phencyclidine and ketamine protect against seizure-related brain damage (abstr). Neurosci Abstr 12:344.

Lampert PW, Gajdusek DC, Gibbs CJ (1972). Subacute spongiform virus encephalopathies. Am J Pathol 68:626–46.

Langlais PJ, Mair RG (1990). Protective effects of the glutamate antagonist MK-801 on pyrithiamine-induced lesions and amino acid changes in rat brain. J Neurosci 10:1664–74.

Lodge D, Anis NA (1982). Effects of phencyclidine on excitatory amino acid activation of spinal interneurons in the cat. Eur J Pharmacol 77:203–4.

Lodge D, Aram JA, Church J, Davies SN, Martin D, O'Shaughnessy CT, Zeman S (1987). Excitatory amino acids and phencyclidine-like drugs. In: Hicks TP, Lodge D, McLennan H, eds. Excitatory amino acid transmission. New York: Alan R. Liss, 83–90.

Lucas DR, Newhouse JP (1957). The toxic effect of sodium L-glutamate on the inner layers of the retina. AMA Arch Ophthalmol 58:193–201.

Mac Dermott AB, Mayer ML, Westbrook GL, Smith SJ, Barker JL (1986). NMDA-receptor activation increases cytoplasmic calcium concentration in cultured spinal cord neurones. Nature 321:519–22.

Martin JB, Kowall NW, Ferrante RJ, Cipolloni PB, Beal MF (1987). Differential sparing of NADPH-diaphorase neurons in quinolinic lesioned rat and primate striatum (abstr). Neurosci Abstr 14:1030.

Masters CL, Kakulas BA, Alpers MP, Gajdusek DC, Gibbs CJ (1976). Preclinical lesions and their progression in the experimental spongiform encephalopathies (kuru and Creutzfeldt-Jakob disease) in primates. J Neuropathol Exp Neurol 35:593–605.

Masu M, Tanabe Y, Tsuchida K, Shigemoto R, Nakanishi S (1991). Sequence and expression of a metabotropic glutamate receptor. Nature 349:760–5.

Maura G, Barzizza A, Lottero P, Raiteri M (1990). The excitatory amino acid-releasing nerve terminals in rat striatum possess D-2 dopamine receptors mediating inhibition of release (Abstr). Neurochem Int 16:53.

Mayer ML, Westbrook GL, Guthrie PB (1984). Voltage-dependent block by Mg^{2+} of NMDA responses in spinal cord neurones. Nature 309:261–3.

McDonald JW, Silverstein FS, Johnston MV (1987). MK-801 protects the neonatal brain from hypoxic-ischemic damage. Eur J Pharmacol 140:359–61.

McDonald JW, Silverstein FS, Johnston MV (1988). NMDA neurotoxicity in 7 D.O. rats offers an in vivo model to rapidly screen neuroprotective drugs: neuroprotective effects of MK-801 and related compounds (Abstr). Neurochem Int 12:37.

McDonald JW, Trescher WH, Johnston MV (1991). The pattern and degree of selective vulnerability to excitotoxic brain injury is dependent upon developmental age. Fidia Res Fnd Sym Series 5:609–14.

Medhamurthy R, Dichek HL, Plant TM, Bernardini I, Cutler GB Jr (1990). Stimulation of gonadotropin secretion in prepubertal monkeys after hypothalamic excitation with aspartate and glutamate. J Clin Endocrinol Metab 71:1390–2.

Meguro H, Mori H, Araki K, Kushiya E, Kutsuwada T, Yamazaki M, Kumanishi T, Arakawa M, Sakimura K, Mishina M (1992). Functional characterization of a heteromeric NMDA receptor channel expressed from cloned cDNAs. Nature 357:70–4.

Miller RF, Slaughter MM (1986). Excitatory amino acid receptors of the retina: diversity of subtypes and conductance mechanisms. Trends Neurosci 9:211–8.

Monyer H, Sprengel R, Schoepfer R, Herb A, Higuchi M, Lomeli H, Burnashev N, Sakmann B, Seeburg PH (1992). Heteromeric NMDA receptors: molecular and functional distinction of subtypes. Science 256:1217–21.

Moriyoshi K, Masu M, Ishii T, Shigemoto R, Mizuno N (1991). Molecular cloning and characterization of the rat NMDA receptor. Nature 354:31–7.

Mosinger JL, Olney JW (1989). Photothrombosis-induced ischemic neuronal degeneration in the rat retina. Exp Neurol 105:110–3.

Mosinger JL, Price MT, Bai HY, Xiao H, Wozniak DF, Olney JW (1991). Blockade of both NMDA and non NMDA receptors is required for optimal protection against ischemic neuronal degeneration in the in vivo adult mammalian retina. Exp Neurol 113:10–17.

Mudd SH, Irreverre F, Laster L (1967). Sulfite oxidase deficiency in man: demonstration of the enzymatic defect. Science 156:1599–1602.

Olney JW (1969a). Glutamate-induced retinal degeneration in neonatal mice. Electron microscopy of the acutely evolving lesion. J Neuropathol Exp Neurol 28:455–74.

Olney JW (1969b). Brain lesions, obesity and other disturbances in mice treated with monosodium glutamate. Science 164:719–21.

Olney JW (1971). Glutamate-induced neuronal necrosis in the infant mouse hypothalamus: an electron microscopic study. J Neuropathol Exp Neurol 30:75–90.

Olney JW (1974). Toxic effects of glutamate and related amino acids on the developing central nervous system. In: Nyhan WN, ed. Heritable disorders of amino acid metabolism. New York: John Wiley & Sons, 501–12.

Olney JW (1984). Excitotoxic food additives—relevance of animal studies to human safety. Neurobehav Toxicol Teratol 6:455–62.

Olney JW (1987). Food additives, excitotoxic. In: Adelman G, ed. Encyclopedia of neuroscience. Boston: Birkhauser, 436–8.

Olney JW (1988a). Endogenous excitotoxins and neuropathological disorders. In: Lodge D, ed. Excitatory amino acids in health and disease. London: John Wiley & Sons, 337–51.

Olney JW (1988b). Revelations in excitotoxicology: What next? In: Cavalheiro EA, Lehmann J, Turski L, eds. Frontiers in excitatory amino acid research. New York: Alan R. Liss, 589–96.

Olney JW, Ho OL (1970). Brain damage in infant mice following oral intake of glutamate, aspartate or cysteine. Nature 227:609–10.

Olney JW, Price MT (1980). Neuroendocrine inteactions of excitatory and inhibitory amino acids. Brain Res Bull 5(suppl 2):361–8.

Olney JW, Ho OL, Rhee V (1971). Cytotoxic effects of acidic and sulphur-containing amino acids on the infant mouse central nervous system. Exp Brain Res 14:61–76.

Olney JW, Sharpe LG, Feigin RD (1972a). Glutamate-induced brain damage in infant primates. J Neuropathol Exp Neurol 31:464–88.

Olney JW, Ho OL, Rhee V, Schainker B (1972b). Cysteine-induced brain damage in infant and fetal rodents. Brain Res 45:309–13.

Olney JW, Misra CH, deGubareff T (1975). Cysteine-S-sulfate: brain damaging metabolite in sulfite oxidase deficiency. J Neuropathol Exp Neurol 34:167–76.

Olney JW, Misra CH, Rhee V (1976). Brain and retinal damage from the lathyrus excitotoxin, β-N-oxalyl-L-α,β- diaminopropionic acid (ODAP). Nature 264:659–61.

Olney JW, deGubareff T, Labruyere J (1979). α-Aminoadipate blocks the neurotoxic action of N-methylaspartate Life Sci 25:537–40.

Olney JW, Labruyere J, Collins JF, Curry K (1981). D-Aminophosphonovalerate is 100-fold more powerful than D-alpha-aminoadipate in blocking N-methylaspartate neurotoxicity. Brain Res 221:207–10.

Olney JW, de Gubareff T, Sloviter RS (1983). "Epileptic" brain damage in rats induced by sustained electrical stimulation of the perforant path. II. Ultrastructural analysis of acute hippocampal pathology. Brain Res Bull 10:699–712.

Olney JW, Collins RC, Sloviter RS (1986a). Excitotoxic mechanisms of epileptic brain damage. In: Delgado-Escueta AV, Ward AA, Woodbury DM, Porte RJ, eds. Basic mechanisms of the epilepsies: molecular and cellular approaches. New York: Raven Press, 857–78.

Olney JW, Price MT, Fuller TA, Labruyere J, Samson L, Carpenter M, Mahan K (1986b). The anti-excitotoxic effects of certain anesthetics, analgesics and sedative-hypnotics. Neurosci Lett 68:29–34.

Olney J, Price M, Shahid Salles K, Labruyere J, Frierdich G (1987a). MK-801 powerfully protects against N-methyl aspartate neurotoxicity. Eur J Pharmacol 141:357–61.

Olney JW, Price MT, Labruyere J, Shahid Salles K, Frierdich G, Mueller M, Silverman E (1987b). Anti-parkinsonian agents are phencyclidine agonists and N-methyl aspartate antagonists. Eur J Pharmacol 142:319–20.

Olney JW, Ikonomidou C, Mosinger JL, Frierdich G (1989). MK-801 prevents hypobaric-ischemic neuronal degeneration in infant rat brain. J Neurosci 9:1701–4.

Olney JW, Zorumski C, Price MT, Labruyere J (1990a). L-Cysteine, a bicarbonate-sensitive endogenous excitotoxin. Science 248:596–9.

Olney JW, Zorumski CF, Stewart GR, Price MT, Wang G, Labruyere J (1990b). Excitotoxicity of L-DOPA and 6-OH-DOPA: Implications for Parkinson's and Huntington's diseases. Exp Neurol 108:269–72.

Olney JW, Price MT, Zorumski CF, Yamada K (1992). Neurotoxicological evidence for a novel benzo-diazepine site within the non-NMDA glutamate receptor complex (abstr). Neurosci Abstr 18:757.

Palmer E, Monaghan DT, Cotman CW (1989). Trans-ACPD, a selective agonist to the PI-coupled excitatory amino acid receptor. Eur J Pharmacol 166:585–7.

Park C, Nehls DG, Ozyurt E, Graham DI, McCulloch J (1987). Ischemic brain damage is reduced by systemic administration of the N-methyl-D-aspartate (NMDA) antagonist, MK-801 (abstr). Neurosci Abstr 13:1029.

Park CK, Nehls DG, Graham DI, Teasdale GM, McCulloch J (1988). Focal cerebral ischaemia in the cat: treatment with the glutamate antagonist MK-801 after induction of ischaemia. J Cereb Blood Flow Metab 8:757–62.

Parker WD, Boyson SJ, Parks JK (1989). Electron transport chain abnormalities in idiopathic Parkinson's disease. Ann Neurol 26:719–23.

Parker WD, Filley CM, Parks JK (1990). Cytochrome oxidase deficiency in Alzheimer's disease. Neurology 40:1302–3.

Perl TM, Bedard L, Kosatsky T, Hockin JC, Todd ECD, Remis RS (1990). An outbreak of toxic encephalopathy caused by eating mussels contaminated with domoic acid. N Engl J Med 322:1775–80.

Plaitakis A (1991). Altered glutamatergic mechanisms and selective motor neuron degeneration in amyotrophic lateral sclerosis: possible role of glycine. Adv Neurol 56:319–26.

Plaitakis A, Caroscio JT (1987). Abnormal glutamate metabolism in amyotrophic lateral sclerosis. Ann Neurol 22:575–9.

Plaitakis A, Nicklas WJ, Desnick RJ (1980). Glutamate dehydrogenase deficiency in three patients with spinocerebellar syndrome. Ann Neurol 7:297–303.

Plaitakis A, Berl S, Yahr MD (1982). Abnormal glutamate metabolism in an adult-onset degenerative neurological disorder. Science 216:193–6.

Plaitakis A, Berl S, Yahr M (1984). Neurological disorders associated with deficiency of glutamate dehydrogenase Ann Neurol 15:144–53.

Plant, TM, Gay VL, Marshall GR, Arslan M (1989). Puberty in monkeys is triggered by chemical stimulation of the hypothalamus. Proc Natl Acad Sci USA 86:2506–10.

Plant TM, Medhamurthy R (1990). Recent studies of the neuroendocrine basis of the prepubertal restraint of pulsatile GnRH release in primates. In: Yen SSC, Vale WW, eds. Neuroendocrine regulation of reproduction. Serono Symposia, 19–28.

Pomara N, Singh R, Deptula D, Chou JC-Y, Schwartz MB, LeWitt PA (1992). Glutamate and other CSF amino acids in Alzheimer's disease. Am J Psychiatry 149:251–4.

Price MT, Olney JW, Cicero TJ (1978). Acute elevations of serum luteinizing hormone induced by kainic acid, N-methyl aspartic acid or homocysteic acid. Neuroendocrinology 26:352–9.

Procter AW, Palmer AM, Francis PT, Lowe SL, Neary D, Murphy E, Doshi R, Bowen DM (1988). Evidence of glutamatergic denervation and possible abnormal metabolism in Alzheimer's disease. J Neurochem 50:790–801.

Ramsay RR, Krueger MJ, Youngster SK, Gluck MR, Casida JE, Singer TP (1990). Interaction of 1-methyl-4-phenylpyridinium ion (MPP+) and its analogs with the rotenone/piericidin binding site of NADH dehydrogenase J Neurochem 56:823–7.

Ransom RW, Stec NL (1988). Cooperative modulation of MK-801 binding to the N-methyl-D-aspartate receptor–ion channel complex by L-glutamate, glycine, and polyamines. J Neurochem 51:830–6.

Reynolds GP, Pearson SJ, Halket J, Sandler M (1988). Brain quinolinic acid in Huntington's disease. J Neurochem 50:1959–60.

Reynolds IJ, Miller RJ (1989). Ifenprodil is a novel type of N-methyl-D-aspartate receptor antagonist: interaction with polyamines. Mol Pharmacol 36:758–65.

Roberts GW, Allsop D, Bruton C (1990). The occult aftermath of boxing. J Neurol Neurosurg Pschiatry 53:373–8.

Romano C, Williams K, Molinoff PB (1991). Polyamines modulate the binding of MK-801 to the solubilized N-methyl-D-aspartate receptor. J Neurochem 57:811–8.

Ross SM, Seelig M, Spencer PS (1987). Specific antagonism of excitotoxic action of uncommon amino acids assayed in organotypic mouse cortical cultures. Brain Res 425:120–7.

Rothman SM (1984). Synaptic release of excitatory amino acid neurotransmitter mediates anoxic neuronal death. J Neurosci 4:1884–91.

Rothman SM (1985). Excitatory amino acid neurotoxicity is produced by passive chloride influx. J Neurosci 6:1483–9.

Rothstein JD, Kuncl RW (1991). Glutamate transport in amytrophic lateral sclerosis: pathophysiological implications. Ann Neurol 30:235–6.

Rothstein JD, Tsai G, Kuncl RW, Clawson L, Cornblath DR, Drachman DB, Pestronk A, Stauch L, Coyle JT (1990). Abnormal excitatory amino acid metabolism in amyotrophic lateral sclerosis. Ann Neurol 28:18–25.

Rothstein JD, Kuncl R, Chaudhry V (1991). Excitatory amino acids in amyotrophic lateral sclerosis: an update. Ann Neurol 30:224–5.

Rothstein JD, Martin LJ, Kuncl RW (1992). Decreased glutamate transport by the brain and spinal cord in amyotrophic lateral sclerosis. N Engl J Med 326:1464–8.

Rowlands GJ, Roberts PJ (1980). Activation of dopamine receptors inhibits calcium-dependent glutamate release from cortico-striatal terminals in vitro. Eur J Pharmacol 62:241–7.

Sandberg M, Butcher SP, Hagberg H (1986). Extracellular overflow of neuroactive amino acids during severe insulin-induced hypoglycemia: in vivo dialysis of the rat hippocampus. J Neurochem 47:178–84.

Schapira AHV, Cooper JM, Detter D, Clark JB, Jenner B, Marsden CD (1990). Mitochondrial complex I deficiency in Parkinson's disease. J Neurochem 54:823–7.

Schoepp DD, Johnson BG (1989). Inhibition of excitatory amino acid–stimulated phosphoinositide hydrolysis in the neonatal rat hippocampus by 2-amino-3-phosphonopropionate. J Neurochem 53:273–8.

Schoepp DD, Johnson BG, Smith ECR, McQuaid LA (1990). Stereoselectivity and mode of inhibition of phosphoinositide-coupled excitatory amino acid receptors by 2-amino-3-phosphonopropionic acid. Mol Pharmacol 38:222–8.

Schwarcz R, Kohler C (1983). Differential vulnerability of central neurons of the rat to quinolinic acid. Neurosci Lett 38:85–90.

Sheardown MJ, Nielsen EO, Hansen AJ, Jacobsen P, Honore T (1990). 2,3-Dihydroxy-6-nitro-7-sulfamoyl-benzo(F)quinoxaline: a neuroprotectant for cerebral ischemia. Science 247:571–4.

Shoffner JM, Watts RL, Juncos JL, Torroni A, Wallace DL (1991). Mitochondrial oxidative phosphorylation defects in Parkinson's disease. J Neurochem 54:823–7.

Simon RP, Swan JH, Griffiths T, Meldrum BS (1984). Blockade of N-methyl-D-aspartate receptors may protect against ischemic damage in the brain. Science 226:850–2.

Singer TP, Ramsay RR (1990). Mechanism of toxicity of MPTP. FEBS Lett 274:1–8.

Sladeczek F, Pin JP, Recasens M, Bockaert J, Weiss S (1985). Glutamate stimulates inositol phosphate formation in striatal neurones. Nature 173:717–9.

Sloviter RS (1983). "Epileptic" brain damage in rats induced by sustained electrical stimulation of the perforant path. I Acute electrophysiological and light microscopic studies. Brain Res Bull 10:675–97.

Sonsalla PK, Nicklas WJ, Heikkila RE (1989). Role for excitatory amino acids in methamphetamine-induced nigrostriatal dopaminergic toxicity. Science 243:398–400.

Spencer PS, Schaumburg HH, Cohn DF, Seth PK (1984). Lathyrism: a useful model of primary lateral sclerosis. In: Rose FC, ed. Research progress in motor neurone disease. London: Pitman, 312–27.

Spencer PS, Ludolph A, Dwived MP, Roy DN, Hugon J, Schaumburg HH (1986). Lathyrism: evidence for role of the neuroexcitatory aminoacid BOAA. Lancet 2:1066–7.

Spencer PS, Nunn PB, Hugon J, Ludolph AC, Ross SM, Roy DN, Robertson RC (1987). Guam amyotrophic lateral sclerosis–parkinsonism–dementia linked to a plant excitant neurotoxin. Science 327:517–22.

Stewart GR, Zorumski CF, Price MT, Olney JW (1990). Domoic acid: a dementia-inducing excitotoxic food poison with kainic acid receptor specificity. Exp Neurol 110:127–38.

Sugiyama H, Ito I, Hirono C (1987). A new type of glutamate receptor linked to inositol phospholipid metabolism. Nature 312:531–3.

Teitelbaum JS, Zatorre RJ, Carpenter S, Gendron D, Evans AC, Gjedde A, Cashman NR (1990). Neurologic sequelae of domoic acid intoxication due to the ingestion of contaminated mussels. N Engl J Med 322:1781–7.

Thal LJ, Mandel RJ, Terry RD, Buzsaki G, Gage FH (1990). Nucleus basalis lesions fail to induce sensile plaques in the rat. Exp Neurol 108:88–90.

Tryphonas L, Iverson F (1990). Neuropathology of excitatory neurotoxins: the domoic acid model. Toxicol Pathol 18:165–9.

Tryphonas L, Truelove J, Nera E, Iverson F (1990). Acute neurotoxicity of domoic acid in the rat. Toxicol Pathol 18:1–9.

Turski L, Bressler K, Rettig K-J, Loeschmann PA, Wachtel H (1991). Protection of substantia nigra from MPP+ neurotoxicity by *N*-methyl-D-aspartate antagonists. Nature 349:414–8.

Urbanski HF (1990). A role for *N*-methyl-D-aspartate receptors in the control of seasonal breeding. Endocrinology 127:2223–8.

Urbanski HF, Ojeda SR (1987). Activation of luteinizing hormone–releasing hormone release advances the onset of female puberty. Neuroendocrinology 46:273–6.

Urbanski HF, Ojeda SR (1990). A role for *N*-methyl-D-aspartate (NMDA) receptors in the control of LH secretion and initiation of female puberty. Endocrinology 126:1774–6.

Verdoorn TA, Burnashev N, Monyer H, Seeburg PH, Sakmann B (1991). Structural determinants of ion flow through recombinant glutamate receptor channels. Science 252:1715–8.

Wang GJ, Labruyere J, Price MT, Olney JW (1990). Extreme sensitivity of infant animals to glutamate toxicity: role of NMDA receptors (abstr). Neurosci Abstr 16:198.

Watkins JC (1978). Excitatory amino acids. In: McGeer E, Olney JW, McGeer P, eds. Kainic acid as a tool in neurobiology. New York: Raven Press, 37–69.

Watkins JC, Evans RH (1981). Excitatory amino acid transmitters. Annu Rev Pharmacol Toxicol 21:165–204.

Watson S, Abbot A (1990). TiPS receptor nomenclature supplement. Trends Pharmacol Sci (suppl):1–30.

Weiss J, Goldberg MP, Choi DW (1986). Ketamine protects cultured neocortical neurons from hypoxic injury. Brain Res. 380:186–90.

Weiss JH, Choi DW (1988). Beta-*N*-methylamino-L-alanine neurotoxicity: requirement for bicarbonate as a cofactor. Science 241:973–5.

Werner P, Voigt M, Keinanen K, Wisden W, Seeburg PH (1991). Cloning of a putative high-affinity kainate receptor expressed predominantly in hippocampal CA3 cells. Nature 351:742–4.

Westbrook GL, Mayer ML (1987). Micromolar concentrations of Zn^{++} antagonize NMDA and GABA responses of hippocampal neurones. Nature 328:640–643.

Wieloch T (1985). Hypoglycemia-induced neuronal damage prevented by an *N*-methyl-D-aspartate antogonist. Science 230:681–3.

Wieloch T, Engelsen B, Westerberg E, Auer R (1985). Lesions of the glutamatergic corticostriatal projections in the rat ameliorate hypoglycemic brain damage in the striatum. Neurosci Lett 58:25–30.

Wilson RC, Knobil E (1982). Acute effects of *N*-methyl-DL-aspartate on the release of pituitary gonadotropins and prolactin in the adult female rhesus monkey. Brain Res 248:177–9.

Wozniak DF, Stewart GR, Sun S, Olney JW (1991). Sensitivity of basal forebrain somatostatinergic neurons to *N*-methyl aspartate neurotoxicity (abstr). Neurosci Abstr. 17:1066.

Yamazaki M, Mori H, Araki K, Mori KJ, Mishina M (1992). Cloning, expression and modulation of a mouse NMDA receptor subunit. Fed Eur Biochem Soc 300:39–45.

Young AB, Greenamyre JT, Hollingsworth Z, Albin R, D'Amato C, Shoulson I, Penney JB (1988). NMDA receptor losses in putamen from patients with Huntington's disease. Science 241:981–3.

Zeevalk G, Olynyk S, Nicklas W (1988). Excitotoxicity in chick retina caused by the unusual amino acids BOAA and BMAA: effects of MK-801 and DIDS (abstr). Neurosci Abstr 14:418.

Zorumski CF, Yamada K, Mennerick S, Olney JW (1992). Electrophysiological evidence for a novel benzodiazepine site within the non-NMDA glutamate receptor complex (abstr). Neurosci Abst 18: 757.

18
The Use of Neurotoxins to Model Neurological Diseases

Thomas J. Walsh
Rutgers University
New Brunswick, New Jersey

Karen Opello
Rutgers University
Piscataway, New Jersey

James David Adams, Jr., and Lori K. Klaidman
University of Southern California School of Pharmacy
Los Angeles, California

INTRODUCTION

Neurotoxicology integrates the best aspects of pharmacology, neuroscience, and toxicology. While borrowing from these disciplines it has established unique approaches, questions, and model systems. For example, it has contributed to 1.) isolating the multitude of environmental factors that damage the nervous system, 2.) characterizing the nature of the insult in both developing and mature organisms, and 3.) identifying the populations at risk. These efforts have symbolized the scope of modern neurotoxicology, but there is now a growing appreciation that neurotoxicology, neurology, and biological psychiatry share common interests that are based on a set of unified conceptual questions. The unifying goals for all of these disciplines are to discern the biology of neural insult, its functional consequences, and the extent and underlying mechanisms of recovery of function.

The most problematic neurological disorder are those associated with the degeneration of brain neurons. Alzheimer's, Huntington's, and Parkinson's diseases manifest constellations of behavioral and neurological symptoms that result from the selective destruction of specific neuronal populations. While research is beginning to disclose the pathophysiology and molecular biology of these disorders, there is a widening gap between our understanding of the biology of these diseases and our ability to prevent or treat them. A concerted effort must be mounted to develop new and appropriate treatments for neurodegenerative disorders. One of the prerequisites for such an effort is to develop animal models that help to focus on the mechanisms of neurodegeneration and the most logical approaches to prevent or modify this process. Selective neurotoxins have played a pivotal role in the development of models of neurological disorders.

NEUROTOXINS AS TOOLS TO MODEL NEURODEGENERATIVE DISORDERS

Toxic chemicals can have both beneficial and injurious effects. Natural toxins enhance the survival of a species by deterring potential predators and by incapacitating prey. In addition, there is a growing list of both natural and synthetic toxins in the environment that are used in industrial settings. These include pesticides, therapeutic drugs, solvents, organic and inorganic metals, air pollutants, radioactive materials, and food additives and contaminants (Casarett et al., 1980). The injurious properties of these compounds are becoming well know, but some toxins can also be used as powerful biological tools. According to one of the founders of toxicology, "all substances are poisons; there is none which is not poison. The right dose differentiates a poison and a remedy" (Paracelsus, 1567). The right compound and dose might also allow us to ask important questions about biology and disease.

Specific neurotoxic compounds have been used to examine morphological, biochemical, and molecular correlates of brain function. Compounds that disrupt specific ion channels (tetrodotoxin, tetraethylammonium), axoplasmic transport processes (colchicine), neuronal populations (kainic acid, MPTP), or neurotransmitter systems (6-hydroxydopamine, 5,7-dihydroxytryptamine, DSP-4) have helped to characterize the fundamental neurobiology of brain cells and the principles of synaptic transmission (McGeer et al., 1987). In efforts to better understand neurodegenerative diseases, neurotoxins have been used to examine the plasticity of brain systems and the extent of neural reorganization following injury, to address basic questions about how the nervous system functions following compromise of a specific transmitter, and finally, to examine the covariation between altered neurotransmitter dynamics and behavior and to develop animal models of neurological disorders (Sanberg and Coyle, 1984). Table 1 presents a list of neurotoxins that have been used to model neurological disorders.

The purpose of this chapter is to discuss how neurotoxins have been used to generate animal models of neurodegenerative disorders. We will address the rationale and goals that guide the development of animal models. We will concentrate on two areas of research: animal models of Parkinson's and Alzheimer's disease. These diseases are two of the most

Table 1 Neurotoxins That Have Been Used to Model
Neurological Diseases

Adult-onset disorders	
AF64A	Alzheimer's disease
Ibotenic acid	
Colchicine	
Ibotenic acid	Huntington's disease
Quinolinic acid	
6-Hydroxydopamine	Parkinson's disease
MPTP	
Methamphetamine	
Kainic acid	Temporal lobe epilepsy
Developmental disorders	
Methylazoxymethanol	Microcephaly
α-Methylphenylalanine	Phenylketonuria
Neonatal 6-hydroxydopamine	Lesch-Nyhan Syndrome

common age-related neurodegenerative disorders, and there has been a concentrated effort to develop models to further understand the disease processes and to generate efficacious therapies.

THE DEFINITION OF ANIMAL MODELS

Kornetsky (1977) defines animal models as "an experimental compromise in which a simple experimental system is used to represent a more complex and less available system." Models are designed to explore the causes, manifestations, and treatment of human diseases. There is a pervasive sentiment that animal models are a necessary approach to understanding human pathology. While they are unable to reproduce the multifactorial causes and symptoms of most neurological diseases, they do provide a viable way to explore specific questions concerning structure and function.

Model systems can be associated with different experimental goals. One can conceptualize at least three types of animal model: 1.) mechanistic, 2.) analogous, and 3.) etiological.

Mechanistic Models

The mechanistic model examines the mechanisms underlying a given phenomenon (e.g., neurodegeneration or mitochondrial dysfunction). These models directly explore the relationship between neural dysfunction and alterations in a given cellular parameter. They provide information about the "phenomena of neurodegeneration." For example, delineating the mechanisms of mitochondrial dysfunction induced by toxins such as MPP^+ and its impact on neuronal integrity could provide insights into a number of diseases that have no known etiology. In fact, a current focus for the study of Parkinson's, Alzheimer's, and Huntington's diseases is mitochondrial dysfunction (Schapira et al., 1990).

Another aspect of the mechanistic model is to examine mechanisms that contribute to a functional phenomenon. For example, chlordecone is an organochlorine insecticide that induces tremor. Investigators have examined the role of specific neurotransmitters and brain sites in this phenomenon to better understand the neurobiology of tremor (Gerhart et al., 1985).

Analogous Models

A second type of model tries to reproduce the biological and functional changes observed in human diseases. By characterizing the disease process and exploring new therapeutic interventions, these models help to relate specific neural alterations to specific symptoms. Which symptoms are associated with injury to which areas? They do not focus on specific etiological factors that predispose to neurodegenerative disorders but rather examine changes in the brain that induce a similar profile of symptoms. In this context, excitotoxins have been widely used to produce models of a variety of neurological diseases, even though excitotoxicity may not be a causative factor in the disease process. Excitotoxins such as kainic acid, ibotenic acid, quinolinic acid, and N-methyl-D-aspartate (NMDA) can be used to produce axon-sparing lesions in specific brain areas. Sanberg and colleagues have used these compounds to reproduce the profile of neuropathology and functional changes observed in Huntington's disease (Sanberg and Coyle, 1984). This model has provided a way to explore new therapeutic strategies for this disorder.

Another way to induce an analogous model is to use toxins that target a class of neurons that are prominently affected in a disease. For example, dopaminergic neurons degenerate in Parkinson's disease, and this results in the classic motor symptoms associated with the disease. The catecholamine neurotoxin 6-hydroxydopamine can be used to induce a similar pattern of damage. This toxin is taken into either dopamine or norepinephrine terminals, depending on pharmacological pretreatment, and it destroys the neuron. There are currently a variety of toxins that selectively injure neurotransmitter-specific neurons. For example, 6-hydroxydopamine and DSP-4 affect catecholamine neurons, 5,7-dihydroxytryptamine affects serotonin neurons, and AF64A affects cholinergic neurons.

Etiological Models

A third type of model addresses specific etiological theories of neurodegenerative disorders. For example, if compound X contributes to disease Y, it should reproduce a similar profile of symptoms in other species. There has been much speculation about the role of aluminum in Alzheimer's disease (AD). If it is a causative factor, it should produce "Alzheimer disease–like" effects in animal models. However, at present there is little supporting evidence for such a hypothesis, because aluminum fails to produce these effects in animals. An implied corollary is that the cellular mechanism of toxicity will reveal pathophysiogical factors involved in the disease process.

Criteria for Establishing Animal Models

The development of a viable animal model of any neurological or psychiatric disorder must be predicated on a set of preestablished criteria. In one of the first attempts to formulate meaningful criteria for animal models, McKinney and Bunney (1969) proposed that models should recapitulate the disease in four dimensions: etiology, symptomatology, treatment efficacy, and underlying pathophysiology. However, this strategy is too exacting for models of disorders whose etiology is obscure and probably combinatorial. A variety of interacting influences might lead to a physiological condition that is conducive to the development of brain changes associated with neurodegenerative diseases (see Walsh and Opello, 1992).

Providing a set of criteria for the development and evaluation of animal models identifies areas for future research and provides an archetype to evaluate the comprehensiveness of existing models. Willner (1991) suggests that animal models should be evaluated in relation to their face validity, predictive validity, and construct validity.

"*Face validity*" refers to the phenomenological similarity between the model and the disease state. Are some of the essential and characteristic behavioral and neurobiological symptoms of the disorder reproduced with acceptable fidelity in the model? For example, AD is associated with the degeneration of cholinergic neurons in the basal forebrain that innervate structures involved in the coordination of memory processes, most notably the hippocampus and cortex. The functional consequence is a loss of presynaptic cholinergic indices and the impairment of memory processes dependent on these brain systems. To have face validity, a model of AD must produce a persistent cholinergic hypofunction and associated memory impairments.

A second consideration is *predictive validity*, which is based on the correspondence between efficacy of therapeutic strategies in the model and in the disease state. L-Dopa and other dopamine agonists can improve the motor impairments observed in models of Parkinson's disease. There is a correspondence between the treatment modalities that are used to manage the disease and those that are efficacious in the model. Therefore, the predictive validity of the model is in part predicated on whether it produces symptoms that are responsive to standard therapy. However, predictive validity is problematic for models of neurological diseases that lack established treatment regimens (i.e., positive controls). There is a conspicuous disparity between the effectiveness of drugs in animal models of AD and in patients with the disease (Sarter et al., 1992). A variety of drugs (cholinergic agonists, cholinesterase inhibitors, nootropics) are effective in reversing cognitive deficits in currently available models of AD but lack clinical efficacy.

The final criterion to consider is the *construct validity* of an animal model. What are the theoretical considerations and the rationale for the development of a specific animal model? A neurodegenerative disease may present a wide array of neurobiological and behavioral changes. Alzheimer's disease is associated with changes in brain systems, neurotransmitters, metabolic processes, cytoskeletal integrity, protein processing, and gene expression. Which of these changes, alone or in combination, should serve as a focus for the development of a model of the disease? Which pathological event most contributes to the behavioral pathology? Since the etiology of AD remains obscure, and in fact may be combinatorial, an animal model must focus on relevant behavioral and neurobiological "target" symptoms. This strategy has frequently been employed in the development of models of AD.

ALZHEIMER'S DISEASE

Characteristics and Demographics

Alzheimer's disease is the most prevalent of the age-related cognitive disorders. In the United States it affects approximately 15% of people over the age of 65, the most rapidly expanding segment of the population (Evans et al., 1989). The cost of institutional care for AD patients in the United States alone has been estimated at 3 billion dollars a year. The etiology of the disorder is unknown, and a variety of factors including advanced age, genetic predispositions, exposure to environmental toxins, neuroactive viruses, and prior brain injury may contribute to the onset of the disease. No effective preventative measures or treatment modalities are currently available.

The morphological changes in AD affect selective brain areas that participate in emotional elaboration and higher-order cognitive functions. The triad of cellular changes that identify the disease—neurofibrillary tangles, granulovacuolar degeneration, and amyloid plaques—are most concentrated in the hippocampus, the association cortex, and several areas of the limbic system. There is also loss of cholinergic neurons in the basal forebrain, which provide the primary cholinergic input to the cortex and the hippocampus (Whitehouse et al., 1985). Other brain areas that can be affected include the locus coeruleus and the raphe nuclei (see Hardy et al., 1985). While these later changes are evident in subpopulations of patients or late in the course of the disease, they have not been shown to relate to the prevailing memory disorder (Mann et al., 1981).

The Cholinergic System in Alzheimer's Disease

A major focus for the study of AD has been the cholinergic system (Bartus et al., 1982). All biochemical markers of presynaptic cholinergic function, including acetylcholine (ACh) synthesis, high-affinity choline transport (HAChT), and ACh release are decreased in the hippocampus and neocortex in AD (Coyle et al., 1983; Rylett et al., 1983). There is also a pronounced loss of cholinergic neurons in the basal forebrain that innervate these regions (Whitehouse et al., 1985). These changes are an important part of the disease process, since there is a significant correlation between the severity of dementia, the number of senile plaques, and the loss of cholinergic markers (Wilcock et al., 1982). Animal studies also support a role for the cholinergic system in memory processes (reviewed in Walsh and Chrobak, 1991).

Cholinergic neurons in the medial septum and vertical limb of the diagonal band project to the hippocampus and synapse on pyramidal cells, granule cells, and interneurons (see Frotscher and Leranth, 1985). While cholinergic synapses may account for only 10% of all the synapses in the hippocampus, the cholinergic component of the septohippocampal pathway exerts a profound influence on this structure by inducing the theta rhythm (see Bland, 1986, for review). Lynch and colleagues have hypothesized that "neuronal activity at this frequency [theta] is optimal for the induction of synaptic plasticity in the hippocampus" (Larson et al., 1986).

Memory Impairments in Alzheimer's Disease

The profile of cognitive changes observed in AD has provided indirect support for the hypothesis that there are at least two memory processes that are responsible for certain types of cognitive operation (Cohen and Squire, 1980; Nissen et al., 1987). One process, referred to as reference memory, seems to support the performance of skills or habits, a class of operations dependent on rules or procedures. The other, referred to as working memory, allows the retention of specific information about events or episodes.

Early in the course of AD there is a profile of selective cognitive deficits in which working memory is disrupted but reference memory is not. For example, patients are impaired in the acquisition and retention of recently presented information but are not impaired in the acquisition of cognitive and perceptual skills (Cohen and Squire, 1980). This dissociation of memory processes is most evident in those situations where a subject can perform a learned perceptual or motor skill in the absence of any recollection of the specific episodes in which it was acquired (Knopman and Nissen, 1987).

Cognitive scientists have attempted to formally characterize the nature of the memory impairments observed in AD using Baddeley's working memory model as a theoretical framework (Baddeley, 1986). Working memory organizes and directs specific cognitive processes to deal with the demands of the situation. Baddeley postulates a tripartite model of working memory including a central executive system that coordinates and directs two peripheral working memory systems: 1.) the articulatory loop system, which retains verbal information, and 2.) the visual-spatial system, which retains nonverbal information. Neuropsychological testing has demonstrated a selective impairment in the central executive system that occurs early in AD. This cognitive change may be related to the loss of cholinergic function, since muscarinic antagonists can produce a similar disruption of working memory, and in particular of the central executive system, in young adults (Nissen et al., 1987; Rusted and Warburton, 1988). Taken together, these observations suggest that an early cognitive change in AD is an impairment of the central executive system, which coordinates working memory processes, and that this impairment may be related to the loss of cholinergic function.

ANIMAL MODELS OF ALZHEIMER'S DISEASE

There is compelling evidence that the memory impairments in AD are dependent on the degree of cholinergic hypofunction. Therefore, a logical strategy for developing an animal model of AD might be to focus on the "target" symptoms of working memory deficits and cholinergic hypofunction. However, the development of a reliable model of AD has proved to be challenging, since the etiology of the disease is obscure and is likely to involve a variety of interacting factors. Therefore, while it is possible to induce some of the behavioral and neurobiological alterations associated with AD, the proximal cause of these changes is probably not analogous to the multitude of etiological factors that contribute to the human condition. Currently, no one model mimics all the major characteristics of the human disease state.

Ethylcholine Aziridinium Ion

The rate-limiting step in the synthesis of ACh is the HAChT system. This system is localized to cholinergic terminals, and its activity is coupled to the activity of the neuron (Jope, 1979). Increasing or decreasing the activity of cholinergic neurons produces parallel changes in the kinetics of the HAChT system (Simon et al., 1976). The unique presence of the HAChT system on cholinergic terminals has inspired investigators to develop compounds that selectively target this site. Most notably, a variety of analogues of choline have been examined as potential cholinergic-specific neurotixins that interact with the HAChT system (see Hanin et al., 1987).

Fisher and Hanin (1980) explored a series of choline analogues and found that one of these compounds, ethylcholine aziridinium ion (AF64A), had cholinotoxic properties that make it useful for both in vivo and in vitro studies. AF64A is a neurotoxic analogue of choline that inhibits the HAChT system. Following intracerebroventricular (ICV) injection, AF64A produces a 30–60% reduction in all indices of presynaptic cholinergic function including 1.) regional concentrations of ACh, 2.) the activity of choline acetyltransferase (ChAT), 3.) HAChT, and 4.) K^+-stimulated release of ACh from slices of hippocampus (see Hanin, 1990, for review of AF64A's neurochemical effects and for relevant references). These effects develop over time, with maximal decreases evident approximately 7 days following treatment and persisting for at least 1 year following injection (Leventer et al., 1987). These changes are regionally selective, with the cholinergic input to the hippocampus being affected and projections to the cortex and the interneurons in the striatum being spared (Chrobak et al., 1988).

The AF64A-induced decreases in cholinergic function are not accompanied by persistent changes in the regional concentrations of catecholamines, serotonin, or glutamate. While AF64A does not produce lasting changes in other transmitter systems, it can produce temporally limited changes that may be secondary to a disruption of normal cholinergic function. For example, administration of hemicholinium-3 or its analogue A-4 before AF64A attenuates the loss of cholinergic and serotonergic markers in the hippocampus (Potter et al., 1987). These compounds are both potent inhibitors of HAChT, with inhibitory rate constants 30–100 times greater than that of AF64A, and they prevent AF64A from gaining access to the HAChT system (Barker and Mittag, 1975). These data indicate that the effects of AF64A on neurotransmitter systems other than ACh are probably secondary to the cholinergic hypofunction.

Mechanism of Toxicity

Current evidence suggests that the effects of AF64A on cholinergic neurons comprise at least three distinct phases. The first stage involves a concentration-dependent interaction with the HAChT system located on cholinergic nerve terminals. At high concentrations

($>$ 22.5 μM) AF64A rapidly alkylates nucleophilic sites on the proteins composing the uptake system. This rapidly inhibits the HAChT system and prevents AF64A from gaining access to the inside of the terminal. However, at low concentrations ($<$ 11 μM) AF64A is taken into the terminal by the HAChT system. Once inside the terminal it can be acetylated by ChAT to yield a putative false transmitter, acetyl-AF64A. Both AF64A and its metabolite initiate a second phase of toxicity, which is described below.

The initial cholinotoxic effects of AF64A are dependent on its interaction with the HAChT system, since they can be prevented by compounds that compete for the HAChT system, such as high levels of choline or hemicholinium-3 (Curti and Marchbanks, 1984). More recently, Chrobak and colleagues (1989) reported that pretreatment of rats with hemicholinium-3 prevented AF64A-induced cholinotoxicity as well as the behavioral impairments induced by the toxin.

The second phase of toxicity involves AF64A's interaction with a variety of enzymes that use choline as a substrate. It binds to these enzymes because of its structural similarity to choline, but its aziridinium ring alkylates their catalytic sites; AF64A inhibits ChAT, choline kinase, choline dehydrogenase, and acetylcholinesterase (AChE) (Barlow and Marchbanks, 1984; Sandberg et al., 1985). This results in a persistent presynaptic cholinergic hypofunction in which all measures of ACh synthesis and release are affected. The effects of AF64A also appear to be specific to enzymes that interact with choline. Sandberg and colleagues (1985) reported that concentrations of AF64A that inhibited ChAT, choline kinase, and AChE activity in the cholinergic cell line N6-108-15 by 95% had no effect on choline-independent enzymes including lactic dehydrogenase, carboxypeptidase A, chymotrypsinogen, and alcohol dehydrogenase.

Recovery of enzymatic activity would involve gene expression, synthesis of new enzyme, and axoplasmic transport of the enzyme to the affected terminal. There is also evidence that AF64A disrupts these necessary "regenerative" processes. Kasa and Hanin (1985) reported that AF64A produced a dose-related blockade of axopasmic transport in both the septohippocampal pathway and a sciatic nerve preparation. These alterations in transport might disrupt axon integrity and prevent any newly synthesized enzyme from gaining access to the nerve terminal. Therefore, the second phase of AF64A toxicity involves an inhibition of choline-specific enzymes and a disruption of cytoskeletal processes that contribute to axoplasmic transport and cell viability.

While the effects of AF64A on cholinergic parameters have been extensively studied, there has been little effort to understand how AF64A kills cells. Following ICV injection, AF64A does produce a dose-related decrease in the number of cholinergic neurons in the medial septum, with different cell groups being uniquely vulnerable (Chrobak et al., 1988; Lorens et al. 1991). Lorens and colleagues reported the following order of susceptibility among the different cholinergic cell groups in the septum: intermediate $>>$ dorsal $>$ midline $>>$ ventral. Is there an inherent selective vulnerability or resistance of distinct cholinergic neurons? Understanding this phenomenon might help to delineate the factors that regulate degeneration of cholinergic neurons in a variety of neurological disorders.

The final phase of AF64A toxicity (i.e., cell death) may be related to the effects of this compound on nucleic acids and their essential intracellular functions. AF64A is structurally similar to several antitumor agents, such as nitrogen mustard, that produce cytotoxic effects through their interactions with DNA, RNA, and other cellular macromolecules. Futscher and colleagues (1992) recently demonstrated that AF64A does produce dose-dependent DNA strand breaks and the premature termination of RNA transcription. Therefore, the final and terminal phase of toxicity may be a disruption of fundamental cellular processes involving the translation and transcription of genes that are necessary for neuronal survival. Finally, there is preliminary evidence that oxidative stress may be a critical component of AF64A-induced cholinotoxicity (Walsh et al., 1992).

AF64A Effects on Working and Reference Memory

A central question concerning the AF64A model is whether the compound produces cognitive changes that resemble the ones observed in AD. Is working memory impaired while reference memory is intact?

A number of reports have shown that AF64A preferentially affects working memory. Spatial tasks are commonly used to assess cognitive function and its neurobiological substrates, since 1.) spatial memory is well developed in rodents, 2.) spatial tasks are available to assess both working and reference memory, and 3.) spatial memory depends on the integrity of the cholinergic septophippocampal pathway.

AF64A was found to produce a dissociation between working and reference memory in a T-maze task that independently assessed both types of memory within the same trial (Chrobak et al., 1986). In this task each trial was initiated by placing the rat into either the left or the right start/goal box of the T maze for 15 seconds. The food-deprived rat was then rewarded with a single chocolate-flavored pellet for turning into and traversing the stem of the maze and for subsequently returning to the alternate start/goal location. This task involves 1.) a trial-independent component (reference memory) that involves an invariant response of running down the stem of the maze and 2.) a trial-dependent response (working memory) in which the animal must maintain a representation of the start location in order to perform accurately (Chrobak et al., 1986).

Rats injected ICV with cerebrospinal fluid (CSF) readily reacquired both components of the task. The AF64A group, however, exhibited a transient decrease in reference memory that recovered within 30 trials and a persistent decrease in working memory that was evident throughout the 75 postoperative trials. Working memory was impaired in this group even when their reference memory performance was comparable to that of controls and close to 100% accurate. These behavioral deficits were associated with a 42% decrease in ChAT activity in the hippocampus with no alterations in the corpus striatum or frontal cortex.

A problem that can arise in studies of spatial memory is that rats can often adopt response strategies that are compatible with completion of the task. In a radial-arm maze task a rat may consistently enter arms 1,2,3 . . . 8 in sequential order without error for each trial. This would clearly minimize or eliminate the working memory aspect of the task. In an effort to minimize this confounding factor, a version of the radial-arm maze task that requires an animal to remember a specific training episode was introduced. In this task barriers are used to force the animals to select a predetermined set of four out of eight arms. Four arms are open and baited with food and four arms are blocked. After entering all four open arms, rats are returned to their home cages for a specified delay period. Following this period they are returned to the maze, and all eight arms are now open, but only those arms that were blocked during the predelay sessions now contain food. This represents a delayed non-match-to-sample (DNMTS) task. The pattern of open and closed arms varies randomly from day to day. Therefore, the animals are presented with a new working memory problem (i.e., episode) each day.

Rats were tested in a series of tasks that assessed both working and reference memory following ICV injection of CSF or 3.0 nmol of AF64A (Chrobak et al., 1988).

Rats were trained in the delay working memory task before surgery and were subsequently tested for 30 postoperative trials with delays of 0, 0.5, 1, 5, 15 or 30 min randomly imposed between the fourth and fifth arm choices. The CSF-injected rats exhibited excellent performance (80–85%) at each of the delays. However, the AF64A-injected group performed at approximately chance levels (50–60%) of accuracy regardless of delay condition. Despite the impairments in the delay task, the AF64A group were able to acquire a position discrimination in which they learned to perform an invariant trial-independent response of always going to the same spatial location in a T maze. All animals required a comparable number of trials to achieve a performance criterion of 70%, 80%, or 90% correct in any 10-trial block in this reference-memory task.

These data demonstrated a dissociation in memory processes, with working memory being impaired but reference memory intact. These behavioral deficits were associated with a 50% decrease in ChAT activity in the hippocampus and no alterations in enzyme activity in the frontal cortex, parietal cortex, cingulate gyrus, amygdala, or corpus striatum. Further, there were no alterations in the regional concentrations of norepinephrine, dopamine, (DOPAC) dihydroxyphenylacetic acid, serotonin, or (5-HIAA) 5-hydroxyindoleacetic acid.

Subsequent studies found that the working memory impairments induced by AF64A were dose-dependent and related to the cognitive demands of the task (Chrobak and Walsh, 1991). Rats were bilaterally injected ICV with 0, 0.75, or 1.5 nmol AF64A and tested with either 0-, 1-, or 2-h delays in the DNMTS task. While none of the groups were impaired at the 0 delay condition, the 1.5-nmol group was impaired at both the 1- and the 2-h delay. However, the 0.75-nmol group was impaired only at the 2-h delay. Therefore, the memory impairments were related to the dose of AF64A *and* to the demand placed on the working memory system by the task. This is particularly interesting because of the delay-dependent memory impairments observed in patients with AD (see Hart et al., 1988).

The working-memory impairments induced by AF64A depend on dose and task demands and appear to be related to a select compromise of the cholinergic innervation of the hippocampus. Chrobak and colleagues (1989) reported that hemicholinium-3 pretreatment prevented both the impairment in the working-memory task and the decrease in HAChT. These data clearly suggest that the behavioral deficits result from the cholinergic hypofunction induced by AF64A.

The Use of AF64A to Model Alzheimer's Disease

There is compelling evidence that a central cholinergic hypofunction is responsible for the profile of cognitive changes seen in AD. Patients with AD exhibit decreases in presynaptic cholinergic indices and a loss of cholinergic neurons in the basal forebrain, both of which are correlated with the degree of cognitive impairment. AF64A does produce a profile of neurobiological and behavioral changes in the rat that closely resembles the changes observed in AD (see Table 2). Following ICV injection, the model recapitulates many of the anatomical, biochemical, and behavioral deficits observed in AD. It provides a very useful analogous model of the disease. We have only addressed data based on the ICV injection of AF64A, since injection directly into tissue has been shown in some cases to produce nonselective histological damage (McGurk et al., 1987). AF64A can be used to address specific questions. It can be used and it can be misused. Direct injection into tissue leads to a very high local concentration of this potent alkylating compound. This can lead to interaction with a variety of noncholinergic cell types and nonspecific damage. The AF64A model can be used to evaluate the efficacy, and assist in the development, of treatment modalities that may prove useful in the prevention, remediation, or management of the disorder. A variety of approaches have been examined in this model, including cholinomimetic drugs (Yamazaki et al., 1991), trophic factors (Emerich and Walsh, 1990), fetal transplants (Emerich et al., 1992), and antioxidants (Walsh et al., 1992). Finally, the neurotoxin AF64A is also a powerful tool that can be used to explore the biology of brain cholinergic systems and their functional properties.

PARKINSON'S DISEASE

Characteristics and Demographics

Parkinson's disease (PD) is a progressive neurodegenerative disorder that affects up to 10% of the population over 65 years of age. The disease is characterized by slow movements, stooped posture, resting tremor, rigidity, and other symptoms. Dopaminergic neurons in the zona compacta of the midbrain are lost in great numbers in PD, and this loss may be accompanied by Lewy body formation. Lewy bodies are eosinophilic bodies found in the cytoplasm of dopaminergic neurons in the midbrain and other sites in PD and other diseases. Dopaminergic neurons in the zona compacta of the substantia nigra project to and synapse in the corpus striatum. The death of dopaminergic neurons in the zona compacta is associated with a loss of dopaminergic terminals and up to an 85% decrease in striatal dopamine concentrations (Hornykiewicz and Kish, 1986). This depletion of dopamine is critical to the disease, since replenishment of striatal dopamine with levodopa provides effective therapy for PD patients. However, the pathology of PD is not limited to the midbrain. Other neurons are lost in PD, including catecholaminergic neurons of the locus coeruleus and cholinergic neurons of the nucleus basalis of Meynert, as well as serotonergic neurons and peptidergic neurons. Parkinson's disease is not always found as a single clinical entity. As many as 50% of PD patients also have Alzheimer's disease (Boller et al., 1980).

Table 2 Similarities Between Alzheimer's Disease and the AF64A Model

	Alzheimer's Disease	AF64A
Anatomy		
Cholinergic cell loss in basal forebrain	+	+
Increased aluminum in brain	+	+
Neuritic placques	+	?
Neurofibrillary tangles	+	?
Chemistry		
Presynaptic cholinergic hypofunction	+	+
No changes in muscarinic receptors	+	+
Decreases in brain nicotinic receptors	+	+
Alterations in cytoskeletal function	+	+
Alterations in β-amyloid expression	+	?
Behavior		
Persistent working/episodic memory impairments	+	+
Deficits related to task demand and degree of cholinergic hypofunction	+	+
Spared reference/skill memory	+	+

+ = effect is observed; ? = has not been determined. Appropriate references are found in Hanin, 1990; Walsh and Chrobak, 1991; Walsh and Opello, 1993.

Pathogenesis of Parkinson's Disease

A number of factors could be involved in the pathogenesis of PD. A genetic component is important in PD, since certain families have an increased incidence of PD. In addition, people with a mutated form of cytochrome P-450 may be more likely to develop PD (Armstrong et al., 1992). Parkinson's disease can also be caused by environmental factors including toxins and possibly foods. The metabolic oxidation of an environmental toxin by cytochrome P-450 may be important in PD. 1-Methyl-4-phenyl-1,2,3,6-tetrahydropyridine (MPTP), which is a contaminant of a designer drug, was shown to cause a syndrome in humans very similar to PD (Davis et al., 1979). Other factors in PD include viral infections, elevated dopamine turnover, compromised cerebral blood flow, and mitochondrial dysfunction. One factor common to most of these putative pathogenetic factors is the formation of reactive oxygen species in dopaminergic neurons.

Sources of Oxidative Stress in Parkinson's Disease

Iron exists in the brain in three forms: bound to ferritin, bound to iron-containing proteins, and chelated to the phosphate groups of lipids and other molecules. Oligodendrocytes contain high levels of iron chelated to the phosphate groups of myelin (Hill and Switzer, 1984). Chelated iron can catalyze the formation of oxygen radicals by the reactions below.

(1) $Fe^{+3} + Lipid\text{-}OOH \rightarrow Fe^{+2} + Lipid\text{-}OO\cdot + H^+$
(2) $Fe^{+2} + Lipid\text{-}OOH \rightarrow Fe^{+3} + Lipid\text{-}O\cdot + OH^-$
(3) $Fe^{+2} \ H_2O_2 \rightarrow Fe^{+3} + OH\cdot + OH^-$

Oxygen radicals can mediate lipid peroxidation and lead to a disruption of membrane integrity and cell death.

Parkinson's Disease and Oxidative Stress

Dopaminergic neurons may be uniquely vulnerable to oxidative stress, since cytosolic dopamine (DA) auto-oxidizes to form oxygen radicals and 6-hydroxydopamine (Graham, 1984). In addition, monoamine oxidase type A (MAO-A) oxidizes DA, producing hydrogen peroxide and other reactive oxygen species (Cohen, 1990). Furthermore, oxidative stress in human DA neurons leads to the formation of neuromelanin, a complex aggregation of oxidized DA, dopa, norepinephrine, serotonin, cysteine, and iron and other metal ions, as well as lipofuscin. Neuromelanin also functions in oxidation-reduction reactions as a free radical species. It is interesting that neuromelanin levels are highest in the DA neurons that are the first to be lost in PD (Mann and Yates, 1982).

Protective mechanisms that normally keep this constant oxidative stress in check are significantly compromised in PD patients. Several compounds that detoxify hydrogen peroxide, such as peroxidase, glutathione, glutathione peroxidase, and catalase, have all been shown to be diminished in the substantia nigra and corpus striatum of patients with PD (Ambani et al., 1975). Decreases in these enzymes could leave the brain vulnerable to OH· formation by reaction 3, above.

Failure of mechanisms that protect against oxidative stress is evidenced in PD patients by elevated levels of iron in the zona compacta. Progressive supranuclear palsy and multiple-system atrophy are also associated with increased iron levels in the zona compacta (Dexter, et al., 1991). Alterations of ferritin levels in PD and other forms of neurodegeneration have also been reported (Dexter, et al., 1991). Increases in iron in the substantia nigra during neurodegeneration may be primarily associated with astrocytes and microglial cells, which are responsible for neuronophagia (Sofic et al., 1991). Increases in iron are in turn associated with increases in chelated ferric iron and total iron content (Sofic et al., 1991). It may be that altered iron and ferritin levels in the brain are secondary to nerve cell death. It is also possible that a number of neurodegenerative processes share similar mechanisms of pathogenesis, since iron and ferritin are affected in a number of diseases.

Compensatory Responses

Interestingly, PD is associated with increases in cytosolic and mitochondrial superoxide dismutase, an enzyme that detoxifies oxygen free radicals (Marttila, et al., 1988; Saggu et al., 1989). This may reflect a compensatory response of the brain to the oxidative stress associated with PD. It has been demonstrated that glutathione levels were normal in the midbrains of PD patients who also suffered from AD (Adams et al. 1991b). Compensatory increases in glutathione levels in these patients were found in the hippocampus. These patients also had compensatory increases in vitamin E levels in the midbrain, a structure known to concentrate vitamin E during neurodegeneration. This suggests that vitamin E, a potent antioxidant that has been shown to slow the progression of PD, may protect the midbrain from peroxidative damage. Vitamin C, another major antioxidant known to penetrate readily into the brain, has also been shown to decrease the progression of PD (Fahn, 1991). Similar results have been found in clinical testing of the antioxidant exifone (Allain et al., 1988).

Parkinson's disease may result from certain initial insults that compromise the defensive mechanisms in dopaminergic neurons. These initial insults could result from oxidative stress induced by environmental toxins. Since dopaminergic neurons are probably in a state of constant oxidative stress and contain neuromelanin and potentially inadequate glutathione levels, it may not be difficult to overpower the defensive mechanisms of these cells.

ANIMAL MODELS OF PARKINSON'S DISEASE

There are a number of toxins that produce long-term depletion of striatal dopamine, over many weeks, in animals. These toxins include amphetamine, methamphetamine, 6-hydroxydopamine, 6-aminodopamine, manganese, and others. All of these agents are associated with the induction of oxidative stress in dopaminergic neurons. It is proposed that amphetamine and methamphetamine deplete dopamine in part by releasing dopamine from its storage vesicles. This increases the levels of intracellular dopamine, which may oxidize to form 6-hydroxydopamine (Wagner and Walsh, 1991). Methamphetamine toxicity is also associated with NMDA receptor stimulation. 6-Hydroxydopamine and 6-amino-dopamine can auto-oxidize inside dopaminergic neurons, forming quinones, with the production of $O_2 \cdot^-$, $OH \cdot$ and H_2O_2 (Cohen, 1985). Manganese has been proposed to produce a syndrome similar to PD in some miners, and is known to accelerate the oxidation of dopamine, with resultant oxygen free radical production (Segura-Aguilar and Lind, 1989).

MPTP Model

It is widely accepted that MPTP is a mitochondrial toxin. If PD is associated with oxygen radical production in dopaminergic neurons, and a number of toxins are known to deplete striatal dopamine in animals through production of oxygen radicals, then why is there any interest in MPTP, which is a mitochondrial toxin?

MPTP produces essentially permanent depletion of striatal dopamine in mice, monkeys, and other animals, and probably humans. Long-term diminished locomotor activity following MPTP administration is also noted in monkeys, mice (Ogawa et al., 1985), and humans. In addition, MPTP administration produces a loss of dopaminergic neurons in the midbrain in mice (Heikkila et al., 1984), monkeys (Chiueh et al., 1985), other animals, and humans (Davis et al., 1979). Eosinophilic inclusion bodies, perhaps similar to Lewy bodies, have been noted in the midbrains of monkeys treated with MPTP (Forno et al., 1986). Therefore, interest in MPTP comes from its ability to produce effects similar to PD.

The acute effects of MPTP are worth exploring, since understanding these effects could provide clues about the initial pathogenesis of PD and possible treatment strategies for PD. Almost nothing is known about what happens early in PD, because preclinical changes are not recognizable and appropriate brain tissue is not available for study.

MPTP destroys dopaminergic neurons in the substantia nigra within a few hours of administration (Fig. 1) (Adams et al., 1989a). Similarly, dopaminergic nerve terminals in the corpus striatum are damaged within hours of administration of MPTP. However, other brain cells are also acutely damaged, such as astrocytic foot processes and endothelial cells (Adams et al., 1989a). Damage to capillary endothelial cells by MPTP is associated with a probable decrease in blood perfusion through the brain and some spillage of blood constituents into the brain parenchyma (Adams et al., 1991a). Damage to astrocytes could be critical to the dopaminergic neurons that depend on astrocytes for trophic factors to sustain them.

The acute effects of MPTP on dopamine and its metabolites, DOPAC and HVA, provide interesting clues about PD (Table 3). MPTP quickly depletes mouse striatal dopamine, DOPAC, and HVA within hours of administration (Adams et al., 1989a). The depletion of striatal dopamine by MPTP is noted for many weeks following MPTP administration. However, the effects of MPTP in the substantia nigra are different, with an initial depletion of dopamine, DOPAC, and HVA, followed by increases in these substances within 1 day of administration (Adams et al., 1989a). These increases demonstrate compensatory increases in the turnover of dopamine in surviving neurons to compensate for the loss of neurons in the substantia nigra. This process of increased dopamine turnover in surviving neurons has also been proposed in PD.

MPTP penetrates readily into the brain, where it is a substrate for MAO-B in endothelial cells, astrocytes, and serotonergic neurons. Monoamine oxidase type B produces 1-methyl-4-phenylpyridine (MPP^+) from MPTP. MPP^+ is neurotoxic and is responsible for most of the toxicity of MPTP, since inhibition of MAO-B by selegiline prevents much of the toxicity of MPTP (Chiba et al., 1985). Inhibition of MAO-A by clorgyline does not inhibit the toxicity of MPTP. MPP^+ is toxic to the astrocytes and endothelial cells that produce it, causing the cells to rupture and release MPP^+ into the brain parenchyma. MPP^+ is actively taken into dopaminergic neurons in competition with dopamine. Dopamine uptake–blocking drugs inhibit the toxicity of MPP^+ (Sundstrom and Jonsson, 1985).

MPTP and Mitochondrial Toxicity

Once inside the neuron, MPP^+ is pumped into mitochondria, along the electrochemical gradient, and there it is concentrated into the millimolar range. NADH dehydrogenase,

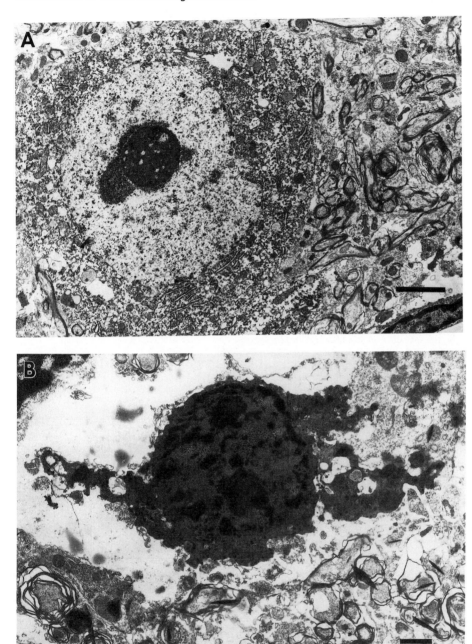

Figure 1   Electron microscopic pictures of control and 1-methyl-4-phenyl-1,2,3,6,-tetrahydropyridine (MPTP)-damaged dopaminergic neurons in the 9-month-old C57 B1/6 male mouse zona compacta. (A) A control dopaminergic neuron stained with a tyrosine hydroxylase antibody and visualized with a peroxidase antiperoxidase system. The neuron demonstrates abundant tyrosine hydroxylase staining in the cytoplasm, but not in the nucleus. (B) A damaged dopaminergic neuron 10 h after the last MPTP treatment. MPTP was given as 4 doses (IP) of 25 mg/kg at 2-h intervals. The neuron still demonstrates tyrosine hydroxylase staining. The cytoplasm is highly condensed and vacuolated. The nucleus is pyknotic. Bar lengths are 1 μ.

Table 3 Effects of MPTP on dopamine (DA), DOPAC, and HVA in the Substantia Nigra and Corpus Striatum— and the Effect of (+)-MK801[a]

Time (h)	DA	DOPAC	HVA
	Substantia Nigra		
Control	21 ± 4	7 ± 2	10 ± 3
5	12 ± 2[b]	2 ± 2	8 ± 1
5 (+)-MK801	8 ± 3[c]	0[c]	7 ± 1[c]
24	62 ± 11[b]	31 ± 9[b]	47 ± 8[b]
	Corpus Striatum		
Control	1120 ± 67	52 ± 4	111 ± 7
5	336 ± 213[b]	4 ± 3[b]	47 ± 8[b]
5(+)-MK801	588 ± 463[c]	16 ± 17[c]	51 ± 55[c]
24	218 ± 68[b]	10 ± 4[b]	48 ± 4[b]

[a]Mice were 8-month-old C57 B1/6 males and were used in groups of 3–5. MPTP was given as 4 doses of 10 mg/kg (IP) at 2-h intervals. (+)-MK801 was given (IP) as a 10 mg/kg dose 10 min before the first dose of MPTP, then as 3 doses of 2.5 mg/kg, 10 min before the final three doses of MPTP. Mice treated with (+)-MK801 along demonstrated results identical to control results. Time refers to the time of sacrifice after the last dose of MPTP. Results are presented as means and standard deviations. Values are picomoles/mg protein.
[b]Significantly different from controls by ANOVA and Newman-Keuls test, $p < 0.05$.
[c]Not different from 5-h data.

also called complex 1, in the mitochondrial electron transport chain is weakly and reversibly inhibited by MPP^+, which can result in decreases in cellular adenosine triphosphate (ATP) levels (Nicklas et al., 1985). The K_m of inhibition of NADH dehydrogenase by MPP^+ is in the millimolar range. Loss of cellular ATP has been heralded as the final cause of death from MPTP toxicity. However, there is no indication that the loss of ATP is permanent. This would require demonstration of increases in hypoxanthine levels. Neurons can survive for many minutes without ATP (Hossman, 1983).

The weak and reversible inhibition of NADH dehydrogenase by MPP^+ is probably self-limiting. The inhibition of NADH dehydrogenase causes the collapse of the mitochondrial membrane potential, which is required for the concentration of MPP^+ by mitochondria. Therefore, MPP^+ will leak out of mitochondria and cease to inhibit NADH dehydrogenase. However, inhibition of NADH dehydrogenase by MPP^+ and other compounds is known to produce oxygen radicals (Hasegawa et al., 1990), perhaps because of a build-up in ubisemiquinone levels. Ubisemiquinone is a reduction product of ubiquinone and is a free radical species capable of reducing oxygen with the production of $O \cdot^-$. MPTP is known to stimulate oxygen radical production by mitochondria (Rossetti et al., 1988). It may be the formation of oxygen radicals in combination with decreases in ATP levels that precipitates the irreversible damage to mitochondria by MPTP.

The mitochondrial toxicity of MPTP has sparked interest in the possible involvement of mitochondria in PD. Several reports have found moderate mitochondrial abnormalities in the brains of PD patients (Schapira et al., 1990). These abnormalities are probably not severe enough to destroy the mitochondria, but they may produce abnormal electron transfer such that large amounts of oxygen radicals may be formed. These oxygen radicals could damage the mitochondria and the entire dopaminergic neuron.

MPTP and Oxidative Stress Mechanisms

There are many mechanisms by which MPTP forms oxygen radicals. One prominent mechanism is that MPP^+ causes the release of dopamine from intracellular vesicles (Rollema et al., 1988). This dopamine is then a substrate for MAO, which forms hydrogen peroxide. Alternatively, dopamine may slowly oxidize to form 6-hydroxydopamine, which readily auto-oxidizes, with the production of oxygen free radicals. This mechanism may be most notable in the corpus striatum, where the stores of dopamine are much higher than in the midbrain.

MPTP may cause a decrease in the perfusion of blood through the brain (Adams et al., 1991a). This may result in the formation of oxygen radicals because of hypoxia and reperfusion. In addition, hypoxia causes dopamine to be released from storage vesicles (Phebus et al., 1986), with resultant production of oxygen radicals as above. Of course, hypoxia may potentiate the mitochondrial toxicity and decrease the mitochondrial uptake of MPP^+ by decreasing ATP levels. Both hypoxia and the mitochondrial toxicity of MPP^+ will result in accumulation of lactate in the brain. Lactate may cause iron to be released from its storage sites in ferritin (Paques et al., 1979). Iron can participate in the reactions shown above to generate oxygen radicals and catalyze lipid peroxidation.

MPP^+ can induce oxidative stress following reduction by cytochrome P-450 reductase, which results in OH· formation (Sinha et al., 1986). Xanthine oxidase, aldehyde dehydrogenase, and lipoamide dehydrogenase can also reduce MPP^+ (Adams et al., 1992). This involves a two-electron reduction of MPP^+. The one-electron reduction potential of MPP^+ is too high for biological reductants to be effective. Instead, a two-electron reduction, also called hydride transfer, is thermodynamically favorable (Oturan et al., 1988). All of the enzymes above are capable of catalyzing hydride transfer to MPP^+, to form 1-methyl-4-phenyl-1,4-dihydropyridine (DHP). The mechanism of hydride transfer and oxidative stress is shown in the reactions below. Any reaction with a positive potential may proceed.

(4)	$MPP^+ + e^-$	$\rightarrow MPP\cdot$	$E = -1\ V$
(5)	$MPP^+ + H^-$	$\rightarrow DHP$	$E = 0.8\ V$
(6)	$DHP + O_2\cdot^-$	$\rightarrow MPP\cdot + OOH^-$	$E = 2.8\ V$
(7)	$MPP\cdot + H_2O_2$	$\rightarrow MPP^+ + OH\cdot + OH^-$	$E = 1.6\ V$
(8)	$MPP\cdot + O_2$	$\rightarrow MPP^+ + O_2\cdot^-$	$E = 0.9\ V$

This mechanisn requires the oxidation of DHP by $O_2\cdot^-$, which is abundant in mitochondria, especially during MPP^+ inhibition of NADH dehydrogenase. The most notable product of this mechanism is OH·, which is readily formed from H_2O_2 and MPP· without the need for iron (Adams et al., 1992). This highly reactive OH· may be responsible for the peroxidation of lipids. It is worth noting that the administration of acetaldehyde to MPTP-treated mice greatly increases the dopaminergic toxicity of MPTP (Corsini et al., 1987). This is undoubtedly due to the flow of electrons from acetaldehyde to aldehyde dehydrogenase to MPP^+, with the production of DHP and eventually OH·.

MPTP and Brain Oxidative Stress

A wealth of data is available demonstrating the in vivo effects of MPTP-induced oxidative stress in the brain (Adams and Odunze, 1991). For instance, MPTP induces lipid peroxidation in the midbrains of vitamin E–deficient mice, but not in normal mice (Adams et al., 1990). This supports the notion of MPTP-induced oxidative stress, since vitamin E–deficient mice are much more susceptible to oxidative stress than normal mice. Lipofuscin, a byproduct of lipid peroxidation, also accumulates in the midbrains of MPTP-treated monkeys (Elsworth et al., 1987). MPP^+ has been demonstrated to stimulate lipid peroxidation in vitro in mouse brain homogenates (Rios and Tapia, 1987). Lipid peroxidation may result from $OH\cdot$ or other free radical attack on lipids.

Glutathione and glutathione disulfide are involved in the toxicity of MPTP. In the corpus striatum, a transient depletion of glutathione has been reported following MPTP administration (Adams et al., 1989b). The midbrains of MPTP-treated mice demonstrate an initial compensatory increase in glutathione (Odunze et al., 1990a) followed by a depletion in glutathione levels (Ferraro et al., 1986). Glutathione disulfide levels have been shown to increase in the midbrains of MPTP-treated mice (Odunze et al., 1990a). These results are consistent with MPTP-induced oxidative stress, in that glutathione disulfide levels increase and glutathione levels may decrease as the result of the action of glutathione peroxidase. Hydrogen peroxide, produced by the dismutation of $O_2{}^{\cdot-}$, is detoxified by glutathione peroxidase, with the concomitant oxidation of glutathione. Depletion of brain glutathione by diethylmaleate makes dopaminergic neurons in the midbrain more susceptible to MPTP toxicity (Adams, et al., 1989b). Finally, the administration to mice of (–)-2-oxo-4-thiazolidine carboxylate, which is known to stimulate glutathione synthesis, increases the brain levels of glutathione and makes them resistant to MPTP toxicity (Wiener et al., 1988). This is consistent with MPTP-induced oxidative stress, which requires glutathione for the detoxification of hydrogen peroxide.

MPTP has been shown to inhibit glutathione disulfide reductase (Adams et al., 1989b). This enzyme is critical to the protection of the brain from oxidative stress, since it reduces glutathione disulfide and effectively recycles glutathione. Increases in glutathione disulfide levels in the brain may be toxic, since glutathione disulfide forms mixed disulfides with proteins and alters the activities of a number of enzymes (Odunze et al., 1990a). Carmustine treatment irreversibly inhibits brain glutathione disulfide reductase and increases the toxicity of MPTP in the midbrain (Adams et al., 1989b). In addition, MPTP treatments deplete brain protein sulfhydryl levels in the corpus striatum, perhaps as a result of protein glutathione disulfide mixed disulfide formation (Odunze et al., 1990a). These data support the importance of glutathione disulfide formed during oxidative stress in the toxicity of MPTP.

Vitamin C administration has been shown to protect the brain from MPTP toxicity (Perry et al., 1985; Sershen et al., 1985). The brain takes up vitamin C from the plasma (Tolbert et al., 1979) and uses vitamin C as a major antioxidant. Vitamin C readily mitigates the toxicity of oxygen free radicals by a number of mechanisms including the regeneration of vitamin E from tocopheryl radical. Vitamin E administration is less reliable at protecting the brain from MPTP toxicity. This may be because vitamin E does not quickly penetrate into the brain. As mentioned before, very little is known about the kinetics of brain vitamin E. However, MPTP administration is known to alter vitamin E levels in many brain regions (Odunze et al., 1990b). Perhaps the most significant alteration is a slow and persistent increase in vitamin E levels in the midbrain following MPTP administration. This increase in vitamin E levels is possibly related to MPTP-induced depletion of ubiquinol levels in the substantia nigra (Fariello et al., 1987). Ubiquinol is an important antioxidant in membranes and is involved in electron transport in mitochondria. The increase in vitamin

E levels may be similar to the compensatory increases in midbrain vitamin E levels seen in PD patients, as discussed above.

Transgenic mice that express higher than normal levels of superoxide dismutase in the brain are resistant to MPTP toxicity (Przedborski et al., 1991). Superoxide dismutase catalyzes the formation of H_2O_2 from $O_2 \cdot^-$ and is known to protect cells from oxidative stress. The protective effects of superoxide dismutase in MPTP toxicity are supportive of an oxidative stress mechanism in MPTP toxicity.

The Use of MPTP to Model Parkinson's Disease

In summary, it is clear that MPTP has at least two major mechanisms of toxicity, mitochondrial and oxidative stress. These two mechanisms function together and are both required for the toxicity of MPTP in dopaminergic neurons. The fact that MPTP does induce oxidative stress in the brain makes it a useful model toxin in the study of PD.

The MPTP model encompasses the goals of each of the three types of animal model described. It has been used in the context of the mechanistic model to examine the effects of mitochondrial dysfunction and oxidative stress on neuron integrity. It has also been used to create an analogous model of PD. MPTP reproduces the cardinal neurobiological features of the disease in several species. Finally, MPTP has been used as an etiological model of PD. MPTP was clearly the causative factor in the development of PD in a number of cases induced by improperly manufactured designer drugs. Whether MPTP or other methyl pyridines in the environment are common factors in PD needs to be determined. However, MPTP has been a valuable tool to explore the causes and biology of PD.

DEVELOPMENTAL DISORDERS

Developmental disorders of the nervous system, including mental retardation, can result from a variety of insults to the developing organism. Genetic factors, metabolic abnormalities, exposure to toxins in the perinatal environment, infections, trauma during delivery, undernutrition, and hypoxia can result in alterations in both cognitive abilities and brain development. Animal models typically focus on one factor that appears to be responsible for retardation. For example, models of fetal alcohol syndrome address the effects of alcohol on the developing nervous system and the functional consequences of that exposure. However, because of the myriad recognized and unrecognized factors that can produce retardation, it is imprudent to develop exclusively animal models that are dependent on the analysis of a single causative factor.

Methylazoxymethanol Model of Microcephaly

Microcephaly is a reduction in brain size that can result from exposure to environmental toxins, malnutrition, and viral infections during critical periods of gestation. Mental retardation and other neurobehavioral deficits are typically associated with microcephaly. Methylazoxymethanol acetate (MAM) is a potent antimitotic agent that has been used to explore the neurobiology of microencephaly and its associated cognitive impairments (Balduini et al., 1986; Shimizu et al., 1991).

By methylating guanine sites in the DNA of a developing organism, MAM halts the active division of cells. Administering MAM at certain gestational periods prevents proliferation of selected cell groups. Cell groups that would normally proliferate at that time point during gestation fail to do so. However, neurons that divide before or after the day(s) of MAM administration are spared.

Prenatal administration of MAM during neurogenesis results in dose- and time-dependent microencephaly (Miner and Davies, 1992). Administered to rats around day 15 of gestation, MAM produces a dramatic, dose-dependent reduction in the formation of cortical, hippocampal, and striatal cell populations. For example, Minger and Davies (1992) report that, following a 15 mg/kg dose of MAM on gestation days 14 and 15, a 40–60% decrease in the number of neurons in the neocortex, with a reduction in cortical volume, was observed. However, the brain stem and basal forebrain regions were entirely spared. In contrast, MAM produces cerebellar atrophy if injected on postnatal day 1 (Balduini, et al., 1986).

Behavioral alterations following prenatal MAM exposure depend on the concomitant cellular and neurochemical changes produced by a particular treatment regimen. Alterations in learning and memory have been observed in a variety of spatial and aversive learning tasks (Banfi et al., 1984). These impairments are consistently accompanied by decreases in hippocampal volume, weight, and cell number, as well as decreases in the thickness of the corpus callosum. In addition, Shimizu et al. (1991) described impaired acquisition and retention of a radial-arm maze task in MAM-treated rats that was associated with a significant decrease in ChAT activity in the hippocampus.

Models of Phenylketonuria

Phenylketonuria (PKU) is an inherited disease transmitted by a recessive autosomal allele that occurs in one of about every 20,000 viable births in the United States (Vorhees et al., 1981). The genetic defect causes a deficiency of the hepatic enzyme phenylalanine hydroxylase that in turn leads to a deficit in the conversion of phenylalanine (Phe) to tyrosine. As a result, there is an increased concentration of Phe in plasma, urine, and the brain. This excess combined with secondary disturbances in other biochemical systems results in moderate to severe mental retardation. Other neurobehavioral changes include language disturbances, agressivity, seizures, hypertonicity, and impaired myelinogenesis (Burri et al., 1990). Fortunately, PKU is treatable by instituting a Phe-restricted diet before postnatal day 120. Despite knowledge of the etiology and nature of the defect and its treatability, it is uncertain how this enzyme deficiency and the resulting biochemical cascade leads to mental retardation. In addition, the current treatment does not lead to optimal intellectual performance. For these reasons, an animal model of PKU is necessary and valuable.

One of several PKU animal models involves transplacental or postnatal delivery of both Phe and p-chlorophenylalanine (PCPA), a potent inhibitor of Phe hydroxylase (Lipton et al., 1967). Phenylketonuria models of this type produce the major characteristics of the disease: 1.) plasma Phe levels higher than 15 mg/dl, 2.) high Phe/tyrosine ratios, and 3.) lasting cognitive impairments (Copenhaver et al., 1974; Anderson, 1976). Furthermore, combined Phe-PCPA administration leads to reductions in levels of serotonin and catecholamines similar in magnitude to those seen in humans with the disease (Vorhees et al., 1981). A problem with the use of PCPA is that this drug also potently inhibits the activity of tryptophan hydroxylase in the brain and therefore alters the activity of serotonergic neurons throughout the nervous system (Koe and Weissman, 1966). However, other drugs with greater selectivity for inhibiting Phe hydroxylase activity have been introduced (Greengard et al., 1976).

A second promising model of PKU is produced by combined administration of Phe and α-methylphenylalanine (α-MPhe). α-Methylphenylalanine is a less potent but more selective inhibitor of Phe hydroxylase than PCPA. When administered in conjunction with Phe it produces plasma Phe levels that are comparable to those seen in the Phe-PCPA model (Vorhees et al., 1981). Perinatal Phe–α-MPhe treatment produces lasting cognitive impairments that resemble those observed in humans (Strupp et al., 1992).

The preceding sections described how compounds can be used to model the developmental disorders microcephaly and PKU. Methylazoxymethanol acetate is a potent antimitotic agent that disrupts the genesis of different brain areas when given at specific gestational ages. This provides a way to examine both the consequence of such an insult and ways to promote recovery of function.

The models of PKU use specific agents that induce a physiological state: increased Phe levels in blood and brain. These models can reproduce the biochemical and functional changes observed in PKU, but they do not examine how increased Phe levels promote developmental abnormalities and retardation. However, both MAM and α-MPhe can be used to study brain development, the factors that disrupt this process, the consequences of such a disruption, and behavioral, pharmacological, and interventive approaches that might promote functional recovery.

CONCLUSIONS

This chapter focused on how selective neurotoxic compounds can be used to unravel the function of the nervous system. Neurotoxins can address basic questions at molecular, biochemical, physiological, and behavioral levels of analysis. They have also been invaluable in developing animal models of Alzheimer's, Parkinson's, and Huntington's diseases and developmental disorders of the nervous system. They are powerful tools that can be used in creative ways by all of the different disciplines that constitute the science of neurotoxicology.

ACKNOWLEDGMENTS

This chapter was written while TJW was supported by grant ESO4262 from the National Institutes of Health and grant BNS-9222097 from the National Science Foundation. JDA was supported by grant NS-29442 from the National Institutes of Health.

REFERENCES

Adams JD, Kalivas PW, Miller CA (1989a). The acute histopathology of MPTP in the mouse CNS. Brain Res Bull 23:1–17.

Adams JD, Klaidman LK, Cadenas E (1992). MPP^+ redox cycling: a new mechanism involving hydride transfer. Ann NY Acad Sci 648:239–40.

Adams JD, Klaidman LK, Odunze IN (1989b). Oxidative effects of MPTP in the midbrain. Res Commun Subst Abuse 10:169–80.

Adams JD, Klaidman LK, Odunze IN, Johannessen JN (1991a). Effects of MPTP on the cerebro-vasculature. Int J Dev Neurosci 9:155–60.

Adams JD, Klaidman LK, Odunze IN, Shen HC, Miller CA (1991b). Alzheimer's and Parkinson's disease brain levels of glutathione, glutathione disulfide and vitamin E. Mol Chem Neuropathol 14:213–26.

Adams JD, Odunze IN (1991). Biochemical mechanisms of MPTP toxicity: Could oxidative stress be involved in the brain? Biochem Pharmacol 41:1099–1105.

Adams JD, Odunze IN, Sevanian A (1990). Induction by MPTP of lipid peroxidation in vivo in vitamin E deficient mice. Biochem Pharmacol 39:R5–R8.

Allain H, Denmat J, Bentue-Ferrer D, Milton D, Pignol P, Reymann JM, Pape D, Sabouraud O, Van Den Driessche J (1988). Randomized, double blind trial of exifone versus cognitive problems in Parkinson's disease. Fund Clin Pharmacol 2:1–12.

Ambani LM, Van Woert MH, Murphy S (1975). Brain peroxidase and catalase in Parkinson's disease. Arch Neurol 32:114–8.

Anderson A (1976). Maternal hyperphenylalaninemia: an experimental model in rats. Dev Psychobiol 9:157–66.

Armstrong M, Daly AK, Cholerton S, Bateman DN, Idle JR (1992). Mutant debrisoquine hydroxylation genes in Parkinson's disease. Lancet 339:1017–8.

Baddeley AD (1986). Working memory. Oxford: Clarendon Press.

Balduini W, Cimino M, Lomardelli G, Abbracchio M, Peruzzi G, Cecchini T, Gazzanelli G, Cattabeni F (1986). Microencephalic rats as a model for cognitive disorders. Clin Neuropharmacol 9:S8–S18.

Banfi S, Dorigotti L, Abbracchio M, Balduini W, Coen E, Ragusa C, Cattabeni F (1984). Methylazoxymethanol microencephaly in rats: neurochemical characterization and behavioral studies with the nootropic oxiracetam. Pharmacol Res Comm 16:67–83.

Barker LA, Mittag TW (1975). Comparative studies of substrates and inhibitors of choline transport and choline acetyltransferase. J Pharmacol Exp Ther 192:86–94.

Barlow P, Marchbanks RM (1984). Effect of ethylcholine mustard on choline dehydrogenase and other enzymes of choline metabolism. J Neurochem 43:1568–73.

Bartus RT, Dean RL, Beer B, Lippa AS (1982). The cholinergic hypothesis of geriatric memory dysfunction. Science 217:408–17.

Bland BH (1986). The physiology and pharmacology of hippocampal formation theta rhythms. Prog Neurobiol 26:1–54.

Boller F, Mizutani T, Roessmann U, Gambetti P (1980). Parkinson disease, dementia and Alzheimer disease: clinicopathological correlations. Ann Neurol 7:329–35.

Burri R, Steffen C, Steiger S, Brodbeck U, Colombo JP, Herschkowitz N (1990). Reduced myelinogenesis and recovery in hyperphenylalanemic rats: correlation between brain phenylalanine levels, characteristic brain enzymes for myelination and brain development. Mol Chem Neuropathol 13:57–69.

Casarett J, Klaassen CD, Amdur MO, eds. (1980). Casarett and Doull's toxicology: the basic science of poisons. New York: Macmillan.

Chiba K, Peterson LA, Castagnoli KP, Trevor AJ, Castagnoli N (1985). Studies on the mechanism of bioactivation of the selective nigrostriatal toxin MPTP. Drug Metab Dispos 13:342–7.

Chiueh CC, Burns RS, Markey SP, Jacobowitz DM, Kopin IJ (1985). Primate model of parkinsonism: selective lesion of nigrostriatal neurons by MPTP produces an extrapyramidal syndrome in rhesus monkeys. Life Sci 36:213–8.

Chrobak JJ, Hanin I, Walsh TJ (1986). AF64A (ethylcholine mustard aziridinium ion), a cholinergic neurotoxin, selectively impairs working memory in a multiple component T-maze task. Brain Res 414:15–21.

Chrobak JJ, Walsh TJ (1991). Dose and delay dependent working/episodic memory impairments following intraventricular administration of ethylcholine aziridinium ion (AF64A). Behav Neural Biol 56:200–12.

Chrobak JJ, Hanin I, Schmechel DE, Walsh TJ (1988). AF64A-induced working memory impairment: behavioral, neurochemical and histological correlates. Brain Res 463:107–17.

Chrobak JJ, Spates MJ, Stackman RW, Walsh TJ (1989). Hemicholinium-3 prevents the working memory impairments and the cholinergic hypofunction induced by ethylcholine aziridinium ion (AF64A). Brain Res 504:269–75.

Cohen G (1985). Oxidative stress in the nervous system. In: Sies H, ed. Oxidative stress. New York: Academic Press, 383–402.

Cohen G (1990). Monoamine oxidase and oxidative stress at dopaminergic synapses. J Neural Transm 32(suppl):229–38.

Cohen NJ, Squire LR (1980). Preserved learning and retention of pattern analyzing skill in amnesia: dissociation of knowing how and knowing that. Science 210:207–9.

Copenhaver JH, Carver MJ, Schalock RL (1974). Experimental maternal hyperphenylalaninemia: biochemical effects and offspring development. Dev Psychobiol 7:175–84.

Corsini CU, Zuddas A, Bonuccelli U, Schinelli S, Kopin IJ (1987). MPTP toxicity in mice is enhanced by pretreatment with diethyldithiocarbamate. Eur J Pharmacol 119:127–8.

Coyle JT, Price DL, DeLong MR (1983). Alzheimer's disease: a disorder of cortical cholinergic innervation. Science 219:1184–90.

Curti D, Marchbanks RM (1984). Kinetics of irreversible inhibition of choline transport in synaptosomes by ethylcholine mustard aziridinium. J Membrane Biol 82:259–68.

Davis GC, Williams AC, Markey SP, Ebert MH, Caine ED, Reichert CM, Kopin IJ (1979). Chronic parkinsonism secondary to intravenous injection of meperidine analogues. Psychiatry Res 1:249–54.

Dexter DT, Carayon A, Javoy-Agid F, Agid Y, Wells FR, Daniel SE, Lees AJ, Jenner P, Marsden CD (1991). Alterations in the levels of iron, ferritin, and other trace metals in Parkinson's disease and other neurodegenerative diseases affecting the basal ganglia. Brain 114:1953–75.

Elsworth JD, Deutch AY, Redmond DE, Sladek JR (1987). Differential responsiveness to MPTP toxicity in sub-regions of the primate substantia nigra and striatum. Life Sci 40:193–202.

Emerich DF, Walsh TJ (1990). Ganglioside AGF2 promotes task-dependent behavioral recovery and attenuates the cholinergic hypofunction induced by AF64A. Brain Res 527:299–307.

Emerich DF, Black B, Kesslak P, Cottman C, Walsh TJ (1992). Transplantation of fetal cholinergic neurons into hippocampus attenuates the cognitive and neurochemical deficits induced by AF64A. Brain Res Bull 28:219–26.

Evans DA, Funkenstein HH, Albert MS, Scherr PA, Cook NR, Chown MJ, Herbert LE, Hennekens CH, Taylor JO (1989). Prevalence of Alzheimer's disease in a community population of older persons. JAMA 262:2551–6.

Fahn S (1991). An open trial of high dosage antioxidants in early Parkinson's disease. Am J Clin Nutr 53:380s–382s.

Fariello RG, Ghirardi O, Peschechera A, Ramacci MT, Angelucci L (1987). Transient nigral ubiquinone depletion after single MPTP administration in mice. Neuropharmacology 26:1799–1802.

Ferraro TN, Golden GT, DeMattei M, Hare TA, Fariello RG (1986). Effect of MPTP on levels of glutathione in the extrapyramidal system of the mouse. Neuropharmacology 25:1071–4.

Fisher A, Hanin I (1980). Minireview: choline analogs as potential tools in developing selective animal models of central cholinergic hypofunction. Life Sci 27:1615–43.

Fisher A, Hanin I (1986). Potential animal models for senile dementia of Alzheimer's type, with emphasis on AF64A-induced cholinotoxicity. Annu Rev Pharmacol Toxicol 26:161–81.

Forno LS, Langston JW, DeLanney LE, Irwin I, Ricaurte GA (1986). Locus ceruleus lesions and eosinophilic inclusions in MPTP treated monkeys. Ann Neurol 20:449–55.

Frotscher M, Leranth C (1985). Cholinergic innervation of the rat hippocampus as revealed by choline acetyltransferase immunocytochemistry: a combined light and electron microscopic study. J Comp Neurol 239:237–46.

Futscher BW, Pieper RO, Barnes DM, Hanin I, Erickson LC (1992). DNA-damaging and transcription terminating lesions induced by AF64A in vitro. J Neurochem 58:1504–9.

Gerhart JM, Hong JS, Tilson HA (1985). Studies on the mechanism of chlordecone-induced tremor in rats. Neurotoxicology 6:211–30.

Graham DG (1984). Catecholamine toxicity: a proposal for the molecular pathogenesis of manganese neurotoxicity and Parkinson's disease. Neurotoxicology 5:83–96.

Greengard O, Yoss MS, Del Valle JA (1976). α-Methylphenylalanine, a new inducer of chronic hyperphenylalaninemia in suckling rats. Science 192:1007–8.

Greiner PO, Bonnet CM, Angignard D, Dupont JM, Herold M, Borzeix MG (1992). Neuropharmacological study of aged MAM-treated rats. Neurobiol Aging 13:527–9.

Hanin I (1990). AF64A-induced cholinergic hypofunction. Prog Brain Res 84:289–99.

Hanin I, Fisher A, Hortnagl H, Leventer SM, Potter PE, Walsh TJ (1987). Ethylcholine mustard aziridinium (AF64A; ECMA) and other potential cholinergic neuron-specific neurotoxins. In: Meltzer HY, ed. Psychopharmacology—the third generation of progress. New York: Raven Press, 341–9.

Hardy J, Adolfsson R, Alafuzoff I, Bucht G, Marcusson J, Nyberg P, Perdahl E, Wester P, Winblad B (1985). Transmitter deficits in Alzheimer's disease. Neurochem Int 7:545–63.

Hart RP, Kwentus JA, Harkins SW, Taylor JR (1988). Rate of forgetting in mild Alzheimer's-type dementia. Brain Cognition 7:31–8.

Hasegawa E, Takeshige K, Oishi T, Murai Y, Minakami S (1990). MPP$^+$ induces NADH dependent superoxide formation and enhances NADH dependent lipid peroxidation in bovine heart submitochondrial particles. Biochem Biophys Res Commun 170:1049–55.

Heikkila RE, Hess A, Duvoisin RC (1984). Dopaminergic neurotoxicity of MPTP in mice. Science 224:1451–3.

Hill JM, Switzer RC (1984). The regional distribution and cellular localization of iron in the rat brain. Neuroscience 11:595–603.

Hornykiewicz O, Kish SJ (1986). Biochemical pathophysiology of Parkinson's disease. Adv Neurol 45:19–34.

Hossman KA (1983). Neuronal survival and revival during and after cerebral ischemia. Am J Emerg Med 1:191–7.

Jope RS (1979). High affinity choline transport and acetyl CoA production in brain and their roles in the regulation of acetylcholine synthesis. Brain Res Rev 180:313–44.

Kasa P, Hanin I (1985). Ethylcholine mustard aziridinium blocks the axoplasmic transport of acetylcholinesterase in cholinergic nerve fibers of the rat. Histochemistry 83:343–5.

Knopman DS, Nissen MJ (1987). Implicit learning in patients with probable Alzheimer's disease. Neurology 37:784–7.

Koe BK, Weissman A (1966). p-Chlorophenylalanine: a specific depletor of brain serotonin. J Pharmacol Exp Ther 154:499–516.

Kornetsky C (1977). Animal models: promises and problems. In: Hanin I, Usdin E, eds. Animal models in psychiatry and neurology. New York: Pergamon Press, 1–7.

Larson J, Wong D, Lynch G (1986). Pattern stimulation at the theta frequency is optimal for the induction of hippocampal long-term potentiation. Brain Res 363:347–50.

Leventer SM, Wulfert E, Hanin I (1987). Time course of ethylcholine aziridinium ion (AF64A)-induced cholinotoxicity in vivo. Neuropharmacology 26:361–5.

Lipton MA, Gordon R, Guroff G, Udenfriend S (1967). p-Chlorophenylalnine-induced chemical manifestation of phenylketonuria in rats. Science 156:248–50.

Lorens SK, Kindel G, Dong XW, Lee JM, Hanin I (1991). Septal choline acetyltransferase immunoreactive neurons: dose-dependent effects of AF64A. Brain Res Bull 26:965–71.

Mann JJ, Stanley M, Neophitides A, de Leon M, Ferris SH, Gershon S (1981). Central amine metabolism in Alzheimer's disease: in vivo relationship to cognitive deficit. Neurobiol Aging 2:57–60.

Mann DMA, Yates PO (1982). Pathogenesis of Parkinson's disease. Arch Neurol 39:545–9.

Marttila RJ, Lorentz H, Rinne UK (1988). Oxygen toxicity protecting enzymes in Parkinson's disease. J Neurol Sci 86:321–31.

McGeer PL, Eccles JC, McGeer EG (1987). Molecular neurobiology of the mammalian brain. New York: Plenum Press.

McGurk SR, Hartgraves SL, Kelly PH, Gordons MN, Butcher LL (1987). Is ethylcholine aziridinium ion a specific cholinergic neurotoxin? Neuroscience 22:215–24.

McKinney WT, Bunney WE (1969). Animal model of depression: review of evidence and implications for research. Arch Gen Psychiatry 21:240–8.

Minger SL, Davies P (1992). Persistent innervation of the rat neocortex by basal forebrain cholinergic neurons despite the massive reduction of cortical target neurons. Exp Neurol 117:124–38.

Nicklas WJ, Vyas I, Heikkila RE (1985). Inhibition of NADH linked oxidation in brain mitochondria by MPP$^+$, a metabolite of the neurotoxin MPTP. Life Sci 36:2503–8.

Nissen MJ, Knopman DS, Schacter DL (1987). Neurochemical dissociation of memory systems. Neurology 37:789–94.

Odunze IN, Klaidman LK, Adams JD (1990a). MPTP toxicity: differential effects in the striatum, cerebral cortex and midbrain on glutathione, glutathione disulfide and protein sulfhydryl levels. Res Commun Subst Abuse 11:123–34.

Odunze IN, Klaidman LK, Adams JD (1990b). MPTP toxicity in the mouse brain and vitamin E. Neurosci Lett 108:346–9.

Ogawa N, Hirose Y, Ohara S, Ono T, Watanabe Y (1985). A simple quantitative bradykinesia test in MPTP treated mice. Res Common Chem Pathol Pharmacol 50:435–41.

Oturan MA, Dostert P, Benedetti MS, Moiroux J, Anne A, Fleury MB (1988). One electron and two electron reductions of MPP$^+$. J Electroanal Chem 242:171–9.

Paracelsus (1567). Von der Besucht. Düllingen, Germany.

Paques EP, Paques A, Crichton RR (1979). A kinetic study of the mechanism of ferritin formation. The effects of buffer, of pH, and of the iron content of the molecule. J Mol Catalysis 5:363–75.

Perry TL, Yong VW, Clavier RM, Jones K (1985). Partial protection from the dopaminergic neurotoxin N-methyl-4-phenyl-1,2,3,6-tetrahydropyridine by four different antioxidants in the mouse. Neurosci. Lett. 60:109–114.

Phebus LA, Perry KW, Clemens JA, Fuller RW (1986). Brain anoxia releases striatal dopamine in rats. Life Sci 38:2447–53.

Potter PE, Tedford CE, Kindel GH, Hanin I (1987). Inhibition of high affinity choline transport attenuates both cholinergic and noncholinergic effects of ethylcholine aziridinium (AF64A). Brain Res 13:238–44.

Przedborski S, Kostic V, Jackson-Lewis V, Carlson E, Epstein CJ, Cadet JL (1991). Quantitative autoradiographic distribution of [^{3}H]-MPTP binding in the brains of superoxide dismutase transgenic mice. Brain Res Bull 26:987–91.

Rios C, Tapia R (1987). Changes in lipid peroxidation induced by MPTP and MPP$^+$ in mouse brain homogenates. Neurosci Lett 77:321–6.

Rollema H, Kuhr WG, Kranenborg G, De Vries J, Van Den Berg C (1988). MPP$^+$ induced efflux of dopamine and lactate from rat striatum have similar time courses as shown by in vivo brain dialysis. J Pharmacol Exp Ther 245:858–66.

Rossetti ZL, Sotgiu A, Sharp DE, Hadjiconstantinou M, Neff NH (1988). MPTP and free radicals in vitro. Biochem Pharmacol 37:4573–4.

Rossor MN, Iversen LL, Reynolds GP, Mountjoy CQ, Roth M (1984). Neurochemical characteristics of early and late onset types of Alzheimer's disease. Br Med J 283:961–4.

Rusted JM, Warburton DM (1988). The effects of scopolamine on working memory in healthy young volunteers. Psychopharmacology 96:145–52.

Rylett RJ, Ball MJ, Colhoun EH (1983). Evidence for high affinity choline transport in synaptosomes prepared from hippocampus and neocortex of patients with Alzheimer's disease. Brain Res 289:169–75.

Saggu H, Cooksey J, Dexter D, Wells FR, Lees A, Jenner P, Marsden CD (1989). A selective increase in particulate superoxide dismutase activity in parkinsonian substantia nigra. J Neurochem 53:692–7.

Sanberg PR, Coyle JT (1984). Scientific approaches to Huntington's disease. CRC Crit Rev Neurobiol 1:1–44.

Sandberg K, Schnaar RL, McKinney M, Hanin I, Fisher A, Coyle JT (1985). AF64A: an active site directed irreversible inhibitor of choline acetyltransferase. J Neurochem 44:439–45.

Sarter kM, Hagan J, Dudchenko P (1992). Behavioral screening for cognition enhancers: from indiscriminate to valid testing: part I. Psychopharmacology 107:144–50.

Schapira AHV, Cooper JM, Dexter D, Clark JB, Jenner P, Marsden CD (1990). Mitochondrial complex 1 deficiency in Parkinson's disease. J Neurochem 54:823–7.

Segura-Aguilar J, Lind C (1989). On the mechanism of the Mn^{+3} induced neurotoxicity of dopamine: prevention of quinone derived oxygen toxicity by DT diaphorase and superoxide dismutase. Chem Biol Interact 72:309–24.

Sershen H, Reith MEA, Hashim A, Lajtha A (1985). Protection against MPTP neurotoxicity by the antioxidant ascorbic acid. Neuropharmacology 24:1257–9.

Shimizu J, Tamaru M, Katsukara T, Matsutani T, Nagata Y (1991). Effects of fetal treatment with methylazoxymethanol acetate on radial maze performance in rats. Neurosci Res 11:209–14.

Simon JR, Atweh S, Kuhar MJ (1976). Sodium-dependent high affinity choline uptake: a regulatory step in the synthesis of acetylcholine. J Neurochem 26:909–22.

Sinha BK, Singh Y, Krishna G (1986). Formation of superoxide and hydroxyl radicals from MPP^+: reductive activation by NADPH cytochrome P450 reductase. Biochem Biophys Res Commun 135:583–8.

Sofic E, Paulus W, Jellinger W, Riederer P, Youdim MBH (1991). Selective increase of iron in substantia nigra zona compacta of parkinsonian brains. J Neurochem 56:978–82.

Strupp BJ, Himmelstein S, Bunsy M, Levitsky D, Kesler M (1992). Cognitive profile of rats exposed to lactational hyperphenylalaninemia: correspondence with human mental retardation. Dev Psychobiol 23:195–214.

Sundstrom E, Jonsson G (1985). Pharmacological interference with the neurotoxic action of MPTP on central catecholamine neurons in the mouse. Eur J Pharmacol 110:293–9.

Tamaru M, Yukari H, Nagayoshi M, Matsutani T (1988). Brain changes in rats induced by prenatal injection methylazoxymethanol. Teratology 37:149–57.

Tolbert LC, Thomas TN, Middaugh LD, Zemp JW (1979). Effect of ascorbic acid on neurochemical, behavioral, and physiological systems mediated by catecholamines. Life Sci 25:2189–95.

Vorhees CV, Butcher RE, Berry HK (1981). Progress in experimental phenylketonuria: a critical review. Neurosci Biobehav Rev 5:177–90.

Wagner GC, Walsh SL (1991). Evaluation of the effects of inhibition of monoamine oxidase and senescence on methamphetamine induced neuronal damage. Int J Dev Neurosci 9:171–4.

Walsh TJ, Opello KD (1992). Neuroplasticity, the aging brain, and Alzheimer's disease. Neurotoxicology 13:101–10.

Walsh TJ, Opello KD (in press). The use of AF64A to model Alzheimer's disease. In: Woodruff M, Nonneman A, eds. Animal models of toxin-induced neurological disorders. New York: Plenum Press.

Walsh TJ, Wortwein G, Stackman RW, Boudy SC (1992). AF64A (ethylcholine aziridinium ion) produces oxidative stress: relation to cholinotoxicity and functional deficits (abstr). Soc Neurosci Abst 18:1140.

Walsh TJ, Chrobak JJ (1991). Animals models of Alzheimer's disease: role of hippocampal cholinergic systems in working memory. In: Dachowski L, Flaherty C, eds. Current topics in animal learning: brain, emotion, and cognition. New Jersey: Lawrence Erlbaum, 347–79.

Whitehouse PJ, Struble RG, Hedreen JC, Clark AW, Price DL (1985). Alzheimer's disease and related dementias: selective involvement of specific neuronal systems. CRC Crit Rev Clin Neurobiol 1:319–39.

Wiener HL, Hashim A, Lajtha A, Sershen H (1988). (–)-2-Oxo-4-thiazolidine carboxylic acid attenuates MPTP induced neurotoxicity. Res Commun Subst Abuse 9:53–60.

Wilcock GK, Esiri MM, Bowen DM, Smith CCT (1982). Alzheimer's disease: correlation of cortical choline acetyltransferase activity with the severity of dementia and histological abnormalities. J Neurol Sci 57:407–17.

Willner P (1991). Behavioural models in psychopharmacology. In: Willner P, ed. Behavioural models in psychopharmacology. Cambridge, England: Cambridge University Press, 3–18.

Yamazaki N, Kato K, Kurihara E, Nagaoka A (1991). Cholinergic drugs reverse AF64A-induced impairment of passive avoidance learning of rats. Psychopharmacology 103:215–22.

19
Molecular Neurotoxicology

Melvin L. Billingsley
Pennsylvania State University College of Medicine
Hershey, Pennsylvania

James P. O'Callaghan
U.S. Environmental Protection Agency
Research Triangle Park, North Carolina

INTRODUCTION

Advances in neurobiology have been fostered by the recent applications of the techniques of molecular biology. Because of the incredible genetic diversity of the mammalian brain, recombinant DNA technology has been used to unravel structural and functional genes of the nervous system (Sutcliffe et al., 1983). For example, receptors have been traditionally classified on the basis of their pharmacologic profiles. By using molecular cloning and gene library screening strategies, deduced amino acid sequences of families of receptors have been identified (Lefkowitz and Caron, 1988). These receptors can then be expressed in heterologous cell types, and their function can be studied in vitro. Thus, the application of molecular techniques has led to a greater understanding of the brain on a more reductionist level.

Neurotoxicology, which is a more integrative discipline, will benefit by advances in molecular neurobiology; however, the appropriate use of these techniques is warranted. In a field as complex as neurotoxicology, approaches ranging from epidemiology, behavior, electrophysiology, neurochemistry, and cell biology will continue to be used along with molecular approaches. In this chapter, we wish to outline some of the areas in which molecular neurotoxicology will provide answers to important issues, and to illustrate pitfalls that can accompany such techniques. We have divided this chapter into subdivisions in which molecular approaches may provide insight into mechanisms of toxicity.

GENERAL ISSUES RELATED TO BIOMARKERS OF NEUROTOXICITY

Several issues should be considered when evaluating the usefulness of biomarkers for neurotoxicity. One key issue to consider in the evaluation of biomarkers is the relationship between the expression of the putative biomarker and "structural damage" to the nervous tissue. For instance, will the loss of expression of a given neuronal protein hallmark permanent neuronal damage and correlate with a loss of Nissl staining (Reuhl and Lowndes, 1992)? Alternatively, how will biomarker expression be altered if the damage is transitory, with loss of synaptic terminals but preservation of perikarya (Crino et al., 1989)? The key focus of this issue strikes at the heart of neurotoxicity—what is a definition of structural damage? Is it necessary to have a loss of Nissl staining on tissue sections and a positive silver stain for degeneration, as well as a loss of biomarker expression, or is alteration in any one of these parameters sufficient to indicate the presence of damage?

A second issue is the question of localization of damage in the central nervous system (CNS) following neurotoxicant administration. One way to state this issue is to ask whether the loss or increased expression of a putative biomarker must be seen only in the region that shows histologically verified structural alterations. If a region shows changes in either histology or biomarkers, but not both, will this be interpreted as a positive response? If a second brain region receiving projections from the site of initial damage shows a change in a biomarker, what additional factors will be needed to interpret correctly whether the second site is truly damaged or only a false positive?

A third issue is more general, and asks whether it is reasonable to expect to have a generic marker of neuronal (or glial) cell damage. Given the diversity of mammalian brain gene expression (25,000–35,000 separate genes), it may be difficult to find a universally positive index of damage (Sutcliffe, 1988). Conversely, silver degeneration stains have produced positive results in many cases of mechanical and chemically induced damage. This suggests that a common "substrate" of degeneration may exist that, if found to be the result of a specific macromolecule, may serve as a useful generic biomarker.

Finally, the issues of false positives and false negatives will be crucial to determine the utility of a given biomarker. For instance, in the cases of several regionally specific biomarkers, pharmacological agents that do not cause toxicity can enhance expression of putative biomarkers (e.g., *c-fos* and *fra*-related antigens) (Murphy et al., 1991). How can these false positives be sorted out? In the case of rapid neurochemical changes such as those caused by organophosphate-induced inhibition of cholinesterases, will biomarkers other than the presence of cholinesterase serve any useful purpose? Several toxicants appear to cause transsynaptic changes that are manifest as a change in specific protein expression in postsynaptic cells; there is no apparent death of the receptive cell (Balaban et al., 1989). Finally, there is the issue of induction of apoptosis, or cell death that occurs in a manner dependent on protein synthesis following removal of a growth factor. (Martin et al., 1988). A toxicant could reduce expression of a key neurotrophic factor, leading to induction of apoptosis in a target cell. These issues indicate some of the complexities that can accompany toxic responses in the nervous system. In the following sections, we hope to use specific examples to allow the reader to consider some of the more general issues related to applications of molecular biologic techniques in neurotoxicology.

PREDICTION OF NEUROTOXICITY USING MOLECULAR APPROACHES

It is difficult to imagine that molecular techniques alone will predict the neurotoxic potential of a given new chemical entity. However, it is likely that molecular approaches will be useful in the development of biomarkers of toxicity. Several candidate gene products have been isolated that may serve as useful markers of nervous system damage. As a general rule, such markers will not be predictive of mechanism, but rather will indicate that some degree of damage has occurred in the CNS.

Three major categories of useful biomarkers of CNS damage can be envisioned. The first category includes neuron-specific proteins that will be lost from damaged neurons following toxic effects. Synapsin I (DeCamilli et al., 1990), synaptic vesicle proteins such as synaptophysin (Jahn et al., 1985), and cytoskeletal proteins such as spectrin, (Riederer et al., 1986), tau protein (Lee et al., 1988), and MAP-2 (Goedert et al., 1991) are examples of neuron-specific proteins. A loss of cellular immunoreactivity or presence of immunoreactivity of neuron-specific proteins in extracellular fluid could serve as a measure of neuronal damage. Technically, it is difficult to determine subtle degrees of damage by measuring the loss of cellular immunoreactivity following administration. Factors that confound such measurements include reactive synaptogenesis, which can lead to transient increases in protein expression, persistence of immunoreactive proteolytic products near the lesion, and increased protein expression by neurons adjacent to the lesion. In general, the protocol used to assess loss of these proteins would be either Western immunoblot of tissue sections or fluid, immunocytochemistry of tissues, or immunoassay of extracellular fluids. Northern blot analysis of mRNA from toxicant-treated brain would not be expected to offer a predictive advantage relative to immunochemical approaches.

A second type of biomarker for neurotoxicology would comprise regionally specific proteins. Such proteins would delineate subsets of neurons on the basis of either their transmitter phenotype (e.g., tyrosine hydroxylase for catecholaminergic neurons) (Zigmond and Stricker, 1989), specific receptor-mediated processes that participate in the presumed toxicity (e.g., excitatory glutamate receptors) (Choi, 1990a), or structural features that are found only in specific neurons, such as cerebellins (Ziai et al., 1988) and SNAP-25 (Oyler et al., 1990). Loss of tyrosine hydroxylase immunoreactivity has been used to document damage to central dopaminergic and noradrenergic processes following administration of toxicants such as 6-hydroxydopamine and 1-methyl-4-phenyl-1,2,3,6-tetrahydropyridine (MPTP) (Spina et al., 1992). In contrast, the presence of *N*-methyl-D-aspartate (NMDA) receptors has been used to predict whether a neuron will be sensitive to excitotoxic insult caused by excess glutamate release (Choi, 1990b). Thus, both the presence of and the subsequent loss of NMDA receptor immunoreactivity can be used to predict vulnerability and to document toxicity. Recently, the loss of SNAP-25, a synaptosomal-associated protein expressed at high levels in the hippocampus, has been used to document the extent of lesions of the perforant pathway from the entorhinal cortex to the hippocampus (Oyler et al., 1991). Thus, this group of proteins can be used to delineate better whether a specific subgroup of neurons has been damaged by a putative neurotoxicant. Protocols that would be useful for assessment of such biomarkers include immunocytochemistry, Western blot analysis of discrete brain regions, in situ hybridization, and Northern blots of discrete brain regions.

A final arbitrary category of biomarkers for neurotoxicology would include proteins that are expressed at much higher levels following neurotoxicant administration. The key advantage of such proteins is that levels of both protein and mRNA rise following toxic insult. Several candidate proteins have been well characterized, including the neuronal expression of immediate early genes such as *c-fos* (Morgan and Curran, 1989) *c-jun* and heat-shock proteins (Gonzalez et al., 1989) and the glial expression of glial fibrillary acidic protein (GFAP) (O'Callaghan, 1988). In the case of *c-fos*, administration of the convulsant metrazol or the excitotoxin kainic acid led to a rapid (1–4 h) rise in hippocampal *c-fos* immunoreactivity, an increased expression of *c-fos* mRNA on Northern blots, and increased in situ hybridization for *c-fos* mRNA. Thus, *c-fos* serves as a marker for neurons that are undergoing metabolic activation, which in some cases may lead to ultimate neuronal death (Sonnenberg et al., 1989; Sakurai-Yamashita et al., 1991). In the case of heat-shock proteins, periods of ischemia in rodents have been observed to increase expression in susceptible neurons (Li et al., 1992). Studies are under way to determine whether such expression can be used as a reliable predictor of ultimate neuronal death, or whether this pattern of expression serves to protect some of the neurons from the effects of the insult.

The "ideal" biomarker would be categorized as follows: 1.) it should increase dramatically following toxicant exposure; 2.) expression should be confined to cells that will undergo degeneration; 3.) it should be elevated in cells distal to the lesion site that will undergo degeneration via secondary mechanisms; and 4.) it should be easily and sensitively assayed. To date, no such marker has been found. It is likely that combinations of markers will be employed to accurately assess the neurotoxic potential of a given compound, and that such markers will be correlated with silver degeneration stains and other classical indices of toxicity.

We would like to focus on the use of GFAP as a marker of neuronal damage and illustrate the positive and negative aspects of its use in neurotoxicity assessment. Overall, GFAP can serve as a good index of neuronal damage induced by trauma, immunologic damage, or toxicant administration (O'Callaghan, 1992). The increases in GFAP generally occur in the region of damage, and the degree of increase reflects the extent of damage. Second, increases in GFAP occur at levels of toxicants below those that would lead to Nissl-verified histological damage; this suggests that GFAP is a sensitive index of damage (Brock and O'Callaghan, 1988). Third, a range of immunoassays and cDNA probes are available to assay changes in GFAP at the cellular and regional level (O'Callaghan, 1991). On the basis of the more general issues listed above, GFAP fulfills several criteria as a useful biomarker.

On the more problematic side, GFAP levels can increase following damage to the blood-brain barrier (Guilian et al., 1988). This issue can be addressed by noting GFAP increases in tissue sections adjacent to regions with disrupted blood-brain barriers. Such increases would give a "false positive" of cellular damage, although damage to the blood-brain barrier is a significant toxicity. Second, increases in GFAP are transient, and the time course of expression varies among toxicants. However, by carefully examining selected times after intoxication, this issue can be addressed. Another major issue is that levels of GFAP change in response to alterations in adrenal and testicular hormones (Nichols et al., 1990; O'Callaghan et al., 1990). Damage to these organs could alter the toxicant-induced response, rendering interpretation difficult. Levels of GFAP are also sensitive to significant increases or decreases in neuronal activity. This change may, in part, be due to expression of neurotransmitter receptors on astrocytes; the functional significance of these receptors is not yet known (Kimmelberg, 1983). Finally, the promotor region of the GFAP gene contains elements that are responsive to cAMP; activation of such promotors via physiologic mechanisms could also lead to a false positive interpretation (Rataboul et al., 1988; Reves et al., 1989). Alterations in astrocyte GFAP levels in the CNS may be part of a normal response to dynamic changes, with toxicant-induced expression representing the most severe end of the activation spectrum.

In summary, molecular techniques have allowed development of methods and molecular probes for the study of toxicant-induced changes in the CNS. Because cDNAs can be readily characterized and used to analyze gene structure and function, it is possible to consider some of the additional complexities (e.g., promoters, enhancers) of biomarker expression that may confound interpretation. As an illustration of an ideal scenario for use of biomarkers, consider the case of toxicant-induced damage to the hippocampal pyramidal fields. The damaged pyramidal hippocampal neurons should stain positive for silver degeneration stains, whereas the dentate gyrus should be negative. General neuronal markers such as synapsin I and spectrin should be significantly reduced at both the immunocytochemical and the immunoblot level. Regional hippocampal markers such as SNAP-25 should also be reduced in damaged pyramidal neurons. Several days after damage, GFAP levels should rise as manifest by increased protein and mRNA. This idealized scenario is shown schematically in Fig. 1.

MOLECULAR BIOLOGIC APPROACHES FOR DETERMINING MECHANISMS OF SELECTIVE NEUROTOXICANTS

One approach from our lab that successfully combined strategies of molecular biology with a current problem in neurotoxicology was attempting to determine the mechanism of the selective neurotoxicity of trimethyltin (TMT). Trimethyltin is an organotin that selectively destroys neurons in disparate regions of the rodent brain. Although the hippocampus and entorhinal cortex are regions of prominent damage, degenerating neurons can be found in

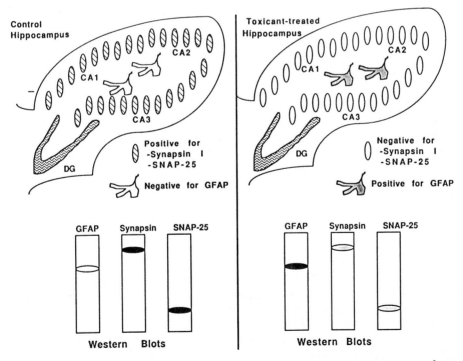

Figure 1 Schematic detection of neurotoxic damage to hippocampus using immunologic methods. In untreated rat hippocampus, CA1-3 pyramidal cells express synapsin I, a general neuronal marker, and SNAP-25, a neuronal marker enriched in the hippocampus. Glial cells are nonreactive for glial fibrillary acidic protein (GFAP). Following toxicant treatment (e.g., trimethyltin, kainic acid), CA1-3 neurons undergo degenerative changes, losing immunoreactivity to both synapsin and SNAP-25. A glial reaction occurs, resulting in greatly increased production of GFAP.

various other regions of the brain (Balaban et al., 1988). There are no readily discernable common features between TMT-sensitive neurons, and pharmacological and metabolic mechanisms have not accounted for the selective toxicity of TMT. Thus, we hypothesized that expression of a specific protein or proteins in sensitive cells may account for the selective toxicity. Although the converse hypothesis, that most cells have proteins that protect them from TMT toxicity, can be entertained, we thought that selective toxicity is more likely to be an "active" process.

Using this hypothesis as a guide, we set out to isolate specific cDNAs from TMT-sensitive cells by employing the subtractive hybridization protocol shown in Fig. 2.

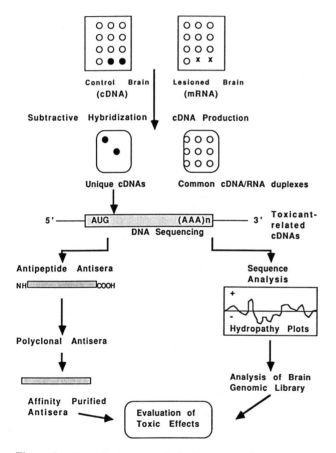

Figure 2   Use of subtractive hybridization techniques in neurotoxicology. The assumption is that gene products in subsets of brain neurons (filled dots) sensitize neurons to effects of toxicants and are lost following toxicant treatment. By subtracting toxicant-treated mRNA from control brain cDNAs, single-stranded cDNAs representing genes unique to the control state can be isolated. Unique cDNAs can be removed from common cDNA/mRNA heteroduplexes with several techniques (hydroxyapatite, avidin-biotin capture, etc.) and cloned into appropriate vectors for screening and, ultimately, analysis of DNA sequence. The peptide sequence predicted from DNA sequences can then be used to develop antipeptide antisera, which can verify effects of the toxicant in tissue. DNA sequence analysis can also be used to predict secondary structure and find homologies. Both cDNA and antibody probes can be used to evaluate toxicant effects and to help determine whether a given cDNA is a biomarker or related to toxicant mechanisms.

Subtractive hybridization allows selective enrichment for population- or treatment-specific gene products. In addition, the resulting cDNAs can be cloned into bacterial or phage vectors, used to derive DNA sequence information, and the resulting sequence can be used to predict protein structure. The predicted peptide structure can then be used to guide the production of antibodies, and the cDNA, if full-length, can be expressed as a fusion protein in either bacterial or eukaryotic systems.

This procedure can result in the isolation of a gene product that could be either a biomarker of TMT damage or a key target for the toxicant. In order to discriminate between such possibilities, an expression vector containing a selectable marker (e.g., neomycin resistance gene) can be introduced into heterologous mammalian cell lines that are insensitive to the toxicant. If the cDNA codes for a mechanistically linked protein, the insensitive heterologous cell line should show increased sensitivity to TMT upon in vitro transfection and expression. If the cDNA is a biomarker, transfected heterologous cells should not show enhanced sensitivity to the toxicant.

Using subtractive hybridization, we isolated a cDNA that is expressed primarily in TMT-sensitive cells (Krady et al., 1990). Screening of the subtracted cDNAs consisted of using Northern blot analysis of mRNA from TMT-treated and control rat brain, coupled with in situ hybridization. A positive cDNA consisted of one that labeled TMT-sensitive cells in control rat brains following in situ hybridization and that showed a near-complete absence on Northern blots from TMT-treated rat brain. The subtracted cDNA was cloned into a bacterial vector and used to screen rat brain cDNA libraries for isloation of a full-length cDNA. The full-length cDNAs as determined using size estimates from Northern blots (~3.0 Kb) were sequenced, and an open reading frame was determined (Toggas et al., 1992). The putative protein encoded by this cDNA, termed "stannin," was found to have no recognizable homologies with other known proteins. Amino acid sequence information was used to develop antipeptide antisera against the putative protein. The affinity-purified antisera recognized a peptide of approximately 10 kDa on immunoblots. Immunoreactivity was seen in TMT-sensitive cells such as hippocampal pyramidal cells and entorhinal cortical neurons. Stannin immunoreactivity in the hippocampus declined following TMT treatments (Toggas et al., 1993). Current studies are focused on development of expression vectors for use in TMT-insensitive mammalian cell lines to help determine whether stannin is a biomarker or mechanistically responsible for TMT toxicity.

This strategy illustrates how molecular technologies can be employed to solve specific questions in neurotoxicity. It may be that cell lines can be created that express high levels of stannin, allowing for the development of model systems for use in determination of organotin toxicity. In addition, it is now possible to broaden the question to ask whether expression of stannin predisposes cells to damage by other heavy metals or ischemic insult. The power of this approach is that molecular probes in the form of cDNAs, fusion proteins, and antisera can be readily developed that greatly aid in performing mechanistic experiments.

However, the use of such sophisticated and labor-intensive technologies must be considered on a case-by-case basis at present. When the mechanisms of neurotoxicity involve differential gene expression, as in the case of glial versus neuronal toxicity, neurotransmitter system–specific damage, and related cases, molecular biologic approaches may afford insight that would be difficult to obtain using traditional biochemical technologies. In the case of the neurotoxicants 6-hydroxydopamine and MPTP, subtractive hybridization would be expected to isolate cDNAs that code for tyrosine hydroxylase, which is a widely accepted biomarker for catecholamine neurons, and cDNAs for catecholamine uptake pumps, which are directly related to the mechanisms of these toxicants.

When the toxicant in question causes immediate interruption of neurochemical systems, as in the case of cholinesterase inhibitors, convulsants such as strychnine, and neurotoxic amphetamine derivatives, more conventional biochemical approaches will continue to prove useful. At the present time, the more reductionistic molecular neurobiologic approaches should be integrated closely with toxicants whose behavioral, cell-biological, and neurochemical profiles are somewhat known.

POTENTIAL USES OF MOLECULAR BIOLOGY IN NEUROTOXICOLOGY

We have focused on two approaches in which molecular approaches can influence neurotoxicology—the development of newer biomarkers of toxicity and, in selected cases, determination of neurotoxicant mechanisms. In the future, however, more sophisticated measures of changes in neuron-specific gene expression will be possible, opening the door for early detection of subtle toxicant effects. In addition, the use of transgenic mice and embryonic stem cell technologies for producing gene "knockouts" in mice is likely to affect neurotoxicology (Palmiter and Brinster, 1986; Capecchi, 1989). Finally, it is now possible to construct hybrid cell lines that express specific neuronal markers, and to use such cell lines to develop in vitro neurotoxicology screens.

The use of polymerase chain reaction (PCR) techniques has rapidly become the approach of choice for rapid and highly sensitive detection of events at the level of single-copy nucleic acids. For measurement of mRNA, a cDNA pool can be constructed and used for initial amplifications (Gilliland et al., 1990). Several recent improvements in this technology have allowed quantitative PCR to be useful in rapid measurement of induced changes in specific genes. By using carefully selected DNA primers, amplification of specific gene products can be developed into quantitative reliable assays. Because only minute samples are required for PCR, subtle, regionally specific changes in a battery of biomarkers could be easily determined in tissue sections. By coupling micropunch dissection techniques, regional variation in gene expression could be determined. In addition, a single tissue sample could be amplified with a battery of primers specific for neuronal, region-specific, and glial genes. Thus, PCR offers the opportunity to increase the sensitivity and selectivity of detection of neurotoxicant-induced changes in specific markers.

In other areas of toxicology, whether a given chemical can increase the incidence of mutagenesis is determined by following induction of alterations in a transgenic mouse expressing high levels of the *H-ras* oncogene. The equivalent system has not been developed for neurotoxicology, but it is possible to envision the creation of strains that would be useful for predicting the onset of a neurotoxic insult. In one instance, it would be possible to couple the GFAP promoter/enhancer region to a colorimetric enzyme such as β-galactosidase. If the transgene was expressed in glial cells, an astrogliotic response resulting from toxicant exposure would result in expression of increasing levels of β-galactosidase. This expression would show up as increasingly blue glial cells surrounding the site of the putative lesion. By using other reporter genes, it would be possible to quantitate gene expression with in vitro techniques. Similarly, it is possible to use this strategy to couple promoter-driven expression of a neuronal marker of damage such as heat shock proteins to other colorimetric reporter genes. Neurons slated for damage would show enhanced expression of the reporter gene. It is possible to create strains that express both a neuronal and a glial transgene, coupled to separate reporter genes. The advantage of these systems is that sensitive histochemistry can be used to demonstrate the cellular site of action and to localize the response to a given brain region.

An alternative strategy is to direct expression of a toxicant-related gene in heterologous tissues using transgenic techniques. For instance, if a specific neuronal gene was directly responsible for neurotoxicity of a given agent, would expression of this gene in kidney cells sensitize them to the toxicant? A compatible approach would be to express a transgene containing an inducible antisense cDNA against the sensitizing protein in toxicant-sensitive neurons. This type of construct would be predicted to suppress toxicity to the specific entity upon induction of the antisense cDNA, since the antisense cDNA would prevent expression of the sensitizing protein.

The third and more far-reaching strategy is to use recent advances in embryonic stem cell technology to produce so-called "gene knockout" murine strains. In this technique, embryonic stem cells are manipulated in vitro so that, via the process of homologous recombination, specific, targeted genes are suppressed. When the modified stem cells are reinjected into the blastocyst, chimeras are created that lack the targeted gene in specific cell populations. Via successive breeding, strains containing specific deletions of neuronal enzymes have been created. Most recently, a murine strain lacking neuronal calmodulin-dependent protein kinase II was created (Silva et al., 1992; Silva et al., 1992). These mice were used to demonstrate that lack of expression of this enzyme in the hippocampus led to learning defects in spatial memory. It is possible to envision how selected strains could be developed that are deficient in the dopamine reuptake protein pump. Such mice should be resistant to the effects of MPTP, in that the molecule is not likely to concentrate in dopamine neurons. In addition, such mice are likely to show other behavioral and phenotypic changes that are related to the altered genotype. Similar models could be created with respect to other neuronal molecules that may participate in neurotoxic responses. Likely candidate genes include deletions of specific excitotoxic receptor subtypes and enzymes that may actively metabolize compounds to reactive species in situ.

Creation of sensitive cell lines for use in neurotoxicology remains a short-term objective (Veronesi, 1992). To date, neuroblastoma- and glia-derived cells have not been consistently useful for prediction of specific neurotoxic insults seen only in whole animals. However, it is possible to envision that engineered cell lines can be created that express neuronal or glial phenotypes and respond to toxicants with more than a necrotic response. By using selective transfections, it may be possible to create cells that are sensitive only to specific neuronal perturbations, such as a hippocampal-derived cell that responds only to one type of excitotoxicant. Furthermore, it is likely that immortalized human and rodent neural lines will continue to be developed, with a goal of having an immortalized line that is not transformed by oncogenic agents and retains the phenotypic characteristics of a neuron.

SUMMARY

We have attempted to outline, using specific examples, how molecular approaches can be used to address issues in neurotoxicology. In the first instance, the search for adequate biomarkers of neuronal damage will continue, and will be aided considerably by techniques of molecular biology (Verity, 1992). However, it is unlikely that a single, perfect marker will be found; use of a battery of such markers is likely. Initially, such biomarkers are likely to be assayed through immunologic approaches, with lesser use of mRNA-directed approaches such as Northern blots and in situ hybridization. However, as techniques of PCR are refined, it is likely that mRNA levels, as determined by PCR amplification of the cognate cDNAs, will become more rapid and sensitive measures of a range of gene products that respond to toxic insults. Finally, the creation of new murine models incorporating both transgenic information and gene knockouts is likely to affect neurotoxicology in the near future.

As with any developing technology, particularly when a reductionist strategy is imposed on a more integrative discipline, initial enthusiasm for the techniques is often followed by disgruntlement. Since methods for neurotoxicological evaluation continue to evolve, it is likely that molecular biological techniques will find a place in the laboratory of the neurotoxicologist. However, the future is best envisioned as one in which behavioral, neurochemical, histological, and molecular techniques are used to complement one another in order to better understand mechanisms of neurotoxicant action.

ACKNOWLEDGMENTS

The authors wish to thank Ms. Christine Patanow for expert technical assistance. This work was supported by Public Health Service grant RO1-ES05450 and Environmental Protection Agency grant R818002-01-0 to M.L.B.

REFERENCES

Balaban CD, Billingsley ML, Kincaid RL. Evidence for trans-synaptic regulation of calmodulin-dependent cyclic nucleotide phosphodiesterase in cerebellar Purkinje cells. J Neurosci 9:2374–81.

Balaban CD, O'Callaghan JP, Billingsley ML (1988). Trimethyltin-induced neuronal damage in the rat: comparative studies using silver degeneration stains, immunocytochemistry and immunoassay for neuronotypic and gliotypic proteins. Neuroscience 26:337–61.

Brock TO, O'Callaghan JP (1988). Quantitative changes in the synaptic vesicle proteins synapsin I and p38 and the astrocyte-specific protein glial fibrillary acidic protein are associated with chemical-induced injury to the rat central nervous system. J Neurosci 7:931–42.

Capecchi MR (1989). Altering the genome by homologous recombination. Science 244:1288–92.

Choi DW (1990a). The role of glutamate neurotoxicity in hypoxic-ischemic neuronal death. Annu Rev Neurosci 13:171–82.

Choi DW (1990b). Cerebral hypoxia: some new approaches and unanswered questions. J Neurosci 10:2493–2501.

Crino PB, Vogt BA, Chen J-C, Volicer L (1989). Neurotoxic effects of partially oxidized serotonin: tryptamine-4,5-dione. Brain Res 504:247–57.

DeCamilli P, Benfenati F, Valtorta F, Greengard P (1990). The synapsins. Annu Rev Cell Biol 6:433–60.

Gilliland G, Perrin S, Bunn HF (1990). Competitive PCR for quantitation of mRNA. In: Innis MA, Gelfand DH, Sninsky JJ, White TJ, eds. PCR protocols: a guide to methods and applications. San Diego: Raven Press, 60–70.

Goedert M, Crowther RA, Garner CC (1991). Molecular characterization of microtubule-associated proteins tau and MAP-2. Trends Neurosci 14:193–9.

Gonzalez MF, Shiraishi K, Hisanaga K, Sagar SM, Mandabach M, Sharp FR (1989). Heat shock proteins as markers of neural injury. Mol Brain Res 6:93–100.

Guilian D, Woodward J, Krebs JF, Lachman LB (1988). Intracerebral injection of interleukin-1 stimulates astrogliosis and neovascularization. J Neurosci 8:2485–90.

Jahn R, Schiebler W, Ouimet C, Greengard P (1985). A 38,000-dalton membrane protein (p38) present in synaptic vesicles. Proc Natl Acad Sci USA 82:4137–41.

Kimmelberg HK (1983). Primary astrocyte cultures—a key to astrocyte function. Cell Mol Neurobiol 3:1–16.

Krady JK, Oyler GA, Balaban CD, Billingsley ML (1990). Use of avidin-biotin subtractive hybridization to characterize mRNA common to neurons destroyed by the selective neurotoxicant trimethyltin. Mol Brain Res 7:287–97.

Lee G, Cowan N, Kirschner M (1988). The primary structure and heterogeneity of tau protein from mouse brain. Science 239:285–8.

Lefkowtiz RJ, Caron MG (1988). Adrenergic receptors. J Biol Chem 263:4993–6.

Li Y, Chopp M, Garcia JH, Yoshida Y, Zhang ZG, Levine SR (1992). Distribution of the 72-kd heat-shock protein as a function of transient focal cerebral ischemia in rats. Stroke 23:1292–8.

Martin DB, Schmidt RE, DiStefano PS, Lowry OH, Carter JG, Johnson EM (1988). Inhibitors of protein synthesis and RNA synthesis prevent neuronal death caused by nerve growth factor deprivation. J Cell Biol 106:829–44.

Morgan JI, Curran T (1989). Stimulus-transcription coupling in neurons: role of cellular immediate-early genes. Trends Neurosci 12:459–62.

Murphy TH, Worley PF, Nakabeppu Y, Christy B, Gastel J, Baraban JM (1991). Synaptic regulation of immediate early gene expression in primary cultures of cortical neurons. J Neurochem 57:1862–72.

Nichols NR, Osterberg HH, Masters JN, Millar SL, Finch CE (1990). Messenger RNA for glial fibrillary acidic protein is decreased in rat brain following acute and chronic corticosterone treatment. Mol Brain Res 7:1–7.

O'Callaghan JP (1988). Neurotypic and gliotypic proteins as biochemical markers of neurotoxicity. Neurotoxicol Teratol 10:445–52.

O'Callaghan JP (1991). Quantification of glial fibrillary acidic protein: comparison of slot-immunobinding assays with a novel sandwich ELISA. Neurotoxical Teratol 13:102–6.

O'Callaghan JP (1992). Assessment of neurotoxicity using assays of neuron- and glia-localized proteins: chronology and critique. In: Tilson HA, Mitchell C, eds. Neurotoxicology. New York: Raven Press, 83–100.

O'Callaghan JP, Brinton RE, McEwen BS (1990). Glucocorticoids regulate the concentration of glial fibrillary acidic protein throughout the brain. Brain Res 512:312–21.

Oyler GA, Higgins GA, Hart RA, Battenberg E, Bloom FE, Billingsley ML, Wilson MC (1990). The identification of a novel synaptosomal associated protein, SNAP-25, differentially expressed by neuronal subpopulations. J Cell Biol 109:3039–52.

Oyler GA, Polli JW, Wilson MC, Billingsley ML (1991). Developmental expression of the synaptosomal associated protein (SNAP-25) in rat brain. Proc Natl Acad Sci USA 88:5247–51.

Palmiter RD, Brinster RL (1986). Germ-line transformation of mice. Annu Rev Genet 20:465–99.

Rataboul P, Faucon Biguet N, Vernier P, De Vitry F, Boulgrand S, Privat A, Mallet J (1988). Identification of a human glial fibrillary acidic protein cDNA: a tool for the molecular analysis of reactive gliosis in the mammalian central nervous system. J Neurosci Res 20:165–75.

Reuhl K, Lowndes HE (1992). Factors influencing morphological expression of neurotoxicity. In: Tilson HA, Mitchell CL, eds. Neurotoxicology. New York: Raven Press, 67–82.

Reves SA, Helman LJ, Allison A, Israel MA (1989). Molecular cloning and primary structure of human glial fibrillary acidic protein. Proc Natl Acad Sci USA 86:5178–82.

Riederer BM, Zagon IS, Goodman SR (1986). Brain spectrin (240/235) and brain spectrin (240/235E): two distinct spectrin subtypes with different location within mammalian neural cells. J Cell Biol 102:2088–97.

Sakurai-Yamashita Y, Sassone-Corsi P, Gombos G (1991). Immunohistochemistry of *c-fos* in mouse brain during postnatal development: basal levels and changing response to metrazol and kainate injection. Eur J Neurosci 3:764–70.

Silva AL, Stevens CF, Tonegawa S, Wang Y (1992). Deficient hippocampal long-term potentiation in α-calcium-calmodulin kinase II mutant mice. Science 257:201–6.

Silva AL, Paylor R, Wehner JM, Tonegawa S (1992). Impaired spatial learning in calcium calmodulin kinase II mutant mice. Science 257:206–11.

Sonnenberg JL, Mitchelmore C, McGregor-Leon PF, Hempstead J, Morgan JI, Curran T (1989). Glutamate receptor agonists increase the expression of Fos Fra and AP-1 DNA binding activity in the mammalian brain. J Neurosci Res 24:72–80.

Spina MB, Squinto SP, Miller J, Lindsay RM, Hyman C (1992). Brain-derived neurotrophic factor protects dopamine neurons against 6-hydroxydopamine and N-methyl-4-phenylpyridinium ion toxicity: involvement of the glutathione system. J Neurochem 59:99–106.

Sutcliffe JG (1988). mRNA in the mammalian central nervous system. Annu Rev Neurosci 11:157–98.

Sutcliffe JG, Milner RJ, Shinnick TM, Bloom FE (1983). Identifying the protein products of brain-specific genes using antibodies to chemically synthesized peptides. Cell 33:671–82.

Toggas SM, Krady JK, Billingsley ML (1992). Molecular neurotoxicology of trimethyltin: identification of stannin, a novel protein expressed in trimethyltin-sensitive cells. Mol Pharmacol 42:44–56.

Toggas SM, Krady JK, Thompson TA, Billingsley ML (1993). Molecular mechanisms of selective neurotoxicants: studies on organotin compounds. Ann NY Acad Sci 679:157–77.

Verity MA (1992). Determination of neurotoxicity using molecular biological approaches. In: Tilson HA, Mitchell C, eds. Neurotoxicology. New York: Raven Press, 1–20.

Veronesi B (1992). The use of cell culture for evaluating neurotoxicity. In: Tilson HA, Mitchell C, eds. Neurotoxicology. New York: Raven Press, 21–49.

Ziai MR, Sangameswaran L, Hempstead JL, Danho W, Morgan JI (1988). An immunochemical analysis of the distribution of a brain-specific polypeptide PEP-19. J Neurochem 51:1771–6.

Zigmond MJ, Stricker EM (1989). Animal models of parkinsonism using selective neurotoxins: clinical and basic implications. Int Rev Neurobiol 31:1–79.

20
Induction of Oxidative Stress in the Brain by Neurotoxic Agents

Stephen C. Bondy
University of California
Irvine, California

INTRODUCTION

The terms "free radicals" and "oxygen radicals" have become commonly used in the past decade as a result of overwhelming data suggesting that oxygen radicals are involved in a variety of disease processes. The works of Freeman and Crapo (1982) and Halliwell and Gutteridge (1985, 1989) especially have addressed the ubiquitous role of free radicals in the biology of disease and tissue injury. Most of the issues considered to date have dealt with the role of free radicals in the mechanisms of carcinogenesis, ischemia, and aging. In the field of toxicology, free radical research has primarily focused on the area of pulmonary and cardiac toxicity and hepatotoxicity.

The liver and the lung have long been known to be vulnerable to oxidative stress. The brain, with its high lipid content, high rate of oxidative metabolism, and somewhat low levels of free radical–eliminating enzymes, also may be a prime target of free radical–mediated damage. The localization of antioxidant systems primarily to glia rather than neurons (Savolainen, 1978; Raps et al., 1989), while providing a first line of defense, may render the neurons especially susceptible to toxicants successfully traversing this barrier.

It has been known for several decades that the mammalian brain contains large amounts of substrates that are susceptible to free radical attack, such as unsaturated lipids and catecholamines. However, Halliwell and Gutteridge (1985) were the first to discuss the potential role of oxygen radicals in the nervous system. The involvement of these reactive species in hyperoxia, ischemia, trauma, stroke, and transition metal–dependent reactions in the brain has since been a topic of considerable interest (Braughler and Hall, 1989; Floyd, 1990).

Several diverse neurotoxic events may lead to excess formation of free radicals. The idea that a variety of drug and chemical pathogeneses are associated with free radical mechanisms has been previously proposed (Kehrer et al., 1988). This may significantly contribute to the properties of many neurotoxic agents. Any imbalance of cellular redox status in favor of greater oxidative activity can lead to several kinds of macromolecular damage, such as disruption of genomic function by alterations to DNA or impairment of membrane properties by attack on protiens or lipids. Lipid-peroxidative events are especially hazardous, since lipoperoxy radicals can initiate oxidative chain reactions (Freeman and Crapo, 1982). Thus, the high lipid content of myelin makes nervous tissue especially susceptible to oxidative stress.

Neurotoxic compounds have characteristic and individual properties and often cause distinctive morphological and biochemical lesions. However, some relatively nonspecific features also constitute part of the overall toxicity of a given agent. Recent attempts to unify the diffuse discipline of neurotoxicology have led to the concept of "final common pathways" that characterize frequently occurring cellular responses to disruption of homeostasis resulting from exposure to xenobiotic agents. The present work considers the possibility that oxygen radicals may be mediators of a "final common pathway" in several mechanisms of neurotoxicity.

Free radicals are defined as species with one or more unpaired electrons. Since oxygen is ubiquitous in aerobic organisms, oxygen-centered free radicals have been implicated in several physiological, toxicological, and pathological phenomena. However, while superoxide anion and hydroxyl radical qualify as oxygen-centered radicals, hydrogen peroxide is a potent cellular toxicant that lacks unpaired electrons. The terms "reactive oxygen species" (ROS) and "oxygen radicals" have been used to describe all oxygen-centered radicals and nonradicals.

The precise nature of oxygen radicals produced in the central nervous system (CNS) is by no means clear. The difficulty of establishing this with certainty is due to the short half-life and rapid interconvertibility of many of the putative key species (LeBel et al., 1992a). Relatively stable species such as superoxide and hydrogen peroxide give rise to less clearly defined, highly active, transient species that are the primary oxidants. Evaluation of the free radical–forming potential of neurotoxic agents, and determination of whether oxygen radicals are common mediators of neurotoxicity, should not be delayed until the identity of critical oxygen radicals is unequivocally clarified.

ENDOGENOUS CAUSES OF GENERATION OF REACTIVE OXYGEN SPECIES

Oxidative phosphorylation

About 2% of the oxygen consumed by mitochondria is incompletely reduced and appears as oxygen radicals (Boveris and Chance, 1973). This proportion may be increased when the efficient functioning of mitochondrial electron transport systems is compromised. This could account for the increased lipid peroxidation found in the brains of mice exposed to nonlethal levels of cyanide (Johnson et al., 1987).

Cytosolic Acidity

Lowered pH resulting from excess glycolytic activity not only may accelerate the process of liberating protein-bound iron in organisms but may also lead to an impairment of oxidative adenosine triphosphate (ATP) generation and to the appearance of the pro-oxidant protonated superoxide (Siesjo, 1988). However, there is evidence that the reduction of pH during ATP depletion maybe protective and enhance cell survival (Kehrer et al., 1990).

Chlordecone, a neurotoxic insecticide, elevates pH within synaptosomes and depresses oxygen radical synthesis (Bondy and McKee, 1990).

Multivalent Presence of Metal Ions with Potential

Liberation of protein-bound iron can occur by enhanced degradation of important iron-binding proteins such as ferritin and transferrin. A small increase in levels of free iron within cells can dramatically accelerate rates of oxygen radical production (Minotti and Aust, 1989). A key feature in establishing the rate of production of oxygen radicals by tissue is the cytosolic concentration of free metal ions possessing the capacity to readily change their valence state. Iron is considered the most important of these, but levels of free manganese and copper may also be significant factors (Aust et al., 1985).

Eicosanoid Production

Enhanced phopholipase activity can lead to the release of arachidonic acid. This polyunsaturated fatty acid contains four ethylenic bonds and is readily auto-oxidizable. In fact, impure preparations of this chemical may explode spontaneously on exposure to air (Halliwell and Gutteridge, 1989). The enzymic conversion of this compound to many bioactive prostaglandins, leukotrienes, and thromboxanes by cyclo-oxygenases and lipoxygenases leads to considerable oxygen radical generation (Freeman and Crapo, 1982; Saunders and Horrocks, 1987). All major catabolic pathways of arachidonic acid involve the utilization of molecular oxygen and the formation of hydroperoxide or epoxide intermediates (Fig. 1). Subsequent metabolism by peroxidases and hydrolases can lead to further formation of free radicals. The physiological relevance of this is illustrated by the finding that antioxidants can protect against arachidonic acid–induced cerebral edema (Asamo et al., 1989).

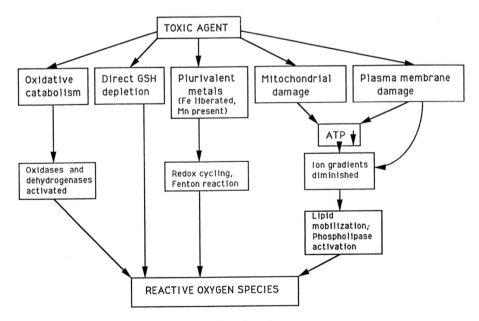

Figure 1   Pathways of neurotoxicant-induced oxidative stress.

Increased levels of cytosolic free calcium may result from either breakdown of the steep concentration gradient of calcium across the plasma membrane or liberation of the large amounts of calcium bound intracellularly within mitochondria or endoplasmic reticulum. This elevation can activate phospholipases and thus stimulate oxygen radical production. In fact, the activation of phospholipase D has been functionally linked to superoxide anion production (Bonser et al., 1989). A reciprocal relation exists, since free radicals can enhance phospholipase A_2 activity within cerebral capillaries (Au et al., 1985). Conversely, phospholipase A_2 may selectively induce oxidative changes to the γ-amino-butyric acid (GABA)-regulated chloride channel and thus increase cell excitability (Schwartz et al., 1988). Such bidirectional mechanisms have the potential to reach a critical level and set in motion an ever-increasing entropic cascade.

Evidence is accumulating for a messenger role for reactive oxygen species within cells. Endothelium-derived relaxing factor has been identified as nitric oxide, a free radical (Bruckdorfer et al., 1990).

Oxidases

Chemical induction of cytochrome P-450–containing mixed-function mono-oxidases can increase the rate of phase I detoxification reactions. The oxidative metabolism of many lipophilic compounds, while necessary for their conjugation and excretion, often involves the transient formation of highly reactive oxidative intermediates such as epoxides (Sevanian et al., 1990). While mixed-function oxidases predominate in the liver, they are also present in the nervous system, largely within neurons (Hansson et al. 1990). At the intracellular level, most of these cerebral oxidases are mitochondrial rather than microsomal, and like the corresponding hepatic enzymes they are inducible (Perrin et al., 1990). Products of such enzymes may include epoxides in which the C-O-C ring strain often results in a potent oxidizing chemical. Xanthine oxidase is a prime generator of superoxide and may be a significant exacerbating factor in several pathological states.

Phagocytosis

Extracellular formation of superoxide anion by phagocytes has long been recognized as a bactericidal mechanism. Similar oxidative activity has been observed in cerebral microglia (Halliwell and Gutteridge, 1989). Astroglial activation is a common event following neural trauma, and reactive astrocytes are active in clearance of cell debris and, ultimately, in the formation of glial scar tissue. Although the phenomenon of reactive oxygen species generation has not been documented in the injured brain during neuronophagia, the ROS-enhancing potential of such events is worthy of further study.

REGULATION OF LEVELS OF REACTIVE OXYGEN SPECIES

Protection against excess levels of oxygen reactive species is effected by a wide range of intracellular mechanisms. Only when such defensive processes are overwhelmed does oxidative damage ensue.

Enzymes

Enzymes such as superoxide dismutase and catalase and peroxidase are able to destroy the superoxide radical and hydrogen peroxide, respectively. While these oxidant species are not in themselves very active, they are able to interact in the presence of trace amounts of iron and, by the Haber-Weiss reaction, give rise to the highly reactive, short-lived hydroxyl radical. Levels of protective enzymes are somewhat low in the brain (Savolainen, 1978), and much of the brain's antioxidant capacity lies within cerebral capillaries and glial cells (Tayarani et al., 1987). Since the cerebral microvasculature is also a major site of lipid peroxidative activity (Hall and Braughler, 1989) and mixed-function oxidase activity (Ghersi-Egea, 1988), this may prevent diffusion of pro-oxidants into neurons. Treatment of neurons with nerve growth factor is able to confer resistance to oxidative damage, apparently by induction of antioxidant enzymes (Jackson et al., 1990).

Metal Chelation

Iron- and copper-sequestering proteins such as ferritin, transferrin, and ceruloplasmin are important means of ensuring extremely low levels of free cytosolic metals with a potential for valence changes. Such metals are crucial cofactors in ROS generation. Lower antioxidant activity in Parkinson's disease has been related to decreased levels of ferritin in the brain (Dexter et al., 1990). Metallothionein is induced by, and can sequester, several metals with a high affinity for–SH groups, such as mercury and cadmium. This protein also acts as an antioxidant because of its high sulfhydryl content and its ability to dismutate superoxide anion.

Soluble Factors

The presence of diffusible antioxidant vitamins and provitamins provides protection against oxygen radicals. Such molecules may be predominantly lipophilic (β-carotene, α-tocopherol, retinoic acid) or water-soluble (ascorbic acid). A major source of reducing power is glutathione, which normally exists at high concentrations intracellularly (1–5 mM) (Halliwell and Gutteridge, 1985). Glutathione is maintained largely in the reduced form by glutathione reductase, acting in conjunction with NADPH. Inhibition of NADPH-generating processes may compromise intracellular levels of glutathione and thus reducing power. However, NADPH is also an essential component of many oxidases, including the mixed-function oxidases.

Glutathione reserves can be depleted by oxidative stress (Maellaro et al., 1990), and such depletion in the brain can cause neurological deficits (Calvin et al., 1986). The brain stem has a rather low glutathione content and a high mixed-function oxidase content relative to other brain regions. It has been proposed that this combination may render the region especially vulnerable to oxidative damage, and that this is relevant to nigral damage in Parkinson's disease (Perry et al., 1982; Ravindranath et al., 1989).

Some serum proteins, notably albumin, can act as free radical scavengers (Halliwell, 1988). However, the low protein content of cerebrospinal fluid makes both albumin and ferritin largely unavailable to the CNS (Halliwell, 1989).

NEUROTOXICANT-INDUCED GENERATION OF REACTIVE OXYGEN SPECIES WITHIN THE BRAIN

While several neurotoxic chemicals can stimulate ROS production within the nervous system, this does not imply that such stimulation represents their primary mechanism of toxic action. Pro-oxidant properties of a chemical may 1.) be the main source of its neurotoxicity, 2.) contribute to its overall harmfulness, or 3.) be an epiphenomenon, only secondarily relating to tissue damage.

The events subserving xenobiotic stimulation of ROS frequently involve an excess activation of one or more of the endogenous ROS-producing processes, or inhibition of the protective systems described above.

Metals

Metals can catalyze formation of excess ROS by several independent mechanisms that, although initiated by a single metal, may act in concert.

The ability of a metal ion to exist in several valence states, and thus to transfer single electrons, is found in many metals, including iron, manganese, and mercury. The neurotoxicity of manganese is thought to be specifically due to its capacity to catalyze the auto-oxidation of catecholamines (Donaldson et al., 1981).

Methylmercury is able to increase cerebellar rates of ROS generation (LeBel et al., 1990). This may reflect both the valence ambiguity of mercury and the deleterious effect of this heavy metal on anabolic processes such as oxidative phosphorylation and protein synthesis (Verity et al., 1975). The latter events may be related to the powerful affinity of mercury for the sulfhydryl groups of proteins and of glutathione. The capacity of methylmercury to elevate cytosolic calcium (Komulainen and Bondy, 1987) may also be relevant to its oxidant properties. Vitamin E is protective against methylmercury- and cadmium-induced neurotoxicity (Chang et al., 1978; Shukla et al., 1988), and deferoxamine pretreatment can also block methylmercury-induced elevation of ROS within the brain (LeBel et al., 1992b).

Thallium owes some of its neurotoxicity to the fact that it can partially substitute for potassium and may interfere with critical functions of potassium. However, the ability of this element to exist in both mono- and trivalent states, and its affinity for glutathione, may account for its enhancement of lipid peroxidation in the corpus striatum (Hasan and Ali, 1981).

Both organic and inorganic lead have been shown to enhance rates of lipid peroxidation or ROS formation (Ramstoek et al., 1980; Rehman, 1984; Ali and Bondy, 1989; LeBel et al., 1990). Lead neither has a major affinity for sulfhydryl groups nor readily undergoes valence flux under physiological conditions. However, calcium flux is deranged in cases of severe lead poisoning (Tonge et al., 1977), and this may form the basis of the oxidant properties of lead. Vitamin E can protect against some of the neural damage induced by triethyllead (Ramstoek et al., 1980).

The induction of hyperactivity by a toxic chemical may be sufficient to lead to enhanced ROS production, probably by way of increasing cytosolic levels of free calcium. This may account for the excess oxidant activity described in the brains of animals treated with organometals such as trimethyltin and triethyllead (Ali and Bondy, 1989, LeBel et al., 1990). In these studies, as with the methylmercury results, the regional distribution of the excess oxidative activity paralleled the sites of known neuropathological changes. This implies that induced oxidative events are likely to be a significant component of the neurotoxicity of these metals rather than an irrelevant epiphenomenon.

Organic Solvents

The ability of various organic solvents to effect excess ROS synthesis has been described for several tissues (Ahmad et al., 1987; Cojocel et al., 1989), but the brain has received little attention in this context. However, the neurotoxicity of two solvents of environmental significance, ethanol and toluene, has been reported, and will be discussed here. A large range of enzymes and other factors may account for an association between solvent exposure and excess oxidative events. Evidence for, and potential mechanisms of solvent-induced ROS production, are listed below.

Glutathione Levels

Reductions and also increases in glutathione levels have been found in the brain following ethanol or toluene dosing (Guerri and Grisolia, 1980; Nordmann, 1987; Natsuki, 1991; Uysal et al., 1989; Mattia et al., 1992). Since compensatory processes can be rapid after induction of excessive ROS, both reductions and increases in cerebral glutathione may be regarded as indices of oxidative stress (Adams et al., 1989).

Lipid Peroxidation

Elevations in lipid peroxidation following ethanol or toluene treatment are found in the brain (Uysal et al., 1989; Mattia et al., 1992). The attenuation of some of these ethanol-induced changes by the lipid-soluble antioxidant vitamins A and E, and the depletion of antioxidant vitamins in the CNS of ethanol-treated rats (Nordmann, 1987; Nadiger et al., 1988), confirm the presence of induced oxidative stress.

Free Iron

Free ionic or incompletely sequestered iron may be essential for the appearance of ethanol-induced ROS. Ethanol may effect the liberation of low-molecular-weight iron in the brain from bound intracellular reserves (Nordmann et al., 1987; Rouach et al., 1990). The superoxide anion can release iron from ferritin (Nordmann et al., 1987), and this may underlie such observations. That the presence of small amounts of low-molecular-weight iron may lead to the formation of ROS is illustrated by the protective effects of iron chelators such as deferoxamine on ethanol-related changes in cerebral oxidative events (Shaw, 1989; Nordmann et al., 1992). It has even been suggested that iron-sequestering chemicals can reduce physical dependence on ethanol (Nordmann et al., 1988).

Lipid Mobilization

Solvent-stimulated lipid mobilization is another phenomenon to be considered as a source of ROS. Ethanol has been shown to activate phospholipases A_1 and A_2 in an isolated cardiac preparation (Choy et al., 1989). This possibility has not yet been reported for corresponding cerebral tissue but is certainly likely. The effect is blocked in the presence of α-tocopherol. Phospholipase activity is also significantly stimulated in synaptosomes isolated from rats exposed to toluene (LeBel and Schatz, 1990). The liberation of arachidonic acid by phospholipase A_2 sets in motion a range of oxidative catabolic processes: the "arachidonic acid cascade." This polyunsaturated fatty acid contains four ethylenic bonds and is readily oxidizable. The enzymatic conversion of this compound to prostaglandins, leukotrienes, and thromboxanes by cyclo-oxygenases and lipoxygenases leads to considerable ROS generation (Saunders and Horrocks, 1987). Toluene alters synaptosomal phospholipid methyltransferase activity, an event that has also been shown to be affected by oxygen radicals (Kaneko et al., 1990).

Acetaldehyde Generation

It has been postulated that acetaldehyde generated during the metabolism of ethanol can initiate oxidative stress by reaction with, and depletion of, protective thiols such as cysteine and glutathione. Microsomal mixed-function oxidases may also be a direct target of acetaldehyde. Binding of this ethanol metabolite to these enzymes, forming a stable adduct, can impair their properties (Lucas et al., 1990). Thus, the P-450 11E1 enzyme induced by ethanol is more likely to be malfunctioning (Behrens et al., 1988). The extent to which acetaldehyde found within the brain after ethanol dosing is generated intrinsically rather than systemically transported from the liver is unclear. The reactivity of acetaldehyde with many biological constituents suggests that it is likely to be synthesized close to the site where it is detected. Following ethanol treatment, however, acetaldehyde levels of brain interstitial fluid are above those present in the CNS (Westcott et al., 1980). This suggests that acetaldehyde can cross the blood-brain barrier. Cysteine and ascorbic acid are protective against the acute behavioral toxicity of acetaldehyde, supporting the significance of acetaldehyde-inducible oxidative stress to the brain (O'Neill and Rahwan, 1976). However, such agents may also have nonantioxidant ameliorative effects, by preventing the formation of adducts of acetaldehyde with protein (Wickramansinghe and Hasan, 1992).

Catabolic Processes

The catabolic steps involved in the degradation of ethanol and toluene are candidates for the origin of excess ROS. Several major classes of enzyme need to be considered in this context.

Mixed-Function Oxidases. Since oxidases utilize molecular oxygen directly, their induction has the potential for enhancing ROS production. Ethanol is known to induce a specific microsomal mixed-function oxidase. P45011E1, in the liver (Ekstrom and Ingelman-Sundberg, 1989). This enzyme is inducible by ethanol and can generate oxidizing species in the absence of substrates as long as NADPH is present (Kuthan and Ulbrich, 1982). Under such conditions, it has been reported to exhibit an unusually high rate of oxidase- and H_2O_2-generating activity (Ekstrom and Ingelman-Sundberg, 1989). More recently, a parallel induction of P4501E11 has been found in the CNS, where it is present in much lower concentration (Hansson et al., 1990). The distinct susceptibility of the cerebellum and the hippocampus to ethanol-induced morphological damage may relate to their relatively high content of cytochrome P-450 11E1 mono-oxygenase.

    The role of mixed-function oxidases in solvent-stimulated ROS generation is also indicated by the finding that the capacity of toluene to stimulate cortical ROS production can be blocked by pretreatment of rats with an inhibitor of mixed-function oxidases, namely metyrapone (Mattia et al., 1991).

    Benzene is not able to induce oxygen radical formation in a manner parallel to that of toluene, either in vitro or in vivo (Mattia et al., 1991). It may be that the lack of activity of benzene in this regard is related to the absence of an attached methyl group available for oxidation. However, it has been suggested that *trans,trans*-muconaldehyde, a minor, potentially toxic metabolite of benzene, plays a role in benzene-induced free radical events (Witz et al., 1985).

Superoxide Dismutase. Increased levels of superoxide dismutase, an inducible enzyme, are generally taken as indirect evidence of an increased oxidant milieu. Since this is a sulfhydryl enzyme, however, depression of its level in a tissue can also reflect oxidative denaturation. Following ethanol treatment, decreases in superoxide dismutase have been found in the brain (Ledig et al., 1981). Ethanol-effected increases in neuronal and glial superoxide dismutase have also been reported (Ledig et al., 1991). As with glutathione, biphasic fluxes of superoxide dismutase levels are common, and a change in either direction may relate to the presence of excess ROS.

Alcohol Dehydrogenase. The relatively nonspecific soluble enzyme alcohol dehydrogenase is considered the primary initial step in the catabolism of ethanol. There is evidence that the activity of several dehydrogenases including alcohol dehydrogenase can bring about ROS formation, even though oxygen is not directly involved (Mattia et al., 1992). The inhibition of ethanol or toluene-effected free radical production by an inhibitor of alcohol dehydrogenase, 4-methylpyrazole (Gonthier et al., 1991; Mattia et al., 1992), suggests that ROS are generated by this enzyme. However, 4-methylpyrazole is also capable of inhibition of mixed-function oxidases (Feierman and Cedarbaum, 1985), so use of this agent does not allow a clear distinction to be made between the two major routes of ethanol breakdown.

Catalase. The evidence for involvement of the soluble enzyme catalase in ethanol degradation is that pretreatment of rats with ethanol can block the inhibition of cerebral catalase normally brought about by 3-amino-1,2,4-triazole (Cohen et al., 1980). This inhibitor can also attenuate some behavioral effects of ethanol, further suggesting the relevance of this route of oxidation to the brain (Aragon et al., 1989). However, such a pathway would be more likely to absorb than to generate free radicals, since hydrogen peroxide is a cosubstrate in this oxidation. Alcohol dehydrogenase is present in the brain only in small amounts (Raskin and Sokoloff, 1970) and may play a lesser role there than in the liver; thus catalase may be on the major primary oxidant pathway of alcohol in the CNS.

Aldehyde Dehydrogenase. The mitochondrial NAD^+-dependent enzyme aldehyde dehydrogenase constitutes the major means of oxidation of acetaldehyde by the liver. It is also present in the brain (Westcott et al., 1980). Electron spin resonance studies reveal that this dehydrogenase is capable of producing hydroxyl ions (Mattia et al., 1992). Benzaldehyde is a potent agent in enhancing oxygen radical formation (Mattia et al., 1992). This suggests that benzaldehyde is an active metabolite responsible for the pro-oxident properties of toluene.

Aldehyde Oxidase and Xanthine Oxidase. Both xanthine oxidase and aldehyde oxidase are molybdenum- and flavin-containing enzymes. The presence of the latter enzyme in the brain is equivocal, but xanthine oxidase, which can also oxidize acetaldehyde, is present in all tissues. This enzyme is derived by the proteolytic modification of xanthine dehydrogenase. Ethanol treatment may also bring about this enzyme conversion (Nordmann et al., 1988), and acetaldehyde appears to be the agent directly responsible for this (Sultatos, 1988). The further oxidation of ethanol is primarily by way of aldehyde dehydrogenase. However, more extended dosing is also likely to effect conversion of xanthine dehydrogenase to the oxidase, thereby increasing the contribution of xanthine oxidase to ethanol catabolism.

Other Toxicants

Further suggestion of the ability of ethanol to enhance induced neural oxidative stress comes from results of studies combining ethanol with other toxicants. Manganese, 6-hydroxydopamine, 1-methyl-4-phenylpyridinium (MPP^+), three agents suspected to owe part of their neurotoxicity to oxidative events confined to the dopaminergic system, interact with ethanol or acetaldehyde in a synergistic manner (Zuddas et al., 1989; Ledig et al., 1991; Oldfield et al., 1991).

A final unsolved issue is the extent to which overall solvent toxicity is related to oxidative stress. The hepatic events consequent to prolonged and high levels of ethanol ingestion, such as lipid mobilization, are very likely to involve harmful pro-oxidant events. Such dramatic changes are generally not seen in nervous tissue in the absence of thiamine deficiency. However, the brain is an organ with very limited potential for cell replacement and can be vulnerable to gradual incremental deficits. Such slowly accumulating lesions, although difficult to quantitate, can be irreversible. These subtle changes may accelerate deficits resulting from normal physiological aging and enhance susceptibility to additional neurological stressors.

Several other solvents such as styrene and xylenes also stimulate CNS production of ROS (Trenga et al., 1991; Mattia and Bondy, unpublished data). The free radical–inducing property of solvents may not enhance their acute toxicity (Kefalas and Stacey, 1989) but has been proposed as effecting more subtle processes such as an acceleration of normal aging processes (Ahmad et al., 1987).

Agents Specifically Acting on Dopaminergic Neurons

Dopaminergic circuitry is especially vulnerable to neurotoxic damage, and this is at least in part due to the readiness with which dopamine is auto-oxidized in the presence of trace amounts of metals with multivalence potential. In addition, dopamine can be enzymically oxidized by monoamine oxidases to 3,4-dihydroxyphenyl acetaldehyde and H_2O_2.

A role for oxidative stress in the processes underlying 1-methyl-4-phenyl-1,2,3,6-tetrahydropyridine (MPTP) neurotoxicity has been proposed in recent years. This compound, a contaminant of an illicitly manufactured meperidine analogue, has been the subject of much interest, since the neurological damage that it can cause closely resembles Parkinson's disease. MPTP is a very specific dopaminergic neurotoxin. There is considerable support for the "mitochondrial theory" of MPTP toxicity, which postulates that MPP^+, the ultimate oxidation product of MPTP, blocks the reoxidation of NADH dehydrogenase by coenzyme Q_{10} and eventually leads to ATP depletion in a rotenone-like fashion (Heikilla et al., 1989). However, there are also several studies that suggest oxygen radicals may play a role in MPTP-induced neuronal damage (Rios and Tapia, 1987; Odunze et al., 1990). Vitamin E has also been shown to protect against neural oxidative stress induced by MPTP (Odunze et al., 1990). Ganglioside GM1, a membrane-stabilizing agent effective within the CNS, may also mitigate some components of oxidative damage to neural tissue. This ganglioside has been reported to protect against MPTP (Hadjiconstantinou et al., 1989) and against directly induced oxidative activity (Bondy et al., 1990).

The conflicting conceptions of the primary locus of action of MPP^+, either by inhibition of a specific mitochondrial enzyme or as an oxidative stressor, may be reconciled by the finding that the metabolic inhibitors rotenone and antimycin can increase the generation rate of oxygen radicals in crude rat synaptosomes and mitochondria (Cino and Del Maestro, 1989; Ali et al., 1992).

Emerging information concerning MPTP has led to several new ideas concerning a very prevalent neurological disorder, Parkinson's disease. These concepts include both the possibility that an environmental agent is contributory to the pathogenesis of parkinsonism (Tanner and Langston, 1990) and the potential for antioxidant therapy for this disorder (Parkinson's Study Group, 1989). Parkinson's disease has been associated with abnormally high levels of superoxide dismutase within the substantia nigra (Saggu et al., 1989), implying an induced response to oxidative stress. A contribution of environmentally prevalent agents such as pyridines to the incidence of this disorder has been proposed. In addition, the potential utility of several antioxidant therapies is currently under investigation (Shoulson, 1989; McCrodden et al., 1990). There is evidence that *n*-hexane may specifically damage dopaminergic neurons and precipitate parkinsonian symptoms in both humans and experimental animals (Pezzoli et al., 1990). The environmental relevance of this is enhanced by the detection of the neurotoxic metabolite of *n*-hexane, 2,5-hexanedione, in the urine of persons not known to have been exposed to organic solvents (Fedtke and Bolt, 1986).

The neurotoxicity of another abused drug, methamphetamine, may in part be due to oxidative stress relating to dopaminergic and serotonergic circuitry (De Vito and Wagner, 1989). This was inferred by the attenuation of metamphetamine-induced neuropathological changes by pretreatment with a variety of antioxidants. Neuronal destruction induced by levodopa and 6-hydroxydopamine is also thought to occur via free radical mechanisms (Olney et al., 1990), and the administration of hydroxyl radical scavengers such as phenylthiazolylthiourea and methimazole is protective against such induced damage (Cohen, 1988).

There are several reports that neuroleptics may elevate lipid peroxidation in the CNS, and it has been proposed that this is a cause of tardive dyskinesia and a result of increased catecholamine metabolism (Lohr et al., 1990).

Metabolic Inhibitors

Cerebral lipid peroxidation can be stimulated by cyanide (Johnson et al., 1987; Ardelt et al., 1989). This illustrates that interruption of the respiratory chain can lead to excess free radical production. While acute cyanide exposure is rapidly lethal, more chronic exposures as a result of excess cyanogenic glycosides (e.g., in cassava) in the diet of some less developed countries can result in ataxic neuropathy (Politis et al. 1980). This may be related to the high levels of unsaturated fatty acids in myelin that form a clear target for ROS-induced lipid peroxidation (Halliwell, 1989).

Excitatory Compounds

Excitatory events are often associated with neurotoxic exposures. Many agents impair effective mitochondrial oxidation of energy-producing substrates. The consequent depletion of ATP as a result of metabolic insult can lead to dissipation of ionic gradients. Entry of calcium into the cell may increase synaptic firing rates, while lowering of the sodium/potassium gradients will increase axonal excitability. Intracellular calcium overload can also set off a cascade of other events, such as phospholipase activation, potentially leading to elevation of free radical production (Pazdernik et al., 1992). Some neurotoxicants (such as β-*N*-oxalyl-L-alanine [ODAP]) are glutamate agonists, while others (such as lindane) act as GABA antagonists. Both types of interaction with neurons can directly depolarize postsynaptic cells.

Recently, evidence suggesting a role for free radicals in excitotoxic events has been accumulating. Excess neuronal activity is known to have the potential to effect neuronal death, especially in the hippocampus. In addition to the frank neuronal hyperactivity apparent in epilepsy, several other neurological disorders are associated with hyperexcitatory events within the brain. These include transient cerebral ischemia followed by restoration of the vascular oxygen supply. Free radicals may play a role in seizure-related brain damage (Nelson and Olson, 1987; Ikeda and Long, 1990), and superoxide anion is generated within the brain during seizure activity (Armstead et al., 1989). Attenuation of convulsive activity by phenytoin or corticosteroids also reduces cerebral levels of lipid peroxidation (Willmore and Triggs, 1984). Free radical generation during cerebral ischemia may underlie delayed neuronal death (Kitagawa et al., 1990; Sutherland et al., 1991).

Various mechanisms have been proposed as forming the basis of such injury induced by oxidative damage. Several reports indicate that there may be a direct relation between activation of various classes of glutamate receptor and free radical formation. D-glutamate and L-glutamate, as well as several glutamate agonists, can directly enhance ROS in isolated cerebral systems (Bondy and Lee, 1993). Glutamate toxicity in a neuronal cell line has been attributed to inhibition of cystine transport and consequent oxidative stress (Murphy et al., 1989). Activation of the N-methyl-D-aspartate (NMDA) receptor site has been implicated in the postischemic elevation of lipid peroxidation in the hippocampud (Haba et al., 1991). There is a report of exacerbation of NMDA toxicity in glutathione-deficient cortical cultures (Bridges et al., 1990).

Calcium stimulation of phopholipase A_2 and thence the arachidonic acid cascade, followed by the consequent activation of ROS by lipoxygenases, may be a means by which excitatory events promote excess generation of ROS (Pellerin and Wolfe, 1991). NMDA agonists are especially potent in the stimulation of nitric oxide synthetase (Kiedrowski et al., 1992), and nitric oxide can interact with superoxide to form the intensely oxidant nitroperoxyl radical. There is evidence suggesting that the free radical nitric oxide mediates the neurotoxicity of glutamate (Dawson et al., 1991). Kainate-induced damage to cerebellar neurons may also be mediated at least in part by induction of superoxide (Dykens et al., 1987). A possible mechanism underlying this may be the induction of nerve growth factor (Ballarin et al., 1991).

The shellfish neurotoxin domoic acid, which predominantly acts as a glutamate agonist at the kainate site (Sutherland et al., 1990), was very potent in enhancing synaptosomal ROS (Bondy and Lee, 1992). When administered to mice, domoic acid has been found to elevate cerebral levels of superoxide dismutase (Bose et al., 1990), which also suggests an ability to promote oxidative stress. Excitants that have not been extensively studied for their ROS-inducing potential include food additives (monosodium glutamate and aspartame) and β-N-oxalyl-L-alanine (ODAP), a glutamergic agonist found in chickling-peas and a suspected cause of neurolathyrism.

Transient ischemia elevates cerebral levels of excitatory amino acids and rates of hydroxyl radical formation (Delbarre et al., 1991). Whether one of these events gives rise to the second is not well established. Excitatory events may stimulate ROS, but there is also evidence that ROS can lead to release of excitatory amino acids (Pellegrini-Giampietro et al., 1990). Peroxidative damage can also impair inhibitory processes as judged by inhibition of GABA-stimulated chloride uptake (Schwartz et al., 1988). Glutamine synthetase appears to be especially sensitive to ROS-induced damage, and this may increase glutamate concentrations (Schor, 1988). A bidirectional cooperation between excess neuronal activity and free radicals may therefore be relatively common (Oh and Betz, 1991), but the functional value of such a potentially synergistic association is unclear. While there is a correlation between excitotoxicity and free radical generation, an unequivocal causal relation remains to be uncovered.

Other Agents

Several antioxidant agents can protect against hexachlorophene-induced cerebral edema and myelin damage (Hanig et al., 1984). The neurotoxicity of this chemical is thus likely to involve its catalysis of free radical formation.

CONCLUSION

The kinds of metabolic change effected by many agents deleterious to nerve tissue often have the potential for inducing excess oxygen radical production (Fig. 1). The resulting oxidative damage may constitute a varying proportion of the total toxicity of a wide range of chemicals. Any chemical disrupting membrane structure or mitochondrial function by diverse means has the potential for induction of oxygen radicals. This is especially true of the broad range of neurotoxic agents causing hyperexcitation.

Intrinsic defensive antioxidant factors must first be overwhelmed before excess ROS can damage cell functioning. This increases the likelihood that initial ROS-related damage is region-specific. Such distinctive vulnerability may have either a chemical or an anatomical basis. An example of the first case involves areas rich in catecholamine neurons. These neurotransmitters are prone to oxidation and can give rise to semi-oxidized products that can result in continued and potentiated oxidative damage. An example of anatomical susceptibility is the hippocampus. The hippocampus is especially vulnerable to excitotoxic damage. This is probably by virtue of its distinctive anatomy, whereby response to repetitive stimuli is continually augmented rather than undergoing increasing suppression, an adaptive response characteristic of most brain regions.

Neurotoxic insult is not an "all-or-none" event, since subtle and insidious gradations of damage can occur. Since broad, low-level exposures to hazardous agents are common, the overall magnitude of the problem across the population is very difficult to estimate. Marginal deficiencies of antioxidant vitamins over extended periods may increase vulnerability to chronic exposure to low levels of free radical–promoting environmental contaminants. The effect of this may be expressed as subclinical events that are very difficult to quantitate but undoubtedly relate to the overall well-being of a person. Environmental factors are a suspected contributory element in many neurodegenerative disorders, and chronic excitotoxicity is the postulated mechanism of action (Hennberry and Spatz, 1991). As life expectancy increases, this is an area of great relevance to an aging population and offers a significant challenge for future research.

ACKNOWLEDGMENT

This work was supported by grant AA8281 from the National Institutes of Health.

REFERENCES

Adams JD, Klaidman LK, Odunze IN (1989). Oxidative effects of MPTP in the midbrain. Res Commun Subst Abuse 10:169–180.

Ahmad FF, Cowan DL, Sun AY (1987). Detection of free radical formation in various tissues after acute carbon tetrachloride administration in the gerbil. Life Sci 41:2469–75.

Ali SF, Bondy SC (1989). Triethyl lead–induced damage in various regions of the rat brain. J Toxicol Environ Health 26:235–42.

Ali SF, LeBel CP, Bondy SC (1992). Reactive oxygen species formation as a biomarker of methylmercury and trimethyltin neurotoxicity. Neurotoxicology 13:637–648.

Aragon CMG, Spivak K, Amit Z (1989). Effects of 3-amino-1,2,4-triazole on ethanol-induced open field activity: evidence for brain catalase mediation of ethanol's effects. Alcohol Clin Exp Res 13:104–8.

Ardelt BK, Borowitz JL, Isom GE (1989). Brain lipid peroxidation and antioxidant protectant mechanisms following acute cyanide intoxication. Toxicology 56:147–54.

Armstead WM, Mirro R, Leffler CW, Busija DW (1989). Cerebral superoxide anion generation during seizures in newborn pigs. J Cerebral Blood Flow Metab 9:175–9.

Asano T, Koide T, Gotch O, Joshita H, Hanamura T, Shigeno T, Tokakura K (1989). The role of free radicals and eicosanoids in the pathogenic mechanism underlying ischemic brain edema. Mol Chem Neuropathol 10:101–33.

Au AM, Chan PH, Fishman RA (1985). Stimulation of phospholipase A_2 activity by oxygen-derived free radicals in isolated brain capillaries. J Cell Biochem 27:449–59.

Aust SD, Morehouse LA, Thomas CE (1985). Role of metals in oxygen radical reactions. J Free Rad Biol Med 1:3–25.

Ballarin M, Ernfors P, Linderfors N, Persson H (1991). Hippocampal damage and kainic acid injection induce a rapid increase in mRNA for BDNF and NGF in the rat brain. Exp Neurol 114:35–43.

Banik NL, Hogan EL, Hsu CY (1987). The multimolecular cascade of spinal cord injury. Neurochem Pathol 7:57–77.

Behrens VJ, Hoerner M, Lasker JM, Lieber LS (1988). Formation of acetaldehyde adducts with ethanol inducible P-450IIEI in vivo. Biochem Biophys Res Commun 154:584–590.

Bondy SC (1990). Intracellular calcium and neurotoxic events. Neurotoxicol Teratol 11:527–31.

Bondy SC, McKee M (1990). Prevention of chemically induced synaptosomal changes. J Neurosci Res 25:229–35.

Bondy SC, McKee M, LeBel CP (1991). Changes in synaptosomal pH and rates of oxygen radical formation induced by chlordecone. Mol Chem Neuropath 13:95–106.

Bondy SC, Lee DK (1993). The relation between excitotoxicity and oxidative stress. Brain Res. 610:224–233.

Bonser RW, Thompson NT, Randall RW, Garland LG (1989). Phospholipase D activation is functionally linked to superoxide generation in the human neutrophil. Biochem J 264:617–20.

Bose R, Sutherland GR, Pinsky C (1990). Excitotoxins and free radicals: accomplices in post-ischemic and other neurodegeneration. Eur J Pharmacol 183:1170–1.

Boveris A, Chance B (1973). The mitochondrial generation of hydrogen peroxide: general properties and the effect of hyperbaric oxygen. Biochem J 134:707–16.

Braughler JM, Hall ED (1989). Central nervous system trauma and stroke. I. Biochemical considerations for oxygen radical formation and lipid peroxidation. Free Rad Biol Med 6:289–301.

Bridges RJ, Koh J, Hatalski CG, Cotman CW (1990). Increased excitotoxic vulnerability of cortical cultures with reduced levels of glutathione. Eur J Pharmacol 192:199–200.

Bruckdorfer KR, Jacobs M, Rice-Evans C (1990). Endothelium-derived relaxing factor (nitric oxide), lipoprotein oxidation, and atherosclerosis. Biochem Soc Trans 18:1061–3.

Calvin HI, Medvedovsky C, Worgul B (1986). Near-total glutathione depletion and age-specific cataracts induced by buthionine sulfoximine in mice. Science 133:553–5.

Cao W, Carney JM, Duchon A, Floyd RA, Chevion M (1988). Oxygen free radical involvement in ischemia and superfusion injury to brain. Neurosci Lett 88:233–8.

Chang LW, Gilbert M, Sprecher J (1978). Modification of methylmercury neurotoxicity by vitamin E. Environ Res 17:356–66.

Choi DW (1990). Cerebral hypoxia: new approaches and unanswered questions. J Neurosci 10:2493–2501.

Choy PC, OK, Man RYK, Chan AC (1989). Phosphatidylcholine metabolism in isolated rat heart: modulation by ethanol and vitamin E. Biochim Biophys Acta 1005:225–32.

Cino M, Del Maestro RF (1989). Generation of hydrogen peroxide by brain mitochondria: the effect of reoxygenation following postdecapatative ischemia. Arch Biochem Biophys 269:623–38.

Cohen G (1988). Oxygen radicals and Parkinson's disease. In: Halliwell B, ed. Oxygen radicals and tissue injury. Oxford: Clarendon Press, 130–5.

Cohen G, Sinet PM, Heikkila R (1980). Ethanol oxidation by rat brain in vivo. Alcohol Clin Exp Res 4:366–70.

Cojocel C, Beuter W, Muller W, Mayer D (1989). Lipid peroxidation: a possible mechanism of trichloroethylene nephrotoxicity. Toxicology 55:131–41.

Daniell LC, Brass EP, Harris RA (1988). Effect of ethanol on intracellular ionized calcium concentrations in synaptosomes and hepatocytes. Mol Pharmacol 32:831–7.

Davies KJA (1987). Protein damage and degradation by oxygen radicals. I. General aspects. J Biol Chem 262:9895–9901.

Dawson VL, Dawson TM, London ED, Bredt, DS, Snyder SH (1991). Nitric oxzide mediates glutamate neurotoxicity in primary cortical culture. Proc. Nat. Acad. Sci. 88:6368–6371.

De Vito MJ, Wagner GC (1989). Metamphetamine induced neuronal damage: a possible role for free radicals. Neuropharmacology 28:1145–50.

Delbarre G, Delbarre B, Calinon F, Ferger A (1991). Accumulation of amino acids and hydroxyl free radicals in brain and retina of gerbil after transient ischemia. J Ocular Pharmacol 7:147–55.

Devasagayam TPA (1989). Decreased peroxidative potential in rat brain microsomal fractions during ageing. Neurosci Lett 103:92–6.

Dexter DT, Carayon A, Vidarlhet M, Ruberg M, Agid F, Agid Y, Lees AJ, Wells FR, Jenner P, Marsden CD (1990). Decreased ferritin levels in brain in Parkinson's disease. J Neurochem 55:16–20.

Dildy JE, Leslie SW (1989). Ethanol inhibits NMDA-induced increase of free intracellular Ca^{2+} in dissociated brain cells. Brain Res 499:383–7.

Donaldson J, Labella FS, Gessa D (1981). Enhanced autoxidation of dopamine as a possible basis of manganese neurotoxicity. Neurotoxicology 2:53–64.

Dykens JA, Stern A, Trenkner E (1987). Mechanism of kainate toxicity to cerebellar neurons in vitro is analogous to reperfusion tissue injury. J Neurochem 49:1222–8.

Ekstrom G, Ingelman-Sundberg M (1989). Activity and lipid peroxidation dependent of ethanol-inducible cytochrome P-450 (P-450IIEI). Biochem Pharmacol 38:1313–9.

Essman WB, Wollman SB (1989). Free radicals, central nervous system processes and brain functions. In: Das DK, Essman WB, eds. Oxygen radicals: systemic events and disease processes. Basel: Karger, 172–91.

Fedtke N, Bolt HM (1986). Detection of 2,5 hexanedione in the urine of persons not exposed to n-hexane. Int Arch Occup Health 57:143–8.

Feierman DE, Cedarbaum AI (1985). Increased content of cytochrome P-450 and 4-methylpyrazole binding spectra after 4-methylpyrazole treatment. Biochem Biophys Res Commun 126:1076–81.

Floyd RA (1990). Role of oxygen free radicals in carcinogenesis and brain ischemia. FASEB J 4:2587–7.

Floyd RA, Zaleska MM, Harmon H (1984). Possible involvement of iron and oxygen free radicals in aspects of aging in brain. In: Armstrong D, ed. Free radicals in molecular biology, aging, and disease. New York: Raven Press, 143–61.

Freeman B, Crapo JD (1982). Biology of disease: free radicals and tissue injury. Lab Invest 47:412–26.

Fridovich I (1989). Oxygen radicals from acetaldehyde. Free Rad Biol Med 7:557–8.

Ghersi-Egea JF, Mim A, Siest G (1988). A new aspect of the protective functions of the blood-brain barrier: activities of four drug metabolizing enzymes in isolated rat brain microvessels. Life Sci 42:2515–23.

Gonthier B, Jeunet A, Barret L (1991). Electron spin resonance study of free radicals produced from ethanol and acetaldehyde after exposure to a Fenton system or to brain and liver microsomes. Alcohol 8:369–75.

Guerri C, Grisolia S (1980). Changes in glutathione in acute and chronic alcohol intoxication. Pharmacol Biochem Behav 13:53–61.

Gutteridge JM, Westermarck T, Santavvori P (1983). Iron and oxygen radicals in tissue damage: implications for neuronal ceroid lipofuscinoses. Acta Neurol Scand 68:365–70.

Haba K, Ogawa N, Mizukawa K, Mori A (1991). Time course of changes in lipid peroxidation, pre- and postsynaptic cholinergic indices, NMDA receptor binding and neuronal death in the gerbil hippocampus following transient ischemia, Brain Res 40:116–22.

Hadjiconstantinou M, Mariani AP, Neff NH (1989). GM$_1$ ganglioside-induced recovery of nigrostriatal dopaminergic neurons after MPTP: an immunohistochemical study. Brain Res 484:297–303.

Hall ED, Braughler JM (1989). Central nervous system trauma and stroke. II. Physiological and pharmacological evidence for involvement of oxygen radicals and lipid peroxidation. Free Rad Biol Med 6:303–13.

Halliwell B (1988). Albumin—an important extracellular antioxidant? Biochem Pharmacol 37:569–71.

Halliwell B (1989). Oxidants and the central nervous system: some fundamental questions. Is oxidant damage relevant to Parkinson's disease, Alzheimer's disease, traumatic injury or stroke? Acta Neurol Scand 126:23–33.

Halliwell B, Gutteridge JMC (1985). Oxygen radicals and the nervous system. Trends Neurosci 8:22–6.

Halliwell B, Gutteridge JMC (1989). Free Radicals in Biology and Medicine. Oxford: Clarendon Press, 266.

Hanig JP, Yoder PD, Krop S (1984). Protection with butylated hydroxytoluene and other compounds against intoxication and mortality caused by hexachlorophene. Food Chem Toxic 22:185–9.

Hansson T, Tindberg N, Ingelman-Sundberg M, Kohler L (1990). Regional distribution of etha-nol-inducible cytochrome P-450 IIEI in the rat central nervous system. Neuroscience 34:451–63.

Hanstein WG (1976). Uncoupling of oxidative phosphorylation. Biochem Biophys Acta 456:129–48.

Hasan M, Ali SF (1981). Effects of thallium, nickel and cobalt administration on the lipid peroxidation in different regions of the rat brain. Toxicol Appl Pharmacol 57:8–13.

Heikkila RE, Sieber BA, Mansino L, Sonsalla PK (1989). Some features of the nigrostriatal dopaminergic neurotoxin 1-methyl-4-phenyl-1,2,3,6-tetrahydropyridine (MPTP) in the mouse. Mol Chem Neuropathol 10:171–83.

Hennberry R, Spatz L (1991). The role of environmental factors in neurodegenerative disorders. Neurobiol Aging 12:75–9.

Ikeda Y, Long DL (1990). The molecular basis of brain injury and brain edema: the role of oxygen free radicals. Neurosurgery 27:1–11.

Jackson GR, Apffel L, Werrbach-Perez K, Perez-Polo JR (1990). Role of nerve growth factor in oxidant-antioxidant balance and neuronal injury. I. Stimulation of hydrogen peroxide resistance. J Neurosci Res 25:360–8.

Johnson JD, Conroy WG, Buxis KD, Isom GE (1987). Peroxidation of brain lipids following cyanide intoxication in mice. Toxicology 46:21–8.

Kaneko M, Panagia V, Paolillo G, Majumder S, Ou C, Challa NS (1990). Inhibition of cardiac phosphatidylethanolamine N-methylation by oxygen free radicals. Biochem Biophys Acta 1021:33–8.

Kefalas V, Stacey NH (1989). Potentiation of carbon tetrachloride-induced lipid peroxidation by trichloroethylene in isolated rat Repatocytes: no role in enhanced toxicity. Toxicol Appl. Pharmacol. 101:158–169.

Kehrer JP, Jones DP, LeMasters JJ, Farber JL, Jaeschke H (1990). Mechanisms of hypoxic cell injury. Toxicol Appl Pharmacol 106:165–78.

Kehrer JP, Mossman BT, Sevanian A, Trush MA, Smith MT (1988). Free radical mechanisms in chemical pathogenesis. Toxicol Appl Pharmacol 95:349–62.

Kiedrowski LE, Costa E, Wroblewski JT (1992). Glutamate receptor agonists stimulate nitric oxide synthase in primary cultures of cerebellar granule cells. J Neurochem 58:335–41.

Kitagawa K, Matsumoto M, Oda T, Nunobe M, Hata R, Handa N, Fukunaga R, Isaka Y, Kimura K, Maeda H, Mikoshiba K, Kamado T (1990). Free radical generation during brief period of cerebral ischemia may trigger delayed neuronal death. Neuroscience 35:551–8.

Komulainen H, Bondy SC (1987). Increased free intrasynaptosomal Ca^{2+} by neurotoxic organometals: distinctive mechanisms. Toxicol Appl Pharmacol 88:77–86.

Kontos HA (1989). Oxygen radicals in CNS damage. Chem Biol Interact 72:229–55.

Kuthan H, Ulbrich V (1982). Oxidase and oxygenase function of the microsomal cytochrome P-450 monoxygenase system. Eur J Biochem 126:583–8.

LeBel CP, Ali SF, McKee M, Bondy SC (1990). Organometal-induced increases in oxygen radical activity: The potential of 2′,7′-dichlorofluorescin diacetate as an index of neurotoxic damage. Toxicol Appl Pharmacol 104:17–24.

LeBel CP, Bondy SC (1990). Sensitive and rapid quantitation of oxygen reactive species in rat synaptosomes. Neurochem Int 17:435–40.

LeBel CP, Bondy SC (1991). Persistent protein damage despite reduced oxygen radical formation in the aging rat brain. Int J Dev Neurosci 9:139–46.

LeBel CP, Schatz RA (1990). Altered synaptosomal phospholipid metabolism after toluene: possible relationship with membrane fluidity, Na^+, K^+-adenosine triphosphatase and phospholipid methylation. J Pharmacol Exp Ther 253:1189–97.

LeBel CP, Ishchiropoulos H, Bondy SC (1992a). Fluorometric detection of reactive oxygen species: characterization of the probe 2′,7′-dichlorofluorescin diacetate. Res Chem Toxicol 5:227–31.

LeBel CP, Ali SF and Bondy SC (1992b). Deteroxamine inhibits methyl mercury-induced increases in reactive oxygen species formation in rat brain. Toxicol Appl. Pharmacol. 112:161–165.

Ledig M, M'Pavia JR, Mandel P (1981). Superoxide dismutase activity in rat brain during acute and chronic alcohol intoxication. Neurochem Res 6:385–91.

Ledig M, Tholey G, Megias-Megias L, Kopp P, Wedler F (1991). Combined effects of ethanol and manganese on cultured neurons and glia. Neurochem Res 16:591–6.

Levy DI, Sucher NJ, Lipton SA (1990). Redox modulation of NMDA receptor–mediated toxicity in mammalian central nervous system neurons. Neurosci Lett 110:291–6.

Lewin R (1987). Drug trial for Parkinson's disease. Science 236:1420.

Lohr JB, Kuczenski R, Bracha HS, Moir M, Jeste DV (1990). Increased indices of free radical activity in the cerebrospinal fluid of patients with tardive dyskinesia. Biol Psychiatry 28:535–9.

Lucas D, Lamboeuf Y, DeSaint-Blanquet G, Menez JF (1990). Ethanol-inducible cytochrome P-450 activity and increase in acetaldehyde bound to microsomes after chronic administration of acetaldehyde or ethanol. Alcohol Alcoholism 25:395–400.

Maellaro E, Cassini AF, Del Bello B, Comporti M (1990). Lipid peroxidation and antioxidant systems in liver injury produced by glutathione depleting agents. Biochem Pharmacol 39:1513–21.

Malis CD, Bonventre JV (1986). Mechanism of calcium potentiation of oxygen free radical injury to renal mitochondria. J Biol Chem 261:14201–8.

Mattia CJ, Adams JD, Bondy SC (1993). Free radical induction in the brain and liver by products of toluene catabolism. Biochem. Pharmacol. 46:103–110.

Mattia CJ, LeBel CP, Bondy SC (1991). Effect of toluene and its metabolites on cerebral oxygen radical formation. Biochem Pharmacol 42:879–82.

McCrodden JM, Tipton KF, Sullivan JP (1990). The neurotoxicity of MPTP and the relevance to Parkinson's disease. Pharmacol Toxicol 67:8–13.

Minotti G, Aust SD (1989). The role of iron in oxygen radical mediated lipid peroxidation. Chem Biol Interact 71:1–19.

Muma NA, Troncoso JC, Hoffman PN, Koo EH, Price DL (1988). Aluminum neurotoxicity: altered expression of cytoskeletal genes. Mol Brain Res 3:115–22.

Murphy TH, Myamato M, Sastre A, Schaar RL, Coyle JT (1989). Glutamate toxity in a neuronal cell line involves inhibition of cystine transport leading to oxidative stress. Neuron 2:1547–58.

Nadiger HA, Marcus SK, Chavdrakala MV (1988). Lipid peroxidation and ethanol toxicity in rat brain: effect of vitamin E deficiency and supplementation. Med Sci Res 16:1273–4.

Natsuki R (1991). Effect of ethanol on calcium uptake and phospholipid turnover by stimulation of adrenoceptors and muscarinic receptors in mouse brain and heart synaptosomes. Biochem Pharmacol 42:39–44.

Nelson SR, Olson JP (1987). Role of early edema in the development of regional seizure-related brain damage, Neurochem Res 12:561–4.

Nordmann R (1987). Oxidative stress from alcohol in the brain. Alcohol Alcoholism 1:75–82.

Nordmann R, Ribiere C, Rouach H (1987). Involvement of iron and iron-catalyzed free radical production in ethanol metabolism and toxicity. Enzyme 37:57–69.

Nordmann R, Ribiere C, Rouach H (1988). Pathophysiological relevance of free radicals to the ethanol-induced disorder in membrane lipids. In: Crastes de Paulet A, Douste-Blazy L, Paoletti R, eds. Free radicals, lipoproteins and membrane lipids. New York: Plenum Press, 309–19.

Nordmann R, Ribiere L, Rouach H (1992). Implication of free radical mechanisms in ethanol-induced cellular injury. Free Rad Biol Med 12:219–40.

O'Neill P, Rahwan RG (1976). Protection against active toxicity of acetaldehyde in mice. Res Commun Chem Pathol Pharmacol 13:125–31.

Odunze IN, Klaidman LK, Adams JD (1990). MPTP toxicity in the mouse brain and vitamin E. Neurosci Lett 108:346–9.

Oh SM, Betz AL (1991). Interaction between free radicals and excitatory amino acids in the formation of ischemic brain edema in rats. Stroke 22:915–21.

Oldfield FF, Cowan DL, Sun AY (1991). The involvement of ethanol in the free radical reaction of 6-hydroxydopamine. Neurochem Res 18:83–7.

Olesen SP (1986). Rapid increase in blood-brain barrier permeability during severe hypoxia and metabolic inhibition. Brain Res 368:24–9.

Oliver CN, Starke-Reed PE, Stadtman ER, Lin GJ, Correy JM, Floyd RA (1990). Oxidative damage to brain proteins, loss of glutamine synthetase activity and production of free radicals during ischemia/reperfusion-induced injury to gerbil brain. Proc Natl Acad Sci USA 87:5144–7.

Olney JW, Ikonomidou C, Mosinger JL, Friedrich G (1989). MK-801 prevents hypobaric-ischemic neuronal degeneration in the infant rat brain. J Neurosci 9:1701–4.

Olney JW, Zorumski CF, Stewart GR, Price MT, Wong G, Labruyere J (1990). Excitotoxicity of 1-DOPA and 6-OH-DOPA: implications for Parkinson's and Huntington's diseases. Exp Neurol 108:269–72.

Opacka J, Opalska B, Kolokowski J, Wronska-Nofer T (1986). Neurotoxic effects of combined exposure to carbon disulphide and ethanol in rats. Toxicol Lett 32:9–11.

Parkinson's Study Group (1989). DATATOP: a multicenter clinical trial in early Parkinson's disease. Arch Neurol 46:1052–60.

Pazdernik TL, Layton M, Nelson SR, Samson FE (1992). The osmotic/calcium stress theory of brain damage: are free radicals involved? Neurochem Res 17:11–21.

Pellegrini-Giampietro DE, Cherici G, Alesiani M, Carla V, Moroni F (1990). Excitatory amino acid release and free radical formation may cooperate in the genesis of ischemia-induced neuronal damage. Neuroscience 10:1035–41.

Pellerin L, Wolfe LS (1990). Release of arachidonic acid by NMDA-receptor activation in the rat hippocampus, Neurochem Res 16:983–9.

Perrin R, Minn A, Ghersi-Egea JF, Grasshot MC, Siest G (1990). Distribution of cytochrome P450 activities towards alkoxyresorufin derivatives in rat brain regions, subcellular fractions and isolated cerebral microvessels. Biochem Pharmacol 40:2145–51.

Perry TL, Godin DV, Hansen S (1982). Parkinson's disease: a disorder due to nigral glutathione deficiency: Neurosci Lett 33:305–10.

Pezzoli G, Ricciardi S, Masotto C, Mariani CB, Cerenzi A (1990). N-hexane induces Parkinsonism in rats. Brain Res 531:355–7.

Phillips SC (1987). Can brain lesions occur in experimental animals by administration of ethanol or acetaldehyde? Acta Med Scand [Suppl] 717:67–72.

Politis MJ, Schaumburg HH, Spencer PH (1980). Neurotoxicity of selected chemicals. In Spencer PS and Schaumburg HH, eds. Experimental and Clinical Neurotoxicology. Baltimore-Williams and Wilkins, 613–630.

Porta EA (1988). Role of oxidative damage in the aging process. In: Chow CK, ed. Cellular antioxidant defense mechanisms. Vol. 3. New York: CRC Press, 1–52.

Ramstoek ER, Hoekstra WG, Ganther HE (1980). Trialkyl lead metabolism and lipid peroxidation in vivo in vitamin E– and selenium-deficient rats as measured by ethane production. Toxicol Appl Pharmacol 54:251–7.

Raps SP, Lai JCK, Hertz L, Cooper AJL (1989). Glutathione is present in high concentrations in cultured astrocytes, but not in cultured neurons. Brain Res 493:398–401.

Raskin NH, Sokoloff L (1970). Alcohol dehydrogenase activity in rat brain and liver. J Neurochem 17:1677–87.

Ravindranath V, Shivakumar R, Anandatheerthavarada HK (1989). Low glutathione levels in aged rats. Neurosci Lett 101:187–90.

Rehman SV (1984). Lead-induced regional lipid peroxidation in brain. Toxicol Lett 21:333–7.

Rios C, Tapia R (1987). Changes in lipid peroxidation induced by 1-methyl-4-phenyl-1,2,3,6-tetrahydropyridine and 1-methyl-4-phenylpyridinium in mouse brain homogenates. Neurosci Lett 77:321–6.

Rouach H, Houze P, Orfanelli MT, Gentil M, Bourdon R, Nordmann R (1990). Effect of acute ethanol administration on the subcellular distribution of iron in rat liver and cerebellum. Biochem Pharmacol 39:1095–1100.

Rouach H, Park MK, Orfanelli MT, Janvier B, Nordmann R (1987). Ethanol-induced oxidative stress in the rat cerebellum. Alcohol Alcoholism [Suppl] 1:207–11.

Sadrzadeh SM, Anderson DK, Panter SS, Hallaway PE, Eaton JW (1987). Hemoglobin potentiates nervous system damage. J Clin Invest 79:662–4.

Saggu H, Cooksey J, Dexter D, Wells FR, Lees A, Jenner P, Marsden CD (1989). A selective increase in particulate superoxide dismutase activity in Parkinsonian substantia nigra. J Neurochem 53:692–7.

Saunders R, Horrocks LP (1987). Eicosanoids, plasma membranes, and molecular mechanisms of spinal cord injury. Neurochem Pathol 7:1–22.

Savolainen H (1978). Superoxide dismutase and glutathione peroxidase activities in rat brain. Res Commun Chem Pathol Pharmacol 21:173–5.

Sawada M, Carlson JC (1987). Changes in superoxide radical and lipid peroxide formation in the brain, heart and liver during the lifetime of the rat. Mech Aging Dev 41:125–37.

Scarpa M, Rigo A, Viglino P, Stevanato R, Bracco F, Battistin L (1987). Age dependence of the level of the enzymes involved in the protection against active oxygen species in the rat brain. Proc Soc Exp Biol Med 185:129–33.

Schisler NJ, Singh SM (1989). Effect of ethanol in vivo on enzymes which detoxify oxygen free radicals. Free Rad Biol Med 7:117–23.

Schmucker DL, Vessey DA, Wang RK, James JL, Maloney A (1984). Age-dependent alterations in the physicochemical properties of rat liver membranes. Mech Aging Dev 27, 207–217.

Schor NF (1988). Inactivation of mammalian brain glutamine synthetase by oxygen radicals. Brain Res 456:17–21.

Schwartz R, Skolnick P, Paul SM (1988). Regulation of γ-aminobutyric acid/barbiturate receptor–gated chloride ion flux in brain vesicles by phospholipase A_2: possible role of oxygen radicals. J Neurochem 50:565–71.

Sevanian A, Nordenbrank K, Kim E, Ernster L, Hochstein P (1990). Microsomal lipid peroxidation: the role of NADPH-cytochrome P450 reductase and cytochrome P450. Free Rad Biol Med 8:145–52.

Shaw S (1989). Lipid peroxidation, iron mobilization and free radical generation induced by alcohol. Free Rad Biol Med 7:541–7.

Shoulson I (1989). Deprenyl and α-tocopherol antioxidative therapy of Parkinsonism (DATATOP). Acta Neurol Scand 126:171–5.

Shukla GS, Srivastava RS, Chandra SV (1988). Prevention of cadmium-induced effects on regional glutathione status of rat brain by vitamin E. J Appl Toxicol 8:355–8.

Siesjo BK (1988). Acidosis and ischemic brain damage. Neurochem Pathol 9:31–88.

Sinha S, Toner N, Chisuick M, Davies J, Bogle S (1987). Vitamin E supplementation reduces frequency of periventricular hemorrhage in very preterm babies. Cancer 1:466–8.

Sokol RJ (1989). Vitamin E and neurologic function in man. Free Rad Biol Med 6:189–207.

Stadtman ER (1990). Metal ion catalyzed oxidation of proteins: biochemical mechanism and biological consequences. Free Rad Biol Med 9:315–25.

Sultatos LG (1988). Effects of acute ethanol administration on the hepatic xanthine dehydrogenase (oxidase) system in the rat. J Pharmacol Exp Ther 246:946–9.

Sutherland RJ, Hoesing JM, Wishaw IQ (1990). Domoic acid, an environmental neurotoxin, produces hippocampal damage and severe memory impairment. Neurosci Lett 120:221–3.

Tadolini B, Cabrini L (1990). The influence of pH on OH· scavenger inhibition of damage to deoxyribose by Fenton reaction. Mol Cell Biochem 94:97–104.

Tanner CM, Langston JW (1990). Do environmental toxins cause Parkinson's disease? A cricital review. Neurology 40 (suppl 3):17–30.

Tauck DL, Ashbeck GA (1990). Glycine synergistically potentiates the enhancement of LTP induced by a sulfhydryl reducing agent. Brain Res 519:129–132.

Tayarani I, Chaudiere J, Lefauconnier JM, Bourre JM (1987). Enzymatic protection against peroxidative damage in isolated brain capillaries. J Neurochem 48:1399–1410.

Tonge JI, Burry AF, Saal JR (1977). Cerebellar calcification: a possible marker of lead poisoning. Pathology 9:289–300.

Trenga CA, Kunkel DD, Eaton DL, Costa LG (1991). Effect of styrene oxide on brain glutathione. Neurotoxicology 12:165–78.

Uysal M, Kutalp G, Odzemirler G, Aykac G (1989). Ethanol-induced changes in lipid peroxidation and glutathione content in rat brain. Drug Alcohol Depend 23:227–30.

Vanella A, Villa RF, Gorini A, Campisi A, Giuffrida-Stella AM (1989). Superoxide dismutase and cytochrome oxidase activities in light and heavy synaptic mitochondria from rat cerebral cortex during aging. J Neurosci Res 22:351–5.

Verity MA, Brown WJ, Cheung M (1975). Organic mercurial encephalopathy: in vivo and in vitro effects of methyl mercury on synaptosomal respiration. J Neurochem 25:759–65.

Vitorica J, Machado A, Satrustegui J (1984). Age-dependent variations in peroxide-utilizing enzymes from rat brain mitochondria and cytoplasm. J Neurochem 42:351–6.

Vlessis AA, Widener LL, Bartos D (1990). Effect of peroxide, sodium, and calcium on brain mitochondrial respiration potential role in cerebral ischemia and reperfusion. J Neurochem 54:1412–8.

Westcott JH, Weiner H, Schutz I, Myers RD (1980). In vivo acetaldehyde in the brain of the rat treated with ethanol. Biochem Pharmacol 29:411–41.

Wickramansinghe SH, Hasan R (1992). In vitro effects of vitamin C, thioctic acid and dehydrolipoic acid on the cytotoxicity of post-ethanol serum. Biochem Pharmacol 43:407–11.

Willmore LJ, Triggs WJ (1984). Effect of phenytoin and corticosteroids on seizures and lipid peroxidation in experimental post-traumatic epilepsy. J Neurosurg 60:467–75.

Witz G, Rao GS, Goldstein BD (1985). Short-term toxicity of trans,trans-muconaldehyde. Toxicol Appl Pharmacol 80:511–6.

Zuddas A, Corsini GU, Schinelli S, Barker JL, Kopin IJ, Di Porzio U (1989). Acetaldehyde directly enhances MPP[+] neurotoxicity and delays its elimination from the striatum. Brain Res 501:11–22.

21
Biochemical and Molecular Bases of Myelinopathy

Pierre Morell
University of North Carolina at Chapel Hill
Chapel Hill, North Carolina

CELLULAR ORIGIN AND STRUCTURE OF MYELIN

The brain and spinal cord may be grossly divided into areas of gray matter, which are enriched in nerve cell bodies and associated dendritic processes, and of white matter, which are greatly enriched in myelinated axons. The glistening "white" appearance of white matter is due to the presence of myelin, which accounts for about half of the dry weight of such brain areas. Nerves of the peripheral nervous system (PNS) are equivalent to white matter in that a section of such a structure looks "white" and consists largely of myelinated axons, the myelin again accounting for about half of the total dry weight. For a general review of the structure, composition, and metabolism of myelin, see Morell et al. (1993) or more detailed commentary on specific topics in two collections of reviews (Morell, 1984; Martenson, 1992).

Myelin is a greatly extended and modified plasma membrane that is spirally arranged and compacted around the axon (Fig. 1). In the PNS, there is a one-to-one relationship between a region of axon and the Schwann cell that myelinates it (Fig. 2). In the central nervous system (CNS), myelin is an extension of the surface membrane of the oligo-dendroglial cell. The morphology of this cell is quite complex, since a single cell can myelinate parts of several dozen axons (Fig. 3). The structural features of myelinating cells and of myelin are the subject of a very considerable literature. Some of these structural features are noted below, since they are essential to an understanding of myelinopathy; indeed, the term "myelinopathy" is in the realm of morphology and is defined by morphological criteria.

The structural features of myelin are dominated by the compacted successive spirals of the extruded plasma membrane. As visualized by electron microscopy, the major "dense" lines alternate with lighter "intraperiod" lines (Fig. 1). The dense line corresponds to the compaction of the cytoplasmic faces, while the "intraperiod" line (which can be resolved into a doublet at high resolution) signals the apposition of the external faces of the

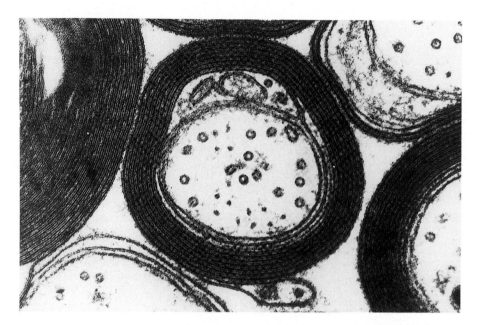

Figure 1   Electron micrograph of a central nervous system myelinated fiber from spinal cord of an adult dog. Note the repeating pattern of the major dense line and the intraperiod line as they spiral around the axon. Neurotubules and neurofilaments are visible in the axon. (Courtesy of Professor Cedric Raine of Albert Einstein College of Medicine, New York, New York.)

membrane. Thus it is the dense line that contains the virtual space (space that would be there were the apposed membranes to separate), which is in contact with the glial cell body cytoplasm. This virtual space also opens out to the lateral loop, inner loop, and outer loop (the columns of cytoplasm demarcating the edges of the compacted cytoplasmic sheet), which are in continuity with the perikaryal cytoplasm. Columns of cytoplasm may penetrate into regions of compacted myelin; these "incisures" are indicated on Figs. 2 and 3.

A single Schwann cell may envelop in myelin a length of axon as great as 1 mm. In the CNS, the length of axon myelinated by a single process of an oligodendroglial cell is somewhat less, but ranges up to several hundred microns. The region of the axon myelinated by a single Schwann cell, or by a single process of an oligodendroglial cell, is referred to as an internodal segment. This terminology arose because the myelinated segments are separated by short regions of axolemma that are not surrounded by compact myelin. These regions, nodes of Ranvier, have a complex structure and composition that is different in the CNS and PNS (and is not detailed in the simple illustrative figures). For purposes of this chapter it is sufficient to consider the nodes as the location at which, if Na^+ channels open, there is influx of this ion from extracellular space into the axoplasm.

FUNCTION OF MYELIN

The role of myelin is to facilitate conduction of waves of depolarization along the axon (for review, see Ritchie, 1984). In an unmyelinated axon, the progression of the wave of depolarization is maintained by a steadily moving local circuit involving ion currents. The signal moves relatively slowly down the axon as succeeding sections of voltage-sensitive

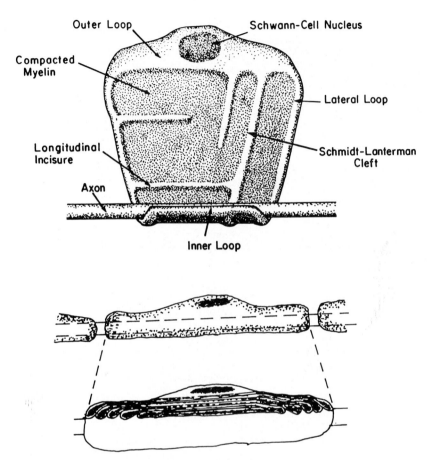

Figure 2 A diagram showing a Schwann cell unrolled from a peripheral nervous system axon. This illustrates the rim of cytoplasm surrounding the compacted structure, the lateral loop, and the inner loop, as well as tubes of cytoplasm that penetrate into the region of compacted myelin, Schmidt-Lanterman clefts, and longitudinal incisures. Below is a longitudinal view of the wrapped sheath and of a cross-section through this.

ion channels are opened. In myelinated nerves, the local circuit generated at a given internode cannot flow through the high-resistance sheath, and therefore it depolarizes the membrane at the next node. Thus, active excitation is discontinuously propagated from node to node (saltatory conduction). In axons above a certain critical size, this mode of conduction is much faster than is the continuous propagation of the impulse characteristic of unmyelinated neurons. Conduction in myelinated axons is also much more energy-efficient than is the case in unmyelinated axons. The presence of myelin causes a rearrangement of ion channels (for review, see Black et al., 1991), and so the loss of the sodium ion gradient occurs only at nodes. Thus, the "running down" of the gradient, and the consequent need to restore the original distribution of ions by energy-requiring mechanisms involving Na^+, K^+-ATPase, is much diminished relative to the situation when the whole axolemmal surface must be depolarized. The end result is that, on the average, myelinated nerves conduct impulses an order of magnitude more rapidly and two orders

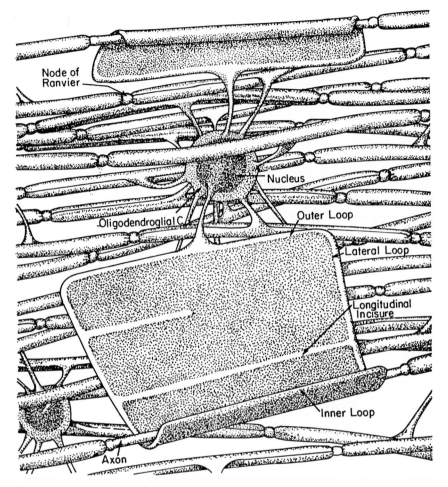

Figure 3 A diagram showing an oligodendroglial cell body of the central nervous system and some of its many myelinating processes. One of these has been unrolled, in a manner similar to the Schwann cell of Fig. 2, to illustrate the rim of cytoplasm around the compacted myelin. Note that longitudinal incisures are present, but Schmidt-Lanterman clefts are not common.

of magnitude more efficiently with respect to loss of ion gradient than is the case for unmyelinated fibers.

The consequences of toxicant-induced demyelination are, functionally, attributable to perturbation of saltatory conduction. If a single internodal segment is missing, the wave of depolarization will usually not traverse the denuded region. In some cases there will eventually be adaptation. The Na^+ channels, initially concentrated at the nodal region, will spread to the denuded region and support conduction of impulses in a manner similar to that in unmyelinated fibers. This may not always be helpful in a physiological sense, however, since the signal moves more slowly across the demyelinated internode and thus arrives at its target out of phase temporally with the signal from completely myelinated axons.

In addition to the essentially passive role of myelin as an insulator, myelin and myelinating glia have other less well defined functions. Ion channels of several types are found in myelinating glial cells (Barres et al., 1990), and there is speculation that these may also be found in myelin. Myelin has receptors for a number of neurotransmitters (for review, see Ledeen, 1992) and other components of signal-transduction systems (e.g., see Braun et al., 1990b), and this hints at some more active relationship between the operation of neurons and their axons and the associated myelinating glia.

COMPOSITION OF MYELIN

Although myelin is an extension of the plasma membrane, its composition is atypical of such membranes. Brain myelin is relatively impoverished in proteins (these constitute 30% or less of the dry weight) and enriched in lipids (70% of dry weight) relative to most other plasma membranes, which contain at least as much protein as lipid. The lipid composition is unusual in that there is a high concentration of plasmalogen and of the galactolipids galactosylceramide and sulfatide, components found only in low concentrations in other tissues. The concentration of galactolipids is sometimes used as an indicator of myelin concentration. Myelin is also enriched in cholesterol relative to other tissues. Some of the literature on myelin lipids is reviewed by Benjamins et al. (1984).

The most prominent proteins of CNS myelin are proteolipid protein and the myelin basic proteins. Proteolipid protein has a sequence-derived molecular weight of 30,000 daltons and is post-translationally modified by acylation, in part accounting for its hydrophobicity. An additional protein, produced by an RNA splice variant of the same gene that codes for proteolipid protein, is known as DM20 (the nomenclature refers to its apparent molecular weight of 20,000 daltons). The quantitatively most significant of the myelin basic proteins has a molecular weight of slightly over 18,000 daltons and undergoes several post-translational modifications, including phosphorylation. A number of other basic protein components of myelin are produced by messages that are splice variants of the same gene; the type and amount of these other proteins is species-specific. Proteolipid protein and the major myelin basic protein have been extensively studied for decades, and much is known about their chemical and biochemical properties (for review, see Lees and Brostoff, 1984). In addition to amino acid sequences, information is available concerning cDNA and genomic sequences, post-transcriptional splicing, and post-translational modification, as related to control of the production of these proteins (for review, see Mikoshiba et al., 1991).

A variety of other, mostly higher-molecular-weight, proteins have also been characterized. A significant literature details the properties and possible functions of myelin-associated glycoprotein (Quarles et al., 1992) and cyclic nucleotide phosphodiesterase (Sprinkle, 1989; see also Braun et al., 1990a). The former is postulated to play a special role at the glial cell–axon interface.

The composition of myelin of the PNS is even more biased than is that of CNS myelin with respect to the ratio of lipid to protein; the lipids comprise almost 80% of dry weight. The lipid composition is similar to that of CNS myelin, although there are some quantitative differences. Protein composition is, however, markedly different from that of CNS myelin. More than half of PNS myelin protein is accounted for by a single 28,000-dalton protein specific to the PNS, P_0 protein, which is very different from any CNS protein (for review, see Smith, 1983; Norton and Cammer, 1984). As with the major CNS proteins, there is currently a rapid accumulation of information at the level of molecular biology (for review, see Uyemura et al., 1992). Peripheral nervous system myelin also contains some myelin basic proteins originating from the same gene as in the CNS, although these are quantitatively less significant. There is also present a gene for a unique basic protein, for historical reasons referred to as P_2 (see Martenson and Uyemura, 1992, for review). Another PNS-specific myelin protein, PMP-22 (Snipes et al., 1992; previously partially characterized by Kitamura et al., 1976), is also present, as are some of the same high-molecularweight proteins as are found in CNS myelin.

Contrary to the earlier view of myelin as a very simple membrane without intrinsic enzyme activities, it has become clear that myelin indeed contains many enzymes (for review, see Ledeen, 1992). Activities shown to be intrinsic components of myelin include many that are involved in metabolism of myelin lipids, including some accounting for several aspects of phosphoinositide metabolism. Proteases, kinases, and phosphates that act on proteins are also present. A number of kinases intrinsic to myelin have been characterized. Present also are activities that could be involved in ion transport (to be discussed later). Of interest is the presence in myelin of an isoform of glutathione-S-transferase (Tansey and Cammer, 1991) that could possibly be involved in the intracellular processing of certain toxicants.

Components of the myelin membrane play a role in development. Myelin of the CNS contains inhibitors of neurite outgrowth (Schwab, 1990), at least in part accounting for lack of functional regeneration following injury to the brain. On the other hand, during nerve degeneration in the PNS, some product of myelin degeneration is responsible for Schwann cell proliferation (Salzer and Bunge, 1980). This specific mitogen, which provokes a necessary step in the remyelination process, may be a peptide resulting from processing of myelin basic protein by macrophages (Baichwal and DeVries, 1989).

DEVELOPMENT OF MYELIN

Myelination follows the phylogenetic development of the nervous system. In humans, motor roots myelinate just past the middle period of pregnancy, but many of the pathways in the brain are not myelinated until the end of the second year of life. Myelin accumulation continues at an ever-slower pace throughout the first two decades. In rats the myelination of the CNS is postnatal. The brain starts forming myelin at 10–12 days of age. Myelination peaks at about 20 days, and almost all pathways appear to be myelinated by a week or so later. Although rats are the animal model most commonly used in studies of myelination, it should be noted that they are unusual in that myelin accumulation, albeit at an ever-decreasing rate, continues throughout adulthood. This is presumably a correlate of a species-specific characteristic; rats continue body growth throughout adulthood.

During development the deposition of myelin occurs with a caudal-rostral gradient; e.g., the spinal cord myelinates earlier than the brain stem, and the forebrain is myelinated relatively later. In any one tract, axons are myelinated with some degree of synchrony over a relatively restricted period of time. At the time of initial myelination, the oligodendroglial cells are depositing relatively vast amounts of myelin, several times the weight of their perikarkyon each day, and myelinating glia account for much of the brain's utilization of energy and biosynthetic resources. Myelination is tightly programmed during development and may be much disrupted by metabolic or toxic insult at critical times (Wiggins, 1986).

The situation with respect to the PNS is analogous to that in the CNS. Various nerves become myelinated at somewhat different times, although this process occurs earlier than myelination of the CNS. A common object of study with respect to PNS myelination is the sciatic nerve of rats; in this structure myelination begins a day or two after birth. Since the developmental spurt in body growth is much later than for the brain, the growth of limbs dictates that rapid myelination continue for a long time. Although the sciatic nerve is well myelinated by 2 weeks of age, the animal continues to grow rapidly and the sciatic nerve becomes proportionally longer as the leg grows. Consequently, myelin keeps being synthesized for deposition to the ever-lengthening myelinating domain (internode) supported by each individual Schwann cell. It is thus easy to establish by morphological criteria whether—following recovery from an experimental demyelinating insult—a particular myelin internode was present originally or whether it has been newly synthesized as the result of a myelination-demyelination cycle. Internodes present from early development and retained to maturity are long because of lengthening during development. In contrast, when Schwann cells remyelinate a demyelinated region they reestablish short myelinating domains (see Chapter 8 by Bouldin and Goodrum in this volume).

METABOLISM OF MYELIN

Although myelin was initially considered to be metabolically inert, it has become clear over the last two decades that many myelin components turn over at significant rates. These half-lives are of the order of days and weeks for different types of phospholipids (Ousley and Morell, 1992) and of weeks for the peptide backbone of myelin proteins (for review, see Benjamins and Smith, 1984). Some components turn over very rapidly; a large proportion of the phosphate moieties of polyphosphoinositides (Deshmukh et al., 1981) and of myelin basic protein (Desjardins and Morell, 1983) equilibrate with injected radioactive phosphate with half-lives of the order of minutes or possibly even faster. How can this happen in the compacted layers of myelin? Explanations for the mechanisms involved rapidly reduce to hand waving. One possibility is that metabolism in the compacted region involves transient invasion of fingers of cytoplasm extending from the lateral loop region. In the PNS myelin such structures can be visualized as Schmidt-Lanterman clefts. This feature is not commonly seen in myelin of the CNS; possibly this structure might exist in vivo but not survive preparation for electron microscopy.

There are other signs of active metabolism compartmentalized within the myelin sheath. Many enzymes of lipid metabolism and some of other pathways are present in purified myelin. There is evidence for binding sites for cholinergic ligands (see Ledeen, 1992, for review of enzymes and receptors in myelin); these are thought to stimulate certain aspects of phospholipid turnover (e.g., Kahn and Morell, 1988). The above comments relate to metabolism in the CNS; the situation in the PNS is similar except that metabolic turnover is somewhat more rapid.

The notion of an energy-dependent process to maintain myelin compaction is often informally discussed, but there is no consensus as to what this means in molecular terms. The mechanism involved must explain how water is excluded from both the intraperiod line (extracellular space) and the dense line (cytoplasmic space). This could, in theory, involve exclusively some direct mechanical force to squeeze membranes together. More likely is a mechanism involving active pumping, possibly of some cation or anion, which would eventually drag water along by osmosis. Ions and accompanying water should be actively pumped from the extracellular space to the cytoplasmic face of myelin. This could involve active processes generally localized along the myelin membrane. Compatible with this view is the demonstration that significant levels of Na^+,K^+-ATPase are present in compacted myelin (Reiss et al., 1981), as is carbonic anhydrase (Cammer et al., 1976).

That proteolipid protein is a proton ionophore (Lin and Lees, 1982) also invites speculation as to the mechanism for water removal.

Intimately related to the mechanism of water clearance from extracellular space is the question of what happens to this water as it enters the cytoplasmic face of the myelin membrane. Ions and water appearing at this location should somehow end up in the cytoplasmic compartment. Such a compartment exists at the lateral loop region, since cytoplasm at that location is in continuity with that in the perikaryon. The uptake of water from the intraperiod line region could be restricted to membrane at the lateral loop region, thus allowing for direct entry of water and ions into cytoplasm. What if ion pumping takes place along the entire internodal length of membrane? As noted above, the idea that compacted regions of myelin have metabolism and transport activity no longer seems as far-fetched as it did a decade ago. The dynamic cytoplasmic inclusions, Schmidt-Lanterman clefts, might be involved. The point of these highly speculative comments is to indicate that there are several somewhat specialized metabolic processes involved in maintenance of myelin structure. These are likely targets of certain toxicants that bring about damage to myelin. In many cases, more specific experiments to test such hypotheses are limited by the paucity of information concerning the structure, function, composition, and metabolism of myelin.

CLASSIFICATION OF DISORDERS OF MYELIN

"Myelinopathy" is a morphologically defined term suggesting damage to white matter or, more specifically, to myelin. Disorders involving myelin can be classified on the bases of different criteria. Some disorders are specific for the CNS, while others preferentially affect the PNS. Basic to gaining insight into mechanisms involved is whether a disorder involving myelin represents primary demyelination or secondary demyelination. The term "primary demyelination" indicates that, following an insult, damage is first observed in myelin or its supporting glial cell. Much of the following discussion will relate to toxicants that bring about such demyelination. The term "segmental demyelination" indicates a primary demyelination in a pattern where certain internodes are bereft of myelin while adjacent segments retain myelin. A second-order distinction, again one made initially on morphological grounds, is that between damage to the myelinating cell (in the PNS this is referred to as a Schwannopathy) and damage directly to myelin.

Secondary demyelination indicates a process in which it is the neuron that appears affected initially, and the demyelination observed is secondary to the dissolution of the underlying axon. Secondary demyelination is an inevitable consequence of serious damage to neurons supporting myelinated axons. The distinction between primary and secondary demyelination is usually made on the basis of ultrastructural criteria as to which element (axon or myelin) seems to bear the initial damage. There is room for some subjectivity in such a classification. Also, there are toxic insults that lack specificity, so that the final picture may well be a mixture of primary and secondary demyelination.

Another class of disorders of myelin does not fit into either of the above classifications; the term "hypomyelination" implies a lack of appropriate accumulation of myelin during development. This can result from disease processes or nutritional disorders, or be the result of toxicant exposure during development.

The term "dysmyelination" is also seen, often used incorrectly and in a rather vague context. The meaningful use of this term is now restricted to description of certain inborn errors of metabolism in which a block in breakdown of a myelin lipid causes accumulation of myelin of abnormal composition, leading eventually to collapse of the structure of myelin. It is not known whether any toxicant has a mode of action leading to such a disturbance.

TOXICANT-INDUCED DISORDERS INVOLVING MYELIN

As noted above, damage to the myelin sheath can be primary, or it can be secondary to damage to neurons. It has been known for many decades that an intact axon is necessary to maintain myelin—it is generally assumed that some kind of continued signaling to the myelinating glial cell is required for maintenance of the myelin sheath. Many aspects of neuorotoxicity as they apply to damage to neurons are covered in other chapters. In all those cases leading to death of neurons, there is destruction of myelin enveloping the associated axons.

This chapter will, however, focus primarily on neurotoxicity that is expressed initially as damage to myelinating glial cells or myelin (primary demyelination). There will be some mention of toxicants that preferentially target myelinated axons (these also may be considered as myelinopathies in the more general sense of targeting white matter). The reader will note that almost all references are to toxicity in animal systems. This raises the issue that because of species variability (based on, for example, differences in ability of the liver to metabolize a toxicant), animal systems may provide information that is not in complete accord with the situation in humans. It is, however, very difficult to draw conclusions as to mechanisms from investigations of human exposure. Studies with human material are usually not possible until the patient dies, in which case the immediate consequences of the toxic insult may be invisible in the midst of the subsequent pathology—thus the impetus for animal studies to examine the development of the pathology and the need for the assumption that the molecular mode of action of the toxicant is similar in humans and other mammals.

Damage initially specific for myelin or its supporting cell is presumably targeted toward some specialized aspect of this system. Certain factors of relevance can be assessed. These include the following:

1. A relatively nonspecific chemical feature, the hydrophobicity of myelin consequent to its high proportion of lipid, explains why certain toxicants accumulate at this site. Hydrophobicity can easily be determined in vitro. An in vivo correlate can be measured by determination of preferential accumulation of the toxicant or relevant metabolite in white matter relative to gray matter. More specifically, subcellular fractionation can be carried out and the actual accumulation of a toxic substance in isolated myelin determined.
2. Myelin has a specialized chemical composition. Thus, myelinating glia have a high activity for synthesis of compounds enriched in myelin. Compounds that preferentially perturb such biosynthetic pathways are potentially neurotoxic.
3. Much of the accumulation of myelin, and the consequent very heavy metabolic load on myelinating cells, occurs during a somewhat restricted developmental period. Thus, even a somewhat generalized metabolic insult, applied at the time of maximal metabolic activity of myelinating cells, may preferentially impair accumulation of myelin. This is likely to be permanent, since the complex developmental program of brain is highly ordered temporally and the window of opportunity for a developmental event to take place normally may be narrower than is the case for other tissues.
4. The highly organized structure of the multilamellar myelin membrane suggests that

its composition with respect to different structural components is very critical; slight changes in composition would be expected to affect fluidity and membrane dimensions. Thus, alterations in fatty acid composition or cholesterol content may result in pathological consequences to myelin before other membrane structures are affected.

5. Some active aspect of metabolism is involved in prevention of myelin edema; the active processes involved in maintaining the multilayered structure of myelin may constitute a target for certain neurotoxicants. Accumulation of fluid at the intraperiod line in response to a toxicant is justification for consideration of this mechanism of action.

6. There are certain metabolic insults that cause damage to "white matter" but are not targeted to a specific feature of myelinating cells as such. In such cases it may be that the structural unit of axon–myelinating cell has some feature that renders it preferentially susceptible to certain toxicants.

7. As with any neurotoxic process, evaluation of pathophysiology must give due consideration to the barrier systems that separate toxic compounds in the circulation from the CNS (blood-brain barrier) and from the PNS (blood-nerve barrier). It is, however, often difficult to establish whether damage to barrier function is causal of or consequent to demyelination.

Some specific myelinopathies are discussed below. The list is not comprehensive, in that damage to myelin has been reported as a neurotoxic consequence of exposure to many compounds. The toxicants discussed below have been selected as illustrative of those for which there are some data, or at least hypothesis, relevant to mechanisms involved as they relate specifically to myelination.

TRIETHYLTIN

The neurotoxicity of triethyltin in humans became apparent when a large number of patients suffered severe consequences, including 100 deaths, as a result of contamination of a medication by triethyltin (Rouzaud and Lutier, 1954; for review, see Watanabe, 1980). Studies with a variety of animals showed neurotoxic symptoms associated with severe brain edema. The most extensive studies have been done with rats. In this model the preferential susceptibility of CNS white matter is readily demonstrable; the swelling of the myelin is due to the presence of vacuoles formed by splitting of the intraperiod line (Aleu et al., 1963). Treatment with triethyltin for several weeks brings about a net loss of over 25% of the brain myelin; this can be measured as a reduction in isolatable myelin (Eto et al., 1971; Smith, 1973). The degraded myelin is actually catabolized, since there is an absolute decrease in brain levels of the myelin-specific lipid cerebroside (Eto et al., 1971). The rapid onset of the toxicity, and its demonstration in culture systems (Graham et al., 1975), suggest that triethyltin itself, rather than a metabolite, is the immediate toxicant. Myelin of the CNS is preferentially vulnerable to triethyltin; drastic chronic treatment will, however, cause splitting of the intraperiod line of PNS myelin as well (Graham and Gonatas, 1973).

The results of metabolic studies fit well with the observed pathology. Under a regimen of chronic dosing with triethyltin, synthesis of myelin lipids is initially depressed and then, after several weeks, increased above control levels. Incorporation of radioactive leucine into brain myelin proteins is also increased above control levels after several weeks of treatment (Smith, 1973). A recent observation by Veronesi et al. (1991) is that mRNA from myelin basic protein is increased within hours of intraperitoneal injection of triethyltin at a dose of either 0.8 mg/kg or 8.0 mg/kg. This suggests the utility of triethyltin as a model to study control of expression of myelin protein genes.

The demonstrated specificity for the neurotoxicity of triethyltin is compatible with the relative hydrophobicity of this molecule, which suggests it should concentrate in myelin. In addition, Lock and Aldridge (1975) identified a high-affinity binding site for triethyltin on rat brain myelin. Occupation of this binding site is not, in itself, specific for damage to myelin; triethyllead binds to the same site yet does not produce myelin edema. With respect to mechanism of toxicity, it appears that triethyltin somehow interferes with maintenance of osmotic regulation at the cellular and organelle level. The above-noted reasons for possible greater accumulation of triethyltin in myelin might account for the relative specificity of the observed pathology.

The failure in osmotic regulation is likely to be a consequence of the interference of triethyltin with oxidative phosphorylation (Aldridge and Cremer, 1955). This could be through an effect directly on the mitochondrial Mg^{2+}-ATPase (Wassenaar and Kroon, 1973). Another aspect of the mechanism involved probably relates to the fact that triethyltin is an ionophore, able to catalyze Cl^-/OH^- exchange (Selwayn et al., 1970). This could bring about collapse of maintenance of the proton gradient required for ATP production, or allow chloride to block the entry into mitochondria of other anionic substrates necessary for oxidative phosphorylation (discussed by Lock, 1976, and Cammer, 1980). Relevant are recent data indicating that an even more specific action of organotins (effect at a lower concentration) is blocking of the uniport mitochondrial inner membrane anion channel (Powers and Beavis, 1991). As noted by Cammer (1980), there is also evidence suggesting the direct action of triethyltin on myelin, presumably involving facilitation of Cl^- entry and therefore influx of water into the intraperiod line region.

An in vivo study by Stine et al. (1988) provided information on developmental aspects. These authors reported that "in vivo brain tin concentrations in five day old rats following a neurotoxic dose of triethyltin are sufficient to inhibit brain mitochondrial ATPase, whereas in adults, tin concentrations are insufficient for inhibition." Their conclusion was that in the neonatal rat triethyltin may cause neuronal cell death, whereas in older animals triethyltin binds to myelin—thus sparing mitochondrial adenosine triphosphatase (ATPase) but targeting myelin and the cells associated with its formation.

The overall picture is that, in young animals, triethyltin enters the brain and acts on mitochondria in all neural cells to limit production or utilization of adenosine triphosphate (ATP). The specificity of triethyltin in causing "neurotoxicity" may be due to the fact that in young animals the brain is growing more rapidly than other organs and has a great requirement for energy both to maintain function and for synthesis of macromolecules for growth. In older animals, in which myelin has already been deposited, treatment with triethyltin clearly causes preferential damage of the myelin sheath. This specificity is related to sequestration of the triethyltin in myelin as a result of hydrophobicity, as well as specific binding of triethyltin to myelin. The accumulation of triethyltin presumably interferes with energy-dependent exclusion of fluid from the intraperiod line (compaction of the extracellular faces of the spiral wrapping of the membranes that form the myelin sheath). The fluid accumulation can be demonstrated using x-ray diffraction techniques to show that triethyltin induces an ordered structure swollen at the intraperiod line (Kirschner and Sapirstein, 1982).

It is of interest that recovery from triethyltin edema is blocked by acetazolamide (Yanagisawa et al., 1990). This drug blocks carbonic anhydrase. This observation can be related to work by Cammer et al. (1976) and Reiss et al. (1981), who have localized carbonic anhydrase within the myelin sheath and suggest that the role of this enzyme in myelin includes its involvement in some aspect of water transport. This hypothesis is related to previous observations that swelling of glial cells (removal of water from the environment) is stimulated by HCO_3^- and blocked by acetazolamide (see Bourke and Kimelberg, 1975, for discussion).

The structure-activity relationship of the trialkyltin compounds has been explored, and it appears that hydrophobicity is essential for targeting to myelin. The above-noted specificity of triethyltin for myelin does not hold for the less hydrophobic trimethyltin, which is selectively damaging to neurons, especially those of the hippocampus (O'Callaghan and Miller, 1984). In an in vitro system triethyltin and trimethyltin differ significantly in their effects on certain membrane channels (Komulainen and Bondy, 1987). The administration of dimethylethyltin and methyldiethyltin results in pathologic consequences resembling, but slightly less specific than, those of trimethyltin and triethyltin, respectively (Aldridge et al., 1987).

Another aspect of preferential susceptibility during development is revealed by chronic dosage of young animals. When rats were administered triethyltin at 1 mg/kg body weight by gavage starting at 2 days of age, the normal developmental accumulation of myelin was decreased by 50%, as was the rate of synthesis of myelin proteins (Blaker et al., 1981). There was specificity for perturbation of myelination, since the decrement in myelin was much greater than the decrement in body or brain weight. Myelin that did accumulate, however, was normal in composition. The observed deficit is not completely specific to myelin, since neonatal rats dosed with triethyltin also had appreciable deficits in proteins that are specific markers for neuronal cytoskeleton, synapses, and astrocytes (O'Callaghan and Miller, 1988). The spectrum of effects may simply reflect the fact that oligodendroglia will be the cell type ordinarily undergoing the greatest proliferation between a few days and a few weeks after birth of the rat. Many neurons will also be affected, since these cells are rapidly extending processes and engaged in biosynthesis of mitochondria. Deficits in myelin accumulation caused by exposure to triethyltin during development persist into adulthood (Toews et al., 1983).

HEXACHLOROPHENE

Hexachlorophene (2,2'-methylenebis(3,4,6-trichlorophenol)) is an antimicrobial agent that for some two decades was extensively used at high concentrations in the formulation of certain soaps and detergents. Publication of data and a review of the literature by the original patenter of this product (Gump, 1969) clarified the dangers in the indiscriminate use of this compound. The potential human neurotoxicity of hexachlorophene was heavily publicized in connection with the practice, at one time common, of bathing newborn babies with solution containing hexachlorophene to prevent bacterial infections (Herter, 1959; for review, see Towfighi, 1980).

Hexachlorophene can be absorbed through the skin, in part a reflection of its hydrophobicity, the same property that is associated with targeting to myelin. The myelin edema, due to splitting of the intraperiod line, is readily observed in human material (Powell et al., 1973). A model neurotoxicity is readily produced in rats. In adult animals the single-oral-dose LD_{50} is about 66 mg/kg (Gaines et al. 1973). Chronic exposure through a diet containing 500 ppm hexachlorophene induces progressive paralysis over several weeks (Kimbrough, 1976). As with triethyltin, hexachlorophene is toxic in young rats, but edema is not a characteristic until after 15 days of age, when myelin membranes have accumulated in sufficient quantity to serve as a hydrophobic reservoir for hexachlorophene, and myelin intraperiod lines are available for fluid accumulation (Nieminen et al., 1973). Both the CNS and the PNS are affected (Towfighi et al., 1974). When adult rats are treated with hexachlorophene, a floating fraction, similar to that found subsequent to triethyltin exposure, is characteristic. The disruption of myelin by treatment of animals with hexachlorophene is, however, presumably somewhat less severe than when exposure is to triethyltin, since there is not a decrease in isolatable myelin (Cammer et al., 1975). As with other neurotoxicants, if the animals are exposed during development there is a somewhat different spectrum of consequences, in this case including a decrement in the normal developmental accumulation of myelin relative to controls (Matthieu et al., 1974).

Much of the literature concerning the effects of hexachlorophene on membranes and on various enzymes in vitro and in vivo has been summarized by Cammer (1980). The general picture presented then still seems appropriate: quite low concentrations of hexachlorophene uncouple oxidative phosphorylation (Cammer and Moore, 1972). It has also been noted that carbonic anhydrase activity is inhibited by hexachlorophene treatment in vitro or in vivo; this seems to be due to direct inhibition of the enzyme (Cammer et al. 1976). This is in contrast to the situation with triethyltin, in which administration of the toxicant brings about some inhibition of carbonic anhydrase activity, but apparently not by direct interaction of toxicant and enzyme. The actions of hexachlorophene in inhibition of energy metabolism and of carbonic anhydrase activity are factors that would decrease the active exclusion of water from the intraperiod line. This, along with the likelihood of concentration of this lipophilic toxicant in myelin and the possibility of its direct action on the membrane, probably accounts for the observed pathology induced by hexachlorophene.

A study of "cell-specific marker enzymes" has been conducted on several regions of the CNS of rats dosed with hexachlorophene, 20 mg/kg p.o. for 53 days. Neuronal-specific enzymes were only slightly altered relative to a significant increase in the nonneuronal enzymes: nonneuronal enolase, glutamine synthetase, and 2′,3′-cyclic nucleotide phosphodiesterase (Kung et al., 1989). The increase in the myelin enriched enzyme 2,′3′-cyclic nucleotide phosphodiesterase might be a compensatory phenomenon; a more acute exposure (40 mg/kg/day p.o. for 9 days) led to a decrease in activity of this marker (Kung et al., 1988). A freeze-fracture study of the effects of hexachlorophene on myelin morphology in *Xenopus* tadpoles has been carried out by Reier et al. (1978); this is a convenient model, since the toxicant is just added to the tank.

LEAD

Exposure of children to lead is a well-known developmental risk factor. Acute exposure of young children to lead results in severe encephalopathy, but this is not particularly myelin-specific, in contrast to the myelin specificity of edema produced by hexachlorophene or triethyltin. Chronic lead intoxication of children or adults can also result in a wallerian type of neuropathy. In humans, lead toxicity is not preferentially targeted to myelin. The segmental demyelination of the PNS in response to exposure to inorganic lead is prominent only in certain animals. A model segmental demyelination can be produced in rats by administration of lead salts in the drinking water or by intraperitoneal injection (Dyck et al., 1977; Lampert and Schochet, 1968; Ohnishi et al., 1977; Schlaepfer, 1969; Krigman et al., 1980). There is swelling of Schwann cell cytoplasm and splitting of myelin—in this case at both the intraperiod and the major dense lines. An early change observed is Schwann cell hypertrophy due to increase in both cytoplasmic and nuclear compartments (Monton and Coria, 1991). This hypertrophy, prominent after 6 weeks on 4% lead acetate in drinking water, was completely reversed after 30 days of recovery.

The mode of action by which lead targets Schwann cells is not clear. Lead has been accused of a multitude of sins with respect to disruption of ion transport and of oxidative phosphorylation. A common denominator for some of these effects may be competition of lead with calcium ions for energy-requiring transport (for review, see Silbergeld, 1984). Proposed mechanisms do not, however, provide a clear-cut rationale for specificity of toxicity for Schwann cells or PNS myelin. In addition to damage to existing myelin, lead seems to inhibit the process of myelination. This can be demonstrated for PNS components under culture conditions; in dorsal root ganglion–Schwann cell cultures, the process of myelination is inhibited by a 1 µM concentration of lead (Windebank, 1986).

The process of myelination in the CNS is somewhat preferentially affected by lead acetate treatment (400 mg/kg body weight per day by gavage) during development; accumulation of brain myelin is decreased significantly relative to controls undergoing the same slight degree of malnourishment as the lead-treated animals (Toews et al., 1980). The decrement in myelin induced by early exposure to inorganic lead persists into adulthood (Toews et al., 1983). In developing rats the interaction of lead treatment and mild malnutrition induced by milk deprivation (and therefore calcium restriction) are synergistic with respect to decreasing the normal developmental accumulation of myelin (Harry et al., 1985); this result is preferential for females as compared with males. Low doses of lead, sufficient to produce some microscopically discernible hemorrhagic encephalopathy in the cerebellum of young rats but not resulting in failure to gain weight normally, did not depress myelination (Sundstrom and Karlsson, 1987).

TRIETHYLLEAD

Despite similarities in the chemistry of trialkyltin and trialkyllead, triethyllead given to adult rats does not target myelin as does triethyltin. The compounds are similar in that triethyllead given to developing animals does block myelin accumulation (Konat and Clausen, 1976). A metabolic study by this group (Konat et al., 1976) also suggests some specificity for myelin in that total protein synthesis in the forebrain was less affected than was synthesis of myelin protein. Protein composition of the myelin that is formed is normal (Konat and Clausen, 1978). In still other studies (Konat and Clausen, 1980; Konat and Offner, 1982), some evidence was obtained for interference in post-translational processing of integral membrane proteins such as those composing myelin. Windebank (1986) used an in vitro model system of dorsal root ganglion neurons that were cultured so as to grow out and be myelinated. Lead produced complete inhibition of myelination at 10^{-6} M; the author suggests that this indicates a preferential effect on myelination.

METHYLMERCURY

Methylmercury is a potent neurotoxicant that affects many neurobiological processes (Chang, 1990). It has been suggested, however, that damage to neurons and that evidenced in myelin may be independently initiated. Subsequent to in vivo treatment of rats with methylmercury, cerebellar slices are diminished with respect to a capacity to incorporate sulfate into the myelin characteristic lipid sulfatide. In vitro studies (Grundt and Neskovic, 1980) indicate that methylmercury inhibits a number of enzymes that are involved in synthesis of myelin lipids. Kawamata et al. (1987) demonstrated that acute dosing with methylmercury (injection of 10 mg of methylmercury chloride/kg body weight each day) inhibits the normal phosphorylation of peripheral myelin proteins.

CUPRIZONE

Cuprizone (biscyclohexanoneoxalyhydrazone) is a copper chelator. When administered to weanling mice it results in a CNS demyelination that is reversible upon removal of Cuprizone from the diet. The loss of myelin, as measured by decrease of galactosylcera-mide, may be as great as 70% in white matter regions of the cerebrum (Carey and Freeman, 1983). The insult is highly species-specific, since it can be induced in rats but not nearly as readily in mice (Love, 1988). In connection with this model, Fujita et al. (1990) studied the regulation of the mRNA for myelin-associated glycoprotein, a molecule located at the myelin-axonal interfaces and thought to be involved in the axon-glial cell recognition process. The mRNA exists in two major splice variants. Both are severely down-regulated during the demyelinating phase. Upon termination of Cuprizone treatment and consequent remyelination, one splice variant reaches normal levels and the other mRNA species actually accumulates above control levels.

A straightforward interpretation of the pathophysiology is that the chelation of copper results in a deficiency in cytochrome oxidase activity, hence retarding the generation of ATP and of energy-driven ion transport. Again, though, it appears there are myelin- or oligodendroglial cell–specific aspects of Cuprizone toxicity. Of particular interest is the observation that chronic Cuprizone application inhibits carbonic anhydrase activity well before demyelination can be observed (Komoly et al., 1987). Cuprizone-induced demye-lination is not obligatorily linked to blood-brain barrier alterations (Bakker and Ludwin, 1987). This is in contrast to the situation in the PNS, when demyelination is obligatorily linked to blood-nerve barrier breakdown (see chapter 8).

ISONIAZID

The drug isoniazid (isonicotinoylhydrazide), used in therapy for tuberculosis, interferes with activity of vitamin B_6–dependent enzymes. This action is largely due to inhibition of synthesis of the active coenzyme by inhibition of pyridoxal phosphokinase. Isoniazid administration can lead to a peripheral neuropathy in both humans (e.g., Ochoa, 1970) and animals. In rats the neuropathy can be induced acutely at a dose of over 1000mg/kg or chronically by presenting isoniazid as 0.25% of the diet. The neuropathy is initially distal and is more severe in motor nerves (reviewed by Blakemore, 1980). The pathology is usually interpreted as involving initial damage to the axon and therefore being of the wallerian type. It is discussed in this chapter because there are changes in myelin and Schwann cell structure early in the course of the pathology (Schlaepfer and Hager, 1964; Sea and Peterson, 1975). This may be related to the nature of the pathological mechanism. Morphologically, an edema is apparent that is unusual because water collects between the myelin and the axon, compressing the axon and causing separation of most of its surface from the encircling myelinating Schwann cell (Jacobs et al., 1979). This may be an example in which the structure of the myelinated unit is a factor in susceptibility to a toxicant.

It has been noted by Blakemore (1980) that in certain species (dogs but not rats) there is also development of CNS lesions, primarily related to oligodendroglial cells and characterized initially by myelin edema and vacuolation resembling that seen with

Cuprizone treatment. There is a difference in the pathogenesis of isoniazid-induced central and peripheral lesions, since the latter, but not the former, can usually be prevented by the simultaneous adminisration of pyridoxine. The molecular basis of targeting for the oligodendroglial cells in certain circumstances is not known.

DIPHTHERIA TOXIN

The human disease diphtheria is induced by *Corynebacterium diphtheriae* infection. Although animals do not normally become infected, the disease can be mimicked by parenteral administration of the toxin. The observation of neuropathy in infected humans and animals receiving the toxin has been followed up by studies after intraneural injection of the toxin. There is prominent segmental demyelination of the injected nerve (Cavanaugh and Jacobs, 1964). The model of intraneural injection of toxin into rat sciatic nerve is useful for morphological studies of primary demyelination and remyelination (Hildebrand, 1989). It has long been known that diphtheria toxin interferes with certain aspects of protein synthesis. There is some evidence, obtained by incubating sciatic nerve with radioactive precursors in the presence of toxin, that there is preferential inhibition of the synthesis of myelin proteins (Pleasure et al., 1973).

TELLURIUM

Although tellurium toxicity in humans is extremely rare, the primary demyelination induced in rats by tellurium feeding is of interest as a model system for correlation of a specific metabolic insult and demyelination. When weanling rats, 20 days of age, are given a diet containing approximately 1% by dry weight of elemental tellurium, there is rapid onset of neuropathy. Within 3 days the animals have severe hind-limb paralysis. The morphological correlate is a segmental demyelination of the sciatic nerve with few observable degenerative changes in axons; nonmyelinating Schwann cells are not affected (Lampert et al., 1970; Duckett et al., 1979; Takahashi, 1981; Said and Duckett, 1981). Only young animals undergo demyelination; adults given tellurium have only relatively subtle perturbations. The largest myelin internodes are the most vulnerable (Bouldin et al., 1988).

Tellurium intoxication also results in profound inhibition of cholesterol synthesis by inhibition of squalene epoxidase (Harry et al., 1989; Wagner-Recio et al., 1991). The block of cholesterol synthesis is systemic; there is some accumulation of squalene (the substrate for the blocked reaction) in all organs, and in the liver, accumulation of squalene accounts for 10% of dry weight after 5 days of treatment. Accumulation is much less dramatic in the sciatic nerve, but it is many times above control levels and can be visualized as lipid droplets within myelinating Schwann cells (Goodrum et al., 1990). Experiments with labeled precursors of lipids and proteins show that squalene accumulation is by far the most dramatic observable perturbation, and thus a block in cholesterol synthesis appears to be the initial and very prominent metabolic event. It is thus tempting to assign the observed demyelination as being directly consequent to the block in cholesterol synthesis. Recent work (Toews et al., 1990) demonstrates that the lack of cholesterol rapidly brings about inhibition, at the level of transcription, of the synthesis of myelin proteins in the PNS. This level of analysis of a toxicant-induced demyelination helps define several questions.

Why does the systemic block in cholesterol biosynthesis have such specificity for pathology of peripheral nerves? A partial explanation is that enzyme activities involved in biosynthesis of cholesterol by the liver, including squalene epoxidase, which is initially blocked by tellurium treatment, are rapidly up-regulated (Toews et al., 1991, and unpublished results from the author's laboratory). This up-regulation, as well as the presence of dietary cholesterol, keeps circulating cholesterol levels normal and allows for transfer of cholesterol to most tissues. Peripheral nerves, however, cannot utilize circulating cholesterol; the source of cholesterol for myelin in nerve is exclusively local biosynthesis (Jurevics and Morell, 1994). Furthermore, control of the rate-limiting enzyme in cholesterol biosynthesis, hydroxymethylglutaryl-CoA reductase, is sufficiently different in liver and nerve so that the compensatory up-regulation seen in the liver does not occur in nerves (Wagner-Recio et al., 1991; Toews et al., 1991). It is not surprising that aspects of the control of cholesterol biosynthesis are different in the liver and the nervous system. In the liver, the feedback mechanisms controlling cholesterol biosynthesis are set by the levels of circulating plasma lipoproteins. Less is known about control of cholesterol biosynthesis in nervous tissue, but it seems reasonable that production of cholesterol should be coupled to the need for myelin synthesis and coordinately controlled with the production of other myelin components. In any case, the shutdown of synthesis of PNS myelin components, coupled with even the slow rate of normal metabolic turnover of myelin, leads to destabilization and breakdown of this structure. It should be emphasized that myelin has rigid requirements for lipid fluidity necessary for maintenance of its highly ordered structure; even relatively slight shifts in composition could easily lead to its destabilization and collapse.

Another question is, Why is the CNS spared? The reason for this is probably that, at the time of tellurium insult in weanling rats, the normal rate of accumulation of myelin, and therefore demand for cholesterol, is at least an order of magnitude higher in the sciatic nerve than in the brain (Rawlins and Smith, 1971). Thus, the lack of cholesterol has a proportionately more severe affect on the PNS than on the CNS. The suggestion that a rapid rate of synthesis of myelin is an important factor receives support from the fact that weanling animals (a time when PNS myelin is accumulating very rapidly) are preferentially susceptible and that this susceptibility drops off very rapidly with further maturation. Other aspects of the use of this model to study the cell-biological aspects of peripheral demyelination are described in Chapter 8.

2′,3′-DIDEOXYCYTIDINE

The nucleoside analogue 2′,3′-dideoxycytidine is clinically relevant as an inhibitor of human immunodeficiency virus reverse transcriptase. The occasional dose-related neuropathy consequent to treatment of human patients has been further investigated with a rabbit model (Anderson et al., 1992). There is species specificity in that the animal model is more specific for damage to myelin than is the human disorder. Dose levels of above 50 mg/kg/day by oral intubation resulted in clinical neuropathy with myelin splitting and intramyelinic edema, as well as demyelination and remyelination in peripheral nerves. There is axonopathy as manifested by a reduction in the number of larger axons. Anderson et al. suggest that "the myelinopathy observed apparently precedes and may precipitate any subsequent axonopathy." One reason to pursue this model is to test the possibility that a pure myelinopathy can precipitate axonopathy. Although it is clear that axonopathy leads to demyelination, whether the converse occurs has not been unambiguously demonstrated. In this context, a question to be resolved is whether the action of dideoxycytidine is indeed specific for Schwann cells or whether there is also some toxicity for neurons that is just expressed later than in Schwann cells. Another aspect of specificity for dideoxycytidine toxicity is possible targeting of the mitochondrial DNA polymerase (Chen and Cheng, 1989), although it is not clear how this would target Schwann cells preferentially. Specificity for Schwann cells relative to oligodendroglia may relate to partial exclusion of dideoxycytidine from brain (Kelley et al., 1987).

VIGABATRIN

Vigabatrin (γ-vinyl-γ-aminobutyric acid) is an enzyme-activated, irreversible inhibitor of γ-aminobutyric acid (GABA) transaminase and is of clinical utility as an antiepileptic drug. It causes vacuolation in CNS myelinated tracts as a result of splitting at the intraperiod line of the myelin sheath (Butler, 1989). The myelin pathology is species-specific, being found in rodents and dogs but not in primates (Cannon et al., 1991). The pathology is not duplicated by presentation of vigabatrin to myelinated rat cerebellar cultures (Hauw et al., 1989). The relationship between the metabolic block, which might perturb levels of the inhibitory transmitter GABA, and specificity for oligodendroglial cells or myelin is not clear. It may be relevant that cultured oligodendroglial cells are depolarized by GABA (Gilbert et al., 1984) and that cell lines of oligodendroglial cell origin have GABA receptors that are different from those on neurons or astrocytes (von Blankenfeld et al., 1991). It might be, however, that the pathology is secondary to a decrease in activity of the underlying axons that is not reflected in alterations in structure.

CARBON MONOXIDE

Carbon monoxide binds to hemoglobin and thus rapidly blocks the availability of oxygen to tissues. Carbon monoxide poisoning has long been known to involve white matter pathology; the human pathology has been reviewed and classified by Lapresle and Fardeau (1967). Although this situation is an anoxic insult, it differs somewhat from hypoxia in that, although oxygen content is greatly reduced, arterial oxygen tension may not be so affected. The observed tissue damage reflects not only hypoxia; carbon monoxide poisoning is usually accompanied by partial ischemia (reviewed by Ginsberg, 1980). A primate model, exposure of juvenile rhesus monkeys to 0.1–0.3% carbon monoxide for various times, has been extensively studied by Ginsberg et al. (1974), who consistently observed severe white matter damage. Nevertheless, there is no evidence that primary damage is to myelin or oligodendroglial cells. An electron microscopic study by Funata et al. (1982) showed that in cats exposed to carbon monoxide, the axonal damage occurred before damage to myelin.

The more general phenomenon of white matter damage during anoxia has been the target of research and speculation. It is clear that certain types of anoxic insult, such as carbon monoxide poisoning, produce white matter damage through a mechanism that is "specific" to white matter in that it is different from the mechanism causing anoxic damage to gray matter. It is thought that anoxia causes damage to neuronal cell bodies by allowing for influx of Ca^{2+} through excitotoxin-gated channels (Choi, 1988). A current hypothesis to account for the damage to white matter also invokes entry of excess Ca^{2+}, but in this case secondary to influx of Na^+ and reverse operation of the Na^+-Ca^{2+} exchange process. Waxman et al. (1991) review evidence that this is because of the density of sodium channels in a restricted area of the axonal membrane, a phenomenon specific for myelinated axons at the nodes of Ranvier. Under ordinary conditions, the Na^+ gradient in the axon is maintained by the Na^+-K^+ pump; this prevents Ca^{2+} from accumulating by maintaining operation of the Na^+-Ca^{2+} exchanger (exchanging intracellular Ca^{2+} for extracellular Na^+). Waxman et al. (1991) suggest that, as energy metabolism declines in anoxia, there is no longer adequate energy-dependent exclusion of Na^+ from the axon in the nodal region. The region of the axon directly below the node of Ranvier, where Na^+ would be expected to enter, may have sufficient accumulation of Na^+ to be preferentially vulnerable to reversal of the Na^+-Ca^{2+} exchanger.

SUMMARY COMMENTS AND FUTURE PERSPECTIVES

Myelinopathy is defined in morphological terms as a process causing damage to white matter. As noted earlier, this classification applies to some degree to a large variety of toxicant-induced disorders, since any event that causes neuronal death will result in damage to the white matter associated with the axons of those neurons. There are, however, a number of situations where damage to myelin or myelinating cells, or to the structure of the myelinated axon, is an initial site of action of a toxicant. This suggests that the toxicant targets some specific aspect of the chemistry, metabolism, or structure of myelin or myelinating glia. Hydrophobicity of a toxicant, promoting its accumulation in myelin, is assumed to be relevant in several of the cases discussed (e.g., triethyltin and hexachlorophene). Interference with active exclusion of water from compacted layers of myelin is clearly an important factor in primary demyelination. Not enough is known about the normal operation of this mechanism to localize the toxicant induced lesions at a molecular level. Processes with which toxicants could interfere include oxidative phosphorylation, inhibition of an enzyme involved with some specialized aspect of ion or water transport, or direct damage to myelin such that the ion gradients generated to pump water cannot be isolated between impermeable membranes. Again, triethyltin and hexachlorophene are examples of toxicants that almost certainly have mechanisms of action relating to movement of water. Specialized aspects of the composition of myelin, and of the metabolic pathways involved in controlling this composition, are also points of vulnerability. In the example of tellurium toxicity, cholesterol biosynthesis and nervous system–specific aspects of its biosynthesis are targeted. Susceptibility of myelintion to metabolic insult during particular developmental phases (corresponding to proliferation of certain precursor cells and to the period of very rapid myelination) is illustrated with several of the toxicants that have different effects when applied during development relative to exposure during adulthood. There is also the interesting class of disorders (e.g., those related to anoxia, such as carbon monoxide poisoning) that may target some aspect of axonal metabolism that is dictated by its being part of the axon-myelin unit.

Further knowledge as to what factors are involved in toxic insults specific to myelin is limited by our knowledge of the metabolic processes preferentially expressed in the synthesis and metabolic support of this structure. It is, for example, conceivable that certain toxicants that are soluble in membranes could preferentially directly disturb the structure of myelin. There are many as yet only partially understood steps in the process of recognition and interaction between myelinating glia and axons and in the specific program of events that leads to up-regulation of myelin synthesis (for a review of events as they relate to Schwann cells, see Gould et al., 1992). It is possible that some of these are preferentially vulnerable to certain toxicants. It is well known that there are metabolic relationships between axons and mature glial cells, presumably including exchanges of some sort of extracellular signals, and that these are necessary to sustain their functional relationship. There is a literature concerning these relationships as they involve non-myelinating Schwann cells (e.g., Villegas, 1978; Jahromi et al., 1992) and some information relating to myelinating Schwann cells (e.g., Gould et al., 1992). These processes are also potential targets for toxicity. As noted earlier, susceptibility of CNS myelin to damage from vigabatrin, which perturbs levels of an inhibitory neurotransmitter, may reflect interference with a neurotransmitter-mediated communication between neurons and oligodendroglia. The history of development of understanding of mechanisms of toxic insult to myelin is parallel to the situation in other areas of neurotoxicology—better understanding of pathological processes is coupled to gains in basic knowledge of normal operation of the nervous system.

ACKNOWLEDGMENTS

The excellent review by Cammer (1980) was of great value to me in developing my views concerning metabolic susceptibility of myelin to toxic insult. I acknowledge discussions with Dr. Wendy Cammer and with Dr. Arrel Toews on topics mentioned herein. My own research in myelin and in toxic insults to myelin has been funded primarily by U.S. Public Health Service grants ESO1104 and NS11615.

REFERENCES

Aldridge WN, Cremer JE (1955). The biochemistry of organo-tin compounds; diethyltin dichloride and triethyltin sulfate. Biochem J 61:406–18.

Aldridge WN, Verschoyle RD, Thompson CA, Brown AW (1987). The toxicity and neuropathology of dimethylethyltin and methyldiethyltin in rats. Neuropathol Appl Neurobiol 13:55–69.

Aleu FP, Katzman R, Terry RD (1963). Fine structure and electrolyte analysis of cerebral edema induced by alkyl tin intoxication. J Neuropathol Exp Neurol 22:403–13.

Anderson TD, Davidovich A, Arceo R, Brosnan C, Arezzo J, Schaumburg H (1992). Peripheral neuropathy induced by 2′,3′-dideoxycytidine. A rabbit model of 2′,3′-dideoxycytidine neurotoxicity. Lab Invest 66:63–74.

Baichwal R, DeVries G (1989). A mitogen for Schwann cells is derived from myelin basic protein. Biochem Biophys Res Commun 164:883–8.

Bakker DA, Ludwin SK (1987). Blood-brain barrier permeability during Cuprizone-induced demyelination. Implications for the pathogenesis of immune-mediated demyelination diseases. J Neurol Sci 78:125–37.

Barres BA, Chun LLY, Corey DP (1990). Ion channels in vertebrate glia. Annu Rev Neurosci 13:441–74.

Benjamins JA, Smith ME (1984). Metabolism of myelin. In: Morell P, ed. Myelin. 2nd ed. New York: Plenum Press, 225–49.

Benjamins JA, Morell P, Hartman BK, Agrawal HC (1984). CNS myelin. In: Lajtha A, ed. Handbook of neurochemistry. New York: Plenum Press, 361–415.

Black JA, Kocsis JD, Waxman SG (1991). Ion channel organization of the myelinated fiber. Trends Neurosci 13:48–54.

Blakemore WF (1980). Isoniazid. In: Spencer PS, Schaumburg HH, eds. Experimental and clinical neurotoxicology. Baltimore: Williams & Williams, 476–89.

Blaker WD, Krigman MR, Thomas DJ, Mushak P, Morell P (1981). Effect of triethyl tin on myelination in the developing rat. J Neurochem 36:44–52.

Bouldin TW, Samsa G, Earnhardt T, Krigman MR (1988). Schwann-cell vulnerability to demyelination is associated with internodal length in tellurium neuropathy. J Neuropathol Exp Neurol 47:41–7.

Bourke RS, Kimelberg HK (1975). The effect of HCO_3^- on the swelling and ion uptake of monkey cerebral cortex under conditions of raised extracellular potassium. J Neurochem 25:323–8.

Braun PE, Bambrick LL, Edwards AM, Bernier L (1990a). 2',3'-cyclic nucleotide 3'-phosphodiesterase has characteristics of cytoskeletal proteins. A hypothesis for its function. Ann NY Acad Sci 605:55–65.

Braun PE, Horvath E, Yong VW, Bernier L (1990b). Identification of GTP-binding proteins in myelin and oligodendrocyte membranes. J Neurosci Res 26:16–23.

Butler WH (1989). The neuropathology of vigabatrin. Epilepsia 30:S3:15–17.

Cammer W (1980). Toxic demyelination: biochemical studies and hypothetical mechanisms. In: Spencer PS, Schaumburg HH, eds. Experimental and clinical neurotoxicology. Baltimore: Williams & Williams, 239–56.

Cammer W, Moore CL (1972). The effect of hexachlorophene on the respiration of liver and brain mitochondria. Biochem Biophys Res Commun 46:1887–94.

Cammer W, Fredman T, Rose AL, Norton WT (1976). Brain carbonic anhydrase: activity in isolated myelin and the effect of hexachlorophene. J Neurochem 27:165–71.

Cammer W, Rose AL, Norton WT (1975). Biochemical and pathological studies of myelin in hexachlorophene intoxication. Brain Res 98:547–59.

Cannon DJ, Butler WH, Mumford JP, Lewis PJ (1991). Neuropathologic findings in patients receiving long-term vigabatrin therapy for chronic intractable epilepsy. J Child Neurol 2:17–24.

Carey EM, Freeman NM (1983). Biochemical changes in Cuprizone-induced spongiform encephalopathy. I. Changes in the activities of 2',3'-cyclic nucleotide 3'-phosphohydrolase, oligodendroglial ceramide galactosyl transferase, and the hydrolysis of the alkenyl group of alkenyl, acyl-glycerophospholipids by plasmalogenase in different regions of the brain. Neurochem Res 8:1029–44.

Cavanaugh JB, Jacobs JM (1964). Some quantitative aspects of diphtheritic neuropathy. Br J Exp Pathol 45:309–22.

Chang LW (1990). The neurotoxicology and pathology of organomercury, organolead, and organotin. J Toxicol Sci 15:S4:125–151.

Chen C, Cheng Y (1989). Delayed cytotoxicity and selective loss of mitochondrial DNA in cells treated with the anti–human immunodeficiency virus compound 2',3'-dideoxycytidine. J Biol Chem 264:11934–7.

Choi DW (1988). Calcium-mediated neurotoxicity: a relationship to specific channel types and role in ischemic damage. Trends Neurosci 11:465–9.

Deshmukh DS, Kuizon S, Bear WD, Brockerhoff H (1981). Rapid incorporation in vivo of intracerebrally injected $^{32}P_i$ into polyphosphoinositides of three subfractions of rat brain myelin. J Neurochem 36:594–601.

DesJardins KC, Morell P (1983). The phosphate groups modifying myelin basic proteins are metabolically labile; the methyl groups are stable. J Cell Biol 97:438–46.

Duckett S, Said G, Streletz LG, White RG, Galle P (1979). Tellurium-induced neuropathy: correlative physiological, morphological and electron microprobe studies. Neuropathol Appl Neurobiol 5:265–78.

Dyck PJ, O'Brien PC, Ohnishi A (1977). Lead neuropathy: 2. Random distribution of segmental demyelination among "old internodes" of myelinated fibers. J Neuropathol Exp Neurol 36:570–5.

Eto Y, Suzuki K, Suzuki K (1971). Lipid composition of rat brain myelin in triethyl tin–induced edema. J Lipid Res 12:570–9.

Fujita N, Ishiguro H, Sato S, Kurihara T, Kuwano R, Sakimura K, Takahashi Y, Miyatake T (1990). Induction of myelin-associated mRNA in experimental remyelination. Brain Res 513:152–5.

Funata N, Okeda R, Takano T, Miyazaki Y (1982). Electron microscopic observations of experimental carbon monoxide encephalopathy in the acute phase. Acta Pathol Jpn 32:219–29.

Gaines TB, Kimbrough RD, Linder RE (1973). The oral and dermal toxicity of hexachlorophene in rats. Toxicol Appl Pharmacol 25:332–43.

Gilbert P, Kettenmann H, Schachner M (1984). τ-Aminobutyric acid directly depolarizes cultured oligodendrocytes. J Neurosci 4:561–9.

Ginsberg MD (1980). Carbon monoxide. In: Spencer PS, Schaumburg HH, eds. Experimental and clinical neurotoxicology. Baltimore: Williams & Williams, 374–94.

Ginsberg MD, Myers RE, McDonagh BF (1974). Experimental carbon monoxide encephalopathy in the primate: II. Clinical aspects, neuropathology, and physiologic correlation. Arch Neurol 30:209–16.

Goodrum JF, Earnhardt TS, Goines ND, Bouldin TW (1990). Lipid droplets in Schwann cells during tellurium neuropathy are derived from newly synthesized lipid. J Neurochem 55: 1928–32.

Gould RM, Kristjan RJ, Mirsky R, Tennekoon G (1992). The cell of Schwann: an update. In: Martenson RE, ed. Myelin: biology and chemistry. Boca Raton, Florida: CRC Press, 123–71.

Graham DI, Gonatas NK (1973). Triethyltin sulfate–induced splitting of peripheral myelin in rats. Lab Invest 29:628–32.

Graham DI, Kim SU, Gonatas NK, Guyotte L (1975). The neurotoxic effects of triethyltin sulfate on myelinating cultures of mouse spinal cord. J Neuropathol Exp Neurol 34:401–12.

Grundt I, Neskovic NM (1980). Comparison of the inhibition by methylmercury and triethyllead of galactolipid accumulation in rat brain. Environ Res 23:282–91.

Gump WS (1969). Toxicological properties of hexachlorophene. J Soc Cosmet Chem 20:173–84.

Harry GJ, Goodrum JF, Bouldin TW, Wagner-Recio M, Toews AD, Morell P (1989). Tellurium-induced neuropathy: metabolic alterations associated with demyelination and remyelination in rat sciatic nerve. J Neurochem 52:938–45.

Harry GJ, Toews AD, Krigman MR, Morell P (1985). The effect of lead toxicity and milk deprivation on myelination in the rat. Toxicol Appl Pharmacol 77:458–64.

Hauw JJ, Boutry JM, Sun P, Sazdovitch V, Duyckaerts C (1989). Effects of vigabatrin and of GABA on myelinated rat cerebellar cultures: preliminary data. Br J Clin Pharmacol 27(suppl): 47S–52S.

Herter WB (1959). Hexachlorophene poisoning. Kaiser Found Med Bull 7:228–30.

Hildebrand C (1989). Myelin sheath remodelling in remyelinated rat sciatic nerve. J Neurocytol 18:285–94.

Jacobs KS, Miller RH, Whittle A, Cavanaugh JB (1979). Studies on the early changes in acute isoniazid neuropathy in the rat. Acta Neuropathol 47:85–92.

Jacobs KS, Lemasters JJ, Reiter LW (1983). Inhibition of ATPase activities of brain and liver homogenates by triethyltin (TET). Dev Toxicol Environ Sci 11:517–20.

Jahromi BS, Robitaille R, Charlton MP (1992). Transmitter release increases intracellular calcium in perisynaptic Schwann cells in situ. Neuron 8:1069–77.

Jurevics HA, Morell P (1994). Sources of cholesterol for kidney and nerve during development. J Lipid Res 35(in press).

Kahn DW, Morell P (1988). Phosphatidic acid and phosphoinositide turnover in myelin and its stimulation by acetylcholine. J Neurochem 50:1542–50.

Kawamata O, Kasama H, Omata S, Sugano H (1987). Decrease in protein phosphorylation in central and peripheral nervous tissues of methylmercury-treated rat. Arch Toxicol 59:346–52.

Kelley JA, Litterst CL, Roth JS, Vistica DT, Opolack DG, Cooney DA, Nadkarni M, Balis FM, Broder S, Johns DG (1987). The disposition and metabolism of 2',3'-dideoxycytidine, an in vitro inhibitor of human T-lymphotrophic virus type III infectivity, in mice and monkeys. Drug Metab Disp 15:595–601.

Kimbrough RD (1976). Hexachlorophene: toxicity and use as an antibacterial agent. In: Hayes WJ Jr, ed. Essays in toxicology. Vol. 7. New York: Academic Press, 99–120.

Kirschner DA, Sapirstein VS (1982). Triethyl tin–induced myelin oedema: an intermediate swelling state detected by x-ray diffraction. J Neurocytol 11:559–69.

Kitamura K, Suzuki M, Uyemura K (1976). Purification and partial characterization of two glycoproteins in bovine peripheral myelin membrane. Biochem Biophys Acta 455:806–16.

Komoly S, Jeyasingham MD, Pratt OE, Lantos PL (1987). Decrease in oligodendrocyte carbonic anhydrase activity preceding myelin degeneration in Cuprizone induced demyelination. J Neurol Sci 79:141–8.

Komulainen H, Bondy SC (1987). Increased free intrasynaptosomal Ca^{2+} by neurotoxic organometals: distinctive mechanisms. Toxicol Appl Pharmacol 88:77–86.

Konat G, Clausen J (1976). Triethyllead-induced hypomyelination in the developing rat forebrain. Exp Neurol 50:124–33.

Konat G, Clausen J (1978). Protein composition of forebrain myelin isolated from triethyllead-intoxicated young rats. J Neurochem 30:907–9.

Konat G, Clausen J (1980). Suppressive effect of triethyllead on entry of proteins into the CNS myelin sheath in vitro. J Neurochem 35:382–7.

Konat G, Offner H (1982). Effect of triethyllead on post-translational processing of myelin proteins. Exp Neurol 75:89–94.

Konat G, Offner H, Clausen J (1976). Triethyllead-restrained myelin deposition and protein synthesis in the developing rat forebrain. Exp Neurol 52:58–65.

Krigman MR, Bouldin TW, Mushak P (1980). Lead. In: Spencer PS, Schaumburg HH, eds. Experimental and clinical neurotoxicology. Baltimore: Williams & Williams, 490–507.

Kung MP, Nickerson PA, Sansone FM, Olson JR, Kostyniak PJ, Adolf MA, Roth JA (1988). Effect of chronic exposure to hexachlorophene on rat brain cell specific marker enzymes. Neurotoxicology 10:201–10.

Kung MP, Nickerson PA, Sansone FM, Olson JR, Kostyniak PJ, Adolf MA, Lein PJ, Roth JA (1989). Effect of short-term exposure to hexachlorophene on rat brain cell specific marker enzymes. Fund Appl Toxicol 11:519–27.

Lampert PW, Schochet SS (1968). Demyelination and remyelination in lead neuropathy: electron microscopic studies. J Neuropathol Exp Neurol 27:527–45.

Lampert P, Garro F, Pentschew A (1970). Tellurium neuropathy. Acta Neuropathol (Berlin) 15:308–17.

Lapresle J, Fardeau M (1967). The central nervous system and carbon monoxide poisoning: II. Anatomical study of brain lesions following intoxication with carbon monoxide (22 cases). Prog Brain Res 24:31–74.

Ledeen RW (1992). Enzymes and receptors of myelin. In: Martenson RE, ed. Myelin: biology and chemistry. Boca Raton, Florida: CRC Press, 531–70.

Lees MB, Brostoff SW (1984). Proteins of myelin. In: Morell P, ed. Myelin. 2nd ed. New York: Plenum Press, 197–217.

Lin L-FH, Lees MB (1982). Interactions of dicyclohexyl-carbodiimide with myelin proteolipid. Proc Natl Acad Sci USA 79:941–5.

Lock EA (1976). The action of triethyltin on the respiration of rat brain cortex slices. J Neurochem 26:887–92.

Lock EA, Aldridge WN (1975). The binding of triethyltin to rat brain myelin. J Neurochem 25:871–6.

Love S (1988). Cuprizone neurotoxicity in the rat: morphologic observations. J Neurol Sci 84:223–37.

Martenson RE, Uyemura K (1992). Myelin P2, a neuritogenic member of the family of cytoplasmic lipid-binding proteins. In: Martenson RE, ed. Myelin: biology and chemistry. Boca Raton, Florida: CRC Press, 509–28.

Martenson RE, ed. (1992). Myelin: biology and chemistry. Boca Raton, Florida: CRC Press.

Matthieu M-M, Zimmerman AW, Webster HdeF, Ulsamer AG, Brady RO, Quarles RH (1974). Hexachlorophene intoxication: characterization of myelin and myelin related fractions in the rat during early postnatal development. Exp Neurol 45:558–75.

Mikoshiba K, Okano H, Tamura T, Ikenaka K (1991). Structure and function of myelin protein genes. Annu Rev Neurosci 140:201–17.

Monton F, Coria F (1991). Reversible Schwann cell hypertrophy in lead neuropathy. Neuropathol Appl Neurobiol 17:231–6.

Morell P, Ed. (1984). Myelin. 2nd Ed. New York: Plenum Press.

Morell P, Quarles RH, Norton WT (1993). Myelin formation, structure, and biochemistry. In: Albers RW, Siegel GW, Molinoff P, Agranoff B, eds. Basic nueorchemistry. 5th Ed. New York: Raven Press, 117–143.

Nieminen L, Bjondahl K, Mottonen M (1973). Effect of hexachlorophene on the rat brain during organogenesis. Food Cosmet Toxicol 11:635–9.

Norton WT, Cammer W (1984). Isolation and characterization of myelin. In: Morell P, ed. Myelin. 2nd ed. New York: Plenum Press, 147–95.

O'Callaghan JP, Miller DB (1984). Neuron-specific phosphoproteins as biochemical indicators of neurotoxicity: effects of acute administration of trimethyltin to the adult rat. J Pharmacol Exp Ther 231:737–43.

O'Callaghan JP, Miller DB (1988). Acute exposure of the neonatal rat to triethyltin results in persistent changes in neurotypic and gliotypic proteins. J Pharmacol Exp Ther 244:368–78.

Ochoa J (1970). Isoniazid neuropathy in man: quantitative electron microscope study. Brain 93:831–50.

Ohnishi A, Schilling K, Brimijoin WS, Lambert EH, Fairbanks VG, Dyck PJ (1977). Lead neuropathy: 1. Morphometry, nerve conduction, and choline acetyltransferase transport: new finding of edema associated with segmental demyelination. J Neuropathol Exp Neurol 36:499–518.

Ousley AH, Morell P (1992). Individual molecular species of phosphatidylcholine and phosphatidylethanolamine in myelin turn over at different rates. J Biol Chem 267:10362–9.

Pleasure DB, Feldman B, Prockop DJ (1973). Diphtheria toxin inhibits the syntiesis of myelin proteolipid and basic proteins by peripheral nerve in vitro. J Neurochem 20:81–90.

Powell H, Searner O, Gluck L, Lampert P (1973). Hexachlorophene myelinopathy in premature infants. J Pediatr 82:976–81.

Powers MF, Beavis AD (1991). Triorganotins inhibit the mitochondrial inner membrane anion channel. J Biol Chem 266:17250–6.

Quarles RH, Colman DR, Salzer JL, Trapp BD (1992). Myelin-associated glycoprotein: structure-function relationships and involvement in neurological diseases. In: Martenson RE, ed. Myelin; biology and chemistry. Boca Raton, Florida: CRC Press, 413–48.

Rawlins FA, Smith ME (1971). Myelin synthesis in vitro: a comparative study of central and peripheral nervous tissue. J Neurochem 18:1861–70.

Reier PJ, Tabira T, Webster HdeF (1978). Hexachlorophene-induced myelin lesions in the amphibian central nervous system: a freeze-fracture study. J Neurol Sci 35:257–74.

Reiss DS, Lees MB, Sapirstein VS (1981). Is Na^+,K^+-ATPase a myelin associated enzyme? J Neurochem 36:1418–26.

Ritchie JM (1984). Physiological basis of conduction in myelinated nerve fibers. In: Morell P, ed. Myelin. 2nd Ed. New York: Plenum Press, 117–41.

Rouzaud M, Lutier J (1954). Oédeme subaigu cérébrométéningé du a une intoxication d'actualité. Presse Médicale 62:1075.

Said G, Duckett S (1981). Tellurium-induced myelinopathy in adult rats. Muscle Nerve 4:319–25.

Salzer JL, Bunge RP (1980). Studies of Schwann cell proliferation. I. An analysis in tissue culture of proliferation during development, wallerian degeneration and direct injury. J Cell Biol 84:739–52.

Schlaepfer WW (1969). Experimental lead neuropathy: a disease of the supporting cells in the peripheral nervous system. J Neuropathol Exp Neurol 28:401–18.

Schlaepfer WW, Hager H (1964). Ultrastructural studies of INH-induced neuropathy in rats. II. Alteration and decomposition of the myelin sheath. Am J Pathol 45:423–33.

Schwab ME (1990). Myelin-associated inhibitors of neurite growth and regeneration in the CNS. TINS 13:452–6.

Sea CP, Peterson RG (1975). Ultrastructure and biochemistry of myelin after isoniazid-induced nerve degeneration in rats. Exp Neurol 48:252–60.

Selwyn MJ, Dawson AP, Stockdale M, Grain N (1970). Chloride-hydroxide exchange across mitochondrial, erythrocyte and artificial lipid membranes mediated by trialkyl and triphenyltin compounds. Eur J Biochem 14:120–6.

Silbergeld EK (1984). Mitochondrial mechanisms of lead nmeurotoxicity. In: Narahashi T, ed. Cellular and molecular neurotoxicology. New York: Raven Press, 153–64.

Smith ME (1973). Studies on the mechanism of demyelination: triethyl tin–induced demyelination. J Neurochem 21:357–72.

Smith ME (1983). Peripheral nervous system myelin properties and metabolism. In: Lajtha A, ed. Handbook of neurochemistry. New York: Plenum Press, 201–23.

Snipes GJ, Suter U, Welcher AA, Shooter EM (1992). Characterization of a novel peripheral nervous system myelin protein (PMP-22/SR13). J Cell Biol 117:225–38.

Sprinkle TJ (1989). 2′,3′-cyclic nucleotide 3′-phosphodiesterase, an oligodendrocyte–Schwann cell and myelin-associated enzyme of the nervous system. Crit Rev Neurobiol 4:235–301.

Stine KE, Reiter LW, Lemasters JJ (1988). Alkyltin inhibition of ATPase activities in tissue homogenates and subcellular fractions from adult and neonatal rats. Toxicol Appl Pharmacol 94:394–406.

Sundstrom R, Karlsson B (1987). Myelin basic protein in brains of rats with low dose lead encephalopathy. Arch Toxicol 59:341–5.

Takahashi T (1981). Experimental study on segmental demyelination in tellurium neuropathy. Hokkaido Igaku Zasshi 856:105–31.

Tansey FA, Cammer W (1991). A Pi form of glutathione-S-transferase is a myelin and oligodendrocyte-associated enzyme in mouse brain. J Neurochem 57:95–102.

Toews AD, Krigman MR, Thomas DJ, Morell P (1980). Effect of inorganic lead exposure on myelination in the rat. Neurochem Res 5:605–16.

Toews AD, Lee SY, Popko B, Morell P (1990). Tellurium-induced neuropathy: a model for reversible reductions in myelin protein gene expression. J Neurosci Res 26:501–7.

Toews AD, Blaker WD, Thomas DJ, Gaynor JJ, Krigman MR, Mushak P, Morell P (1983). Myelin deficits produced by early postnatal exposure to inorganic lead or triethyltin are persistent. J Neurochem 41:816–22.

Toews AD, Goodrum JF, Lee SY, Eckermann C, Morell P (1991). Tellurium-induced alterations in HMG-CoA reductase gene expression and enzyme activity: differential effects in sciatic nerve and liver suggest tissue-specific regulation of cholesterol synthesis. J Neurochem 57:1902–6.

Towfighi J (1980). Hexachlorophene. In: Spencer PS, Schaumburg HH, eds. Experimental and clinical neurotoxicology. Baltimore: Williams & Williams, 440–55.

Towfighi J, Gonatas NK, McCree L (1974). Hexachlorophene-induced changes in central and peripheral myelinated axons of developing and adult rats. Lab Invest 31:712–21.

Uyemura K, Kitamura K, Miura M (1992). Structure and molecular biology of PO protein. In: Martenson RE, ed. Myelin: biology and chemistry. Boca Raton, Florida: CRC Press, 413–48.

Veronesi B, Jones K, Gupta S, Pringle J, Mezei C (1991). Myelin basic protein–messenger RNA (MBP-mRNA) expression during triethyltin-induced myelin edema. Neurotoxicology 12:265–76.

Villegas J (1978). Cholinergic systems in axon–Schwann cell interactions. TINS 1:66–8.

Von Blankenfeld G, Trotter J, Kettenmann H (1991). Expression and developmental regulation of a GABA$_A$ receptor in cultured murine cells of the oligodendrocyte lineage. Eur J Neurosci 3:310–6.

Wagner-Recio M, Toews AD, Morell P (1991). Tellurium blocks cholesterol synthesis by inhibiting squalene metabolism: preferential vulnerability to this metabolic block leads to peripheral nervous system demyelination. J Neurochem 57:1891–1901.

Wassenaar JS, Kroon AM (1973). Effects of triethyltin on different ATPases, 5′-nucleotidase and phosphodiesterases in grey and white matter of rabbit brain and their relation with brain edema. Eur Neurol 10:349–70.

Watanabe I (1980). Organotins (triethyltin). In: Spencer PS, Schaumburg HH, eds. Experimental and clinical neurotoxicology. Baltimore: Williams & Williams, 545–57.

Waxman SG, Ransom BR, Stys PK (1991). Non-synaptic mechanisms of Ca(2+)-mediated injury in CNS white matter. Trends Neurosci 14:461–8.

Wiggins RC (1986). Myelination: a critical stage in development. Neurotoxicology 7:103–20.

Windebank AJ (1986). Specific inhibition of myelination by lead in vitro; comparison with arsenic, thallium, and mercury. Exp Neurol 94:203–12.

Yanagisawa K, Ishigro H, Kaneko K, Miyatake T (1990). Acetazolamide inhibits the recovery from triethyl tin intoxication: putative role of carbonic anhydrase in dehydration of central myelin. Neurochem Res 15:483–6.

22
Role of Ion Channels in Neurotoxicity

Toshio Narahashi
Northwestern University Medical School
Chicago, Illinois

INTRODUCTION

Role of Ion Channels in the Nervous System

Classification

Ion channels play vital roles in a variety of normal physiological functions of all kinds of cells. In inexcitable cells, the activity of ion channels is essential for hormone release, cell-to-cell communication, and intracellular calcium homeostasis, to mention a few functions. In excitable cells, ion channels are the critical sites for generation of action potentials, neurotransmitter release, and muscle contraction. Thus it is not surprising to see the increasing evidence that ion channels are the target sites of a variety of chemicals, including therapeutic drugs, toxicants, and natural toxins.

Ion channels may be classified into two large groups: one includes voltage-activated ion channels in which the gating mechanism is controlled by the membrane potential; and the other comprises transmitter-activated ion channels in which the gating mechanism is operated by binding of the neurotransmitter to its receptor. The voltage-activated channels include sodium channels, potassium channels, and calcium channels, and the transmitter-activated channels include those activated by acetylcholine (ACh), glutamate, γ-aminobutyric acid (GABA), glycine, serotonin, dopamine, norepinephrine, and histamine.

The chemicals that cause neurotoxicity comprise a wide variety of agents. Practically all therapeutic drugs are toxic if given at excessive doses, and many of them cause toxicity to the nervous system. Thus, some of the therapeutic drugs that exert potent and/or specific effects on ion channels are discussed in this chapter. Many environmental toxicants are also toxic to the nervous system. Here the term "toxicants" is defined as synthetic toxic chemicals, as opposed to "toxins," which are natural toxic substances. Some of the natural toxins exert potent and specific actions on ion channels. Both environmental neurotoxicants and natural neurotoxins are included in this chapter.

Role of Ion Channels in Action Potentials

Action potentials are generated as a result of opening and closing of certain types of ion channel. For example, in most nerve fibers, opening of sodium channels generates an upstroke of action potential, and closing of sodium channels and opening of potassium channels cause a downstroke of action potential. In cardiac cells, both sodium and calcium channels are involved in the generation of action potentials, and opening of potassium channels terminates the action potential. Propagation of action potentials is mediated by local circuit currents flowing across the nerve membrane that in turn cause opening of the ion channels involved. When an action potential arrives at the nerve terminal, the membrane depolarization opens calcium channels, which in turn causes calcium ions to flow in, thereby triggering release of neurotransmitter.

Role of Ion Channels in Synaptic and Neuromuscular Transmission

As described in the preceding section, opening of calcium channels at the nerve terminal causes release of neurotransmitter. The released transmitter binds to the receptor on the postsynaptic membrane, causing opening of the ion channel associated with that receptor. The ions that carry current through the open channel vary depending on the receptor-channel complex. For example, in the ACh-activated channel, it is mainly sodium and potassium ions that carry the current. In the N-methyl-D-aspartate (NMDA)-activated channel, sodium and calcium carry the current, and in the GABA-activated channel, the current carrier is chloride. The current flowing through the open channel in the postsynaptic membrane causes the excitable membrane that surrounds the postsynaptic membrane to be depolarized, thereby generating action potentials. In inhibitory synapses, such as those in GABAergic system, the current through the postsynaptic membrane may cause a hyperpolarization, a depolarization, or no change in membrane potential, depending on the relative levels of the chloride equilibrium potential and the resting membrane potential. The resultant increase in conductance of inhibitory postsynaptic membrane causes short-circuiting of the surrounding membrane, thereby curtailing the effectiveness of the depolarizing current flowing through the nearby excitatory postsynaptic membrane. This results in inhibition of synaptic transmission.

Approaches and Methods

Since the action potential is generated as a result of complex behavior of ion channels, it is virtually impossible to elucidate the mechanism by which a test compound alters the function of the ion channels by simply observing the action potential. Other difficulties pertain to the fast speed at which excitation takes place. Conventional isotope flux measurements and imaging techniques are too slow to detect and analyze millisecond-order events associated with action potential. Thus it is imperative to record electrical events in order to measure opening and closing of ion channels. The most straightforward and powerful technique is "voltage clamp," whereby currents carried by certain ions through open channels can be recorded and analyzed (Narahashi, 1992a). The voltage clamp technique was first developed by Cole (1949) and was extensively used in the detailed kinetic analyses of sodium and potassium channels of squid giant axons (Hodgkin and Huxley, 1959a,b,c,d; Hodgkin et al., 1952). The technique was then applied to other forms of excitable cells: for the first time to skeletal muscle end plates by Takeuchi and Takeuchi (1959), to central neurons by Hagiwara and Saito (1959), and to the nodes of Ranvier by Dodge and Frankenhaeuser (1958).

Although perfect and straightforward, the classical voltage clamp technique has limitations to its application to various types of excitable cells. It requires "space clamp" conditions in which the membrane potential and current density must be kept uniform through the entire preparation. The space clamp condition can be easily established in large-diameter nerve fibers like squid giant axons, in muscle end plates, and in large neurons without many branches. However, it is extremely difficult, if not impossible, to establish the space clamp condition in some other types of cell, such as cardiac cells that form syncytium and small neurons to which intracellular microelectrodes are difficult to apply.

A breakthrough for this formidable obstacle was made by Neher and Sakmann (1976), who successfully applied a patch electrode to the external surface of denervated skeletal muscle to record currents flowing through individual open channels associated with ACh receptors. This technique, called "patch clamp," was further improved to record single channel currents more accurately (Hamill et al., 1981). This was accomplished by establishing a "gigaohm seal" around the rim of the glass capillary electrode tip. Furthermore, methods were developed whereby a small membrane patch could be isolated from a cell at the tip of the electrode. This provides the flexibility of having either "outside-out" or "inside-out" membrane patch. Methods were also developed to record currents flowing through the entire cell membrane—"whole-cell" patch clamp as opposed to "single-channel" patch clamp. Thus the patch clamp technique, including both whole-cell and single-channel versions, is now applicable to practically any type of cell as long as cell diameter is slightly larger than the electrode tip diameter. Ion channel activities have been studied with a variety of cell types, including central nervous system (CNS) neurons, neuroblastoma cells, skeletal muscle myocytes, cardiac myocytes, smooth muscle cells, lymphocytes, red blood cells, glial cells, and secretory cells, to mention a few. This revolutionary patch clamp technique has made it possible to use any cell types for channel study, thereby broadening the scope of applicability to neurotoxicology as well.

Role of Ion Channels in Neurotoxicity: General Considerations

As briefly outlined in the preceding sections, ion channels play pivotal roles in normal physiological function of the nervous system. Thus it is quite natural to imagine the importance of ion channels in neurotoxicity as well. However, the development of ion channel neurotoxicology has been hampered to some extent for several reasons. First of all, the application of sophisticated electrophysiological techniques, such as voltage clamp, to neurotoxicology depended largely on the development of the techniques. Voltage clamp was not an easy technique when it was developed in the late 1940s and early 1950s. After it was firmly established by Hodgkin et al. (1952) for the study of ion channels of squid giant axons, it took 7 years for the first studies of interactions of local anesthetics with sodium and potassium channels to be published by Taylor (1959) and Shanes et al. (1959). Furthermore, it was not until 1964 that voltage clamp was applied for the first time to the toxicological study of tetrodotoxin (TTX) block of sodium channels (Narahashi et al., 1964). Second, most neurotoxicologists have been working on behavioral, biochemical, or histological aspects of toxic action. Third, neurophysiologists who have been well trained in advanced electrophysiological techniques are in general not interested in neurotoxicology or even do not recognize the potential usefulness of some neurotoxins and neurotoxicants as chemical tools as described below ("Voltage-Activated Ion Channels and Neurotoxicity"). However, studies of ion channel neurotoxicology are now about to flourish, thanks to the development of patch clamp techniques.

Modulation of Voltage-Activated Ion Channels

The types of chemical modulation of voltage-activated ion channels may be divided into two large categories: suppression and augmentation of channel activity (Catterall, 1980; Narahashi, 1984a). Changes in cellular function as a result of such modulation vary depending on the ion channel involved. For instance, suppression or block of sodium channels will naturally lead to block of action potential. Augmentation of sodium channel activity will cause hyperexcitation. On the other hand, suppression of potassium channels will prolong the falling phase of the action potential, thereby causing hyperexcitation. Block of calcium channels will bring up a variety of changes in cellular function, depending on the exact role of the calcium channel in question; these changes include depression of neuronal discharges, suppression of cardiac muscle contraction, and block of synaptic transmission, to mention a few. In any event, it is clear that alteration of voltage-activated ion channels will result in serious dysfunction of neurons.

Modulation of Transmitter-Activated Ion Channels

Transmitter-activated ion channels can also be modified to either suppression or augmentation. For example, suppression of any ion channels associated with the excitatory postsynaptic membrane will result in a decrease in synaptic transmission. Their augmentation will facilitate synaptic transmission. Suppression of ion channels associated with the inhibitory postsynaptic membrane will cause hyperexcitation, and their augmentation will cause depression of the nervous system.

VOLTAGE-ACTIVATED ION CHANNELS AND NEUROTOXICITY

Sodium Channels

Natural Toxins

Blockers.

Tetrodotoxin and saxitoxin. Tetrodotoxin (Fig. 1) blocks the neuronal sodium channel selectively at low concentrations. The first evidence in support of this notion was obtained by Narahashi et al. (1960) through intracellular microelectrode experiments with frog skeletal muscle fibers. The action potential was blocked by TTX without any change in resting membrane potential or resting membrane resistance or delayed rectification, which is indicative of delayed potassium channel activity. Voltage clamp experiments with lobster giant axons that were conducted shortly afterward clearly demonstrated the validity of this hypothesis (Narahashi et al., 1964). This pioneering study was extended by Narahashi and his colleagues to include various aspects of TTX block of sodium channels and confirmed by other investigators (see Narahashi, 1974, 1988a).

In short, TTX blocks the sodium channels with a K_i in the nanomolar order without any effect on other channels (Fig. 2); it is effective only from the external surface of the membrane; TTX block is voltage dependent; and the TTX molecule binds to or near the external mouth of the sodium channel on a one-to-one stoichiometric basis. Single-channel patch clamp experiments with neuroblastoma N1E-115 cells have clearly shown that in the presence of 3 nM TTX, which is close to its K_i value, the number of sodium channel openings is reduced to approximately 50% of that of control, although the mean current amplitude and mean open time remain unchanged (Fig. 3), and that TTX blocks the sodium channel on a one-to-one stoichiometric basis (Quandt et al., 1985). These results indicate that the sodium channels bound by TTX molecules are blocked, while those not bound by

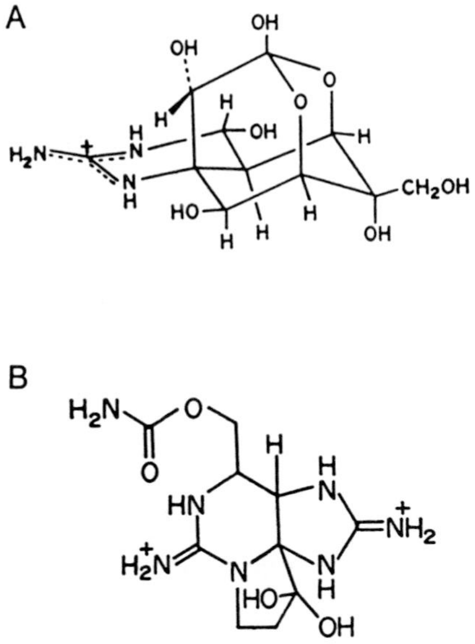

A

B

Figure 1 Structures of tetrodotoxin (A) and saxitoxin (B). (From Narahashi, 1988b.)

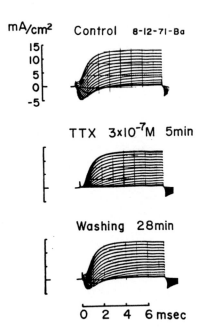

Figure 2 Block of sodium currents by tetrodotoxin (TTX). In the control, the membrane current associated with a step depolarization to various levels is composed of a transient inward or outward sodium current and a steady-state potassium current. Tetrodotoxin blocks the sodium currents without any effect on the potassium currents, and the effect is reversible after washing with TTX-free solution.

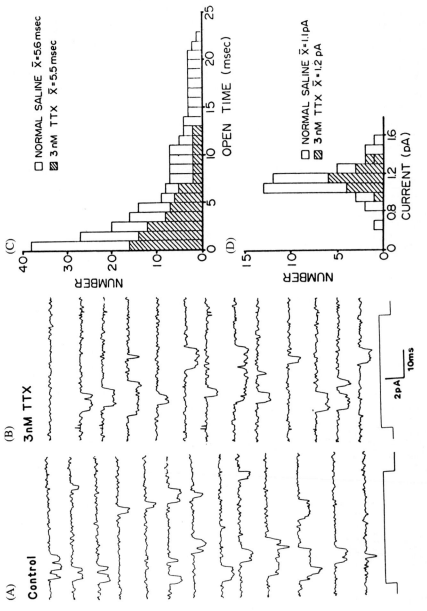

Figure 3 Effects of tetrodotoxin on single sodium channel currents. (A) Examples of current records obtained from an outside-out membrane patch in normal saline solutions in response to depolarizations from a holding potential of –90 to –30 mV as shown at the bottom. Temperature 10°C. (B) Same as A, but after application of 3 nM tetrodotoxin (TTX) to the external membrane surface. (C) Open time distributions before and after exposure to TTX. (D) Amplitude histograms before and after exposure to TTX. (A and B from Quandt et al. (1985); C and D from Narahashi, 1986.)

TTX molecules are not blocked and are capable of generating the normal sodium currents. Because of its highly specific and potent action, TTX has been used extensively as a useful chemical tool in the laboratory since the discovery of its action. The discovery of selective TTX block of sodium channels has made an additional contribution to neuroscience: it has paved the way for the use of chemicals as tools, an idea that was almost inconceivable before.

Saxitoxin (STX, Fig. 1) is the toxic component isolated from the dinoflagellate *Gonyaulax catenella* and was found to exert the same sodium channel–blocking action as TTX (see Narahashi, 1974, 1988a). Saxitoxin has also been used extensively as a chemical tool in the laboratory.

There are many ways to use TTX or STX as a tool to study neurophysiology, neuropharmacology, and neurotoxicology. One of the simplest and most straightforward methods is to block the sodium channel current, allowing the pure potassium channel current to flow. Thus it is possible to perform detailed kinetic analyses of potassium channels. Tetrodotoxin and STX can also be used for the study of neurotransmitter release. Because TTX and STX do not affect transmitter release nor the postsynaptic membrane channels, the relationship between nerve terminal depolarization and transmitter release can be studied with a synaptic or neuromuscular preparation in the presence of TTX or STX. Tetrodotoxin and STX have been used to estimate the density of sodium channels in various neuronal preparations through measurement of their binding to the channel. Whenever the experimental protocol requires elimination of the sodium channel activity, TTX or STX proves useful. They are also very useful to tag the sodium channel component in experiments to study the molecular structure of the channel.

Conotoxins. The venom from the marine snail *Conus geographus* contains conotoxin GIIIA (geographutoxin I), conotoxin GIIIB (geographutoxin II), and conotoxin GIIIC, which block skeletal muscle sodium channels without any effect on neuronal sodium channels (see Wu and Narahashi, 1988). This group of toxins is also called μ-conotoxins. μ-Conotoxin is the first neurotoxin that has been found to discriminate between the nerve and muscle sodium channels.

Modulators. Channel modulators may be defined as chemicals that alter the kinetic behavior of the channel by various mechanisms. Certain chemicals inhibit the inactivation mechanism, thereby causing a prolonged current to flow. Some others alter the activation kinetics in such a way as to slow the activation and/or deactivation process; this alteration also results in a prolonged current. There are also chemicals that cause a shift of voltage dependence of the activation or inactivation mechanism. A combination of any of these changes is possible. Thus, seemingly the same end point could occur as a result of alteration of different mechanisms of channel gating.

Batrachotoxin. Batrachotoxin (BTX) is one of the toxic principles contained in skin secretions of the Colombian poison arrow frog *Phyllobates aurotaenia* (Fig. 4). Batrachotoxin causes hyperexcitation in animals, and this is due to drastic modulation of sodium channel kinetics in nerves, skeletal muscle, and cardiac muscle (Albuquerque et al., 1971; Khodorov, 1985; Narahashi, 1974, 1984a). In squid giant axons, BTX inhibits sodium channel inactivation, thus producing a prolonged sodium current, and the activation voltage of the sodium channel is shifted in the hyperpolarizing direction, allowing the sodium channel to open at large negative potentials (Tanguy and Yeh, 1991). Single sodium channels of neuroblastoma cells are kept open for unusually long periods in the presence of BTX (Quandt and Narahashi, 1982) (Fig. 5). These changes in sodium channel gating

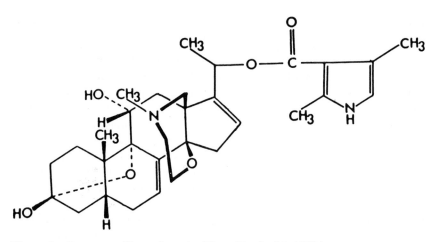

Figure 4   Structure of batrachotoxin. (From Narahashi, 1973.)

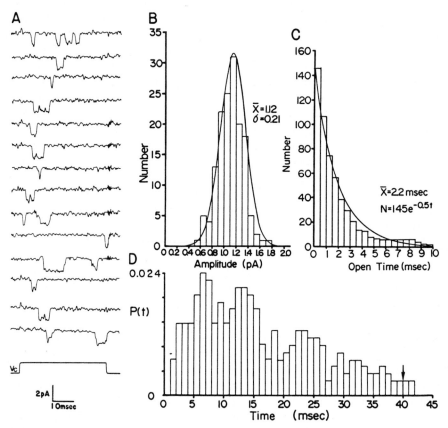

Figure 5   Single sodium channel activity of neuroblastoma cell membranes under normal conditions (A–D) and in the presence of batrachotoxin (BTX) (E–H). The mean open time is greatly prolonged from 2 ms in control (C) to 60–150 ms with BTX (G). The mean current amplitude is decreased from 1.1 pA in control (B) to 0.8 pA with BTX (F). The probability of channel openings during a 40-ms depolarizing pulse in control (D) is greatly changed by BTX, with which the probability is maintained constant during a 160-ms depolarizing pulse (H). These time courses mimic the whole-cell sodium currents. (From Quandt and Narahashi, 1982.)

kinetics cause a sizable membrane depolarization (Narahashi et al., 1971). Because of the ability of BTX to keep the sodium channel open for long periods, it has been used extensively as a chemical tool, especially in bilayer models into which the sodium channel proteins are incorporated; it is easy to measure single sodium channel currents under this condition when their open times are prolonged.

Grayanotoxins. Grayanotoxins (GTXs) are toxins contained in the leaves of plants that belong to the family Ericaceae, e.g., *Leucothoe, Rhododendron, Andromeda,* and *Kalmia.* Like BTX, GTXs also cause hyperexcitation in animals as a result of modulation of the sodium channel (Narahashi, 1974, 1984a). The mechanism of action of GTXs is also very similar to that of BTX. Grayanotoxins inhibit sodium channel inactivation and shift the activation voltage in the hyperpolarizing direction; these changes in sodium channel gating kinetics cause a large depolarization.

Veratridine. Veratridine is one of the veratrum alkaloids contained in plants that belong to the tribe Veratreae and the family Liliaceae. Veratridine causes hyperexcitation and membrane depolarization in the nerve as a result of modulation of sodium channel gating kinetics (Narahashi, 1974; Narahashi and Herman, 1992). The mean open time of single sodium channels is prolonged, the single sodium channel conductance is decreased, and a prolonged whole cell sodium current flows. Veratridine has also been used extensively as a tool to keep the sodium channel open for a long time.

Other modulators. Several other toxins and chemicals are known to modulate

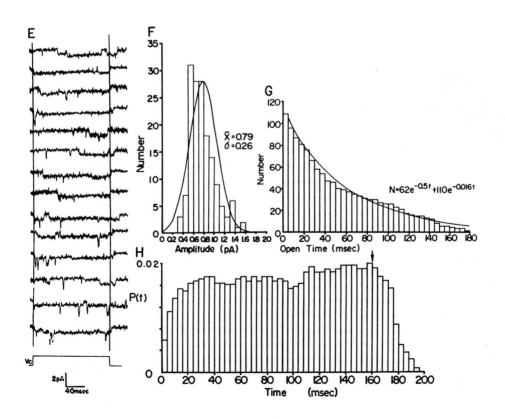

sodium channel gating kinetics (Narahashi, 1974; Narahashi and Herman, 1992; Wu and Narahashi, 1988). They include ciguatoxin, which is produced by the dinoflagellate *Gambrierdiscus toxicus* and contained in tropical fish; aconitine, contained in the plant *Aconitum napellus*; brevetoxins, produced by the dinoflagellate *Ptychodiscus brevis*; *Goniopora* toxin, contained in stony corals of the genus *Goniopora*; sea anemone toxins, including *Anemonia sulcata* toxin II, *Condylactis gigantea* toxin, and anthopleurin A from *Anthopleura xanthogrammica*; and scorpion toxins, such as toxins I, III, IV, V, VI, and VII and varI-3 from *Centruroides sculpturatus*, toxin IIα from *Leiurus quinquestriatus*, toxins M_7 and 2001 from *Buthus eupeus*, toxins V and XII from *Buthus tamulus*, toxins I and II from *Androctonus australis*, toxin II from *Centruroides suffusus*, and toxins γ and TsIV-5 from *Tityus serrulatus*.

Environmental Neurotoxicants

A variety of environmental neurotoxicants are known to affect the sodium channels, including insecticides, heavy metals, and solvents. However, the most potent of them are the insecticides pyrethroids and DDT, which exert their toxic effect through modulation of the sodium channels.

Pyrethroids and DDT. The mechanisms of action of pyrethroids and DDT on the nervous system have been studied very extensively during the past 40 years, and they represent the case where interactions of environmental neurotoxicants with ion channels have been most thoroughly established to explain the symptoms of poisoning in animals, including mammals and insects. Many review articles have been published (Narahashi, 1971, 1976, 1981, 1985, 1987a, 1988b, 1989, 1992b; Ruigt, 1984; Soderlund and Bloomquist, 1989; Vijverberg and van den Bercken, 1990; Woolley, 1981). Despite the difference in chemical structures, pyrethroids and DDT exert very similar, if not completely identical, actions on the nervous system.

DDT is one of the synthetic insecticides developed during World War II and was used extensively until the 1960s. However, environmental concerns, including its long-term residual toxicity, prompted the synthesis of derivatives of pyrethrins, natural insecticides contained in the flowers of *Chrysanthemum cinerariaefolium*. Pyrethrins are ideal insecticides with high insecticidal activity, low mammalian toxicity, and biodegradability. A large number of pyrethrin derivatives have been synthesized and evaluated for their insecticidal activity and mammalian toxicity, and at least two dozen or so are now being used as insecticides. Pyrethroids may be classified into two large groups based primarily on their chemical structure: the pyrethroids without a cyano group at the α position are called type I, and those with an α cyano group are called type II (Fig. 6). Although type I and type II pyrethroids cause somewhat different symptoms of poisoning in mammals, they both modify the gating kinetics of sodium channels in a similar manner. DDT resembles type I pyrethroids in this respect.

Modification of whole-cell sodium current by pyrethroids and DDT. Both pyrethroids and DDT cause hyperexcitability in animals expressed in various forms, such as ataxia, convulsions, tremors, hypersensitivity, and choreoathetosis. As expected from these symptoms of poisoning, repetitive discharges are observed in various regions of the nerve and muscle system, including nerve fibers, synapses, and neuromuscular junctions. The mechanisms underlying these repetitive discharges are somewhat different in different regions of the nerve, yet all of them originate from prolonged flow of sodium currents through the open sodium channels.

Voltage clamp experiments with lobster, crayfish, and squid giant axons, exposed to

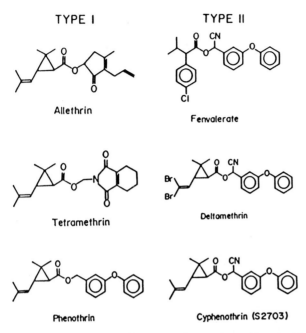

TYPE I

Allethrin

Tetramethrin

Phenothrin

TYPE II

Fenvalerate

Deltamethrin

Cyphenothrin (S2703)

Figure 6 Structures of type I and type II pyrethroids. (From Narahashi, 1985.)

type I pyrethroids or DDT, have clearly shown that the sodium current associated with a step depolarizing pulse is markedly prolonged and that the sodium tail current associated with a step repolarization is also increased and prolonged. The effects of allethrin, a type I pyrethroid, on a squid giant axon are shown in Fig. 7. The prolonged sodium current will increase and prolong the depolarizing after-potential from which repetitive after-discharges are produced. This is the basis for hyperactivity generated by type I pyrethroids and DDT in nerve fibers. Type I pyrethroids also cause membrane depolarization, the degree of which varies depending on the kind of pyrethroid and the kind of nerve preparation. The depolarization is due to prolonged flow of sodium current and a shift of the sodium channel activation voltage in the hyperpolarizing direction; these changes allow a prolonged sodium current to flow at the normal resting potential, thereby causing a depolarization.

Type II pyrethroids also modify the sodium channel gating kinetics in a manner similar to that caused by type I pyrethroids and DDT, yet there are some quantitative differences between the two types of pyrethroid. In the axons exposed to type II pyrethroids, the peak amplitude of the sodium current is suppressed to some extent, a prolonged sodium current flows during a step depolarizing pulse, the tail sodium current is greatly prolonged and decays more slowly than that observed in the presence of type I pyrethroids, and the sodium channel activation voltage is shifted in the hyperpolarizing direction. The time constant of tail current decay is often as long as minutes. These changes in sodium channel gating kinetics cause a membrane depolarization greater than that produced by type I pyrethroids. As a result of the large membrane depolarization, no repetitive after-discharges are induced in nerve fibers. However, membrane depolarization of sensory neurons generates massive discharges toward the CNS, which in turn cause paresthesia and synaptic disturbances.

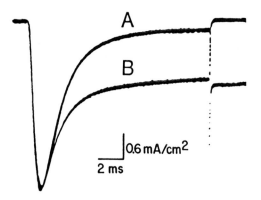

Figure 7 Effects of 1 μM (+)-*trans* allethrin, a type I pyrethroid, on the sodium current of a squid giant axon. The membrane was step depolarized to –20 mV from a holding potential of –100 mV in K-free external and internal perfusates. In the control (A), the peak transient sodium current is followed by a small slow current during a depolarizing step, and the tail sodium current upon step repolarization decays quickly. After application of allethrin (B), the peak transient sodium current remains unchanged, but the slow current and tail current are increased in amplitude and the latter decays very slowly. (From Narahashi, 1984b.)

A diagram illustrating the sites of action of type I and type II pyrethroids on the nervous system is shown in Fig. 8.

Modification of single sodium channels by pyrethroids. Single-sodium-channel patch clamp experiments with neuroblastoma N1E-115 cells have disclosed several important features of pyrethroid action (Chinn and Narahashi, 1986, 1989; Holloway et al., 1989; Yamamoto et al., 1983). An example of a single-channel experiment with deltamethrin is shown in Fig. 9. First of all, the mean open time of sodium channels is greatly prolonged by pyrethroids. The normal sodium channels are kept open for only a few milliseconds during a step depolarization, and pyrethroids allow them to open for several hundred milliseconds to as long as several seconds. This contributes to the prolonged whole-cell sodium current in the presence of pyrethroids. Second, the channels are kept open even after termination of the depolarizing pulse; this explains the prolonged tail current. Third, although normal sodium channels open only near the beginning of a depolarizing pulse, the sodium channel exposed to pyrethroids can open with long delays during a depolarizing pulse. This accounts for the inhibition of sodium channel inactivation and contributes to the prolonged whole-cell sodium current. Fourth, single-sodium-channel conductance remains unchanged in the presence of pyrethroids. Type I and type II pyrethroids exert basically the same effects on single sodium channels. However, the prolongation of channel open time is much more pronounced with type II than with type I pyrethroids.

In summary, these changes in single-channel behavior indicate that pyrethroids slow the gating kinetics of channel opening (activation), channel closing (deactivation), and channel inactivation. It remains to be seen exactly how these changes in gating kinetics take place. A variety of experiments designed to locate the site of action of pyrethroids suggest that the pyrethroid molecules get access to the gating machinery through the membrane lipid phase (see below).

Closed- vs. open-channel modification. One of the important questions about channel block or modulation is whether the drug in question binds or interacts with the

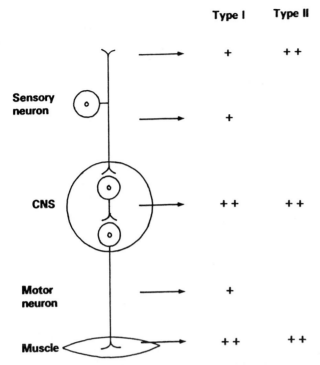

Figure 8 Sites of action of type I and type II pyrethroids on the nervous system. Plus signs indicate degree of generation of repetitive activity. Type I, but not type II, pyrethroids generally initiate repetitive discharges in nerve fibers. Both initiate repetitive activity at synapses and neuromuscular junctions, owing partly to repetitive discharges at the nerve terminals and partly to membrane depolarization of the terminals, which would cause massive release of transmitter. Type II pyrethroids are more potent than type I pyrethroids on the sensory receptors because of their stronger depolarizing effect. (From Narahashi, 1992b.)

channel in its open or closed state. If it is open-channel block or modulation, there is a possibility that the drug penetrates and binds to an intrachannel site. On the other hand, if it is closed-channel block or modulation, the drug must bind to a site outside the channel. Open-channel block or modulation can also result in use-dependent block or modulation, which requires opening of the channel. A possible scheme of opening and closing of normal and pyrethroid-modified sodium channels is illustrated in Fig. 10. In order to answer this question, two types of experiment have been performed.

Since the slow tail current of pyrethroid-treated axons is indicative of the activity of the modified sodium channels, the rate at which the sodium channel reaches the modified open state can be measured from the time course of development of the slow tail current amplitude following various durations of depolarization. In tetramethrin-treated squid giant axons, the time course of the development of the slow tail current is expressed by two exponential functions (Lund and Narahashi, 1981). Therefore, the modified open state may be reached by two separate routes, one via open-channel modification and the other via closed-channel modification. If the rate at which the sodium channel reaches the modified open state is independent of pyrethroid concentration, it is compatible with closed channel modification. The data indicate that a large fraction of sodium channels are modified by

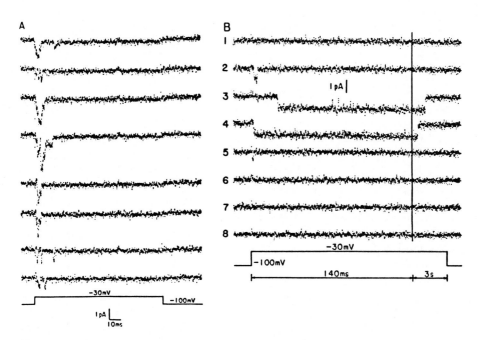

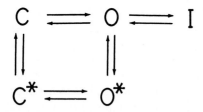

Figure 9 Effects of deltamethrin on single sodium channel currents of a neuroblastoma cell (N1E-115). (A) Currents from a cell before drug treatment in response to 140-ms depolarizing steps from a holding potential of –100 to –30 mV with a 3-s interpulse interval. Records were taken at a rate of 100 μs per point. (B) Currents after exposure to 10 μM deltamethrin. The membrane patch was depolarized for 3140 ms from a holding potential of –100 to –30 mV. The interpulse interval was 3 s. The time scale changes during the voltage step as indicated in the Figure. During the first 140 ms, data records were taken at a rate of 100 μs per point, and after the vertical line records were taken at a rate of 10 ms per point. (From Chinn and Narahashi, 1986.)

pyrethroids in the closed state while a small fraction is modified in the open state (de-Weille et al., 1988). The latter may be limited by channel inactivation.

The pyrethroid-induced closed-channel modification is also supported by single-channel experiments (Holloway et al., 1989). This hypothesis predicts that the probability of observing prolonged openings of the pyrethroid-modified channels is independent of the duration of depolarizing pulse applied as stimulus. This was actually the case.

In summary, sodium channels are modified by pyrethroids while they are in the

$$C \rightleftharpoons O \rightleftharpoons I$$
$$C^* \rightleftharpoons O^*$$

Figure 10 Scheme of opening and closing of normal and pyrethroid-modified sodium channels. C, O, and I indicate normal closed, open, and inactivated channels, respectively. C* and O* indicate pyrethroid-modified closed and open channels, respectively. (From Narahashi, 1989.)

closed configuration, but the affinity of pyrethroids increases as the channels open. Thus, an additional fraction of sodium channels is modified by stimulation. This notion also accounts for use-dependent modification of the channels by pyrethroids (Lund and Narahashi, 1983; Salgado et al., 1989).

Site of action in the sodium channel. A few different approaches have been used to determine the site of action of pyrethroids in the sodium channel. One approach is to measure relative cation permeabilities of the open sodium channel in squid giant axons before and during application of pyrethroids. Tetramethrin has virtually no effect on the cation permeability ratios for sodium, lithium, ammonium, guanidine, and formamidine. Since the relative permeability of the sodium channel to various cations is controlled by the selectivity filter located near the external orifice of the channel (Hille, 1971), it is concluded that tetramethrin does not alter its function (Yamamoto et al., 1986).

Open sodium channels are known to be blocked, in a manner dependent on the membrane potential, by certain permeating cations, such as sodium, lithium, ammonium, guanidine, formamidine, calcium, and magnesium (Yamamoto et al., 1984, 1985). This cation block is interpreted as being due to binding of the permeating cation to a site inside the channel, thus reflecting the profile of energy barriers inside the channel. The cation block remains unchanged after exposure of tetramethrin. It is concluded that tetramethrin does not interfere with or bind to these intrachannel sites (Yamamoto et al., 1986).

The aforementioned results exclude as the pyrethroid-binding sites the intrachannel sites that regulate cation permeation and block. Pyrethroid molecules are highly hydrophobic and drastically modify the gating kinetics of the sodium channel. Therefore, it is possible for the pyrethroid molecules to get access to the gating machinery via the lipid phase of the membrane. One way of determining the site of action of pyrethroids in the sodium channel is to examine the interactions or competition between pyrethroids and other chemicals known to bind to specific sites in the channel.

n-Octylguanidine has been shown to block the open sodium channel from inside the membrane (Kirsch et al., 1980) in a manner similar to that of local anesthetics (Strichartz, 1973; Courtney, 1975, 1980; Courtney et al., 1978; Hille 1977; Khodorov et al., 1976; Yeh, 1978, 1980), pancuronium (Yeh and Narahashi, 1977), 9-aminoacridine (Yeh, 1979), and strychnine (Shapiro, 1977). These chemicals enter the sodium channel via the open gates located at the inner orifice. Experiments with internally perfused squid giant axons have clearly shown that phenothrin does not affect the octylguanidine block of the sodium channel (deWeille et al., 1988). Thus, pyrethroids appear to bind to a site different from the intrachannel binding site of octylguanidine and presumably of local anesthetics.

Batrachotoxin and GTXs depolarize the nerve membrane (Narahashi et al., 1971; Albuquerque et al., 1973; Seyama and Narahashi, 1973; Narahashi and Seyama, 1974) by inhibiting sodium channel inactivation and by shifting the sodium channel activation potential in the hyperpolarizing direction (Khodorov, 1978, 1985; Khodorov and Revenko, 1979; Seyama and Narahashi, 1981; Tanguy and Yeh, 1991; Tanguy et al., 1984). It appears that the BTX and GTX molecules bind to an intrachannel site to which the inactivation gate normally binds, causing inactivation. In the internally perfused squid giant axon, tetramethrin produces a characteristic tail current in the presence of GTX I. Thus GTX I and tetramethrin act on the sodium channel independently, suggesting that they bind to different channel sites (Takeda and Narahashi, 1988).

Tetrodotoxin is another useful tool to locate the site of action of pyrethroids in the sodium channel as it binds to the external orifice of the channel, thereby occluding the flow of sodium current. The dose-response relationships for tetramethrin modification of squid axon sodium channels in the absence and presence of TTX clearly indicate that TTX suppresses the maximal response in a concentration-dependent manner without changing the ED_{50} value for tetramethrin modification, indicating noncompetitive antagonism. It is concluded that tetramethrin and TTX do not share the same binding site (Lund and Narahashi, 1982).

In summary, pyrethroids do not act on an intrachannel site or on the TTX-binding site near the external orifice of the channel. Pyrethroids most likely get access to the channel-gating machinery via the lipid phase of the membrane.

Stereospecificity and site of action of pyrethroid isomers. Any pyrethroid exists in several isomers, because there are two or more chiral centers in the molecule. The insecticidal activity of each isomer varies greatly and has been shown to be positively correlated with its potency in modifying the sodium channel (Lund and Narahashi, 1983). The (−)-*trans* and (−)-*cis* forms of tetramethrin have little or no activity on the sodium channel, whereas the (+)-*trans* and (+)-*cis* forms are highly potent. Dose-response analyses of the antagonism between (+)- and (−)-isomers have led to a scheme depicting three sites of action of tetramethrin in the sodium channel (Fig. 11). There is a *trans* site to which (+)-*trans* and (−)-*trans* forms bind with high and low affinity, respectively. A *cis* site is for the *cis* isomers, and both (+)-*cis* and (−)-*cis* tetramethrin bind to it with high affinity. A third negative allosteric side, when bound by (−)-*trans* isomer with high affinity and by (−)-*cis* isomer with low affinity, modulates the activity of the *trans* and *cis* sites (Lund and Narahashi, 1982). The exact locations of these three sites in the molecular model of the sodium channel remain to be established.

Minimum effective concentrations. Pyrethrins and pyrethroids are known to stimulate nerve preparations at very low concentrations ranging from 50 pM to 10 nM (Narahashi, 1989). These studies were based on observations of repetitive discharges. However, most voltage clamp experiments were performed with higher concentrations of pyrethroids, usually in the micromolar order. This raised a question as to whether the voltage clamp data on sodium channel modification were relevant to toxicity in animals.

A satisfactory answer to this question was obtained in due consideration of the threshold phenomenon. Repetitive after-discharges are induced by a single stimulus in pyrethroid-treated nerve preparations when the depolarizing after-potential reaches the threshold for excitation. Calculations indicate that in order for the depolarizing after-po-

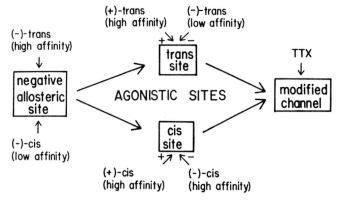

Figure 11 Hypothetical model for the interactions of tetramethrin with the sodium channel. TTX = tetrodotoxin. (From Lund and Narahashi, 1982.)

tential to reach the threshold, only a very small fraction of the sodium channel population, 0.1% or less, needs to be modified by tetramethrin (Lund and Narahashi, 1982). This concentration is in the order of ED_1 or less in the dose-response relationship for modification of sodium channels. Thus, the effect of tetramethrin in modifying the sodium channel is greatly amplified through the threshold phenomenon. This concept of toxicity amplification applies to the effect of any other chemicals as long as a threshold phenomenon is involved. Traditional comparison of in vitro ED_{50} values with the concentrations in the serum or body fluid of animals or patients could be very misleading.

Pyrazoles. The dihydropyrazole RH3421, methyl 1-(N-(α,α,α-trifluoro-p-tolyl) carbamoyl-3-(4-chlorophenyl)-4-methyl-2-pyrazolin-4-yl)carboxylate, possesses some insecticidal activity. It blocks $^{22}Na^+$ uptake by mouse brain vesicles stimulated by veratridine or BTX (Deecher and Soderlund, 1991). Crayfish giant axons are blocked by dihydropyrazoles as a result of their binding to the sodium channel (Salgado, 1990).

Phenylpyrazoles, which also have insecticidal and herbicidal activity, exert different actions on nerve membranes. The membrane is depolarized, but this is not mediated via the sodium channel or glutamate receptor channel complex. The depolarization leads the nerve to death (Klis et al., 1991).

Therapeutic Drugs

Certain therapeutic drugs act on the sodium channel, thereby causing therapeutic or toxic effects. In fact, many drugs, when given at very high concentrations, suppress the activity of sodium channels, but therapeutic or toxic significance at such high concentrations is questionable. Only brief outlines of interactions of certain therapeutic drugs with the sodium channel are given here.

Local Anesthetics. Local anesthetics have been studied for a long time for their action on the sodium channel. In fact, they were studied by voltage clamp techniques in the late 1950s, when no other pharmacological or toxicological studies had been performed with these techniques. Shanes et al. (1959) and Taylor (1959) conducted voltage clamp experiments with squid giant axons to examine the effects of procaine and cocaine on the sodium and potassium channels. Both local anesthetics block both channels, and the sodium channel block is directly responsible for conduction block, which is the basis for local anesthesia. However, their potencies are not high, requiring millimolar concentrations to affect the channels. Local anesthetics have since been studied extensively for their effects on the sodium channel. Although these local anesthetic studies are not toxicological, a brief highlight is given below, as they have contributed significantly to the basic concept of drug-channel interactions, which is applicable to neurotoxicology.

Site of action of local anesthetics in the sodium channel. Most local anesthetics are tertiary amines with a pK_a value between 7 and 9. Thus they exist in both the charged cationic form and the uncharged molecular form at neutral pH. The question of which form is active in blocking nerve conduction had been a matter of controversy for a number of years. Older experiments were based on recording action potentials extracellularly from nerve bundles and comparing the blocking potency of local anesthetics at different pH values. Most studies indicated that the blocking potency increased with increasing the pH. It was concluded that the uncharged form was responsible for conduction block (see Narahashi and Frazier, 1971; Ritchie and Greengard, 1966). However, there were many data that conflicted with this hypothesis. More elaborate and careful experiments were performed by Ritchie and Greengard (1966), who claimed that it was the charged cationic form that was active, on the basis of the role of the nerve sheath as a diffusion barrier for local anesthetics. However, some experimental data were still incompatible with this notion. One important point that was missed previously was the role of the nerve membrane as a diffusion barrier for local anesthetics. Elaborate experiments with internally perfused squid giant axons were successful in solving this problem.

With internally (and externally) perfused squid giant axons, it is easy to apply a test compound to either side of the membrane at well-defined concentrations and to change and control the pH of both phases. Such experiments with compounds 6211 ($pK_a = 6.3$) and 6603 ($pK_a = 9.8$), tertiary amine lidocaine derivatives, have clearly indicated that the compounds penetrate the nerve membrane in the uncharged molecular form, are ionized inside the cell, and block the sodium and potassium channels in the charged cationic form from inside the nerve membrane (Fig. 12) (Narahashi et al., 1970). Additional evidence in support of this notion was obtained by using the quaternary derivatives of lidocaine, QX312 and QX572 (Frazier et al., 1970). The permanently charged quaternary derivatives, although different in structure from the charged cationic form of the tertiary anesthetics, were effective in blocking the channels only when applied inside the preparation.

Use dependence of local anesthetic block. Local anesthetics and other sodium channel–blocking agents have been studied extensively for the mechanism of use-dependent block of sodium channels since the pioneering work by Strichartz (1973). When applied at a certain concentration, a local anesthetic blocks the sodium channel to some extent as tested by the first depolarizing stimulus. When repetitive depolarizing pulses are applied, block may be intensified in a manner dependent on the stimulus frequency, exhibiting use-dependent block (Fig. 13). This is due to several factors, including whether block requires channel opening, whether the channel can close with the local anesthetic molecule trapped inside, whether the rate of recovery from channel inactivation is slowed by the local anesthetic, and whether the local anesthetic has a higher affinity for the inactivated

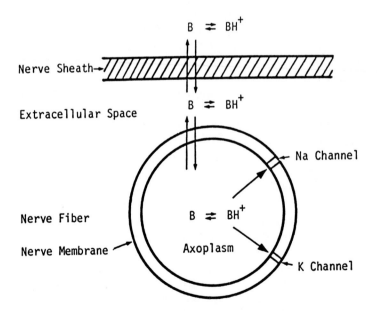

Figure 12 Schematic drawing for the site of action and active form of local anesthetic. It penetrates the nerve sheath and nerve membrane in the uncharged form (B) and blocks Na and K channels from inside of the nerve membrane in the charged form (BH^+).

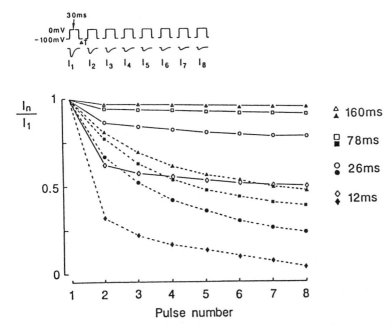

Figure 13 The time course of change in the amplitude of sodium current elicited by a train of depolarizing pulses. Eight consecutive pulses to 0 mV (30-ms duration) were delivered with various pulse intervals ranging from 12 ms to 3 s from a holding potential of –100 mV. The peak current amplitude for each pulse in the train (I_n) was normalized to that of the first pulse (I_1) and is plotted as a function of the pulse number. Open symbols, control; closed symbols, in the presence of 1 μM chlorpromazine. Numerals attached to the symbols or traces indicate interpulse intervals (ΔT). (From Ogata et al., 1990.)

state than the resting state of the channel. Therefore, use dependence of block (or modulation in general) is an important parameter to elucidate the mechanism of action of any blocking or modulating agents (Hille, 1977).

Psychotropic Drugs. Some psychotropic drugs, including chlorpromazine, haloperidol, and imipramine, have been shown to block both sodium and calcium channels in neurons and cardiac myocytes (Ogata and Narahashi, 1989, 1990; Ogata et al., 1989a,b, 1990). Chlorpromazine block of cardiac sodium channels appears to be responsible for its toxicity to cardiac tissue. Block of neuronal sodium and calcium channels by these psychotropic drugs may also be related to their toxicity. Chlorpromazine blocks the sodium channel of neuroblastoma N1E-115 cells and cardiac myocytes in a use-dependent manner (Fig. 13). It has a much higher affinity for the inactivated state of the channel than for the resting state. By contrast, chlorpromazine block of calcium channels is not use dependent. Thus these actions mimic, to some extent, local anesthetic block of neuronal sodium channels.

Potassium Channels

Until 10–15 years ago, the delayed rectifying potassium channel was the only potassium channel that had been studied extensively. More recent developments of advanced electrophysiological techniques such as patch clamp have made it possible to study other neuronal potassium channels in great detail. It is also important to recognize that some of the potassium channel agents have potential application to therapy for cardiovascular and other disorders. Several reviews have been published recently (Cook, 1988; Castle et al., 1989; Adams and Nonner, 1990; deWeille and Lazdunski, 1990; Dreyer, 1990; Inoue and Yoshii, 1992; Meves, 1992).

Voltage-Activated Potassium Channels

Delayed Rectifying Potassium Channels. Delayed rectifying potassium channels are present in various excitable cells and are responsible for the falling phase of the action potential. Tetraethylammonium (TEA) is the first chemical agent that was discovered to block this potassium channel (Tasaki and Hagiwara, 1957). Tetraethylammonium and its longer-chain derivatives such as nonyltriethylammonium block the outward potassium current without affecting the inward potassium current in a manner dependent on current direction (Armstrong, 1969, 1971; Armstrong and Binstock, 1965). In squid axons, TEA is effective only when applied inside, whereas in the node of Ranvier and skeletal muscle it is effective from either side of the membrane. Although TEA is not particularly potent, requiring 20–40 mM to block the potassium channel, it has been used extensively as a tool to eliminate potassium channel activity.

4-Aminopyridine (4-AP) blocks the delayed rectifying potassium channel (Pelhate and Pichon, 1974; Yeh et al., 1976). It is effective from either side of the membrane, with a K_i of 30 μM, but block is dependent on the membrane potential and the duration of depolarization (Fig. 14). 3,4-Diaminopyridine is more potent, with a K_i of 5.8 and 0.7 μM for external and internal applications, respectively (Kirsch and Narahashi, 1978). Thus, aminopyridines have been used as tools, yet caution must be exercised because of their voltage- and time-dependent nature of block.

Cesium ions block the delayed rectifying potassium channel in a manner dependent on the direction of current flow: internal Cs^+ is effective against outward currents, whereas external Cs^+ is effective against inward currents (Chandler and Meves, 1965; Adelman and Senft, 1966). Barium ions also block this potassium channel from both sides of the membrane (Armstrong and Taylor, 1980; Eaton and Brodwick, 1980).

Some natural toxins are known to block the delayed rectifying potassium channel. Noxiustoxin, isolated from the venom of the Mexican scorpion *Centruroides noxius*, blocks this potassium channel in its open state, with a K_i of 400 nM (Carbone et al., 1982, 1987).

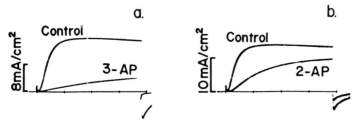

Figure 14 Patterns of squid axon K current in 2- and 3-aminopyridine (2-AP, 3-AP). Membrane currents during a clamp pulse to +100 mV before and after external application of 1 mM 3-AP (a) or 1 mM 2-AP (b). External solution contained 300 nM tetrodotoxin in each case. (From Yeh et al., 1976.)

Mast cell degranulating (MCD) peptide blocks the $f1$ component of the delayed rectifying potassium current (Bräu et al., 1990). Dendrotoxin, isolated from the green mamba *Dendroaspis angusticeps*, and dendrotoxin I, isolated from the black mamba *Dendroaspis polylepis*, are known to block the transient A-current and voltage-activated transient Ca^{2+}-dependent potassium current (Halliwell et al., 1986; Bourque, 1988), but they block the delayed rectifying potassium current more potently (Penner et al., 1986).

Inward Rectifying Potassium Channels. Inward rectifying or anomalous rectifying potassium channels are blocked by Ba^{2+} (Hagiwara et al., 1978; Ohmori et al., 1981), Cs^+ (Hagiwara et al., 1976), and H^+ (Hagiwara et al., 1978; Moody and Hagiwara, 1982).

Transient Potassium Channels (A-Currents). Transient potassium current, or A-current, is produced by membrane depolarization. It is an outward current, attains a peak, and decays (Hagiwara et al., 1961; Connor and Stevens, 1971). A-current appears to modulate the neuron's firing rate. Some agents block A-current, but none selectively. Aminopyridines block A-current (Thompson, 1977, 1982; Gustafsson et al., 1982), but they also block delayed rectifying potassium channels and transient Ca-dependent potassium channels. Charybdotoxin, isolated from the venom of the Mideastern scorpion *Leiurus quinquestriatus* var. *hebraeus*, is known as a specific blocker of the Ca-activated potassium channel, but it also blocks A-currents (MacKinnon et al., 1988). Dendrotoxin exerts a slow and weak blocking action on A-currents (Halliwell et al., 1986; Dolly et al., 1984).

Transient Calcium-Dependent Potassium Channels. Transient calcium-dependent potassium channels are activated by membrane depolarization in a manner dependent on intracellular calcium concentration. They are blocked by removal of Ca^{2+} from the extracellular fluid, by block of calcium channels by Co^{2+}, Mn^{2+}, or Cd^{2+}, or by replacement of Ca^{2+} by Ba^{2+}. These channels are found in various cells including magnocellular neurosecretory cells of the rat supraoptic nucleus (Bourque, 1988). They are insensitive to TEA but blocked by 4-aminopyridine and dendrotoxin.

M-Currents. M-current is found in various types of cell (Brown, 1988) and appears to modulate the frequency and pattern of discharges (Adams, 1982). M-current is inhibited by a variety of muscarinic ACh receptor agonists, including ACh, muscarine, methacholine, and oxotremorine, and by other agents, such as t-luteinizing hormone releasing hormone (t-LHRH), substance P, substance K, eledoisin, kassinin, physalaemin, and Ba^{2+} ions (Brown, 1988).

Calcium-Activated Potassium Channels

Calcium-activated potassium channels are activated and modulated by an increase in intracellular Ca^{2+} concentration. The channels are classified into three groups based on single-channel conductance: 1) "big" or "maxi" channels with a high conductance of 100–250 pS; 2) "intermediate" channels with an 18–50 pS conductance; and 3) "small" channels with a 10–14 pS conductance (Cook, 1988; Dreyer, 1990). Big and intermediate potassium channels are opened by both membrane depolarization and an increase in intracellular Ca^{2+} concentration. Small potassium channels are opened by an increase in intracellular Ca^{2+} concentration only.

Several blockers acting on calcium-activated potassium channels are known. Apamin, isolated from the venom of the honeybee *Apis mellifera*, blocks the small Ca^{2+}-activated potassium channels (Blatz and Magleby, 1986; Hugues et al., 1982; Seagar et al., 1984). The apamin-sensitive small channels are insensitive to TEA, whereas large channels are blocked by TEA and charybdotoxin but not by apamin (Miller et al., 1985; Romey and

Lazdunski, 1984; Romey et al., 1984; Pennefather et al., 1985). Charybdotoxin is a potent blocker of the big and intermediate Ca^{2+}-activated potassium channels (Miller et al., 1985; Hermann and Erxleben, 1987). Leiurotoxin I, also isolated from the venom of the *Leiurus* scorpion, blocks the small Ca^{2+}-activated potassium channels (Chicchi et al., 1988).

Adenosine Triphosphate–Sensitive Potassium Channels

The adenosine triphosphate (ATP)-sensitive potassium channel is inhibited by an increase in intracellular ATP concentration and is found in various cells, including cardiac cells, skeletal muscle, pancreatic β-cells, arterial smooth muscle, and cortical neurons (deWeille and Lazdunski, 1990; Noma, 1983; Noma and Shibasaki, 1988; Ashcroft, 1988; Rorsman and Trube, 1990; Rorsman et al., 1990; Bean and Friel, 1990). This channel plays important roles in a variety of physiological functions. For example, in pancreatic β cells, the chain of events is as follows: glucose metabolism → ATP → closing of the channel → membrane depolarization → opening of the voltage-activated Ca channels → Ca^{2+} influx → insulin release (Ashcroft, 1988). In cardiac cells: ischemia → decrease in ATP → opening of the channel → membrane hyperpolarization → shortening of the action potential → decrease in consumption of the high-energy phosphate → prevention of the cell from irreversible damage (Noma and Shibasaki, 1988).

Tolbutamide and glyburide are hypoglycemic sulfonylureas and are used in the treatment of diabetes. Their mechanism of action has been disclosed recently: they block the ATP-sensitive potassium channel, thereby eliciting insulin secretion (Rorsman et al., 1990; Quast and Cook, 1989).

Potassium Channel Openers

Chemical agents that open potassium channels have received much attention recently because of potential therapeutic applications to the treatment of cardiovascular disorders (Quast and Cook, 1989; Edwards and Weston, 1990). They include cromakalim, pinacidil, nicorandil, minoxidil, diazoxide, and RP52891. The idea behind this is that opening of potassium channels leads to relaxation of blood vessels. However, potential side effects include cardiac dysrhythmias and cell death in the brain as a result of release of excitatory amino acids triggered by potassium accumulation in the interstitial space. A recent single-channel study has shown that cromakalim opens the ATP-sensitive potassium channel (Standen et al., 1989). However, pinacidil also has a blocking action on the voltage-activated calcium channel and Ca^{2+}-activated potassium channel.

Calcium Channels

Calcium channels play a variety of important roles in nerve and muscle activity, including release of neurotransmitters and hormones, generation of action potentials, control of pacemaker and bursting activity, and excitation-contraction coupling. Because of their widespread distribution and activity, calcium channels are considered potential target sites for a number of therapeutic drugs, neurotoxins, and environmental neurotoxicants. For example, verapamil, diltiazem, and dihydropyridines have been developed into useful drugs in the treatment of cardiovascular disorders (Janis et al., 1987; Janis and Triggle, 1991).

Studies of calcium channels have been greatly accelerated since the development of patch clamp techniques (Hamill et al., 1981). Since calcium channels are particularly important in the activity of neurons, cardiac muscle, and smooth muscle, all of which are difficult to study by using the classical voltage clamp techniques, patch lamp techniques provided us with powerful and straightforward approaches to the analysis of calcium channel function. Calcium channels are traditionally classified into four large groups, transient or T-type, long-lasting or L-type, N-type, and P-type (Hosey and Lazdunski, 1988; Narahashi and Herman, 1992; Tsien et al., 1991). However, this classification should not be taken as a rigorous definition, since detailed physiological and pharmacological characteristics of one type of calcium channels are somewhat different among different types of cell and different species of animal.

T-type, or type I, calcium channels are defined by two physiological characteristics (Fig. 15): 1) they are inactivated during a depolarization, and 2) they are opened at relatively large negative potentials (low voltage–activated). Their distribution is widespread, including neuroblastoma cells, dorsal root ganglion neurons, endocrine cells, cardiac cells, and vascular smooth muscle. T-type calcium channels play an important role in generating slow depolarizing responses that in turn elicit bursts of impulses and in pacemaker activity of cardiac cells. N-type calcium channels are also inactivated during a depolarization, but more slowly than T-type calcium channels, and they are activated at relatively small negative potentials (high voltage–activated). They appear to be involved in neurotransmitter release and other neuronal functions. L-type calcium channels are not significantly inactivated during a depolarization and are activated at relatively small negative potentials (high voltage–activated). They are found in a variety of cells, including neuroblastoma cells, dorsal root ganglion neurons, cardiac cells, vascular smooth muscle, and endocrine cells. Their physiological roles are still to be determined but are likely to include excitation-contraction coupling in muscles, release of neurotransmitters and hormones, and modulation of excitability. P-type calcium channels were first discovered in Purkinje cells. They are activated at small negative potentials (high voltage–activated) and are characterized by sensitivity to certain toxins such as funnel-web spider toxin (FTX) (Llinás et al., 1992).

T-Type Calcium Channels

No specific and potent blockers of T-type calcium channels have been discovered yet. Phenytoin blocks T-type calcium channels of neuroblastoma cells without much effect on

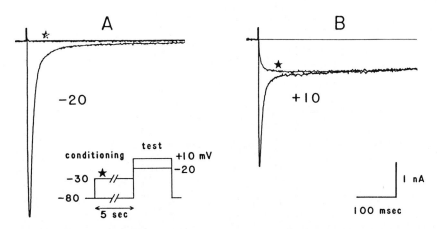

Figure 15 Selective inactivation of the transient component of calcium channel current by a conditioning depolarization. Membrane currents associated with step depolarizations to –20 mV (A) or +10 mV (B) following a 5-s conditioning pulse to –30 mV (asterisks) from a holding potential of –80 mV or without the prepulse. Leakage currents have been subtracted. Temperature, 33.1°C. (From Narahashi et al., 1987.)

L-type calcium channels (Fig. 16), but the potency is not high, requiring 30 μM to block the current by 50% (Twombly et al., 1988). The pyrethroid insecticide tetramethrin blocks T-type calcium channels of neuroblastoma cells (Yoshii et al., 1985) and the sinoatrial node (Hagiwara et al., 1988). Octanol blocks T-type calcium channels selectively in inferior olivary neurons (Llinás and Yarom, 1986), but in neuroblastoma cells it blocks both T- and L-type calcium channels (Twombly and Narahashi, 1989). There are other chemicals that block T-type calcium channels nonselectively, including ethanol (Twombly et al., 1990) and polyvalent cations, such as La^{3+}, Pb^{2+}, Cd^{2+}, Ni^{2+} and Co^{2+} (Narahashi et al., 1987).

The role of calcium channels in the action of pyrethroids remains to be established. Permethrin stimulation of electrical activity of neurosecretory cells of the stick insect at a very low concentration of 50 pM was interpreted as being due to stimulation of calcium channels (Orchard and Osborne, 1979; Osborne, 1980; Gammon and Sander, 1985), because these cells were thought to generate action potentials by inward calcium currents (Osborne, 1980). However, the observed stimulation of the cells by permethrin does not necessarily indicate its actions on calcium channels. Both sodium and calcium channels are usually present in various regions of the cell, and repetitive discharges observed could have been derived from the stimulation of sodium channels (Narahashi, 1989).

N-Type Calcium Channels

ω-Conotoxin GVIA, isolated from the venom of the marine snail *Conus geographus*, blocks N-type calcium channels of dorsal root ganglion and sympathetic neurons (McCleskey et

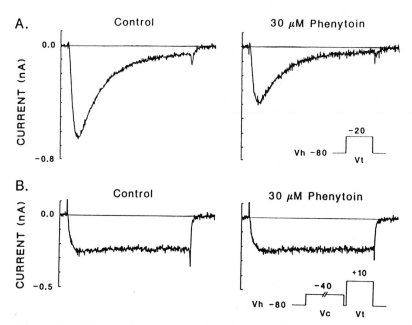

Figure 16 Effect of phenytoin on isolated type I and type II calcium channel currents. (A) Type I currents were elicited by applying 200-ms depolarizing test pulses to –20 mV from a holding potential (Vh) of –80 mV (inset). These currents were reduced in amplitude after 10 min of exposure to 30 μM phenytoin. (B) Type II currents were isolated with 5-s conditioning pulses (Vc) to –40 mV, followed by 200-ms test pulses (Vt) to +10 mV. Phenytoin did not alter the amplitude of these currents. (From Twombly et al., 1988.)

al., 1987), dorsal root ganglion × neuroblastoma hybrid (F-11) cells (Boland and Dingledine, 1990), sensory neurons (Kasai et al., 1987), and human neuroblastoma (IMR32) cells (Carbone et al., 1990). Although ω-conotoxin blocks some L-type calcium channels, all N-type calcium channels so far studied are sensitive to it. Lead is a potent blocker of N-type calcium channels, albeit not selectively (Reuveny and Narahashi, 1991).

L-Type Calcium Channels

Several groups of chemicals are known to block L-type calcium channels (Janis et al., 1987). They include phenylalkylamines, such as verapamil and D600, dihydropyridines, such as nifedipine, nimodipine, and nitrendipine, and benzothiazepines such as diltiazem. Several others are also known to block L-type calcium channels, albeit not selectively: benzodiazepines (diazepam, chlordiazepoxide) (Watabe et al., 1986; Reuveny et al., 1993); barbiturates (phenobarbital and pentobarbital) (Twombly et al., 1987); ethanol (Twombly et al., 1990); the polyvalent cations Co^{2+}, Ni^{2+}, Cd^{2+}, Pb^{2+}, and La^{3+} (Narahashi et al., 1987; Reuveny and Narahashi, 1991); and chlorpromazine (Ogata and Narahashi, 1990). Leucine-enkephalin is a potent and selective blocker of L-type calcium channels with a K_i of 8.8 nM, and block occurs via δ opioid receptors (Fig. 17) (Tsunoo et al., 1986). It should be emphasized that the potencies of these agents in blocking L-type calcium channels vary considerably among different cell types (Narahashi and Herman, 1992).

P-Type Calcium Channels

P-type calcium channels are not sensitive to dihydropyridines or ω-conotoxin GVIA but are blocked by funnel-web spider toxin FTX (Llinás et al., 1989, 1992; Jackson and Parks, 1989).

Calcium Channel Activators

Bay K 8644, a dihydropyridine, is well known to increase the amplitude of the whole-cell L-type calcium channel current (Fox et al., 1987). At the single-channel level, Bay K 8644 prolongs the mean open time and shifts the activation voltage in the hyperpolarizing direction without changing the single-channel conductance. This compound has been used as a tool to increase L-type calcium channel currents.

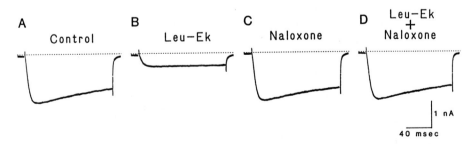

Figure 17 Naloxone antagonism of leucine-enkephalin (Leu-EK)-induced block of Ca^{2+} channels. (A) Ca^{2+} channel currents were evoked by a depolarization from a holding potential of −80 mV to +10 mV. (B) Record was taken 3 min after exposure to 25 nM Leu-EK. Then, Leu-EK was washed out with a saline solution containing 1 μM naloxone. (C) Record was taken 5 min after naloxone treatment. (D) Record was taken 3 min after reapplication of 25 nM Leu-EK in the presence of naloxone. Dotted lines represent zero current level. (From Tsunoo et al., 1986.)

TRANSMITTER-ACTIVATED ION CHANNELS AND NEUROTOXICITY

Acetylcholine Receptor Channels

Acetylcholine receptor (AChR) channels have been studied for a number of years, since the pioneering work by Takeuchi and Takeuchi (1959, 1960), who applied voltage clamp techniques for the first time to skeletal muscle end plate channels. Nicotinic AChR channels have since been studied extensively for their physiological and pharmacological properties, and many reviews have been published (Adams, 1981; Albuquerque et al., 1988a,b; Colquhoun, 1981; Galzi et al., 1991; Karlin, 1991; Luetje et al., 1990; Mathie et al., 1988; Peper et al., 1982; Lambert, 1983; Whittaker, 1990; Narahashi, 1987b, 1992c). However, our knowledge about neuronal nicotinic AChR channels and muscarinic AChR channels is quite limited, and more patch clamp studies are needed. Acetylcholine receptor channels are an important target site of a variety of therapeutic and environmental agents, and most studies have been performed using end plate channels.

Acetylcholine Receptor Channel Blockers

Receptor Blockers. Several chemicals are known to block AChRs, thereby suppressing the activity of the channel. A classical example is *d*-tubocurarine. However, recent studies have shown that this agent also blocks the AChR channel directly. One of the most important AChR blockers is α-bungarotoxin (α-BuTX), isolated from the venom of the snake *Bungarus multicinctus* (Chang and Lee, 1963). It blocks the nerve evoked end plate potential by binding to the AChR without any effect on the end plate membrane potential and the nerve conduction. However, it was not until the early 1970s that α-BuTX was used as a tool to study the AChR (Changeux et al., 1970; Miledi et al., 1971). Nicotine, which has been used as an insecticide, blocks the end plate current and causes the end plate depolarization, with apparent K_a values of 5 μM and 60 μM, respectively (Wang and Narahashi, 1972). The lower K_a value for block of end plate current is probably due to receptor desensitization. Nicotine also blocks the AChR channel directly by binding to the open channel (Aracava et al., 1988).

Channel Blockers. Lidocaine was the first agent shown to block the end plate AChR channel directly (Steinbach, 1968a,b). It binds to the channel while it is open. Since then, a large number of chemicals have been shown to block the end plate AChR channel directly: other local anesthetics (procaine, QX-314, QX-222), antimuscarinic agents (atropine, scopolamine, quinuclidinyl benzilate), general anesthetics (pentobarbital, thiopental, ketamine, halothane), other CNS agents (phenytoin, diazepam, phencyclidine), antibiotics (polymyxin B, clindamycin), antiviral agents (amantadine), anticholinesterases (neostigmine, physostigmine), ganglionic blocking agents (trimethaphan, hexamethonium, tetraethylammonium), depolarizing neuromuscular blocking agents (decamethonium, nicotine), natural toxins (perhydrohistrionicotoxin, gephyrotoxin, anatoxin a), antiplasmodiums (quinacrine), and guanidine derivatives (Albuquerque et al., 1988a,b; Spivak and Albuquerque, 1982; Peper et al., 1982; Lambert, 1983; Narahashi, 1987b). Extensive analyses of the mechanisms of action of some of these agents have disclosed unique state dependence, voltage dependence, and use dependence of block (Farley et al., 1981; Adams, 1977; Vogel et al., 1984; Spivak et al., 1982; Neher and Steinbach, 1978). It should be emphasized that many anticholinesterases block the ACh-activated channels in their open configuration. This action contributes to their toxicity.

Neuronal nicotinic AChRs are not sensitive to α-BuTX (Brown and Fumagalli, 1977; Kato and Narahashi, 1982). Another component of the venom from *Bungarus multicinctus*, κ-bungarotoxin, has a potent blocking action on certain neuronal AChRs (Chiappinelli, 1983; Mathie et al., 1988).

Channel Openers. Anatoxins, isolated from the blue-green algae *Anabaena flosaquae*, open the end plate AChR channels (Aracava et al., 1988). Openings occur in clusters separated by long silent periods.

Excitatory Glutamate Receptor Channels

The excitatory glutamate receptor channel system is widely distributed in the mammalian CNS, invertebrate CNS, and invertebrate neuromuscular junctions. Whereas the importance of its physiological function has been known for many years, it was not until the 1980s that extensive studies were commenced by using patch clamp techniques. Although L-glutamate is an endogenous neurotransmitter, several other amino acids are now known to stimulate the receptors in somewhat different manners. Thus this system is often called the excitatory amino acid (EAA) receptor-channel complex.

There are several reasons for the popularity of this area of study: 1) it is related to neurotoxicity, including ischemic brain damage; 2) it is related to epileptic discharge; 3) it is related to long-term potentiation; and 4) some classes of drugs act on this system. Several excellent reviews have been published during the past few years (Collingridge and Lester, 1989; Johnson and Jones, 1990; MacDonald and Nowak, 1990; Mayer and Miller, 1990; Monaghan et al., 1989; Olney, 1990; Wong and Kemp, 1991; Wroblewski and Danysz, 1989).

Classification and Characterization of Glutamate Receptor Channels

The EAA receptor-channel complex is traditionally classified into four groups, i.e., NMDA, kainate, quisqualate or AMPA (α-amino-3-hydroxy-5-methyl-4-isoxazole propionic acid), and AP4 (2-amino-4-phosphonobutanoate) receptors. Recently, an additional ACPD (*trans*-1-amino-cyclopentyl-1,3-decarboxylate) receptor has been proposed (Monaghan et al., 1989). The NMDA, kainate, and AMPA receptors have been studied most extensively, and our knowledge about the AP4 and ACPD receptors is limited. Examples of currents induced by quisqualate, kainate, and NMDA in rat hippocampal neurons in primary culture are shown in Fig. 18.

The NMDA receptor-channel complex is activated by NMDA, L-glutamate, L-aspartate, and ibotenate, modulated by glycine, and blocked by a host of divalent cations and chemicals, including Mg^{2+}, Zn^{2+}, CPP (3-3(2-carboxypiperazine-4-yl)propyl-1-phosphate), AP5 (2-amino-5-phosphonovalerate), PCP (phencyclidine), and ketamine. The glycine site in the NMDA receptor-channel complex is strychnine resistant, and glycine binding is an absolute requirement for the channel to open (Benveniste et al., 1990; Vyklicky et al., 1990). The channel thus opened is highly permeable to Ca^{2+}, with a Ca^{2+} permeability $(P_{Ca})/Na^+$ permeability (P_{Na}) ratio of 10.6 (Mayer and Westbrook, 1987) and a P_{Ca}/P_{Cs} ratio of 6.2 (Iino et al., 1990). Thus, receptor activation would lead to a massive influx of Ca^{2+}, which in turn causes a series of events including the activation of phospholipase C, increase in inositol triphosphate synthesis, and the release of Ca^{2+} from intracellular stores. These events are thought to lead to neurotoxicity.

The kainate receptor-channel complex is activated by several agonists, with the potency order domoate > kainate > quisqualate > > L-glutamate. It is blocked by CNQX (6-cyano-7-nitro-quinoxaline-2,3-dione) and DNQX (6,7-dinitro-quinoxaline-2,3-dione). The open channel is permeable to cations, but Ca^{2+} is much less permeant than Na^+, with a

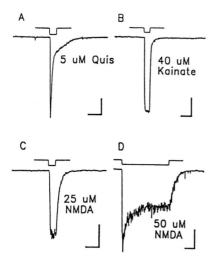

Figure 18   Currents induced by 5 μM quisqualate (A), 40 μM kainate (B), 25 μM NMDA (with 5 μM glycine) (C), and 50 μM NMDA (with 1 μM glycine) (D) in rat hippocampal neurons. Holding potential –80 mV. Current calibrations: 500 pA (A) and 200 pA (B, C, and D). Time calibrations: 500 ms (A, B, and C) and 2 sec (D).

P_{Ca}/P_{Na} of 0.15. The AMPA receptor-channel complex is activated by several agonists, with the potency order quisqualate ≥ AMPA > L-glutamate > kainate. It is blocked by CNQX and DNQX. The channel is permeable to cations with a P_{Ca}/P_{Na} of 0.15.

The role of glycine in the activity of NMDA receptor channels deserves further comment. Glycine augments the NMDA-induced current (Johnson and Ascher, 1987). It has recently been shown that glycine is absolutely required for activation of the NMDA receptor channels, on the basis of the inability of high concentrations of NMDA to induce currents in the presence of 7-chlorokynurenic acid, a selective glycine receptor antagonist (Vyklicky et al., 1990). Glycine is potent in augmenting NMDA-induced current, with an EC_{50} of 134 nM (Vyklicky et al., 1990), causing a problem in designing experiments, as it is very difficult to eliminate a small contamination of NMDA samples with glycine. Models have been developed in which NMDA receptor channels can be opened or desensitized only when bound by glycine, and in which the NMDA receptor has four independent sites, two for glycine and two for glutamate or NMDA (Benveniste et al., 1990).

Block by Divalent Cations

A variety of divalent cations have been shown to block the NMDA receptor channel. Some of them, including Mg^{2+} and Zn^{2+}, have been studied extensively, and they can serve as useful tools for elucidating the mechanism of action of various drugs on the NMDA receptor-channel. Mg^{2+} causes open channel block in a voltage-dependent manner, block being intensified with hyperpolarization (Nowak et al., 1984; Mayer et al., 1984). On the basis of Woodhull's equation (Woodhull, 1973), the Mg^{2+} binding site is located at midpoint in the channel pore. However, Mg^{2+} is also effective in blocking NMDA receptor channels when applied to the internal membrane surface, and the binding site is different from that calculated from the data on the external application of Mg^{2+} (Johnson and Ascher, 1990). Thus reservations must be made concerning the application of Woodhull's calculation to determine the geographical binding site. At large hyperpolarized membrane potentials (–150 mV to –200 mV), Mg^{2+} block is relieved, resulting in an N-shaped current-voltage (I-V) curve (Mayer and Westbrook, 1987). This relief may occur because Mg^{2+} is driven out of the inner orifice of the channel by hyperpolarizing inward current. In single-channel experiments, Mg^{2+} was seen to cause fast block (flickering block) (MacDonald and Nowak, 1990). However, the simple sequential-block model proposed by Neher and Steinbach (1978) for local anesthetic block of acetylcholine-activated channels does not apply here, because the characteristics of Mg^{2+} block fail to meet all the criteria of the sequential block. More complex models are required.

Zn^{2+} also blocks NMDA receptor channels. Unlike Mg^{2+} block, Zn^{2+} block is voltage independent, suggesting that its binding site is located on or near the external orifice of the channel (Westbrook and Mayer, 1987). The action of Zn^{2+} is not limited to NMDA receptor channels and is more complex, because it augments the currents induced by kainate, quisqualate, or L-glutamate in glycine-free conditions (Mayer et al., 1989). Furthermore, depending on the presence or absence of Mg^{2+}, Zn^{2+} either suppresses or increases the currents induced by L-glutamate, AMPA, or kainate (Rassendren et al., 1990). At the single-channel level, Zn^{2+} (1–10 μM) decreases the probability of channel openings in a voltage-independent manner, and at higher concentrations (10–100 μM) Zn^{2+} decreases the single-channel current amplitude, suggesting fast block (Christine and Choi, 1990).

Other divalent cations have also been found to block NMDA receptor channels, with the potency sequence $Ni^{2+} > Co^{2+} > Mg^{2+} > Mn^{2+} > Ca^{2+}$. Ions that give up their water slowly are considered blockers (e.g. Ni^{2+}, Co^{2+}, Mg^{2+}), whereas ions that dehydrate more quickly are considered to be permeant (e.g. Ca^{2+}, Ba^{2+}, Cd^{2+}, Sr^{2+}) (Collingridge and Lester, 1989). However, this classification is rather arbitrary, because many of these divalent cations can permeate and block (e.g. Ca^{2+}, Mg^{2+}, Cd^{2+}).

Block by Drugs and Chemicals

Ketamine and PCP have received much attention for their blocking action on NMDA receptor channels. Both block the NMDA-induced current in a voltage-dependent and use-dependent manner, without effect on the kainate- or quisqualate-induced current (Honey et al., 1985; MacDonald et al., 1987; Miljkovic and MacDonald, 1987). Its K_i values are estimated to be 1.5 μM at –60 mV and 49 μM at +40 mV, and the binding site appears to be located close to the cytoplasmic surface (Mayer et al., 1988). However, this interpretation about the binding site has been questioned recently (MacDonald and Nowak, 1990). Ketamine reduces the mean open time, and its action and recovery from it are slow, suggesting that ketamine enters the open channel and is trapped within the channel unless NMDA agonists reopen the channel (Mayer et al., 1988; MacDonald et al., 1987).

Dizocilpine (MK-801), an anticonvulsant, blocks the NMDA-induced current selectively (Wong et al., 1986). Binding and unbinding of MK-801 occur only if the channel is activated, and recovery from block in the presence of NMDA is strongly voltage dependent, being faster at positive potentials (Huettner and Bean, 1988). At the single-channel level, it shortens the mean open time, decreases the frequency of openings, and decreases the burst time, characteristics of open-channel block (Huettner and Bean, 1988).

Some antidepressants, neuroleptic drugs, and phencyclidine-like drugs have been shown to block NMDA receptor channels. These include imipramine, chlorimipramine, desmethylimipramine, nortriptyline, protriptyline, chlorpromazine, dextromethorphan, cyclazocine, and (±)-SKF 10,047 (Reynolds and Miller, 1988; Sills and Loo, 1989).

Desipramine blocks NMDA-induced current in a voltage-dependent manner, with a K_i of 10 μM, but has no effect on kainate- or quisqualate-induced current (Sernagor et al., 1989). Promazine reduces single-channel open time and appears to act as an open-channel blocker (Sernagor et al., 1989). Haloperidol at low concentrations (0.1–1 μM) augments NMDA-induced current by increasing the frequency of single-channel openings; it decreases the current at higher concentrations (1–30 μM) (Rocha et al., 1989; Siqueira-Rocha et al., 1990). Pentobarbital decreases currents induced by kainate, quisqualate, L-aspartate, and NMDA in a voltage-dependent manner, block being intensified with hyperpolarization (Miljkovic and MacDonald, 1987; Collingridge and Lester, 1989). It appears to act on the channel. Infenprodil, an anti-ischemic drug, blocks the NMDA receptor channel complex (Wong and Kemp, 1991).

The EAA receptor-channel system has been shown to be affected by pyrethroids. The binding of [^{3}H]kainate to mouse brain homogenates was inhibited by pyrethroids with IC_{25} values ranging from 80 nM for deltamethrin to 8 μM for *cis*-permethrin (Staatz et al., 1982). The glutamate sensitivity of the muscle of housefly larvae was suppressed by 1 μM cypermethrin (Seabrook et al., 1988). In view of the reasonably high potencies for these actions, the EAA system merits further study.

Ethanol also blocks the NMDA-activated channels without much effect on the kainate- and quisqualate-activated channels (Lovinger et al., 1989). Ethanol is not potent, with 61% suppression at 50 mM. It has also been shown that ethanol has a dual effect on NMDA-activated channels (Lima-Landman and Albuquerque, 1989). At low concentrations (1.74–8.65 mM), ethanol increases the probability of openings without changing the mean open time, whereas at higher concentrations (86.5–174 mM) it decreases both the probability of openings and the mean open time.

Spider and wasp toxins have been shown to block glutamate receptor channels (Blagbrough et al., 1992). Argiopine, a spider toxin, blocks the NMDA response selectively in rat cortical neurons (Kemp et al., 1989). Philanthotoxin-433 and argiotoxin-636 block glutamate-induced responses in crayfish and locust muscles when the channels are open (Usherwood and Blagbrough, 1989).

Role of Polyamines in Ischemic Neuronal Damage

Cerebral ischemia is associated with an increase in putrescine levels (Koenig et al., 1990; Paschen et al., 1988; Roehn et al., 1990). The postischemic overshoot in putrescine formation may be related to alterations in cellular calcium homeostasis: mitochondrial calcium uptake and NMDA-dependent calcium influx are increased (Jensen et al., 1989; McGurk et al., 1990). Polyamines bind to calcium channels (Pullan et al., 1990). Polyamines also inhibit protein kinase C (Qi et al., 1983), the activation of which inhibits the L-type calcium channels (Linden and Routtenberg, 1989). Thus, polyamines appear to play an important role in ischemia through interaction with calcium channels. Recent experiments have indeed shown that putrescine augments the L-type calcium channel current (Herman et al., 1993).

The activation of the NMDA receptor causes an increase in ornithine decarboxylase (ODC) activity that in turn increases putrescine (Koenig et al., 1990). Spermine and spermidine increase the binding of [^{3}H]-MK-801 to the NMDA receptor channel, but putrescine is without effect (Williams et al., 1990). Spermine and spermidine augment the NMDA-induced current in a manner additive to glycine potentiation, and the effect is not reversed by putrescine; on the contrary, putrescine has agonist-like actions of its own, potentiating the NMDA-induced current (Sprosen and Woodruff, 1990).

Inhibitory Amino Acid Receptor Channels

There are three major types of inhibitory amino acid receptor channel system, i.e., GABA$_A$, GABA$_B$, and glycine systems. In arthropods, GABA is an inhibitory transmitter at neuromuscular junctions. In mammals, glycine is the major inhibitory transmitter in the spinal cord and brain stem, and GABA is an inhibitory transmitter in the spinal cord, cortex, midbrain, and cerebellum. The GABA$_A$ system is present primarily on the postsynaptic side, whereas the GABA$_B$ system is on both the presynaptic and the postsynaptic sides.

Drugs Acting on GABA$_A$ Receptor Channels

A large number of chemicals and drugs are known to interact with the GABA$_A$ receptor-channel complex. At least five binding sites have been identified on the basis of the affinity of these drugs: the GABA site, the benzodiazepine site, the barbiturate site, the picrotoxin site, and chloride channel (Olsen et al., 1988, 1991). γ-Aminobutyric acid and muscimol bind to the GABA site, thereby opening the chloride channel. This site is blocked by bicuculline and a few other drugs. Benzodiazepines are known to bind to the benzodiazepine site, leading to a potentiation of the action of GABA. This site is inhibited by Ro15-1788. β-Carboline 3-carboxylate esters act as allosteric inhibitors or inverse agonists of the benzodiazepine site, thereby acting as convulsants or proconvulsants. Barbiturates potentiate the action of GABA and open the chloride channel through binding to the barbiturate site. Picrotoxin, pentylenetetrazol, lindane, dieldrin, and tert-butylbicyclo-phosphorothionate (TBPS) block the chloride channel. There are other agents that potentiate the action of GABA, but their binding site remains to be established. They are ethanol (Huidobro-Toro et al., 1987; Mehta and Ticku, 1988; Suzdak et al., 1986; Ticku et al., 1986; Nishio and Narahashi, 1990), longer-chain alcohols (Nakahiro et al., 1991), the inhalational general anesthetics halothane, enflurane, and isoflurane (Nakahiro et al., 1989), and Hg^{2+} ions (Arakawa et al., 1991). The anthelmintic and insecticidal avermectin B$_{1a}$ is a potent partial agonist; it activates the receptor-channel complex, inhibits binding of [^{3}H]muscimol and [^{35}S]TBPS, and potentiates binding of [^{3}H]flunitrazepam (Abalis et al., 1986).

Patch clamp studies have disclosed some aspects of the mechanisms underlying the drug–GABA$_A$ receptor-channel interactions. Pentobarbital prolongs the mean open time without changing the single-channel conductance or the frequency of channel openings, thereby increasing the GABA-induced whole-cell current (Mienville and Vicini, 1989). Picrotoxin and pregnenolone sulfate decrease the frequency of channel openings, leading to a block of GABA-induced whole-cell current (Mienville and Vicini, 1989). Diazepam increases the GABA-induced whole-cell current by prolonging the mean open time without changing the probability of openings (Twyman et al., 1989).

The GABA$_A$ receptor-channel complex is a pentameric protein comprising five subunits of various combinations (Olsen, 1992; Olsen and Tobin, 1990; Fritschy et al., 1992). At present six α, four β, four γ, one δ, and one ρ subunits are known to exist. Each subunit contains four domains. The distributions of various subunits among different cell types and the affinities of each subunit or of combinations of subunits for GABA$_A$ modulators remain largely to be established.

Effects of Pyrethroids on GABA$_A$ Receptor Channels

Type II pyrethroids that possess a cyano group at the α position have been shown to block the GABA$_A$ receptor-channel complex (Abalis et al., 1986; Bloomquist et al., 1986; Crofton et al., 1987; Eshleman and Murray, 1990; Gammon and Sander, 1985; Lawrence and Casida, 1983; Lawrence et al., 1985; Lummis et al., 1987; Ramadan et al., 1988a). The GABA hypothesis has been a matter of extensive debate, partly because the potency and efficacy of the action are low. Patch clamp experiments with rat dorsal root ganglion neurons have unequivocally shown that while 10 μM deltamethrin greatly prolongs the sodium current, as expected, the GABA-induced chloride current recorded from the very same cell remains totally unchanged (Fig. 19) (Ogata et al., 1988). However, more recent patch clamp experiments with rat hippocampal neurons have indicated that there is a transient increase in GABA-induced chloride current following application of pyrethroids (Frey and Narahashi, 1989; Frey et al., 1989). Thus more careful and extensive studies along this line are warranted. The transient stimulation of the GABA system may be responsible for certain phases of symptoms of poisoning in animals.

It has been claimed that the peripheral benzodiazepine receptors are a target for both type I and type II pyrethroids (Devaud and Murray, 1988). A significant correlation was found between the proconvulsant effects of the pyrethroids and their respective IC_{50} values as inhibitors of [3H]Ro5-4864 binding. However, other investigators claimed that the correlation between their potencies in inhibiting [3H]Ro5-4864 binding and their toxicities was poor (Ramadan et al., 1988b).

Effects of Lindane and Cyclodienes on GABA$_A$ Receptor Channels

Whereas the action of lindane and cyclodienes to stimulate synaptic transmission was demonstrated more than 30 years ago (Yamasaki and Ishii (Narahashi), 1954; Yamasaki and Narahashi, 1958), it was not until the early 1980s that the GABA receptor-channel complex was suggested as being their target site. Lindane and cyclodienes were shown to antagonize the action of GABA in stimulating $^{36}Cl^-$ uptake by various nerve and muscle preparations (Abalis et al., 1986; Bloomquist and Soderlund, 1985; Bloomquist et al., 1986; Ghiasuddin and Matsumura, 1982). These insecticides also inhibited the binding of [35S]TBPS

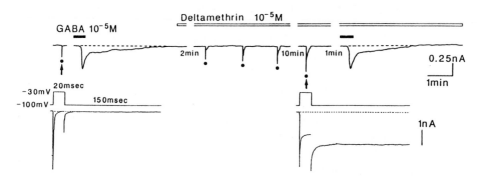

Figure 19 Effects of deltamethrin on the sodium current and the γ-aminobutyric acid (GABA)-induced inward current. The membrane was held at –100 mV. In the upper tracings, the membrane current was registered on a pen-recorder. At points indicated by dots, 20-ms depolarizing pulses to –30 mV were applied to generate sodium currents. At the two points indicated by upward arrows, the sodium currents were recorded on an oscilloscope with an expanded time scale. GABA (10 μM) and deltamethrin (10 μM) were applied during periods indicated by black and white horizontal bars, respectively. Whereas the GABA-induced current remained unchanged by deltamethrin, the sodium current underwent drastic changes causing prolongation of currents during and after the depolarizing pulse. (From Ogata et al., 1988.)

(Bermudez et al., 1991; Cole and Casida, 1986; Llorens et al., 1990; Lummis et al., 1990; Matsumura and Ghiasuddin, 1983; Matsumoto et al., 1988; Olsen et al., 1989; Thompson et al., 1990).

The first patch clamp experiments for these insecticides have clearly demonstrated that the GABA-induced chloride current is suppressed by lindane and cyclodienes (Fig. 20) (Ogata et al., 1988). Noise analyses conducted recently by Bermudez et al. (1991) with cockroach neurons have shown that lindane and dieldrin decrease the frequency of GABA-chloride channel openings without changing the mean open time. Whereas dieldrin had no significant effect on the single-channel conductance, lindane decreased it. The latter effect of lindane was not observed by Zufall et al. (1989), who found no effect in crayfish stomach muscle. Thus there still remains an important controversy regarding the effect of lindane on single channels.

These studies of lindane and cyclodienes have paved the avenue toward the mechanism of interactions of these insecticides on the GABA receptor-channel complex. A number of questions remain to be answered. The points in question include 1) changes in whole-cell and single-channel current characteristics; 2) the exact site of action on the GABA receptor-channel complex (e.g., GABA site, barbiturate site, benzodiazepine site, channel site, etc.); 3) the effects of lindane isomers, such as α-, β-, and δ-BHC; 4) voltage dependence and use dependence of action; 5) interactions of these insecticides with various divalent cations (e.g., Zn^{2+}, Cu^{2+}) and trivalent cations (La^{3+}, other lanthanides) that are known to modulate the GABA receptor channel complex (Ma and Narahashi, 1993; Yan and Narahashi, 1992); and 6) species and tissue specificity of insecticide–GABA system interactions.

Drugs Acting on GABA$_B$ Receptor Channels

The activation of the GABA$_B$ receptor opens a potassium channel and closes a calcium channel. This system appears to be involved in various physiological functions, such as inhibition of transmitter and hormone release, mediation of slow inhibitory postsynaptic potentials, increase in gastric motility, suppression of hippocampal epileptiform activity, and relaxation of bronchi and the urinary bladder (Bowery, 1989). The potency and selectivity of the agents that act on the GABA$_B$ system vary greatly. For instance, (–)-β-hydroxy-GABA acts on both the GABA$_A$ and the GABA$_B$ system equally. Kojic amine stimulates the GABA$_B$ system and antagonizes the GABA$_A$ system. δ-Aminovaleric acid suppresses the GABA$_B$ system while stimulating the GABA$_A$ system. 3-Aminopropyl-phosphinic acid and (–)-baclofen are selective agonists of the GABA$_B$ system, and muscimol

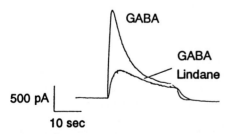

Figure 20 Effects of lindane on γ-aminobutyric acid (GABA)-activated chloride current in a rat hippocampal neuron. GABA 15 μM applied by puffer generates an inward chloride current (upward deflection) that decays to a slow phase. Lindane 50 μM co-applied with GABA greatly suppressed the current. (From Narahashi et al., 1992.)

stimulates the $GABA_A$ system more potently than the $GABA_B$ system. Much remains to be studied concerning the role of the $GABA_B$ system in neurotoxicity.

Adenosine Triphosphate–Activated Channels

Ion channels that can be activated by ATP were first described by Krishtal et al. (1983) in mammalian sensory neurons. Many other tissues have since been found to be endowed with ATP-activated channels, including vascular smooth muscle (Benham et al., 1987; Benham and Tsien, 1987), vas deferens (Nakazawa and Matsuki, 1987; Friel, 1988), cultured skeletal muscle (Hume and Honig, 1986), and cardiac muscle (Friel and Bean, 1988). Details of the ATP-activated channels are reviewed by Bean and Friel (1990).

When applied at micromolar concentrations, ATP induces an inward current at a holding potential of –80 mV. In frog sensory neurons, the ATP-induced current is hardly desensitized during application, whereas in some other preparations, such as frog atrial cells, rat dorsal root ganglion neurons, and rat vas deferens, the current is desensitized. The current reverses its polarity at 0 mV, indicating that the channel is nonselective to cations (Bean and Friel, 1990).

Little information has been accumulated regarding the pharmacology or toxicology of the ATP-activated cation channels. α,β-Methylene ATP inhibits ATP-activated current in cardiac atrial cells (Friel and Bean, 1988) and in cardiac sympathetic neurons (Fieber and Adams, 1988). However, it has no antagonistic effect on vas deferens cells (Friel, 1988). Adenosine 5'-(β,γ-methylene)triphosphonate acts as a competitive antagonist, with a K_i of 21 μM in sensory neurons (Krishtal et al., 1988).

REFERENCES

Abalis IM, Eldefrawi ME, Eldefrawi AT (1986). Effects of insecticides on GABA-induced chloride influx into rat brain microsacs. J Toxicol Environ Health 18:13–23.

Adams DJ, Nonner W (1990). Voltage-dependent potassium channels: gating, ion permeation and block. In: Cook NS, ed. Potassium channels: structure, classification, function and therapeutic potential. Chichester, U.K.: Ellis Horwood, 40–69.

Adams PR (1977). Voltage jump analysis of procaine action at frog endplate. J Physiol 268:291–318.

Adams PR (1981). Acetylcholine receptor kinetics. J Membrane Biol 58:161–74.

Adams PR (1982). Voltage-dependent conductances of vertebrate neurones. Trends Neurosci 5:116–9.

Adelman WJ Jr, Senft JP (1966). Voltage clamp studies on the effect of internal cesium ion on sodium and potassium currents in the squid giant axon. J Gen Physiol 50:279–93.

Albuquerque EX, Daly J, Witkop B (1971). Batrachotoxin: chemistry and pharmacology. Science 172:995–1002.

Albuquerque EX, Seyama I, Narahashi T (1973). Characterization of batrachotoxin-induced depolarization of the squid giant axons. J Pharmacol Exp Ther 184:308–14.

Albuquerque EX, Alkondon M, Deshpande SS, Cintra WM, Aracava Y, Brossi A (1988a). The role of carbamates and oximes in reversing toxicity of organophosphorus compounds: a perspective into mechanisms. In: Lunt GG, ed. Neurotox '88: molecular basis of drug and pesticide action. Amsterdam: Elsevier, 349–73.

Albuquerque EX, Daly JW, Warnick JE (1988b). Macromolecular sites for specific neurotoxins and drugs on chemosensitive synapses and electrical excitation in biological membranes. In: Narahashi T, ed. Ion channels. Vol. 1. New York: Plenum Press, 95–162.

Aracava Y, Swanson KL, Rozental R, Albuquerque EX (1988). Structure-activity relationship of (+)anatoxin-a derivatives and enantiomers of nicotine on the peripheral and central nicotinic acetylcholine receptor subtypes. In: Lunt GG, ed. Neurotox '88: molecular basis of drug and pesticide action. Amsterdam: Elsevier, 157–84.

Arakawa O, Nakahiro M, Narahashi T (1991). Mercury modulation of GABA-activated chloride channels and non-specific cation channels in rat dorsal root ganglion neurons. Brain Res 551:58–63.

Armstrong CM (1969). Inactivation of the potassium conductance and related phenomena caused by quaternary ammonium ion injection in squid axons. J Gen Physiol 54:553–75.

Armstrong CM (1971). Interaction of tetraethylammonium ion derivatives with the potassium channels of giant axons. J Gen Physiol 58:413–37.

Armstrong CM, Binstock L (1965). Anomalous rectification in the squid giant axon injected with tetraethylammonium chloride. J Gen Physiol 48:859–72.

Armstrong CM, Taylor SR (1980). Interaction of barium ions with potassium channels in squid giant axons. Biophys J 30:473–88.

Ashcroft FM (1988). Adenosine-5'-triphosphate-sensitive potassium channels. Annu Rev Neurosci 11:97–118.

Bean BP, Friel DD (1990). ATP-activated channels in excitable cells. In: Narahashi T, ed. Ion channels. Vol. 2. New York: Plenum Press, 169–203.

Benham CD, Tsien RW (1987). A novel receptor-operated Ca^{2+}-permeable channel activated by ATP in smooth muscle. Nature 328:275–8.

Benham CD, Bolton TB, Byrne NG, Large WA (1987). Action of externally applied adenosine triphosphate on single smooth muscle cells from rabbit ear artery. J Physiol 387:473–88.

Benveniste M, Clements J, Vyklicky L Jr, Mayer ML (1990). A kinetic analysis of the modulation of N-methyl-D-aspartic acid receptors by glycine in mouse cultured hippocampal neurones. J Physiol 428:333–57.

Bermudez I, Hawkins CA, Taylor AM, Beadle DJ (1991). Actions of insecticides on the insect GABA receptor complex. J Receptor Res 11:221–32.

Blagbrough IS, Brackley PTH, Bruce M, Bycroft BW, Mather AJ, Millington S, Sudan HL, Usherwood PNR (1992). Arthropod toxins as leads for novel insecticides: an assessment of polyamine amides as glutamate antagonists. Toxicon 30:303–22.

Blatz AL, Magleby KL (1986). Single apamin-blocked Ca-activated K^+ channels of small conductance in cultured rat skeletal muscle. Nature 323:718–20.

Bloomquist JR, Soderlund DM (1985). Neurotoxic insecticides inhibit GABA-dependent chloride uptake by mouse brain vesicles. Biochem Biophys Res Comm 133:37–43.

Bloomquist JR, Adams PM, Soderlund DM (1986). Inhibition of γ-aminobutyric acid–stimulated chloride flux in mouse brain vesicles by polychlorocycloalkane and pyrethroid insecticides. NeuroToxicology 7(3):11–20.

Boland LM, Dingledine R (1990). Multiple components of both transient and sustained barium currents in a rat dorsal root ganglion cell line. J Physiol 420:223–45.

Bourque CW (1988). Transient calcium-dependent potassium current in magnocellular neurosecretory cells of the rat supraoptic nucleus. J Physiol 397:331–47.

Bowery N (1989). GABAB receptors and their significance in mammalian pharmacology. Trends Pharmacol Sci 10:401–7.

Bräu ME, Dreyer F, Jonas P, Repp H, Vogel W (1990). A K^+ channel in *Xenopus* nerve fibres selectively blocked by bee and snake toxins: binding and voltage-clamp experiments. J Physiol 420:365–85.

Brown DA (1988). M currents. In: Narahashi T, ed. Ion Channels. Vol. 1. New York: Plenum Press, 55–94.

Brown DA, Fumagalli L (1977). Dissociation of α-bungarotoxin binding and receptor block in the rat superior cervical ganglion. Brain Res 129:165–8.

Carbone E, Wanke E, Prestipino G, Possani LD, Maelicke A (1982). Selective blockage of voltage-dependent K^+ channels by a novel scorpion toxin. Nature 296:90–1.

Carbone E, Prestipino G, Spadavecchia L, Franciolini F, Possani LD (1987). Blocking of the squid axon K^+ channel by noxiustoxin: a toxin from the venom of the scorpion *Centruroides noxius*. Pflügers Arch 408:423–31.

Carbone E, Sher E, Clementi F (1990). Ca currents in human neuroblastoma IMR32 cells: kinetics, permeability and pharmacology. Pflügers Arch 416:170–9.

Castle NA, Haylett DG, Jenkinson DH (1989). Toxins in the characterization of potassium channels. Trends Pharmacol Sci 12:59–65.

Catterall WA (1980). Neurotoxins that act on voltage-sensitive sodium channels in excitable membranes. Annu Rev Pharmacol Toxicol 20:15–43.

Chandler WK, Meves H (1965). Voltage clamp experiments on internally perfused giant axons. J Physiol 180:788–820.

Chang CC, Lee CY (1963). Isolation of neurotoxins from the venom of *Bungarus multicinctus* and their mode of neuromuscular blocking action. Arch Intern Pharmacodyn 144:241–57.

Changeux J-P, Kasai M, Lee CY (1970). Use of a snake venom toxin to characterize the cholinergic receptor protein. Proc Natl Acad Sci USA 67:1241–7.

Chiappinelli VA (1983). Kappa-bungarotoxin: a probe for the neuronal nicotinic receptor in avian ciliary ganglion. Brain Res 277:9–22.

Chicchi GG, Gimenez-Gallego G, Ber E, Garcia ML, Winquist R, Cascieri MA (1988). Purification and characterization of a unique, potent inhibitor of apamin binding from *Leiurus quinquestriatus hebraeus* venom. J Biol Chem 263:10192–7.

Chinn K, Narahashi T (1986). Stabilization of sodium channel states by deltamethrin in mouse neuroblastoma cells. J Physiol 380:191–207.

Chinn K, Narahashi T (1989). Temperature-dependent subconducting states and kinetics of deltamethrin-modified sodium channels of neuroblastoma cells. Pflügers Arch 413:571–9.

Christine CW, Choi DW (1990). Effect of zinc on NMDA receptor–mediated channel currents in cortical neurons. J Neurosci 10:108–16.

Cole KS (1949). Dynamic electrical characteristics of the squid axon membrane. Arch Sci Physiol 3:253–8.

Cole LM, Casida JE (1986). Polychlorocycloalkane insecticide–induced convulsions in mice in relation to disruption of the GABA-regulated chloride ionophore. Life Sci 39:1855–62.

Collingridge GL, Lester RAJ (1989). Excitatory amino acid receptors in the vertebrate central nervous system. Pharmacol Rev 40:143–210.

Colquhoun D (1981). How fast do drugs work? Trends Pharmacol Sci 2:212–7.

Connor JA, Stevens CF (1971). Voltage clamp studies of a transient outward membrane current in gastropod neural somata. J Physiol 213:21–30.

Cook NS (1988). The pharmacology of potassium channels and their therapeutic potential. Trends Pharmacol Sci 9:21–8.

Courtney KR (1975). Mechanism of frequency-dependent inhibition of sodium currents in frog myelinated nerve by the lidocaine derivative GEA 968. J Pharmacol Exp Ther 195:225–36.

Courtney KR (1980). Structure-activity relations for the frequency-dependent sodium channel block in nerve by local anesthetics. J Pharmacol Exp Ther 213:114–9.

Courtney KR, Kendig JJ, Cohen EN (1978). The rates of interaction of local anesthetics with sodium channels in nerve. J Pharmacol Exp Ther 207:594–604.

Crofton KM, Reiter LW, Mailman RB (1987). Pyrethroid insecticides and radioligand displacement from the GABA receptor chloride ionophore complex. Toxicol Lett 35:183–90.

Deecher DC, Soderlund DM (1991). RH 3421, an insecticidal dihydropyrazole, inhibits sodium channel–dependent sodium uptake in mouse brain preparations. Pesticide Biochem Physiol 39:130–7.

Devaud LL, Murray TF (1988). Involvement of peripheral-type benzodiazepine receptors in the proconvulsant actions of pyrethroid insecticides. J Pharmacol Exp Ther 247:14–22.

DeWeille JR, Lazdunski M (1990). Regulation of the ATP-sensitive potassium channel. In: Narahashi T, ed. Ion Channels. Vol. 2. New York: Plenum Press, 205–22.

DeWeille JR, Vijverberg HPM, Narahashi T (1988). Interactions of pyrethroids and octylguanidine with sodium channels of squid giant axons. Brain Res 445:1–11.

Dodge FA, Frankenhaeuser B (1958). Membrane currents in isolated frog nerve fibre under voltage clamp conditions. J Physiol 143:76–90.

Dolly JO, Halliwell JV, Black JD, Williams RS, Pelchen-Matthews A, Breeze AL, Mahraban F, Othman IB, Black AR (1984). Botulinum neurotoxin and dendrotoxin as probes for studies on transmitter release. J Physiol (Paris) 79:280–303.

Dreyer F (1990). Peptide toxins and potassium channels. Rev Physiol Biochem Pharmacol 115:93–136.

Eaton DC, Brodwick MS (1980). Effects of barium on the potassium conductance of squid axon. J Gen Physiol 75:727–50.

Edwards G, Weston AH (1990). Structure-activity relationship of K^+ channel openers. Trends Pharmacol Sci 11:417–22.

Eshleman AJ, Murray TF (1990). Dependence on gamma-aminobutyric acid of pyrethroid and 4′-chlorodiazepam modulation of the binding of t-[^{35}S]butylbicyclophosphorothionate in piscine brain. Neuropharmacology 29:641–8.

Farley JM, Watanabe S, Yeh JZ, Narahashi T (1981). Endplate channel block by guanidine derivatives. J Gen Physiol 77:273–93.

Fieber LA, Adams DJ (1988). Pharmacological antagonism of ACh and ATP receptor-channels in rat cultured parasympathetic neurons (abstr). Soc Neurosci Abstr 14:639.

Fox AP, Nowycky MC, Tsien RW (1987). Single-channel recordings of three types of calcium channels in chick sensory neurones. J Physiol 394:173–200.

Frazier DT, Narahashi T, Yamada M (1970). The site of action and active form of local anesthetics. II. Experiments with quaternary compounds. J Pharmacol Exp Ther 171:45–51.

Frey JM, Narahashi T (1989). Deltamethrin alters pentobarbital-induced chloride currents in cultured hippocampal neurons (abstr). Soc Neurosci Abstr 15:1151.

Frey J, Dichter M, Narahashi T (1989). Effects of lindane and fenvalerate on GABA-activated chloride currents in cultured hippocampal neurons (abstr). Toxicologist 9:149.

Friel DD (1988). An ATP-sensitive conductance in single smooth muscle cells from the rat vas deferens. J Physiol 401:361–80.

Friel DD, Bean BP (1988). Two ATP-activated conductances in bullfrog atrial cells. J Gen Physiol 91:1–27.

Fritschy J-M, Benke D, Mertens S, Oertel WH, Bachi T, Möhler H (1992). Five subtypes of type A γ-aminobutyric acid receptors identified in neurons by double and triple immunofluorescence staining with subunit-specific antibodies. Proc Natl Acad Sci USA 89:6726–30.

Galzi J-L, Revah F, Bessis A, Changeux J-P (1991). Functional architecture of the nicotinic acetylcholine receptor: from electric organ to brain. Annu Rev Pharmacol Toxicol 31:37–72.

Gammon DW, Sander G (1985). Two mechanisms of pyrethroid action: electrophysiological and pharmacological evidence. NeuroToxicology 6(2):63–86.

Ghiasuddin SM, Matsumura F (1982). Inhibition of gamma-aminobutyric acid (GABA)-induced chloride uptake by gamma-BHC and heptachlor epoxide. Comp Biochem Physiol 73C:141–4.

Gustafsson B, Galvan M, Grafe P, Wigström H (1982). A transient outward current in a mammalian central neurone blocked by 4-aminopyridine. Nature 299:252–4.

Hagiwara N, Irisawa H, Kameyama M (1988). Contribution of two types of calcium currents to the pacemaker potentials of rabbit sino-atrial node cells. J Physiol 395:233–53.

Hagiwara S, Saito N (1959). Voltage-current relations in nerve cell membrane of *Onchidium verruculatum*. J Physiol 148:161–79.

Hagiwara S, Kusano K, Saito N (1961). Membrane changes of *Onchidium* nerve cell in potassium-rich media. J Physiol 155:470–89.

Hagiwara S, Miyazaki S, Rosenthal NP (1976). Potassium current and the effect of cesium on this current during anomalous rectification of the egg cell membrane of a starfish. J Gen Physiol 67:621–38.

Hagiwara S, Miyazaki S, Moody W, Patlak J (1978). Blocking effects of barium and hydrogen ions on the potassium current during anomalous rectification in the starfish egg. J Physiol 279:167–85.

Halliwell JV, Othman IB, Pelchen-Matthews A, Dolly JO (1986). Central action of dendrotoxin:

selective reduction of a transient K conductance in hippocampus and binding to localized acceptors. Proc Natl Acad Sci USA 83:493–7.

Hamill OP, Marty A, Neher E, Sakmann B, Sigworth FJ (1981). Improved patch-clamp techniques for high-resolution current recording from cells and cell-free membrane patches. Pflügers Arch 391:85–100.

Hermann A, Erxleben C (1987). Charybdotoxin selectivity blocks small Ca-activated K channels in *Aplysia* neurons. J Gen Physiol 90:27–47.

Herman MD, Reuveny E, Narahashi T (1993). The effect of polyamines on voltage-activated calcium channels in N1E-115 mouse neuroblastoma cells. J Physiol 462:645–60.

Hille B (1971). The permeability of the sodium channel to organic cations in myelinated nerve. J Gen Physiol 58:599–619.

Hille B (1977). Local anesthetic: hydrophilic and hydrophobic pathways for the drug-receptor reaction. J Gen Physiol 69:497–515.

Hodgkin AL, Huxley AF (1952a). Currents carried by sodium and potassium ions through the membrane of the giant axon of *Loligo*. J Physiol 116:449–72.

Hodgkin AL, Huxley AF (1952b). The components of membrane conductance in the giant axon of *Loligo*. J Physiol 116:473–96.

Hodgkin AL, Huxley AF (1952c). The dual effect of membrane potential on sodium conductance in the giant axon of *Loligo*. J Physiol 116:497–506.

Hodgkin AL, Huxley AF (1952d). A quantitative description of membrane current and its application to conduction and excitation in nerve. J Physiol 117:500–44.

Hodgkin AL, Huxley AF, Katz B (1952). Measurement of current-voltage relations in the membrane of the giant axon of *Loligo*. J Physiol 116:424–48.

Holloway SF, Narahashi T, Salgado VL, Wu CH (1989). Kinetic properties of single sodium channels modified by fenvalerate in mouse neuroblastoma cells. Pflügers Arch 414:613–21.

Honey CR, Miljkovic Z, MacDonald JF (1985). Ketamine and phencyclidine cause a voltage-dependent block of responses to L-aspartic acid. Neurosci Lett 61:135–9.

Hosey MM, Lazdunski M (1988). Calcium channels: molecular pharmacology, structure and regulation. J Membrane Biol 104:81–105.

Huettner JE, Bean BP (1988). Block of N-methyl-D-aspartate-activated current by the anticonvulsant MK-801: selective binding to open channels. Proc Natl Acad Sci USA 85:1307–11.

Hugues M, Schmid H, Romey G, Duval D, Frelin C, Lazdunski M (1982). The Ca^{2+}-dependent slow K^+ conductance in cultured rat muscle cells: characterization with apamin. EMBO J 1:1039–42.

Huidobro-Toro JP, Bleck V, Allan AM, Harris RA (1987). Neurochemical actions of anesthetic drugs on the γ-aminobutyric acid receptor-chloride channel complex. J Pharmacol Exp Ther 242:963–9.

Hume RI, Honig MG (1986). Excitatory action of ATP on embryonic chick muscle. J Neurosci 6:681–90.

Iino M, Ozawa S, Tsuzuki K (1990). Permeation of calcium through excitatory amino acid receptor channels in cultured rat hippocampal neurones. J Physiol 424:151–65.

Inoue M, Yoshii M (1992). Modulation of ion channels by somatostatin and acetylcholine. Prog Neurobiol 38:203–30.

Jackson H, Parks TN (1989). Spider toxins: recent applications in neurobiology. Annu Rev Neurosci 12:405–14.

Janis RA, Triggle DJ (1991). Drugs acting on calcium channels. In: Hurwitz L, Partridge LD, Leach JK, eds. Calcium channels: their properties, functions, regulation, and clinical relevance. Boca Raton, Florida: CRC Press, 195–249..

Janis RA, Silver PJ, Triggle DJ (1987). Drug action and cellular calcium regulation. Adv Drug Res 16:309–591.

Jensen JR, Lynch G, Baudry M (1989). Allosteric activation of brain mitochondrial Ca^{2+} uptake by spermine and by Ca^{2+}: brain regional differences. J Neurochem 53:1182–7.

Johnson JW, Ascher P (1987). Glycine potentiates the NMDA response in cultured mouse brain neurones. Nature 325:529–31.

Johnson JW, Ascher P (1990). Voltage-dependent block by intracellular Mg^{2+} of N-methyl-D-aspartate-activated channels. Biophys J 57:1085–90.

Johnson KM, Jones SM (1990). Neuropharmacology of phencyclidine: basic mechanisms and therapeutic potential. Annu Rev Pharmacol Toxicol 30:707–50.

Karlin A (1991). Explorations of the nicotinic acetylcholine receptor. In: Harvey Lectures, series 85. New York: Wiley-Liss, 71–107.

Kasai H, Aosaki T, Fukada J (1987). Presynaptic Ca-antagonist ω-conotoxin irreversibly blocks N-type Ca channels in chick sensory neurons. Neurosci Res 4:228–35.

Kato E, Narahashi T (1982). Low sensitivity of the neuroblastoma cell cholinergic receptors to erabutoxins and α-bungarotoxin. Brain Res 245:159–62.

Kemp JA, Priestley T, Woodruff GN (1989). Selective antagonism of N-methyl-D-aspartate responses in rat cultured cortical neurones by the spider toxin, argiopine. J Physiol 410:26P.

Khodorov BI (1978). CHemicals as tools to study nerve fiber sodium channels: effects of batrachotoxin and some local anesthetics. In: Tosteson DC, Yu AO, Latorre R, eds. Membrane transport processes. Vol. 2. New York: Raven Press, 153–74.

Khodorov BI (1985). Batrachotoxin as a tool to study voltage-sensitive sodium channels of excitable membranes. Prog Biophys Mol Biol 45:57–148.

Khodorov BI, Revenko SV (1979). Further analysis of the mechanisms of action of batrachotoxin on the membrane of myelinated nerve. Neuroscience 4:1315–30.

Khodorov BI, Shishkova L, Peganov E, Revenko S (1976). Inhibition of sodium currents in frog Ranvier node treated with local anesthetics. Role of slow sodium inactivation. Biochim Biophys Acta 433:409–35.

Kirsch GE, Narahashi T (1978). 3,4-Diaminopyridine: a potent new potassium channel blocker. Biophys J 22:507–12.

Kirsch GE, Yeh JZ, Farley JM, Narahashi T (1980). Interaction of n-alkylguanidines with the sodium channels of squid axon membrane. J Gen Physiol 76:315–35.

Klis SFL, Vijverberg HPM, van den Bercken J (1991). Phenylpyrazoles, a new class of pesticides: an electrophysiological investigation into basic effects. Pesticide Biochem Physiol 39:210–8.

Koenig H, Goldstone AD, Lu CY, Trout JJ (1990). Brain polyamines are controlled by N-methyl-D-aspartate receptors during ischemia and recirculation. Stroke 21(suppl):III98–102.

Krishtal OA, Marchenko SM, Pidoplichko VI (1983). Receptor for ATP in the membrane of mammalian sensory neurones. Neurosci Lett 35:41–5.

Krishtal OA, Marchenko SM, Obukhov AG, Volkova TM (1988). Receptors for ATP in rat sensory neurons: the structure-function relationship for ligands. Br J Pharmacol 95:1057–62.

Lambert JJ (1983). Drug-induced modification of ionic conductance at the neuromuscular junction. Annu Rev Pharmacol Toxicol 23:505–39.

Lawrence LJ, Casida JE (1983). Stereospecific action of pyrethroid insecticides on the γ-aminobutyric acid receptor–ionophore complex. Science 221:1399–1401.

Lawrence LJ, Gee KW, Yamamura HI (1985). Interactions of pyrethroid insecticides with chloride ionophore–associated binding sites. NeuroToxicology 6(2):87–98.

Lima-Landman MTR, Albuquerque EX (1989). Ethanol potentiates and blocks NMDA-activated single-channel currents in rat hippocampal pyramidal cells. FEBS Lett 247:61–7.

Linden DL, Routtenberg A (1989). *Cis*-fatty acids, which activate protein kinase C, attenuate Na^+ and Ca^{2+} currents in mouse neuroblastoma cells. J Physiol 419:95–119.

Llinás R, Yarom Y (1986). Specific blockage of the low threshold calcium channel by high molecular weight alcohols (abstr). Soc Neurosci Abstr 12:174.

Llinás R, Sugimori M, Lin J-W, Cherksey B (1989). Blocking and isolation of a calcium channel from neurons in mammals and cephalopods utilizing a toxin fraction (FTX) from funnel-web spider poison. Proc Natl Acad Sci USA 86:1689–93.

Llinás R, Sugimori M, Hillman DE, Cherksey B (1992). Distribution and functional significance of the P-type, voltage-dependent Ca^{2+} channels in the mammalian central nervous system. Trends Neurosci 15:351–5.

Llorens J, Sunol C, Tusell JM, Rodriguez-Farre E (1990). Lindane inhibition of [^{35}S]TBPS binding to the GABA$_A$ receptor in rat brain. Neurotoxicol Teratol 12:607–10.

Lovinger DM, White G, Weight FF (1989). Ethanol inhibits NMDA-activated ion current in hippocampal neurons. Science 243:1721–4.

Luetje CW, Patrick J, Séguéla P (1990). Nicotine receptors in the mammalian brain. FASEB J 4:2753–60.

Lummis SCR, Chow SC, Holan G, Johnston GAR (1987). γ-Aminobutyric acid receptor ionophore complexes: differential effects of deltamethrin, dichlorodiphenyltrichloroethane, and some novel insecticides in a rat brain membrane preparation. J Neurochem 48:689–94.

Lummis SC, Buckingham SD, Rauh JJ, Sattelle DB (1990). Blocking actions of heptachlor at an insect central nervous system GABA receptor. Proc Roy Soc Lond B240:97–106.

Lund AE, Narahashi T (1981). Kinetics of sodium channel modification by the insecticide tetramethrin in squid axon membranes. J Pharmacol Exp Ther 219:464–73.

Lund AE, Narahashi T (1982). Dose-dependent interaction of the pyrethroid isomers with sodium channels of squid axon membranes. Neurotoxicology 3:11–24.

Lund AE, Narahashi T (1983). Kinetics of sodium channel modification as the basis for the variation in the nerve membrane effects of pyrethroids and DDT analogs. Pesticide Biochem Physiol 20:203–16.

Ma JY, Narahashi T (1993). Differential modulation of GABA$_A$ receptor-channel complex by polyvalent cations in rat dorsal root ganglion neurons. Brain Res 607:222–32.

MacDonald JF, Nowak LM (1990). Mechanisms of blockade of excitatory amino acid receptor channels. Trends Pharmacol Sci 11:167–72.

MacDonald JF, Miljkovic Z, Pennefather P (1987). Use-dependent block of excitatory amino acid currents in cultured neurons by ketamine. J Neurophysiol 58:251–6.

MacKinnon R, Reinhart PH, White MM (1988). Charybdotoxin block of *Shaker* K$^+$ channels suggests that different types of K$^+$ channels share common structural features. Neuron 1:997–1001.

Mathie A, Cull-Candy SG, Colquhoun D (1988). The mammalian neuronal nicotinic receptor and its block by drugs. In: Lunt GG, ed. Neurotox '88: molecular basis of drug and pesticide action. Amsterdam: Elsevier, 393–403.

Matsumoto K, Eldefrawi ME, Eldefrawi AT (1988). Action of polychlorocycloalkane insecticides on binding of [^{35}S]t-butylbicyclophosphorothionate to *Torpedo* electric organ membranes and stereospecificity of the binding site. Toxicol Appl Pharmacol 95:220–9.

Matsumura F, Ghiasuddin SM (1983). Evidence for similarities between cyclodiene type insecticides and picrotoxinin in their action mechanisms. J Environ Health Sci B18:1–14.

Mayer ML, Miller RJ (1990). Excitatory amino acid receptors, second messengers and regulation of intracellular Ca^{2+} in mammalian neurons. Trends Pharmacol Sci 11:254–60.

Mayer ML, Westbrook GL (1987). Permeation and block of N-methyl-D-aspartic acid receptor channels by divalent cations in mouse cultured central neurones. J Physiol 394:501–27.

Mayer ML, Westbrook GL, Guthrie PB (1984). Voltage-dependent block by Mg^{2+} of NMDA responses in spinal cord neurones. Nature 309:261–3.

Mayer ML, Westbrook GL, Vyklicky L Jr (1988). Sites of antagonist action on N-methyl-D-aspartic acid receptors studied using fluctuation analysis and a rapid perfusion technique. J Neurophysiol 60:645–63.

Mayer ML, Vyklicky L Jr, Westbrook GL (1989). Modulation of excitatory amino acid receptors by group IIB metal cations in cultured mouse hippocampal neurones. J Physiol 415:329–50.

McCleskey EW, Fox AP, Feldman DH, Cruz LJ, Olivera BM, Tsien RW, Yoshikami D (1987). ω-Conotoxin: direct and persistent blockade of specific types of calcium channels in neurons but not muscle. Proc Natl Acad Sci USA 84:4327–31.

McGurk JF, Bennett MVL, Zukin RS (1990). Polyamines potentiate responses of N-methyl-D-aspartate receptors expressed in *Xenopus* oocytes. Proc Natl Acad Sci USA 87:9971–4.

Mehta AK, Ticku MK (1988). Ethanol potentiation of GABAergic transmission in cultured spinal cord neurons involves γ-aminobutyric acid$_A$–gated chloride channels. J Pharmacol Exp Ther 246:558–64.

Meves H (1992). Potassium channel toxins. In: Herken H, Hucho F, eds. Handbook of experimental pharmacology, vol. 102, selective neurotoxicity. Berlin: Springer-Verlag, 739–74.

Mienville JM, Vicini S (1989). Pregnenolone sulfate antagonizes GABA$_A$ receptor–mediated currents via a reduction of channel opening frequency. Brain Res 489:190–4.

Miledi R, Molinoff P, Potter LT (1971). Isolation of the cholinergic receptor protein of *Torpedo* electric tissue. Nature 229:554–7.

Miljkovic Z, MacDonald JF (1987). Pentobarbital block of excitatory amino acid currents. In: Hicks TP, Lodge D, McLennan H, eds. Excitatory amino acid transmission. New York: Alan R. Liss, 59–62.

Miller C, Moczydlowski E, Latorre R, Philipps M (1985). Charybdotoxin: a protein inhibitor of single Ca^{2+}-activated K^+ channels from mammalian skeletal muscle. Nature 313:316–8.

Monaghan DT, Bridges RJ, Cotman CW (1989). The excitatory amino acid receptors: their classes, pharmacology, and distinct properties in the function of the central nervous system. Annu Rev Pharmacol Toxicol 29:365–402.

Moody WJ, Hagiwara S (1982). Block of inward rectification by intracellular H^+ in immature oocytes of the starfish *Mediaster aequalis*. J Gen Physiol 79:115–30.

Nakahiro M, Yeh JZ, Brunner E, Narahashi T (1989). General anesthetics modulate GABA receptor channel complex in rat dorsal root ganglion neurons. FASEB J 3:1850–4.

Nakahiro M, Arakawa O, Narahashi T (1991). Modulation of γ-aminobutyric acid receptor-channel complex by alcohols. J Pharmacol Exp Ther 259:235–40.

Nakazawa K, Matsuki N (1987). Adenosine triphosphate–activated inward current of isolated smooth muscle cells from rat vas deferens. Pflügers Arch 409:644–6.

Narahashi T (1971). Effects of insecticides on excitable tissues. In: Beament JWL, Treherne JE, Wigglesworth VB, eds. Advances in insect physiology. Vol. 8. New York: Academic Press, 1–93.

Narahashi T (1973). Drugs affecting axonal membranes. In: Dikstein S, ed. Fundamentals of cell pharmacology. Springfield, Illinois: Thomas, 395–424.

Narahashi T (1974). Chemicals as tools in the study of excitable membranes. Physiol Rev 54:813–89.

Narahashi T (1976). Effects of insecticides on nervous conduction and synaptic transmission. In: Wilkinson CF, ed. Insecticide biochemistry and physiology. New York: Plenum Press, 327–52.

Narahashi T (1981). Mode of action of chlorinated hydrocarbon pesticides on the nervous system. In: Khan MAQ, ed. Halogenated hydrocarbons: health and ecological effects. Elmsford, New York: Pergamon Press, 222–42.

Narahashi T (1984a). Pharmacology of nerve membrane sodium channels. In: Baker PF, ed. Current topics in membranes and transport, vol. 22, the squid axon. New York: Academic Press, 483–516.

Narahashi T (1984b). Drug-ionic channel interactions: single channel measurements. Ann Neurol 16(suppl):S39–51.

Narahashi T (1985). Nerve membrane ionic channels as the primary target of pyrethroids. Neuro-Toxicology 6(2):3–22.

Narahashi T (1986). Nerve membrane ionic channels as the target of toxicants. Toxic interfaces of neurones, smoke and genes. Arch Toxicol Suppl 9:3–13.

Narahashi T (1987a). Neuronal target sites of insecticides. In: Hollingworth RM, Green MB, eds. Sites of action for neurotoxic pesticides. American Chemical Society symposium series, no. 356. Washington, DC: American Chemical Society, 226–50.

Narahashi T (1987b). Pharmacology of acetylcholine activated ion channels: contemporary approaches. In: Dun N, Perlman RL, eds. Neurobiology of acetylcholine. New York: Plenum Press, 339–51.

Narahashi T (1988a). Mechanism of tetrodotoxin and saxitoxin action. In: Tu AT, ed. Handbook of natural toxins, vol. 3, marine toxins and venoms. New York: Marcell Dekker, 185–210.

Narahashi T (1988b). Molecular and cellular approaches to neurotoxicology: past, present and future. In: Lunt GG, ed. Neurotox '88. Molecular basis of drug and pesticide action. Amsterdam: Elsevier, 269–88.

Narahashi T (1989). The role of ion channels in insecticide action. In: Narahashi T, Chambers JE, eds. Insecticide action: from molecule to organism. New York: Plenum Press, 55–84.

Narahashi T (1992a). Mechanisms of neurotoxicity. Electrophysiological studies. Cellular electrophysiology. In: Abou-Donia MB, ed. Neurotoxicology. Boca Raton, Florida: CRC Press, 155–89.

Narahashi T (1992b). Nerve membrane Na^+ channels as targets of insecticides. Trends Pharmacol Sci 13:236–41.

Narahashi T (1992c). An overview of toxins and drugs as tools to study excitable membrane ion channels. II. Transmitter-activated channels. In: Rudy B, Iverson LE, eds. Methods in enzymology: ion channels. Orlando, Florida: Academic Press, 643–58.

Narahashi T, Frazier DT (1971). Site of action and active form of local anesthetics. In: Ehrenpreis S, Solnitzky OC, eds. Neuroscience research. Vol. 4. New York: Academic Press, 65–99.

Narahashi T, Herman MD (1992). An overview of toxins and drugs as tools to study excitable membrane ion channels. I. Voltage-activated channels. In: Rudy B, Iverson LE, eds. Methods in enzymology: ion channels. Orlando, Florida: Academic Press, 620–43.

Narahashi T, Seyama I (1974). Mechanism of nerve membrane depolarization caused by grayanotoxin I. J Physiol 242:471–87.

Narahashi T, Deguchi T, Urakawa N, Ohkubo Y (1960). Stabilization and rectification of muscle fiber membrane by tetrodotoxin. Am J Physiol 198:934–8.

Narahashi T, Moore JW, Scott WR (1964). Tetrodotoxin blockage of sodium conductance increase in lobster giant axons. J Gen Physiol 47:965–74.

Narahashi T, Frazier DT, Yamada M (1970). The site of action and active form of local anesthetics. I. Theory and pH experiments with tertiary compounds. J Pharmacol Exp Ther 171:32–44.

Narahashi T, Albuquerque EX, Deguchi T (1971). Effects of batrachotoxin on membrane potential and conductance of squid giant axons. J Gen Physiol 58:54–70.

Narahashi T, Tsunoo A, Yoshii M (1987). Characterization of two types of calcium channels in mouse neuroblastoma cells. J Physiol 383:231–49.

Narahashi T, Frey JM, Ginsburg KS, Roy ML (1992). Sodium and GABA-activated channels as the targets of pyrethroids and cyclodienes. In: Chambers PL, Chambers CM, Bolt HM, Preziosi P, eds. Toxicology from discovery and experimentation to the human perspective. Amsterdam, The Netherlands: Elsevier, 429–36.

Neher E, Sakmann B (1976). Single-channel currents recorded from membrane of denervated frog muscle fibres. Nature 260:779–802.

Neher E, Steinbach JH (1978). Local anaesthetics transiently block currents through single acetylcholine-receptor channels. J Physiol 277:153–76.

Nishio M, Narahashi T (1990). Ethanol enhancement of GABA-activated chloride current in rat dorsal root ganglion neurons. Brain Res 518:283–6.

Noma A (1983). ATP-regulated K^+ channels in cardiac muscle. Nature 305:147–8.

Noma A, Shibasaki T (1988). Intracellular ATP and cardiac membrane currents. In: Narahashi T, ed. Ion Channels. Vol. 1. New York: Plenum Press, 183–212.

Nowak L, Bregestovski P, Ascher P, Herbet A, Prochiantz A (1984). Magnesium gates glutamate-activated channels in mouse central neurones. Nature 307:462–5.

Ogata N, Narahashi T (1989). Block of sodium channels by psychotropic drugs in single guinea pig cardiac myocytes. Br J Pharmacol 97:905–13.

Ogata N, Narahashi T (1990). Potent blocking action of chlorpromazine on two types of calcium channels in cultured neuroblastoma cells. J Pharmacol Exp Ther 252:1142–9.

Ogata N, Vogel SM, Narahashi T (1988). Lindane but not deltamethrin blocks a component of GABA-activated chloride channels. FASEB J 2:2895–900.

Ogata N, Yoshii M, Narahashi T (1989a). Psychotropic drugs block voltage-gated ion channels in neuroblastoma cells. Brain Res 476:140–4.

Ogata N, Nishimura M, Narahashi T (1989b). Kinetics of chlorpromazine block of sodium channels in single guinea pig cardiac myocytes. J Pharmacol Exp Ther 248:605–13.

Ogata N, Yoshii M, Narahashi T (1990). Differential block of sodium and calcium channels by chlorpromazine in mouse neuroblastoma cells. J Physiol 420:165–83.

Ohmori H, Yoshida S, Hagiwara S (1981). Single K^+ channel currents of anomalous rectification in cultured rat myotubes. Proc Natl Acad Sci USA 78:4960–4.

Olney JW (1990). Excitotoxic amino acids and neuropsychiatric disorders. Annu Rev Pharmacol Toxicol 30:47–71.

Olsen RW (1992). GABA$_A$-benzodiazepine receptor subtypes. Biotech Update 7:145–53.

Olsen RW, Tobin AJ (1990). Molecular biology of GABA$_A$ receptors. FASEB J 4:1469–80.

Olsen RW, Bureau M, Ransom RW, Deng L, Dilber A, Smith G, Krestchatisky M, Tobin AJ (1988). The GABA receptor–chloride ion channel protein complex. In: Kito S, Segawa T, Kuriyama K, Tohyama M, Olsen RW, eds. Neuroreceptors and signal transduction. New York: Plenum Press, 1–14.

Olsen RW, Szamraj O, Miller T (1989). t-[^{35}S]Butylbicyclophosphorothionate binding sites in invertebrate tissues. J Neurochem 52:1311–8.

Olsen RW, Sapp DM, Bureau MH, Turner DM, Kokka N (1991). Allosteric actions of central nervous system depressants including anesthetics on subtypes of the inhibitory γ-aminobutyric acid$_A$ receptor-chloride channel complex. Ann NY Acad Sci 625:145–54.

Orchard I, Osborne MP (1979). The action of insecticides on neurosecretory neurons in the stick insect, *Carausius morosus*. Pesticide Biochem Physiol 10:197–202.

Osborne MP (1980). Action of pyrethroids upon neurosecretory tissue in the stick insect, *Carausius morosus*. In: Mathieu J, ed. Pyrethroid insecticide: chemistry and action. Roussel Uclaf, Romainville, France, 18–21.

Paschen W, Schmidt-Kastner R, Hallmayer J, Djuricic B (1988). Polyamines in cerebral ischemia. Neurochem Pathol 9:1–20.

Pelhate M, Pichon Y (1974). Selective inhibition of potassium current in the giant axon of the cockroach. J Physiol 242:90P.

Pennefather P, Lancaster B, Adams PR, Nicoll RA (1985). Two distinct Ca-dependent K currents in bullfrog sympathetic ganglion cells. Proc Natl Acad Sci USA 82:3040–4.

Penner R, Petersen M, Pierau Fr-K, Dreyer F (1986). Dendrotoxin: a selective blocker of a non-inactivating potassium current in guinea-pig dorsal root ganglion neurons. Pflügers Arch 407:365–9.

Peper K, Bradley RJ, Dreyer F (1982). The acetylcholine receptor at the neuromuscular junction. Physiol Rev 62:1271–1340.

Pullan LM, Keith RA, LaMonte J, Strempo RJ, Salama AI (1990). The polyamine spermine affects omega-conotoxin binding and function at N-type voltage-sensitive calcium channels. J Autonomic Pharmacol 10:213–9.

Qi DF, Schatzman RC, Mazzei GJ, Turner RS, Raynor RL, Liao S, Kuo JF (1983). Polyamines inhibit phospholipid-sensitive and calmodulin-sensitive Ca^{2+}-dependent protein kinases. Biochem J 213:281–8.

Quandt FN, Narahashi T (1982). Modification of single Na^+ channels by batrachotoxin. Proc Natl Acad Sci USA 79:6732–6.

Quandt FN, Yeh JZ, Narahashi T (1985). All or none block of single Na^+ channels by tetrodotoxin. Neurosci Lett 54:77–83.

Quast U, Cook NS (1989). Moving together: K^+ channel openers and ATP-sensitive K^+ channels. Trends Pharmacol Sci 10:431–5.

Ramadan AA, Bakry NM, Marei ASM, Eldefrawi AT, Eldefrawi ME (1988a). Action of pyrethroids on GABA$_A$ receptor function. Pesticide Biochem Physiol 32:97–105.

Ramadan AA, Bakry NM, Marei ASM, Eldefrawi AT, Eldefrawi ME (1988b). Actions of pyrethroids on the peripheral benzodiazepine receptor. Pesticide Biochem Physiol 32:106–13.

Rassendren F-A, Lory P, Pin J-P, Nargest J (1990). Zinc has opposite effects on NMDA and non-NMDA receptors expressed in *Xenopus* oocytes. Neuron 4:733–40.

Reuveny E, Narahashi T (1991). Potent blocking action of lead on voltage-activated calcium channels in human neuroblastoma cells SH-SY5Y. Brain Res 545:312–4.

Reuveny E, Twombly DA, Narahashi T (1993). Chlordiazepoxide block of two types of calcium channels in neuroblastoma cells. J Pharmacol Exp Ther 264:22–8.

Reynolds IJ, Miller RJ (1988). Tricyclic antidepressants block N-methyl-D-aspartate receptors: similarities to the action of zinc. Br J Pharmacol 95:95–102.

Ritchie JM, Greengard P (1966). On the mode of action of local anesthetics. Annu Rev Pharmacol 6:405–30.

Rocha ES, Ramoa A, Albuquerque EX (1989). Modulation of NMDA response by haloperidol and m-nitro-PCP (abstr). Soc Neurosci Abstr 15:534.

Roehn G, Kocker M, Oschlies U, Hossmann K-A, Paschen W (1990). Putrescine content and structural defects in isolated fractions of rat brain after reversible cerebral ischemia. Exp Neurol 107:249–55.

Romey G, Lazdunski M (1984). The coexistence in rat muscle cells of two distinct classes of Ca^{2+}-dependent K^+ channels with different pharmacological properties and different physiological functions. Biochem Biophys Res Commun 118:669–74.

Romey G, Hugues M, Schmid-Antomarchi H, Lazdunski M (1984). Apamin: a specific toxin to study a class of Ca^{2+}-dependent K^+ channels. J Physiol (Paris) 79:259–64.

Rorsman P, Trube G (1990). Biophysics and physiology of ATP-regulated K^+ channels (K_{ATP}). In: Cook NS, ed. Potassium channels: structure, classification and therapeutic potential. Chichester, U.K.: Horwood, 96–116.

Rorsman P, Berggren P-O, Bokvist K, Efendic S (1990). ATP-regulated K^+ channels and diabetes mellitus. News Pharmacol Sci 5:143–7.

Ruigt GSF (1984). Pyrethroids. In: Kerkut GA, Gilbert LI, eds. Comprehensive insect physiology, biochemistry and pharmacology. Vol. 12. Oxford: Pergamon Press, 183–263.

Salgado VL (1990). Mode of action of insecticidal dihydropyrazoles: selective block of impulse generation in sensory nerves. Pesticide Sci 28:389–411.

Salgado VL, Herman MD, Narahashi T (1989). Interactions of the pyrethroid fenvalerate with nerve membrane sodium channels: temperature dependence and mechanism of depolarization. NeuroToxicology 10:1–14.

Seabrook GR, Duce IR, Irving SN (1988). Effects of the pyrethroid cypermethrin on L-glutamate-induced changes in the input conductance of the ventrolateral muscles of the larval house fly, *Musca domestica*. Pesticide Biochem Physiol 32:232–9.

Seagar M-J, Granier C, Couraud F (1984). Interactions of the neurotoxin apamin with a Ca^{2+}-activated K^+ channel in primary neuronal cultures. J Biol Chem 259:1491–5.

Sernagor E, Kuhn D, Vyklicky L Jr, Mayer ML (1989). Open channel block of NMDA receptor responses evoked by tricyclic antidepressants. Neuron 2:1221–7.

Seyama I, Narahashi T (1973). Increase in sodium permeability of squid axon membranes by α-dihydrograyanotoxin II. J Pharmacol Exp Ther 184:299–307.

Seyama I, Narahashi T (1981). Modulation of sodium channels of squid nerve membranes by grayanotoxin I. J Pharmacol Exp Ther 219:614–24.

Shanes AM, Freygang WH, Grundfest H, Amatniek E (1959). Anesthetic and calcium action in the voltage clamped squid giant axon. J Gen Physiol 42:793–802.

Shapiro BI (1977). Effects of strychnine on the sodium conductance of the frog node of Ranvier. J Gen Physiol 69:915–26.

Sills MA, Loo PS (1989). Tricyclic antidepressants and dextromethorphan bind with higher affinity to the phencyclidine receptor in the absence of magnesium and l-glutamate. Mol Pharmacol 36:160–5.

Siqueira-Rocha E, Albuquerque EX, Ramoa AS (1990). Effects of sigma ligands on NMDA-induced single channel currents (abstr). Soc Neurosci Abstr 16:86.

Soderlund DM, Bloomquist JR (1989). Neurotoxic actions of pyrethroid insecticides. Annu Rev Entomol 34:77–96.

Spivak CE, Albuquerque EX (1982). Dynamic properties of the nicotinic acetylcholine receptor ionic channel complex: activation and blockade. In: Hanin I, Goldberg AM, eds. Progress in cholinergic biology: model cholinergic synapses. New York: Raven Press, 323–57.

Spivak CE, Maleque MA, Oliveira AC, Masukawa LM, Tokuyama T, Daly JW, Albuquerque EX (1982). Actions of histrionicotoxins at the ionic channel of the nicotinic acetylcholine receptor and at the voltage-sensitive ion channels of muscle membranes. Mol Pharmacol 21:351–61.

Sprosen TS, Woodruff GN (1990). Polyamines potentiate NMDA induced whole-cell currents in cultured striatal neurons. Eur J Pharmacol 179:477–8.

Staatz CG, Bloom AS, Lech JJ (1982). Effect of pyrethroids on [^{3}H]kainic acid binding to mouse forebrain membranes. Toxicol Appl Pharmacol 64:566–9.

Standen NB, Quayle JM, Davies NW, Brayden JE, Huang Y, Nelson MT (1989). Hyperpolarizing vasodilators activate ATP-sensitive K^+ channels in arterial smooth muscle. Science 245:177–80.

Steinbach AB (1968a). Alteration by Xylocaine (lidocaine) and its derivatives of the time course of the endplate potential. J Gen Physiol 52:144–61.

Steinbach AB (1968b). A kinetic model for the action of Xylocaine on receptors for acetylcholine. J Gen Physiol 52:162–80.

Strichartz G (1973). The inhibition of sodium currents in myelinated nerve by quaternary derivatives of lidocaine. J Gen Physiol 62:37–57.

Suzdak PD, Schwartz RD, Skolnick P, Paul SM (1986). Ethanol stimulates γ-aminobutyric acid receptor–mediated chloride transport in rat brain synaptoneurosomes. Proc Natl Acad Sci USA 83:4071–5.

Takeda K, Narahashi T (1988). Chemical modification of sodium channel inactivation: separate sites for the action of grayanotoxin and tetramethrin. Brain Res 448:308–12.

Takeuchi A, Takeuchi N (1959). Active phase of frog's end-plate potential. J Neurophysiol 22:395–411.

Takeuchi A, Takeuchi N (1960). On the permeability of end-plate membrane during the action of transmitter. J Physiol 154:52–67.

Tanguy J, Yeh JZ (1991). BTX modification of Na channels in squid axons. I. State dependence of BTX action. J Gen Physiol 97:499–519.

Tanguy J, Yeh JZ, Narahashi T (1984). Interaction of batrachotoxin with sodium channels in squid axons (abstr). Biophys J 45:184a.

Tasaki I, Hagiwara S (1957). Demonstration of two stable potential states in the squid giant axon under tetraethylammonium chloride. J Gen Physiol 40:859–85.

Taylor RE (1959). Effect of procaine on electrical properties of squid axon membrane. Am J Physiol 196:1071–8.

Thompson RG, Menking DE, Valdes JJ (1990). Comparison of lindane, bicyclophosphate and picrotoxin binding to the putative chloride channel sites in rat brain and *Torpedo* electric organ. Neurotoxicol Teratol 12:57–63.

Thompson SH (1977). Three pharmacologically distinct potassium channels in molluscan neurones. J Physiol 265:465–88.

Thompson S (1982). Aminopyridine block of transient potassium current. J Gen Physiol 80:1–18.

Ticku MK, Lowrimore P, Lehoullier P (1986). Ethanol enhances GABA-induced ^{36}Cl-influx in primary spinal cord cultured neurons. Brain Res Bull 17:123–6.

Tsien RW, Ellinor PT, Horne WA (1991). Molecular diversity of voltage-dependent Ca^{2+} channels. Trends Pharmacol Sci 12:349–54.

Tsunoo A, Yoshii M, Narahashi T (1986). Block of calcium channels by enkephalin and somatostatin in neuroblastoma-glioma hybrid NG108–15 cells. Proc Natl Acad Sci USA 83:9832–6.

Twombly DA, Narahashi T (1989). Calcium channel blocking actions of octanol (abstr). Soc Neurosci Abstr 15:355.

Twombly DA, Herman MD, Narahashi T (1987). Phenobarbital block of voltage-dependent calcium channels in neuroblastoma cells (abstr). Soc Neurosci Abstr 13:102.

Twombly DA, Yoshii M, Narahashi T (1988). Mechanisms of calcium channel block by phenytoin. J Pharmacol Exp Ther 246:189–95.

Twombly DA, Herman MD, Kye CH, Narahashi T (1990). Ethanol effects on two types of voltage-activated calcium channels. J Pharmacol Exp Ther 254:1029–37.

Twyman RE, Rogers CJ, Macdonald RL (1989). Differential regulation of γ-aminobutyric acid receptor channels by diazepam and phenobarbital. Ann Neurol 25:213–20.

Usherwood PNR, Blagbrough IS (1989). Antagonism of insect muscle glutamate receptors—with particular reference to arthropod toxins. In: Narahashi T, Chambers JE, eds. Insecticide action. from molecule to organism. New York: Plenum Press, 13–31.

Vijverberg HPM, van den Bercken J (1990). Neurotoxicological effects and the mode of action of pyrethroid insecticides. Crit Rev Toxicol 21(2):105–126.

Vogel SM, Watanabe S, Yeh JZ, Farley JM, Narahashi T (1984). Current-dependent block of endplate channels by guanidine derivatives. J Gen Physiol 83:901–18.

Vyklicky L Jr, Benveniste M, Mayer ML (1990). Modulation of N-methyl-D-aspartic acid receptor desensitization by glycine in mouse cultured hippocampal neurones. J Physiol 428:313–31.

Wang C, Narahashi T (1972). Mechanisms of dual action of nicotine on end-plate membranes. J Pharmacol Exp Ther 182:427–41.

Watabe S, Yoshii M, Ogata N, Narahashi T (1986). Clonazepam differs from diazepam and nitrazepam in blocking two types of calcium channels (abstr). Soc Neurosci Abstr 12:1193.

Westbrook GL, Mayer ML (1987). Micromolar concentrations of Zn^{2+} antagonize NMDA and GABA responses of hippocampal neurons. Nature 328:640–3.

Whittaker VP (1990). The contribution of drugs and toxins to understanding of cholinergic function. Trends Pharmacol Sci 11:8–13.

Williams K, Dawson VL, Romano C, Dichter MA, Molinoff PB (1990). Characterization of polyamines having agonist, antagonist, and inverse agonist effects at the polyamine recognition site of the NMDA receptor. Neuron 5:199–208.

Wong EHF, Kemp JA (1991). Sites for antagonism on the N-methyl-D-aspartate receptor channel complex. Annu Rev Pharmacol Toxicol 31:401–25.

Wong EHF, Kemp JA, Priestly T, Knight AR, Woodruff GN, Iversen LL (1986). The anti-convulsant MK-801 is a potent N-methyl-D-aspartate antagonist. Proc Natl Acad Sci USA 83:7104–8.

Woodhull AM (1973). Ionic blockage of sodium channels in nerve. J Gen Physiol 61:687–708.

Woolley DE (1981). The neurotoxicity of DDT and possible mechanisms of action. In: Prasal KN, Vernadakis A, eds. Mechanisms of neurotoxic substances. New York: Raven Press, 95–141.

Wroblewski JT, Danysz W (1989). Modulation of glutamate receptors: molecular mechanisms and functional implications. Annu Rev Pharmacol Toxicol 29:441–74.

Wu CH, Narahashi T (1988). Mechanism of action of novel marine neurotoxins on ion channels. Annu Rev Pharmacol Toxicol 28:141–61.

Yamamoto D, Quandt FN, Narahashi T (1983). Modification of single sodium channels by the insecticide tetramethrin. Brain Res 274:344–9.

Yamamoto D, Yeh JZ, Narahashi T (1984). Voltage-dependent calcium block of normal and tetramethrin-modified single sodium channels. Biophys J 45:337–44.

Yamamoto D, Yeh JZ, Narahashi T (1985). Interactions of permeant cations with sodium channels of squid axon membranes. Biophys J 48:361–8.

Yamamoto D, Yeh JZ, Narahashi T (1986). Ion permeation and selectivity of squid axon sodium channels modified by tetramethrin. Brain Res 372:193–7.

Yamasaki T, Ishii (Narahashi) T (1954). Studies on the mechanism of action of insecticides. X. Nervous activity as a factor of development of γ-BHC symptoms in the cockroach. Botyu-Kagaku (Scientific Insect Control) 19:106–12.

Yamasaki T, Narahashi T (1958). Nervous activity as a factor of development of dieldrin symptoms in the cockroach. Studies on the mechanism of action of insecticides XVI. Botyu-Kagaku (Scientific Insect Control) 23:47–54.

Yan M, Narahashi T (1992). Potentiation of GABA-induced chloride current by lanthanides (abstr). Soc Neurosci Abstr 18:249.

Yeh JZ (1978). Sodium inactivation mechanism modulates QX-314 block of sodium channels in squid axons. Biophys J 24:569–74.

Yeh JZ (1979). Dynamics of 9-aminoacridine block of sodium channels in squid axons. J Gen Physiol 73:1–21.

Yeh JZ (1980). Blockage of sodium channels by stereoisomers of local anesthetics. In: Fink BR, ed. Molecular mechanisms of anesthesia. New York: Raven Press, 35–44.

Yeh JZ, Narahashi T (1977). Kinetic analysis of pancuronium interaction with sodium channels in squid axon membranes. J Gen Physiol 69:293–323.

Yeh JZ, Oxford GS, Wu CH, Narahashi T (1976). Dynamics of aminopyridine block of potassium channels in squid axon membrane. J Gen Physiol 68:519–35.

Yoshii M, Tsunoo A, Narahashi T (1985). Effects of pyrethroids and veratridine on two types of Ca channels in neuroblastoma cells (abstr). Soc Neurosci Abstr 11:518.

Zufall F, Franke C, Hatt H (1989). Similarities between the effects of lindane (gamma-HCH) and picrotoxin on ligand-gated chloride channels in crayfish muscle membrane. Brain Res 503:342–5.

Part V
Developmental Neurotoxicology
Introductory Overview

William Slikker, Jr.
National Center for Toxicological Research/FDA
Jefferson, Arkansas

The Congressional designation of the 1990s as the Decade of the Brain underscores the tremendous opportunities offered by the current and anticipated advances in brain research and the enormous cost of mental disorders to the national economy. In the United States, brain-related disorders account for more hospitalizations than any other major disease group, including cancer and cardiovascular diseases. One of four Americans will suffer from a brain-related disorder at some point in his lifetime, and the cost to the national economy for treatment, rehabilitation, and related consequences is an estimated $400 billion each year. According to the Congressional Office of Technology Assessment's recent report on neurotoxicity, among the known or suspected causes of brain-related disorders are exposure to chemicals including pesticides, therapeutic drugs, food additives, foods, cosmetic ingredients, and naturally occurring substances (Office of Technology Assessment, 1990). The discipline of neurotoxicology is devoted to developing a better understanding of the extent, causes, and underlying mechanisms of brain-related disorders.

Nowhere is the pain and suffering from brain-related disorders felt more than by the very young members of our society who must live with their disabilities for a lifetime. Of the 250,000 malformed or impaired children born each year in the United States, approximately half suffer from a nervous system or behavioral deficit. In two-thirds of the cases (66%), the causes of these developmental anomalies are unknown, and they are probably multifactorial. Genetic abnormalities account for 25%, but the remaining 9% of the births of impaired children, roughly 22,000 each year, are believed to be the result of environmental causes. It is estimated that one of ten school-age children suffers from some type of functional deficit. With a focus on the pre- and postnatal periods, developmental neurotoxicology has become an important and energized subdiscipline, with the potential of tremendous impact on the health of young Americans.

The following chapters describe many of the basic principles and current concepts of the area of developmental neurotoxicology. William Slikker, Jr., reviews the maternal, placental and embryonic/fetal factors influencing the placental transfer and pharmacokinetics of neuroactive agents. Evidence is presented in support of the hypothesis that developmental neurotoxicants achieve significant concentrations in the developing nervous system after maternal administration. Known human developmental neurotoxicants are used as examples to demonstrate, in animal models, that these agents are detectable in the nervous system target of toxicity.

Hazel Murphy and Pat Levitt summarize the anatomical and physiological development of the nervous system. The special features of a developing nervous system that enhance its susceptibility to neurotoxicants are discussed. The possible role of cell adhesion molecules in developmental neurotoxicity is discussed by Dr. Laura Lagunowich. In their chapter, Jane Adams and Merle Paule compare the cognitive effects of various developmental neurotoxicants in several species of primates. The principles of extrapolating experimental results from one species to another are discussed, and the utility of examining clinical issues through animal-modeling studies is explored.

Charles Vorhees discusses the various biomarkers of neurotoxicity that can be described in terms of the behavioral and functional ontogeny of the developing organism. The fundamentals, as well as the regulatory implications of developmental behavioral neurotoxicity, are described. Bernard Weiss and Kenneth Reuhl define and discuss the issue of silent toxicity as it pertains to developmental neurotoxicity in the last chapter of this section. With the use of both neurodegenerative diseases and neurotoxic agents, the hypothesis that delayed residual or silent neurotoxicity exists is explored. Experimental designs and models that can be used to describe the extent and mechanisms behind silent neurotoxicity are discussed. As a whole, these chapters provide a review of the challenging discipline of developmental neurotoxicology.

Reference

U.S. Congress, Office of Technology Assessment. (April, 1990) "Neurotoxicity: Identifying and Controlling Poisons of the Nervous System," OTA-BA-436, Washington, DC: U.S. Government Printing Office.

23
Placental Transfer and Pharmacokinetics of Developmental Neurotoxicants

William Slikker, Jr.
National Center for Toxicological Research/FDA
Jefferson, Arkansas

INTRODUCTION

The ability of an agent to induce neurotoxicity in the developing animal may be due to either its direct or its indirect effects. An agent may produce toxicity in the maternal organism or the placenta that in turn may be reflected by neurotoxicity in the conceptus. Alternatively, an agent may directly interact with the nervous system of the conceptus to produce neurotoxicity. In the latter case, the agent or its metabolite must cross the placenta and the blood-brain barrier of the conceptus in order to produce neurotoxicity. It is the complicated journey of the direct-acting developmental neurotoxicant that is the focus of this chapter.

Chemical Passage

En route between the site of maternal administration and the nervous system of the conceptus are two specialized sets of membranes that chemicals must cross. Both the placenta and the fetal blood-brain barrier have their origins in the conceptus and have anatomical and functional features that influence chemical transfer to the developing conceptus. These two sets of membranes share two additional features: both undergo considerable change with development and exhibit substantial species differences.

Placenta

Morphologically, the placenta may be defined as the fusion or opposition of fetal membranes to the uterine mucous membrane (Kaufmann and King, 1982). As in many species, the human actually exhibits two placentas, the early yolk-sac placenta (days 13 to 80 of gestation) overlapping developmentally with the later chorioallantoic placenta (days 21 to term) (Garbis-Berkvens and Peters, 1987). The human yolk-sac placenta consists of endoderm (inner lining) and mesothelium (outer lining), both with microvilli. The interposed mesenchyma contains vessels and blood-forming tissues from day 16 onward. This temporary but physiologically important structure is believed to have several absorptive and secretory functions, including nutrient transfer and synthesis of proteins such as alpha-fetoprotein, and there is evidence for hemoglobin synthesis and porphyrin metabolism (Garbis-Berkvens and Peters, 1987). Differences between the yolk-sac placenta of the human and that of the rat include an opposite layering of the endoderm and mesothelium in the rat inverted visceral yolk sac, and lack of direct contact between the human yolksac and the maternal circulation as observed in the rat.

The human chorioallantoic placenta consists of two morphologically and physiologically distinguished cell layers, the mononucleated, inner layer of cytotrophoblasts producing the multinucleated, outer layer of syncytiotrophoblasts (Garbis-Berkvens and Peters, 1987). During the first trimester, the placenta develops fetal cotyledons consisting of a special maternal artery that discharges blood into loose centers of fetal lobules with numerous villi. These villi arise from cytotrophoblast cell proliferation into the maternal decidual tissue. As pregnancy progresses, the syncytiotrophoblast layer (in direct contact with maternal blood and relatively thick in early pregnancy) becomes progressively thinner (Garbis-Berkvens and Peters, 1987). The cytotrophoblast layer becomes more discontinuous and the endothelium of the embryonic/fetal vessles within the villi becomes thinner. Thus, as pregnancy progresses, there is closer contact between the fetal blood and the placental cell layer most important to placental function and maternal-embryonic/fetal exchange, the syncytiotrophoblast. On the macroscopic level, the effects of gestational age can be exemplified by comparing the tremendous change in the ratio of placental/fetal weight (at 10 weeks, ratio = 4; at 40 weeks, ratio = 0.2; Hytten and Leitch, 1971).

Merely on the basis of the number of layers of cells between fetal and maternal circulations, it is tempting to define similarities and differences of chemical placental transfer by anatomy alone. Neither the functional nor the anatomical thickness of the placenta, however, is consistently related to the number of layers separating the conceptus from the mother. It must be realized that any substance in the maternal circulation can, to some extent, be transferred across the placenta unless it is metabolized or detoxified before or during its placental passage (Garbis-Berkvens and Peters, 1987).

From a functional perspective, one may define species differences by focusing on the placental transfer of a series of nonmetabolized model compounds of increasing molecular weight by the isolated, dually perfused placenta. As reported by Illsley et al. (1985), placental transfer, as defined by a clearance ratio, decreases as the molecular weight of the model compounds increases. Under these very controlled conditions without maternal or fetal involvement, differences between species in placental transfer were evident, with sheep being more different from humans than were guinea pigs. Thus, while anatomical differences between species, alone may not fully predict rates of placental transfer of chemicals, functional assessments have been shown to be useful in defining the exposure of the conceptus after maternal dose administration.

Blood-Brain Barrier

The central nervous system (CNS) and cerebrospinal fluid (CSF) are separated from the blood by the blood-brain barrier. The choroid plexus and the blood vessels of the brain and subarachnoid membrane are the interfaces between the blood and the CSF and brain (Rapoport, 1976). Peripheral nerves also exhibit a barrier composed of the blood vessels that surround nerve bundles. Intercellular diffusion is restricted at all these barrier sites by cells with tight junctions. The cells of the blood vessels are endothelial, whereas those of the choroid plexus and arachnoid and perineurium (peripheral nerves) are epithelial (Rapoport, 1976). These barrier cells are connected by tight junctions that block paracellular diffusion and contain few transfer vesicles (Lefauconnier et al., 1986). Because of these features, blood-borne solutes must course through two different membranes and the cytoplasm of the endothelial cells before reaching the extracellular space of the brain. Molecules pass through membranes by passive diffusion as a function of the lipid-solubility of their un-ionized form. Ionized forms of these molecules do not trasverse membranes but are in equilibrium with their un-ionized forms on the basis of the pH of the environment and their dissociation constants. Additional regulators of chemical blood-brain transfer include astrocytic processes that ensheathe cerebral capillaries, specific carriers located on cell membranes, and cytoplasmic metabolic enzymes (Rapoport, 1976; Lefauconnier et al., 1986; Heistad, 1984).

After a review of the pharmacokinetic principles that govern the delivery of a chemical to the nervous system of the conceptus after maternal administration, the effects of known human developmental neurotoxicants on the developing nervous system will be discussed. Whether animal models have been developed to mimic these developmental effects observed in humans will also be discussed. The developmental pharmacokinetics and relative embryonic/fetal-maternal exposure to each agent or chemical class will be discussed with use of available literature values. These data will then be used to test the general hypothesis that neurotoxicants readily cross the placenta and enter the developing nervous system.

PHARMACOKINETICS

A chemical must pass through and may interact with several anatomical compartments on its journey from the site of maternal administration to the nervous system of the developing conceptus. Therefore, these primary anatomical sites will be used as focal points for discussion of the principles of pharmacokinetics as they relate to developmental neurotoxicants.

Maternal Considerations

One of the primary reasons for applying pharmacokinetic principles to the study of developmental neurotoxicology is to determine the concentration of chemicals at the suspected site of action as a function of time. Maternal factors act either to enhance or to diminish the concentration of an active chemical in the nervous system of the conceptus. For example, maternal detoxification would tend to decrease the concentration of the active agent, whereas maternal bioactivation would enhance its concentration. Maternal factors including absorption, distribution, serum binding, and elimination also influence the concentration of active agent at the target site. Because of the physiological changes that occur during pregnancy, the influence of these maternal factors on chemical delivery may also change during gestation. (Noschel et al., 1980; Cummings, 1983; Bogaert and Thiery, 1983; Juchau and Faustman-Watts, 1983; Juchau, 1983). These issues have recently been reviewed (Juchau and Faustman-Watts, 1983; Juchau, 1983; Levy, 1981; Brock-Utne et al., 1980; Krauer et al., 1980).

Placental Transfer

Factors that influence the placental transfer of chemicals include uterine/placental blood flow, placental permeability, and placental metabolism (Mirkin and Singh, 1976; Miller et al., 1976; Waddell and Marlowe, 1981; Mihaly and Morgan, 1984). These factors also are not static during pregnancy but may change as gestation progresses. In addition, placental morphology varies among species, so that interspecies extrapolation is not always straight-forward. Several recent reviews have discussed the factors affecting placental transfer of chemicals (Waddell and Marlowe, 1981; Mihaly and Morgan, 1984; Juchau, 1980a,b; Welsch, 1982). This discussion will focus on how these factors may influence the delivery of chemicals to the nervous system of the conceptus.

Blood Flow

Chemical delivery to the developing conceptus relies primarily on blood flow to the placenta. Although chemicals may transfer from mother to fetus via the amniotic fluid after crossing the amnion, the majority of agents attain access to the conceptus via placental passage (Nau and Liddiard, 1978). Rodents and lagomorphs, which are widely used in developmental toxicity testing, have placentation that changes from a fully inverted and persistent yolk-sac type to a chorioallantoic placenta on about day 11.5 of gestation (Everett, 1935; Beck, 1976; Beck, 1981). Buelke-Sam et al. (1982) examined the absolute and relative blood flow to the rat placenta over gestational ages 11–20 days and found that relative blood flow increased eightfold from day 11 to day 20 of gestation. Chemical exposure of the conceptus is based primarily on the equilibrium achieved between the unbound drug concentration in the maternal and fetal plasma. Therefore, over time, this eightfold increase in relative placental blood flow may not result in a dramatic difference in chemical concentration in the conceptus. In addition to the changes in placental blood flow that occur in the uncompromised rat during gestation, changes in blood flow as a result of chemical exposure must also be considered. Experimentally induced changes in blood flow have been shown to alter normal development of the conceptus (Greiss and Gobble, 1967; Barr and Brent, 1978; Millicovsky and DeSesso, 1980). Vasoactive agents such as serotonin (Robson and Sullivan, 1966; Craig, 1966), prostaglandins (Rankin, 1978), and cigarette smoke (Lehtovirta and Forss, 1978) inhibit uteroplacental blood flow and may induce deleterious fetal effects.

Permeability

Placental permeability to a chemical is influenced by both placental characteristics such as thickness, surface area, carrier systems, and lipid/protein content of the membranes and by characteristics of the chemical agent such as degree of ionization, lipid solubility, protein binding, and molecular weight (Mirkin and Singh, 1976; Mihaly and Morgan, 1984; Welsch, 1982). It is now recognized that almost any maternally administered compound has the potential to cross the placenta. The rate of placental transfer is rapid for nonionized, lipid-soluble chemicals of low molecular weight (less than 1000) and is largely controlled by placental blood flow (Mirkin and Singh, 1976; Mihaly and Morgan, 1984). However, charged molecules such as tubocurarine have been shown to enter the fetus (Kivalo and Saarikoski, 1972, 1976). Likewise, highly ionized chemicals that are at normal blood pH, such as the salicylates, also readily cross the placenta (Wilson et al., 1977). The question is thus not whether a compound crosses the placenta, but at what rate.

The degree of plasma protein binding of a chemical also influences its rate of placental transfer, since it is generally only the free drug that crosses the membranes of the placenta (Krauer et al., 1980; Welsch, 1982). Protein binding is usually reversible, and there is a finite number of binding sites; thus, binding is saturable and equilibrium may be described by the law of mass action (Krauer et al., 1980; Miller et al., 1976). As long as binding is reversible, it does not prevent the chemical from crossing membranes but only slows the rate at which the transfer occurs (Levine, 1973).

Biotransformation

Chemical biotransformation has been subdivided into two major phases. Phase I reactions include oxidation, reduction, hydrolysis, or other reactions that modify chemicals in such a way that phase II reactions may occur. Phase II reactions involve the conjugation of chemicals with an endogenous moiety, such as glucuronic acid or sulfate (Williams, 1959). The overall effect of these biotransformations is to increase chemical polarity, resulting in more rapid excretion, biological inactivation, or both. In some cases, however, biotransformation results in the formation of a more potent or toxic agent capable of producing deleterious effects.

Placental metabolism may be the most decisive of several factors influencing the delivery of chemicals to the developing conceptus. Placental biotransformation of a chemical occurring before fetal delivery may dramatically alter the chemical profile observed in the conceptus from that in the maternal organism (Slikker et al., 1982b). Equilibrium factors, which may clearly influence the rate of placental transfer, can result in quantitative differences of exposure; placental metabolism, however, can qualitatively alter the exposure of the conceptus to potentially toxic chemicals.

Placental metabolism is less well characterized than hepatic metabolism, but existing data suggest that placental metabolic capacity is severely limited as compared with adult hepatic capacity (Mirkin and Singh, 1976; Juchau, 1980b). For example, even though evidence for the presence of several forms of placental cytochrome P-450 have been reported (Juchau, 1975; Zachariah and Juchau, 1977), none of them appear to be inducible by phenobarbital-type agents (Juchau, 1980a). Likewise, conjugation reactions involving synthetic donor molecules, such as glucuronidation, sulfation, and acetylation, have either not been observed at all or observed only at very low levels in the placenta as compared with the liver (Juchau, 1980b).

Embryonic/Fetal Considerations

The biotransformation of chemicals affects the concentration of biologically active agents at the cellular locus of action. Chemical biotransformation may result in the formation of either an active, potentially toxic metabolite (bioactivation) or an inactive metabolite (detoxification). Knowledge of the activities of chemical-metabolizing enzymes in various tissues aids in the understanding of tissue susceptibilities and in the ability to extrapolate between species. As with most systems during development, however, the various chemical-metabolizing systems undergo quantitative if not qualitative changes. Nevertheless, tremendous progress has been made in describing and comparing chemical metabolism in the developing conceptus of various species (Neims et al., 1976; Pelkonen, 1977; Dutton, 1978; Nau and Neubert, 1978; Pelkonen, 1980). The ontogeny and regulatory factors of chemical metabolism have recently been reviewed, and the expression of fetal P-450 isozymes is believed to be under both developmental and tissue-specific regulatory factors. (Leakey, 1983; Dutton and Leakey, 1981; Eltom et al., 1992).

Delivery

The majority of chemicals entering the fetal circulation do so via the umbilical vein after passage through the placenta. A portion of the blood flow entering the liver of the conceptus is shunted via the ductus venosus directly to the inferior vena cava and to the heart for total body distribution (Rudolph and Heymann, 1967). As in the adult, approximately 16% of this cardiac output is directed toward the fetal brain (Behrman et al., 1970). The remaining umbilical flow enters hepatic tissue and exits to the vena cava via the portal vein (Dawes, 1968). Therefore, a fraction of the blood-borne chemical first passes through the developing liver, while another fraction passes directly to the remaining tissues of the developing conceptus (Power and Longo, 1975). Other routes of chemical entry to the conceptus are possible, such as penetration through the placental membranes directly into amniotic fluid and then into the conceptus (Castelazo-Ayala et al., 1972). During pregnancy, the human fetus is known to swallow (deglutition) a portion of the amniotic fluid (and urinate into it as well). This route of chemical exposure would be inherently slower and of much smaller magnitude than that occurring via the umbilical circulation (Reynolds, 1972).

Once chemicals are in the fetal circulation, factors that control the distribution and elimination of chemicals in adults are also present, including plasma protein binding, lipid/water partitioning, renal excretion in later gestation, and, to a greater or lesser extent, chemical biotransformation (Mirkin and Singh, 1976).

Biotransformation

Chemical biotransformation by the developing conceptus has been extensively reviewed (Rane and Tomson, 1980; Leakey, 1983; Juchau and Faustman-Watts, 1983; Juchau, 1983; Neims et al., 1976; Pelkonen, 1977; Dutton, 1978; Nau and Neubert, 1978; Pelkonen, 1980; Dutton and Leakey, 1981; Dvorchik, 1981; Slikker et al., 1988). Even though data have been collected with a variety of techniques and some "data gaps" exist because of technical or ethical reasons, several general conclusions may be drawn from the literature:

1.   During prenatal development, the activities of most, but not all, systems that catalyze both phase I and phase II reactions are lower than in the adult of the species.
2.   As in the adult, the conceptus exhibits substrate specificity in its ability to metabolize chemicals. This suggests the existence of several sets of enzymes or isozymes that may or may not be the same as in the adult.
3.   These enzyme systems may be inhibited or induced by pretreatment with a variety of chemicals.
4.   Enzyme activity generally increases with gestational age. However, the ontogeny of each individual enzyme may be different, and the controlling mechanisms of maturation of enzyme activity are incompletely understood.
5.   Prenatal human and nonhuman primates exhibit higher levels of many metabolizing enzymes (especially P-450s) than do other commonly used laboratory models.
6.   As in the adult, the liver of the conceptus appears to have the greatest capacity for chemical metabolism, although the fetal adrenal gland, kidney, and lung do exhibit metabolic capabilities.

Elimination

Just as placental transfer of chemicals is the predominant pathway from the maternal system to the conceptus, placental transfer is also the predominant route for embryonic/fetal chemical elimination, and the same pharmacokinetic rules apply; those agents that are nonionized and lipid-soluble will leave the conceptus as determined by the concentration gradient from conceptus to mother. If, however, a chemical has been conjugated by the fetus (e.g., glucuronidation, sulfation) or otherwise metabolized to a more polar form, the rate of return to the maternal circulation will be slower than for the parent compound (Dancis, 1958; Levitz et al., 1960; Goebelsmann, 1968; Goebelsmann et al., 1972).

Central Nervous System Considerations

The blood-brain barrier, much like the placenta, is not an impermeable barrier at all, but a regulatory interface between blood and the nervous system. The regulatory function of this interface is superimposed on baseline permeability restrictions and controls the immediate environment of the glial and neuronal cells (Rapoport, 1976). The description of the role of the CSF, choroid plexus, and cerebrovascular endothelium in the regulatory capacity of the blood-brain barrier is beyond the scope of this chapter but has been described in detail elsewhere (Rapoport, 1976). With a focus on developmental neurotoxicity, there are two areas of special concern: the circumventricular organs (CVOs) of the brain, which lie outside the normal protection of the blood-brain barrier, and the developmental changes that alter susceptibility to neurotoxicant exposure.

The CVOs are highly vascularized structures that are in contact with the brain median ventricular system, and therefore, with CSF, but lack the usual protection of the blood-brain barrier. These structures include the subfornical organ, pineal gland, median eminence, choroid plexus, suprapineal recess, neurohypophysis, area postrema, sub-commisural organ, and supraoptic crest (Mark and Farmer, 1984). Agents that generally do not have access to most brain areas because of the blood-brain barrier pass readily into the CVOs, owing, at least in part, to the fenestrated endothelial walls and widened perivascular spaces of the CVO blood vessels (Price et al., 1981). Several agents, such as glutamate and 6-hydroxydopamine, that normally require direct brain injection to produce neurotoxicity have been shown to induce CVO damage when administered systemically (Olney et al., 1977; Palazzo et al., 1978).

The ontogeny of the blood-brain barrier in the developing animal is complicated in that several of its aspects mature at different rates. These include the tight junctions between endothelial cells of the cerebral blood vessels, astrocytic processes or end-feet that may completely ensheathe cerebral capillaries, several transport mechanisms (e.g., small ion, glucose, amino acids, certain monocarboxylic acids, deoxynucleosides, vitamins), and metabolism by endothelial and choroid plexus enzymes (Saunders, 1977). Determining the impact of each one of these features on the functionality of the blood-brain barrier during development is confounded by the concomitant dramatic changes in brain mass and CSF volume and turnover (Rapoport, 1976).

One of the major components of the blood-brain barrier, the tight junctions between endothelial cells, appears early in fetal development and does not subsequently undergo detectable changes (Saunders, 1977). In contrast, the development of astrocytic processes appears to correlate with the physiological data reflecting the maturation of barrier function (Johanson, 1980). Certain transport functions also exhibit a maturational component. The selective, carrier-mediated transport of 19 amino acids was studied in the developing rat. The transport systems were present in the early neonatal rat, but entry rates for most of the amino acids decreased with age (Banos et al., 1971). The capacity to move lactate across the blood-brain barrier in the neonatal rat is several times greater than in the adult (Cremer et al., 1979). In contrast, the carrier-mediated influx of glucose into the rat brain is low at birth and increases to maximal levels in the young adult (Daniel et al., 1978). Although little is known about developmental changes, there is evidence for two nucleoside transport systems: a facilitated diffusion system for certain nucleosides excluding thymidine, deoxyuridine, and deoxycytidine at the blood-brain barrier; and an active transport system at the blood-CSF barrier (the choroid plexus) for thymidine and deoxycytidine (Spector and Eells, 1984). Enzymes such as NADH tetrazolium reductase and ATPase increase and alkaline phosphatases decreases in cerebral capillaries with fetal development. Both dopa-decarboxylase and monoamine oxidase are present in the vascular endothelium of the immature brain and become more effective with age (Rapoport, 1976). In general, little information is available concerning the ontogeny of many features of the blood-brain barrier and choroid plexus because of the technical problems associated with studying these phenomena. The available information does suggest that, with the exception of the tight junctions, several features of the blood-brain barrier responsible for controlling brain exposure to chemicals change with maturation. Whether these maturational changes alter CNS susceptibility to neurotoxicants, however, will continue to be determined on a case-by-case basis until a more comprehensive data base is available.

PHARMACOKINETIC MODELS

Compartmental Models

Pharmacokinetic models, which allow for the mathematical description of chemical distribution within the fetomaternal unit, can be helpful in defining aspects of embryonic fetal exposure. Models have been described by several authors, and, depending on the extent of fetal or placental metabolism, the following generalizations can be made:

1. If a chemical is transferred to the conceptus by simple diffusion and no significant fetal or placental metabolism or fetal renal excretion occurs, then, under steady-state conditions, the pharmacokinetic parameters and concentration of unbound chemical in maternal blood can be used to predict the upper limits of unbound chemical in the conceptus (Gillette, 1979).
2. If the chemical is slowly diffusible, the maximum concentration of the chemical in maternal blood may occur much earlier than the maximum concentration in the conceptus. Maternal blood concentrations, however, can be used to predict the area under the curve and thus the average concentration of the unbound chemical in fetal tissue, again assuming no fetal or placental metabolism or excretion by the fetal kidney (Gillette, 1979). Maternal blood concentrations then provide upper limits for the concentration of chemical in the conceptus.
3. If the chemical is rapidly metabolized by the conceptus or the placenta, relative to the rate of diffusion across the placenta, then it is not possible to predict concentrations of the chemical in the conceptus solely on the basis of maternal blood concentrations (Slikker et al., 1982a; Slikker et al., 1982b; Gillette, 1979).

Unfortunately, a number of factors limit the application of these generalities to real-life situations. Among these is the binding of chemicals to plasma or serum protein (Levy, 1981). Such binding can alter the distribution and elimination of chemicals. Protein binding of individual compounds may change during pregnancy and may vary between mother and fetus or neonate (Levy, 1981; Levy, 1976; Gillette, 1977; Murphy, 1979; Hamar and Levy, 1980). It must be remembered, however, that protein binding is usually a reversible equilibrium interaction and that some of the free (unbound) chemical will therefore always be available for transfer and/or target tissue interaction. Other factors affecting maternal/fetal chemical concentrations are pH, electrochemical gradients across the placenta, and active or unidirectional placental transport processes (Levy, 1981; Waddell and Marlowe, 1981).

Physiologically Based Models

Physiologically based pharmacokinetic (PBPK) models are useful tools for calculating the disposition of a chemical and its metabolites in various organs in the body over time (Bischoff et al., 1971; Luecke et al., 1980). Because PBPK models employ parameters associated with anatomical structures and physiological states, they may have advantages over the classical, abstract compartmental models. By the use in the PBPK model of information such as organ size, blood flow, metabolic conversion rate of parent compound to metabolite, and protein-binding affinities, many of the limitations of the compartmental models can be overcome.

A necessity of pharmacokinetic models for developmental neurotoxicants is the ability to link the mathematical model to the ever-changing stage of development of the conceptus during pregnancy. Several recent PBPK models have been developed to incorporate size and functional changes of the maternal, placental, and embryonic/fetal systems into the model (O'Flaherty et al., 1992; Lutz et al., 1977; Luecke et al., 1992). With the input of physiological parameters from the literature (e.g., Snyder, 1974), local concentrations of toxicants at the presumed site of action as a function of the particular stage of development of that particular tissue can be estimated and compared between species. However, developmental PBPK models to predict the fate of neurotoxicants in fetal brain regions as a function of development have yet to be developed and validated.

NEUROACTIVE AGENTS AND DEVELOPMENTAL TOXICITY

Human Developmental Neurotoxicants

A list of human developmental neurotoxicants is shown in Table 1 and is a composite of identified agents from published and unpublished sources (Shepard, 1985; Smith et al., 1983; Beckman and Brent, 1984; Hoar, 1984; Slikker, 1987; Slikker et al., 1988; J. Schardein and C. Kimmel, personal communication). It is interesting to note that the majority of the known human developmental toxicants are also developmental neurotoxicants (see below). This list of known human developmental neurotoxicants is not the product of any systematic testing scheme, but rather has been generated primarily from case reports of alert physicians and epidemiologists. These neurotoxicants represent a wide range of drugs and environmental chemicals that can serve as a diverse reference to test hypotheses regarding the role of neurotoxic chemical delivery to the developing CNS. Each agent is discussed in terms of its neurotoxicity in the developing human and in animal surrogates, and of its ability to reach the target, the developing CNS.

Alcohol

In 1968, Lemoine et al. described a series of abnormalities in 127 children born to alcoholic mothers. This study showed an increased incidence of prenatal growth deficiency, a 25% incidence of malformations, and evidence of psychomotor dysfunction. In 1973, Jones and Smith described 11 infants with a similar constellation of features that they subsequently termed the fetal alcohol syndrome (Jones and Smith, 1973; Jones et al., 1973). Heavy

Table 1 Human Developmental Neurotoxicants and Associated Animal Model Data

Human developmental neurotoxicants	Effect	Animal model	Embryo or fetal brain concentrations[a]
Alcohol	Facial, CNS, neural	Mouse, dog, rat, sheep, pig-tailed monkey, pig	+
Anticonvulsants, (phenytoin, primidone, phenobarbital, carbamazepine)	Craniofacial, digital, neural	Mouse (certain strains), rat	+
Diones	Facial, cardiac, neural	Rat, primate	ND
Valproic acid	Neural tube, facial	Hamster, primate	ND
Chemotherapeutic agents			
Antimetabolites (e.g., methotrexate)	Skull, limb, CNS, digit	Rat, sheep, mouse rabbit, cat	+
Alkylators (e.g., cyclophosphamide)	Multiple	Rat, mouse, rabbit primate, ferret	+
Cocaine	Behavioral	Rat	+
Lead	CNS, behavioral	Rat, mouse, primate	+ (postnatal)
Methylmercury	Neural	Rat, mouse, cat, primate	+
Nicotine (smoking)	CNS, behavioral	Rat, mouse	+
PCB, PBB	Pigment, skeletal, behavioral	Rat, primate	+
Retinoids	CNS, ear, cardiac	Mouse, primates (2 species), hamster	+

[a]+, embryo or fetal brain concentrations reported in the literature; ND, no data on fetal brain concentrations found in the literature.
CNS = central nervous system; PCB = polychlorinated biphenyl; PBB = polybrominated biphenyl.

alcohol consumption during pregnancy poses a high risk (40–50%) of adverse pregnancy outcome, including spontaneous abortion and malformed and/or growth-retarded live-born infants (Kline et al., 1980; Jones et al., 1974).

A variety of animal models have been used to demonstrate dose-related responses to prenatal exposure to alcohol, including mice (Chernoff, 1977), rats (Abel and Dintcheff, 1978), dogs (Ellis and Pick, 1980), and monkeys (Clarren et al., 1987). Although many end points of developmental toxicity are similar between these species and man, the most consistent finding is growth retardation. The assessment of alcohol's effects in animal models has been confounded by the fact that a voluntary reduction in dietary intake commonly accompanied experimental alcohol administration (Goad, 1982). As demonstrated by Goal et al. (1984), however, alcohol is fetotoxic even in well-nourished animals. In vitro whole embryo culture techniques have demonstrated that both ethanol and its oxidized metabolite, acetaldehyde, produce direct, concentration-dependent embryotoxic effects (Brown et al., 1979; Campbell and Fantel, 1983). These data indicate that animal models are predictive of the toxic effects of alcohol in the developing human.

Alcohol is a low-molecular-weight, lipid-soluble chemical that crosses cellular membranes readily. Studies by Hill et al. (1983) clearly demonstrated that after intravenous maternal administration of ethanol to the pregnant monkey, the fetal: maternal plasma ratio quickly achieved unity and maintained it for the duration of the experiment.

Anticonvulsants

The anticonvulsants listed in Table 1 may be loosely lumped together because of the generality of their developmental neurotoxic effects. Impairment of mental performance and/or microcephaly have been reported in children of mothers who used several different anticonvulscants alone or in combination for control of epilepsy during pregnancy (Shepard, 1985; Adams et al., 1990).

Prenatal exposure to the anticonvulsant trimethadione, for example, has been associated with a spectrum of effects including developmental delay, speech difficulty, and craniofacial anomalies, termed the fetal trimethadione syndrome (Goldman and Yaffe, 1978). Specific anomalies associated with the trimethadione syndrome are V-shaped eyebrows, and low-set ears, and these, as well as lack of phalangeal hypoplasia, distinguish this syndrome from that produced by phenytoin. Although the mechanisms underlying its developmental toxicity are unknown, the therapeutic effects of trimethadione are mediated via its major metabolite, dimethadione (Rall and Schleifer, 1990).

The anticonvulsant valproic acid has been associated with neural tube defects including spina bifida in children whose mothers used the drug during pregnancy (Martinez-Frios, 1990). Although animal models have been difficult to develop because of limited sensitive periods and pharmacokinetic considerations, mouse, rat, rabbit, and primate models have been useful in mimicking many human developmental toxicities (Vorhees, 1987; Roberts et al., 1991; Nau et al., 1991).

Phenytoin is also believed to be a human developmental toxicant, causing craniofacial anomalies and mental deficiency in human infants exposed in utero (Hanson et al., 1976). Rodent models have been developed, and data from both clinical and animal studies suggest that maternal serum phenytoin concentrations correlate with developmental toxicity (Roberts et al., 1991).

These relatively low-molecular-weight and/or lipid-soluble agents all have profound effects on the adult CNS and readily gain access to the brain (Rall and Schleifer, 1990). Information regarding embryonic/fetal brain concentrations of these agents is limited, but the developmental neurotoxicity data do suggest that the developing brain is a target (Adams et al., 1990)

Chemotherapeutic Agents

Therapeutic agents used to treat cancer include several antimetabolites and alkylating chemicals. Methotrexate will be used as a representative of the antimetabolite group.

Folic acid antagonists such as methotrexate produce their cytotoxic effects by binding with great affinity to dihydrofolate reductase, thus blocking one-carbon transfer reactions (Calabresi and Parks, 1980). When consumed during early pregnancy, methotrexate causes abortion and/or fetal malformations including craniofacial anomalies and growth retardation (Beckman and Brent, 1984). As reviewed by Hendrickx et al. (1983), the embryotoxicity of methotrexate is similar in the mouse, rat, rabbit, and rhesus monkey. Some of these effects are similar to those observed clinically (e.g., craniofacial anomalies and cleft palate). Wilson et al. (1979) point out, however, that the degree and type of embryotoxicity was not closely correlated with the level or duration of concentration of methotrexate in the embryos of two different species, the rat and monkey.

Cyclophosphamide, a representative of the alkylating agents, has been implicated as a human teratogen. Exposed infants had multiple malformations including ectrodactyly and cleft palate (Hendrickx et al., 1983). Similar malformations have been reported in the offspring of a variety of animal models including rats, mice, rabbits, and monkeys

(Hendrickx et al., 1983; Shepard, 1985). Cyclophosphamide is toxic to the developing cultured rat embryo only when an oxidative metabolic system is present (Fantel, 1982). More recent studies by Mirkes et al. (1984) conclude that two metabolites of cyclophosphamide, phosphoramide mustard and acrolein, can mediate cyclophosphamide teratogenesis, but that acrolein must be metabolically generated at the locus of action within the embryo to be active.

Cocaine

Cocaine use during pregnancy has been reported to lead to premature births (Ney et al., 1990), fetal growth retardation (Zuckerman et al., 1989), and depressed interactive abilities and impairment of organizational abilities in newborns and children (Chasnoff et al., 1985, 1987). However, polypharmacy and nutritional and general health status must be considered in assessing the clinical outcome after prenatal cocaine exposure. Studies in rodents have supported the hypothesis that cocaine is a developmental neurotoxicant. Spear and co-workers have demonstrated both behavioral and neurochemical alterations in rat pups after maternal exposure to cocaine (Spear et al., 1989; Scalzo et al., 1990). Dow-Edwards and collaborators have described neurochemical alterations in rat pups after neonatal cocaine exposure (Dow-Edwards et al., 1988). Controversy continues, however, as to the relative importance of direct cocaine effects on the developing rat pup versus maternal and nutritional effects of cocaine (Wiggins and Ruiz, 1990).

The disposition of cocaine has been described in the pregnant rat (Wiggins et al., 1989; Spear et al., 1989), guinea pig (Sandberg and Olsen, 1992), sheep (Woods et al., 1989), and monkey (Binienda et al., 1993), and to a limited extent in humans (Mittleman et al., 1989). The ratio of fetal:maternal area under the concentration time curve or single time point comparisons for cocaine usually ranges from 0.1 to 0.5. Brain concentrations are generally higher than blood concentrations, however, and fetal:maternal brain ratios for cocaine range from 0.2 to 1. Thus, as expected for a low-molecular-weight, lipid-soluble compound such as cocaine, the nervous system of the conceptus is a readily exposed target.

Lead

Clinical studies have clearly indicated that the developing CNS is susceptable to lead toxicity, as evidenced by disruptions in cognitive development and learning and changes in reflexive and electrophysiological end points and social-interaction behavior. Longitudinal studies have confirmed associations between umbilical cord blood lead levels and cognitive function in children. Blood lead levels of 10–15 μg/dl have been linked to behavioral deficits (Davis et al., 1990).

Animal studies in primates and rodents have produced results similar to those observed in humans. The ability of animals to perform complex behavioral tasks believed to measure cognition and learning shows disruption at blood lead levels of 15–20 μg/dl (Davis et al., 1990).

Methylmercury

Human exposure to methylmercury during gestation has been associated with cerebral palsy and microcephaly in the offspring (Minamata disease) (Harada, 1978). Results from experimental animal studies have been consistent with clinical findings in that CNS defects have been demonstrated in the mouse, rat, and cat (Reuhl and Chang, 1979). Mercury inactivates sulfhydryl enzymes by forming covalent bonds with sulfur and thus interferes with cellular metabolism and function (Klaassen, 1980).

Long-term exposure to low doses of methylmercury in the developing rat can alter brain concentrations of neurotransmitters (Lindstrom et al., 1991). Methylmercury readily crosses the placenta and is able to produce developmental toxicity. Thus it is in contrast to the inorganic mercurials, which do not cross the placenta and are generally without effect (Miller and Shaikh, 1983). In the developing brain methylmercury concentrations of less than 3 μg/g have been associated with neurobehavioral toxicity in both the developing human and laboratory animal models (Burbacher et al., 1990).

Nicotine

Epidemiological studies have indicated that smoking tobacco during pregnancy is associated with decreased birth weight, increased mortality, and neurobehavioral deficits in offspring (Picone et al., 1982; Brooke et al., 1989; Streissguth et al., 1984). Although there is a heterogeneity in the persistence of the impairments, a variety of abnormalities have been observed in offspring of women smokers, including deficits in cognitive function (Dunn and McBurney, 1977; Naeye and Peters, 1984), learning impairment (Butler and Goldstein, 1973), impaired attention and orientation (Jacobson et al., 1984), and poor impulse control (Rantakallio, 1983).

In animal models, dose-related effects of nicotine include intrauterine growth retardation and behavioral and neurochemical alterations (Navarro et al., 1989a; Slotkin et al., 1987a). Lower doses of nicotine (0.5 mg/kg/day, over days 1–20 of gestation) did not result in the decreased birth weight noted at higher doses but did induce altered avoidance learning in 60-day-old rat progeny. Recently, Erikkson and Fredirkisson (1992) reported that neonatal mice exposed to nicotine at 132 μg/kg/day for 5 days starting at 10 days of age were hyperactive at 4 months of age and had altered swim maze learning at 7 months of age. Along with other studies, these data indicate that developmental neurotoxicity is associated with nicotine exposure in several animal models including the rat, mouse, and guinea pig (Johns et al., 1982).

Although the mechanism responsible for nicotine's neurotoxicity is not fully understood, developmental neurochemical studies provide evidence that nicotinic receptors and their interaction with the developing cholinergic and catecholaminergic systems may be important for its observed neurobehavioral developmental toxicity (Levin, 1992; Navarro et al., 1989b; Slotkin et al., 1987b).

In the mouse, nicotine has been found to accumulate in the placenta (and to a lesser extent in the fetus) relative to maternal plasma (Tjalve et al., 1968). As a result, the ratio of embryonic:maternal plasma nicotine concentration was 5.4 on gestational day 9 in the pregnant mouse (Roberts et al., 1989). In the late-gestational rat (gestational day 19), the fetal brain–maternal plasma nicotine concentration ratio was 3.5 (Mosier and Jansons, 1972).

Polychlorinated Biphenyls

The consumption of polychlorinated biphenyl (PCB)-contaminated cooking oil by pregnant women in Japan and Taiwan resulted in the birth of newborns with dark-brown staining of the skin and low birth weights (Shepard, 1985). A variety of clinical studies as recently summarized by Tilson et al. (1990) have indicated that neurobehavioral deficits in children can be attributed to exposure to PCBs in utero.

In animals models, PCBs have a low potential for producing gross physical malformations, but neurotoxic and immunotoxic effects have been reported (Loose et al., 1979; Tilson et al., 1979). Rodent studies indicate that rat pups exposed prenatally to PCBs exhibit alteration of postnatal behaviors including active-avoidance learning and retention of a visual discrimination task (Lilienthal and Winneke, 1991). Although maternal concentrations were not reported, brain concentrations of PCBs in littermates of these pups at birth attained 0.21 μg/g for all PCB congeners combined.

Retinoids

The isomer of vitamin A *cis*-retinoic acid (isotretinoin) produces a variety of congenital defects involving craniofacial and CNS structures in human infants exposed to this agent in utero (Lammer et al., 1985). The effects in infants and children of prenatal exposure to *cis*-retinoic acid have recently been described and include mental retardation and learning and attention deficits (Adams and Lammer, 1991). The results of this clinical study and others using animal models provide evidence that developmental CNS toxicants can produce neuropsychological deficits in the absence of anatomically detectable pathology in the CNS.

Studies in a variety of animal models have corroborated the human findings. Early studies with pregnant rats and monkeys, more than a decade before clinical cases were reported, showed vitamin A (all-*trans*-retinoic acid) to be a developmental neurotoxicant (Hutchings et al., 1973; Vorhees et al., 1979). Human and monkey studies have described embryonic/fetal exposure to vitamin A and metabolites after maternal administration of either *cis*-retinoic or all-*trans*-retinoic acid (Eckhoff et al., 1991; Creech Kraft et al., 1989). Although fetal brain concentrations have not been systematically evaluated, preliminary data indicate that the brain of the early monkey fetus is a target for maternally administered all-*trans*-retinoic acid (Eckhoff et al., 1991; Slikker and Eckhoff, unpublished observation, 1991).

CONCLUSION

On the basis of the physicochemical properties of neuroactive chemicals and the cellular similarities of the involved membranes, a hypothesis that neuroactive agents readily cross the placenta and enter the developing nervous system has arisen. The ability of neuroactive agents to affect the adult nervous system suggests that these chemicals have physicochemical characteristics that allow them to cross the blood-brain barrier. These characteristics, including lipid-solubility, degree of ionization, molecular size, transporter binding, and receptor interactions, are consistent with some of the chemical properties controlling placental transfer. Although the anatomical aspects of the blood-brain and placental barriers are considerably different, they share physiological similarities. Neither is an impermeable barrier, but a regulatory, multicellular interface between blood and other tissue. The properties of these interfaces are similar in that both involve cells with lipid bilayer membranes and metabolic, transport, and uptake capabilities. Therefore, it is not surprising that a general belief has developed that the maternal administration of neuroactive chemicals will result in significant in utero exposure to the developing conceptus.

To test the hypothesis that neuroactive agents would be active during development, the ability of a number of known human developmental neurotoxicants to reach the embryonic or fetal brain was examined. Although data were not available for every developmental neurotoxicant listed, every chemical class or individual agent had been detected in the developing embryonic or fetal brain of at least one relevant animal model. In some instances (e.g., nicotine), the fetal brain concentrations were actually many times higher than respective maternal blood concentrations. In other cases (e.g., methylmercury and PCBs), the concentrations in the conceptus were less than in the maternal system, but at least were detectable. Thus, there is ample evidence that the majority of known developmental neurotoxicants have the ability to achieve significant concentrations in their target tissue, the developing nervous system.

REFERENCES

Abel EL, Dintcheff BA (1978). Effects of prenatal alcohol exposure on growth and development in rats. J Pharmacol Exp Ther. 207:916–21.

Adams J, Lammer EJ (1991). Relationship between dysmorphology and neuro-psychological function in children exposed to isotretinoin "in utero." In: Fujii E, Barr CJ, eds. Functional neuroteratology of short-term exposure to drugs. Tokyo University Press, 159–170.

Adams J, Vorhees CV, Middaugh LD (1990). Developmental neurotoxicity of anticonvulsants: human and animal evidence on phenytoin. Neurotoxicol Teratol 12:203–14.

Banos G, Daniel PM, Moorhouse SR, Pratt OE (1971). The entry of amino acids into the brain of the rat during the postnatal period. J Physiol 213:45–6.

Barr M, Brent RL (1978). Uterine vascular interruption and combined radiation and surgical procedures. In: Wilson JG, Fraser FC, eds. Handbook of teratology. Vol. 4. New York: Plenum Press, 275–304

Beck F (1976). Comparative placental morphology and function. Environ Health Perspect 18:5–12.

Beck F (1981). Comparative placental morphology and function. In: Kimmel CA, Buelke-Sam J, eds. Developmental toxicity. New York: Raven Press, 35–54.

Beckman DA, Brent RL (1984). Mechanisms of teratogenesis. Annu Rev Pharmacol Toxicol 24:483–500.

Behrman RE, Lees MH, Peterson EN, DeLannoy CW, Seeds AE (1970). Distribution of the circulation in the normal and asphyxiated fetal primate. Am J Obstet Gynecol 106:956–69.

Binienda Z, Bailey JR, Duhart HM, Slikker W Jr, Paule MG (1993). Transplacental pharmacokinetics and maternal/fetal plasma concentrations of cocaine in pregnant macaques near term. Drug Metab Disp 21(2):364–368.

Bischoff KB, Dedrick RL, Zaharko DS, Longstreth JA (1971). Methotrexate pharmacokinetics. J Pharm Sci 60:1128–33.

Bogaert MC, Thiery M (1983). Pharmacokinetics and pregnancy. Eur J Obstet Gynecol Reprod Biol 16:229–35.

Brock-Utne JG, Downing JW, Mankowitz E (1980). Drugs and the fetomaternal unit. S Afr Med J 58(9):366–9.

Brooke OG, Anderson HR, Bland JM, Peacock JL, Stewart DM (1989). Effects on birth weight of smoking, alcohol, caffeine, socioeconomic factors, and psychosocial stress. Br Med J 298:795–801.

Brown NA, Goulding EH, Fabro S (1979). Ethanol embryotoxicity: direct effects on mammalian embryos in vitro. Science 206:573–5.

Buelke-Sam J, Holson JF, Nelson CJ (1982). Blood flow during pregnancy in the rat: II. Dynamics of and litter variability in uterine flow. Teratology 26:279–88.

Burbacher TM, Rodier PM, Weiss B (1990). Methylmercury developmental neurotoxicity: a comparison of effects in humans and animals. Neurotoxicol Teratol 12:191–202.

Butler NR, Goldstein H (1973). Smoking in pregnancy and subsequent child development. Br Med J 4:573–5.

Calabresi P, Parks RE Jr (1980). Antiproliferative agents and drugs used for immunosuppression. In: Gilman AG, Goodman LS, Gilman A, eds. The pharmacological basis of therapeutics. 6th ed. New York: Macmillan, 1273

Campbell MA, Fantel AG (1983). Teratogenicity of acetaldehyde in vitro: relevance to the fetal alcohol syndrome. Life Sci 32:2641–7.

Castelazo-Ayala L, Karchmer S, Shor-Pinsker V (1972). The biochemistry of amniotic fluid during normal pregnancy. Correlation with maternal and fetal blood. In: Hodari AA, Mariona F, eds. Physiological biochemistry of the fetus. Springfield, Illinois: Charles C, Thomas, 32–53.

Chasnoff IJ, Burn WJ, Schnoll SH, Burns KA (1985). Cocaine use in pregnancy. N Engl J Med 313:666–9.

Chasnoff IJ, Burns KA, Burns WJ (1987). Cocaine use in pregnancy: perinatal morbidity and mortality. Neurotoxicol Teratol 9:291–293.

Chernoff GF (1977). The fetal alcohol syndrome in mice: an animal model. Teratology 15:223–36.

Clarren SK, Bowden DM, Astley SJ (1987). Pregnancy outcomes after weekly oral administration of ethanol during gestation in the pig-tailed macaque. Teratology 35:345–54.

Craig JM (1966). Mechanism of serotonin induced abortion in rats. Arch Pathol Lab Med 81:257–63.

Creech Kraft J, Nau H, Lammer E, Olney A (1989). Human embryo retinoid concentrations after maternal intake of isotretinoin. N Engl J Med 321:262 (letter).

Cremer JE, Cunningham VJ, Pardridge WM, Braun, LD, Oldendorf, WH (1979). Kinetics of blood-brain barrier transport of pyruvate, lactate and glucose in suckling, weanling and adult rats. J Neurochem 334:439–45.

Cummings AJ (1983). A survey of pharmacokinetic data from pregnant women. Clin Pharm 8:344–54.

Dancis J, Money WL, Condon GP, Mortimer L (1958). The relative transfer of estrogens and their glucuronides across the placenta in the guinea pig. J Clin Invest 37:1373–8.

Daniel PM, Lover ER, Pratt OE (1978). The effect of age upon the influx of glucose into the brain. J Physiol 274:141–8.

Davis JM, Otto DA, Weil DE, Grant LD (1990). The comparative developmental neurotoxicity of lead in humans and animals. Neurotoxicol Teratol 12:215–29.

Dawes GS (1968). Umbilical blood flow and vascular resistance: changes with age. In: Dawes GS, ed. Foetal and neonatal physiology. Chicago: Year Book Medical Publishers, 69.

Dow-Edwards DL, Freed LA, Milhorat TH (1988). Stimulation of brain metabolism by perinatal cocaine exposure. Dev Brain Res 42:137–41.

Dunn HG, McBurney AK (1977). Cigarette smoking and the fetus and child. Pediatrics 60:772 (letter).

Dutton GJ (1978). Developmental aspects of drug conjugation, with special reference to glucuronidation. Annu Rev Pharmacol Toxicol 18:17–35.

Dutton GJ, Leakey JEA (1981). The perinatal development of drug-metabolizing enzymes: What factors trigger their onset? Prog Drug Res 25:189–273.

Dvorchik BH (1981). Nonhuman primates as animal models for the study of fetal hepatic drug metabolism. In: Soyka LF, Redmond GP, eds. Drug metabolism in the immature human. New York: Raven Press, 146–62.

Eckhoff C, Bailey JR, Slikker W Jr, Nau H (1991). Placental transfer of retinoids following high-dose vitamin A during early pregnancy in the monkey. Teratology 43:371–408.

Ellis FW, Pick JR (1980). An animal model of the fetal alcohol syndrome in beagles. Alcohol Clin Exp Res 4:123–34.

Eltom SE, Babish JG, Schwark WS (1992). The postnatal development of drug-metabolizing enzymes in hepatic, pulmonary and renal tissues of the goat. J Vet Pharmacol Ther 16(2):152–163.

Erikkson P, Fredirkisson A (1992). Exposure to nicotine during a defined period in neonatal life induces changes in behavior response to nicotine and swim-maze performance in adult mice. In: Joan M. Crammer, ed. Tenth International Neurotoxicology Conference Proceedings. Little Rock, AR, p. 28.

Everett JW (1935). Morphological and physiological studies of the placenta in the albino rat. J Exp Zool 70:243–85.

Fantel AG (1982). Culture of whole rodent embryos in teratogen screening. In: Leagtor MS, ed. Proceedings of the consensus workshop on in vitro teratogenesis testing: teratogenesis, carcinogenesis, and mutagenesis. Vol. 2. New York: Alan R. Liss, 231–42.

Garbis-Berkvens JM, Peters PW (1987). Comparative morphology and physiology of embryonic and fetal membranes. In: Nau H, Scott WJ, eds. Pharmacokinetics in teratogenesis. Vol. 1. Boca Raton, FL: CRC Press, 14–44.

Gillette JR (1977). Factors that affect drug concentrations in maternal plasma. In: Wilson JG, Fraser JG, eds. Handbook of teratology. Vol. 3. New York: Plenum Press, 35–78.

Gillette JR (1979). Chairman's introductory statement: Prenatal development of drug metabolism. In: Estabrook RW, Lindenlaub E, eds. The induction of drug metabolism. Vol. 14. Stuttgart: Schattauer Verlag, 501–6.

Goad PT (1982). Final report for experiment numbers 313, 6037, 6067. In: Developmental Toxicity of Ethanol, Jefferson, AK: NCTR, p. 26.

Goad PT, Hill DE, Slikker W Jr, Kimmel CA, Gaylor DW (1984). The role of maternal diet in the developmental toxicology of ethanol. Toxicol Appl Pharmacol 73:256–67.

Goebelsmann U, Wiqvist N, Diczfalusy E (1968). Placental transfer of oestriol glucosiduronates. Acta Endocrinol 59:426–32.

Goebelsmann U, Roberts JM, Jaffe RB (1972). Placental transfer of ^{3}H-oestriol-3-sulphate-16-glucosiduronate and ^{3}H-oestriol-16-glucosiduronate-^{14}C. Acta Endocrinol 70:132–42.

Goldman AS, Yaffe SJ (1978). Fetal trimethadione syndrome. Teratology 17:103–6.

Greiss FC, Gobble FL (1967). Effect of sympathetic nerve stimulation on the uterine vascular bed. Am J Obstet Gynecol 92:962–7.

Hamar C, Levy G (1980). Serum protein binding of drugs and bilirubin in newborn infants and their mothers. Clin Pharmacol Ther 28:58–63.

Hanson JW, Myrianthopoulos NC, Sedgwick Harvey MA, Smith DW (1976). Risks to the offspring of women treated with the hydantoin anticonvulsant, with emphasis on the fetal hydantoin syndrome. J Pediatrics 89:662–8.

Harada M (1978). Congenital minamata disease. Teratology 18:285–8.

Heistad DD (1984). The blood-brain barrier. Fed Proc 43:185.

Hendrickx AG, Binkerd PE, Rowland JM (1983). Developmental toxicity and nonhuman primates. In: Kalter H, ed. Issues and reviews in teratology. New York: Plenum Press, 149–80.

Hill DE, Slikker W Jr, Goad PT, Bailey JR, Sziszak TJ, Hendrickx AG (1983). Maternal, fetal, and neonatal elimination of ethanol in nonhuman primates. Dev Pharmacol Ther 6:259–68.

Hoar RM (1984). Reproduction/teratology. Fund Appl Toxicol 4:S335–40.

Hutchings DE, Gibbon J, Kaufman MA (1973). Maternal vitamin A excess during the early fetal period: effects on learning and development in the offspring. Dev Psychol 6:445–57.

Hytten FE, Leitch I, eds. (1971). The product of conception. In: The physiology of human pregnancy. Oxford: Blackwell Scientific Publications, 322.

Illsley NP, Hall S, Penfold P, Stacey TE (1985). Diffusional permeability of the human placenta. Contr Gynecol Obstet 13:92–7.

Jacobson SW, Fein GG, Jacobson LJ, Schwartz PM, Dowler JK (1984). Neonatal correlates of prenatal exposure to smoking, caffeine, and alcohol. Infant Behav Devel 7:253–65.

Johanson CE (1980). Permeability and avacularity of the developing brain: cerebellum vs cerebral cortex. Brain Res 190:3–16.

Johns JM, Louis TM, Becker RF, Means LW (1982). Behavioral effects of prenatal exposure to nicotine in guinea pigs. Neurobehav Toxicol Teratol 4:365–9.

Jones KL, Smith DW (1973). Recognition of the fetal alcohol syndrome in early infancy. Lancet 2:999–1101.

Jones KL, Smith DW, Ulleland CN, Streissguth AP (1973). Pattern of malformation in offspring of chronic alcoholic mothers. Lancet 1:1267–71.

Jones KL, Smith DW, Streissguth AP, Myrianthopoulos NC (1974). Outcome in offspring of chronic alcoholic women. Lancet 1:1076–8.

Juchau MR (1975). Mixed-function oxidation in the human placenta. In: Morselli PL, Garattini S, Sereni F, eds. Basic therapeutic aspects of perinatal pharmacology. New York: Raven Press,

Juchau MR (1980a). Extrahepatic drug biotransformation in the placenta. In Gram TE, ed.

Extrahepatic metabolism of drugs and other foreign compounds. New York: S.P. Medical and Scientific Books, 211–38.

Juchau MR (1980b). Drug biotransformation in the placenta. Pharmacol Ther 8:501–24.

Juchau MR (1983). Disposition of chemical contaminants in maternal-embryonic/fetal systems. In: Saxena J, ed. Hazard assessment of chemicals current developments. Vol. 2. New York: Academic Press, 95–132.

Juchau MR, Faustman-Watts E (1983). Pharmacokinetic considerations in the maternal-placental-fetal unit. Clin Obstet Gynecol 26:379–90.

Kaufmann P, King BF (1982). Structural and functional organization of the placenta. Basel: Karger.

Kivalo I, Saarikoski S (1972). Placental transmission and foetal uptake of ^{14}C-dimethyltubocurarine. Br J Anaesth 44:557 (Abstract).

Kivalo I, Saarikoski S (1976). Placental transfer of ^{14}C-dimethyltubocurarine during caesarean section. Br J Anaesth 48:239–242.

Klaassen CD (1980). Heavy metals and heavy-metal antagonists. In: Gilman AG, Goodman LS, Gilman A, eds. The pharmacological basis of therapeutics. 6th ed. New York: Macmillan, 1623.

Kline J, Shrout P, Stein Z, Susser M, Warburton D (1980). Drinking during pregnancy and spontaneous abortion. Lancet 2:176–180.

Krauer B, Krauer F, Hytten FE (1980). Drug disposition and pharmacokinetics in the maternal-placental-fetal-unit. Pharmacol Ther 10:301–28.

Lammer EJ, Chen DT, Hoar RM, Agnish ND, Benke PS, Braun JT, Curry CJ, Fernhoff PM, Grix AW Jr, Lott LT, Richard JM, Sun SC (1985). Retinoic acid embryopathy. N Engl J Med 313:837–41.

Leakey JEA (1983). Ontogenesis. In: Caldwell J, ed. Biological basis of detoxication. New York: Academic Press, 77–103.

Lefauconnier JM, Tayarani Y, Bernard G (1986). Blood-brain barrier permeability to excitatory amino acids. Adv Exp Med Biol 203:191–8.

Lehtovirta P, Forss M (1978). The acute effect of smoking on intervillous blood flow of the placenta. Br J Obstet Gynecol 85:729–31.

Lemoine P, Harousseau H, Borteyru J, Menuet J (1968). Les enfants de parents alcooliques. Anomalies observées. A propos de 127 cas. Quest Med 25:476–82.

Levin ED (1992). Nicotinic systems and cognitive functions. Psychopharmacology 108(4):417–431.

Levine RR (1973). Pharmacology: drug actions and reactions. Boston: Little, Brown.

Levitz M, Condon GP, Money WL, Dancis J (1960). The relative transfer of estrogens and their sulfates across the guinea pig placenta: sulfurylation of estrogens by the placenta. J Biol Chem 235:973–7.

Levy G (1976). Clinical implications of interindividual differences in plasma protein binding of drugs and endogenous substances. In: Benet LZ, ed. The effect of disease states on drug pharmacokinetics. Washington, D.C.: American Pharmaceutical Association, 137.

Levy G (1981). Pharmacokinetics of fetal and neonatal exposure to drugs. Obstet Gynecol 58(suppl 5):9S–16S.

Lilienthal H, Winneke G (1991). Sensitive periods for behavioral toxicity of polycholorinated biphenyls: determination by cross-fostering in rats. Fund Appl Toxicol 17:368–75.

Lindstrom H, Luthman J, Oskarsson A, Sundberg J, Olson L (1991). Effects of long-term treatment with methyl mercury on the developing rat brain. Environ Res 56:158–69.

Loose LD, Silkworth JB, Mudzinski SP, Pittman KA, Benitz K-F, Mueller W (1979). Modification of the immune response by organochlorine xenobiotics. Drug Chem Toxicol 2:111–32.

Luecke RH, Thomason L, Wosilait WD (1980). Physiological flow model for drug elimination in the rat. Comput Prog Biomed 2(2):88–98.

Luecke RH, Wosilait WD, Young JF (1993). A mathematical analysis for teratological sensitivity. J Math Comput Model (in press).

Lutz RJ, Dedrick RL, Mathews HB, Eling TE, Anderson MW (1977). A preliminary pharmacokinetic model for several chlorinated biphenyls in the rat. Drug Metab Disp 5:386–97.

Mark MH, Farmer PM (1984). The human subfornical organ: an anatomic and ultrastructural study. Ann Clin Lab Sci 14:427–42.

Martinez-Frias ML (1990). Clinical manifestation of prenatal exposure to valproic acid using case reports and epidemiologic information. Am J Med Genet 37:277–82.

Mihaly GW, Morgan DJ (1984). Placental drug transfer: effects of gestational age and species. Pharmacol Ther 23:253–66.

Miller RK, Koszalka TR, Brent RL (1976). The transport of molecules across placental membranes. In: Post G, Nicolson GL, eds. The cell surface in animal embryogenesis and development. New York: Elsevier/North-Holland, 145–223.

Miller RK, Shaikh ZA (1983). Prenatal metabolism: metals and metallothionein. In: Clarkson T, Nordberg G, Sager P, eds. Reproductive and developmental toxicity of metals. New York: Plenum Press, 153–204.

Millicovsky G, DeSesso JM (1980). Differential embryonic cardiovascular responses to acute maternal uterine ischemia: an in vivo microscopic study of rabbit embryos with either intact or clamped umbilical cords. Teratology 22:335–43.

Mirkes PE, Greenaway JC, Rogers JA, Brundrett RB (1984). Role of acrolein in cyclophosphamide teratogenicity in rat embryos in vitro. Toxicol Appl Pharmacol 72:281–91.

Mirkin BL, Singh S (1976). Placental transfer of pharmacologically active molecules. In: Mirkin BL, ed. Perinatal pharmacology and therapeutics. New York: Academic Press, 1–69.

Mittleman RG, Cofino JC, Hearn WL (1989). Tissue distribution of cocaine in a pregnant woman. J Forensic Sci 34:481–6.

Mosier HD Jr, Jansons RA (1972). Distribution and fate of nicotine in the rat fetus. Teratology 6:303–12.

Murphy BEP (1979). The influence of serum proteins on the metabolism of cortisol by human placenta. J Steroid Biochem 10:387–92.

Naeye RL, Peters EC (1984). Mental development of children whose mothers smoked during pregnancy. J Am Coll Obstet Gynecol 64:601–7.

Nau H, Hauck RS, Ehlers K (1991). Valproic acid–induced neural tube defects in mouse and human: aspects of chirality, alternative drug development, pharmacokinetics and possible mechanisms. Pharmacol Toxicol 69:310–21.

Nau H, Liddiard C (1978). Placental transfer of drugs during early human pregnancy. In: Neubert D, Merker H-J, Nau H, Langman J, eds. Role of pharmacokinetics in prenatal and perinatal toxicology. Stuttgart: Thieme, 465–81.

Nau H, Neubert D (1978). Development of drug-metabolizing monooxygenase systems in various mammalian species including man. Its significance for transplacental toxicity. In: Neubert D, Merker H-J, Nau H, Langman J, eds. Role of pharmacokinetics in prenatal and perinatal toxicology. Stuttgart: Thieme, 13–44.

Navarro HA, Seidler FJ, Eylers JP, Baker FE, Dobbins SS, Lappi SE, Slotkin TA (1989a). Effects of prenatal nicotine exposure on development of central and peripheral cholinergic neurotransmitter systems. Evidence for cholinergic trophic influences in developing brain. J Pharmacol Exp Ther 252:894–900.

Navarro HA, Seidler FJ, Schwartz RD, Baker FE, Dobbins SS, Slotkin TA (1989b). Prenatal exposure to nicotine impairs nervous system development at a dose which does not affect viability or growth. Brain Res Bull 23:187–92.

Neims AH, Warner M, Loughnan PM, Arandam JV (1976). Developmental aspects of the hepatic cytochrome P-450 monooxygenase system. Annu Rev Pharmacol 16:427–445.

Ney JA, Dooley SL, Keith LG, Chasnoff IJ, Socol ML (1990). The prevalence of substance abuse in patients with suspected preterm labor. Am J Obstet Gynecol 162:1562–7.

Noschel H, Peiker G, Boigt R, Meinhold P, Muller B, Schroder S, Bonow A (1980). Research on pharmacokinetics during pregnancy. Arch Toxicol Suppl 4:380–4.

O'Flaherty EJ, Scott W, Schreiner C, Beliles RP (1992). A physiologically based kinetic model of rat and mouse gestation: disposition of a weak acid. Toxicol Appl Pharmacol 112:245–56.

Olney JW, Rhee V, DeGubareff T (1977). Neurotoxic effects of glutamate on mouse area postrema. Brain Res 120:151–7.

Palazzo MC, Brizzee KR, Hofer H, Mehler WR (1978). Effects of systemic administration of 6-hydroxydopamine on the circumventricular organs in nonhuman primates. Cell Tiss Res 191:141–50.

Pelkonen O (1977). Transplacental transfer of foreign compounds and their metabolism by the foetus. Prog Drug Metab 2:119–61.

Pelkonen O (1980). Biotransformation of xenobiotics in the fetus. Pharmacol Ther 10:261–81.

Picone AP, Allen LH, Olsen PN, Ferris ME (1982). Pregnancy outcome in North American women. II. Effects of diet, cigarette smoking, stress, and weight gain on placentas, and on neonatal physical and behavioral characteristics. Am J Clin Nutr 36:1214–24.

Power GG, Longo LD (1975). Fetal circulation times and their implications for tissue oxygenation. Gynecol Invest 6:342–55.

Price MT, Olney JW, Lowry OH, Buchsbaum S (1981). Uptake of exogenous glutamate and aspartate by circumventricular organs but not other regions of brain. J Neurochem 36:1774–80.

Rall TW, Schleifer LS (1990). Drugs effective in the therapy of the epilepsies. In: Gilman AG, Rall TW, Nies AS, Taylor P, eds. The pharmacological basis of therapeutics. 8th Ed. New York: Pergamon Press, 436–62.

Rane A, Tomson G (1980). Prenatal and neonatal drug metabolism in man. Eur J Clin Pharmacol 18:9–15.

Rankin JHG (1978). Role of prostaglandins in the maintenance of the placental circulation. In: Coceani F, Olley PM, eds. Advances in prostaglandin and thromboxane research. Vol. 4. New York: Raven Press, 261–9.

Rantakallio P (1983). A follow-up study up to the age of 14 of children whose mothers smoked during pregnancy. Acta Paediatr Scand 72:747–53.

Rapoport MD (1976) Blood-brain barrier in physiology and medicine. New York: Raven Press, 1–86.

Reuhl KR, Chang LW (1979). Effects of methylmercury on the development of the nervous system: a review. Neurotoxicology 1:21–55.

Reynolds WA (1972). Fetal sources of amniotic fluid,. An enigma. In: Hodari AA, Mariona F, eds. Physiological biochemistry of the fetus. Springfield, Illinois: Charles C. Thomas, 3–31.

Rosa FW (1983). Teratogenicity of isotretinoin. Lancet 2:513 (Letter).

Roberts LG, LaBorde JB, Slikker W Jr (1991). Phenytoin teratogenicity and midgestational pharmacokinetics in mice. Teratology 44:497–505.

Roberts LG, Luck W, Holder CL, Scott WJ, Nau H, Slikker W Jr (1989). Embryo-maternal distribution of basic compounds in the CD-1 mouse: doxylamine and nicotine. Toxicol Appl Pharmacol 97:134–140.

Roberts LG, LaBorde JB, Slikker W Jr (1991). Phenytoin teratogenicity and midgestational pharmacokinetics in mice. Teratology 44:497–505.

Robson JM, Sullivan FM (1966). Analysis of actions of 5-hydrotryptamine in pregnancy. J Physiol 184:717–32.

Rudolph AM, Heymann MA (1967). The circulation of the fetus in utero. Circ Res 21:163–84.

Sandberg JA, Olsen GD (1992). Cocaine and metabolite concentrations in the fetal guinea pig after chronic maternal cocaine administration. J Pharmacol Exp Ther 260:587–91.

Saunders NR (1977). Ontogeny of the blood-brain barrier. Exp Eye Res 25(suppl):523–50.

Scalzo FM, Ali SF, Frambes NA, Spear LP (1990). Weanling rats exposed prenatally to cocaine exhibit an increase in striatal D2 dopamine binding associated with an increase in ligand affinity. Pharmacol Biochem Behav 37:371–3.

Shepard TH (1985). Catalog of teratogenic agents. 5th Ed. Baltimore, London: Johns Hopkins University Press.

Slikker W Jr (1987). The role of metabolism in the testing of developmental toxicants. Regul Toxicol Pharmacol 7:390–413.

Slikker W Jr, Bailey JR, Newport GD, Lipe GW, Hill DE (1982a). Placental transfer and metabolism of 17α-ethynylestradiol-17β in the rhesus monkey. J Pharmacol Exp Ther 223:483–9.

Slikker W Jr, Bailey JR, Leakey JEA (1988). Ontogeny of hepatic drug metabolizing enzymes in the rhesus monkey: comparisons of in vitro and in vivo conditions. In: Neubert D, Merker H-J, Hendrickx, eds. Nonhuman primates—developmental biology and toxicology 413–426, Berlin and Vienna: Veberreuter Wissenschaft.

Slikker W Jr, Hill DE, Young JF (1982b). Comparison of the transplacental pharmacokinetics of 17β-estradiol and diethylstilbestrol in the subhuman primate. J Pharmacol Exp Ther 221:173–82.

Slotkin TA, Orband-Miller L, Queen KL, Whitmore WL, Seidler FJ (1987a). Development of [^{3}H]nicotine binding sites in brain regions of rats exposed to nicotine prenatally via maternal injections or infusions. J Pharmacol Exp Ther 242:232–7.

Slotkin TA, Orband-Miller L, Queen KL, Whitmore WL, Seidler FJ (1987b). Effects of prenatal nicotine exposure on biochemical development of rat brain regions: maternal drug infusions via osmotic minipumps. J Pharmacol Exp Ther 240:602–11.

Smith MK, Kimmel GL, Kochhar DM, Shepard TH, Speilberg SP, Wilson JG (1983). A selection of candidate compounds for in vivo teratogenesis test validation. Teratogen Carinogen Mutagen 3:461–80.

Snyder WS (chairman) (1974). Report of the Task Group on Reference Man, International Commission on Radiological Protection. Pergamon Press.

Spear LP, Kirstein CL, Bell J, Yoottanasumpun V, Greenbaum R, O'Shea J, Hoffman H, Spear NE (1989). Effects of prenatal cocaine exposure on behavior during the early postnatal period. Neurotoxicol Teratol 11:57–63.

Spear LP, Frambes NA, Kirstein CL (1989). Fetal and maternal brain and plasma levels of cocaine and benzoylecgonine following chronic subcutaneous administration of cocaine during gestation in rats. Psychopharmacology 97:427–31.

Spector R, Eells J (1984). Deoxynucleoside and vitamin transport into the central nervous system. Fed Proc 43:196–200.

Streissguth AP, Martin DC, Barr HM, Sandman BM, Kirchner GL, Darby BL (1984). Intrauterine alcohol and nicotine exposure: attention and reaction time in 4-year-old children. Dev Psychol 20:533–41.

Tilson HA, Davis GJ, McLachlan JA, Lucier GW (1979). The effects of polychlorinated biphenyls given prenatally on the neurobehavioral development of mice. Environ Res 18:466–74.

Tilson HA, Jacobson JL, Rogan WJ (1990). Polychlorinated biphenyls and the developing nervous system: cross-species comparison. Neurotoxicol Teratol 12:239–48.

Tjalve H, Hansson E, Schmitterlow CG (1968). Passage of ^{14}C-nicotine and its metabolites into mice foretuses and placentae. Acta Pharmacol Toxicol 26:539–55.

Vorhees CV (1987). Teratogenicity and developmental toxicity of valproic acid in rats. Teratology 35:195–202.

Vorhees CV, Brunner RL, Butcher RE (1979). Psychotropic drugs as behavioral teratogens. Science 205:1220–5.

Waddell WJ, Marlowe C (1981). Transfer of drugs across the placenta. Pharmacol Ther 14:375–90.

Welsch F (1982). Placental and fetal uptake of drugs. J Vet Pharmacol Ther 5:91–104.

Wiggins RC, Rolsten C, Ruiz B, Davis CM (1989). Pharmacokinetics of cocaine: basic studies of route, dosage, pregnancy and lactation. Neurotoxicology 10:367–82.

Wiggins RC, Ruiz B (1990). Development under the influence of cocaine. I. A comparison of the effects of daily cocaine treatment and resultant undernutrition on pregnancy and early growth in a large population of rats. Metab Brain Dis 5(2):85–99.

Williams RT (1959). Detoxication mechanisms. 2nd Ed. London: Chapman & Hall.

Wilson JG, Ritter EJ, Scott WJ, Fradkin R (1977). Comparative distribution and embryotoxicity of acetylsalicyclic acid in pregnant rats and rhesus monkeys. Toxicol Appl Pharmacol 41:67–78.

Wilson JG, Scott WJ, Ritter EJ, Fradkin R (1979). Comparative distribution and embryotoxicity of methotrexate in pregnant rats and rhesus monkeys. Teratology 19:71–79.

Woods JR, Plessinger MA, Soctt K, Miller RN (1989). The pharmacokinetics of cocaine: fetal lamb studies. Ann NY Acad Sci 562:267–79.

Zachariah PK, Juchau MR (1977). Inhibition of human placental mixed-function oxidations with carbon monoxide: reversal with monochromatic light. J Steroid Biochem 8:221–8.

Zuckerman B, Frank DA, Hingson R, Amaro R, Levenson SM, Kayne H, Parker S, Vinci R, Aboagye K, Fried LE, Cabral H, Timperi H, Bauchner H (1989). Effects of maternal marijuana and cocaine on fetal growth. N Engl J Med 320:762–8.

24
Events in Central Nervous System Development as the Bases for Susceptibility to Neurotoxicity

Pat Levitt
University of Medicine and Dentristy of New Jersey
Piscataway, New Jersey

E. Hazel Murphy
Medical College of Pennsylvania
Philadelphia, Pennsylvania

INTRODUCTION

The central nervous system (CNS) arises from a rather simple epithelium to form a highly complex organ whose function depends on the appropriate formation of neural circuits. Both genetic and environmental factors guide the formation of the CNS by controlling the cellular interactions that drive the events that occur during CNS development (for review, see Sidman and Rakic, 1973; Purves and Lichtman, 1985; Jacobson, 1991). While the precise mechanisms that control the intrinsic and extrinsic determinants of neural development remain unclear, neurobiologists have found a number of factors that can alter the normal course of events during brain formation. A major focus of developmental neurobiologists has been to define clearly how specific events that underlie pattern formation in the brain are controlled and the specific extrinsic factors that, when introduced to the developing system, are most likely to result in anomalous cell-cell interactions. The descriptions of the past 30 years, together with the introduction of newer technologies, have resulted in a greater understanding of the temporal and spatial patterns of each critical event in neural development, including cell genesis, migration, morpho-differentiation, molecular differentiation, and synaptogenesis. These events will be summarized in the context of introducing the reader to aspects of neuronal development that may be particularly susceptible to aberrant environmental factors.

BASICS OF CENTRAL NERVOUS SYSTEM DEVELOPMENT

Neural Tube and Neural Crest

The principal cell types of the CNS, neurons and macroglia (astrocytes and oligodendrocytes),[a] arise from a pseudostratified epithelium that has its origins as an ectodermal sheet. Through interactions with the underlying mesoderm, the central ectoderm is induced to fold and form an elongated tube. The folds rise up to fuse dorsally and centrally, with cells pinching off along the length of the tube to form the neural crest. This cell group undergoes a complex series of migrations throughout the embryo and ultimately forms the peripheral autonomic and sensory nervous system, Schwann cells, and connective tissue elements in the head region. Cell interactions, defined by the migratory routes selected by the neural crest cells, ultimately regulate the phenotypic choices made by the neural crest cells. This area of investigation has made particularly outstanding advances in terms of understanding the molecular components in the environment that regulate neural crest differentiation, but will not be discussed in this review (Patterson, 1990; Fraser and Bonner-Fraser, 1991; Weston, 1991; Anderson, 1993a,b).

The neural tube first closes at the level of the future mesencephalon and then zips in both an anterior and a posterior direction, in the rodent taking about 2 days to complete the process. The tube that forms is composed of a lumen, which will be the future ventricular system, and an epithelium, named the germinal or ventricular zone (Boulder Committee, 1970). The cells of the epithelium are fusiform, each having a process that attaches to the luminal surface, but with nuclei distributed at different levels of the epithelium. Not all cells reach the outer surface, providing the pseudostratified classification. This epithelium contains the stem cell population that gives rise to all brain cells.

The early-formed neural tube already shows structural signs of specialization between regions. Caudally, the rhombencephalon—the future pons and medulla—exhibits discrete constrictions that form the rhombomere segments of the brain stem. It is quite striking that these structural differences are mimicked by molecular heterogeneity that may account for the regional specification of the early neural tube. Homeobox gene expression corresponds to different brain segments and appears to regulate the expression of segment-specific traits (Holland and Hogan, 1988; Patel et al., 1989; Chisaka et al., 1992; Martinez and Alvarado-Mallart, 1990; Bally-Cuif et al., 1992; McMahon et al., 1992; McMahon, 1993). Most striking has been the revelation that the boundaries, which do not appear to exhibit physical restrictions, nonetheless form borders between groups of developing cells that are destined for distinct regions of the brain stem (Fraser et al., 1990; Guthrie and Lumsden, 1991). These descriptive studies on early pattern formation in the CNS revealed a surprising organization within the neuroepithelium, one suggesting that significant differences may exist between populations of cells at levels of the neural tube that give rise to each of the major brain subdivisions. Such early distinctions could be regulated by intrinsic differential expression of genes, such as homeobox genes, but are most likely to involve additional epigenetic regulation. This has been shown elegantly with transplants of fetal tissue in which specific gene expression by cells originally from the metencephalon can be regulated by new environmental interactions (Martinez and Alvarado-Mallart, 1990; Bally-Cuif et al., 1992). While

---

[a]The microglial cell has its origins embryonically from mesodermal cells. The blood-borne monocyte and microglial cell share many of the same unique cell surface antigens, and it is believed that a shared stem cell in bone marrow gives rise to both. Carbon particle and dye labeling studies have shown that the future microglial cells invade the CNS parenchyma at the time of angiogenesis and remain as the resident phagocytic population, increasing in number during a protracted period of development (Ling and Wong, 1993).

each region of the neural tube may be destined to form a unique brain region, basic cellular events in all regions govern the formation of the specific pattern that each region expresses.

Cellular Events That Produce Neurons and Glia

Early in neural tube formation, cell nuclei are stratified across the thickness of the tissue and comprise the ventricular zone. Their processes extend to the connective tissue covering, the pia mater, and form a cell-free zone called the marginal zone. At this stage, all cells are actively engaged in the cell cycle and undergo a series of stereotyped cytokinetic movements during cell proliferation. Their nuclear position in the epithelium reflects, to some extent, the phase of the cell cycle, with nuclei closest to the ventricular surface undergoing mitosis and those farthest from that surface engaging in DNA synthesis (Sauer, 1935; Sauer and Chittenden, 1959). It is unclear how this movement is regulated in the tube and, most important, how cells know when to exit the cycle. Perhaps one of the key issues of developmental neurobiology is the behavior of the different stem cell populations, from potential intrinsic differences to unique susceptibility to environmental alterations. What is clear is that all neuronal and macroglial populations arise from the proliferative pools in the tube and that anomalous behavior by a specific group of stem cells will therefore almost certainly result in subsequent CNS damage.

Convention notes that neurons are permanently postmitotic, being maintained in the G_1 phase of the cell cycle upon completion of final mitosis (Miale and Sidman, 1961). The time of exit has been defined as the "birthdate" of the neuron, the point in its history that represents the onset of differentiation. Both neurons and glia have defined birthdates, although glial cells maintain an ability to divide under certain physiological conditions. Recent cell culture studies indicate that mature, postmitotic neurons can be induced to reenter the cell cycle and generate new populations of neurons (Reynolds and Weiss, 1992). Such events have not been documented in vivo, and it remains clear that almost all neuronal populations in the adult brain arise from stem cells in the ventricular zone of the neural tube.

The first documented differences in neuronal groups are the distinct times at which cells destined for different parts of the brain are born. In large, gyrencephalic animals, development is protracted and temporal patterns of neurogenesis are quite apparent (for reviews, see Sidman and Rakic, 1973; Bayer and Altman, 1991; Jacobson, 1991). This is not the case in lissencephalic vertebrates, such as rats, in which such temporal gradients exist but are less obvious. Nonetheless, time of origin has served as a means to follow specific populations of neurons through their developmental course. This is done through the specific labeling of cells in their final DNA synthesis, or S-phase, with the radiolabeled base[3]H-thymidine (for examples, see Sidman et al., 1959; Taber-Pierce, 1973; Rakic, 1974; Bayer and Altman, 1991) or more recently, with the base analogue bromodeoxyuridine (BrdU) (Miller and Nowakowski, 1988; Nowakowski et al., 1989). Those cells that incorporate the analogues in S-phase, but continue in the cell cycle to divide, will dilute the label, eventually to undetectable levels if they divide more than a few times. When permanently incorporated in a cell that exits the cycle, however, the label can be used to document the site of origin and movement of neurons to their final destinations in the brain. For example, injection of labeled thymidine into the embryo, followed by sacrifice at various times (e.g., 2 h to 2 weeks in the rodent), will allow the investigator to trace the migratory paths selected by specific groups of labeled cells.

One of the best examples of how time of origin has led to a basic understanding of how specific brain areas form is the cerebral cortex, where the laminar features are generated over time by differential movement of groups of neurons born at different times (Hicks and D'Amato, 1968; Rakic, 1974; Smart and Smart, 1982; Luskin and Shatz, 1985; Bayer and Altman, 1991). In all mammals, neurons destined for deep layers of the cortex undergo their final mitosis before those destined for more superficial layers. Neurogenesis begins during fetal development and in many mammals can be completed before birth. In a few instances, however, the neurons forming the most superficial layers continue to be generated early postnatally (McConnell, 1985). Temporal differences in cell production are maintained during the period of cell movement, as the first-generated neurons settle in their final position before subsequent generations of neurons. Patterns of cell production, such as those described in the cerebral cortex, have been observed in most brain regions (see Jacobson, 1991). The basic observation that different populations of neurons in the same structure are produced at different stages of development means that changes in environmental stimuli that may occur over time can have profoundly different effects on the formation of each brain region.

Because macroglial cells only transiently leave the cell cycle during development, and this occurs rather late, it was believed at one time that most neurons are generated before the onset of gliogenesis. While the onset of astroglial and oligodendroglial maturation follows the beginning of neuronal differentiation, recent examination of glial cell development indicates that there are special populations of these nonneuronal cells from the earliest stage of neurogenesis (Schmechel and Rakic, 1979; Levitt and Rakic, 1980; Levitt et al., 1981, 1983).

Cell Migration as a Basic Component of Brain Histogenesis

Migration of neural crest cells through a complex milieu to attain their final position in the embryo is a well-known feature of peripheral nervous system development. Cell movement in the CNS, while not always appreciated as a critical developmental event, is of paramount importance in distributing cell populations throughout the neuraxis. In almost all instances, cells arising from the progenitor pools in the ventricular zone must migrate long distances to acquire their final position in the developing CNS. This movement occurs along well-defined routes, organized by specialized, early-developing nonneuronal cells known as radial glia. These specialized epithelial cells were first noted by Ramón y Cajal and were thought to form a support or scaffold for the rather fragile developing CNS. It was not until the late 1960s that the radial epithelial, or glial, cell was rediscovered as a potentially significant element in brain formation (Astrom, 1967; Mugnaini and Forstronen, 1967). Electron microscopy and Golgi impregnation methods revealed a remarkable arcade of radially aligned processes emanating from the glial cell bodies sitting along the ventricular zone. Rakic documented close associations between migrating neurons and the radial processes and suggested that the glial fibers served as a temporary scaffold for cells moving to their final destination (Rakic, 1971a,b, 1972). Detailed Golgi and immunocytochemical analysis revealed that the radial glial cell was present throughout the neuraxis and, except in the cerebellar cortex, underwent transformation into mature astrocytes (Schmechel and Rakic, 1979; Levitt and Rakic, 1980).

While recent time-lapse video microscopy studies indicate that the radial glial fiber does not serve as the sole path by which neurons achieve their final position, most studies indicate that the vast majority of migrating cells follow these radial guides (O'Rourke et al., 1992). The mechanisms underlying this specific cell-cell interaction, and how cell migration in the CNS is regulated, have been the subject of intensive investigation. Neurologically mutant mice were identified years ago in which specific defects in migratory behavior of neurons were highlighted, particularly in laminated structures such as the cerebral and cerebellar cortices. Analysis of these mutant animal models suggested that interactions between migrating neurons and radial glial cells are probably defective (for reviews, see Caviness and Rakic, 1978; Hatten and Mason 1986; Caviness et al., 1989), particularly in relation to adhesion (Hatten, 1990, 1993). The initial descriptions of the neurological mutant weaver mouse (wv/wv) indicated a fatal outcome to cerebellar granule neurons that failed to migrate. Abnormal architecture of the midline Bergmann glia pointed to this defect as the prime culprit, but the primary gene anomaly was correctly defined by use of mouse chimeras, animals produced by the rather spectacular method of joining embryos of two different genotypes (usually a mutant and wild-type [+/+] combination; see Mullen and Herrup, 1979, for review of method) at the eight cell stage. Chimeras of wv/wv – +/+ demonstrated that granule neurons that are genotypically weaver were unable to migrate even in the midst of wild-type normal glial fibers (Goldowitz and Mullen, 1982; Goldowitz, 1989). Cell culture experiments showed similarly that wv/wv granule neurons failed to migrate normally, even when combined with normal glial cells (Hatten et al., 1986). In addition, mutant glial cells were able to mediate normal migratory behavior of the wild-type neurons, indicating again a defect in the mutant granule neurons. Chimeric analysis of neonates indicated that the proliferative cells giving rise to granule neurons may be defective in their behavior (Smeyne and Goldowitz, 1989). Subsequent culture studies more clearly defined the cellular anomaly in the weaver neurons (Gao et al., 1992). It appears that progenitor cells that give rise to the postmitotic neuron are defective, but can be positively influenced by populations of normal cells. The postmitotic weaver neurons lack the ability to extend processes that probably are needed for facilitating cell association with the glial guides. This important neuron-glia association in cell migration is probably controlled in part by special adhesion molecules (Hatten, 1993). Antibody perturbation studies, using probes against HNK-1, a ubiquitous carbohydrate antigen, can modify granule neuron migration (Kunemund et al., 1988). It is probably the case that a number of different adhesive and other molecular factors regulate cell movement. In fact, recent experiments suggest that simple changes in ion flux can be quite important in controlling neuronal migration.

Ion regulation of cell adhesion and process extension is clearly an important factor in neuronal differentiation (for review see Kater and Mills, 1991). Cell movement also appears to be highly regulated by specific ionic interactions. Recently, Komuro and Rakic (1992, 1993) initiated investigations, using a model tissue slice preparation of the cerebellar cortex, to explore factors that could modulate neuronal migration. It is perhaps of greatest interest that they found that a specific subtype of calcium channel, the N-type, is capable of regulating neuronal movement along radial glial fibers in the slice preparation. Specific blockers of this channel can simply stop the movement of neurons along their glial guides. The specificity is interesting, because it suggests that certain types of intracellular signaling, mediated by a channel with specific kinetic features, are critical in this developmental event, and that it is not regulated simply by general passage of calcium ions. In fact, N-methyl-D-aspartate (NMDA) antagonists have been found to be as effective in blocking cell migration (Komuro and Rakic, 1993), suggesting a specific receptor-mediated effect of calcium in this important morphogenetic event. The work highlights the potential susceptibility of cell migration in the nervous system, because one could imagine that even minor disturbances in extracellular fluid content could have profound effects on cell migration. Modification of membrane-membrane interactions, which are clearly regulated by macromolecular adhesion components and ion fluxes, could lead to altered migratory behavior, events that often occur after neurotoxic exposure (see below).

Axon Targetting

Perhaps our most significant gains in understanding specific neurodevelopmental processes are in the area of axon pathfinding and target recognition. Sperry's concept of neurotropism (1963), with specific chemical interactions underlying the formation of well-defined neural connections in the brain, has gained critical support with the application of molecular techniques. Evidence has mounted that targeting may be a balance between growth-enhancing and growth-inhibiting molecular systems, each mediated by a unique set of molecules. The first evidence that the neurons of the brain produce a large number of distinct molecules that label certain pathways and cell populations came from monoclonal antibody studies. While success was most obvious in invertebrates (Zipser and McKay, 1981; Goodman et al., 1984), the use of developing brain material as an immunogen led to the production of antibodies that labeled functional subsets of cells, axons, and pathways (for reviews see Rutishauser and Jessell, 1988; Valentino et al., 1985; Levitt, 1985). Many of these antibodies recognize cell surface molecules, many of which display adhesive properties and comprise the Ig superfamily of neural adhesion proteins (Jessell, 1988; Edelman and Crossin, 1991; Grumet, 1991). In vitro cell culture analysis has demonstrated that cell adhesion molecules, including integrin membrane receptors for extracellular matrix molecules, can mediate specific axon outgrowth (Lagenaur and Lemmon, 1987; Rathjen et al., 1987; Jessell, 1988; Reichardt and Tomaselli, 1991). In some instances, when given a choice, neurites will actually select certain macromolecules over others. These types of experiment have served as indirect evidence that axon pathfinding and target recognition can be mediated by such differential adhesion. Production of mutations in Drosophila has supported this idea, because elimination of certain adhesive molecules, particularly those that have homology to vertebrate counterparts, results in abnormal pathfinding (Elkins et al., 1990). A molecule with characteristics of an adhesive protein (Zukhareva and Levitt, 1992), but with expression patterns more selective than most (Levitt, 1984), has been examined for the mediation of axonal targeting. The limbic system–associated membrane protein (LAMP) is required for the formation of the septohippocampal circuit in vitro (Keller and Levitt, 1989; Keller et al., 1989), and more recently has been shown to modulate the growth of mossy fibers in the neonatal hippocampus in situ (Barbe and Levitt, 1992a). This is a cell surface protein that is expressed in cortical and subcortical areas of the limbic system, including the frontal cortex, basal forebrain, hippocampus, limbic thalamus, hypothalamus, amygdala, and other areas. Limbic system–associated membrane protein is one of the few examples of a membrane protein in the vertebrate brain that can control specific afferent-target interactions (see also Baier and Bonhoeffer, 1992). It is interesting that alteration of LAMP expression does not result in major structural anomalies or defects in fiber outgrowth, but rather in a change in circuit formation. This is perhaps an important site of regulation that could be particularly prone to modifications due to toxin exposure.

A number of examples now exist that highlight the importance of controlling growth through inhibitory substances (for review see Schwab et al., 1993). Axon pathfinding can be readily guided not only by actively growth-enhancing molecules, but by antigens that prevent growth through certain regions or across certain pathways. Even extracellular molecules, such as matrix proteoglycans, can be very critical in modulating the growth of developing axon systems (Reichardt and Tomaselli, 1991). Some proteoglycans, such as those in the heparin sulfate family, may be very important for binding neurotrophic molecules and presenting them to stimulate growth or neuron survival (Unsicker, et al., 1993). Others, which may fall into the chondroitin sulfate family, have been shown to be refractory to growth under certain conditions (Snow et al., 1991). Finally, it has been postulated that neuron populations have specific stop signals, surface molecules that can actually halt ongoing axon movement and could result in synapse formation (Raper and Grunewald, 1990; Baird et al., 1992). Our current concept of axon targeting to the appropriate terminal area seems to include a number of different molecular interactions, facilitating growth along correct pathways (positive) and limiting extension into certain areas (negative), followed by the ability to make choices in terms of turns and penetration into targets (positive), with a final controlling feature that must include the ability to impart cessation of growth (negative stop signals).

Synaptogenesis and the Formation of Final Connectivity Patterns

In truth, we know very little about the molecular features that lead to synapse formation in the CNS. It is clear that all of the events must proceed relatively normally in order for the final outcome to include appropriate synapse formation. In most systems in the brain, target innervation of specific groups of afferents occurs in a very specific manner, with few examples of inappropriate or exuberant targeting. Perhaps the cerebral cortex is again a convenient region on which to focus this discussion, because it exhibits almost all the different types of targeting and growth and much experimental manipulation has been done in an attempt to identify the mechanisms that govern these events in the cortex.

Certainly, the cerebral cortical projection systems serve as a principal example of controlled overgrowth, with cortico-cortical and subcortically projecting systems building transient interactions for a specific period of postnatal development. Such transient or exuberant corticofugal projections, which have been reported in most vertebrate species examined thus far, are eliminated during normal development (Innocenti and Frost, 1979; Rhoades et al., 1984; Stanfield, 1984). Projections into the cerebral cortex, in contrast, develop in a very specific fashion from their inception prenatally, forming the basis for specific target recognition in this brain region. Thalamocortical axons grow through the internal capsule prenatally, reaching underneath the developing cortex even before their potential neuronal targets, the layer IV neurons, are produced (Rakic, 1977; Ghosh et al., 1990; de Carlo and O'Leary, 1992; Erzurumlu and Jhaveri, 1992). It has been shown that the thalamic axons use a temporary neuronal scaffold, called the subplate, for targeting temporary, though functional, synapse formation (Chun and Shatz, 1989a,b; Goodman and Shatz, 1993). These subplate neurons are among the first produced in the developing cortex (Kostovic and Rakic, 1980, 1990; Luskin and Shatz, 1985) and may carry both axon-targeting and stop signals to achieve this specific afferent patterning (Ghosh et al., 1990; Ghosh and Shatz, 1992). The means by which the afferent axons break these connections and form new, permanent ones in the cortex proper remain a mystery, but one likely to involve cell death of the subplate cells and secretion of chemoattractants from the overlying cortex. These temporary connections are not usually considered abnormal or exuberant, because the axons targeted the appropriate areas of the cortex to form these temporary projections. The terminal arborizations of the axons may, however, be exuberant and dependent on appropriately patterned neural activity for their refinement (Bear et al., 1987; Zahs, 1989; see discussion below).

Cortical neurons, in contrast to afferent neurons in the thalamus, clearly form projections with brain regions that ultimately are lost. It is the latter event, and the fine reorganization of specific synaptic relationships of the projections into the cerebral cortex, that are critical for proper final circuit formation. A number of laboratories have investigated these events, revealing some important areas of potential regulation. In the cortico-cortical system, neurons that project to a larger terminal area are not lost during development, but instead seem to abandon specific collaterals to that region. The underlying control of this decision may come in the form of specific activity patterns.

When activity patterns result in co-activation of pre- and postsynaptic elements, synapses are stabilized (for reviews see Stryker and Harris, 1986; Reiter and Stryker, 1988; Constantine-Paton et al., 1990; Grigonis and Murphy, 1993; Jessell and Kandel, 1993). In the absence of such co-activation, axon collaterals fail to achieve synaptic contact and are eliminated. This pattern of selective stabilization of appropriate projections and elimination of inappropriate connections may be disrupted by elimination of neural activity (for reviews see Shatz, 1990; Stryker, 1991; Goodman and Shatz, 1993) or by inducing abnormal patterns of neural activity (Cline et al., 1987; Murphy and Grigonis, 1988; Grigonis and Murphy, 1991; Goodman and Shatz, 1993).

MOLECULAR INFLUENCES ON BRAIN DEVELOPMENT

The Positive Effects of Neurotrophins and Neurotransmitters

We have noted above that certain macromolecular features of neural development have taken center stage. These mostly include cell surface proteins that control cell interactions leading to migration, axon growth, and synapse formation. Clearly, diffusible molecules are also critical in nervous system development. The size of the family of neurotrophin and neurocytokine growth factors, which target cells in the nervous system, has exploded recently, mostly because of molecular cloning approaches that have documented families of secreted factors and their receptors (for reviews see Thoenen, 1991; Altin and Bradshaw, 1992; Patterson and Landis, 1992; Schlessinger and Ulrich, 1992; Patterson and Nawa, 1993). It is important to note that it is in the area of receptor research that an almost unbelievable relationship between neurotrophin activities in the brain and cytokines in the immune system has emerged. Clearly, growth factors, including molecules first discovered in non-neural tissues, and neurotrophins can modulate the behavior of CNS and neural crest stem cells (Stemple et al., 1988; Cattaneo and McKay, 1990; DiCicco-Bloom et al., 1990), cytodifferentiation, including dendritic and axon outgrowth, and perhaps their most critical feature, cell survival. Cell death remains a mystery in CNS development, not in terms of the actual occurrences throughout the neuraxis, but rather the reason for using such a strategy to generate a mature brain. Cell death is an important natural aspect of development, occurring in most regions of the CNS (Cunningham, 1982; Cowan et al., 1984; Oppenheim, 1991). It has been suggested that trophic factors regulate naturally occurring cell death, although only two examples demonstrate that administration of factors will save CNS neurons that would normally die (Oppenheim et al., 1992). The issue of trophin-cell interactions becomes more complicated with the analysis of receptor expression. Laboratories have recently begun to map the expression of the tyrosine kinase family of receptors (*trk* A,B,C) during development, and the low-affinity NGF (p75), EGF, and IGF receptor mRNAs have been mapped by in situ hybridization (for reviews, see Fallon and Loughlin, 1993; Hefti et al., 1993). We note these rather descriptive discoveries because to date, most of the evidence that cytokines and trophins are active developmentally comes from in vitro analysis. We believe these will be very important families of molecules to investigate, particularly in relation to most of the major developmental events that have been reviewed above. One basic strategy that laboratories will begin to use to discern their roles in development is gene knockouts. While this strategy is theoretically sound and potentially exciting in its outcome, knockout strategies of single genes in

Drosophila (for example, Elkins et al., 1990) and mice (for example, Grant et al., 1992) often fail to yield a discernible mutant phenotype. There are excellent examples where this approach has worked, but the relatively surprising finding that many single knockouts fail to generate an altered phenotype may reflect the rather remarkable redundancy of developing systems in the groups of molecules used to modulate specific developmental events.

This brings us to what has previously been considered the unconventional role of neurotransmitters in neural development. Again, little evidence has accumulated from studies in vivo that suggests important roles for neurotransmitters, but certainly model cell culture systems have been developed that indicate great potential. Neurotransmitter systems exhibit a variety of developmental profiles, from the very early monoamine systems in the brain stem (for review, see Levitt, 1982), which innervate a large number of areas in the brain (for reviews of anatomy, see Moore and Bloom, 1978, 1979; Steinbusch, 1981; Moore and Card, 1984), to the late-expressing neuropeptides and amino acid transmitters in cerebral cortical neurons. The very early development of central monoamine and acetylcholine systems led to hypotheses concerning their role in controlling cell proliferation and dendritic growth. Some experimental evidence exists for both (Blue and Parnavelas, 1982; Coyle et al., 1986; Hohmann et al., 1988), but the most convincing studies have been in vitro (for reviews, see Lauder, 1988; Mattson, 1988; Leslie, 1993; Lauder, 1993). Catecholamines appear to affect cell survival, although it may be through the nonspecific production of toxic free radicals (Rosenberg, 1988). Dopamine and serotonin both have been shown to greatly modify axon and dendritic outgrowth, probably through second messenger systems (for reviews see Mattson, 1988; Lipton and Kater, 1989). Neuropeptides such as thyrotropin releasing hormone (TRH) and vasoactive intestinal polypeptide (VIP) are neurotrophic, and perhaps the most convincing culture evidence for a role of neurotransmitters comes from the work involving glutamate, whose excitotoxic effects on certain populations of neurons, through specific NMDA and non-NMDA receptors, has been well documented (for reviews, see Lipton and Kater, 1989; Leslie, 1993). Clearly, glutamate involvement, through the mediation of specific patterns of activity, could potentially have a substantial impact on survival of specific neuron populations, cell motility, fiber outgrowth, and final connectivity patterns. An important example of how activity clearly plays a role in the developmental plasticity in the brain comes from studies in the visual cortex. Both the cholinergic and the monoaminergic systems are critical in regulating the response of the visual cortex to visual deprivation during a critical period of development (Bear and Singer, 1986; Cline et al., 1987; Constantine-Paton et al., 1990). Alteration of any of these systems, through their afferents or receptors, results in marked changes in the final response of the visual projections and their target neurons.

Targets of Neurotoxins and Teratogens

Each of the events that we have reviewed is a potential target of substances that can result in severely altered brain development. Clearly, a more in-depth understanding of the molecular features that regulate each histotypic event is needed in order to predict the types of substance that can lead to malformations and permanent changes in brain organization. In the cerebral cortex, alcohol has effects on cell proliferation and migration (Miller, 1986, 1988; Miller and Potempa, 1990) and morphological differentiation of neurons (West et al., 1981; Stoltenburg-Didinger and Spohr, 1983; West et al., 1986), events that are controlled by cytokines, adhesion molecules, and ions. What do all of these factors have in common? Certainly, all work through specific membrane channels and receptors that control signaling between the cell and its environment. Membrane integrity is, therefore, a critical point of control for neurons and glia during development, as well as in the mature brain.

It is relatively simple to extrapolate membrane effects to more specific substances. For example, those drugs that interfere with neurotransmitter function could potentially alter any of the developmental events on which we have focused, from proliferation to synapse formation. In our laboratories, we recently have noted a potentially critical role for the dopamine system in neuronal differentiation. We base this on the rather striking, anomalous effects of prenatal cocaine exposure (Jones et al., 1992) on cerebral cortical development. A cortical region that receives a very dense dopaminergic innervation, the anterior cingulate cortex, exhibits profound, permanent decreases in and altered patterns of growth of apical dendrites. Analysis of dendritic growth in the visual cortex, an area lacking a significant dopamine input, reveals a normal pattern. Some groups have found that cocaine exposure in rodents can lead to changes in cell-proliferative behavior (Gressens et al., 1992), temporal development of monoamines (Akbari et al., 1992), and dopamine receptor binding (Scalzo et al., 1990). We have found perhaps a more disturbing effect of cocaine exposure. Intravenous administration during the latter two-thirds of gestation in the rabbit failed to result in major brain abnormalities yet generated pyramidal neurons in certain cerebral cortical regions that have stunted and twisted dendrites. In these regions, the number of γ-aminobutyric acid (GABA) immunoreactive interneurons was also increased (Wang and Murphy, 1993). One very profound aspect of these recent findings is the lack of these changes induced by cocaine in regions lacking a significant dopamine innervation. These changes appear long-lasting and form the basis for future detailed studies of the specific interactions of the dopamine system with corticogenesis and cell differentiation.

SUMMARY

The descriptive anatomical studies of Ramón y Cajal (1890, 1909, 1911) provided the groundwork for a century of accumulated, detailed information about the developmental events that underlie brain formation. Experimental approaches have become increasingly more sophisticated over the last 10–15 years and now allow us to postulate specific cellular and molecular mechanisms that regulate events from decisions of neuronal lineage to synaptic stabilization. These advances will be pivotal in designing studies to investigate specific factors that modify brain development and, most important, to identify strategies for repairing the outcomes of developmental perturbations.

REFERENCES

Akbari HM, Kramer HK, Whitaker-Azmitia PM, Spear LP, Azmitia EC (1992). Prenatal cocaine exposure disrupts the development of the serotonergic system. Brain Res 572:57–63.
Altin JG, Bradshaw RA (1992). Nerve growth factor and related substances: structure and mechanism of action. In: Laughlin SE, Fallon JH, eds. Neurotrophic factors. New York: Academic Press, 129–80.
Anderson DJ (1993a). Cell and molecular biology of neural crest lineage diversification. Curr Opin Neurobiol 3:8–13.

Anderson DJ (1993b). Molecular control of cell fate in the neural crest: the sympathoadrenal lineage. Annu Rev Neurosci 16:129–58.

Astrom K-E (1967). On the early development of the isocortex in fetal sheep. Prog Brain Res 26:1–59.

Baier H, Bonhoeffer F (1992). Axon guidance by gradients of a target-derived component. Science 255:472–5.

Bally-Cuif L, Alvarado-Mallart RM, Darnell DK, Wassef M (1992). Relationship between Wnt-1 and En-2 expression domains during early development of normal and ectopic met-mesencephalon. Development 115:999–1009.

Baird DH, Baptista CA, Wang L-C, Mason CA (1992). Specificity of a target cell–derived stop signal for afferent axonal growth. J Neurobiol 23:579–91.

Barbe MF, Levitt P (1991). The early commitment of fetal neurons to limbic cortex. J Neurosci 11:519–33.

Barbe MF, Levitt P (1992a). Attraction of specific thalamic afferents by cerebral grafts is dependent on the molecular fate of the implant. Proc Natl Acad Sci USA 89:3706–10.

Barbe MF, Levitt P (1992b). Disruption in vivo of the developing hippocampal mossy fiber circuit by antibodies to the limbic system–associated membrane protein (abstr). Neurosci Abstr 18:38.

Bayer S, Altman J (1991). Neocortical development. New York: Raven Press.

Bear MF, Cooper LN, Ebner FF (1987). A physiological basis for a theory of synapse modification. Science 237:42–8.

Bear MF, Singer W (1986). Modulation of visual cortical plasticity by acetylcholine and noradrenaline. Nature 320:172–6.

Blue ME, Parnavelas JG (1982). The effect of neonatal 6-hydroxydopamine treatment on synaptogenesis in the visual cortex of the rat. J Comp Neurol 205:199–205.

Boulder Committee (1970). Embryonic vertebrate central nervous system: revised terminology. Anat Rec 166:257–61.

Cattaneo E, McKay R (1990). Proliferation and differentiation of neuronal stem cells regulated by nerve growth factor. Nature 347:762–5.

Caviness VS Jr, Misson JP, Gadisseux J-F (1989). Abnormal neuronal migration patterns and disorders of neocortical development. In: Galaburda A, ed. From reading to neuron. Cambridge, Massachusetts: MIT Press, 405–42.

Caviness VS Jr, Rakic P (1978). Mechanisms of cortical development: a view from mutations in mice. Annu Rev Neurosci 1:297–326.

Chisaka O, Musci TS, Capecchi MR (1992). Developmental defect of the ear, cranial nerves and hindbrain resulting from the targeted disruption of the mouse homeobox gene Hox-1.6. Nature 355:516–20.

Chun JJM, Shatz CJ (1989a). Interstitial cells of the adult neocortical white matter are the remnant of the early generated subplate neuron population. J Comp Neurol 282:555–69.

Chun JJM, Shatz CJ (1989b). The earliest-generated neurons of the cat cerebral cortex: characterization by MAP2 and neurotransmitter immunohistochemistry during fetal life. J Neurosci 9:1648–67.

Cline HT, Debski EA, Constantine-Paton M. (1987). N-methyl-D-aspartate receptor antagonist desegregates eye-specific stripes. Proc Natl Acad Sci USA 84:4342–5.

Constantine-Paton M, Cline HT, Debski E (1990). Patterned activity, synaptic convergence, and the NMDA receptor in developing visual pathways. Annu Rev Neurosci 13:129–54.

Cowan WM, Fawcett JW, O'Leary DM, Stanfield BB (1984). Regressive events in neurogenesis. Science 225:1258–65.

Coyle JT, Oster-Granite ML, Gearhart JD (1986). The neurobiologic consequences of Down syndrome. Brain Res Bull 16:773–87.

Cunningham TJ (1982). Naturally occurring death and its regulation by developing neural pathways. Intl Rev Cytol 74:163–86.

De Carlos JA, O'Leary DDM (1992). Growth and targeting of subplate axons and establishment of major cortical pathways. J Neurosci 12:1194–1211.

DiCicco-Bloom E, Townes-Anderson E, Black IB (1990). Neuroblast mitosis in dissociated culture: regulation and relationship to differentiation. J Cell Biol 110:2073–86.

Edelman GM, Crossin KL (1991). Cell adhesion molecules: implications for a molecular histology. Annu Rev Biochem 60:155–90.

Elkins T, Zinn K, McAllister L, Hoffmann FM, Goodman CS (1990). Genetic analysis of a drosophila neural cell adhesion molecule: interaction of fasciclin I and Abelson tyrosine kinase mutations. Cell 60:565–75.

Erzurumlu RS, Jhaveri S (1992). Emergence of connectivity in the embryonic rat parietal cortex. Cereb Cortex 2:336–52.

Fallon JH, Loughlin SE (1993). Functional implications of the anatomical localization of neurotrophic factors. In: Loughlin SE, Fallon JH, eds. Neurotrophic factors. New York: Academic Press, 1–24.

Ferri RT, Levitt P (1993). Cerebral cortical progenitors are fated to produce region-specific neuronal populations. Cereb Cortex 3:187–198.

Fraser S, Bronner-Fraser ME (1991). Migrating neural crest cells in the trunk of the avian embryo are multipotent. Development 112:913–20.

Fraser S, Keynes R, Lumsden A (1990). Segmentation in the chick embryo hindbrain is defined by cell lineage restrictions. Nature 344:431–5.

Gao W-Q, Liu X-L, Hatten ME (1992). The weaver gene encodes a nonautonomous signal for CNS neuronal differentiation. Cell 68:841–54.

Ghosh A, Shatz CJ (1992). Involvement of subplate neurons in the formation of ocular dominance columns. Science 255:1441–3.

Ghosh A, Antonini A, McConnell SK, Shatz CJ (1990). Requirement for subplate neurons in the formation of the thalamocortical connections. Nature 347:179–81.

Goldowitz D (1989). The weaver granuloprival phenotype is due to intrinsic action of the mutant locus in the granule cell: evidence from homozygous weaver chimeras. Neuron 2:1565–75.

Goldowitz D, Mullen RJ (1982). Granule cell as a site of gene action in the weaver mouse cerebellum: evidence from heterozygous mutant chimeras. J Neurosci 2:156–72.

Goodman CS, Bastiani MJ, Doe CQ, du Lac S, Helfand SL, Kuwada JY, Thomas JB (1984). Cell recognition during neuronal development. Science 225:1271–9.

Goodman CS, Shatz CJ (1993). Developmental mechanisms that generate precise patterns of neuronal connectivity. Cell 72/Neuron 10(suppl):77–98.

Grant SGN, O'Dell TJ, Karl KA, Stein PA, Soriano P, Kandel ER (1992). Impaired long-term potentiation, spatial learning and hippocampal development in fyn mutant mice. Science 258:1903–10.

Gressens P, Kosofsky BE, Evrard P (1992). Cocaine-induced disturbances of corticogenesis in the developing murine brain. Neurosci Lett 140:113–6.

Grigonis AM, Murphy EH (1991). The organization of callosal connections in the visual cortex of the rabbit following neonatal enucleation, dark rearing and strobe rearing. J Comp Neurol 312:561–72.

Grigonis AM, Murphy EH (1993). The effects of epileptic cortical activity on the development of callosal projections. Dev. Brain Res. (in press).

Grumet M (1991). Cell adhesion molecules and their subgroups in the nervous system. Curr Opin Neurobiol 1:370–6.

Guthrie S, Lumsden A (1991). Formation and regeneration of rhombomere boundaries in the developing chick hindbrain. Development 112:221–9.

Hatten ME (1990). A common mechanism for glial-guided neuronal migration in different regions of the developing brain. TINS 13:179–83.

Hatten ME (1993). The role of migration in central nervous system neuronal development. Curr Opin Neurobiol 3:38–44.

Hatten ME, Liem RKH, Mason CA (1986). Weaver mouse cerebellar granule neurons fail to migrate on wild-type astroglial processes in vitro. J Neurosci 6:2676–83.

Hatten ME, Mason CA (1986). Neuron-astroglia interactions in vitro and in vivo. TINS 9:168–74.

Hefti F, Denton TL, Knusel B, Lapchak PA (1993). Neurotrophic factors: what are they and what are they doing? In: Loughlin SE, Fallon JH, eds. Neurotrophic factors. New York: Academic Press, 25–49.

Hicks SP, D'Amato CJ (1968). Cell migrations to the isocortex in the rat. Anat Rec 160:619–34.

Hohmann CF, Brooks AR, Coyle JT (1988). Neonatal lesions of the basal forebrain cholinergic neurons result in abnormal cortical development. Dev Brain Res 42:253–64.

Holland PWH, Hogan BL (1988). Genes Dev 2:773–82.

Horton HL, Levitt P (1988). A unique membrane protein is expressed on early developing limbic system axons and cortical targets. J Neurosci 8:4653–61.

Innocenti GM, Frost DO (1979). Effects of visual experience on the maturation of the efferent system to the corpus callosum. Nature 280:231–4.

Jacobson M (1991). Developmental neurobiology. New York: Plenum Press.

Jessell TM (1988). Adhesion molecules and the hierarchy of neural development. Neuron 1:3–13.

Jessell TM, Kandel ER (1993). Synaptic transmission: a bidirectional and self-modifiable form of cell-cell communication. Cell 72/Neuron 10(suppl):1–30.

Jones L, Fischer I, Levitt P (1992). Effects of prenatal cocaine on the development of cerebral cortex of dutch belted rabbits (abstr). Neurosci Abstr 18:421.

Kater SB, Mills LR (1991). Regulation of growth cone behavior by calcium. J Neurosci 11:891–9.

Keller F, Levitt P (1989). Developmental and regeneration-associated regulation of the limbic system–associated membrane protein (LAMP) in explant cultures of the rat brain. Neuroscience 28:455–74.

Keller F, Rimvall K, Barbe MF, Levitt P (1989). A membrane protein associated with the limbic system mediates the formation of the septohippocampal pathway *in vitro*. Neuron 3:551–61.

Komuro H, Rakic P (1992). Selective role of N-type calcium channels in neuronal migration. Science 257:806–9.

Komuro H, Rakic P (1993). Modulation of neuronal migration by NMDA receptors. Science 260:95–7.

Kostovic I, Rakic P (1980). Cytology and time of origin of interstitial neurons in the white matter in infant and adult human and monkey telencephalon. J Neurocytol 9:219–42.

Kostovic I, Rakic P (1990). Developmental history of the transient subplate zone in the visual and somatosensory cortex of the macaque monkey and human brain. J Comp Neurol 297:441–70.

Kunemund V, Jungalwala FB, Fischer G, Chou DKH, Keilhauer G, Schachner M (1988). The L2/HNK-1 carbohydrate of neural cell adhesion molecules is involved in cell interactions. J Cell Biol 106:213–23.

Lagenaur C, Lemmon V (1987). An L1-like molecule, the 8D9 antigen, is a potent substrate for neurite extension. Proc Natl Acad Sci USA 84:7753–7.

Lauder JM (1988). Neurotransmitters as morphogens. Prog Brain Res 73:365–87.

Lauder JM (1993). Neurotransmitters as growth regulatory signals: role of receptors and second messenger systems. TINS 16:233–240.

Leslie FM (1993). Neurotransmitters as neurotrophic factors. In: Loughlin SE, Fallon JH, eds. Neurotrophic factors. New York: Academic Press, 565–98.

Levitt P (1982). Central monoamine neuron systems: their organization in the developing and mature primate brain and the genetic regulation of their terminal fields. In: Friedhoff AJ, Chase TN, eds. Gilles de la Tourette syndrome. New York: Raven Press, 49–59.

Levitt P (1984). A monoclonal antibody to limbic system neurons. Science 223:299–301.

Levitt P (1985). Relating molecular specificity to normal and abnormal brain development. Ann NY Acad Sci 450:239–46.

Levitt P, Cooper ML, Rakic P (1981). Coexistence of neuronal and glial precursor cells in the ventricular zone of the fetal monkey cerebrum: an ultrastructural immunoperoxidase analysis. J Neurosci 1:27–39.

Levitt P, Cooper ML, Rakic P (1983). Early divergence and changing proportions of neuronal and glial precursor cells in the primate cerebral ventricular zone. Dev Biol 96:472–84.

Levitt P, Ferri RT, Barbe MF (1993). Progressive acquisition of cortical phenotypes as a mechanism for specifying the developing cerebral cortex. Perspect Dev Neurobiol 1:65–74.

Levitt P, Rakic P (1980). Immunoperoxidase localization of glial fibrillary acidic protein in radial glial cells and astrocytes of the developing rhesus monkey brain. J Comp Neurol 193:815–40.

Levitt P, Rakic P (1982). The time of genesis, embryonic origin and differentiation of the brainstem monoamines neurons in the rhesus monkey. Dev Brain Res 4:4630–4.

Ling E-A, Wong W-C (1993). The origin and nature of ramified and amoeboid microglia: a historical review and current concepts. Glia 7:9–18.

Lipton SA, Kater SB (1989). Neurotransmitter regulation of neuronal outgrowth, plasticity and survival. TINS 12:265–70.

Luskin MB, Shatz CJ (1985). Neurogenesis of the cat's visual cortex. J Comp Neurol 242:611–31.

Martinez S, Alvarado-Mallart R-M (1990). Expression of the homeobox Chick-en in chick/quail chimeras with inverted mes-metencephalic grafts. Dev Biol 139:432–6.

Mattson MP (1988). Neurotransmitters in the regulation of neuronal cytoarchitecture. Brain Res Rev 13:179–212.

McConnell SK (1985). Migration and differentiation of cerebral cortical neurons after transplantation in the brains of ferrets. Science 229:1268–71.

McMahon AP (1993). Cell signalling in induction and anterior-posterior patterning of the vertebrate central nervous system. Curr Opin Neurobiol 3:4–7.

McMahon AP, Joyner AL, Bradley A, McMahon JA (1992). The midbrain-hindbrain phenotype of Wnt-1-/Wnt-1–mice results from stepwise deletion of Engrailed-expressing cells by 9.5 days postcoitum. Cell 69:581–95.

Miale IL, Sidman RL (1961). An autoradiographic analysis of histogenesis in the mouse cerebellum. Exp Neurol 4:277–96.

Miller MW (1986). Effects of alcohol on the generation and migration of cerebral cortical neurons. Science 233:1308–11.

Miller MW (1988). Effects of prenatal exposure to ethanol on the development of cerebral cortex: I. Neuronal generation. Alcoholism 12:440–9.

Miller MW, Nowakowski RS (1988). Use of bromodeoxyuridine-immunohistochemistry to examine the proliferation, migration and time of origin of cells in the central nervous system. Brain Res 457:44–52.

Miller MW, Potempa G (1990). Numbers of neurons and glia in mature rat somatosensory cortex: effects of prenatal exposure to ethanol. J Comp Neurol 293:92–102.

Moore RY, Bloom FE (1978). Central catecholamine neuron systems: anatomy and physiology of the dopamine systems. Annu Rev Neurosci 1:129–69.

Moore RY, Bloom FE (1979). Central catecholamine neuron systems: anatomy and physiology of the norepinephrine and epinephrine systems. Annu Rev Neurosci 2:113–68.

Moore RY, Card JP (1984). Noradrenaline-containing systems. In: Bjorklund A, Hokfelt T, eds. Handbook of chemical neuroanatomy, vol 2: classical transmitters in the CNS, part I. Amsterdam: Elsevier, 123–56.

Mugnaini E, Forstronen PF (1967). Ultrastructural studies on the cerebellar histogenesis. I. Differentiation of granule cells and development of glomeruli in the chick embryo. Z Zellforsch 77:115–43.

Mullen RJ, Herrup K (1979). Chimeric analysis of mouse cerebellar mutants. In: Breakefield XO, ed. Neurogenetics: genetic approach to the nervous system. Amsterdam: Elsevier/North Holland, 173–96.

Murphy EH, Grigonis AM (1988). Postnatal development of the visual corpus callosum: the influence of activity of the retinofugal projections. Behav Brain Res 30:151–63.

Nowakowski RS, Lewin SB, Miller MW (1989). Bromodeoxyuridine immunohistochemical determination of the lengths of the cell cycle and the DNA-synthetic phase for an anatomically defined population. J Neurocytol 18:311–8.

Oppenheim RW (1991). Cell death in the developing nervous system. Annu Rev Neurosci 14:453–501.

Oppenheim RW, Wei Y-Q, Prevette D, Yin QW (1992). Brain-derived neurotrophic factor rescues developing avian motoneurons from cell death. Nature 360:755–7.

O'Rourke NA, Dailey ME, Smith SJ, McConnell SK (1992). Diverse migratory pathways in the developing cerebral cortex. Science 255:373–6.

Patel NH, Martin-Blanco E, Coleman KG, Poole SJ, Ellis MC, Kornberg TB, Goodman CS (1989). Expression of engrailed proteins in arthropods, annelids and chordates. Cell 58:955–68.

Patterson PH (1990). Control of cell fate in a vertebrate neurogenic lineage. Cell 62:1035–8.

Patteson PH, Landis SC (1992). Phenotype specifying factors and the control of neuronal differentiation decisions. In: Hendry IA, Hill CE, eds. Development, regeneration and plasticity of the autonomic nervous system. Chur, Switzerland: Harwood Academic Publishers, 231– 65.

Patterson PH, Nawa H (1993). Neuronal differentiation factors/cytokines and synaptic plasticity. Cell 72/Neuron 10(suppl):123–73.

Purves D, Lichtman JW (1985). Principles of neural development. Sunderland, Massachusetts: Sinauer Associates.

Rakic P (1971a). Guidance of neurons migrating to the fetal monkey neocortex. Brain Res 33:471–6.

Rakic P (1971b). Neuron-glia relationship during granule cell migration in developing cerebellar cortex. A Golgi and electron microscopic study in macacus rhesus. J Comp Neurol 141:283–312.

Rakic P (1972). Mode of cell migration to the superficial layers of fetal monkey neocortex. J Comp Neurol 145:61–84.

Rakic P (1974). Neurons in the rhesus monkey visual system: systematic relation between time of origin and eventual disposition. Science 183:425–7.

Rakic P (1977). Prenatal development of the visual system in the rhesus monkey. Phil Trans R Soc Lond (B) 278:245–60.

Ramón y Cajal S (1890). Sur l'origine et les ramifications des fibres nerveuses de la moelle embryonnaire. Anat. Anz. 5, 85–119.

Ramón y Cajal S (1909). Histologie du Système Nerveux de l'Homme et des Vertèbres, vol. 1. Maloine, Paris. Reprinted in Consejo Superior de Investigaciones Cientificas, Instituto Ramón y Cajal, Madrid, 1952.

Ramón y Cajal S (1911). Histologie du Système Nerveux de l'Homme et des Vertèbres, vol. 2. Maloine, Paris. Reprinted in Consejo Superior de Investigaciones Cientificas, Instituto Ramón y Cajal, Madrid, 1954.

Raper JA, Grunewald EB (1990). Temporal retinal growth cones collapse on contract with nasal retinal axons. Exp Neurol 109:70–4.

Rathjen FG, Wolff JM, Frank R, Bonhoeffer F, Rutishauser U (1987). Membrane glycoproteins involved in neurite fasciculation. J Cell Biol 104:343–53.

Reichardt LF, Tomaselli KJ (1991). Extracellular matrix molecules and their receptors. Annu Rev Neurosci 14:531–70.

Reiter HO, Stryker MP (1988). Neural plasticity without postsynaptic action potentials: less active inputs become dominant when kitten visual cortical cells are pharmacologically inhibited. Proc Natl Acad Sci USA 85:3623–7.

Reynolds BA, Weiss S (1992). Generation of neurons and astrocytes from isolated cells of the adult mammalian central nervous system. Science 255:1707–10.

Rhoades RW, Mooney RD, Fox SE (1984). Afferent input and development of visual callosal connections in hamster. In: Stone J, Rappaport E, eds. Development of visual pathways in mammals. New York: Alan R. Liss, 231–42.

Rosenberg PA (1988). Catecholamine toxicity in cerebral cortex in dissociated cell culture. J Neurosci 8:2887–94.

Rutishauser U, Jessell TM (1988). Cell adhesion molecules in vertebrate neural development. Physiol Rev 68:819–857.

Sauer F (1935). The cellular structure of the neural tube. J Comp Neurol 63:13–23.

Sauer F, Chittenden AC (1959). Deoxyribonucleic acid content of cell nuclei in the neural tube of the chick embryo: evidence for intermitotic migration of nuclei. Exp Cell Res 16:1–6.

Scalzo FM, Ali SF, Framdes NA, Spear LP (1990). Weanling rats exposed prenatally to cocaine exhibit an increase in striatal D2 dopamine binding associated with an increase in ligand affinity. Pharmacol Biochem Behav 37:371–3.

Schlessinger J, Ullrich A (1992). Growth factor signaling by receptor kinases. Neuron 9:383–91.

Schmechel DE, Rakic P (1979). A Golgi study of radial glial cells in developing monkey telencephalon: morphogenesis and transformation into astrocytes. Anat Embryol 156:115–52.

Schwab ME, Kapfhammer JP, Bandtlow CE (1993). Inhibitors of neurite growth. Annu Rev Neurosci 16:565–96.

Shatz CJ (1990). Impulse activity and the patterning of connections during CNS development. Neuron 5:745–56.

Sidman RL, Miale IL, Feder N (1959). Cell proliferation and migration in the primitive ependymal zone; an autoradiographic study of histogenesis in the nervous system. Exp Neurol 1:322–333.

Sidman RL, Rakic P (1973). Neuronal migration with special reference to developing human brain: a review. Brain Res 62:1–35.

Smart IHM, Smart M (1982). Growth patterns in the lateral wall of the mouse telencephalon. I. Autoradiographic studies of the histogenesis of the isocortex and adjacent areas. J Anat 134:273–98.

Smeyne RJ, Goldowitz D (1989). Development and death of external granular layer cells in the weaver mouse cerebellum: a quantititative study. J Neurosci 9:1608–20.

Snow DM, Watanabe M, Letourneau PC, Silver J (1991). A chondroitin sulfate proteoglycan may influence the direction of retinal ganglion cell outgrowth. Development 113:1473–85.

Spear LP, Kirstein CL, Frambes NA (1990). Cocaine effects on the developing central nervous system: behavioural, psychopharmacological, and neurochemical studies. Ann NY Acad Sci 660:290–307.

Sperry RW (1963). Chemoaffinity in the orderly growth of nerve fiber patterns and connections. Proc Natl Acad Sci USA 50:703–10.

Stanfield BB (1984). Postnatal re-organization of cortical projections: the role of collateral elimination. TINS 7:37–41.

Steinbusch HWM (1981). Distribution of serotonin-immunoreativity in the central nervous system of the rat—cell bodies and terminals. Neuroscience 6:557–618.

Stemple DL, Mahanthappa NK, Anderson DJ (1988). Basic FGF induces neuronal differentiation, cell division and NGF-dependence in chromaffin cells: a sequence of events in sympathetic development. Neuron 1:517–25.

Stoltenburg-Didinger G, Spohr HL (1983). Fetal alcohol syndrome and mental retardation: spine distribution of pyramidal cells in prenatal alcohol-exposed rat cerebral cortex; a Golgi study. Dev Brain Res 11:119–23.

Stryker MP (1991). Activity-dependent re-organization of afferents in the developing mammalian visual system. In: Lam DM-K, Shatz CJ, eds. Development of the visual system. Cambridge, Massachusetts: MIT Press, 267–88.

Stryker MP, Harris WA (1986). Binocular impulse blockade prevents the formation of ocular dominance columns in cat visual cortex. J Neurosci 6:2117–33.

Taber-Pierce E (1973). Time of origin of neurons in the brain stem of the mouse. Prog Brain Res 40:53–65.

Thoenen H (1991). The changing scene of neurotrophic factors. TINS 14:165–70.

Unsicker K, Grothe G, Ludecke G, Otto D, Westermann R (1993). Fibroblast growth factors: their roles in the central and peripheral nervous system. In: Loughlin SE, Fallon JH, eds. Neurotrophic factors. New York: Academic Press, 313–38.

Wang XH, Murphy EH (1993). Prenatal cocaine exposure results in region specific changes in the development of the GABAergic system in rabbit neocortex. Soc Neurosc Abst 19:50.

West JR, Hamre KM, Cassell MD (1986). Effects of ethanol exposure during the third trimester equivalent on neuron number in rat hippocampus and dentate gyrus. Alcohol (New York) 10:190–7.

West JR, Hodges CC, Black AC (1981). Prenatal exposure to ethanol alters the organization of hippocampal mossy fibers in rats. Science 211:957–9.

Weston JA (1991). Sequential segregation and fate of developmentally restricted intermediate cell populations in the neural crest lineage. Curr Top Dev Biol 25:133–53.

Valentino KL, Winter J, Reichardt LF (1985). Applications of monoclonal antibodies to neuroscience research. Annu Rev Neurosci 8:199–232.

Zacco A, Cooper V, Hyland-Fisher S, Chantler PD, Horton HL, Levitt P (1989). Isolation, biochemical characterization and ultrastructural localization of the limbic system associated membrane protein (LAMP), a protein expressed on neurons comprising functional neural circuits. J Neurosci 10:73–90.

Zahs KR (1989). Influence of neural activity on the development and plasticity of the cat's visual cortex. In: Landmesser LT, ed. The assembly of the nervous system. New York: Alan R. Liss, 259–78.

Zipser B, McKay RDG (1981). Monoclonal antibodies distinguish identifiable neurons in the leech. Nature 289:549–54.

Zukhareva V, Levitt P (1992). Homophilic binding and phosphatidyl inositol linkage of the limbic system–associated membrane protein (LAMP) are consistent with a role in specific recognition events in the developing brain. Mol Biol Cell 3:197a.

25
Concepts on Cell Adhesion Molecules and Their Possible Roles in Neurotoxicity

Laura A. Lagunowich
Regeneron Pharmaceuticals, Inc.
Tarrytown, New York

"You know it's there, but you just don't know where, but just because you can never reach it doesn't mean that it's not worth looking for."
—*The Phantom Tollbooth, Norton Juster*

The identification of specific molecular targets of toxicity has long been the goal of developmental neurotoxicologists. However, a simple identification of a molecular or metabolic mechanism becomes far more complex in light of the dynamic processes surrounding the development of the central nervous system. This development of the nervous system is dependent on specific mechanisms occurring in a programmed manner to generate a mature functional tissue. These mechanisms include cell division, differentiation, adhesion, migration and death and the numerous factors that modulate these events (Fig. 1).

Essential for brain development are numerous morphoregulatory molecules that control cell-cell interactions, cell sorting, and pattern formation. The specific spatial and temporal expression of these morphoregulatory molecules is imperative for proper neural histogenesis. The role of adhesion molecules as mediators of proper histogenesis was first described by Moscona in 1952. It was observed that cells of dissociated animal tissues can assemble autonomously and reform the original tissue-like structure. Since that time, several investigators have continued to explore the mechanism(s) that mediate this cell-cell sorting and tissue histogenesis (Townes and Holtfreter, 1955). During embryogenesis, cell-cell interactions are imperative for initiation of several critical morphogenetic processes. These interactions may be instrumental in immediate binding events or may mediate long-range morphogenetic events that control and are controlled by underlying cytoskeletal/intracellular systems.

Following the pioneering work of Moscona and of Townes and Holtfreter in the 1950s, great strides have been made toward the identification, characterization, and classification

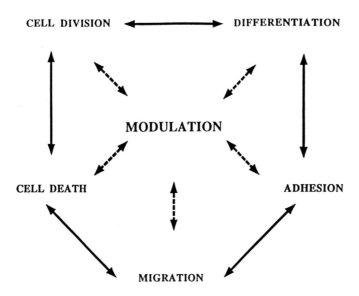

Figure 1   Schematic representation of tissue development.

of several distinct adhesion molecules in the developing embryo. The first two classes of adhesion molecules to be characterized were the calcium-independent adhesion molecules and the calcium-dependent molecules. The distinction between these molecules is based on a dependence on calcium for function and for protection from proteolysis. The calcium-independent and calcium-dependent molecules are further classified on the basis of the tissue in which they were first identified. This designation does not imply, however, that they are limited to those tissues.

THE CELL ADHESION MOLECULES

The initial identification of the neural cell adhesion molecule NCAM (Rutishauser et al., 1976) was followed by the subsequent observation that it mediated calcium-independent adhesions among neural cells. This left unresolved the molecular nature of the components mediating the calcium-dependent adhesions that had been functionally and immunologically distinguished from calcium-independent adhesions among these same cells (Takeichi et al., 1979; Grunwald et al., 1980; Brackenbury et al., 1981; Magnani et al., 1981; Thomas et al., 1981). Methods for the ultimate identification of these molecules were derived from early observations 1.) that the tissues of certain invertebrates and amphibian embryos may be dissociated simply by chelation of divalent cations, 2.) that avian and mammalian tissue generally requires the use of proteolytic enzymes for efficient tissue dissociation, and 3.) that the proteolytic dissociation of these tissues is more efficient in the absence of calcium (Moscona, 1952; Steinberg, 1958; Steinberg et al., 1973). Calcium-dependent modulation of the sensitivity of cell surface proteins and cell adhesive properties to digestion by trypsin was used to identify a calcium-dependent cell adhesion molecule in a fibroblastic cell line (Takeichi, 1977). These methods were subsequently used to identify embryonic chick retina calcium-dependent adhesion proteins (Grunwald et al., 1980) and N-cadherin (Hatta and Takeichi, 1986). Other members of the growing family of biochemically related proteins collectively called cadherins have been identified in a wide variety of tissues and species. Immunochemical, biochemical, and molecular genetic analyses of these proteins in a variety of species and tissues have revealed a high degree of structural and functional conservation among the members of the cadherin family.

NCAM

The first neural cell adhesion molecule to be identified was NCAM. The existence and function of the molecule as a developmentally regulated CAM was first recognized by Rutishauser et al. (1976). Purification and characterization required several years of study (Rutishauser et al., 1983; Rutishauser and Jessel, 1988). With the introduction of new immunologic and molecular genetic techniques, and with the relative abundance of the molecule, the characterization of NCAM has advanced rapidly.

The NCAM molecule is a glycoprotein of a single polypeptide chain with significant homogeneity of the protein and carbohydrate moieities. NCAM has been identified in SDS/PAGE (sodium dodecyl sulfate/polyacrylamide gel electrophoresis) as having three major variants. The amount of each varies between tissues and at specific developmental times. The three major forms of NCAM are identified on the basis of their relative molecular weight as determined by gel electrophoresis. The three forms are designated NCAM 180, 140, and 120. The differences in the molecular weight can be attributed to a difference in the length of the polypeptide chain of the molecule. NCAM 180 and 140 are transmembrane proteins that contain unique immunoglobulin-like domains (hence their designation in the Ig-super-gene family). These specific immunoglobulin domains are loops of amino acids joined by a disulfide bond. The NCAM molecule is also modified post-translationally by phosphorylation and sulfation (Hoffman and Edelman, 1983). A single gene has been identified for NCAM, and the differences in NCAM forms seem to be due to differential splicing. The NCAM 120 molecule does not contain a transmembrane domain or a cytoplasmic domain. It is linked to the surface of cells via an inositol phosphate linkage (Edelman et al., 1990)

One of the unique characteristics of the NCAM molecule is its differential glycosylation during development. These variations in glycosylation are due to differences in the amount of sialic acid on the molecule. The more highly glycosylated form, the one expressed early in development, has a sialic acid content of approximately 30%. Because of the expression of this highly glycosylated form in early development, it is often referred to as E-NCAM. The high level of sialic acid on cells that are moving and sorting seems to play a repulsive role. Cells that have a high amount of E-NCAM are less adhesive, and it is only when this high–sialic acid molecule switches to the lower–sialic acid form that NCAM-mediated adhesion occurs. This change from a high sialic acid content to a low sialic acid content (approximately 10%) is a closely orchestrated transition that occurs at specific developmental stages (Rutishauser and Jessel, 1988).

Because of a widespread distribution of NCAM in early neural morphogenesis, it seems evident that this molecule is critical for the development of proper tissue architecture. Specific tissues expressing NCAM during development include the neural plate, morphogenetically active structures such as the notochord, neural crest, somites, and placodes, some epidermis and mesenchyme, and the mesonephros. NCAM can also be found on glial cells, and a muscle-specific isoform of NCAM has been isolated (Dickson et al., 1987). Distribution of NCAM during development indicates that the molecule is uniformly distributed along the axon. In the visual system the molecule can be seen to be preferentially distributed at the radial glia end feet. NCAM in vivo has a role in the guidance of axons to their targets and in the innervation of skeletal muscle by motor neurons (for review see Rutishauser and Jessel, 1988). The unique characteristics of the NCAM molecule, during both embryogenesis and adult life, make its role in mediating a molecular or metabolic response to a toxic insult a key area of investigation.

NEUROTOXICITY AND NCAM: SOME EXAMPLES

The effect of lead on specific cell adhesion molecules in brain development has only recently been described. Cookman et al. (1987) reported that low-level chronic lead exposure during development inhibited the normal conversion of the highly sialated form of NCAM (E-NCAM) to its less sialated form in the adult. This inhibition of conversion seems to be mediated by an effect of lead on the sialyltransferase resident in the Golgi apparatus (Breen and Regen, 1988). These investigators concluded that inhibition of NCAM conversion may affect synaptogenesis in the cerebellum and that disruption of cell adhesion molecules can lead to significant morphological defects in the developing nervous system.

In addition, preliminary studies have demonstrated that methylmercury (MeHg), a known cerebellar toxicant (Reuhl and Chang, 1979), affects NCAM. It has been shown by biochemical analysis of cerebella from neonatal mice pups that the administration of methylmercury to newborn mice inhibits the conversion of embryonic NCAM to the adult form of NCAM. Following postnatal intraperitoneal injection of methylmercury for a period of 4 days beginning on postnatal day 1 there was a significant difference in the amount of embryonic NCAM in the cerebellum of these mice. In the treated mice the highly sialated form of NCAM persisted, while in the control animals the embryonic form had begun to disappear and the less sialated form appeared. Not only does methylmercury affect one of the cell adhesion molecules orchestrating brain development; it also affects the necessary post-translational modifications of normal NCAM expression (Lagunowich et al., 1991; Graff et al., 1992).

To correlate these findings to an established in vitro model it was shown that sublethal concentrations of methylmercury diminish NCAM staining on neurons derived from embryonal carcinoma cells. Parallel biochemical studies indicated a significant reduction in NCAM protein in these cells. The recovery of NCAM following methylmercury toxicity was also assessed by immunohistochemistry and by biochemical analysis. These experiments revealed that while NCAM was detectable biochemically after 2 hours of recovery, no NCAM was detected on neurites until 4 hours of recovery. This slower reappearance on the cell surface suggests that recovery of NCAM after methylmercury exposure requires the insertion into the membrane of newly synthesized NCAM. These experiments illustrate the differential effect of heavy metal toxicity on the different cell adhesion molecules in the developing nervous system (Graff et al., 1993).

Further experiments have been conducted to evaluate whether toxic injury altered the profile of NCAM in damaged neural areas. Following treatment with trimethyltin (TMT), a known neurotoxin, the hippocampi of exposed animals were assessed for NCAM content. Decreased amounts of one isoform of NCAM (180) were evident in injured animals 24 hours after exposure. Complete loss of NCAM 180 was detected 48 hours after TMT injection. This loss of NCAM 180 may represent an attempt to recapitulate normal embryonic development and thus repair the damaged tissue. Further study will have to be done to clarify this very specific effect on the NCAM molecule following injury (Dey et al., 1993).

THE CADHERINS

The cadherin gene family of Ca^{2+}-dependent cell adhesion molecules was originally composed of a rather limited number of transmembrane glycoproteins. Each member was found to regulate cell adhesion of particular cell types and was thus thought to be fundamental for the organization of the multicellular organisms. This gene family continues to grow, since more and more cadherin molecules are being identified.

To date, the members of the cadherin family include N-cadherin, first identified in the brain and retina of the chick—thus its designation N, for neural. However, it was later found to be associated with other non-neural tissues as well (Takeichi et al., 1979; Volk and Geiger, 1986; Grunwald et al., 1980). E-cadherin (also known as uvomorulin) is designated E for epithelium, where it was first identified. E-cadherin was later found to play a pivotal role in compaction of the developing mouse embryo (Kemler et al., 1977). P-cadherin was isolated in the 1980s from mouse placenta and has been further characterized and been shown to play a role in early implantation events (Nose and Takeichi, 1986). The calcium-dependent adhesion molecule that was identified in abundance in the chicken liver was called L-CAM (Bertolotti et al., 1980). Recently added to these well-described molecules are the newest members of this diversified family. These new adhesion molecules include M-cadherin (mouse myoblasts; Donalies et al., 1991), R-cadherin (retina and brain; Inuzuka et al., 1991), T-cadherin (a truncated form of cadherin; Ranscht and Bronner, 1991), B-cadherin (esp. choroid plexus and optic tectum; Napolitano et al., 1991), and, in *Xenopus*, EP-cadherin (unfertilized eggs and cleavage-stage embryos; Ginsberg et al., 1991) and U-cadherin (cleavage-stage embryos; Muller et al., 1992). This list of adhesion molecules is in no way complete, and with sophisticated molecular-biology techniques new molecules are being isolated all the time. To further this discussion of adhesion molecules as targets of toxicity we will elaborate on N-cadherin, the molecule that mediates, in part, the normal development and histogenesis of the central nervous system.

N-cadherin was the first calcium-dependent adhesion molecule to be associated with specific developmental events in nervous system. Structurally, N-cadherin possesses a high degree of structural homology to the other members of this family, with the most highly conserved sequence being the intracellular domain. This high homology within the cytoplasmic domain of the molecule indicates its functional importance in developmental processes. The molecular weight of N-cadherin in neural tissues is 130 kD, with an isoelectric point of 4.8. In non-neural tissues such as the lens and the heart the molecular weight is slightly higher (135 kD), and this is most likely due to differential glycosylation of the molecule in these tissues. The identification of N-cadherin as a molecule mediating calcium-dependent adhesion in dissociated cells occurred almost simultaneously in three independent laboratories. N-cadherin was identified in 1979 by Takeichi et al. in extracts of chicken embryonic brain and retina. In 1980 Grunwald and associates identified a protein in chick retina, which they named gp130/4.8, thhat possessed characteristics similar to those of N-cadherin. Volk and Geiger in 1986 identified a protein in chicken heart and lens that they referred to as A-CAM (on the basis of its localization to the adherent junctions in these tissues). It was later determined that these three molecules were in fact the same calcium-dependent adhesion protein (Lagunowich et al., 1991; Crittenden et al., 1987). Much has been discovered about the structure and function of this molecule in normal developmental processes.

N-cadherin is a 130-kD protein that has a transmembrane domain and a cytoplasmic domain (Fig. 2). N-cadherin has a calcium binding site on the extracellular domain that is

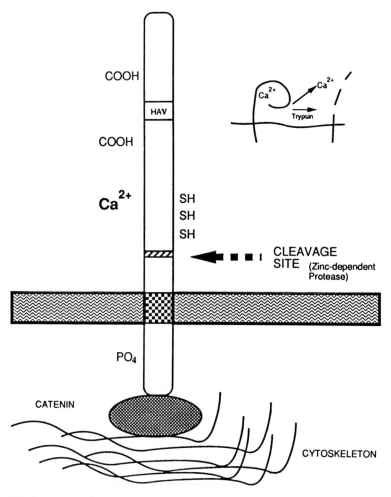

COOH

HAV

COOH

Ca^{2+} SH
               SH
               SH

◀ ■ ■ ■ ▮   CLEAVAGE
               SITE (Zinc-dependent
                         Protease)

PO$_4$

CATENIN

CYTOSKELETON

Figure 2   N-cadherin.

responsible for imparting a specific conformation to this molecule. This conformation protects N-cadherin from proteolytic digestion by trypsin. Little is known at this time about the structure of the calcium-binding region, although in another cadherin (E-cadherin) it has been predicted that this calcium-binding region is associated with six repeated units that could represent putative Ca^{2+}-binding sites. (Ringwald et al., 1987). Also on the extracellular domain of N-cadherin are numerous glycosylation sites that, depending on the amount of glycosylation present, impart the changes in molecular weight seen between tissues (Volk and Geiger, 1986) The amino acid sequence responsible for the homophilic binding of N-cadherin has been identified as an HAV sequence near the N-terminus of the molecule (Blaschuk et al., 1990). A relatively unexplored area of the structure of N-cadherin is in the sulfation of the molecule post-translationally (Lagunowich and Grunwald, 1991). Sulfation experiments have demonstrated that only a portion of the total population of N-cadherin is sulfated, and that the bulk of the sulfate label seems to be associated with a population of N-cadherin molecules that have a slower electrophoretic mobility and more acidic isoelectric point than the less heavily sulfated portion. It has been suggested that a change in the net charge of a protein alters its ability to function in cell adhesion in a manner similar to the sialic acid on NCAM. It is possible that the sulfation on N-cadherin is a mechanism modulating the molecule's adhesive function. It is also possible that a sulfated domain on N-cadherin mediates the interaction with specific receptors. As it has been suggested that sulfation affects various aspects of protein function, it is necessary to investigate further this modification on N-cadherin. This sulfated domain of N-cadherin must be considered, in the light of specific toxicants, to act primarily at sulfhydryl groups.

More closely scrutinized has been the role that phosphorylation and proteolytic degradation play in the regulation of this molecule. It has been shown that N-cadherin is a phosphoprotein and that phosphorylation of N-cadherin occurs in both a tissue-specific and an age-specific fashion during chick development. Within the neural retina N-cadherin appears to be relatively underphosphorylated during early developmental stages, when it is relatively abundant and widely distributed, and more heavily phosphorylated later in development, when it is expressed at much lower levels and in a spatially restricted manner. It is of interest that this apparent change in phosphorylation state correlated with an abundance of pericellularly distributed N-cadherin early in development and a localization to the zonula adherens junctional region later in development. Of further significance is that N-cadherin becomes associated with the cytoskeleton, via a linking molecule known as catenin, and that this linkage may be mediated by the cytoplasmic phosphorylation of N-cadherin (Lagunowich and Grunwald, 1991). It had been observed in vitro that N-cadherin is cleaved via some mechanism to generate a soluble 90-kD fragment. Recently it has been described that this 90-kD fragment is produced in vivo, and endogenous release seems to be mediated by a zinc-dependent metalloprotease. This endogenous metalloprotease that is responsible for degradation of N-cadherin does so in the presence of calcium, and thus may have a different substrate specificity than trypsin on the molecule (Roark et al., 1992). The 90-kD fragment of N-cadherin has been shown to retain biological activity and can promote the outgrowth of neurites in vitro (Paradies and Grunwald, 1993) This may be due to the fact that the 90-kD fragment incorporates the identified homophilic binding domain (HAV sequence).

N-cadherin has been shown to play a functionally important role in normal nervous system development. In the nervous system, N-cadherin has been shown to play a role in cell-cell sorting and in normal retina histogenesis. Later in development N-cadherin plays a role in the maintenance of the mature tissue via its association with the adherent junctions. Further studies have demonstrated a functional role for this molecule in the guidance of growth cones during neurite extension (Takeichi et al., 1979; Hatta and Takeichi, 1986; Matsunaga et al., 1988a,b). Antibodies against N-cadherin have been shown to disrupt the development of normal cytoarchitecture (Matsunaga et al., 1988b). Antibodies can also inhibit neurite outgrowth on muscle, astroglial cells, and Schwann cells (Bixby et al., 1987, 1988; Tomaselli et al., 1988). Expression of N-cadherin has been shown to be one of the first differences to distinguish ectoderm (epidermis) from other surrounding tissues. This expression of N-cadherin in the ectoderm may in fact be an inductive event that stimulates the development of the neural plate (Detrick et al., 1990). N-cadherin plays a continued role in early neural development by mediating the closure of the neural tube. Studies have shown that a misexpression of N-cadherin either spatially or temporally results in embryos displaying neural tube defects (Detrick et al., 1990). These studies were indicative that N-cadherin expression or misexpression in the nervous system alters the normal developmental program (Edelman and Thiery, 1985; Takeichi, 1988). These well-described structural and functional characteristics that occur at developmentally specific times allow questions to be raised regarding the interaction of specific toxicants at these structural sites.

NEUROTOXICITY AND N-CADHERIN: LEAD AS AN EXAMPLE

Relatively little is known about the interaction of environmental toxicants with the cadherin molecule, and at this time we can only speculate on possible mechanisms of interaction. The well-described biochemical and functional characteristics of the cadherin molecules suggest possible sites of interference by toxicants. A central characteristic that may be a provocative target for toxicant interaction is the extracellular calcium site. Divalent cations such as lead may be able to displace or replace calcium on the adhesion molecule, with a subsequent disruption of the structure and function of the molecule. Lead ingestion has been shown to have a particularly devastating impact on early neurodevelopmental events (for review see Lansdown and Yule, 1986). The extensive dynamic processes occurring at these times during development make this a period highly susceptible to toxic injury with serious and widespread consequences. Possible mechanisms underlying these dysmorphogenic events include cell adhesion molecules that regulate the cell-cell interactions during early neural processes. While the morphological and histological changes in the brain following developmental lead exposure have been investigated, the molecular changes involved in lead toxicity are still poorly understood. Lead has the ability to compete directly with calcium binding sites and in some instances to completely dislodge calcium in biological systems. Because of the known characteristics of these adhesion molecules and the essential role they play in nervous system development, they are provocative targets for metal toxicity.

Furthermore, lead has been shown to have significant deleterious effects on early nervous system processes. Lead crosses the placenta and may cause miscarriage, high rate of fetal loss, and sterility (Angle and McIntire, 1964; Rom, 1976). Much of the investigation surrounding lead exposure has been concerned with transplacental passage of the metal, embryotoxicity, and teratogenic effects of lead during the later stages of pregnancy and into the early postnatal period. Less is known about how lead affects the embryo at earlier stages of pregnancy and during the preimplantation period. There is evidence that lead affects the cleavage rate of mouse embryos (Jacquet et al., 1976). Other investigators have demonstrated that treatment of chick embryos with lead leads to hydrocephalus and anterior meningoceles (Karnofsky and Ridgway, 1952; Butt et al., 1952).

An as yet unexplored area of lead toxicity is that of interference with calcium-dependent adhesion molecules. Studies indicate (Lagunowich and Reuhl, 1992) that lead can affect the function of N-cadherin in vitro but does not interfere with the expression of the molecule at the cell surface. Because of the significance of these molecules in brain development and the ability of lead to replace calcium in biochemical processes (Pounds, 1984), it is essential to investigate the effect of lead on the N-cadherin molecule in early brain development. Preliminary studies have established a relationship between exposure to lead and functional perturbation of N-cadherin, a calcium-dependent adhesion molecule. Studies were conducted that used the established in vitro aggregation assays with calcium as the traditional "functional" cation and substituted other similar divalent cations to study the effect on cell adhesion.

Small aggregates of neural retina from 10-day chick embryos were cultured in vitro for 24 hours in the presence of 1 mM calcium or 1 mM–1 μM lead acetate. In the calcium-containing medium they aggregated into histotype groups, as described previously (Grunwald et al., 1980; Lagunowich and Grunwald, 1989). These aggregates were quite stable and resistant to mechanical dissociation. When neural retina aggregates were cultured in the presence of lead (at all concentrations) the tissues gradually became looser and more friable. The peripheries of the aggregates became dissociated, and upon trituration these aggregates were readily dispersed into smaller clumps. The appearance of these aggregates was in clear contrast to the aggregates seen in the calcium-containing medium (Fig. 3). This change in aggregate morphology is essentially identical to the change seen when aggregates are cultured in the presence of N-cadherin–blocking antibodies (Matsunaga et al., 1988b).

As a means of examining the nature of the interference of lead with the calcium-dependent adhesion molecule on neural retina cells, the proteolytic sensitivity in the presence of lead was determined. In this study, as in previous reports, N-cadherin was protected from proteolytic degradation by trypsin in the presence of 1 mM calcium (Lagunowich and Grunwald, 1989). However, when lead was substituted for calcium at concentrations from 1 mM to 1 μM there was no protection from proteolysis by trypsin. To investigate further the role of lead in promoting trypsin proteolysis, cells were preincubated with decreasing concentrations of lead and then trypsinized in the presence of calcium. These results indicate that lead alone is not enough to stimulate endogenous proteolysis of N-cadherin (which would indicate a different mechanism of interference) but rather may be interacting with the molecule in a manner that changes its conformation, making it susceptible to trypsin. When cells are "rescued" from lead by calcium and then treated with trypsin,

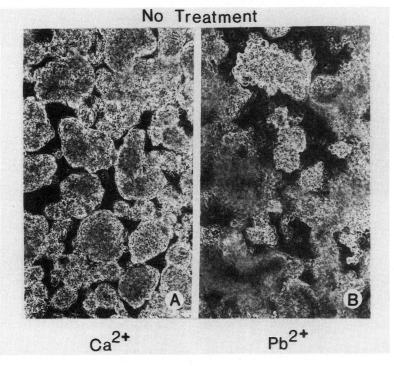

Figure 3 Effect of low-level lead on retinal aggregate morphology. Cells were obtained from 10-day embryonic neural retinas, mechanically dissociated, and placed into culture in the presence of 1 mM calcium (A) or 10 μM lead acetate (B) for 24 h.

control levels of N-cadherin are detected by immunoblot analysis. The ability of retinal cells to form histotypic aggregates following trypsinization in the presence of calcium and of lead and during culture in lead- and calcium-containing medium was investigated using rotation-mediated aggregation cultures. Cells were prepared from tissues by calcium-free trypsinization (TRP-cells), which removes surface-associated cell adhesion molecules, by trypsinization in the presence of calcium (CaT cells), which preserves an intact calcium-dependent adhesive system, or by trypsinization in the presence of lead acetate (PbT cells), to determine whether the calcium-dependent adhesive system is preserved under these conditions. The results indicate that CaT cells from 10-day embryo retinas are able to from large aggregates in calcium-containing medium even in the absence of new protein synthesis. However, when these cells were placed into lead-containing medium they no longer maintained their tight, rounded appearance. TRP cells are able to form large aggregates only when protein synthesis occurs and not in the presence of the protein-synthesis inhibitor. TRP cells were unable to reaggregate when placed into lead-containing medium. PbT cells are unable to form large aggregates in medium containing lead, but do form aggregates in medium containing calcium when protein synthesis is not inhibited. Twenty-four hours following trypsinization all the cells that were cultured in calcium-containing medium, without cycloheximide, had formed large histotypic aggregates. Only the cells that had been calcium-trypsinized and cultured in calcium medium with cycloheximide were able to form and maintain aggregates. All cells cultured in lead-containing medium, with or without cycloheximide, had lost (or never acquired) the histotypic morphology of the retinal aggregates. Parallel biochemical analyses indicated the presence of N-cadherin in all CaT cell populations and all PbT populations, as well as in the cells that were trypsinized and cultured without cycloheximide. Additional studies indicate that in ovo exposure to lead results in a delay in the maturation and closure of the neural tube. Control embryos showed normal maturation and development, while embryos exposed to lead and to a blocking antibody showed similar, if not identical, delays in maturation and neural fold fusion (Lagunowich et al., 1993). These data suggest that while lead does not interfere with the expression of N-cadherin on the cell surface, it does interfere with its function. Collectively, these data suggest that certain morphologic defects following lead exposure may be mediated by a disturbance of the proper function of the calcium-dependent adhesion molecule.

FURTHER SPECULATION AND FUTURE DIRECTIONS

As can be seen from the above examples, the area of cell adhesion molecules as targets of toxicity is just beginning to evolve. Although still in its genesis, it is an area that has real potential for identifying a potential starting point to address mechanisms involved in or related to toxic injury. We have only begun to touch on some of the areas of molecular changes in response to a toxic injury, and much more work is needed to put these small pieces of information into a cohesive dialogue about toxicity. We know nothing about the effect of toxicants on cell adhesion molecule–cytoskeleton interaction. We have to begin to question the interference of toxicants with specific post-translational modifications. Endogenous proteolysis of calcium-dependent adhesion molecules (a decrease or increase in the natural occurrence) should be considered a potential site of toxic injury. Since this proteolysis is mediated by a zinc-dependent protease, it seems likely that a divalent cation could interfere with the normal function of the protease. Of relevant importance when discussing the role of cell adhesion molecules in mediating a response to toxic injury is the consideration of the specific developmental window at which the insult occurs. The dynamic process of early brain development may be far more susceptible to toxicity, and thus the high expression of cell adhesion molecules, than the more developed brain. With understanding of the normal expression and regulation of the proteins that mediate brain morphogenesis it is more likely that a mechanism of toxicity can be identified. Developmental biologists continue to discover new adhesion molecules—there will probably be five new ones described by the time this chapter is published—and more and more critical developmental functions are being attributed to these molecules and their role in the complexity of morphogenesis. The task of identifying a single molecule or mechanism of toxicity may seem overwhelming in light of all the nuances of development, but just because the task is difficult, or the molecule or mechanism is elusive, the developmental neurotoxicologist is not precluded from looking for the answer.

REFERENCES

Angle CR, McIntire MS (1964). Lead poisoning during pregnancy. Am J Dis Child 108:436–9.

Bertolloti R, Rutishauser U, Edelman GM (1980). A cell surface molecule involved in aggregation of embryonic liver cells. Proc Natl Acad Sci USA 77:4381–5.

Bixby JL, Pratt RS, Lilien J, Reichardt LF (1987). Neurite outgrowth on muscle cell surfaces involves extracellular matrix receptors as well as Ca^{2+}-dependent and independent cell adhesion molecules. Proc Natl Acad Sci USA 84:2555–9.

Bixby JL, Lilien J, Reichardt L (1988). Identification of the major proteins that promote neuronal process outgrowth on Schwann cells *in vitro*. J Cell Biol 107:353–62.

Blaschuk OW, Sullivan R, David S, Pouliot Y (1990). Identification of a cadherin cell adhesion recognition sequence. Dev Biol 139:227–9.

Brackenbury R, Rutishauser U, Edelman GM (1981). Distinct calcium-independent and calcium-dependent adhesion systems of chicken embryonic cells. Proc Natl Acad Sci USA 78:387–91.

Breen KC, Regen CM (1988). Lead stimulates Golgi sialyltransferase at times coincident with the embryonic to adult conversion of the neural cell adhesion molecule (N-CAM). Toxicology 49:71–6.

Butt EM, Pearson HE, Simonsen DG (1952). Production of meningoceles and cranioschisis in chick embryos with lead nitrate. PSEBM 79:247–249.

Cookman GR, King W, Regen CM (1987). Chronic low-level lead exposure impairs embryonic to adult conversion of the neural cell adhesion molecule. J Neurochem 49:399–403.

Crittenden SL, Pratt RS, Cook JS, Balsamo J, Lilien J (1987). Immunologiclly unique and common domains within a family of proteins related to the retina Ca^{2+}-dependent cell adhesion molecule, NCalCAM. Development 101:729–40.

Detrick RJ, Dickey D, Kintner C (1990). The effects of N-cadherin misexpression on morphogenesis in Xenopus embryos. Neuron 4:493–506.

Dey MP, Graff RD, Lagunowich LA, Reuhl KR (1993). TMT causes selective loss of the 180 kD form of the neural cell adhesion molecule (NCAM) in adult mouse hippocampus. (abstr) Toxicologist 13:167.

Dickson G, Gower HJ, Barton CH, Prentice HM, Elsom LL, Moore SE, Cox RD, Quinn C, Putt W, Walsh F (1987). Human muscle neural cell adhesion molecule (N-CAM): identification of a muscle-specific sequence in the extracellular domain. Cell 50:1119–30.

Donalies M, Cramer M, Ringwald M, Starzinski-Powitz A (1991). Expression of M-cadherin, a member of the cadherin multi-gene family, correlates with differentiation of skeletal muscle cells. Proc Natl Acad Sci USA 88:8024–8.

Edelman GM, Thiery JP, eds. (1985). The cell in contact: adhesions and junctions as morphogenetic determinents. New York: John Wiley & Sons.

Edelman GM, Cunningham B, Thiery JP (1990). Morphoregulatory Molecules. New York: John Wiley & Sons.

Ginsberg D, DeSimone D, Geiger B (1991). Expression of a novel cadherin (EP-cadherin) in unfertilized eggs and early Xenopus embryos. Development 111:315–25.

Graff RD, Lagunowich LA, Reuhl KR (1992). Alterations in N-CAM expression by methylmercury: *in vivo* and *in vitro* correlation. Toxicologist 12:312.

Graff RD, Elzer JA, Lagunowich LA, Reuhl KR (1993). Methylmercury alters expression of the neural cell adhesion molecule (NCAM) in cultured neurons. Toxicologist (in press).

Grunwald GB, Geller RL, Lilien J (1980). Enzymatic dissection of embryonic cell adhesive mechanisms. J Cell Biol 85:766–76.

Hatta K, Takeichi M (1986). Expression of N-cadherin molecules associated with early morphogenetic events in chick development. Nature 320:447–9.

Hoffman S, Edelman G (1983). Kinetics of homophilic binding by embryonic and adult forms of the neural cell adhesion molecule. Proc Natl Acad Sci USA 80:5762–6.

Inuzuka H, Redies C, Takeichi M (1991). Differential expression of R- and N-cadherin in neural and mesodermal tissues during early chicken development. Development 113:959–67.

Jacquet P, Leonard A, Gerber GB (1976). Action of lead on early divisions of the mouse embryo. Toxicology 6:129–32.

Karnofsky DA, Ridgway L (1952). Production of injury to the central nervous system of the chick embryo by lead salts. J Pharmacol Exp Ther 104:176–86.

Kemler R, Babinet C, Eisen H, Jacob F (1977). Surface antigen in early differentiation. Proc Natl Acad Sci USA 74:4449–52.

Lagunowich LA, Grunwald GB (1989). Expression of calcium-dependent cell adhesion during ocular development: a biochemical, histochemical and functional analysis. Dev Biol 135:158–71.

Lagunowich LA, Grunwald GB (1991). Tissue and age-specificity of post-translational modifications of N-cadherin during chick embryo development. Differentiation 47:19–27.

Lagunowich LA, Bhambhani S, Graff RD, Reuhl KR (1991). Cell adhesion molecules in the cerebellum: targets of methylmercury toxicity? (abstr) Soc Neurosci Abstr 17:715.

Lagunowich LA, Reuhl KR (1992). Lead interferes with calcium-dependent adhesion molecules on neural cells *in vitro*. (abstr) Toxicologist 12:315.

Lagunowich LA, Stein AP, Reuhl KR (1993). N-cadherin mediated aggregation and neurulation are disrupted by exposure to lead. (abstr) Toxicologist 13:168.

Lansdown R, Yule W (1986). The lead debate: the environment, toxicology and child health. London and Sydney: Croom Helm.

Magnani JL, Thomas WA, Steinberg MS (1981). Two distinct adhesion mechanisms in embryonic chick neural retina cells. I. A kinetic analysis. Dev Biol 81:96–105.

Matsunaga M, Hatta K, Nagafuchi A, Takeichi M (1988a). Guidance of optic nerve fibers by N-cadherin adhesion molecules. Nature 334:62–4.

Matsunaga M, Hatta K, Takeichi M (1988b). Role of N-cadherin cell adhesion molecules in the histogenesis of neural retina. Neuron 1:289–95.

Moscona AA (1952). Cell suspensions from organ rudiments of chick embryos. Exp Cell Res 3:535–9.

Muller AHJ, Angres B, Hausen P (1992). U-cadherin in Xenopus oogenesis and oocyte maturation. Development 114:533–43.

Napolitano EW, Venstrom K, Wheeler EF, Reichardt LF (1991). Molecular cloning and characterization of B-cadherin, a novel chick cadherin. J Cell Biol 113:893–905.

Nose A, Takeichi M (1986). A novel cadherin cell adhesion molecule: its expression patterns associated with implantation and organogenesis of mouse embryos. J Cell Biol 103:2649–58.

Paradies NE, Grunwald GB (1992). Purification and characterization of an endogenous proteolytically-derived soluble fragment of N-cadherin which retains adhesive function (abstr). Neurosci Abstr. 18:1325.

Pounds JG (1984). Effect of lead intoxication on calcium homeostasis and calcium-mediated cell function: a review. Neurotoxicology 5:295–332.

Rauscht B, Bronner MF (1991). T-cadherin expression alternates with migrating neural crest cells in the trunk of the avain embryo. Development 111:15–22.

Reuhl KR, Chang L (1979). Effects of methylmercury on the development of the nervous system: a review. Neurotoxicology 1:21–55.

Ringwald M, Schuh R, Vestweber D, Eistetter H, Lottspeich F, Engel J, Dolz R, Jahnig F, Epplen J, Mayer S, Muller C, Kemler R (1987). The structure of cell adhesion molecule uvomorulin. Insights into the molecular mechanism of Ca^{2+}-dependent cell adhesion. EMBO J 6:3647–53.

Roark EF, Paradies NE, Lagunowich LA, Grunwald GB (1992). Evidence for endogenous proteases, mRNA level and insulin as multiple mechanisms of N-cadherin down-regulation during retinal development. Development 114:973–84.

Rom WN (1976). Effects of lead on the female and reproduction: a review. Mt Sinai J Med 43:542–52.

Rutishauser U, Thiery JP, Brackenbury R, Sela B, Edelman GM (1976). Mechanism of adhesion among cells from neural tissues of the chick embryo. Proc Natl Acad Sci USA 73:577–81.

Rutishauser U, Grumet M, Edelman E (1983). N-CAM mediates initial interactions between spinal cord neurons and muscle cells in culture. J Cell Biol 97:145–52.

Rutishauser U, Jessell TM (1988). Cell adhesion molecules in vertebrate development. Physiol Rev 68:819–57

Steinberg MS (1958). On the chemical bonds between animal cells. A mechanism for type specific association. Am Nat 92:65–81.

Steinberg MS, Armstrong PB, Granger RE (1973). On the recovery of adhesiveness by trypsin-dissociated cells. J Membr Biol 13:97–128.

Takeichi M (1977). Functional correlation between cell adhesive properties and some cell surface proteins. J Cell Biol 75:464–474.

Takeichi M, Ozaki MS, Tokunaga K, Okada TS (1979). Experimental manipulation of cell surface to affect cellular recognition mechanisms. Dev Biol 70:195–205.

Takeichi M (1988). The cadherins: cell-cell adhesion molecules controlling animal morphogenesis. Development 102:639–55.

Thomas WA, Thomson J, Magnani JL, Steinberg MS (1981). Two distinct adhesion mechanisms in embryonic neural retina cells. III. Functional specificity. Dev Biol 8:379–85.

Tomaselli K, Neugebauer KM, Bixby JL, Lilien J, Reichardt L (1988). N-cadherin and integrin: two receptor systems that mediate neuronal process outgrowth on astrocyte surfaces. Neuron 1:33–43.

Townes P, Holtfreter J (1955). Directed movements and selective adhesion of embryonic amphibian cells. J Exp Zool 128:53–120.

Volk T, Geiger B (1986). A-CAM: a 135-kD receptor of intercellular adherens junctions. I. Immunoelectron localization and biochemical studies. J Cell Biol 103:1441–50.

26
Interspecies Comparison of the Evaluation of Cognitive Developmental Effects of Neurotoxicants in Primates

Merle G. Paule
National Center for Toxicological Research/FDA
Jefferson, Arkansas

Jane Adams
University of Massachusetts
Boston, Massachusetts

INTRODUCTION

This review examines the characteristics of studies focusing on the "cognitive" effects of exposure to selected developmental neurotoxicants in human and nonhuman primates, evaluates the quality of these data for making interspecies comparisons, and makes suggestions for designing studies that will facilitate the extrapolation of data across species. As discussed by Eckerman and Bushnell (1992), the term "cognition," as it applies to animal behavior, will be used here to refer to processes thought to include aspects of attention, learning, and memory. Behavioral data obtained using animal models have often been discussed as just that, i.e., with little or no attempt to try to bridge the gap between animal and human behavior or brain function. It is likely that the lack of attempts by animal researchers to interpret animal behavioral data in terms familiar to researchers outside the discipline has slowed the acceptance and use of such procedures by other scientists, including toxicologists. While it is not the intent of this chapter to resolve issues of terminology and theory between behaviorists and cognitivists, it is recognized that the use of metaphor can be important for a coherent discussion of the topics that follow.

We will first consider the nature of the current human data base and discuss the types of information needed to determine adequately whether or not cognitive functioning has been compromised by developmental exposure to a neurotoxic agent. Next we examine methodological approaches and resulting data from studies using nonhuman primates. Because of the paucity of studies on the effects of other compounds in nonhuman primates, this discussion will be restricted to studies of the developmental consequences of exposure to lead and methylmercury. Next, we address the strengths and weaknesses of the data from selected studies of human and nonhuman primates with respect to examination of the validity of extrapolating effects across species. Finally, we will discuss research approaches that may provide information relevant to improving confidence in extrapolating findings between species with respect to cognitive functioning following exposure to toxicants.

CHARACTERISTICS OF HUMAN STUDIES THAT HAVE EXAMINED COGNITIVE END POINTS IN CHILDREN EXPOSED TO DEVELOPMENTAL TOXICANTS

While it is clear that the most compelling information relevant to risk assessment is derived from the study of known human exposures, such studies almost always suffer from a lack of the experimental rigor that can be obtained in the experimental (generally, animal) laboratory. The characteristics of studies concerning human developmental neurotoxicants vary greatly between studies of agents that are generally used voluntarily (e.g., prescription, licit, and illicit drugs) and those that are not (e.g., environmental compounds). Adams et al. (1990) evaluated the human literature on the antiepileptic drug diphenylhydantoin and identified a common set of shortcomings that often compromise the results of human studies. These included small sample sizes; inadequate definition of exposure levels in relation to developmental stage at exposure; restriction of outcome assessments to early infancy; restriction of assessment methodologies; inadequate assessment of the effects of variables such as parental education, occupation, other drug or medication use, and general health and liefstyle characteristics; and inadequate use of appropriate controls. Similarly, Day (1992) examined the characteristics of the human literature concerning the fetal alcohol syndrome and other alcohol-related effects and identified methodological problems in case and control selection procedures; ascertainment of alcohol use with respect to quantity, duration, frequency, and pattern; comparable ascertainment of the use of other substances; assessment of substance use with respect to gestational stage; and measurement and utilization of appropriate covariates of alcohol use.

When attention is focused on the characteristics of human studies of environmental agents, however, a different picture emerges. Table 1 reviews certain characteristics of human studies of the developmental neurotoxicity of lead and methylmercury, agents for which data in nonhuman primates are also available. As is evident, features differ between the selected literature on methylmercury and lead. Accordingly, the two data bases are discussed separately.

Methylmercury

Human studies focussing on the cognitive consequences of methylmercury exposure have examined reasonably large samples of children (>80) from "disaster areas" and therefore have primarily reported the effects of exposure to only high levels. Burbacher et al. (1990a) have published an excellent overview of this literature that examines dose-response issues relevant to neuropathological as well as intellectual and other behavioral end points.

With respect to methodological issues, it can be seen in Table 1 that published studies have focused on a narrow range of assessments, typically general mental ability and/or gross motor system function. With respect to the assessment of cognitive function, an over-reliance on measures of general mental ability or on performance on single tests of

Table 1 Characteristics of Selected Studies of the Neurobehavioral Effects of Human Developmental Exposure to Methylmercury and Lead

Study	Exposure level and period	Age at test	Reported examinations		
			General mental ability	Specific abilities	Appropriate covariates
Methylmercury					
Harada, 1977	Prenatal poisoning, 12–20 ppm for brain[a]	Early childhood	Yes	No	Not discussed
Marsh, 1987	Prenatal exposure, <3–20 ppm, brain[a]	Early childhood	Yes	No	Not discussed
Lead					
Boston Longitudinal Study					
Bellinger et al., 1987	Prenatal, <3 vs 6.5 vs >10 μg/dl; 24 months, 6.8 μg/dl	6, 12, 18, 24 months	Yes, Bayley Scales of Infant Development	No	Yes, numerous
Bellinger et al., 1991	Same subjects as above	5 yr	Yes, McCarthy Test of Children's Abilities	Yes, on subscales	Yes, numerous
Bellinger et al., 1992	Same subjects as above	10 yr	Yes, WISC-R and K-TEA	Yes, on subtests	Yes, numerous
Cincinnati Longitudinal Study					
Dietrich et al., 1987	Prenatal, 5–8 μg/dl	1 yr	Yes, Bayley scales	No	Yes, numerous
Dietrich et al., 1991	Prenatal, 5–8 μg/dl; postnatal, 10–17 μg/dl	4 yr	Yes, K-ABC	Yes, K-ABC subtests	Yes, numerous
Port Pirie Longitudinal Study					
McMichael et al., 1988	Prenatal 0.3–0.7 μmol/L; postnatal, 0.6–1.4 μmol/L	4 yr	Yes, McCarthy Test of Children's Abilities	Yes, on subscales	Yes, numerous

[a]Doses estimated by Burbacher et al., 1990a.
WISC-R = Wechsler Intelligence Scale for Children-Revised; K-TEA = Kaufman Test of Educational Achievement; K-ABC = Kaufman Assessment Battery for Children.

psychomotor function is evident. A global dichotomous approach has typically been taken in the identification of cognitive and/or motor dysfunction, whereby investigators have focused on the incidence of mental retardation or cerebral palsy, without examining other degrees or types of impairment. With respect to cognitive function, this is problematic because many children may have general mental abilities within the normal range but nevertheless have learning disabilities specific to one or more areas of processing. Such disabilities may represent toxicant-induced effects that would generally go undetected. Similar arguments apply to subtle aspects of neuromotor functioning.

Lead

The lead studies listed in Table 1, like those for methylmercury, have also been conducted using relatively large samples of children (>170). Unlike the situation for methylmercury, however, most studies concerning the cognitive consequences of lead exposure have examined the effects of levels relevant to those typically found in the environment. These studies of "low" lead exposure have gone beyond the discussion of effects on general mental ability and have carefully examined the nature of the resulting dysfunctions. One general finding is that low-level lead exposure does not increase the incidence of mental retardation, but does reduce the general mental ability scores of groups of exposed children and may compromise certain cognitive processes more than others. Notably, Dietrich et al. (1991) reported specific weaknesses in visual-spatial and visual-motor integration skills at age 4 that were associated with postnatal blood lead levels. Similar findings for preschool children have been reported by Bellinger and co-workers (1992) and McMichael and co-workers (1988). Bellinger et al. (1992) have also reported specific weaknesses in language-based functions in the same sample of children when examined at 10 years of age. Whether or not this developmental difference will also be observed in the Cincinnati sample (Dietrich et al., 1991) and the Port Pirie sample (McMichael et al., 1988) remains to be determined. Thus, as Bellinger et al. (1992) point out, evidence is not yet sufficient to determine whether early developmental exposure to lead produces a specific "behavioral signature."

The children in the Boston, Cincinnati, and Port Pirie studies differ with respect to familial socioeconomic characteristics, important variables with regard to cognitive vulnerability to early lead exposure. As noted in Table 1, these studies have all examined the effects of a range of covariates and have reported effects that persist after adjustment for the influences of numerous covariates representing demographic, reproductive, obstetric, and neonatal status and postnatal environmental quality. Following relevant statistical adjustments, the effects of lead have been shown to interact considerably with social class, so that children from economically less advantaged environments show cognitive deficits at lower blood lead levels than do children from families of higher socioeconomic status (see Dietrich et al., 1991). Such factors may also interact with the nature of the specific functional deficits that are most salient at different ages.

One must keep in mind that low-level exposure to lead is not associated with an increase in mental retardation but may cause deficits in the performance of specific functions. Other agents, such as alcohol, do increase the incidence of mental retardation, and thus fetal alcohol exposure might be expected to result in deficits in most measures. In order to address the specificity of reduced ability in a particular functional domain studied in isolation, the performance of children exposed to a developmental neurotoxicant should, at a minimum, be compared with the performance of both mentally retarded and normal children. Comparison of performance to mental age–matched controls is also helpful.

It is essential to determine whether functional deficits are global and generalize to all areas of processing or whether such deficits represent specific weaknesses in one or more areas of processing and exist alongside normal or even above-average strengths in other areas. This is especially true if one is to develop hypotheses about the neurological basis of noted dysfunctions. An emphasis on disparities in function across areas of processing, each mediated by somewhat "modular" neural substrates, is representative of the developmental neuropsychological approach to the definition of cognitive processing abilities.

A NEUROPSYCHOLOGICAL FRAMEWORK FOR THE EXAMINATION OF COGNITIVE DYSFUNCTION INDUCED BY EXPOSURE TO DEVELOPMENTAL NEUROTOXICANTS

It is important to consider the different types of cognitive process that should be examined if one is to obtain representative samples of a child's cognitive abilities. Research on heterogeneous populations of nonretarded learning-disabled children has identified a common set of cognitive developmental aberrations of multiple etiologies that appear to be present in children (see Pennington, 1991). A parsimonious approach to examining the neurobehavioral characteristics of children exposed to developmental neurotoxicants might be to use test batteries capable of identifying children with deficits similar to those noted in children with learning disabilities. While classification systems and corresponding approaches differ across educational, psychological, psychiatric, and neuropsychological perspectives, the interests of developmental neurotoxicologists in relating dysfunction to underlying neural substrates are compatible with a nosology derived within a neuropsychological framework.

One such classification system, formally presented by Pennington (1991), is representative of the approach taken by many developmental neuropsychologists. Investigators differ with respect to the use of specific labels for each functional category, and debate continues about the validation of primary vs. secondary symptomatology within subtypes (and about the number of specific subtypes); however, it has been argued that Pennington's model represents the "best-known profiles constituting developmental differences" (Denckla, 1991). In Pennington's presentation of the neuropsychological model, learning disabilities are classified according to specific dysfunction in one or more of five major domains of higher-order brain-based functioning: 1.) phonological processing (including dyslexia and other language-based learning disorders); 2.) executive control functions (including attentional/inhibitory deficits as well as the more rigorously defined attention deficit/hyperactivity disorder); 3.) spatial cognition (including the "nonverbal learning disability" category); 4.) long-term memory (including acquired memory deficits); and 5.) social cognition (dissociable from deficits in spatial cognition, autism being the more extreme form). The majority of children in learning-disabled samples have specific weaknesses in the first or second functional domains (phonological processing and/or executive control functions), and these areas appear to be the most vulnerable to dysfunction resulting from genetic/chromosomal disorders as well as postnatal illnesses (for review see Pennington, 1991). Next in prevalence are disorders of spatial cognitive processing.

In studies aimed at assessing the influence of exposure to a developmental neurotoxicant, it would seem strategic to use test batteries capable of assessing functioning in these three areas that appear to be most vulnerable to insult. Multiple methods are available for examining functioning within each of these three domains, with different methods tapping different functions and corresponding substrates with varying degrees of specificity, reliability, and validity at different ages (for discussion, see Pennington, 1991; Lezak, 1983; Kaplan et al., 1991).

Table 2 provides a sample of tests that would be appropriate for young school-aged children. It should be recognized that this list is a sample and that many other appropriate tests are available. Also, all of the measures are somewhat apical and have been assigned to domains on the basis of historical data, loadings in factor analyses, or published intercorrelations (see Pennington, 1991; Lezak, 1983; Kaplan et al., 1991). These tests are generally considered to reflect functioning in the assigned domain with varying degrees of specificity.

Given the demonstrated vulnerability of motor and sensory systems to the effects of neurotoxicants, assessments of motor and sensory functioning should also be important components of any general testing battery (see review on lead by Laughlin, 1986). Clearly, disturbances in motor or sensory systems could compromise acquisition and/or performance of cognitive tasks (see discussion by Mactutus, 1985). The impact of identified dysfunctions of this type must be considered in or separated from interpretations of performance on other types of task. These considerations are, obviously, also very important for work in animal models.

Table 2 An Example of a Neuropsychological Testing Battery Appropriate for Use in Young Children

Domain measured	Tests[a]	Age/grade range of norms
Language-based	Vocabulary (WISC-III)	6–16
	Comprehension (WISC-III)	6–16
	Similarities (WISC-III)	6–16
	Word attack (Woodcock-Johnson)	G1–12
Executive control	Digit span	6–16
	Symbol search (WISC-III)	6–16
	Wisconsin card sorting test	6–adult
	Continuous performance tasks	5–adult
Spatial cognition	Block design (WISC-III)	6–16
	Object assembly (WISC-III)	6–16
	Beery visuomotor integration	4–15
General mental ability	Based on above WISC-III subtests plus picture completion, picture arrangement, coding, and arithmetic	6–16
"Academic achievement"	Reading recognition (PIAT)	G1–12
	Reading comprehension (PIAT)	G1–12
	Spelling (PIAT and WRAT)	G1–12
	Math (PIAT)	G1–12
	Spelling (WRAT)	G1–12

[a]WISC-III = Wechsler Intelligence Scale for Children; PIAT = Peabody Individual Achievement Test; Woodcock-Johnson = Woodcock-Johnson Psycho-educational Battery—Revised.

As discussed previously, few human studies (with the exception of some on lead exposure) have used batteries of neuropsychological tests to investigate the effects of a developmental toxicant in disrupting specific aspects of cognitive function. A neuropsychological testing approach makes it possible to address the strength/weakness profiles of affected children, and thereby provides suggestive information about abnormalities in specific brain systems believed to mediate such functions. This knowledge then permits the development of hypotheses about particular neural substrates that may have been affected by the toxic insult. When coupled with more "bottom-up" observations derived from available clinical and experimental neuropathology data (especially those obtained from nonhuman primates), the resulting picture would be likely to implicate certain neural pathways or structures as important substrates for specific aspects of function.

CHARACTERISTICS OF STUDIES THAT HAVE EXAMINED COGNITIVE ENDPOINTS IN NONHUMAN PRIMATES EXPOSED TO DEVELOPMENTAL TOXICANTS

Table 3 reviews the characteristics of selected studies published since 1985 that have examined the developmental neurotoxicity of methylmercury and lead in nonhuman primates. This presentation is by no means exhaustive, but it is offered as representative. The number of monkeys used in typical developmental toxicity studies ranges from about 4 to 12 animals per treatment group. Methods appear to have been carefully selected through informed consideration of the human developmental cognitive literature, and their predictive validity to human cognitive processing has been empirically demonstrated in many cases (for discussion, see Burbacher et al., 1986; Gunderson et al., 1986; Rice, 1987). The studies presented indicate that, in the majority of cases, single tests have been used to assess cognitive compromise. It is difficult to judge the degree of severity of the reported group differences in performance and, therefore, difficult to determine the appropriate interpretation of the data for human risk evaluation. While it may sometimes be reasonable to assume that severely impaired performance might generalize across domains of processing (just as mentally retarded children may show impairments on multiple tasks), empirical findings are not always presented that address the severity or the specificity of the "deficit." While such studies can identify specific deficits in the form of processing assessed by the single test, they do not necessarily provide information about the specificity or generality of cognitive deficits across a variety of areas of processing. Therefore, interpretations of such findings as suggestive of increased human risk (for example, for mental retardation or mental deficiency or for a specific type of processing difficulty) must be made with great caution. This is especially true for certain clinical disorders such as attention deficit that are rigorously defined by diagnostic criteria demanding that the attentional deficit not be a symptom of a more general disorder such as mental retardation (American Psychiatric Association, 1987). Investigators working with laboratory animals generally recognize these difficulties and have been quite cautious in the interpretation of their findings.

To facilitate interpretation, it would be helpful to have information about general correlations in performance across tests and/or comparisons of performance across tests in animals with similar exposure histories. This is recognized and has been responsibly addressed by Rice (1992) and Burbacher et al. (1990b). Rice (1992) compared the performance of animals exposed to lead postnatally across multiple measures and with

Table 3 Characteristics of Selected Studies of the Cognitive Effects of Developmental Exposure to Methylmercury and Lead in Nonhuman Primates

Study	Species	Exposure level	Exposure period	Sample size[a]	Performance on single test reported	Performance on multiple tests compared
Burbacher et al., 1990b	Macaca fascicularis	MeHg: 0.96 ppm maternal; 1.56 ppm neonatal	Throughout gestation	12	Yes, indices of social behavior	Yes, to address possible confounding in interpretation
Burbacher et al., 1986	Macaca fascicularis	MeHg: 0.9–1.16 ppm maternal; 1.6 ppm neonatal	Throughout gestation	12	Yes, with longitudinal evaluation on object permanence tasks	No
Gunderson et al., 1986	Macaca fascicularis	MeHg: 1.0–1.3 ppm maternal; 1.7 ppm neonatal	Throughout gestation	10	Yes, visual recognition memory	No
Gunerson et al., 1988	Macaca fascicularis	MeHg: 1.0–1.3 ppm maternal; 1.7 ppm neonatal	Throughout gestation	9	Yes, visual recognition memory	No
Laughlin et al., 1991	Macaca mulatta	Lead: yr 1: 60–80 μg/dl; yr 2: 30–40 μg/dl	Neonatal day 5–365 with dietary manipulations	4	No	Yes, multiple measures of social behavior

Reference	Species	Dose	Exposure period	N		Effects
Levin and Bowman, 1986	*Macaca mulatta*	Lead: variable, pulsed; 0.7 mg/kg/d chronic 1 yr	Neonatal	5	No	Yes, Hamilton search task and delayed spatial alternation
Levin and Bowman, 1989	*Macaca mulatta*	Lead: variable, 1 mg/kg/d 1 yr; 32–70 µg/dl whole blood	Neonatal	25	Yes, delayed spatial alternation	No
Lilienthal et al., 1986	*Macaca mulatta*	Lead: 0, 350, or 600 ppm (ca. 0, 6, or 10 mg/kg)	Pre- and postnatal	17	Yes, learning set formation (also activity)	No
Rice, 1987	*Macaca fascicularis*	Lead: 2.2, 10.9, 13.1, or 33 µg/100 ml whole blood[b]; MeHg: 0.7–0.9 ppm in blood[b]	Day 1–200 r 270; Day 1–200	≥4; 5	In previous publications (Gilbert and Rice, 1987; Rice 1979, 1984, 1985, 1988, 1990; Rice and Gilbert 1985, 1990)	Lead: discrimination learning; reversal learning; spatial and nonspatial matching-to-sample fixed interval and differential reinforcement of low rate responding (FI & DRL) schedules of reinforcement; MeHg: visual perception of spatial frequency
Rice, 1992	*Macaca fascicularis*	Lead: 33 µg/dl[b]	Day 1–270	≥4	In previous publications	Yes, as above at 3 different ages

[a]The number represents the size of the exposed group only.
[b]These values represent sustained levels measured after the end of treatment administration.

testing at different ages. Burbacher et al. (1990b) addressed the specificity of effects on social behavior in monkeys exposed to methylmercury by examining correlations in performance on social and cognitive measures. Low correlations between impairments on the two types of function were demonstrated empirically and showed that social-behavior deficits were not confounded by generalized behavioral deficits.

The typical use of single-test methodological approaches does not necessarily preclude the examination of multiple indices of performance to characterize responses indicative of different aspects of processing or behavior. Thus, one can examine indices of attention to a given task as well as of correctness of performance of that task. Rice (1987) has pointed out the importance of examining rates of acquisition of task performance and within-subject variations in performance on schedule-controlled operant behavior, in addition to the more typical functional end points (e.g., total number of correct responses, total number of errors, and responses to criterion). Rice (1987) also suggests that these end points may be more sensitive in the detection of functional toxicity, particularly at low exposure levels, but this has yet to be demonstrated.

COMPARISON OF DEFICITS IN COGNITIVE FUNCTION FOLLOWING DEVELOPMENTAL EXPOSURE TO LEAD AND METHYLMERCURY—HUMAN VS. NONHUMAN-PRIMATE DATA

The available data concerning the cognitive effects of lead and methylmercury in humans and nonhuman primates make it very difficult to compare and contrast their effects across primate species. Human lead studies have examined the effects of prenatal plus postnatal exposure, whereas studies of nonhuman primates have generally restricted exposures to the postnatal period. Animal and human studies of methylmercury have been more similar with respect to the timing of dosing.

Testing methods for humans and nonhuman primates have also been different. Nevertheless, the methodologies used in primate studies have been demonstrated empirically to have predictive validity for comparable types of performance in humans. For example, Gunderson et al. (1986) carefully discussed the similarities in performance on similar tests of visual recognition memory by normal human and macaque infants as well as by high-risk infants of both species. Burbacher et al. (1986) have also presented information on the stages of development of Piagetian object permanence in macaque and human infants.

The validity of certain methodologies used with nonhuman primates has also been addressed more directly in studies where humans have performed similar tasks. For example, human adults with Alzheimer's-type dementia have been shown to have impaired performance of object-discrimination and non–matching-to-sample tasks that are frequently used with nonhuman primates. These observations demonstrate a high sensitivity for these tasks in assessing human amnestic disorders (Irle et al., 1987). Similarly, Kessler et al. (1986) found impairments in performance of object-discrimination tasks by humans with Korsakoff's psychosis, a disorder resulting from alcohol abuse and related thiamine deficiency.

With respect to the developmental effects of lead and methylmercury (or any other agent one might choose) on specific types of cognitive process, studies are simply not available that allow one to directly compare equivalent types of performance by comparably exposed humans and nonhuman primates. In general, however, studies of humans as well as nonhuman primates clearly demonstrate lead and methylmercury effects on "cognitive function" (see Burbacher et al., 1990a, for methylmercury; and Davis et al., 1990, and Rice, 1987, 1992, for lead).

With regard to specific aspects of cognitive function, only the lead literature permits equitable comparisons, and these comparisons do not implicate similar functional anomalies in humans and animals. As discussed above, preliminary data suggest that preschool children exposed prenatally and postnatally to low levels of lead (blood levels of 10–15 μg/dl) have deficits in spatial cognition that are associated with postnatal blood lead levels. Rice (1992) has suggested that monkeys exposed to higher levels of lead during the first year of life demonstrate weaknesses in a different domain. The monkeys have been reported to demonstrate more deficits in sustained performance of visual tasks performed under intermittent schedules of reinforcement than in other tasks.

Interestingly, these lead effects in nonhuman primates have been interpreted as reflecting differential test sensitivity as opposed to substrate differences in vulnerability. Generally speaking, animal researchers have tended to invoke this type of interpretation when effects on performance differ across tasks. In contrast, clinical researchers tend to focus on differential substrates or functional vulnerabilities more than on issues of "test sensitivities." It is important to acknowledge that whatever the focus of interpretation, the detectability of effects may vary with the quality of the normative or control data, the age of the subjects in relation to transitional stages of development relevant to the particular function of interest, and whether floor or ceiling effects bias the outcome of the test. While interpretation of human data may be reliable when methods include only "well-constructed" tests with empirically documented specificity, methodological characteristics deserve more scrutiny when effects are seen in tests with suboptimal construction features, less specificity, or poorly documented specificity. Age differences in the strengths of processing different types of information must also be considered.

Another issue of importance in the interpretation of the effects of lead exposure on later cognitive function is the relevance of the age at which exposure was measured. Human data suggest that antenatal blood levels are useful predictors of subsequent infant function (Bellinger et al., 1988; Dietrich et al., 1987; McMichael et al., 1988) and that blood lead levels measured at 2 years of age are better predictors of cognitive function at the ages of 4, 5, and 10 years than are levels obtained at the time of behavioral assessment (Bellinger et al., 1992; McMichael et al., 1988; Dietrich et al., 1991). There is a clear indication that an inverse relationship exists between blood lead concentration and cognitive function. These studies have also shown that postnatal blood lead levels tend to peak at 2 years of age. Therefore, the authors have suggested the possibility that the central nervous system may demonstrate an age-specific vulnerability at 2 years of age to disruptions relevant to later cognitive function. To our knowledge, this issue has not yet been examined in nonhuman primate models, studies of which have tended to focus on group differences. This may be due to the smallness of the sample sizes employed relative to the needs of the correlational analyses.

As previously discussed, several studies of the developmental effects of lead show that effects interact considerably with social class, so that children from economically less advantaged environments show cognitive deficits at lower blood lead levels than do children from families of higher socioeconomic status (see discussion by Dietrich et al., 1991). Animal models of differing levels of socioeconomic status have not yet been formally developed. However, differing degrees of environmental enrichment or different rearing procedures may provide a background against which to explore the cognitive effects of developmental neurotoxicants such as lead. Relevant to this topic, Rice (1992) has presented data that show attenuated task-specific effects of lead in 7-year-old monkeys that had an enriched environment (i.e., infant behavioral-testing experience).

RECOMMENDATIONS FOR THE FACILITATION OF THE EXTRAPOLATION OF ANIMAL DATA TO HUMANS

As shown by the experience with methylmercury and lead, it is evident that exposures to developmental neurotoxicants have occurred and probably will continue to occur among humans. However, studies in human populations after accidental or unintended exposures suffer from a plethora of experimental problems, not the least of which is providing data after the fact. Others include unknown exposure levels and durations; restricted assessment possibilities; concomitant exposures to other, sometimes several, neuroactive compounds; and multiple potentially confounding variables, including socioeconomic status, that result in poor or absent controls. In order to maximize scientific rigor and control and to minimize or prevent human exposure, it is preferable to gather such information from animal models. In fact, the primary method of predicting, a priori, the adverse effects of chemicals in humans (i.e., risk assessment) involves the extrapolation of data obtained from laboratory animals to humans. Obviously, the greater the phylogenetic difference between humans and the animals from which the data are obtained, the greater the likelihood of encountering important physiological differences that will affect how chemicals are absorbed, distributed, and metabolized and otherwise interact with the organism. The greater the physiological differences, the greater the likelihood that the observed chemical effects will be different and the greater the uncertainty of the extrapolation process. Thus, it is best to use data from animals as human-like as possible. Since many of our closest animal relatives, the great apes, are endangered and present substantial problems for housing, care, and assessment, the next-best animal surrogates are other, more manageable nonhuman primates such as monkeys and baboons. Specific issues concerning the validity, ethics, and importance to public health of using nonhuman primates as experimental subjects have been clearly discussed elsewhere (Evans, 1990).

In addition to the physiological differences between humans and the species for which data are collected to assess risk for developmental neurotoxicity, there have been (almost without exception) differences in the end points used to study specific brain functions (as in the lead and methylmercury studies). For example, water and radial-arm maze performance is often used as a means of studying learning behavior in rodent animal models; humans, however, generally do not function in water or radial-arm mazes. Although most animal researchers would support the thesis that aspects of water and radial-arm maze performance are relevant to learning, others find it difficult to interpret just how data collected with such procedures are related to the human situation. Recent efforts have been directed at developing "dry" water and radial-arm mazes for use with children (Overman et al., 1992; Peuster et al., 1991), so that at least similar end points can be monitored across species. The task now will be to demonstrate the significance of water and radial-arm maze performance by humans. Here we wish to discuss how one might better design studies of complex brain function in nonhuman primates (and other animals) to facilitate the use of data obtained from laboratory models to predict adverse effects on cognitive functions in humans.

As mentioned, an obstacle to the direct extrapolation of "cognitive" data obtained with nonhuman primates to humans has derived from the fact that, historically, cognitive processes in animals have been studied largely by monitoring behaviors whose specific relationships, or lack thereof, with cognitive processes in humans are unknown. The concept of face validity then has to be invoked when such measures in animals are used as surrogates for measures of cognitive processes in humans. Therefore, in the process of interpreting the effects of toxicants on animal behavior and predicting likely outcomes for human exposures (i.e., extrapolation), a certain leap of faith has traditionally been required, such that substantial uncertainty remains in the risk-assessment process.

In the area of behavioral pharmacology, a discipline that has benefited greatly from the use of animal behavior models, such problems in extrapolation have been addressed by the empirical demonstration of correlations between drug effects on specific animal behaviors and their clinical efficacies (e.g., Cook and Sepinwall, 1975). For example, the ability of the benzodiazepines and other compounds to increase "punished" responding in animal models correlates well with their antianxiety properties in humans. Research in behavioral pharmacology has, however, been driven by the need for product development and has thus been well supported by the private sector. Research in behavioral toxicology, on the other hand, does not generally lead to product development, and could lead to a termination of that process. Thus, in comparison with those in behavioral pharmacology, research efforts in behavioral toxicology have been much slower.

Major efforts need to be focused on the collection of basic research data that will demonstrate how given behaviors in animals do or do not relate to given behaviors in humans. Additionally, efforts must be greatly expanded to study the effects of reference compounds, such as reversibly acting psychoactive drugs and chemicals (as well as prototypic neurotoxicants), on select animal behaviors. These effects can then be compared with the effects of specific brain lesions in the same animal model and with their effects in humans, when these are known. This approach allows assessment of the predictive validity of given animal behaviors, even in the absence of data demonstrating their relationship (or lack thereof) to specific human behaviors. For example, the acute effects of marijuana smoke and δ-9-tetrahydrocannabinol (THC; the active ingredient in marijuana smoke) on several operant behaviors have been determined in rhesus monkeys. Some of the behaviors monitored in these studies that have used an operant test battery (OTB) (Schulze et al., 1988, 1989a) have face validity in modeling short-term memory and time-estimation behaviors in humans. In those studies, time estimation behavior was shown to be very sensitive to disruption by the acute intravenous administration of THC, whereas behavior in the short-term memory task was very sensitive to the acute effects of both marijuana smoke and THC. Those data, along with those from several other studies of acute and chronic drug effects on OTB performance by monkeys (Ferguson and Paule, 1992, 1993; Paule et al., 1992a; Schulze et al., 1989b; Schulze and Paule, 1990; 1991; Schulze et al., 1992) have demonstrated the predictive validity of these tasks: data obtained from the monkey are analogous to those obtained from humans performing tasks thought to depend on similar brain functions. The observation that performance in a given task is more sensitive to the effects of a given compound than is performance in another task suggests, as mentioned previously, that differing neural substrates are involved in the performance of different tasks.

Most efforts in nonhuman-primate behavioral toxicology utilize behaviors that have face validity with respect to important cognitive functions in humans. For example, schedule-controlled operant behaviors (see Cory-Slechta, 1992) have been utilized in monkeys (e.g., Rice, 1987) to model aspects of intellectual functioning that include learning, memory, distractibility, and adaptability. Importantly, these techniques can be used with animals as soon as they can self-feed (Rice 1979; Rice and Gilbert, 1990) and therefore can be used early, as well as late, in developmental studies of the effects of prenatal or early neonatal exposures to toxicants. Additionally, these behaviors can be readily automated and are often presented as versions of tasks that have been administered using the Wisconsin General Test Apparatus (WGTA; e.g., see Mishkin and Delacour, 1975) in studies designed to explore brain structure/function relationships in monkeys. An example of such a task is a derivation of one that was mentioned earlier: the delayed matching-to-sample task that is often used to model short-term memory (e.g., Evans et al., 1986; Paule 1990; Rice 1984). Thus, data exist for nonhuman primates performing analogous short-term memory tasks: comparisons of the effects of brain lesions on performance of the WGTA version of the task with drug effects in the automated version may prove valuable in helping to determine possible anatomical sites of action for given neuroactive compounds.

Few attempts to measure behaviors that have exact human equivalents have yet been made in the animal laboratory. Thus, in tasks designed to model short-term memory in animals, the specific behavioral topographies have generally been different from those used to assess short-term memory in humans: levers and push-buttons are often used for animals, computer touch screens (Sahakian et al., 1988) and paper-and-pencil or verbal responses for humans. Therefore, even though animal behavioral tasks often have face and predictive validity, the actual behaviors measured in them have not been, by virtue of the different manipulanda used in task performance, exactly the same as those that would normally be used with humans. There are a few exceptions to this observation (e.g., Ringo et al., 1986, comparing picture memory in both humans and monkeys), but new computer-assisted designs are helping to eliminate such differences in a variety of tasks (e.g., Washburn et al., 1989; Hopkins et al., 1990; Schulze et al., 1988; Chavoix et al., 1991). Until the importance of such differences is determined, or until they are eliminated, uncertainty in the extrapolation of animal data to humans will remain.

In attempts to address this issue, efforts at the National Center for Toxicological Research (NCTR) and Arkansas Children's Hospital have focused over the past few years on using a standardized operant test battery (the NCTR OTB) to quantitate behaviors thought to be dependent on specific complex brain functions in rhesus monkeys (e.g., Paule et al., 1988a; Paule, 1990; Schulze et al., 1988) and humans (Paule et al., 1988b; 1990; Paule and Cranmer, 1990). The operant tasks employed in the OTB and the brain functions modeled include incremental repeated acquisition for assessment of learning; delayed matching-to-sample for short-term memory and attention; temporal response differentiation for time-estimation; conditioned position responding for color and position discrimination; and progressive ratio for motivation. Compelling similarities in OTB performance by children and nonhuman primates have been demonstrated (Paule et al., 1990): the OTB performance of well-trained 4-year-old rhesus monkeys is essentially the same as that of children aged 4 to 10 years, depending on the task. In these studies, both children and nonhuman primates were required to perform these tasks with the use of identical operant-behavioral panels and manipulanda, the only difference being that monkeys responded for banana-flavored food pellets and children responded for nickels.

Importantly, these studies have also demonstrated that several OTB behaviors in children (including those that model short-term memory and attention, learning, and color and position discrimination) correlate significantly with measures of human full-scale, verbal, and performance IQ scores as determined by performance on the Weschler Preschool Primary Scale of Intelligence, the Peabody Picture Vocabulary Test–Revised, and the Developmental Test of Visual-Motor Integration, respectively (Paule et al., 1992b; Paule 1993). Accuracy and response rate in the time-estimation task, for example, correlate significantly with performance IQ; certain measures of learning-task performance have correlation coefficients of over 0.5 with performance IQ, and correlations of near 0.6 have been noted for aspects of performance in the color- and position-discrimination task. Thus, certain measures of schedule-controlled operant behavior should be predictive of IQ in children and, by analogy, should provide a means for estimating nonhuman equivalents of IQ. Likewise, operant behavioral measures in animals should be useful as biomarkers for predicting the adverse effects of chemicals on measures of intellectual capacity or cognitive ability in humans. It is likely that many schedule-controlled operant behaviors, in addition to those utilized in the NCTR OTB, as well as other types of behavior will also correlate significantly with the more traditional measures of human intellectual capacity. For example, Sen et al. (1983) have shown that simple and choice visual and auditory reaction times correlate with measures of IQ in adult humans. Fagan and McGrath (1981) and Fagan and Singer (1983) have shown that recognition memory in infants is predictive of later intelligence, and a nonhuman animal model employing similar visual-exploration tasks was developed by Levin et al. (1986) and used to study the developmental effects of lead exposure in rhesus monkeys (Levin et al., 1988). Thus, the concern expressed by Winneke (1992) that no direct counterparts to IQ exist in animals may not be fully warranted.

Future efforts should be directed at further exploration of the correlations between specific behaviors of interest to laboratory animal researchers and measures of human behavior deemed important measures of intellectual capacity or achievement. Those behaviors that are found to be associated with performance in instruments that have proved to be useful clinically or in educational settings should then be widely exploited by experimentalists. Additionally, it will be important to develop the same tasks that are used in humans, or at least analogous ones, for use in animals. These should clearly include those used in the traditional neuropsychological arena (see Table 2) and measures of modality-specific memory, right-left discriminations, etc. Such an approach has also been advocated by Vorhees (1992). These efforts will serve to validate additional animal behaviors and demonstrate their relevance to human brain function. Data from such studies will go a long way toward eliminating the uncertainty of using animal behaviors as biomarkers for detecting chemical effects and extrapolating such data to humans. A more thorough understanding of species differences and similarities will provide the crucial information for determining when extrapolation across species is appropriate.

Tasks that are identical or analogous to those performed by humans and nonhuman primates need to be developed for a variety of other laboratory animals, including rodents. Toward this end an automated schedule-controlled operant behavioral system for use with rats, nonhuman primates, humans, and other species is under development at the NCTR, and experiments have been initiated to determine the effects of reference compounds on selected rodent OTB behaviors. Results from these studies will be used to determine the applicability of rodent behavioral data in predicting the cognitive effects of chemicals (assessing risk) in nonhuman primates and humans. The process of cross-species validation needs to proceed empirically in tandem with the development of multispecies behavioral tasks. It will be important that the behavioral tasks chosen be readily automatable, since this will help to minimize the human resources needed to collect the necessary data and minimize the interaction of experimenter with subject. While important and informative, "hands-on" procedures for assessing the cognitive status of young nonhuman primates, such as those that need to be used in nursery-type environments, will probably be too resource-intensive to be applied on the broad scale necessary for the task at hand.

Evidence continues to mount in support of the contention that specific complex behaviors in animals have direct relevance to aspects of important complex brain functions in humans. The automation of such tasks should greatly increase our ability to collect the empirical data necessary to determine the relevance (correlation) of a given behavior in one species to the same or other behaviors in other species and to other behaviors in the same species. Batteries of specific behaviors need to be developed with a view toward using behavioral end points to determine the effects (developmental or otherwise) of chemicals on the integrity of multiple cognitive functional domains in animals. Toxicant effects on these specific animal behaviors can then be used with diminished uncertainty in risk assessments for effects on important human brain functions.

REFERENCES

Adams J, Vorhees CV, Middaugh LD (1990). Developmental neurotoxicity of anticonvulsants: human and animal evidence on phenytoin. Neurotoxicol Teratol 12:203–14.

Bellinger D, Leviton A, Waternaux C, Needleman H, Rabinowitz M (1987). Longitudinal analyses of prenatal and postnatal lead exposure and early cognitive development. N Engl J Med 316:1037–43.

Bellinger D, Leviton A, Waternaux C, Needleman H, Rabinowitz M (1988). Low-level lead exposure, social class, and infant development. Neurotoxicol Teratol 10:497–503.

Bellinger D, Sloman J, Leviton A, Rabinowitz M, Needleman HL, Waternaux C (1991). Low-level lead exposure and children's cognitive function in the preschool years. Pediatrics 87:219–27.

Bellinger D, Stiles KM, Needleman HL (1992). Low level lead exposure, intelligence, and academic achievement: a long term follow-up study. Pediatrics 90:855–61.

Burbacher TM, Grant KS, Mottet NK (1986). Retarded object permanence development in methylmercury exposed Macaca fascicularis infants. Dev Psychol 22:771–6.

Burbacher TM, Rodier PM, Weiss B (1990a). Methylmercury developmental neurotoxicity: a comparison of effects in humans and animals. Neurotoxicol Teratol 12:191–201.

Burbacher TM, Sackett GP, Mottet NK (1990b). Methylmercury effects on the social behavior of Macaca fascicularis infants. Neurotoxicol Teratol 12:65–71.

Chavoix C, Hagger C, Sirigu A, Gravelle M, Aigner T (1991). An automated delayed nonmatching-to-sample task to assess visual recognition memory in humans (abstr). Soc Neurosci Abstr 17:476.

Cook L, Seppinwall J (1975). Reinforcement schedules and extrapolations to humans from animals in behavioral pharmacology. Fed Proc 34:1889–97.

Cory-Slechta DA (1992). Schedule-controlled behavior in neurotoxicology. In: Tilson HA, Mitchell CL, eds. Neurotoxicology. New York: Raven Press, 271–94.

Davis JM, Otto DA, Weil DE, Grant LD (1990). The comparative developmental neurotoxicity of lead in humans and animals. Neurotoxicol Teratol 12:215–29.

Day N (1992). The effects of prenatal alcohol exposure. In: Zagon I, Slotkin T, eds. Maternal substance abuse and the developing nervous system. Orlando, Florida: Academic Press, 27–44.

Denckla MB (1991). Forward. In: Pennington BF, ed. Diagnosing learning disabilities. New York: The Guilford Press, vii-x.

Dietrich KN, Kraft KM, Bornschein RL, Hammond PB, Berger O, Succop PA, Bier M (1987). Low level fetal lead exposure effect on neurobehavioral development in early infancy. Pediatrics 80:721–30.

Dietrich KN, Succop PA, Berger OG, Hammond PB, Bornschein RL (1991). Lead exposure and the cognitive development of urban preschool children: the Cincinnati lead study cohort at age 4 years. Neurotoxicol Teratol 13:203–11.

Eckerman DA, Bushnell PJ (1992). The neurotoxicology of cognition: attention, learning, and memory. In: Tilson HA, Mitchell CL, eds. Neurotoxicology. New York: Raven Press, 213–70.

Evans HL, Bushnell PJ, Reuhl KR, Graefe JF (1986). Cognitive dysfunction and neuropathological changes in macaque monkeys induced by trimethyltin (TMT). Toxicologist 6:215.

Evans HL (1990). Nonhuman primates in behavioral toxicology: issues of validity, ethics and public health. Neurotoxicol Teratol 12:531–6.

Fagan JF, McGrath SK (1981). Infant recognition memory and later intelligence. Intelligence 8:1–9.

Fagan JF, Singer LT (1983). Infant recognition memory as a measure of intelligence. In: Lipsitt LP, ed. Advances in infancy research. Vol. 2. Norwood, New Jersey: Ablex, 31–78.

Ferguson SA, Paule MG (1992). Acute effects of chlorpromazine in a monkey operant behavioral test battery. Pharmacol Biochem Behav 42:333–41.

Ferguson SA, Paule MG (1993). Acute effects of pentobarbital in a monkey operant behavioral test battery. Pharmacol Biochem Behav (in press).

Gilbert SG, Rice DC (1987). Low level lifetime lead exposure produces behavioral toxicity (spatial discrimination reversal) in adult monkeys. Toxicol Appl Pharmacol 91:484–90.

Gunderson VM, Grant KS, Burbacher TM, Fagan JF, Mottet NK (1986). The effect of low level prenatal methylmercury exposure on visual recognition memory in infant crab-eating macaques. Child Dev 57:1076–83.

Gunderson VM, Grant-Webster KS, Burbacher TM, Mottet NK (1988). Visual recognition memory deficits in methylmercury-exposed Macaca fascicularis infants. Neurotoxicol Teratol 10:373–9.

Harada Y (1977). Congenital Minamata disease. In: Tsubak R, Irukayama K, eds. Minamata disease: methylmercury poisoning in Minamata and Niigata. Tokyo: Kodansha, 209–39.

Hopkins WD, Washburn DA, Rumbaugh DM (1990). Processing of form stimuli presented unilaterally in humans, chimpanzees *(Pan troglodytes)*, and monkeys *(Macaca mulatta)*. Behav Neurosci 104:577–82.

Irle E, Kessler J, Markowitsch HJ, Hofmann W (1987). Primate learning tasks reveal strong impairments in patients with presenile or senile dementia of the Alzheimer type. Brain Cogn 6:429–49.

Kaplan E, Fein D, Morris R, Delis D (1991). Manual for WAIS-R as a neuropsychological instrument. San Antonio: The Psychological Corporation.

Kessler J, Irle E, Markowitsch HJ (1986). Korsakoff and alcoholic subjects are severely impaired in animal tests of associative memory. Neuropsychologia 24:671–80.

Laughlin NK (1986). Animal models of the behavioral effects of early lead exposure. In: Riley EP, Vorhees CV, eds. Handbook of behavioral teratology. New York: Plenum Press, 291–320.

Laughlin NK, Bushnell PJ, Bowman RE (1991). Lead exposure and diet: differential effects on social development in the rhesus monkey. Neurotoxicol Teratol 13:429–40.

Levin ED, Bowman RE (1986). Comparative sensitivity of the Hamilton search task and delayed spatial alternation in detecting long-term effects of neonatal lead exposure in monkeys. Neurobehav Toxicol Teratol 8:219–24.

Levin ED, Bowman RE (1989). Longterm effects of chronic postnatal lead exposure on delayed spatial alternation in monkeys. Neurotoxicol Teratol 10:505–10.

Levin ED, Boehm KM, Hagquist WW, Bowman RE (1986). A visual exploration apparatus for infant monkeys. Am J Primatol 10:195–9.

Levin ED, Schneider ML, Ferguson SA, Schantz SL, Bowman RE (1988). Behavioral effects of developmental lead exposure in rhesus monkeys. Dev Psychobiol 21:371–82.

Lezak MD (1983). Neuropsychological assessment. New York: Oxford University Press.

Lilienthal H, Winneke G, Brockhaus A, Malik B (1986). Pre- and postnatal lead exposure in monkeys: effects on activity and learning set formation. Neurobehav Toxicol Teratol 8:265–72.

Mactutus CF (1985). Conceptual and procedural considerations for developmental assessment of learning and memory (dys)function following neurotoxicant exposure. Neurobehav Toxicol Teratol 7:703–8.

Marsh DO (1987). Dose-response relationships in humans: methylmercury epidemics in Japan and Iraq. In: Ecules CU, Annau Z, eds. The toxicity of methylmercury. Baltimore: Johns Hopkins University Press, 45–53.

McMichael AJ, Baghurst PA, Wigg NR, Vimpani GV, Robertson EF, Roberts RJ (1988). Port Pirie cohort study: environmental exposure to lead and children's abilities at the age of 4 years. N Engl J Med 319:468–75.

Mishkin M, Delacour J (1975). An analysis of short-term visual memory in the monkey. J Exp Psychol Anim Behav Proc 104:326–34.

Overman WH, Carter L, Thompson S (1992). Development of place memory in children as measured in a dry Morris maze (abstr). Soc Neurosci Abstr 18:332.

Paule MG, Schulze GE, Slikker W Jr (1988a). Complex brain function in monkeys as a baseline for studying the effects of exogenous compounds. Neurotoxicology 9:463–70.

Paule MG, Cranmer JM, Wilkins JD, Stern HP, Hoffman EL (1988b). Quantitation of complex brain function in children: preliminary evaluation using a nonhuman primate behavioral test battery. Neurotoxicology 9:367–78.

Paule MG (1990). Use of the NCTR operant test battery in nonhuman primates. Neurotoxicol Teratol 12:413–8.

Paule MG, Cranmer JM (1990). Complex brain function in children as measured in the NCTR monkey operant test battery. In: Johnson BL, ed. Advances in neurobehavioral toxicology: applications in environmental and occupational health. Chelsea, Michigan: Lewis, 433–47.

Paule MG, Forrester TM, Maher MA, Cranmer JM, Allen RR (1990). Monkey versus human performance in the NCTR operant test battery. Neurotoxicol Teratol 12:503–7.

Paule MG, Allen RR, Bailey JR, Scallet AC, Ali SF, Brown RM, Slikker W Jr (1992a). Chronic marijuana smoke exposure in the rhesus monkey. II: Effects on progressive ratio and conditioned position responding. J Pharmacol Exp Ther 260:210–22.

Paule MG, Blake DJ, Allen RR, Casey PH (1992b). NCTR operant test battery (OTB) performance in children: correlation with IQ (abstr). Soc Neurosci Abstr 18:332.

Paule MG (1993). Analysis of brain function using a battery of schedule-controlled operant behaviors. In: Weiss B, O'Donoghue J, eds. Toxicological interpretation of neurobehavioral data. New York: Raven Press (in press).

Pennington BF (1991). Diagnosing learning disabilities. New York: The Guilford Press.

Peuster A, Overman AH, Caulfield S, Hakan R (1991). Radial arm maze measures development of spatial memory in young children (abstr). Soc Neurosci Abstr 17:1044.

Rice DC (1979). Operant conditioning of infant monkeys (Macaca fascicularis) for toxicity testing. Neurobehav Toxicol 1(suppl 1):85–92.

Rice DC (1984). Behavioral deficit (delayed matching to sample) in monkeys exposed from birth to low levels of lead. Toxicol Appl Pharmacol 75:337–45.

Rice DC (1985). Chronic low level lead exposure from birth produces deficits in discrimination reversal in monkeys. Toxicol Appl Pharmacol 77:201–10.

Rice DC (1987). Methodological approaches to primate behavioral toxicological testing. Neurotoxicol Teratol 9:161–9.

Rice DC (1988). Schedule-controlled behavior in infant and juvenile monkeys exposed to lead from birth. Neurotoxicol 9:75–88.

Rice DC (1990). Lead-induced behavioral impairment on a spatial discrimination reversal task in monkeys exposed during different periods of development. Toxicol Appl Pharmacol 106:327–333.

Rice DC (1992). Behavioral effects of lead in monkeys tested during infancy and adulthood. Neurotoxicol Teratol 14:235–45.

Rice DC, Gilbert SG (1985). Low lead exposure from birth produces behavioral toxicity (DRL) in monkeys. Toxicol Appl Pharmacol 80:421–6.

Rice DC, Gilbert SG (1990). Automated behavioral procedures for infant monkeys. Neurotoxicol Teratol 12:429–39.

Ringo JL, Lewine JD, Doty RW (1986). Comparable performance by man and macaque on memory for pictures. Neuropsychologia 24:711–7.

Sahakian BJ, Morris RG, Evenden JL, Heald A, Levy R, Philpot M, Robbins T (1988). A comparative study of visuospatial memory and learning in Alzheimer-type dementia and Parkinson's disease. Brain 111:695–718.

Schulze GE, McMillan DE, Bailey JR, Scallet AC, Ali SF, Slikker W Jr, Paule MG (1988). Acute effects of delta-9-tetrahydrocannabinol (THC) in rhesus monkeys as measured by performance in a battery of cognitive function tests. J Pharmacol Exp Ther 245:178–86.

Schulze GE, McMillan DE, Bailey JR, Scallet AC, Ali SF, Slikker W Jr, Paule MG (1989a). Acute effects of marijuana smoke on complex operant behavior in rhesus monkeys. Life Sci 45:465–75.

Schulze GE, Slikker W Jr, Paule MG (1989b). Multiple behavioral effects of diazepam in rhesus monkeys. Pharmacol Biochem Behav 34:29–35.

Schulze GE, Paule MG (1990). Acute effects of *d*-amphetamine in a monkey operant behavioral test battery. Pharmacol Biochem Behav 35:759–65.

Schulze GE, Paule MG (1991). Effects of morphine sulfate on operant behavior in rhesus monkeys. Pharmacol Biochem Behav 38:77–83.

Schulze GE, Gillam MP, Paule MG (1992). Effects of atropine on operant test battery performance in rhesus monkeys. Life Sci 51:487–97.

Sen A, Jensen AR, Sen AK, Arora I (1983). Correlation between reaction time and intelligence in psychometrically similar groups in American and India. Appl Res Ment Retard 4:139–52.

Vorhees CV (1992). Developmental neurotoxicology. In: Tilson HA, Mitchell CL, eds. Neurotoxicology. New York: Raven Press, 295–329.

Washburn DA, Hopkins WD, Rumbaugh DM (1989). Automation of learning-set testing: the video-task paradigm. Behav Res Meth Instr Comp 21:281–4.

Winneke G (1992). Cross species extrapolation in neurotoxicology: neurophysiological and neurobehavioral aspects. Neurotoxicology 13:15–26.

27
Behavioral and Functional Ontogeny: Biomarkers of Neurotoxicity

Charles V. Vorhees
University of Cincinnati and Children's Hospital Research Foundation
Cincinnati, Ohio

INTRODUCTION

Behavioral teratology is the study of developmental disabilities of prenatal origin. Within the larger field of neurotoxicology, behavioral teratology has the distinction of having been the first area to be incorporated into regulatory requirements for new drug approval. These regulatory guidelines, first issued by Japan and Great Britain more than 15 years ago, are important events in the progress of the field (Vorhees, 1986a). The importance lies in the recognition that this is a significant form of toxicity and that the state of knowledge in the field was sufficient to make its evaluation feasible. The intent of the guidelines was to provide protection against drugs that might cause in utero brain injury. In approaching the task of how this would be accomplished, the regulatory authorities made most of the test specifications behavioral. This was also done under later guidelines from the European Community and the U.S. Environmental Protection Agency (EPA). There are four reasons for this approach.

First, behavioral assessment reflects the integrated output of the central nervous system (CNS). Therefore, if behavior is abnormal it is reasonable to infer that some underlying brain process is disrupted. Behavior is perhaps the best overall gauge of brain abnormality, because the CNS is too complex to be comprehensively assessed by highly specific, site-directed biochemical or histological techniques.

Second, behavior can be used to measure the magnitude of a dysfunction regardless of its location within the brain and therefore provides quantitative information concerning the severity of the effect and qualitative information on the type of dysfunction that is present (e.g., expressive vs. receptive language disorder).

Third, since functional assessment is noninvasive, it can be measured repeatedly. In humans this is especially important, since invasive procedures may not be possible.

Fourth, functional assessment often detects adverse effects that cannot be detected with current cellular or molecular techniques. Despite great progress in cellular and

733

molecular biology, behavioral methods remain the standard for documenting both the extent and the temporal onset of the effects of neurotoxins, such as lead's effects on cognitive function.

This is not to say that functional assessment exists in isolation. Increasingly, neuroimaging techniques are becoming important. Hartman (1988) has suggested that the combination of neuropsychological, psychometric, neuroimaging, and neurophysiological methods of assessment is needed to provide a complete understanding of neurotoxic effects in humans. A similar view has recently been suggested for understanding neurotoxic effects in animals (Vorhees, 1992).

The four factors outlined above explain why behavioral methods have been used for the detection of potential neurotoxins. The next issue to consider is why the developing brain is vulnerable, perhaps uniquely vulnerable, to damaging influences. Four characteristics make the developing CNS susceptible: its structural complexity; the protracted time over which its development occurs; the slow maturation of the blood-brain barrier as a defense against exogenous influences; and the slow-to-develop metabolic capacities that functionalize (usually detoxify) exogenous agents. Before discussing the details of each of these, one semantic point requires clarification. In recent years the term "behavioral teratology" has increasingly been replaced with the slightly more general term developmental neurotoxicology.[*] This term has the advantage of including both pre- and postnatal development and not appearing to exclude nonbehavioral effects. Behavioral teratology was never exclusionary (see Vorhees, 1989) but was sometimes taken to be so.

The first factor contributing to the vulnerability of the CNS is its complexity. It has been estimated that one-third of all the genes in the human genome are expressed in nervous system tissue. This proportion is thought to be higher than for any other tissue and illustrates the huge number of gene regulation and expression processes that are required to orchestrate a fully developed and functionally integrated nervous system. It should be obvious that the more processes are involved in the formation and functioning of a structure, the more possibilities there are for something to go awry.

One of the first stages of nervous system vulnerability occurs during early organogenesis, when neurons are rapidly proliferating. A timetable for dates of neuronal birth in different brain regions for rodents has been synthesized from the literature by Rodier (1980). This time-course map is illustrated in Fig. 1, with scales for the mouse and the rat shown along the abscissa. Proliferating cells can be interfered with by agents that act on any step in the cell cycle, and there are a wide variety of drugs and physical agents (e.g., ionizing radiation) that are known to have antimitotic/antiproliferative effects. Neurogenesis is followed by cell migration, in which nascent neurons (neuroblasts) travel to their final destinations within the brain through intervening cell layers, guided by radial glia (Kimelberg and Norenberg, 1989). During this stage, interference by exogenous agents can cause ectopic cell masses because of migration errors or improper layering, even if cells reach the vicinity of their intended destinations. Neuronal migration is followed by differentiation, in which cells are morphologically transformed into specific neuron types. The processes include neurite outgrowth through elongation of axonal and dendritic

---

[*] Herein, a compound that induces neurotoxicity or developmental neurotoxicity will be termed a neurotoxin or developmental neurotoxin. This follows the precedent of current usage in neuroscience as illustrated by authors such as Koob and Bloom (1988), D'Amato et al. (1986), and many others, by Dorland's Medical Dictionary, and by lexicographers at Merriam-Webster (Dr. R. W. Pease, personal communication), rather than the more cumbersome term "neurotoxicant."

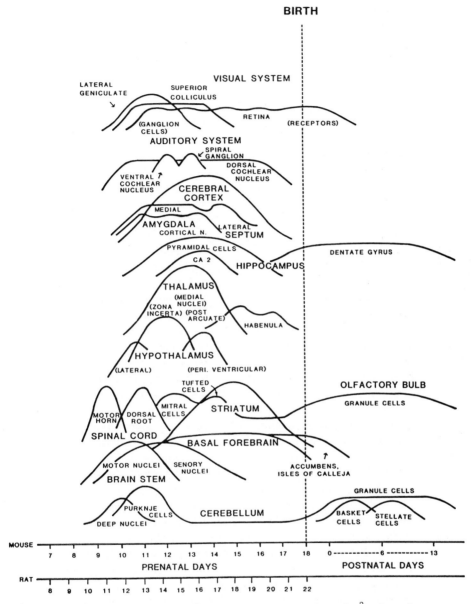

Figure 1   Stages of neurogenesis in different regions of rodent brain by ^{3}H-thymidine incorporation. Adapted originally from Rodier (1980) and reprinted here with modifications from Vorhees (1987).

processes at growth cones. Neurite growth consists of process extension, substrate adhesion, and actin-driven traction and movement. A central question is how neuronal processes find and maintain their targets. Neuroglia play a role in this process by guiding neuronal migration along radial glia, as mentioned above (Kimelberg and Norenberg, 1989). Mounting evidence also supports the role of retrograde transport of growth factors, which not only provide critical tropic or guidance information, but also provide a tonic trophic influence to sustain already established pathways (Crutcher, 1986). Another process is arborization of dendritic spines. This is a crucial process, since these are the sites of synapse formation. Insults during any of these differentiation processes can lead to abnormal cellular morphology and disorganized fiber tracts. This in turn can result in a loss of integration and a system that functions improperly, as has been demonstrated for the visual system when one or both eyes are sutured closed during critical periods of development (Kalil, 1989).

Neurotransmitter expression also occurs during synaptogenesis. Inappropriate signals from exogenous agents may cause shifts in genetic messages that trigger specific neurotransmitters to be synthesized and released in particular neurons. While this process is known to possess some plasticity, disruption may cause one neurotransmitter to be over- or underrepresented, leading to signaling disproportions and the potential for functional disequilibria. Normal development culminates in integration of synaptic function. Such processes appear to depend on waves of synchronized endogenous neuronal discharges. This has been demonstrated most clearly within developing retinal ganglion cell areas, where waves of firing spread across particular regions, but between regions and between the eyes the discharges are asynchronous. This pattern appears important in the formation of the functional layers in the lateral geniculate and visual cortex. Such layering is known to be critical for proper development of vision (Shatz, 1992).

All of these developmental processes, proliferation, migration, differentiation, synaptogenesis, and functional integration, are regulated by a complex array of developmental genes that are influenced by tissue-specific factors and experience-linked neuronal feedback. Gene regulation, tissue-specific factors, and feedback loops are potential targets of exogenous agents. Thus, an agent such as retinoic acid is thought to interfere with development by disrupting the normal function of this morphogen's endogenous concentration gradient, thereby distorting signals critical to normal pattern formation in several tissues, including the CNS.

The second factor accounting for the developing CNS's vulnerability may be traced to its extended timetable of development. Organogenesis for most tissues occurs during early development: embryogenesis. For example, the window of vulnerability for cardiac development begins and ends in humans within an 8-week period following implantation. However, for the CNS the comparable processes extend from embryogenesis, through fetogenesis, to postnatal development to 4–6 years in human beings. Such protracted development presents a broader window for potential interaction and interference from environmental agents than exists for most other organs or systems.

A third factor contributing to the risk confronting the immature CNS is the incompletely developed blood-brain barrier. The adult CNS is a privileged site within the body, so that entry of molecules into most of the brain is restricted by the blood-brain barrier, except in some periventricular nuclei (Goldstein and Betz, 1986). The blood-brain barrier is formed from special tight-junction neuroepithelial cells. The tight junctions prevent crossing of many molecules except those that are small, uncharged, or lipophilic, or for which there is a selective and specific CNS transporter. The selectivity of the blood-brain barrier protects the CNS from many environmental agents that gain access to the systemic circulation. However, the blood-brain barrier is immature during embryonic, fetal, and neonatal development in many mammals (Risau and Wolburg, 1990). The consequence of this is the inability of the developing brain to exclude many blood-borne molecules that would be restricted from the adult brain. Once in the developing brain, exogenous agents have access to the many complex processes of neuronal development outlined above.

Further complicating the situation is the fact that the capacity of the embryo and fetus to clear exogenous materials is lower than that of adults. This brings us to the fourth factor contributing to the vulnerability of the developing CNS. Early in development, both liver and brain P-450 metabolizing enzymes are immature. Once an agent enters the embryonic or fetal circulation it may remain there longer than in the adult, making repeated passes through the brain. When an agent is in the fetal CNS, the immaturity of P-450 enzymes in the brain itself reduces the ability of neural tissue to detoxify and eliminate it (Tyndale et al., 1991).

The situation is not entirely one-sided. Although the developing brain has characteristics that make it especially vulnerable to interference, it has defenses as well. The first of these is that more neurons are produced than are needed, and this surplus pool may serve as a reservoir against losses sustained from exogenous agents. Normally, the excess cells are reduced to sustainable numbers through apoptosis (Altman, 1992). This process is thought to be controlled by a cell's target tissues (Purves and Lichtman, 1985), but if cells are killed by a drug, apoptosis is reduced and the right final cell number may still be achieved. In addition to excess cell production, cells have an array of repair mechanisms that can be triggered to help them maintain their developmental course even when exposed to disruptive influences.

Repair mechanisms are often sufficient to rescue an organism from death, but not necessarily from residual injury. This occurs when the damage exceeds the reserve and repair capacities but is not so massive as to be lethal. In this situation one might expect the disability to be obvious, as it is when limbs sustain similar kinds of injury and limb defects such as ectrodactaly or polydactaly are seen. This is not the case in the brain, where effects can be difficult to characterize. This difference apparently occurs because of the brain's adaptive capacity and because many complex CNS functions are not pre-wired, but are acquired by accrual of component abilities; for example, the brain's ability to handle language depends on its capacity to acquire fundamental semantic, grammatical, and lexical abilities first. Higher-level abilities (and hence disabilities) do not become evident until after the prerequisite lower-level skills are acquired and integrated. Therefore, adaptation and skill acquisition may make underlying dysfunctions invisible at birth and during early life, with dysfunction becoming apparent only when the higher-level integration of these skills is required for a function such as expressive language. Such effects may be described as latent, since they require years to become evident. The residual damage the organism sustained during insult may also be difficult to detect by other means, such as gross pathology. Brain mass and cytoarchitecture often appear unchanged despite the presence of severe functional disorder. While new techniques of quantitative histology and immunocytochemistry and other approaches can sometimes reveal more specific effects, it has repeatedly been observed that identifying the neuropathological substrate of behavioral abnormalities in developing organisms is difficult.

Four reasons have been outlined for the view that the developing CNS is more vulnerable to irreversible injury than the adult CNS. To summarize, these were structural and functional complexity, protracted developmental period, the incomplete development of the blood-brain barrier, and immaturity of the metabolic capacity that enables exogenous agents to be detoxified. However, all of these factors are theoretical. Is there any empirical basis to support these suppositions? There is in fact considerable empirical evidence that the developing CNS is more vulnerable than the adult brain to insult, and this evidence has been described in several recent reports (Office of Technology Assessment, 1990; National Research Council, 1992) and review papers (Vorhees, 1992; Kimmel et al., 1990;

Riley and Vorhees, 1986). These represent but a few examples of the evidence available. Most of the prime examples are reviewed by Kimmel et al. (1990). They provide an extensive compilation of evidence on the effects of early exposure to methylmercury, anticonvulsants, lead, ethanol, polychlorinated biphenyls, ionizing radiation, and drugs of abuse.

Despite the value of behavioral analysis for detecting, characterizing, and formulating the neurotoxic profile of an injurious agent, functional methods have their pitfalls. Because behavior is the final common pathway of CNS output, it is subject to the influence of intervening variables. This influence presents some intrinsic problems for reliably detecting changes in function. Variability, which is the hallmark of individuality, is simultaneously a "background noise" to one seeking to detect deleterious changes due to neurotoxicity. Another difficulty is that functional changes generally do not provide direct guidance to the site of injury; i.e., they do not point directly to the structures of the brain that have been altered. Finally, the interpretation of functional changes, while always meaningful within species, is sometimes difficult to translate across species, since analogous species-typical patterns of behavior may be incompletely understood across species.

In spite of some methodological and interpretive problems, functional analysis remains a mainstay of neurotoxicity detection and of all analyses of brain disorder. While there remains debate about the best specific methods to be used, the number of neurotoxic disorders known (Office of Technology Assessment, 1990; National Research Council, 1992) is sufficient to dictate that currently available methods be used in animals to provide the first line of defense against the introduction of neurotoxins to humans and for understanding the mechanisms by which neurotoxins act on the brain.

BEHAVIORAL ONTOGENY

If dysfunction is the leading indicator of CNS injury during development, what types of behavior can or should be used to assess behavioral ontogeny? This question is answered below by reviewing the broad categories of behaviors that may be applied to investigations of the developing CNS. For those interested in more complete information on what effects have been found for the major known developmental neurotoxins, see Riley and Vorhees (1986).

Transient Aspects of Behavioral Development: The Appearance and Disappearance of Age-Specific Behaviors

There are numerous examples of behaviors that appear and disappear during the course of development. In humans, the most obvious ones include the sucking reflex, which appears prenatally and gradually declines after weaning, and crawling, an intermediate stage of ambulation that appears during the first half-year and dissipates with the emergence of walking at approximately the end of the first year of life.

Similar transiently expressed behaviors exist in rodents. Rats, for example, pass through consistent stages of ambulatory development. These have been well documented and include stages such as head elevation, shoulder elevation, pelvic elevation, pivoting, crawling, and ultimately development of full quadrupedal forward ambulation (Altman and Sudarshan, 1975). Pivoting is a case in point. Pivoting may be seen as early as 4–5 days of age in rats, and it increases rapidly to a peak at 7–9 days, then gradually diminishes as quadrupedal ambulation emerges (Vorhees et al., 1979b). Pivoting is one of the clearest examples of a transient developmental behavior.

Another example occurs as a component of the emergence of swimming behavior. The stages of swimming ontogeny have been well documented. Schapiro et al. (1970) were the first to describe quantitatively two aspects of swimming development: head position (or body angle) and use of the limbs, later called paddling. An even more detailed delineation of limb use was later developed by Bekoff and Trainer (1979). Later, the system developed by Schapiro et al. (1970) was refined, the definitions were made more precise, and a third component was added, termed swimming direction (Vorhees et al., 1979a,b; Vorhees, 1986b). In the present context, limb use is particularly interesting because it is a behavior that exhibits patterns seen only during early development. On day 6 of age, rats placed in water often exhibit asynchronous movement of the limbs that may result in small turning movements but seldom produce forward motion. Within a few days, however, they begin to paddle with all four limbs in an alternating, coordinated pattern that propels them forward. Paddling with all limbs begins to disappear by around day 16, and the animals then switch to a behavior termed forelimb inhibition (Vorhees, 1986b). This marks the emergence of more adult-style swimming in which only the hind limbs are used for forward propulsion, and the forelimbs are held stationary tucked under the jaw except during turning, at which time lateral stroking motions of the forelimbs are seen. All three aspects of swimming ontogeny, organized by stages, are illustrated in Fig. 2.

Still another example of an early but transient behavior is olfactory-guided homing in infant rats (Gregory and Pfaff, 1971). Rats show a developmentally stage-specific preference for home-cage scent that emerges around day 7 of age and remains potent through weaning. A similar preference is shown for the scent of littermates (Altman et al., 1974).

Rats also exhibit a variety of nursing behaviors, including establishing maternal contact, nipple locating and attachment, sucking, milk withdrawal, and cessation of sucking (Blass and Teicher, 1980). Several aspects of these behaviors are developmentally specific and increase during early developmental stages and then decrease with later development.

There is also a developmental course for maternal retrieval behavior in rats, and this is under the control of maternal and neonatal olfactory and auditory cues. One of the auditory cues consists of ultrasonic emission or calls. The emission of the ultrasonic calls can be directly investigated and used as a marker for normal and abnormal development (Damassa et al., 1982). Analyses can include both emergence of calls and the shift to adult forms of calling (Adams, 1982; Amsel et al., 1977). The reader is referred to two excellent reviews on the topic of age-specific behaviors as markers of neurotoxicity (Spear, 1984; Spear et al., 1985). Both of these papers provide additional examples not discussed herein.

Use of Age-Specific Behaviors as Biomarkers of Developmental Disorder

With some of the examples of behavioral ontogeny discussed above, the value of developmental analyses will be illustrated. Schapiro et al. (1970) showed that early treatment with thyroxine accelerated and treatment with cortisol delayed swimming ontogeny in rats, including limb-use patterns. Vorhees et al. showed that a variety of prenatal drug exposures induce delays in swimming development (Vorhees et al., 1979a; Vorhees, 1983).

Rice extended the scoring system of Vorhees to mice, and showed that early exposure to methimazole, an antithyroidogenic agent, produced large and systematic delays in the development of all aspects of swimming ontogeny (Rice and Millan, 1986).

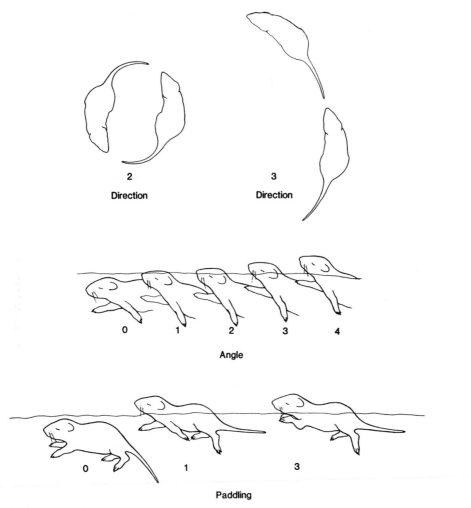

Figure 2 Stages of swimming ontogeny in rodents. Top: stages of swimming direction (stage 1, no turning or alternating right and left, and stage 0, floating or sinking, are not illustrated). Middle: stages of swimming angle; note especially the position of the ears in relation to the water line. Bottom: stages of paddling (stage 2, intermittent forelimb inhibition, is not illustrated). (From Vorhees, 1986b).

There are numerous other behaviors that exhibit transient patterns of expression during development. For example, shock-elicited wall-climbing behavior develops during the second postnatal week of life in rats and dissipates during the third postnatal week. It is thought to be under predominately catecholaminergic control (Spear et al., 1985). Spear et al. (1989) showed that the normal developmental pattern of shock-elicited wall-climbing is impaired in offspring prenatally exposed to cocaine.

Another developmentally stage-specific pattern occurs with sensory preconditioning. When young rats during their second postnatal week are exposed to two neutral olfactory stimuli, one of which is later paired with foot-shock, they learn more readily than older rats to avoid places associated with the stimulus paired with shock (Heyser et al., 1990).

This response has also been found to be impaired in rats prenatally exposed to cocaine (Heyser et al., 1990).

Pivoting has been used less frequently, but it has been shown that changes in pivoting occur in rats prenatally exposed to psychotropic drugs (Vorhees et al., 1979a) or after exposure to anticonvulsants (Vorhees, 1983).

It is evident from this sampling that developmentally specific behaviors can be useful markers of neurotoxicity. Unfortunately, this category of behaviors remains underutilized. The key to further development of this area may lie in research determining the predictive value of such effects, an issue discussed further in the next section.

Predictive Value of Changes in Early Behavior

While transiently expressed behavioral patterns have not been investigated extensively for their predictive value, at least one example can be cited that provides a glimpse at the potential of this line of investigation. In a series of investigations, Vorhees et al. (Vorhees, 1983, 1987; Weisenberger et al., 1990) have shown that prenatal exposure of rats to the anticonvulsant drug phenytoin induces a syndrome characterized by heightened pivoting, delayed swimming ontogeny, delayed air-righting ontogeny, hyperactivity, abnormal circling, and impaired maze learning. What is interesting is that abnormal circling behavior, which in the adult offspring is the most dramatic single symptom of the disorder, is not detectable in the animals when they are young (before weaning). However, increased pivoting is the earliest behavioral abnormality detectable in phenytoin-exposed offspring (Vorhees, 1983). Most important, the pivoting increase found in the phenytoin-exposed offspring presages all later behavioral abnormalities in these animals (Vorhees, 1983, 1987). This suggests that early behavioral markers, even if they are of transiently expressed behaviors, such as pivoting, may prove useful as predictors of later adverse outcomes. If borne out by further research, such early behavioral markers could be of considerable value in estimating neurotoxic liability and might be more efficent than other current methods.

EMERGENCE OF ADULT BEHAVIORS

Emergent Behaviors as Indices of Neurotoxicity

The previous section discussed a subgroup of behaviors that emerge during ontogeny and then disappear as more complex adult patterns unfold. Because these immature behavioral patterns are no longer recognizable in adult performance, the early manifestations may be regarded as transient. The more common case, however, is the emergence of adult patterns in a linear progression from similar antecedent behaviors. This section will describe examples from this class of behaviors. Because the unfolding of most adult forms of behavior may be staged, the rates of attainment of the adult skills can be used as markers of developmental disruption.

One of the classic developmental patterns is that associated with the maturation of ambulation. Once quadrupedal ambulation emerges in rats, around day 10–12, it quantitatively increases each day until it peaks between 16 and 20 days (Moorcroft et al., 1971; Campbell and Raskin, 1978). Thereafter, there is first a rapid decline in the amount of ambulation with advancing age, followed by a very gradual decline that plateaus to nearly asymptotic levels of performance during adulthood. However, this pattern does not obtain under all circumstances. Rats given repeated trials in an open field show a progressive increase in activity across trials with advancing age, instead of a plateau, if testing is begun before day 70 (Bronstein, 1972). In a figure-eight–shaped apparatus, however, there is a preweaning peak in ambulation regardless of whether repeated or single trials are given (Ruppert et al., 1985). Furthermore, other aspects of motor activity, including nose-poke frequency and rearing, show progressive increases with advancing age beginning from day 16 onward, until adult levels are reached (File, 1978). Thus, the progressive increase in various components of motor activity represents a series of stages that can be profiled after treatment and examined for shifts in the slope or position of the plotted normal developmental curve over time.

Another example is the mammalian startle reflex (Davis, 1984). The acoustic startle reflex emerges around day 12 in rats and progressively increases in amplitude (Parisi and Ison, 1979). This increase is at least partially a function of increasing body mass, which influences the measurement of startle in most devices. However, a large part of the increase stems from increases in strength and speed due to recruitment of additional muscles into the response, increased nerve conduction velocities, and increased coordination of muscle groups. A related phenomenon, modification of the startle response using prepulse signals, also exhibits a gradual ontological emergence that begins with the absence of the effect and evolves into the full adult response over a period of several weeks in rats (Parisi and Ison, 1979).

The dynamic or air-righting reflex is yet another example, and it follows a similar course to that seen with startle. The pattern begins with an inability to perform the reflex and progresses to the appearance of the entire reflex pattern within a week. Thereafter, the response exhibits a progressive increase in speed until performance reaches asymptotic levels, which requires another week or more (Elmazar and Sullivan, 1981; Vorhees, 1987).

Spontaneous alternation behavior also exhibits a systematic ontological pattern that has been well documented in rats (Egger et al., 1973). Rats alternate below 50% of the time early in life (during the second week of postnatal development), i.e., they make the same choice repeatedly. Fifty percent alternation frequency emerges at about the time of weaning, and alternation in the adult range (67–75%), depending on the way the procedure is structured, is evident by day 30. Thereafter only small additional increases are seen up to 100 days of age, and no changes occur thereafter.

Passive-avoidance retention also shows a reliable ontological emergence (Potash and Ferguson, 1977). Acquisition of the simplest response is present in weanling rats. However, this learning is a direct function of the criterion used, so that more stringent criteria result in slower acquisition. Nevertheless, with enough training young rats can master even more stringent criteria and retain the response for long periods. Interestingly, young rats given more stringent initial criteria show good retention, but perform less well than adults on retention when the initial learning criterion was set lower. Thus, there is a complex relationship in passive avoidance between age and initial learning and the interaction of these with retention of the response.

Even a basic reflex such as cold-induced shivering shows a developmental profile. Shivering appears in mice at about day 5, and the magnitude of the response increases linearly until about 20 days of age, then plateaus at adult levels (Arjamaa and Lagerspetz, 1979).

Virtually every adult behavior shows a normal pattern of developmental emergence, as exemplified by the cases listed above, and it would be impossible to list all of them. Suffice it to note that any of these can be carefully mapped and used as an index of developmental neurotoxicity by comparing normal and deviant patterns of maturation. The ultimate issue in using such markers is the extent to which deflections from normal maturational rates provide information for predicting, detecting, and characterizing neurotoxic responses. Let us consider each of these in turn.

Predictiveness

It is now evident that some developmental deviations have predictive power. For example, it has been shown that delays in air-righting not only predict other behavioral dysfunctions following prenatal exposure to phenytoin (Elmazar and Sullivan, 1981; Vorhees, 1987), but the degree of the delay predicts the magnitude of the later dysfunction. For example, the most severely air-righting–delayed phenytoin-exposed offspring were those that went on to exhibit the neurological symptoms of abnormal circling and hyperactivity (Minck et al., 1991). There are other examples, but this serves to illustrate the point that early behaviors can have strikingly potent prognostic value when the function examined taps CNS capacities intricately involved in the ultimate dysfunction.

Detection

As an approach to detection, examining behavior developmentally has the advantage that one can sample function closer to the time of exposure to the test agent. If the exposure is prenatal, early postnatal assessment allows one to determine whether there are immediate consequences for CNS function. If such effects are found, continued monitoring allows one to determine whether the effect is a delay or a permanent alteration of function. If the effect is a delay it may be of value to document the end of the effect and to determine whether the delay predicts adverse adult effects, as noted in the previous section, or predicts nonspecific or increased general risk, without suggesting a specific dysfunction. Finally, the end of the delay may signal that the effect has no significant sequelae. However, a word of caution is in order. Developmental delay should not be taken to mean that no adverse effect has occurred, simply because the developmental index in question ultimately reaches adult levels of performance. Returning to the example of phenytoin, recall that all phenytoin-exposed offspring eventually acquired the adult air-righting response, but that did not indicate that the underlying neurological impairment was transient. Quite to the contrary, the animals most delayed in air-righting went on to develop the most severe neurological symptoms, and these symptoms were permanent (Minck et al., 1991).

Characterization

Finally, developmental analysis may be valuable for understanding or characterizing a behavioral dysfunction. In the example of phenytoin, the drug induced a dose-dependent increase in impairment, and the most extreme effect was manifest as the neurological symptom of abnormal circling. Circling appears to be a vestibular-motor impairment that is evident in the adult offspring, and air-righting was a developmental marker that predicted this outcome. Presumably, the reason that air-righting had predictive value was that it contained task demands that were dependent on vestibular functions. Nevertheless, if air-righting had been examined only in adulthood, phenytoin-exposed offspring would have shown little or no effect, apparently because of compensation by other systems. By examining the behavior as it emerged, even small to moderate delays could be seen in this normally tightly controlled developmental sequence. Only by looking at the developmental profile of this reflex did the full extent of the dysfunction emerge in the severely, moderately, and mildly affected offspring. It was even possible to determine differences in specific aspects of the reflex that were affected in severely versus mildly affected phenytoin-exposed offspring (Vorhees, Minck, and Acuff-Smith, unpublished data).

The Analysis of Behaviors into Components: The Role of Development in Understanding Component Processes

In what are among the most elegant and thorough analyses of the components of a complex reflex behavior, two groups of investigators have examined the air-righting response. With high-speed videotape cameras, the ontogeny of the reflex in rats was subjected to detailed examination (Laouris et al., 1990). It was shown that the speed of the reflex is a function of free-fall height. During development, the latency to begin the response dramatically shortens with advancing age, and the speed of rotation accelerates with age as well. The beginnings of the reflex can be detected as early as postnatal day 9 in rats, and the response is fully present by day 18. Further increases in speed occur for several additional days after day 18. The most rapid phase of development of the reflex within this period occurs during a window between days 10 and 14. The initial movement is rotation of the head by twisting of the neck. This is seen most clearly in young animals on days 9–11 and is termed the cervical reflex. Subsequently, there is shoulder rotation followed by pelvic rotation. This overall pattern is always followed in normal animals and constitutes a rostral-to-caudal progression along an axial plane. When rats were harnessed so that they could not rotate their necks independent of their shoulders, they were delayed, but surprisingly by only about 1 day. By day 13, irrespective of fall height, harnessed rats were able to right as well as freely moving controls. This suggests that rats can initiate the reflex either with their head and neck or alternatively with their shoulders. In fact, Pellis et al. (1991) showed that in adult rats, shoulder rotation normally precedes neck rotation.

Studies in a variety of animals show that the triggering of the reflex varies by species. In rats, the reflex is triggered exclusively by the labyrinths (see Pellis et al., 1991). Vision, although capable of triggering an air-righting response in cats, cannot perform this function in rats. However, visual input does modulate the response in rats. Pellis et al. (1989) showed that in blindfolded rats, the latency and speed of the reflex is constant irrespective of free-fall distance, whereas in visually unobstructed animals the latency and speed of rotation are closely linked to height of the fall.

Subsequently, Pellis and associates (1991) showed that cortical input is not influential in visual modulation of the reflex, whereas input from the superior colliculus is. In fact, superior colliculus lesions were unique in blocking visual modulation of the reflex with or without intact vision.

These experiments illustrate how reflexes can be carefully dissected and analyzed into component processes that act jointly to produce the coordinated sequence of behavior recognized as the air-righting reflex. The value of such an approach for developmental neurotoxicology is that it may provide a useful avenue for exploring the underlying mechanism of dysfunction for effects induced by various neurotoxins. An example will be provided below. First, however, several additional examples of component process analysis warrant mentioning.

Pellis et al. (1989) have performed a detailed analysis of the surface- or contact-righting response similar to that described above for air-righting. They showed that contact-righting is very different from air-righting in several key ways, including an important contribution mediated through the lateral hypothalamus. Lateral hypothalamus lesions severely delay contact-righting even while sparing air-righting. However, both reflexes are delayed by labyrinthine lesions, although the effect on contact righting is relatively small (1–2 days) as compared with the effect on air-righting. Furthermore, there are potent proprioceptive components of contact-righting that lead to recovery of function of the reflex over time. What is even more remarkable about this recovery is that it proceeds in a sequentially reversed pattern; i.e., while the normal ontological pattern is rostral-caudal, the postlesion pattern is caudal-rostral. Pellis et al. (1989) discovered, however, that with longer recovery times, there is an ultimate reversion from the pelvic-first to a cephalic-first initiation of the reflex. Eventually, all animals develop the standard cephalic-first dominance pattern—a striking example of recovery of function.

Similar component-process analyses have been conducted by Davis (1984) on the acoustic startle reflex, and more recently by several investigators on spontaneous motor activity (Paulus and Geyer, 1991; Kernan et al., 1989; Sanberg et al., 1985; Vorhees et al., 1992). While these examples represent but a sampling of the variety of component research available, they provide a flavor for the kinds of more specific analyses that are possible. The value of these approaches in understanding particular neurotoxins is yet to be shown for some of these behaviors, but this simply reflects the fact that most of these methods are too new to have been applied to known developmental neurotoxins. One exception is phenytoin and the analysis of activity using video-tracking analysis (Vorhees et al., 1992). As is shown in Fig. 3, the phenytoin circlers exhibit multiple-activity abnormalities. These alterations are not only quantitative, but also qualitative (spatial) and temporal, whereas phenytoin-exposed noncirclers appear normal. This is obviously fertile ground for future research.

To provide an example of drug-induced changes in air-righting, let us return to the case of prenatal exposure to phenytoin. Prenatal phenytoin exposure induces, among other effects, a marked air-righting delay, and furthermore, the delay may be resolved into separate curves for those offspring that later develop abnormal circling and those that do not (Minck et al., 1991). This may be seen in Figs. 4 and 5. Through high-speed photography, several stages of the response in control and phenytoin-exposed offspring are shown. Note that the severely affected phenytoin-exposed animal in these multiple-exposure photographs does not fail to right simply because it is slow to complete the normal rostral-caudal axial rotation sequence. Rather, it fails to right because it does not initiate either shoulder or head-neck rotation. These data suggest that the site of damage in these exposed animals may be in the labyrinthine-vestibular pathway. No evidence yet exists to support this, but it at least provides a testable hypothesis for future investigation, and therein lies the potential value of component-process analyses. They provide a wedge by which overall behavioral effects can be described that goes well beyond identification and characterization of effects. With component analysis, hypotheses about mechanisms can be generated and tested, and through a process of elimination can lead to fuller understanding of the compound's neurotoxicity.

Longitudinal Analysis of Behavior: Ontogeny and Life-Span Models

The concept of "growing into a deficit" has been around for a long time (Isaacson, 1975). This concept arose from lesion studies, in which deficits did not become evident until behaviors normally expected to develop by a certain age were absent or deficient. However, few data exist with chemically induced developmental neurotoxins either to support or to refute the applicability of this concept within behavioral teratology. A related concept is that early insults to the CNS may not become evident until old age, when the brain's

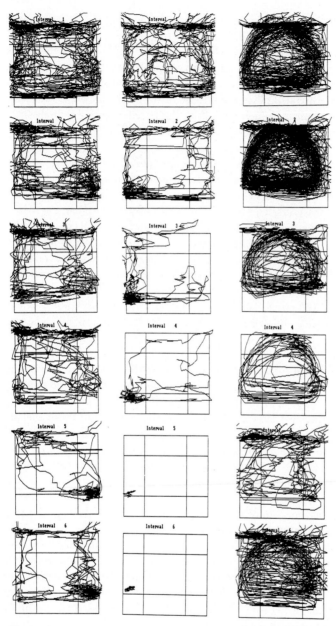

Figure 3 Video tracking tracing from adult female rats exposed prenatally to phenytoin or control. Each interval represents 10 minutes. Left column, control rats; center column, phenytoin-exposed noncircler; right column, phenytoin-exposed circler. Phenytoin (acid) was administered on days E7–18 at 200 mg/kg once per day. Note that the phenytoin-exposed circler not only is more active, but fails to show the potent central-avoidance pattern typical of controls. It also shows little corner preference and is generally boundary-insensitive. Finally, the phenytoin-exposed circler shows diminished habituation across time intervals, and even shows a kind of rebound during the last interval. (From Vorhees et al, 1992).

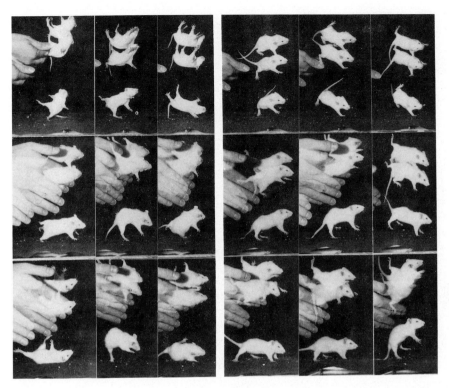

Figure 4 Stop-action multiple-exposure photographs of rats in free fall from a height of 30 cm displaying the air-righting reflex. Left panel: rat exposed prenatally to phenytoin (200 mg/kg/day E7–18). Right panel: control rat. Rows 1, 2, and 3: postnatal age (days) 16, 20, and 24, respectively. Columns 1, 2, and 3: trials 1, 2 and 3, respectively, given on the same day. Note how on day 16 the phenytoin-exposed rat fails to initiate head or shoulder rotation.

reserve and compensatory capacities are reduced (Weiss and Spyker, 1974). The paucity of data on this subject is not difficult to understand when one considers its ramifications. To determine whether latent effects are induced, one must undertake the formidable task of a long-term study. To follow a group of animals systematically from birth to senescence while keeping extraneous variables under tight control is quite difficult. Even for rodents, this entails conducting studies lasting 2–3 years. Not only is the time commitment onerous, but the costs are large and the payoff a matter of conjecture. Thus, such experiments are high-risk ventures and are seldom performed.

An interesting example of these rare longitudinal experiments comes from the work of Martin and her colleagues. They injected gravid rats with 3 mg/kg of nicotine, 5 mg/kg of methamphetamine, or saline throughout gestation and continued the treatment during lactation with direct injection of the drugs to the offspring. The authors found that early nicotine exposure shortened life expectancy, while early methamphetamine exposure induced several effects, including slightly delayed developmental landmark attainment, reduced growth (up to 15 months of age), and increased running-wheel activity (up to 12 months of age) (Martin et al., 1976, 1979). In a follow-up report, the same animals were followed to 39 months of age. The increased running-wheel activity seen previously in

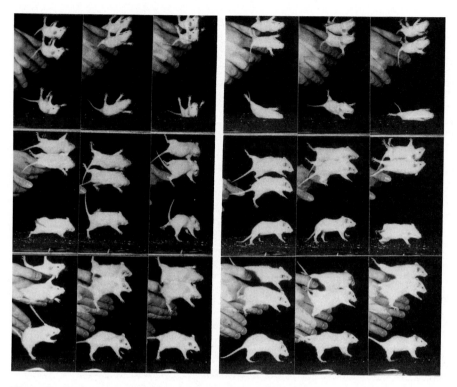

Figure 5 Stop-action multiple-exposure photographs of rats in free fall from a height of 30 cm displaying the air-righting reflex. Left panel: rat exposed prenatally to phenytoin (200 mg/kg/day E7–18) and exhibiting circling later in life. Right panel: phenytoin-exposed rat from the same litter as in the left panel, but not exhibiting circling later in life. Rows 1, 2, and 3: postnatal age (days) 16, 20, and 24, respectively. Columns 1, 2, and 3: trials 1, 2, and 3, respectively, given on the same day. Note how on day 16 the phenytoin-exposed circler fails to initiate head or shoulder rotation, whereas the phenytoin-exposed noncircler initiates rotation but fails to complete it before impact. Compare the latter performance to that of the control animal at the same age in the right top portion of Fig. 4.

methamphetamine-treated offspring at ages up to 12 months persisted to 39 months, while no effect of nicotine was seen. No significant interaction with advanced age was found (Martin and Martin, 1981). These data provide no evidence of a worsening deficit with age, as has been hypothesized might occur in aging animals. These authors also found that a similar set of treatments altered saccharin preference in the offspring when they were tested as adults, as a result of early nicotine or methamphetamine exposure. The shift in saccharin preference persisted in the groups to between 15 and 33 months of age. Again, no evidence was obtained suggesting that age caused either an exaggeration or a lessening of the saccharin preference (Martin et al., 1983).

In a long-term experiment on the effects of prenatal phenytoin, Vorhees and Minck (1989) followed offspring to 16 months of age and evaluated litter-mates for water-maze learning either during early adulthood or at an advanced age. At both ages the phenytoin offspring showed the typical phenytoin-induced severe learning deficit for a complex maze task, but no evidence was obtained suggesting that the effect was either exacerbated or ameliorated with age. Indeed, re-test of the early-tested litter-mates using reversal trials showed that the impairment had not changed in any detectable way during the interval between 2 and 16 months; i.e., they were severely impaired at 2 months and were still severely impaired at 16 months.

It has been reported that mice exposed prenatally to methylmercury exhibit an increase in neurological symptoms at 2.5–3 years of age (Weiss and Spyker, 1974; Spyker, 1975). These symptoms included postural abnormalities, muscular wasting, weight loss, and appetite changes leading to reduced or excess food consumption. It was suggested that the worsening symptoms of the methylmercury-exposed offspring at later ages represented "early aging." There is little evidence to support this supposition. About the only conclusion that the data support is that long-term effects were obtained that were not evident earlier in life. While the amount of evidence available on effects of early exposure to neurotoxins on aging remains limited, at this time it may be concluded that the available data neither support nor refute a general theory of aging as a stage of development that is likely to reveal latent effects caused by early insult. If anything, the current evidence supports a more limited view, namely, that aging may reveal new symptoms with some compounds and not with others. Predicting when the former will occur is at present beyond our reach and will probably not be possible until more is known about mechanisms of aging and about how neurotoxins function to alter basic cellular processes.

The concept of longitudinal or life-span assessment is appealing and may have some promise for understanding the course of neurotoxin-induced developmental illness. However, much work remains to be done in this area. The limits of the data are not only in the number of compounds that have been investigated, but also in the depth of information plumbed in these studies. Most have not been very systematic, relying more on descriptions of how the animals look or walk than on quantitative results of tests of particular functions such as complex learning.

MECHANISMS UNDERLYING DEVELOPMENTAL NEUROTOXICITY

Perhaps two of the most striking developmental neurotoxin-induced syndromes are the fetal retinoid and fetal alcohol syndromes. These syndromes, which involve both malformations and CNS dysfunctions, are particularly relevant to considerations of mechanisms because of new evidence that has been developed in the last few years about the effects of retinoids on embryonic development, whereby they function as a morphogen in the control of limb and CNS pattern formation, and their effects on gene regulation, whereby they act as hormone-like agents. The newer cellular and molecular information will be briefly described, and then links will be drawn to their possible roles in retinoid- and ethanol-induced embryopathies of the CNS.

Newer data provide evidence that retinoids have hormone-like regulatory roles in cell function and act as morphogens during development. When retinoids are administered experimentally to animals they produce a spectrum of CNS effects, including pronounced behavioral dysfunctions (see Vorhees and Butcher, 1982). These findings are summarized in Table 1. As can be seen, a wide variety of effects were found, including effects on higher cognitive functions such as learning. In this entire literature, only one experiment failed to find such effects. In this case effects were found, but not on higher CNS functions (Kutz et al., 1989). This may well have been due to excess offspring mortality in the group exposed to the highest dose, a dose proved by others to be the prime one for inducing functional effects. More recently cognitive deficits comparable to those seen in most animal

Table 1 Summary of Retinoid-Induced Behavioral Dysfunctions in Rats Following Prenatal Exposure

Author	Agent	Strain	Exposure period	Function	Effect
Malakhovskii (1969, 1971)	Retinyl ester	Albino	9	Activity	↓
				Aggression	↓
				Active avoidance	↑ Errors
Butcher et al. (1972)	Retinyl acetate	SD	8–10	Biel maze	↑ Errors
Hutchings et al. (1973)	Retinol	Wistar	13–14[a]	S⁺/S⁻ Oper.	↓ Acquisition
					↓ S⁻ Extinction
Hutchings and Gaston (1974)	Retinol	Wistar	16–17[a]	S⁺/S⁻	↓ Responding
Vorhees (1974)	Retinyl palmitate	F344	8–10	Y-maze	↓ Avoidance
Coyle and Singer (1975)	Retinyl palmitate	Wistar	8–10	Biel maze	↑ Errors
				Henderson puzzle box	↑ Time
Vorhees et al. (1978)	Retinyl palmitate	SD	5–7, 8–10, 11–13, 14–16, 17–19	T-maze	↑ Time 11–13
				Activity	↑ 8–10
				Biel maze	↑ Errors 8–10, 11–13
Vorhees et al. (1979)	Retinyl palmitate	SD	7–20	Cliff avoidance	Delayed
				Surface righting	Delayed
				Negative geotaxis	Delayed
				Swimming ontogeny	Delayed
				Pivoting	↓
				Early activity	↑ Rearing
				Alternation	—
				Biel maze	↑ Errors
				Active avoidance	↑ Avoid
				Passive avoidance	—
				Rotorod	↓

Reference	Compound	Strain	Dose (days)	Endpoint	Effect
Mooney et al. (1981)	Retinyl palmitate	SD	7–9[a]	Head elevation	Delayed
				Shoulder elevation	Delayed
				Hindleg elevation	Delayed
				Air righting	Delayed
				Crawling	Delayed
				Head pointing	Delayed
				Cliff avoidance	Delayed
				Rearing	Delayed
				Wire climbing	—
				Walking	Delayed
				Negative geotaxis	—
				Pivoting	Delayed
				Surface righting	—
				Eye opening	Delayed
				Hair emergence	—
Adams (1982)	Retinyl palmitate	SD	8–10	Negative geotaxis	—
				Ultrasound	← Vocalization
Nolen (1986)	*trans*-Retinoic acid	SD	8–10, 11–13, 14–16	Negative geotaxis	Delayed
				Auditory startle	Delayed
				Open field activity	←
				M-Maze	← Latency
				Running wheel	←→
				Active avoidance	→
Saillenfait and Vannier (1988)	Retinyl palmitate	SD	6–20	Surface righting	Delayed
				Swimming ontogeny	Delayed
				Pupil constriction	—
				Auditory startle	—
				Negative geotaxis	Delayed
				Open field activity	←→
				Rotorod	→
				24-h activity	Nocturnal
				M-maze	—

Table 1 Continued

Author	Agent	Strain	Exposure period	Function	Effect
Kutz et al. (1989)	Retinyl acetate	SD	6-19	Pinna detachment	Delayed
				Eye opening	Delayed
				Incisor eruption	Delayed
				Surface righting	—
				Cliff avoidance	—
				Grasp holding	—
				Negative geotaxis	—
				Swimming	—
				ontogeny	
				Open field activity	—
				S$^+$/S$^-$ Operant	

[a]Dating method corrected from authors' original date so that all pregnancies are uniformly dated, as evidence of conception is set equal 'o day zero of gestation.
SD = Sprague-Dawley.

studies, as shown in Table 1, have been seen in humans following exposure to 13-*cis*-retinoic acid (isotretinoin) (Adams and Lammer, 1991).

Isotretinoin is a highly effective drug for the treatment of acne, and it is specifically indicated for the treatment of cystic acne. Consequently, the drug has been prescribed for many thousands of people in North America, perhaps even overprescribed. The drug's embryotoxicity in all species examined, including humans (Lammer et al., 1985), is also well known. Indeed, the animal data correctly predicted the cognitive deficits later seen in humans (Vorhees, 1986c). How might retinoids work? Retinoids are typically ingested in food in the form of retinyl esters, which are then converted to retinol and subsequently to retinal. A percentage of retinal is in turn converted to retinoic acid. Retinoic acid is carried in plasma to its target cell, which it enters and is transported to the cell nucleus (Wolf, 1991). In the nucleus, retinoic acid binds to specific nuclear receptors, designated RAR and RXR, of which there are now known to be at least 3 subtypes (α, β, γ) of each (Wolf, 1990; Mangelsdorf et al., 1990). The RARs and RXRs, when bound to retinoic acid or perhaps 9-*cis*-retinoic acid in the case of RXRs, form heterodimers that regulate retinoic acid response elements (RAREs) on the promoter regions of several genes (Gudas, 1992; Linney, 1992). All the genes involved are not known, but known genes with RAREs are *ADH3*, *RARβ₂*, *CRABP-1*, and the genes for the calcium channel, oxytocin, and laminin (Gudas, 1992; Linney, 1992). Furthermore, RXR can also bind to the thyroid response element (TRE) along with the thyroid receptor (TR) to form a heterodimer that regulates genes containing thyroid promoter regions. There is extensive overlap between the RXR, TR, and vitamin D_3 receptors. In fact, only small differences in the repeat motif spacing on the TRE convert it to either a RARE or a VDRE (vitamin D_3 response element) (Umesono et al., 1991; Yu et al., 1991). Such findings suggest that the effects of thyroxine and retinoids on brain development and behavior probably occur through complex hormone receptor–mediated gene regulation pathways to alter developmental events in the CNS and other tissues. It is clear that in this area information is rapidly emerging that will shed new light on the mechanisms by which thyroid hormone, retinoic acid, and vitamin D_3 play critical roles in normal development and may eventually help explain why agents that act on these processes have such profound effects on brain function.

It has been suggested recently that the fetal alcohol syndrome may be caused by ethanol's effects on the retinoid pathway, on the basis of evidence that retinoic acid activates the alcohol dehydrogenase gene *ADH3* (see above). This is crucial, since alcohol dehydrogenase catalyzes the conversion of retinol to retinal, the first step in the retinol to retinoic acid pathway (Duester et al., 1991). Thus, high doses of ethanol may restrict the normal production of retinoic acid, leading to a shortage of this agent and disruptions in its function in pattern formation, differentiation, and gene regulation.

REGULATORY IMPLICATIONS OF DEVELOPMENTAL NEUROTOXICITY

Developmental neurotoxicity assessment, under the heading of "behavioral teratogenicity," has been required in some countries since 1974. The history of such guidelines has been reviewed previously (Vorhees, 1986a). During the intervening 19 years, a number of changes have occurred, and no attempt will be made here to review them all. Changes up through the spring of 1991 were reviewed recently (Vorhees, 1992). Several changes have occurred since then that warrant further discussion; however, the previous review (Vorhees, 1992) should be consulted by those wishing more background on the present discussion.

Guidelines that incorporate developmental neurotoxicity evaluations are those covering developmental or reproductive toxicity. In North America they are generally referred to as developmental and reproductive toxicity guidelines, and in Europe they are referred to inclusively as reproductive toxicity guidelines.

There are two broad categories of safety assessment that all countries have instituted. The first comprises assessments of safety of drugs and foods. These may be traced back to the early twentieth century and the original U.S. Food and Drug Act of 1906 (Office of Technology Assessment, 1990). Beginning in the 1970s, new safety standards were introduced to regulate chemicals in the environment and workplace that were the result of pollution or workplace exposure during the manufacture of commercial products. These have been referred to generically as environmental agents. For most of the history of safety assessment, considerations pertaining to drug safety have set the standards that other areas have followed. In more recent years this pattern has begun to change, and aspects of this shift will be discussed below.

The evaluation of drugs for safety was the first area of government toxicity regulation. Preclinical safety evaluation originally consisted of testing for general toxicity, carcinogenicity, and reproductive effects. After the thalidomide disaster, preclinical testing for reproductive effects was divided into three separate segments, with some overlap, each designed to cover a different set of reproductive and developmental events. Segment 1 was designed to cover preconception, fertility, and preimplantation events, segment 2 was designed to cover organogenesis, and segment 3 was designed to cover fetal and postnatal development to the age of weaning.

When the FDA revised its reproductive and developmental toxicity test guidelines in 1966 to form the present three-segment approach, most other countries followed suit. However, although each country followed the overall FDA approach, they also made changes. The problem from the outset was that these changes introduced variations that made it increasingly difficult to adhere strictly to every country's requirement using a single study design. Studies designed for one country were often unsuitable for another. For example, many companies had to perform multiple segment 2 studies to satisfy different national regulatory standards. As the cost of developing new drugs increased, the necessity of performing multiple overlapping developmental toxicity studies was increasingly seen as a source of unnecessary and costly regulation. It was recognized that many of the differences in guidelines between countries did not represent substantial differences in what was discovered about each drug's toxicity. But for political and policy reasons, most countries were reluctant to accept toxicity studies conducted under another country's guidelines. Several attempts to resolve these guideline differences were undertaken, but none succeeded until the efforts by a committee initiated by the European Community (EC) entitled "Guideline on Detection of Toxicity to Reproduction for Medicinal Products" (European Drafting Group, 1992). Perhaps the greater success of this effort was due to good timing, since international competitiveness has become a central policy theme of many industrialized nations. Regulatory reform was widely seen as a means to enhance international competitiveness. Or perhaps this committee's success grew out of the push arising from the EC's own unification, which made trans-European guideline unification a necessary part of EC economic integration. This committee's success many also have grown out of the way the organizers operated, because they sought to develop a very broad consensus among industrial, academic, and governmental scientists throughout Europe, North America, and Japan before seeking regulatory-agency endorsements. This allowed common ground to be formulated first outside of normal governmental structures.

Whatever the reasons, through an extensive series of drafts, meetings, and discussions a guideline was developed that has progressed to the point that it now appears positioned for adoption by EC, U.S., and Japanese regulatory authorities.

In the last review of the proposed international "Guideline on Detection of Toxicity to Reproduction for Medical Products," draft number 9 was summarized and critiqued (Vorhees, 1992). Herein, draft number 13 of this document is reviewed in some detail.

The international guideline, in its first nine drafts, began with the same basic strategy, using the approach dominant today in most industrialized nations, i.e., the three-segment approach outlined above and introduced by the FDA more than 25 years ago. However, draft 9 of the international proposal deviated from those of most nations in defining the three segments so that the exposure periods were non-overlapping. The guideline retained many other mainstream features, including dual-species testing for segment 2, recommending rodents (rats) as the primary species in all segments, the use of three compound-dose groups and controls, an exposure route for drug delivery that mimics the expected route of exposure for humans, etc. Draft 9 added emphasis on pharmacokinetics and, in a gesture to the improved segment 2 design introduced by the Japanese, proposed a modified segment 2 study design of having two identical cohorts of animals, one for near-term necropsy and examination for malformations, and one for delivery and follow-up for examination of growth and functional assessment. Of relevance to the present discussion, behavioral assessments were included in segments 2 and 3, as has been done in the Japanese guidelines for many years.

The newest version of the international guideline, draft 13, has a number of changes as compared with draft 9. The overall strategy has remained the same. However, in an effort to add flexibility and resolve the remaining areas of disagreement among the participants, draft 13 has had large sections of text removed that spelled out the particulars of study design. These details have now been placed in an extended set of notes that follow the main text. The effect of this is to produce a shorter and more conceptually oriented text. The text lays out the main themes and broad purposes of each segment of the guideline, including some of the options that may be considered under different circumstances.

This approach has succeeded in making the guidelines more flexible. To the extent that flexibility will be translated into improved study design and better safety assessment, such a change is obviously desirable. To the extent that too much flexibility ends up being nebulous, such a change is counterproductive. This is a real possibility, because the designation of tests needed to fulfill the guideline has become ephemeral. There is an implication in the current document not only that the choice of which tests to use is left to the discretion of the company, but that even whether a test is done is left to its discretion. The presumption is that each test included and those omitted would have to be justified, but that if a company could persuasively argue, for example, that a drug was not "expected" to produce CNS effects, it might be permitted to skip behavioral testing altogether. The problem with this is that although there are sometimes logical-sounding reasons for not "expecting" a particular agent to induce a particular effect, these predictions are often erroneous. If such logic were the only standard used to conduct safety testing, there would be teratogens on the market today that were in fact caught by current testing requirements. In fact, the history of teratogenesis can be characterized as one of unexpected effects. It is this very problem that caused thalidomide to reach the market with its "unexpected" effects on embryonic development. The requirement that all drugs receive a mandatory set of preclinical tests for toxicity is at the core of the food, drug, and cosmetics law that has proved to be so effective at preventing new teratogens from reaching the market over the last 25 years; and it is this aspect of the process that the international guideline seems to have weakened by making everything negotiable. Thus flexibility, when taken too far, has a palpable cost, and that cost may end up being measured in terms of reduced product safety.

Draft 13 of the international guideline continues the segmental approach noted above. However, the division of the segments has changed since draft 9. As noted, in draft 9 three non-overlapping segments were devised, whereas in draft 13, overlap has been reinstated. In draft 13, the first segment (the fertility and early embryonic development test) advises exposure from before conception through implantation, as in draft 9, and the second segment is the embryofetal segment, including exposure during organogenesis, also as in draft 9. The third segment (the pre- and postnatal development test), is different. It advises exposure from implantation to weaning, much beyond what was proposed in draft 9. Note that the pre- and postnatal test's exposure period overlaps extensively with the embryofetal test's exposure period. Note also that whereas in draft 9 neurobehavioral function was included in two of the segments, those with at least some of the exposure occurring during organogenesis, now such assessment occurs only under one segment (the pre- and postnatal study). The change was caused by the fact that the embryofetal segment has now been reduced to a strict structural-malformations study and that the postnatal cohort originally included has been deleted. The inclusion of a postnatal cohort is mentioned as an option, but its elimination as the "most probable option" is worrisome. Eliminating behavioral testing from segment 2 sets the stage for a drastic reduction in the ability to develop convergent data. Previously, developmental neurotoxicity data across two independent experiments would have been obtained and could be compared, but under the latest revision only one set of behavioral data will be collected. It is difficult to be sanguine about this change.

Beyond the problem of which segments indicate neurotoxicity, the new pre- and postnatal study provides less information on which functions are to be assessed. In draft 9, the guideline specified assessments of "sensory function, reflexes, motor activity, and learning/memory." In draft 13, the guideline specifies, in list fashion, "physical development" (note 18), "sensory functions and reflexes" (note 18), and "behavior" (note 18) (European Drafting Group, 1992). Note 18 begins with the oft-quoted high correlation observed between body weight and physical landmarks of development. The note states that because of this correlation, body weight is the best indicator of physical development, implying that physical landmark data are redundant. The statement reflects no awareness that this correlation has never been proved to be causative, and that the nature of the link between these variables is unknown. This classic error of inference is predicated on the fallacy that what changes together under normal development will similarly co-occur under the influence of experimental treatments. The erroneousness of this prediction is exemplified by methylmercury, which has been shown to accelerate eye opening and incisor eruption in rats exposed prenatally while reducing growth, an association exactly opposite to that seen in controls (Geyer et al., 1985; Vorhees, 1985). If the supposed correlation between physical landmarks and body weight does not hold for a classic neurotoxin such as methylmercury, the concept is seriously flawed. Note 18 reflects no awareness of this well-known finding. This demonstrates the danger of drawing inferences based on data taken from controls or even from studies on experimental compounds in which no neurotoxicity occurred. It also demonstrates a lack of cognizance of the relevant literature.

Note 18 goes further by stating that reflexes are "dependent on physical development." This claim contradicts a significant fraction of the published literature that has found striking exceptions to this tendency. Exceptions disprove hypotheses, and therefore the supposition that the acoustic startle reflex is "dependent" on physical development is unfounded. By contrast, note 18 strongly endorses two sexual-maturity physical landmarks of development: vaginal patency and preputial separation. While these landmarks are no doubt valuable, the basis for elevating these above neurological assessments in a portion of the test guideline designed to assess nervous system function is perplexing.

The note ends with a peculiar paragraph stating that most functional tests have historically been directed towards assessments of "behavior." The meaning of this is unclear. The reference to "behavior" is so general as to be meaningless, because it permits almost any interpretation one wishes. The text goes on to note that despite much research, the Drafting Committee could make no recommendations about which tests of "behavior" might be suitable. In lieu of such recommendations, they default to a position that encourages assessment of "sensory functions, motor activity, learning and memory" (European Drafting Group, 1992). The central question that plagues this document is why it has retreated from its previous stance, in which these functions were required. Furthermore, while the new draft succeeds in increasing the guideline's flexibility, it also introduces a subtext (note 18) that is biased in its appraisal of current knowledge in the field of neurobehavioral assessment. Rather than representing the mainstream, the present document reads like the personal views of a select group. This is a discouraging development and one that will be a setback to the task of advancing neurological risk assessment.

Despite all the problems outlined above, there is one plus in the international proposed guideline; i.e., it would be universally applied to all new pharmaceuticals throughout the industrialized world. This means that for the first time even drugs submitted to the FDA would be required to include nervous system functional assessment, a far cry from the current state of affairs. It is a sad commentary that the FDA, which once stood between the public and thalidomide, has since been immobilized when it comes to providing protection against the risk of brain injury.

Environmental agents represent an entirely different situation, and accordingly, regulatory guidelines for them have had an entirely different history. For environmental agents the U.S. Environmental Protection Agency (EPA) has been the leader in developing standards for neurotoxicity assessment. In 1991, the EPA took another step forward and put in place a test guideline for the detection of developmental neurotoxicity. This new guideline has recently been reviewed. The reader is referred to Driscoll (1991) for a thorough summary of what the guideline calls for and the rationale behind it, and to Vorhees (1992) for a critique of its deficiencies.

Several features of the EPA developmental neurotoxicity guideline stand out. First, it is truly developmental in concept; i.e., the approach to testing is longitudinal, so that effects are followed over time to determine their persistence, using normal development as the referent. Second, the EPA guideline provides clear categories of CNS functions that are to be assessed. Moreover, the guideline provides standards for each functional category. Thus, instead of merely calling for assessment of motor activity, it calls for automated activity in a controlled environment and demonstration of a normal habituation curve. In the case of tests for learning, it goes beyond simply stating that tests for learning should be done, and states that a learning curve must be demonstrated. And instead of simply requiring a test for memory, the EPA guideline requires that control for nonassociative factors to be included to ensure that proper interpretation of the data will be possible.

Third, the EPA guideline is fairly comprehensive, inasmuch as it requires tests subsumed under the functional observational battery and physical landmarks of both male and female development, motor activity, startle reflex, learning, and memory. The latter four categories must be tested repeatedly at different ages, and a window of time for the performance of each assessment is provided. Neuropathological assessments are also described in the guidelines.

This development is promising, but it has a major shortcoming. The EPA has established this guideline as an entity separate from its main guideline for detecting developmental toxicity. This means that compounds will be tested for developmental toxicity without ever receiving assessment for developmental neurotoxicity. Developmental-neurotoxicity assessment will be required only when some other piece of information is available that suggests the possibility of CNS effects. This situation represents a tortured view of development, in which the nervous system is placed apart from the rest of the organism. In this view, the development of all the organ systems of the body is in one sphere and the development of the nervous system in another, a kind of metaphysical dualism. This way of organizing the world appears to have a more political than scientific basis.

This matters because it creates situations in which a chemical is tested for developmental toxicity, found to be acceptable, and approved, only to be discovered later to possess neurotoxicity. When this happens, it will stand in stark relief against the fact that a developmental-neurotoxicity guideline that could have caught the effect sat on the shelf unused. This is not farfetched, since all that need happen is that the developmental toxicity study find no indication in examinations for body weight, skeletal defects, and visceral malformations that the brain was damaged, and the compound would bypass developmental-neurotoxicity scrutiny without so much as a raised eyebrow. The dualistic approach tacitly assumes that if an agent is neurotoxic it will produce an effect on some other organ system. If that were true, methylmercury- and lead-induced developmental neurotoxicity would never have been discovered. This is not to suggest that the agency actually believes in such dualism, but rather that its regulatory actions lack congruence. The EPA should reexamine the situation and reorganize the developmental studies, merging the developmental-toxicity and developmental-neurotoxicity guidelines into one unified protocol. In creating the developmental neurotoxicity guideline, the EPA has taken a significant step forward. Now it remains for the agency to cycle back to this issue and finish the job it started by melding these two guidelines into one.

CONCLUSIONS

Developmental neurotoxicity (behavioral teratology) has evolved from a fledgling subspecialty, more than 20 years ago, to a substantive area of research and safety assessment. The developing nervous system is a structure especially vulnerable to perturbation, a fact that arises from its organizational complexity, protracted developmental period, and gradual accrual of protective barriers. This vulnerability has been amply demonstrated in human disorders and in experimental animals and suggests that CNS development deserves a prominent place in the safety assessment of foods, drugs, and environmental agents. Neurobehavioral methods are critical to the process of detecting and characterizing developmental neurotoxins. A sampling of the categories of behaviors for accomplishing such a task was presented, and it was shown that many promising techniques exist. Continued progress in this area could yield significant benefits for the improvement of public health and the prevention of medical disorders. Accordingly, it is suggested that the developing nervous system be used as a sort of "miner's canary," that is, as an early-warning signal for toxic reactions in other organ systems. In the past, the brain has been relegated to a minor role in safety assessment; it is now time to change this practice and place it in a prominent role as a central index of toxicity.

ACKNOWLEDGMENT

The author wishes to express his sincere appreciation to Drs. E. Mollnow and K. D. Acuff-Smith for their critical comments on this manuscript. The writing of this chapter was made possible through the research support to the author's laboratory provided by National Institutes of Health investigator grants HD21806 and DA06733, center grant ES06096, and training grant ES07051.

NOTE ADDED IN PROOF

Since this chapter was written, the International Conference on Harmonization (ICH) of Technical Requirements for the Registration of Pharmaceuticals for Human Use has issued its final guideline, "Detection of Toxicity to Reproduction for Medical Products." Draft 13 was reviewed herein (pp. 753–758), but the guideline was not finalized and officially adopted by the ICH until June 24, 1993, after this chapter was written. The ICH has now recommended adoption of the finalized guideline by the regulatory bodies of the European Union, United States, and Japan. Action by these governmental neurotoxicity has remained unchanged since draft 13. However, a few points bear mentioning.

The developmental neurotoxicity specifications are now contained in Note 21. This note, similar to its predecessor, states that body weight is the best indicator of physical development in comparison to physical landmarks of development. Note 21 continues to state that reflexes, which it lists as surface righting, auditory startle, air righting, and response to light, are also dependent on physical development, a position that continues to overstate the evidence, especially when neurotoxicity is present. Further, in referring to tests of behavior, note 21 goes on to state that "Even though a great deal of effort has been expended in this direction it is not possible to recommend specific test methods." This statement, implying as it does that great effort expended on test development has not resulted in establishment of tests worthy of recommendation, is false and misleading and reflects the biases of the ICH, not the state of knowledge in this area. Finally, note 21 indicates that finding tests for the assessment of sensory functions, motor activity, learning, and memory is encouraged. By implication, 'encouraged' may be taken to mean 'not required' and 'finding' can be taken to mean 'invention' since the committee, in its diligence, was unable to find even a single method in the literature worthy of mention. On this, the committee's position is disingenuous.

REFERENCES

Adams J (1982). Ultrasonic vocalizations as diagnostic tools in studies of developmental toxicity: an investigation of the effects of hypervitaminosis. A. Neurobehav Toxicol Teratol 4:299–304.

Adams J, Lammer EJ (1991). Relationship between dysmorphology and neuro-psychological function in children exposed to isotretinoin "in utero." In: Fujii T, Boer GJ, eds. Functional neuroteratology of short-term exposure to drugs. Tokyo: Teikyo University Press, 159–68.

Altman J, Brunner RL, Bulut FG, Sudarshan K (1974). The development of behavior in normal and brain-damaged infant rats, studied with homing (nest-seeking) as motivation. In: Vernadakis A, Weiner N, eds. Drugs and the developing brain. New York: Plenum Press, 321–48.

Altman J (1992). Programmed cell death: the paths to suicide. Trends Neurosci 15:278–80.

Altman J, Sudarshan K (1975). Postnatal development of locomotion in the laboratory rat. Anim Behav 23:896–920.

Amsel A, Radek CC, Graham M, Letz R (1977). Ultrasound emission in infant rats as an indicant of arousal during appetitive learning and extinction. Science 197:786–8.

Arjamaa O, Lagerspetz KYH (1979). Postnatal development of shivering in the mouse. J Therm Biol 4:35–9.

Bekoff A, Trainer W (1979). The development of interlimb co-ordination during swimming in postnatal rats. J Exp Biol 83:1–11.

Blass EM, Teicher MH (1980). Suckling. Science 210:15–22.

Bronstein PM (1972). Open-field behavior of the rat as a function of age: cross-sectional and longitudinal investigations. J Comp Physiol Psychol 80:335–41.

Butcher RE, Brunner RL, Roth T, Kimmel CA (1972). A learning impairment associated with maternal hypervitaminosis-A in rats. Life Sci 11:141–5.

Campbell BA, Raskin LA (1978). Ontogeny of behavioral arousal: the role of environmental stimuli. J Comp Physiol Psychol 92:176–84.

Coyle IR, Singer G (1975). The interaction of post-weaning housing conditions and prenatal drug effects on behaviour. Psychopharmacologia 41:237–44.

Crutcher KA (1986). The role of growth factors in neuronal development and plasticity. CRC Crit Rev Clin Neurobiol 2:297–333.

Damassa DA, Clifton DK, Whitmoyer DI (1982). A system for the detection and analysis of ultrasonic calls. Physiol Behav 28:579–81.

D'Amato RJ, Lipman ZP, Snyder SH (1986). Selectivity of the Parkinsonian neurotoxin MPTP: toxic metabolite MPP+ binds to neuromelanin. Science 231:987–9.

Davis M (1984). The mammalian startle response. In: Eaton RC, ed. Neural mechanisms of startle behavior. New York: Plenum Press, 287–351.

Driscoll CD (1991). Screening for developmental neurotoxicity: approaches and controversy. J Am Coll Toxicol 10:697–703.

Duester G, Shean ML, McBride MS, Stewart MJ (1991). Retinoic acid response element in the human alcohol dehydrogenase gene ADH3: implication for regulation of retinoic acid synthesis. Mol Cell Biol 11:1638–46

Egger GJ, Livesey PJ, Dawson RG (1973). Ontogenetic aspects of central cholinergic involvement in spontaneous alternation behavior. Dev Psychobiol 6:289–99.

Elmazar MMA, Sullivan FM (1981). Effect of prenatal phenytoin administration on postnatal development of the rat: a behavioral teratology study. Teratology 24:115–24.

European Drafting Group (1992). Guideline on detection of toxicity to reproduction for medicinal products. Draft No. 13, July 1992. Berlin: International Federation of Teratology Societies.

File SE (1978). The ontogeny of exploration in the rat: habituation and effects of handling. Dev Psychobiol 11:321–8.

Geyer MA, Butcher RE, Fite K (1985). A study of startle and locomotor activity in rats exposed prenatally to methylmercury. Neurobehav Toxicol Teratol 7:759–65.

Goldstein GW, Betz AL (1986). The blood-brain barrier. Sci Am 255:74–83.

Gregory EH, Pfaff DW (1971). Development of olfactory-guided behavior in infant rats. Physiol Behav 6:573–6.

Gudas LJ (1992). Retinoids, retinoid-responsive genes, cell differentiation, and cancer. Cell Growth Differentiation 3:655–62.

Hartman DE (1988). Neuropsychological toxicology: identification and assessment of neurotoxic syndromes. New York: Pergamon Press.

Heyser CJ, Chen W-J, Miller J, Spear NE, Spear LP (1990). Prenatal cocaine exposure induces deficits in Pavlovian conditioning and sensory preconditioning among infant rat pups. Behav Neurosci 104:955–63.

Hutchings DE, Gibbon J, Kaufman MA (1973). Maternal vitamin A excess during the early fetal period: effects on learning and development in the offspring. Dev Psychobiol 6:445–57.

Hutchings DE, Gaston J (1974). The effects of vitamin A excess administered during the mid-fetal period on learning and development in rat offspring. Dev Psychobiol 7:225–33.

Isaacson RL (1975). The myth of recovery from early brain damage. In: Ellis NR, ed. Aberrant development in infancy: human and animal studies. Potomac, Maryland: Lawrence Erlbaum Associates, 1–26.

Kalil RE (1989). Synapse formation in the developing brain. Sci Am 261:76–85.

Kernan WJ Jr, Mullenix PJ, Hopper DL (1989). Time structure analysis of behavioral acts using a computer pattern recognition system. Pharmacol Biochem Behav 34:863–9.

Kimelberg HK, Norenberg MD (1989). Astrocytes. Sci Am 260:66–76.

Kimmel CA, Rees DC, Francis EZ, eds. (1990). Qualitative and quantitative comparability of human and animal developmental neurotoxicity. Neurotoxicol Teratol 12:173–292.

Koob GF, Bloom FE (1988). Cellular and molecular mechanisms of drug dependence. Science 242:715–23.

Kutz SA, Troise NJ, Cimprich RE, Yearsley SM, Rugen PJ (1989). Vitamin A acetate: a behavioral teratology study in rats. Drug Chem Toxicol 12:259–75.

Lammer EJ, Chen DT, Hoar RM, Agnish ND, Benke PJ, Braun JT, Curry CJ, Ernhoff PM, Grix AW, Lott IT, Richard JM, Sun SC (1985). Retinic acid embryopathy. N Engl J Med 313:837–41.

Laouris Y, Kalli-Laouris J, Schwartze P (1990). The postnatal development of the air-righting reaction in albino rats. Quantitative analysis of normal development and the effect of preventing neck-torso and torso-pelvis rotations. Behav Brain Res 37:37–44.

Linney E (1992). Retinoic acid receptors: transcription factors modulating gene regulation, development, and differentiation. Curr Top Dev Biol 27:309–50.

Malakhovskii VG (1969). Behavioral disturbances in rats receiving teratogenic agents antinatally. Bull Exp Biol Med (USSR) 68:1230–2.

Malakhovskii VG (1971). Antenatal effect of pyrimethamine and vitamin A on behavior of the rat progency. Bull Exp Biol Med (USSR) 71:254–6.

Mangelsdorf DJ, Ong ES, Dyck JA, Evans RM (1990). Nuclear receptor that identifies a novel retinoic acid response pathway. Nature 345:224–9.

Martin JC, Martin DC (1981). Voluntary activity in the aging rat as a function of maternal drug exposure. Neurobehav Toxicol Teratol 3:261–4.

Martin JC, Martin DC, Radow B, Day HE (1979). Life span and pathology in offspring following nicotine and methamphetamine exposure. Expl Aging Res 5:509–22.

Martin JC, Martin DC, Radow B, Sigman G (1976). Growth, development and activity in rat offspring following maternal drug exposure. Expl Aging Res 2:235–51.

Martin JC, Martin DC, Sigman G, Day-Pfeiffer H (1983). Saccharin preferences in food deprived aging rats are altered as a function of perinatal drug exposure. Physiol Behav 30:853–8.

Minck DR, Acuff-Smith KD, Vorhees CV (1991). Comparison of the behavioral teratogenic potential of phenytoin, mephenytoin, ethotoin, and hydantoin in rats. Teratology 43:279–93.

Mooney MP, Hoyenga KT, Blick-Hoyenga K, Morton JRC (1981). Prenatal hypervitaminosis A and postnatal behavioral development in the rat. Neurobehav Toxicol Teratol 3:1–4.

Moorcroft WH, Lytle LD, Campbell BA (1971). Ontogeny of starvation-induced behavioral arousal in the rat. J Comp Physiol Psychol 75:59–67.

National Research Council, National Academy of Science (1992). Environmental neurotoxicology. Washington, D.C.: National Academy Press.

Nolen GA (1986). The effects of prenatal retinoic acid on the viability and behavior of the offspring. Neurobehav Toxicol Teratol 8:643–54.

Office of Technology Assessment, United States Congress (1990). Neurotoxicology: identifying and controlling poisons of the nervous system. Washington, D.C.: Congress of the United States.

Parisi T, Ison JR (1979). Development of the acoustic startle response in the rat: ontogenetic changes in the magnitude of inhibition by prepulse stimulation. Dev Psychobiol 12:219–30.

Paulus MP, Geyer MA (1991). A temporal and spatial scaling hypothesis for the behavioral effects of psychostimulants. Psychopharmacology 104:6–16.

Pellis SM, Pellis VC, Chen Y-C, Barzci S, Teitelbaum P (1989). Recovery from axial apraxia in the lateral hypothalamic labyrinthectomized rat reveals three elements of contact-righting: cephallocaudal dominance, axial rotation, and distal limb action. Behav Brain Res 35:241–51.

Pellis SM, Pellis VC, Morrissey TK, Teitelbaum P (1989). Visual modulation of vetiburlarly-triggered air-righting in the rat. Behav Brain Res 35:23–6.

Pellis SM, Pellis VC, Teitelbaum P (1991). Air righting without the cervical righting reflex in adult rats. Behav Brain Res 45:185–8.

Pellis SM, Whishaw IQ, Pellis VC (1991). Visual modulation of vestiburlarly-triggered air-righting in rats involves the superior colliculus. Behav Brain Res 46:151–6.

Potash M, Ferguson HB (1977). The effect of criterion level on the acquisition of retention of a 1-way avoidance response in young and old rats. Dev Psychobiol 10:347–54.

Purves D, Lichtman JW (1985). Principles of neural development. Sunderland, Massachusetts: Sinau.

Rice SA, Millan DP (1986). Validation of a developmental swimming test using Swiss Webster mice perinatally treated with methimazole. Neurobehav Toxicol Teratol 8:69–75.

Riley EP, Vorhees CV, eds. (1986). Handbook of behavioral teratology. New York: Plenum Press.

Risau W, Wolburg H (1990). Development of the blood-brain barrier. Trends Neurosci 12:174–8.

Rodier PM (1980). Chronology of neuron development: animal studies and their clinical implications. Dev Med Child Neurol 22:525–45.

Ruppert PH, Dean KF, Reiter LW (1985). Development of locomotor activity of rats pups in figure-eight mazes. Dev Psychobiol 18:247–60.

Saillenfait AM, Vannier B (1988). Methodological proposal in behavioural teratogenicity testing: assessment of propoxyphene, chlorpromazine, and vitamin A as positive controls. Teratology 37:185–99.

Sanberg PR, Hagenmeyer SH, Henault MA (1985). Automated measurement of multivariate locomotor behavior in rodents. Neurobehav Toxicol Teratol 7:87–94.

Schapiro S, Salas M, Vukovich K (1970). Hormonal effects on ontogeny of swimming ability in the rat: assessment of central nervous system development. Science 168:147–51.

Shatz CJ (1992). The developing brain. Sci Am 267:61–7.

Spear LP (1984). Age at the time of testing reconsidered in neurobehavioral teratology research. In: Yanai J, ed. Neurobehavioral teratology. Amsterdam: Elsevier, 315–28.

Spear LP, Enters EK, Linville DG (1985). Age-specific behaviors as tools for examining teratogen-induced neural alterations. Neurobehav Toxicol Teratol 7:691–5.

Spear LP, Kirstein CL, Bell J, Yoottanasumpun V, Greenbaum R, O'Shea J, Hoffmann H, Spear NE (1989). Effects of prenatal cocaine exposure on behavior during the early postnatal period. Neurotoxicol Teratol 11:57–63.

Spyker JM (1975). Assessing the impact of low level chemicals on development: behavioral and latent effects. Fed Proc 34:1835–44.

Tyndale RF, Sunahara R, Inaba T, Kalow W, Gonzalex FJ, Niznik HB (1991). Neuronal cytochrome P450IID1 (debrisoquine/sparteine-type): potent inhibition of activity by (–)-cocaine and nucleotide sequence identity to human hepatic P450 gene CYP2D6. Mol Pharmacol 40:63–8.

Umesono K, Murakami KK, Thompson CC, Evans RM (1991). Direct repeats as selective response elements for the thyroid hormone, retinoic acid, and vitamin D_3 receptors. Cell 65:1255–66.

Vorhees CV (1974). Some behavioral effects of maternal hypervitaminosis A. Teratology 10:269–74.

Vorhees CV (1983). Fetal anticonvulsant syndrome in rats: Dose- and period-response relationships of prenatal diphenylhydantoin, trimethadione, and phenobarbital exposure on the structural and functional development of the offspring. J Pharmacol Exp Ther 227:274–87.

Vorhees CV (1985). Behavioral effect of prenatal methylmercury in rats: a parallel trial to the Collaborative Behavioral Teratology Study. Neurobehav Toxicol Teratol 7:717–25.

Vorhees CV (1986a). Comparison and critique of government regulations for behavioral teratology. In: Riley EP, Vorhees CV, eds. Handbook of behavioral teratology. New York: Plenum Press, 49–66.

Vorhees CV (1986b). Methods for assessing the adverse effects of foods and other chemicals on animal behavior. Nutr Rev 44(suppl):185–92.

Vorhees CV (1986c). Retinoic acid embryopathy. N Engl J Med 315:262–3.

Vorhees CV (1987). Fetal hydantoin syndrome in rats: dose-effect relationships of prenatal phenytoin on postnatal development and behavior. Teratology 35:287–303.

Vorhees CV (1989). Behavioral teratology: what's not in a name: a reply to Cattabeni and Abbracchio. Neurotoxicol Teratol 11:325–7.

Vorhees CV (1992). Developmental neurotoxicology. In: Tilson HA, Mitchell CL, eds. Neurotoxicology: target organ toxicology series. New York: Raven Press, 295–329.

Vorhees CV, Brunner RL, McDaniel CR, Butcher RE (1978). The relationship of gestational age to vitamin A induced postnatal dysfunction. Teratology 17:271–6.

Vorhees CV, Butcher RE (1982). Behavioral teratogenicity. In: Snell K, ed. Developmental Toxicity. New York: Praeger Press, 247–98.

Vorhees CV, Minck DR (1989). Long-term effects of prenatal phenytoin exposure on offspring behavior in rats. Neurotoxicol Teratol 11:295–305.

Vorhees CV, Acuff-Smith KD, Minck DR, Butcher RE (1992). A method for measuring locomotor behavior in rodents: Contrast-sensitive computer-controlled video tracking activity assessment in rats. Neurotoxicol Teratol 14:43–9.

Vorhees CV, Brunner RL, Butcher RE (1979a). Psychotropic drugs as behavioral teratogens. Science 205:1220–5.

Vorhees CV, Butcher RE, Brunner RL, Sobotka TJ (1979b). A developmental test battery for neurobehavioral toxicity in rats: a preliminary analysis using monosodium glutamate, calcium carrageenan and hydroxyurea. Toxicol Appl Pharmacol 50:267–82.

Vorhees CV, Minck DR (1989). Long-term effects of prenatal phenytoin exposure on offspring behavior in rats. Neurotoxicol Teratol 11:295–305.

Weisenburger WP, Minck DR, Acuff KD, Vorhees CV (1990). Dose-response effects of prenatal phenytoin exposure in rats: effects on early locomotion, maze learning, and memory as a function of phenytoin-induced circling behavior. Neurotoxicol Teratol 12:145–52.

Weiss B, Spyker JM (1974). Behavioral implications of prenatal and early postnatal exposure to chemical pollutants. Pediatrics 53:851–9.

Wolf G (1990). Recent progress in vitamin A research: nuclear retinoic acid receptors and their interaction with gene elements. J Nutr Biochem 1:284–9.

Wolf G (1991). The intracellular vitamin A–binding proteins: an overview of their functions. Nutr Rev 49:1–12.

Yu VC, Selsert C, Andersen B, Holloway JM, Devary OV, Naar AM, Kim SY, Boutin J-M, Glass CK, Rosenfeld MG (1991). RXRβ: A coregulator that enhances binding of retinoic acid, thyroid hormone, and vitamin D receptors to their cognate response elements. Cell 67:1251–6.

28
Delayed Neurotoxicity: A Silent Toxicity

Bernard Weiss

University of Rochester School of Medicine and Dentistry
Rochester, New York

Kenneth Reuhl

Rutgers University
Piscataway, New Jersey

INTRODUCTION

Silent toxicity is a concept with many dimensions and definitions. In its most general sense it refers to a toxic process whose manifestations lurk undetected. In some contexts, it may be used to describe a process with a long latency between original exposure and measureable effect. In others, it may refer to a progressive, cumulative accretion of damage that eventually blooms into detectability. In still others, it encompasses the combined actions of the toxic exposure and another variable, such as aging or a pharmacological challenge, that unveils underlying damage. From a nosological point of view, it may describe a situation in which toxicity remains covert because of inadequate measures.

These illustrations of the concept suggest why it is especially applicable to neurotoxicity. Toxicologists are accustomed to regard carcinogenesis as the prototype of silent toxicity because of its extended latency, often bridging decades, and because of the widely assumed multistage nature of the disease. Neurotoxicity, too, reflects many aspects of a multistage process, and bears other similarities to cancer. The similarities are striking when cancer and neurodegenerative diseases are compared (Weiss, 1991).

THE CANCER PROTOTYPE

Figure 1 shows the hypothetical development of a breast tumor given a specified doubling time after the original carcinogenic event, which itself may be the culmination of a cascade of preceding events. It makes the point quite graphically that clinical detection of the tumor is usually feasible only after the underlying process has accumulated a long subclinical history. Many neurodegenerative diseases must follow a similar progression.

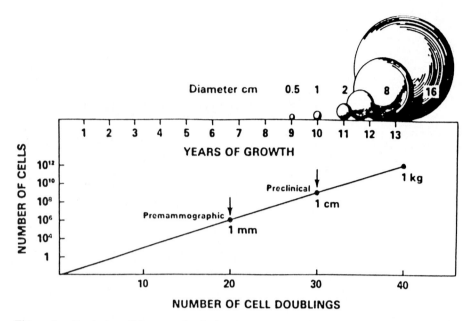

Figure 1   Depiction of the growth of a breast tumor, showing the typically long latency to clinical emergence. Tumor diameter is based on a presumed doubling time of 100 days. (From Gullino, 1977.)

Parkinson's disease, Alzheimer's disease, amyotrophic lateral sclerosis, and other afflictions are presumed also to emerge clinically once they reach an advanced stage. For example, most authorities claim that the course of Parkinson's disease remains covert until perhaps 80–90% of dopaminergic cells in the substantia nigra have succumbed.

Because of this silent progression, the incidence of neurodegenerative diseases, like that of most cancers, accelerates with age. As noted in Table 1, this is one of the cogent parallels between neurodegenerative disease and cancer. Both quantitative and biological models of carcinogenesis typically assume a sequence of stages to explain the conversion of a molecular event acting on DNA into a tumor. Potential triggering events for neurodegenerative diseases are rarely discussed in an analogous way, perhaps because of the lack of a recognized mechanism such as genetic transformation.

Table 1   Analogies Between Carcinogenesis and Neurodegenerative Diseases

1. Age-specific incidence rises sharply with age.
   Is the damage superimposed on or entwined with aging?
2. Clinical signs emerge late in the course of the disease.
   What is the mathematical form of the progression?
   What is the rate of advance once detected?
3. Marked geographic variations are observed.
   What is the role of diet?
   What other environmental variables are critical?
4. Events early in life may underlie the progression.
   Is there a triggering event?
   Is there a cascade of events (a multistage process)?

A second parallel listed in Table 1, the emergence of clinical manifestations late in the course of the disease process, is largely attributable to the reserve and compensatory capacity of the central nervous system. For many of its functions, though hardly all, the brain is a remarkably redundant system. Its redundancy can mask intrinsic damage or deficient function, a problem for assessment and prediction. A neurotoxic process or event initiated by low-dose exposure may lie unnoticed until other events or processes, long afterward, have eroded the redundant margin. Such a possibility is one argument for longitudinal studies.

Environmental etiologies for many cancers are assumed, as listed in Table 1. Individual patterns of behavior, such as cigarette smoking, form one class of environmental agents. Here, the mechanistic connection is unassailable. Marked geographical variations in cancer incidence provoke more subtle questions. Maps from the National Cancer Institute display remarkable differences from one area to another that are difficult to explain by any single variable. Wide differences in the incidence or prevalence of neurodegenerative disease, except for specific cases such as the amyotrophic lateral sclerosis/Parkinsonism Dementia (ALS/PD) syndrome in the western Pacific area, similarly resist direct explanation. Multiple sclerosis displays a striking elevation in prevalence in temperate as compared with tropical latitudes, and even concentrated geographical clusters, suggesting an environmental source that exerts its influence over a long latent period.

Finally, as noted in Table 1, both cancer and neurodegenerative diseases may be the result of an event or events that occurred much earlier in life and lay quiescent for periods as long as decades. Some victims of the ALS-PD syndrome had emigrated from areas such as Guam, its best-known locus, decades before they were diagnosed with the disease (Zhang et al, 1990). It is presumed that, during the earlier periods of their lives, they had been exposed to factors, such as diet, that triggered the degenerative process.

Mathematical models of carcinogenesis are typically formulated to explain the long latencies noted in both experimental and epidemiological investigations. The power functions seen when incidence is plotted against age were major determinants of the multistage model of carcinogenesis, in fact. Peto et al. (1975), however, noted the confounding of age and duration, and offered experimental results supporting duration rather than age itself as the principal variable. Similar modeling and experimental approaches have not been applied to neurotoxicology. They might elicit useful insights, however.

MODEL DISEASES

What Spencer (1990) has termed nature's experiments may help clarify some of the issues posed to neurotoxicology by agents and exposure patterns that engender, at least superficially, long silent periods.

Parkinson's Disease

Damage to and impaired function of the dopamine nigrostriatal system is now presumed to underlie the clinical features of Parkinson's disease (PD). The brains of PD patients show marked erosion in the population of the dopamine-containing pigmented neurons of the substantia nigra (SN) pars compacta, which results in the lowering of dopamine levels throughout the forebrain. Parkinson's disease is also presumed to be preceded by an extended silent period because, as noted earlier, a substantial decline in cell number has to occur before clinical signs erupt, and because the decline is presumed to occur gradually. Marsden (1990) estimated that the process may begin 30 years before its clinical eruption. One source of these assumptions is the loss of SN cells with age in the brains of persons free of clinical PD (McGeer et al, 1988). The decrease in dopamine levels with aging has also been observed in animals. Such findings correspond to data showing an accelerating prevalence of PD with age; white men 45–54 years of age have an estimated prevalence of 43.3 per 100,000, while the prevalence for ages 65 and over is close to 700 per 100,000. It seems reasonable to postulate a connection between the two observations.

Calne et al. (1986) formulated one variant of such a connection. They offered the hypothesis that PD, Alzheimer's disease, and motor neuron disease (amyotrophic lateral sclerosis; ALS) arise from environmentally induced damage to the nervous system but remain clinically silent until the attrition of nerve cell populations with age renders the earlier damage manifest. Because symptoms may not appear until decades after the original damage, they proposed that greater attention be directed to the environment in early life, both to evaluate causation and to devise strategies for prevention.

One rationale for the emphasis on environmental factors in PD is the lack of convincing evidence for a genetic etiology. Even twin studies fail to indicate the kind of concordance to be expected were there a marked genetic influence (Martilla et al., 1988). Moreover, clusters of PD have been reported for which there is no explanation other than the environment. One example is a Canadian study demonstrating a marked difference between rural and urban populations in the prevalence of early-onset PD; one hypothesis proposed to account for the difference points to the sources of drinking water—wells rather than municipal water supplies (Rajput et al., 1986). Even when PD has been observed in families, age differences among the members at the time of onset suggest a common environment rather than common genes as the arbiter. The most compelling source was the discovery of an agent, MPTP (1-methyl-4-phenyl-1,2,3,6-tetrahydropyridine), that selectively damages dopamine-containing cells in primate SN and that can induce a PD syndrome in humans (for review see Langston, 1989). The remarkable specificity of MPTP released a flood of speculation about environmental contributions to PD and to other neurodegenerative diseases as well. Some of the recent data implicate residence, at least early in life, in rural areas of both North America and Nigeria where wells provided the drinking water. Exposure to toxicants such as manganese and other metals (Zayed et al., 1990) and to chemicals used in orchards (Hertzman et al., 1990) also shows associations with PD incidence.

Parkinson's disease is a prototype for neurotoxicity both because of MPTP and because enough is known about dopamine function to support a hypothesized neurotoxic process based on its actions. First, striatal dopamine suffers a loss, in humans, of 5–8% per decade (Carlsson and Winblad, 1976). Second, experimental evidence indicates that nigrostriatal lesions incite compensatory responses in the remaining cells to produce more dopamine (Zigmond et al., 1990). Measurements of the dopamine metabolite homovanillic acid indicate that elevated dopamine turnover also occurs in the brains of patients who have suffered from PD (Hornykiewicz et al, 1989). Figure 2 (Weiss, 1991) shows how much additional dopamine would have to be synthesized by the remaining cells as other cells become dysfunctional. Animal studies suggest that these remaining cells may be able to produce a compensatory five- to tenfold increase in output as the original population of dopamine-producing cells wanes.

This increase in output is not necessarily without cost, however. Several authors hypothesize that the metabolic byproducts of dopamine oxidation may themselves be potent

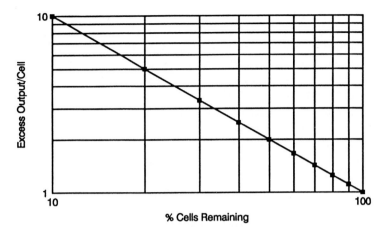

Figure 2   Plot demonstrating the amount of additional dopamine that would have to be synthesized by each remaining cell as other cells die off. For example, if 80% of the original population of cells has succumbed, each of the remaining cells would have to raise its rate of synthesis fivefold.

neurotoxicants. Toxic oxygen species are one such by-product. One metabolic pathway for dopamine proceeds via monoamine oxidase, which produces one mole of hydrogen peroxide for each mole of dopamine oxidized (Langston, 1989). In addition to its direct action, hydrogen peroxide is converted to hydroxyl radicals, another source of oxidative stress (cf, Bondy, this volume). Graham (1984) noted that quinones formed by the autoxidation of dopamine may also be toxic.

McGeer et al. (1988) and others report that PD is an active degenerative process, not simply an acceleration of the natural cell erosion accompanying aging. But it can be argued that once loss has proceeded beyond a certain degree, the compensatory elevation in dopamine synthesis begins to deposit toxic by-products in excess of the capacity of mechanisms capable of disposing and neutralizing them. The observation that glutathione (GSH) levels fall with age suggests one way in which aging might predispose the onset of PD. Although GSH levels must fall substantially before toxicity appears (Uhlig and Wendel, 1992), the combination of decreased GSH concentrations and increased metabolic demands might prove synergistic. Their joint actions could contribute to a mechanistic explanation for the increased incidence of neurodegenerative diseases with aging and for the rates at which clinically manifested syndromes progress.

The aging brain may also prove less resistant to toxic byproducts. Date et al. (1990) noted that MPTP treatments produced permanent damage in older mice (aged 12 months), which was succeeded by at least partial recovery in younger mice (aged 2–3 months). Both aging and earlier injury, then, could set the stage for an active degenerative process provoked by excessive rates of dopamine synthesis. Should disposal of the enhanced production of toxic metabolites be unable to match these production rates, and were disposal rates governed by zero-order kinetics, injury to susceptible cells would accelerate. Some form of such a process was hypothesized by Bernheimer et al. (1973): "The idea suggests itself that clinically manifest Parkinsonism represents the second, decompensated stage of a biochemical disturbance characterized by a progressive [dopamine] deficiency in the striatum."

Alzheimer's Disease

The predominant risk factor for Alzheimer's disease (AD), as for PD, is age. Although family history, indicating a genetic role, modulates the risk, the prevalence of the disease rises sharply beyond the age of 65. Because no environmental contributions as compelling as MPTP have been identified, intrinsic factors such as amyloid proteins rather than extrinsic factors have attracted the bulk of current research. Some extrinsic contributions are now materializing, however. The most intriguing emerged from a study in Shanghai by Zhang et al. (1990) that implicated lack of education in elderly women as a significant risk factor. The authors speculated that lack of education might diminish what they termed a brain "reserve." A history of head trauma is another extrinsic factor and is especially pertinent because psychometric testing indicates residual deficits in head injury victims despite apparent clinical recovery. Heart disease and myocardial infarction also elevate the risk of AD in older patients. A form of AD closely coupled to environmental chemical exposure is the ALS-PD syndrome observed in the western Pacific. It has been ascribed to the consumption of cycad seeds (Spencer, 1990) and to imbalances in mineral intake, particularly of calcium and aluminum (Garruto and Yase, 1986).

The rising incidence of AD with age suggests a long latent period before overt expression of the underlying damage, mostly in the form of intellectual impairment. The underlying damage takes the form of neuronal and synaptic loss in critical brain areas. Pursuit of the molecular foundations of this process, now a subject of intense scrutiny, has increasingly targeted amyloid and its precursor protein, APP. One question that could help illuminate some of those posed to neurotoxicology is how the intrinsic and extrinsic factors are joined.

In parallel with their hypothesis about the possible environmental pathogenesis of PD, Calne et al. (1985) postulated that some forms of AD may also be the product of natural aging combined with some other process, possibly one instigated by an environmental neurotoxicant. Exposure to such a toxicant would further erode the reserve capacity of the nervous system, and the combination would then shift brain functional competence to an age index at which much more damage and impairment is visible. The detection of AD correlates, such as amyloid deposits and neurofibrillary tangles, in the brains of persons who demonstrated no overt signs of diminished function, supports such a hypothesis. Further support comes from the risk factors noted earlier. Lack of education has a counterpart in the animal literature, which shows that enriched environments early in life multiply the richness of synaptic connections (Rosenzweig and Bennett, 1978). Head trauma leading to neuronal death, and cerebral ischemia inducing neuronal damage, are other ways in which reduced reserve capacity might lead to an earlier onset of signs correlated with aging. Dementia pugilistica is surely the outcome of cumulative small-scale head injuries. Choi (1992) speculates that such minute traumas might release excitotoxic amino acids that amplify, in an insidious way, the acute damage.

Some of the speculations about the mechanistic undercurrents of PD point to toxic by-products, as described above. They note how compensatory processes such as elevated dopamine production can seed pathogenetic products. Might similar processes apply to AD? Such a possibility was offered by Greenamyre (1991) in response to the proposition that enhanced neuronal activitation might counteract the degenerative process that marks AD. He proposed that neuronal activation, rather than proving beneficial, might simply accelerate the process because of the expanded release of glutamate; he characterized this as a "use it and lose it" hypothesis.

Amyotrophic Lateral Sclerosis

Motor neuron disease or ALS is more rare than either PD or AD, striking 1–2 people in 100,000. It, too, acts in a remarkably selective manner, destroying the motor neurons of the central nervous system. Although some small percentage of cases can be traced to genetic origins, the most common form of the disease seems to lack a genetic explanation, and it has been speculated that it arises from some unidentified environmental factor. Such a factor to explain the bulk of cases remains to be identified, but, at least for some variants of ALS, an environmental contribution seems compelling.

Silent or subclinical poliomyelitis was advanced as a candidate by Martyn et al. (1988). They compared standardized mortality ratios for ALS during the years 1968–1978 with notification rates for polio during 1931–1939 in 142 defined areas of England and Wales. Most infectious diseases, such as scarlet fever, yielded insignificant correlations between rates during the 1930s and ALS rates 40 years later. For poliomyelitis, in contrast, the regression analysis yielded a coefficient of 0.42. Moreover, no relationship with polio rate could be discerned for any other leading cause of death.

The authors suggested that at least some forms of ALS represent the delayed consequence of a previous subclinical infection with polio virus. Such an early infection, particularly if it occurs during the first few years of life, would be unlikely to produce paralysis, but can lead to loss of critical nerve cells. Later in life, as additional neurons are lost through aging or through excessive demands on the intact neurons, compensation for the original loss, as by collateral sprouting of dendrites, begins to ebb and clinical signs finally emerge.

Some observers note similarities between this hypothesis and the post-polio syndrome, which describes the recurrence of polio signs three or four decades after the original infection. Although ALS and the post-polio syndrome currently represent two distinctive diagnostic groups, the proposed underlying mechanisms overlap substantially. The suggestion by Martyn et al. (1988) that compensatory demands may prod remaining intact neurons into excessive activity has a counterpart in the recommendation of clinicians that post-polio patients minimize certain kinds of physical stresses to conserve their current capacities. It also has a counterpart in Greenamyre's "use it and lose it" hypothesis, noted above, for AD. In fact, recent data also implicate glutamate in the genesis, or at least the progression, of ALS. On the basis of synaptosomal preparations from ALS patients, control patients, and patients with other neurodegenerative diseases, Rothstein et al. (1992) concluded that ALS is associated with a defect in glutamate transport. Such a defect may foster high levels of extracellular glutamate, resulting in neurotoxic reactions in susceptible regions such as the spinal cord and motor cortex. An accompanying editorial by Choi (1992) underscored the role that excitotoxicity is now hypothesized to play in many neurodegenerative diseases.

These three major neurological diseases—PD, AD, and ALS—embody striking parallels with what we generally consider to be neurotoxic responses. All have been connected with nerve cell damage arising from some presumed toxic process rather than with what might be termed a passive or spontaneous erosion of cells with age, for example. It also has been speculated that all three, or at least some variants of them, are possibly rooted in events occurring earlier in life. Finally, they have generated hypotheses about the contribution of environmental factors, including chemicals, to their etiology.

EXAMPLES FROM NEUROTOXICOLOGY

The neurotoxicology literature provides both parallels and contrasts with that devoted to neurodegenerative diseases. The parallels lie in the attribution of processes to account for the late emergence of signs. The contrasts lie in the identification of the responsible agent and the measurement of its effects.

Lead

Recognized as a poison since antiquity, lead has emerged as a model agent for neurobehavioral toxicology because of the different guises in which its toxicity appears. Gross neurotoxicity, such as encephalopathy, is a minor concern in the advanced industrial societies because of protective measures adopted in years past. Subtle neurotoxicity is the predominant concern and the focus both of current research and of regulation.

As a prototype of silent toxicity, lead offers three distinctive although related phenomena. First, lead toxicity offers an example of an adverse effect complex whose manifestations are detectable only after the application of psychological tests. Second, a shift through time is observed in how these adverse effects are expressed. Finally, changing patterns of correlations between indices of exposure and their later consequences have been noted.

The evolution of our current understanding of lead toxicity is acknowledged to have begun with the report of Byers and Lord (1943). It noted that children allegedly recovered from an episode of lead poisoning exhibited, despite the absence of clinical signs, evidence of lingering damage. The indications included hyperactivity and learning disabilities. Between 1943 and 1979, studies of lead toxicity in children turned increasingly to what are now considered the critical variables. A publication by Needleman et al. (1979) completed the movement to the new orientation. In this now-seminal paper, the investigators demonstrated that even in children showing no demonstrable clinical signs of lead toxicity, an index of lead exposure based on concentrations in shed deciduous teeth correlated with scores on an intelligence test and other psychological tests. Silent damage, so to speak, was given a voice.

Needleman et al. followed many of these children, tested originally as first- and second-grade pupils, through high school. In their late teens, the expression of adverse effects assumed another facade (Needleman et al., 1990). Tooth lead concentrations in the early school grades now showed correlations with indices such as the proportion of students graduating from high school or prevalence of reading difficulties. These relationships could have been mediated by IQ or by the problem classroom behaviors, such as impaired attention, noted earlier (Needleman et al., 1979) as correlating with tooth lead levels. Changes in the profile of neurotoxic effects with time, particularly as a consequence of damage early in life, should not be surprising; such changes have been observed, as will be noted later, after experimental lesions.

A different kind of shift, representing a displacement in time, also has been observed with lead. Several groups of investigators undertook longitudinal studies to document how lead might modify the course of neurobehavioral development. Bellinger et al. (1987) have been following a population of infants from birth. The sample was separated into three exposure groups based on mean umbilical cord blood concentrations: low (1.8 μg/dl), medium (6.5 μg/dl), and high (14.5 μg/dl). For the first 2 years, each child was assessed at 6-month intervals with the Bayley Scales of Infant Development. During this time, the gap in scores on the Mental Development Index of the Bayley Scales between the high- and low-lead groups widened, perhaps because items for the later ages are more sensitive to lead effects.

The children were tested again at about 57 months of age. At this time, the major predictor of test scores derived from the WISC-R (Wechsler Intelligence Scale for Children-Revised) turned out to be blood lead levels at age 24 months rather than cord blood concentrations. That a significant correlation appeared is itself surprising given that the mean value was about 7 μg/dl.

Most of the attacks on the human data are based on the contention that important variables remained inadequately controlled. Because parental intelligence, social and economic status, home environment, and many other factors can all contribute to children's IQ performance, confounding can always be raised as an issue. Analogous findings in animal experiments offer the most cogent sources of support for the human data. A long series of experiments by Rice and Gilbert and their collaborators are among those that convincingly confirm the epidemiological results of Needleman et al. (1979, 1990), Bellinger et al. (1987), and others. Conducted in primates, these experiments demonstrate that lead exposure early in life, even at modest blood levels, induces persistent behavioral outcomes. One example is the finding by Rice and Karpinski (1988) based on delayed-alternation performance. In such a situation, the subjects must alternate between two response locations, such as left and right levers, to secure reinforcements, but are given the opportunity to make the response only after a programmed delay. Lead-treated monkeys often persisted in responding on the same lever, despite the lack of reinforcement.

Methylmercury

A voluminous literature testifies to the neurotoxic potency of methylmercury in the fetal brain. The data come from both human and animal research and extend across the entire domain of toxicology from epidemiology to molecular biology. Because methylmercury is such a potent neural poison, gross damage to the nervous system is easy to inflict, which explains why the preponderance of methylmercury research in the laboratory is based on high doses delivered over short periods of time. Most assessments of the functional consequences are also based on restricted periods of time and, moreover, on relatively simple behavioral criteria. Given that dietary consumption of fish accounts for the overwhelming bulk of human exposure to methylmercury, and that chronic consumption is the primary exposure schedule, most of the questions about health risks arise from concerns about subtle functional deficits attributable to neurotoxicity in the developing brain. The available evidence indicates that the consequences of early neurotoxic damage may remain unexpressed for considerable periods.

The calamitous episode of methylmercury poisoning in Iraq in the winter of 1971–1972 (Bakir et al., 1973) yielded an opportunity to study carefully the offspring of mothers who had consumed the contaminated grain. It first became apparent there that even in children who showed no clinical signs of dysfunction during infancy, underlying damage could emerge in forms such as delayed walking (Cox et al., 1989). In children exposed only through breast milk, some manifestations of impaired development became apparent only after they reached 5 years of age (Amin-Zaki et al., 1981). Speech development, because it cannot be observed until at least 2 years of age, was another marker of methylmercury exposure apparent only late in development.

Quantitative psychological testing provides further suggestions of latent damage. Two studies conducted in New Zealand by Kjellstrom et al. (1986, 1989) relied on developmental milestones and intelligence-type tests to assess the relationship between maternal consumption of methylmercury (indexed by hair levels) and developmental status in the offspring. None of the children displayed any evidence of clinical dysfunction, but the higher maternal hair levels were correlated with reduced test scores.

As in humans, the developing brain in laboratory species ranging from monkeys to mice appears to be far more susceptible than the mature brain (reviewed by Reuhl and Chang, 1979; Chang, 1987; Burbacher et al., 1990). Corresponding functional consequences have also been documented (reviewed by Ecles and Annau, 1987). They range from overt motor dysfunction to altered avoidance performance to changes in schedule-controlled operant behavior.

Despite this extensive literature, we remain relatively ignorant about several crucial issues. Most particularly, how is prenatal damage reflected later in the life cycle? Reuhl et al. (1981a,b) observed that residual damage due to prenatal exposure was clearly detectable in the mature brain. Perhaps the most convincing and direct experimental support for the hypothesis that the total effects of early methylmercury exposure many not erupt until advanced age comes from the work of Cranmer (Spyker, 1975). She treated pregnant mice with methylmercury, then maintained selected offspring until late in life. Some of these mice began to evince neurological deficits, such as tremor and ataxia, only after they reached 10–15 months of age. Furthermore, 12- to 15-month-old mice, which appeared normal when observed in the home cage, maintained themselves on a rotating vertical grid only with difficulty. As the exposed mice approached 2.5–3 years of age, the relative incidence of neurological deficits and other signs of deterioration rose steeply. Several peculiar and unexpected syndromes, such as abnormal weight loss and gain, also appeared.

Ionizing Radiation

Mental retardation is accepted as one possible aftermath of exposure to ionizing radiation during gestation. The Hiroshima and Nagasaki populations provide the clearest epidemiological evidence because of the wide range of doses received and because the exposure occurred acutely. Because of recently revised and more accurate estimates of dose, Otake and Schull (1984) were able to correlate dose and risk for different periods during gestation. Their analyses indicate the most vulnerable period to lie between 8 and 15 weeks after conception.

The implications of their findings transcend the bounds of this population. Their analysis suggests that the frequency of clinically defined mental retardation may double, on the basis of a linear regression on dose, with each rad increment of exposure to ionizing radiation during the 8- to 15-week period. This interval is critical for brain development because it includes two waves of cell migration to sites in the neocortex. But another question is evoked by the data. Is it conceivable that, owing to individual differences in susceptibility and timing, other persons incurred less interference with brain development than that required to produce mental retardation? Intelligence test scores obtained after the survivors reached school age, even excluding cases of mental retardation, also showed a significant regression on dose. The loss of IQ points (based on a Japanese test) came to 7–10 points for each gray of absorbed energy by the 8- to 15-week group. It reached 13–21 points for the group exposed between gestational weeks 16 and 25.

These survivors are now in their late forties. Can the early developmental impact still be traced? Will aging add to or magnify the earlier damage? Such questions are probably too politically sensitive to pursue, but some animal data imply that a phenomenon similar to the post-polio syndrome cannot be dismissed. Wallace et al. (1972) exposed neonatal rats to varying regimens of ionizing radiation. Gross motor deficits were apparent early in life, but tended to fade as the rats grew to adulthood. Once they reached about 2.5 years of age, however, some of the animals that earlier had seemed indistinguishable from controls began to manifest ataxia, tremor, gait disorders, and decreased activity. Brain weight and total dose were linearly correlated, and at the higher doses the decrease in brain weight was substantial; but even at the lower doses, which produced only small decreases, behavioral manifestations were detectable. This report indicates that before senescence, the brains of these rats were capable of compensating for the earlier damage, but that they lost that capacity with advanced age and its constriction of compensatory capacity.

Pharmaceuticals

The term "behavioral teratology" actually was first applied to the subsequent functional effects of prenatal exposure to centrally active drugs (Werboff, 1970). Only later was it adopted by experimenters working in toxicology. Drugs continue to provide useful information, however, and underscore the importance of longitudinal investigations.

Benzodiazepines, because of their widespread use, have been the focus of many investigations. A recent review by Bignami et al. (1992) reported on a program devoted to behavioral development in mice. One experiment examined maternal aggression in mice exposed to oxazepam during gestation. Lactating mice with such an exposure history displayed a marked enhancement of aggressive responses toward males intruding into the nest area. Such a tendency, of course, would remain latent until the dams reached breeding age and became pregnant.

An even more complex outcome of prenatal benzodiazepine treatment appeared in a study by Miranda et al. (1990). They administered diazepam to pregnant rats, then followed the offspring until advanced age. During this time, they measured several indices of brain metabolism in animals ranging from 3 to 26 months of age. One of their indices consisted of levels of thiobarbituric acid–reactive substances, an index chosen because certain of these products increase with age. The major component is malondialdehyde (MDA), a product of lipid peroxidation. Different brain regions showed different patterns of MDA levels over time and as a function of dose. After prenatal treatment with the lower dose (1.0 mg/kg), MDA levels tended to be high at 3 months of age, to fall sharply by 18 months of age, and to rise again to the formerly high levels at 26 months of age. The authors concluded that "the processes of development and aging themselves can interact with the consequences of prenatal [diazepam] exposure on metabolism in a manner that indicates the possible presence of important biological transition phases during the lifespan of an organism" (Miranda et al. 1990).

Lesions

Early brain development is usually regarded as a period during which damage is more easily compensated for than in adulthood. The immature brain is held to display greater "plasticity" than the mature brain. The publications of Margaret Kennard (for example, 1940) made such an assertion on the basis of experiments with monkeys who were subjected to acute motor cortex lesions during infancy. They also drew support from other studies in other species. Only later did the flaws in design and reasoning become apparent.

Much of the plasticity doctrine is the product of observations based on trauma to the brain regions subserving language. Children apparently emerge from episodes that obliterate language in adults still capable of acquiring language skills. Such phenomena have led to generalizations about other kinds of damage that are contradicted by a substantial body of evidence. Isaacson (1975), among others, has questioned the validity of such generalizations, arguing that the concept of "recovery" is complex rather than unidimensional. He pointed out, in just one of many examples, that lesions of the medullary pyramids in monkeys produce about equivalent impairment in finger dexterity in adults and infants. He also noted that recovery is task-dependent. Moreover, damage inflicted on the infant brain often leads to marked structural anomalies that may, in part, reflect compensatory processes but that may carry other handicaps. Aberrant histology, which often results from early lesions, carries a potential for functional disruption that may be subtle but still significant.

At least some portion of the plasticity doctrine is attributable to truncated observational periods. Even Kennard's monkeys began to display increased motor deficits as they matured. Isaacson notes that when the dorsolateral prefrontal cortex of infant monkeys was ablated, they failed to show the deficits in delayed-response performance, at 1 year of age, that follow ablations in adults. These findings proved misleading. Goldman (1971) produced either dorsolateral or orbitofrontal lesions in a group of monkeys between 48 and 85 days of age. When tested between 12 and 18 months of age on tasks sensitive to prefrontal lesions made in adulthood, the monkeys with lateral prefrontal lesions showed less impairment than monkeys with similar lesions made in young adulthood. Animals with orbitofrontal lesions showed deficiencies as great as those shown by monkeys operated on in adulthood. The situation reversed when the animals were tested at 24 months of age. Monkeys who had received dorsolateral lesions during infancy were now impaired, but the animals with orbitofrontal lesions were not. Later, Goldman (1974) found a progressive diminution in delayed response capacity in the monkeys with dorsolateral lesions as they grew older.

The emergence of behavioral deficits long after brain damage sustained during infancy is not confined to delayed-response problems. Human infants with unilateral brain damage localized to the parietal lobe did not exhibit coordination problems at first; but, as they grew more mature, increasingly severe clinical signs emerged (Lennenberg, 1968). And, as noted earlier, pyramidal tract lesions in monkeys hinder fine movements later on (Lawrence and Hopkins, 1970). In rats, lesions of the lateral preoptic area produce later anomalies of drinking behavior (Almli et al., 1976). Lesions designed to interfere with neurotransmitter systems may display similar phenomena. Young rats received unilateral lesions produced either by 6-hydroxydopamine or by electrolysis (Schallert, 1988). The lesions were aimed at an area carrying dopaminergic neurons and projections. Within 1–3 months following surgery, most rats had recovered their ability to respond to a von Frey hair applied to several regions on each side of the body. After about the age of 18 months, the contralateral sensorimotor impairment reappeared. One obvious explanation for these results is the decline in nigrostriatal dopamine function with age, but other systems, such as the cerebellum, also show marked changes with age, and the interactions among them are surely quite complex.

One hypothetical mechanism for such effects was offered by Goldman (1974). She suggested that delayed impairment may depend on the degree of functional maturity of the specific brain region underlying the behavioral function. Only when the region, with maturation, becomes essential for the specific behavior do the deficits become manifest.

It is almost as if the animal had to grow into the lesion before its effects become detectable. The basic lesson to be derived from this literature is that most of the questions about delayed effects and silent toxicity cannot be addressed without longitudinal experimental designs.

Even lesions in adults may demonstrate what Finger (1978) terms lesion momentum. At one time, before the introduction of effective drugs for the treatment of schizophrenia, some authorities proposed that excision of certain parts of the frontal lobe could ameliorate the disabling signs of the disease. Hamlin (1970) traced the subsequent history of a group of schizophrenic patients subjected to surgery. Table 2 is a summary of the results. It shows that ablation of the superior frontal cortex resulted in a progressive decline in scores on the Wechsler Adult Intelligence Scale, a deterioration not experienced by the other two groups of patients.

MECHANISMS OF SILENT DAMAGE

The delay between exposure to the eliciting toxicant and consequent expression of toxicity is a major obstacle to the identification and mechanistic study of these agents. From a theoretical perspective, two mechanistic paradigms for silent toxicity appear most likely.

Critical Thresholds

Different anatomical regions of the brain are highly specialized to serve specific functions. Although great numerical redundancy of neurons within these regions is common, once a sufficient number of neurons have been injured or killed, the function subserved by a region may become impaired or even irretrievably lost. A point exists at which the number of neurons remaining after insult may be minimally sufficient to support a particular structure's function, and a second point beyond which the number of surviving neurons is no longer sufficient to maintain normal functioning. This point may be termed the "event

Table 2 Intellectual Function After Frontal Lobe Surgery in Schizophrenics

	Changes in mean Wechsler scores after 8 and 14 years		
	1948 base	1956 change	1962 change
Controls			
Young	66.7	+5.9	+4.5
Old	75.8	+1.2	−4.4
Orbital topectomy			
Young	50.2	+4.3	+11.2
Old	65.3	+0.5	+4.4
Superior topectomy			
Young	91.3	−12.5	−24.2
Old	68.3	−6.0	−16.0

Source: Hamlin, 1970.

threshold," and corresponds to the time at which a previously silent injury becomes clinically apparent.

The concept of a critical threshold is amendable to testing using a variety of pharmacological methods and sensitive behavioral measures. Administration of drugs to reversibly inhibit or enhance the activity of specific neural pathways has been used by behavioral pharmacologists to evaluate functional reserve and to "unmask" neurological deficit (Zigmond and Stricker, 1981). Physiological methods may also be used to reveal subclinical damage. The principle of the event threshold is clearly demonstrated in Parkinson's disease. Normal dopaminergic function of the nigrostriatal pathway may be maintained with a loss of as many as 80% of the neurons in the substantia nigra. When more than this number of neurons are lost, the patient becomes clinically parkinsonian, often with disconcerting rapidity.

As illustrated in Fig. 3, there are several patterns of neuronal loss that might underlie delayed expression of injury. Toxic insult during development or adult life may acutely kill a certain number of neurons, resulting in loss of functional reserve. Normal attrition of surviving neurons proceeds, but is acting on a smaller population of cells. The animal consequently attains the critical threshold prematurely (Fig. 3, line A). Table 3 lists the elements of such a multistage process.

A second pattern would be an increased rate of cell loss arising from toxicant exposure, a process sometimes referred to as accelerated aging. This pattern may occur in instances of chronic exposure to low concentrations of toxicants that continually stress the cell, rendering it susceptible to the additive effect of multiple, sublethal "hits" (Fig. 3, line B).

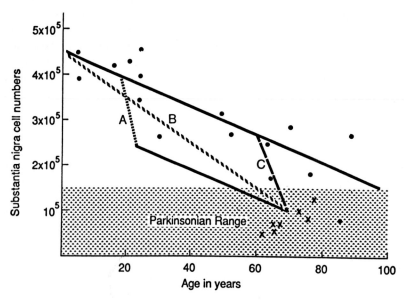

Figure 3 Impact of different histories on cell numbers in human substantia nigra. Controls are represented by solid dots and cases of Parkinson's disease by Xs. The upper line represents the presumed course of normal aging. Line B represents an acceleration of the normal process. Line A represents an early event that depletes the original cell population. Line C represents a later event or active disease. The hatched area shows the range of cell numbers believed to characterize parkinsonian patients. (From McGeer et al., 1988.)

Finally, cells compromised by a toxicant may receive a subsequent stress sufficient to initiate decompensation and sudden loss of functional integrity (Fig. 3, line C). A precipitous drop in competency can appear with secondary emotional or physical demands. Latent tremor, for example, is frequently exacerbated under conditions of excitement or exertion, and subtle decrements in complex functions such as memory can be detected under similar types of stress. This type of clinical decompensation may be temporarily relieved following removal of the stress, providing sufficient neurons remain to support function at a basal level. It is likely, however, that some types of systemic stress (or repeated insult) may result in increased incidence cell dysfunction and death.

Accelerated cell death or enhanced aging is another concept whose intuitive attractiveness belies the difficulty in confirming its existence. The concept underlies many theories of neurodegenerative disease (Brizzee, 1987; Coleman and Flood, 1987). Enhanced morbidity and mortality of treated animals relative to control animals is often observed in long-term studies of toxicants, but is difficult to attribute to any single process. In all likelihood, accelerated cell death is multifactorial, encompassing many cell-injury processes (Finch, 1992).

Failure of Compensatory Response

Following injury, the brain undergoes a series of adaptive and compensatory responses, the nature of which depends on the toxic insult. These responses vary in magnitude from subtle alterations of gene expression and protein synthesis to reactive gliosis following neuronal death. Disturbance of these responses may contribute to the delayed expression of toxic damage and will influence the severity of the defect. Methylmercury is an example of a toxicant whose many effects include a failure of compensatory response. Congenital exposure of rats to methylmercury can cause alterations in the pattern and character of dendritic spines of pyramidal neurons of the cerebral cortex. In treated animals, the dendritic spines retain the morphology of an early developmental state and apparently fail to mature or to compensate for abnormalities in synaptic partners (Stoltenburg-Didinger and Markwort, 1990). Abnormal dendritic structure indicates a potentially abnormal synaptic network, the impact of which might not be detected for some years. Similar types of changes are seen following developmental exposure to lead and other toxic metals.

The failure of normal neuronal compensatory response to changes in microenvironment may contribute to a number of degenerative conditions such as Alzheimer's disease. Coleman and Flood (1987) sketched two paths that might be taken by neurons in the aging brain. Along one path, neurons develop a richer network of dendritic arborizations, presumably to compensate for those cells that die in the course of aging. Along another path, arborizations retract and the cells become functionally inert and finally die. The balance between these two divergent processes might be altered by the kind of damage detected by Stoltenburg-Didinger and Markwort (1990).

Altered Imprinting

Neural commitment, differentiation, and function are dependent on the cell's receiving appropriate cues for genetic expression. These cues are of two types: endogenous cues, which include the proper temporal sequence of gene expression and subsequent modification of the gene product, and exogenous cues, such as hormones, which provide the neuron information regarding which genes and proteins to express.

The role of direct genotoxicity in silent neurotoxicity is still highly speculative. It is clear that individual genetic susceptibilities may function cooperatively with toxic exposures

Table 3 Potential Elements of a Multistage Neurodegenerative Process

1. Erosion of cell numbers
2. Increased transmitter production
3. Accumulation of toxic metabolic products
4. Functional exhaustion
5. Death

to foster the expression of injury. It is also recognized that toxicants such as heavy metals may bind to DNA and alter protein expression. Human childhood genetic neurodegenerative disorders may not present until adulthood (Coker, 1991), but these are usually metabolic diseases associated with the accumulation of abnormal storage products and/or neuronal death. Exposure to carcinogens such as N-ethyl-N-nitrosourea during gestation is an effective method of inducing adult-onset tumors in experimental animals (Kleihues et al., 1976). However, relatively few examples can be found where direct genotoxicity during development leads to noncarcinogenic neurological effects later in life.

More intriguing are chemicals that affect the endocrine system, and whose toxicity is not manifested until a later stage of life. Rodier (1991) studied rats treated with methazoxymethanol acetate at developmental stages during which hypothalamic neurons responsible for growth hormone release were forming. She found alterations in normal size and weight consistent with a deficiency of growth hormone. Delay in somatic growth is seen following prenatal exposure to alcohol in humans (Streissguth et al., 1985) and with some heavy metals (Vorhees, 1985). Damage or loss of neurons whose major activities do not begin until puberty would be expected to have major effects on these critical life stages.

Evidence in support of this supposition is sparse, largely because longitudinal assessment of developmental neurotoxicity is not routinely included in the risk assessment of most chemicals. In studies including longitudinal examinations, findings consistent with neuroendocrine disturbances have been observed. Spyker (1975) reported rapid onset of obesity in mice more than a year after congenital exposure to methylmercury. The presence of hormone receptors and hormone regulatory systems throughout the brain and the ability of hormones to directly regulate neuronal gene expression indicate that neuroendocrine mechanisms may play a crucial, if frequently unappreciated, role in neurotoxic expression by toxicants that either have hormone-mimicking characteristics (such as polychlorinated biphenyls) or target hormone-sensitive regions (such as trimethyltin's effect on the hippocampus). Prospective studies designed to assess neuroendocrine effects, combined with detailed morphometric analysis (Rodier, 1990), will be needed to address this question adequately.

Many paradigms of injury leading to silent toxicity can be described, and many different mechanisms could operate simultaneously and even independently. Even schizophrenia is now being viewed as the product of damage preceding a long latent period. One of the proponents of this view (Waddington, 1993) described the hypothesis in terms evoking the concepts of behavioral teratology: "The neurodevelopmental hypothesis [of schizophrenia] . . . takes as the primary event changes in utero that disrupt the development of fundamental aspects of brain structure and function and that might produce the typical symptoms some two decades later, perhaps only after functional maturation or completion of other, associated, systems or processes—for example, myelination or synaptic pruning" (p. 531).

ACKNOWLEDGMENTS

Preparation supported in part by National Institute of Environmental Health Sciences grants ES 01247 and ES 05433 to Bernard Weiss.

REFERENCES

Almli CR, Golden GT, McMullen NT (1976). Ontogeny of drinking behavior of preweanling rats with lateral preoptic damage. Brain Res Bull 1:437–42.

Amin-Zaki L, Majeed MA, Greenwood MR, Elhassani SB, Clarkson TW, and Doherty RA (1981). Methylmercury poisoning in the Iraqi suckling infant: a longitudinal study over five years. J Appl Toxicol 1:210–14.

Bakir F, Damlugi SF, Amin-Zaki L, Murtadha M, Khalidi A, Al-Rawi NJ, Tikriti S, Dhahir HI, Clarkson TW, Smith J, and Doherty RA (1973). Methylmercury poisoning in Iraq. Science 181:230–41.

Bellinger D, Leviton A, Waternaux C, Needleman H, Rabinowitz M (1987). Longitudinal analyses of prenatal and postnatal lead exposure and early cognitive development. N Engl J Med 316:1037–43.

Bernheimer H, Birkmayer W, Hornykiewicz O, Jellinger K, Steitelberger F (1973). Brain dopamine and the syndromes of Parkinson and Huntington. Clinical and morphological correlations. J Neurol Sci 20:415–55.

Bignami G, Alleva E, Chiarotti F, Laviola G (1992). Selective changes in mouse behavioral development after prenatal benzodiazepine exposure: a progress report. Prog Neuro-Psychopharmacol Biol Psychiatry 16:587–604.

Brizzee KR (1987). Neuron numbers and dendritic extent in normal aging and Alzheimer's disease. Neurobiol. Aging 8:579–80.

Burbacher TM, Rodier PM, Weiss B (1990). Methylmercury developmental neurotoxicity: a comparison of effects in humans and animals. Neurotoxicol Teratol 12:191–202.

Byers RK, Lord EE (1943). Late effects of lead poisoning on mental development. Am J Dis Child 66:471–94.

Calne DB, Eisen A, McGeer E, Spencer P (1986). Alzheimer's disease, Parkinson's disease, and motoneurone disease: abiotrophic interaction between ageing and environment? Lancet 2:1067–70.

Calne DB, Langston JW, Martin WRW, Stoessl AJ, Ruth TJ, Adam MJ, Pate BD, Schulzer M (1985). Positron emission tomography after MPTP: observations relating to the cause of Parkinson's disease. Nature 317:246–8.

Carlsson A, Winblad B (1976). Influences of age and time interval between death and autopsy on dopamine and 3-methoxytyramine levels in human basal ganglia. J Neural Transmission 38:271–6.

Chang LW (1987). The experimental neuropathology of methyl mercury. In: Eccles CU, Annau Z, eds. The toxicity of methyl mercury. Baltimore: John Hopkins University Press, 54–72.

Choi DW (1992). Amyotrophic lateral sclerosis and glutamate—too much of a good thing? N Engl J Med 326:1493–5.

Coker SB (1991). The diagnosis of childhood neurodegenerative disorders presenting as dementia in adults. Neurology 41:794–8.

Coleman PD, Flood DG (1987). Neuron numbers and dendritic extent in normal aging and Alzheimer's disease. Neurobiol Aging 8:521–45.

Cox C, Clarkson TW, Marsh DO, and Amin-Zaki L (1989). Dose-response analysis of infants prenatally exposed to methylmercury: An application of a single compartment model to single-strand hair analysis. Environment Res 49:318–32.

Date I, Notter MFD, Felten SY, Felten DL (1990). MPTP-treated young mice but not aging mice show partial recovery of the nigrostriatal dopaminergic system by stereotaxic injection of acidic fibroblast growth factor (aFGF). Brain Res 526:156–60.

Eccles CU, Annau Z (1987). Prenatal exposure to methyl mercury. In: Eccles CU, Annau Z, eds. The toxicity of methyl mercury. Baltimore: John Hopkins University Press, 104–13.

Finch CE (1992). Mechanisms in senescence: some thoughts in April 1990. Exp Gerontol 27:7–16.

Finger S (1978). Recovery from brain damage. New York: Plenum Press.

Garruto RM, Yase Y (1986). Neurodegenerative disorders of the Western Pacific: The search for mechanisms of pathogenesis. Trends Neurosci 9:368–74.

Goldman PS (1974). An alternative to developmental plasticity: heterology of CNS structures in infants and adults. In: Stein DG, Rosen JJ, Butters N, eds. Plasticity and recovery of function in the central nervous system. New York: Academic Press, 149–74.

Goldman PS (1971). Functional development of the prefrontal cortex in early life and the problem of neuronal plasticity. Exp Neurol 32:366–87.

Graham DG (1984). Catecholamine toxicity: a proposal for the molecular pathogenesis of manganese neurotoxicity and Parkinson's disease. Neurotoxicology 5:83–96.

Greenamyre JT (1991). Neuronal bioenergetic defects, excitotoxicity and Alzheimer's disease: "use it and lose it." Neurobiol Aging, 12:334–6.

Greenamyre JT (1986). The role of glutamate in neurotransmission and in neurologic disease. Arch Neurol 43:1058–63.

Gullino PM (1977). Natural history of breast cancer. Cancer 30:2697–703.

Hamlin RM (1970). Intellectual functions 14 years after frontal lobe surgery. Cortex 6:299–307.

Hertzman C, Wiens M, Bowering D, Snow B, Calne D (1990). Parkinson's disease: a case-control study of occupational and environmental risk factors. Am J Indust Med 17:349–55.

Hornykiewicz O (1989). Ageing and neurotoxins as causative factors in idiopathic Parkinson's disease—a critical analysis of the neurochemical evidence. Prog Neuro-Psychopharmacol Biol Psychiatry 13:319–28.

Isaacson RL (1975). The myth of recovery from early brain damage. In: Ellis NR, ed. Aberrant development in infancy. Human and animal studies. Hillsdale, New Jersey: Lawrence Erlbaum Associates, 1–25.

Kennard MA (1940). Relation of age to motor impairment in man and in subhuman primates. Arch Neurol Psychiatry 44:377–97.

Kennard MA (1938). Reorganization of motor functions in the cerebral cortex of monkeys deprived of motor and premotor areas in infancy. J Neurophysiol 1:477–97.

Kjellstrom T, Kennedy P, Wallis S, Mantell C (1986). Physical and mental development of children with prenatal exposure to mercury from fish. Stage 1. Preliminary tests at age 4. (Report no. 3080). Solna, Sweden: National Swedish Environmental Research Board.

Kjellstrom T, Kennedy P, Wallis S, Stewart A, Friberg L, Lind B, Wutherspoon T, Mantell (1989). Physical and mental development of children with prenatal exposure to mercury from fish. Stage 2. Interview and psychological tests at age 6. (Report no. 3642). Solna, Sweden: National Swedish Environmental Protection Board.

Klihues P, Lantos PL, Magee PN (1976). Chemical carcinogenesis in the nervous system. Int Rev Exp Pathol 15:153–232.

Langston JW (1989). Current theories on the cause of Parkinson's disease. J Neurol Neurosurg Psychiatry (suppl) 13–7.

Lawrence DG, Hopkins DA (1970). Bilateral pyramidal lesions in infant rhesus monkeys. Brain Res 24:543–4.

Lennenberg EH (1968). The effect of age on the outcome of central nervous system disease in children. In: Isaacson RL, ed. The neuropsychology of development. New York: John Wiley & Sons.

Marsden CD (1990). Parkinson's disease. Lancet 335:948–52.

Martilla RJ, Kaprio J, Koskenvuo M, Rinne UK (1988). Parkinson's disease in a nationwide twin study. Neurology 38:1217–19.

Martyn CN, Barker DJP, Osmond C (1988). Motoneuron disease and past poliomyelitis in England and Wales. Lancet 1:1319–22.

McGeer PL, Itagaki S, Akiyama H, McGeer EG (1988). Rate of cell death in Parkinsonism indicates active neuropathological process. Ann Neurol 24:574–6.

Miranda R, Ceckler T, Guillet R, Kellogg C (1990). Aging-related changes in brain metabolism are altered by early developmental exposure to diazepam. Neurobiol Aging 11:117–22.

Needleman HL, Gunnoe C, Leviton A, Reed M, Peresie H, Maher C, Barrett P (1979). Deficits in psychological and classroom performance of children with elevated dentine lead levels. N Engl J Med 300:689–95.

Needleman HL, Schell A, Bellinger D, Leviton A, Allred EN (1990). The long-term effects of exposure to low doses of lead in childhood. An 11-year follow-up report. N Engl J Med 322:83–8.

Otake M, Schull WJ (1984). In utero exposure to A-bomb radiation and mental retardation: a reassessment. Br J Radiol 57:409–14.

Peto R, Roe FJC, Lee PN, Ling L, Clack J (1975). Cancer and aging in mice and men. Br J Cancer 32:411–26.

Rajput AH, Uitti RJ, Stern W, Laverty W (1986). Early onset Parkinson's disease in Saskatchewan—environmental considerations for etiology. Can J Neurol Sci 13:312–6.

Reuhl KR, Chang LW (1979). Effects of methylmercury on the development of the nervous system. Neurotoxicology 1:21–55.

Reuhl KR, Chang LW, Townsend JW (1981). Pathological effects of in utero methylmercury exposure on the cerebellum of the golden hamster. I. Early effects upon the neonatal cerebellar cortex. Environ Res 26:281–306.

Reuhl KR, Chang LW, Townsend J (1981b). Pathological effects of in utero methylmercury exposure on the cerebellum of the golden hamster. II. Residual effects on the adult cerebellum. Environ Res 26:307–27.

Rice DC, Karpinski KF (1988). Lifetime low-level lead exposure produces deficits in delayed alternation in adult monkeys. Neurotoxicol Teratol 10:207–14.

Rodier PM (1990). Developmental neurotoxicology. Toxicol Pathol 18:89–95.

Rodier PM (1991). Prenatal injury to the hypothalamus and its effects on postnatal growth. In: Fujii T, Boer GJ, eds. Functional neuroteratology of short-term exposure to drugs. Tokyo: Teikyo University Press, 39–54

Rosenzweig MR, Bennett EL (1978). Experiental influences on brain anatomy and brain chemistry. In: Gottlieb G, ed. Studies on the development and behavior of the nervous system. Volume 4. Early influences. New York: Academic Press, 289–327.

Rothstein JD, Martin LJ, Kuncl RW (1992). Decreased glutamate transport by the brain and spinal cord in amyotrophic lateral sclerosis. N Engl J Med 326:1464–8.

Schallert T (1988). Aging-dependent emergence of sensorimotor dysfunction in rats recovered from dopamine depletion sustained early in life. Ann NY Acad Sci 515:108–20.

Spencer PS (1990). Chemical time bombs: environmental causes of neurodegenerative diseases. In: Russell RW, Ebert PE, Pope AM, eds. Behavioral measures of neurotoxicity. Washington, D.C.: National Academy Press, 268–84.

Spyker JM (1975). Behavioral teratology and toxicology. In: Weiss B, Laties VG, eds. Behavioral toxicology. New York: Plenum Press, 311–44.

Spyker JM (1975). Assessing the impact of low level chemicals on development: behavioral and latent effects. Fed Proc 34:1835–44.

Stoltenburg-Didinger G, Markwort S (1990). Prenatal methylmercury exposure results in dendritic spine dysgenesis in rats. Neurotoxicol Teratol 12:573–6.

Streissguth AP, Clarren SK, Jones KL (1985). Natural history of the fetal alcohol syndrome. Lancet 2:85–91.

Uhlig S, Wendel A (1992). The physiological consequences of glutathione variations. Life Sci 51:1083–94.

Vorhees CV (1985). Behavioral effects of methylmercury in rats: a parallel trial to the collaborative behavioral teratology study. Neurobehav Toxicol Teratol 7:717–25.

Waddington JL (1993). Schizophrenia: developmental neuroscience and pathobiology. Lancet 341:531–37.

Wallace RB, Daniels CE, Altman J (1972). Behavioral effects of neonatal irradiation of the cerebellum. III. Qualitative observations in aged rats. Dev Psychobiol 5:35–41.

Weiss B (1988). Neurobehavioral toxicity as a basis for risk assessment. Trends Pharmacol Sci 9:59–62.

Weiss B, Simon W (1975). Quantitative perspectives on the long-term toxicity of methylmercury and similar poisons. In: Weiss B, Laties VG, eds. Behavioral toxicology. New York: Plenum Press, 429–38.

Weiss B (1991). Cancer and the dynamics of neurodegenerative processes. Neurotoxicology 12:379–86.

Werboff J (1970). Developmental psychopharmacology. In: Clark WG, del Giudice J, eds. Principles of psychopharmacology. New York: Academic Press, 343–53.

Zayed J, Ducic S, Campanella G, Panisset JC, Andre P, Masson H, Roy M (1990). Facteurs environnmentaux dans l'étiologie de la maladie de Parkinson. Can J Neurol Sci 17:286–91.

Zhang M, Katzman R, Salmon D, Jin H, Cai G, Wang Z, Qu G, Grant I, Yu E, Levy P, Klauber MR, Liu WT (1990). The prevalence of dementia and Alzheimer's disease in Shanghai, China: impact of age, gender, and education. Ann Neurol 27:428–37.

Zhang ZX, Anderson DW, Lavine L, Mantel N (1990). Patterns of acquiring parkinsonism-dementia on Guam 1944 through 1985. Arch Neurol 47:1019–24.

Zigmond MJ, Striker EM (1981). Behavioral tests for detection of subclinical brain damage: an experimental model. In: Merikangas JR, ed. Brain-behavior relationships. Lexington, Massachusetts: D.C. Heath, 93–112.

Zigmond MJ, Abercrombie ED, Berger TW, Grace AA, Stricker EM (1990). Compensations after lesions of central dopaminergic neurons: some clinical and basic implications. Trends Neurol Sci 13:290–6.

Index

About the Editor

LOUIS W. CHANG is a Professor in the Departments of Pathology, Pharmacology, and Toxicology, and Director of Graduate Studies in Experimental Pathology at the University of Arkansas for Medical Sciences, Little Rock. Dr. Chang also serves as a Visiting Professor at both Beijing Medical University and the Institute of Occupational Medicine, Chinese Academy of Preventive Medicine, Beijing, and is a Scientific Advisor and Honor Professor at the National Institute for the Control of Pharmaceutical and Biological Products, Beijing, People's Republic of China. Dr. Chang is a member of the Society of Toxicology, the American Association of Neuropathologists, the American Association of Pathologists, the Society for Neuroscience, and the International Society of Neuropathology, among others. He received the B.A. degree (1966) in chemistry and biology from the University of Massachusetts at Amherst, the M.S. degree (1969) in neuroanatomy and histochemistry from Tufts University School of Medicine, Boston, Massachusetts, and the Ph.D. degree (1972) in pathology from the University of Wisconsin Medical School, Madison. Dr. Chang also received training in neurocytology from Harvard Medical School, Boston, Massachusetts, and in in vitro and biochemical neurotoxicology from the Brain Research Institute at the University of California School of Medicine, Los Angeles.